MW00397590

WILLIAM H. BELL, D.D.S.

Professor
Department of Surgery
Division of Oral and Maxillofacial Surgery
Center for Correction of Dento-Facial Deformities
The University of Texas Health Science Center
Dallas, Texas

WILLIAM R. PROFFIT, D.D.S., Ph.D.

Professor and Chairman
Department of Orthodontics
University of North Carolina
School of Dentistry
Chapel Hill, North Carolina

RAYMOND P. WHITE, Jr., D.D.S., Ph.D.

Dean and Professor of Oral Surgery
University of North Carolina
School of Dentistry
Chapel Hill, North Carolina

W. B. SAUNDERS COMPANY
Philadelphia, London, Toronto

Volume II

SURGICAL CORRECTION OF DENTOFACIAL DEFORMITIES

W. B. Saunders Company: West Washington Square
Philadelphia, PA 19105

1 St. Anne's Road
Eastbourne, East Sussex BN21 3UN, England

1 Goldthorne Avenue
Toronto, Ontario M8Z 5T9, Canada

Library of Congress Cataloging in Publication Data

Bell, William H

Surgical correction of dentofacial deformities.

1. Jaws—Surgery. 2. Jaws—Abnormities and deformities. 3. Face—Abnormities and deformities. I. Proffit, William R., joint author. II. White, Raymond P., joint author. III. Title. [DNLM: 1. Abnormalities—Surgery. 2. Surgery, Oral. 3. Face—Surgery. WU600 B435s]

RD526.B44 617'.522 76–27050

ISBN 0–7216–1675–5

Vol. I ISBN 0-7216-1675-5
Vol. II ISBN 0-7216-1707-7
2-Vol. Set ISBN 0-7216-1671-2

Surgical Correction of Dentofacial Deformities

Last digit is the print number: 9 8 7 6 5 4 3

CONTRIBUTORS

JAMES L. ACKERMAN, D.D.S.

Professor of Orthodontics, University of Pennsylvania, Philadelphia, Pennsylvania; Director, Dental Program, Children's Hospital of Philadelphia, Philadelphia, Pennsylvania.

JOSEPH C. AINSWORTH, III, D.D.S.

Private practice in orthodontics, Irving, Texas.

PATRICK A. ALESSANDRA, D.D.S.

Private practice in orthodontics, Houston, Texas.

RICHARD G. ALEXANDER, D.D.S.

Private practice in orthodontics, Arlington, Texas.

MORGAN L. ALLISON, D.D.S.

Professor, Department of Oral and Maxillofacial Surgery, Ohio State University Dental College, Columbus, Ohio.

JOSE P. AMPIL, D.D.S.

Assistant Professor, The University of Texas Health Science Center at Dallas, Center for Correction of Dento-Facial Deformities, Department of Surgery, Division of Oral and Maxillofacial Surgery, Dallas, Texas.

RONALD D. BAKER, D.D.S.

Professor and Chairman, Department of Oral and Maxillofacial Surgery, School of Dentistry, University of North Carolina, Chapel Hill, North Carolina.

WILLIAM E. BEAUMONT, JR., D.D.S.

Private practice in orthodontics, Clarksville, Tennessee.

WILLIAM H. BELL, D.D.S.

Professor, The University of Texas Health Science Center at Dallas, Center for Correction of Dento-Facial Deformities, Department of Surgery, Division of Oral and Maxillofacial Surgery, Dallas, Texas.

RICHARD R. BEVIS, D.D.S., Ph.D.

Professor, Division of Orthodontics, School of Dentistry, University of Minnesota, Minneapolis, Minnesota.

DALE S. BLOOMQUIST, D.D.S., M.D.

Associate Professor, Department of Oral and Maxillofacial Surgery, University of Washington, School of Dentistry, Seattle, Washington.

CHARLES L. BOLENDER, D.D.S.

University of Washington, School of Dentistry, Seattle, Washington.

JOSEPH N. BONELLO, D.D.S.

Private practice in orthodontics, Pittsburgh, Pennsylvania.

DONALD C. BOOTH, D.M.D.

Professor, Department of Oral and Maxillofacial Surgery, Boston University, School of Graduate Dentistry, Boston, Massachusetts.

JOHN A. BRAMMER, D.D.S.

Resident, Department of Surgery, Division of Oral and Maxillofacial Surgery, Center for Correction of Dento-Facial Deformities, The University of Texas Health Science Center, Dallas, Texas.

IRVING D. BUCHIN, D.D.S.

Private practice in orthodontics, Forest Hills, New York.

H. RICHARD BUCK, D.D.S.

Private practice in orthodontics, Austin, Texas.

ROBERT L. BUCKLES, D.D.S.

Private practice in oral and maxillofacial surgery, Plano, Texas.

THOMAS J. BYRNE, D.D.S.

Private practice in orthodontics, St. Louis, Missouri.

DONALD C. CHASE, D.D.S.

Professor and Chairman, Department of Oral and Maxillofacial Surgery, University of Tennessee, School of Medicine, Knoxville, Tennessee.

M. MICHAEL COHEN, JR., D.M.D.

Professor, Department of Oral and Maxillofacial Surgery, School of Dentistry, University of Washington; Professor, Department of Pediatrics, School of Medicine, University of Washington, Seattle, Washington.

CLIFFORD L. CONDIT, JR., D.D.S.

Private practice in orthodontics, Houston, Texas.

THOMAS D. CREEKMORE, D.D.S.

Private practice in orthodontics, Houston, Texas.

ALEXANDER DELL, D.D.S.

Private practice in orthodontics, Houston, Texas.

VICTOR S. DIETZ, D.D.S.

Private practice in orthodontics, Boston, Massachusetts.

ALBERT M. D'ONOFRIO, D.D.S.

Private practice in orthodontics, New Haven, Connecticut.

JEROME EISENFELD, Ph.D.

Visiting Professor, Department of Medical Computer Science, University of Texas Health Science Center at Dallas, Southwestern Medical School, Dallas, Texas.

BRUCE N. EPKER, D.D.S., Ph.D.

Director, Dentofacial Deformities Program, John Peter Smith Hospital, Fort Worth, Texas.

RICHARD A. FINN, D.D.S.

Resident, Oral and Maxillofacial Surgery, Parkland Memorial Hospital, The University of Texas Health Science Center at Dallas, Dallas, Texas.

RAYMOND J. FONSECA, D.M.D.

Associate Professor, Department of Oral and Maxillofacial Surgery, University of Iowa School of Dentistry, Iowa City, Iowa.

PHILIP N. FREEMAN, D.D.S.

Private practice in oral and maxillofacial surgery, Campbellsville, Kentucky.

LAWRENCE A. FRIEDMAN, D.D.S.

Private practice in periodontics, Houston, Texas.

WILLIAM J. GONYEA, Ph.D.

Associate Professor, Department of Cell Biology, The University of Texas Health Science Center at Dallas, Dallas, Texas.

JACK L. GUNTER, M.D.

Private practice in plastic and reconstructive surgery, Dallas, Texas.

DAVID J. HALL, D.D.S.

Assistant Professor, Department of Orthodontics, School of Dentistry, University of North Carolina, Chapel Hill, North Carolina.

H. DAVID HALL, D.D.S., M.D.

Professor and Chairman, Department of Oral and Maxillofacial Surgery, Vanderbilt University, School of Medicine, Nashville, Tennessee.

FRANZ HARLE, D.D.S., M.D.

Professor, Department of Maxillofacial Surgery, University of Freiberg, Freiberg, West Germany.

JAMES R. HAYWARD, D.D.S.

Professor and Chairman, Department of Oral and Maxillofacial Surgery, School of Dentistry, The University of Michigan, Ann Arbor, Michigan.

DEREK HENDERSON, D.D.S., M.D.

Professor and Chief, St. Thomas Hospital, Department of Oral and Maxillofacial Surgery, London, England.

STEPHEN C. HILL, D.D.S.

Assistant Professor, The University of Texas Health Science Center at Dallas, Center for Correction of Dento-Facial Deformities, Department of Surgery, Division of Oral and Maxillofacial Surgery, Dallas, Texas.

JACK HITTSON, D.D.S.

Private practice in orthodontics, Garland, Texas.

KARL-ERIK HOGEMEN, D.D.S., M.D.

Professor and Director, Department of Plastic Surgery, University Hospital, Malmo, Sweden.

THOMAS H. HOHL, D.D.S.

Assistant Professor, Department of Oral and Maxillofacial Surgery, School of Dentistry, University of Washington, Seattle, Washington.

I. T. JACKSON, M.D.

Professor, Department of Surgery, The Mayo Clinic, Rochester, Minnesota.

JOE D. JACOBS, D.M.D.

Assistant Professor, Department of Orthodontics, Baylor College of Dentistry, Dallas, Texas.

JAMES W. KENNEDY, D.D.S.

Assistant Professor, Department of Oral and Maxillofacial Surgery, University of Texas, Dental Branch, Houston, Texas; private practice in oral and maxillofacial surgery, Houston, Texas.

RALPH B. KERSTEN, M.D.

Professor, Department of Surgery, University of Minnesota School of Medicine, Minneapolis, Minnesota; Director, Division of Cleft Palate, University of Minnesota School of Medicine, Minneapolis, Minnesota.

O. L. KIMBROUGH, D.D.S.

Private practice in orthodontics, Midland, Texas.

HARRY C. KIZER, D.D.S.

Private practice in orthodontics, Dallas, Texas.

MARKELL W. KOHN, D.D.S.

Professor and Chairman, Department of Oral and Maxillofacial Surgery, University of Kentucky Medical Center School of Dentistry, Lexington, Kentucky.

HARRY L. LEGAN, D.D.S.

Assistant Professor, The University of Texas Health Science Center at Dallas, Center for Correction of Dento-Facial Deformities, Department of Surgery, Division of Oral and Maxillofacial Surgery, Dallas, Texas.

JAMES L. LORD, D.D.S.

Private practice in prosthodontics, Seattle, Washington.

KEVIN L. MCBRIDE, D.D.S.

Assistant Clinical Professor, The University of Texas Health Science Center at Dallas, Division of Oral and Maxillofacial Surgery, Dallas, Texas; Chief, Oral and Maxillofacial Surgery, Section Dental Service, Veterans Administration Hospital, Dallas, Texas.

WILLIAM R. MCNEILL, D.D.S., M.S.

Associate Professor, Department of Orthodontics, School of Dentistry, University of Washington, Seattle, Washington.

CHARLES W. MILLER, D.D.S.

Private practice in orthodontics, Columbus, Ohio.

Francis Miller, D.D.S.

Staff Orthodontist, Section Dental Service, Veterans Administration Hospital, Dallas, Texas.

David J. Mishelevich, M.D., Ph.D.

Professor and Chairman, Department of Medical Computer Science, University of Texas Health Science Center at Dallas, Southwestern Medical School, Dallas, Texas.

Peter J. Paulus, D.D.S.

Private practice in orthodontics, Fort Worth, Texas.

Frank Pavel, Jr., D.D.S.

Private practice in oral and maxillofacial surgery, San Diego, California.

Larry J. Peterson, D.D.S., M.S.

Associate Professor, Department of Oral and Maxillofacial Surgery, Schools of Medicine and Dental Medicine, University of Connecticut, Farmington, Connecticut; Attending Staff, John N. Dempsey Hospital of the University of Connecticut, Farmington, Connecticut.

Rodney M. Phillips, D.D.S.

Private practice in oral and maxillofacial surgery, Beaumont, Texas.

David Poswillo, D.D.S., Ph.D.

Professor and Chairman, Department of Oral and Maxillofacial Surgery, The University of Adelaide, Adelaide, South Australia.

Donald R. Poulton, D.D.S.

Professor, Department of Orthodontics, University of California, San Francisco, California.

William R. Proffit, D.D.S., Ph.D.

Professor and Chairman, Department of Orthodontics, University of North Carolina, School of Dentistry, Chapel Hill, North Carolina.

Martin L. Sherling, D.D.S.

Private practice in orthodontics, Dallas, Texas.

Douglas P. Sinn, D.D.S.

Assistant Professor, The University of Texas Health Science Center at Dallas, Center for Correction of Dento-Facial Deformities, Department of Surgery, Division of Oral and Maxillofacial Surgery, Dallas, Texas.

Harold C. Slavkin, D.D.S., Ph.D.

Professor and Chairman, Department of Biochemistry, Laboratory for Developmental Biology, University of Southern California, School of Dentistry, Los Angeles, California.

Larry Snider, D.D.S.

Private practice in oral and maxillofacial surgery, Lakewood, California.

Noel G. Stoker, D.D.S.

Chief, Department of Oral and Maxillofacial Surgery, Valley Medical Center, Fresno, California.

William C. Terry, D.D.S.

Professor, Department of Oral and Maxillofacial Surgery, University of North Carolina School of Dentistry, Chapel Hill, North Carolina.

WILLIAM B. THETFORD, D.D.S.

Private practice in orthodontics, Nashville, Tennessee.

GAYLORD S. THROCKMORTON, Ph.D.

Assistant Professor, Department of Cell Biology, The University of Texas Health Science Center at Dallas, Dallas, Texas.

DAVID S. TOPAZIAN, D.D.S.

Private practice in oral and maxillofacial surgery, Milford, Connecticut.

RICHARD G. TOPAZIAN, D.D.S.

Professor and Chairman, Department of Oral and Maxillofacial Surgery, Schools of Dental Medicine and Medicine, University of Connecticut, Farmington, Connecticut; Attending Staff, John N. Dempsey Hospital of the University of Connecticut, Farmington, Connecticut.

TIMOTHY A. TURVEY, D.D.S.

Assistant Professor, Department of Oral and Maxillofacial Surgery, University of North Carolina School of Dentistry, Chapel Hill, North Carolina.

PAUL VEDTOFFEE, D.D.S.

Private practice in oral and maxillofacial surgery, Copenhagen, Denmark.

DANIEL E. WAITE, D.D.S.

Professor and Chairman, Department of Oral and Maxillofacial Surgery, University of Minnesota, School of Dentistry, Minneapolis, Minnesota.

ROBERT V. WALKER, D.D.S.

Professor and Chairman, University of Texas Health Science Center at Dallas, Center for Correction of Dento-Facial Deformities, Department of Surgery, Division of Oral and Maxillofacial Surgery, Dallas, Texas.

WILLIAM R. WALLACE, D.D.S.

Professor and Chairman, Department of Oral and Maxillofacial Surgery, Ohio State University Dental College, Columbus, Ohio.

WILLIAM C. WARE, D.D.S.

Professor and Chairman, Department of Oral and Maxillofacial Surgery and Oral Biology, School of Dentistry, University of California, San Francisco, California.

KERMIT N. WELCH, D.D.S.

Private practice in orthodontics, Houston, Texas.

ROGER A. WEST, D.D.S.

Associate Professor, Department of Oral and Maxillofacial Surgery, University of Washington School of Dentistry, Seattle, Washington.

RAYMOND P. WHITE, JR., D.D.S., Ph.D.

Professor and Dean, School of Dentistry, University of North Carolina, Chapel Hill, North Carolina.

NANN A. WICKWIRE, D.D.S.

Professor, Department of Orthodontics, College of Dentistry, University of Florida, Gainesville, Florida.

CRAIG E. WILLIAMS, D.D.S.
Private practice in oral and maxillofacial surgery, Dallas, Texas.

KARIN WILMAR, D.D.S., Ph.D.
Orthodontist, Faculty of Odontology, School of Dentistry, University of Lund, Malmo, Sweden.

PAUL L. WINELAND, D.D.S.
Private practice in oral and maxillofacial surgery, Milford, Connecticut.

WILLIAM E. WYATT, D.D.S.
Private practice in orthodontics, Hurst, Texas.

PREFACE

When we finished our training 20–25 years ago (in Houston, Seattle, and Richmond respectively), there were only a handful of surgical procedures to treat dentofacial deformity patients. Most corrections were accomplished in the mandible via an extraoral approach. Orthodontists had virtually no interest in surgery except for prognathism, and surgeons had very little interest in orthodontics. With an empirical basis for surgical techniques, all done without orthodontics and virtually no surgery about the maxilla, it is not surprising that most patients received compromised or unsuccessful treatment. Key publications in the American literature by Obwegeser, Trauner, Köle, Murphey and Walker, and Mohnac catalyzed great interest in new methods of surgical treatment and led to two decades of impressive progress. Our present state of the art and science includes more than 100 surgical procedures, most of which are performed intraorally; an improved understanding of the biologic and surgical principles; orthodontic involvement in the majority of patients treated; and worldwide interest in the correction of dentofacial deformities.

Our present orthognathic surgical techniques are the harvest of yesterday's research. Many questions concerning the future of research and treatment of dentofacial deformity patients remain unanswered. We hope that this book not only will provide answers to clinical questions but, equally important, also will stimulate further research and progress in treatment methods.

Surgical Correction of Dentofacial Deformities is the work of many surgeons and orthodontists involved in the treatment of dentofacial deformities. The impetus to write such a book arose from the need for all individuals involved in treating dentofacial deformities to plan, work, and treat patients together. If optimum function, stability and esthetics are to be achieved in most individuals with such deformities, collaboration between specialists in medicine and dentistry is mandatory.

Our objective has been to write a comprehensive clinical reference on the interdisciplinary art and science of correcting dentofacial deformities by surgery and orthodontics. This work actually combines an atlas of surgical and orthodontic procedures with sound diagnostic and biologic guidelines for their application. When orthognathic surgical procedures are properly planned and executed in concert with orthodontics, and when the patient receives proper postoperative care, virtually all dentofacial deformity patients can be treated effectively.

We were privileged to develop this book during a time when treatment methods for patients with problems of dentofacial deformity were expanding rapidly. This made the project exciting, but it also complicated our work beyond expectation. We owe an enormous debt to the many contributors to the work. They have waited with unusual patience throughout the gestation of these volumes and it is in large part to them that we owe its currentness and clinical insight. Each of us is influenced by our teachers and peers and we hope that this work in some small way begins to repay our debt to these special individuals.

William H. Bell
William R. Proffit
Raymond P. White

ACKNOWLEDGMENTS

For whatever this book achieves, much is owed to many individuals. We are all a product of our teachers, mentors, parents, environment, and colleagues and of the talents and challenges that God provides.

Dr. Sumpter Arnim, a very fascinating and inquisitive individual with a great thirst for life, ignited in me the flame of curiosity for scientific things. This flame, which has burned for over 25 years, has provided me with a number of very interesting, challenging, and exciting professional experiences. The writing of this book has been one of the most challenging. I will always be indebted to Dr. Arnim. To men like Dr. Barnet M. Levy and Dr. Robert V. Walker, I am similarly indebted—both of these men have provided me the opportunity and environment both to continue animal and clinical investigations and to keep one foot in the clinical arena. Both endeavors I dearly love.

For the past eight years, I have had the privilege of working with eight outstanding oral and maxillofacial surgery residents in our Research Laboratory at the University of Texas Southwestern Medical School: Drs. John J. Dann, Raymond J. Fonseca, Steven A. Schendel, James W. Kennedy, Heidi Opdebeeck, Richard A. Finn, John A. Brammer, and Gregory B. Scheideman will each have something very special and unique to contribute to the art and science of our specialty as we will know it in the future. Each of these individuals has had a special part in providing background information for this book. I am proud to say that during the past five years, they have either authored or co-authored 50 original investigations. I mention these facts for two reasons: first, I am indebted to each of them; secondly, I believe that all clinical training programs can and should have the same benefits that our program has derived from such a commitment to research.

I want to extend special thanks to the many dental and medical colleagues who have entrusted the surgical care of their patients to us during the developmental phase of orthognathic surgery. By their support and close collaboration, these colleagues have made possible some of the present surgical advances. Good friends such as Dr. Patrick A. Alessandra and Dr. Thomas Creekmore were two of the first to provide such help.

I am also deeply indebted to my surgical colleagues: Kevin L. McBride, D.D.S., Douglas P. Sinn, D.D.S., Wayne H. Speer, D.D.S., and Robert V. Walker, D.D.S. for their valued assistance.

Special thanks must be extended to the many unsung heroes who have helped prepare the manuscript—manuscript editors Lillian Rodberg and Patrice Smith, our secretaries, and my wife, Sherry. Personal thanks are also due to our publisher, the W. B. Saunders Company, which includes Mr. Carroll Cann, Mr. Raymond Kersey, Mr. Robert Reinhardt, Mrs. Laura Tarves, and Ms. Julia Lawley for their undaunted support and patience during the development of this work.

Many surgical principles described in the book are based upon animal investigations that have been supported for approximately 15 years by the National Institute of Dental Research (Grant DE-03794-08). Special thanks are extended to Mrs. Rebecca McCulloch and Mrs. Margaret Colmenars for their untiring technical assistance with these animal investigations. Special thanks are also extended to the Stryker Corporation, 420 Alcott Street, Kalamazoo, Michigan and the Dow Corning Corporation (manufacturer of Proplast), Midland, Michigan for financial support of the medical illustrations.

The many illustrations are a testimonial to the talent of medical illustrator William O. Winn, and the photographs to the skill of Marcus Bennett and other medical photographers.

Finally, considering the demands on time which this book has imposed, I must acknowledge the patience, cooperation and sacrifice on the part of my family during the past five years. To the special people in my life, Sherry, Bryan, Adam, Christine, and Elizabeth, to my mother Mrs. Madeline Bell, and to my brother Harry L. Bell.

WILLIAM H. BELL

In any complex endeavor, it certainly is true that no one can do it alone. We particularly want to add our acknowledgment of the many contributors to this book; our surgical and orthodontic colleagues in Lexington, Richmond, and Chapel Hill; and our faithful secretaries, who know perhaps better than anyone the true amount of work involved.

WILLIAM R. PROFFIT
RAYMOND P. WHITE

CONTENTS

SURGICAL CORRECTION OF DENTOFACIAL DEFORMITIES

Chapter 11

MANDIBULAR EXCESS

William H. Bell, Raymond P. White, Jr., H. David Hall, and William R. Proffit

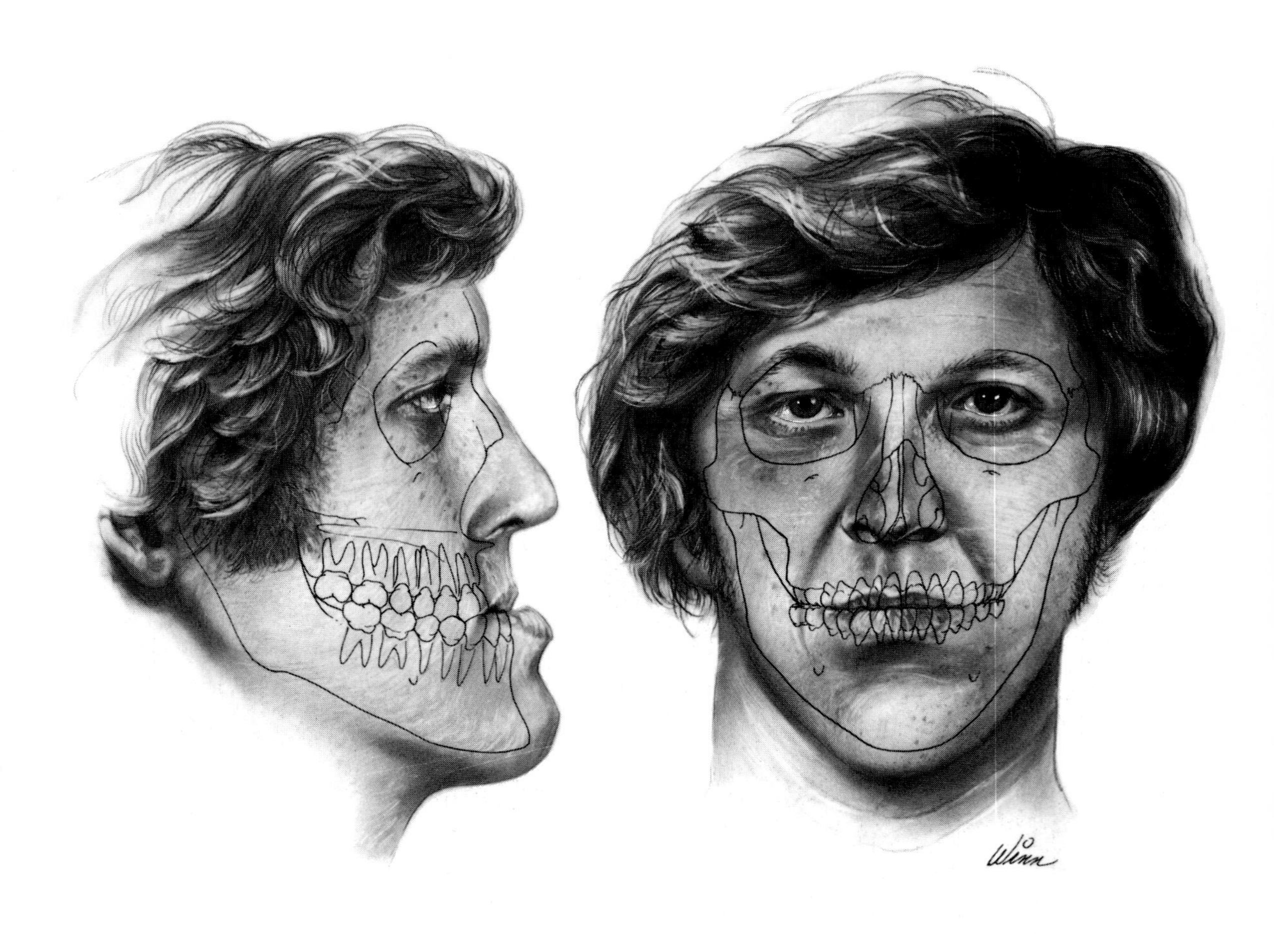

Dentofacial deformity in the lower third of the face resulting from excess mandibular growth is not as common as mandibular deficiency. Data from a recently completed U.S. Public Health Service survey of youths aged 12 to 17 indicate that in about 14 per cent of youths in the United States the mandibular first molar is mesially related to the maxillary first molar.[31] Those who consider a reverse horizontal overlap in the incisor area to be a more accurate indicator of mandibular excess believe that 2.5 per cent of youths in the United States exhibit the problem. A severe problem may exist in the 40 per cent of individuals in this category who exhibit a reverse horizontal overlap greater than 1.0 mm. Orthognathic surgery in conjunction with orthodontic treatment probably would be required for correction in this latter group, estimated to number 340,000.

It is possible that the U.S. Public Health Service Survey understates the problem of mandibular excess. The TPI diagnostic system used in this epidemiologic approach underestimates severe jaw deformity problems. In addition, at age 17 — the upper limit used in the survey — not all individuals would have reached their full growth. The problem of mandibular excess may express itself late in the growth period and therefore be under-represented because of the age range of the selected sample.

Historically, the problem of mandibular excess received the attention of orthodontists and oral surgeons early in the 20th century. Recognizing that orthodontic treatment alone would not solve the problem, Edward Angle suggested that the only possible way to correct a true mandibular protrusion was through a combination of orthodontics and surgery.[2] Because the body of the mandible was surgically accessible, a section of bone could be removed through a skin incision and the mandible shortened.

The early surgical procedures were carried out before the development of antibiotic agents and without the understanding of surgical principles that exists today. In spite of these deficiencies and an occasional prolonged postoperative course, wounds healed, orthodontic treatment was completed, and the individual patient's occlusion and profile were improved.[46] By midcentury, the cooperation gained between the oral surgeon and the orthodontist served as the basis for the general acceptance of combined orthodontic and surgical treatment of mandibular problems as the treatment of choice.[7] This cooperative approach is a major contribution of North American dentistry to the field of facial deformity correction and has been extended to the treatment of midfacial problems in the 1970s.

The cause of mandibular excess is disparate vertical and horizontal growth in the lower third of the face as compared with the upper face. Treatment approaches have been devised to redirect the growth of the skeletal mandible and to encourage growth of the midface to prevent the condition from developing. The *prevention* of mandibular excess lies in this realm, and the subject is discussed briefly in the section of this chapter that describes orthodontic approaches. Problems encountered in some patients treated surgically before mandibular growth was complete have engendered a cautious approach to early treatment of affected patients. Similarity in appearance between siblings and their parents indicates genetics is a major factor in development of mandibular excess.

Part A: Bilateral Mandibular Excess

SYSTEMATIC DESCRIPTION OF THE DEFORMITY

Esthetic Features

Mandibular excess is characterized by a prominent lower third of the face. Skeletal mandibular excess must be differentiated from conditions in which the lower jaw appears excessively large as a result of midfacial deficiency (for example, in the patient with a cleft lip and palate) and from an apparent excess due to an unusually large chin area. Facial structures must be evaluated carefully, since a large mandible will make a correctly proportioned midface seem deficient. Additional information on maxillary deficiency and chin surgery may be found in Chapters 9 and 14, respectively.

The facial appearance typical of mandibular excess can be altered by changing the vertical, sagittal, and horizontal positions of the mandible. A decrease in anterior facial height accentuates the prominence of the lower third of the face, and an increase in anterior facial height de-emphasizes the prominence of the chin area (Fig. 11–1). In the frontal view, the patient with mandibular excess exhibits a broad lower third of the face as well as obvious overdevelopment of the lower jaw. In severe cases, lip incompetence may be seen. The reverse horizontal overlap of the incisor teeth does not provide adequate support for either the upper or the lower lip. The alar base of the nose may appear normal or narrow. Correction of lip posture and nasal deformity is as important a consideration in planning treatment as is treatment of the bony mandible itself.

Asymmetry of the lower third of the face often accompanies mandibular excess. The skeletal midline must be determined with the lower jaw in its physiologic rest position. Occasionally it is helpful to mark the midline of the face directly on the patient's skin to evaluate the degree of asymmetry that is present. A shift of the lower jaw may be detected only as the patient moves from rest position to maximum intercuspation of the teeth. The dental midline of the upper and lower jaws should be determined clinically, and discrepancies between the dental and skeletal midline

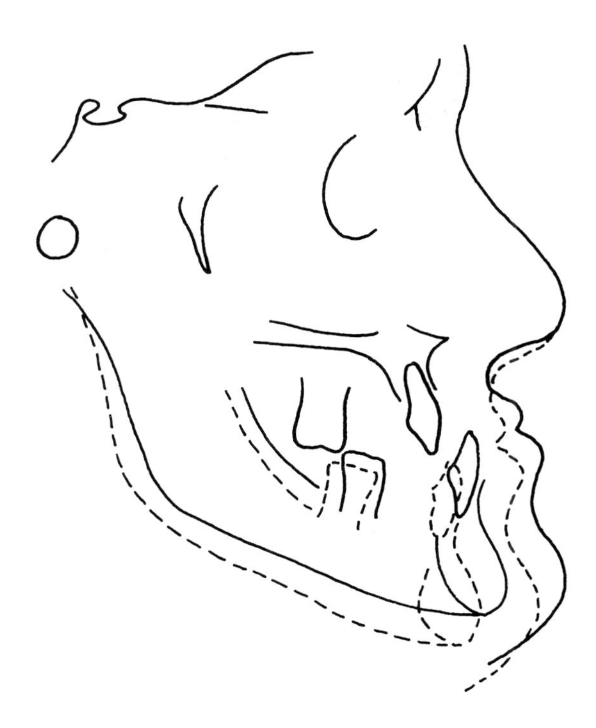

Figure 11–1. Altering the position of the lower jaw can change the chin prominence. The dashed line illustrates the position of the lower jaw when the anterior facial height is increased.

should be noted. Once it is established clinically, the skeletal midline should be marked directly on the diagnostic dental casts.

A prominent lower third of the face will be obvious from the profile view with the patient in natural head position. Mandibular excess is accentuated by decreased anterior facial height caused by missing posterior teeth or by an excessive freeway space. In these instances the abnormal dental relationships allow the lower jaw to overclose. A better evaluation of the facial profile is possible if the proper occlusal vertical dimension of the teeth is initially established by prosthodontic approaches. Temporary wax or acrylic bite wafers will hold the jaws apart during the evaluation phase (see Chapter 19). The mandibular plane may be steep (particularly if excess height of the anterior face accompanies the mandibular excess), or it may be parallel to the palatal plane. An obtuse gonial angle and a steep mandibular plane are considered esthetic defects that are difficult to correct with any type of jaw surgery. The patient who exhibits both anterior vertical excess and horizontal excess in the lower third of the face may have an anterior open bite. In such patients, eruption of anterior teeth could not compensate adequately for the jaw discrepancy.

The relationship of the chin, the lips, and the nose can be evaluated accurately by masking one of the anatomic structures while evaluating the relationship of the other two. A prominent chin button is the most characteristic feature seen in the profile view. In almost all instances, the excess in the lower third of the face gives the middle third of the face the appearance of being deficient. (The middle third of the face must be evaluated carefully to determine its correct position anatomically.) The labiomental fold is diminished or absent, and an acute nasolabial angle may accompany the deformity. It is important to evaluate the submental area. Any correction made in the lower jaw will affect this area as well as the proportions of the face. If there is little demarcation between the submental area and the vertical plane of the anterior aspect of the neck, this problem will be accentuated by shortening the mandible. Such unesthetic changes that are a consequence of this type of ramus surgery may be offset by advancement genioplasty or subapical osteotomy.

Analysis of Dental Casts, Radiographs, and Other Records

INTRA-ARCH ALIGNMENT AND SYMMETRY

In true mandibular excess, maxillary teeth are usually found in a position anterior to their skeletal base. The maxillary anterior teeth are protrusive and facially inclined and the maxillary dental arch takes a V shape in the anterior aspect. The mandibular anterior teeth may be upright in relation to the basal supporting bone of the mandible, or they may be inclined lingually. The mandibular incisors may be crowded. Frequently, one tooth (an incisor or canine) is crowded out of the dental arch lingually.

TRANSVERSE RELATIONSHIP OF TEETH AND JAWS

Frequently, a posterior crossbite is found. Although the crossbite may be due to a wide mandible, the maxillary posterior teeth may be inclined buccally or a transverse deficiency may exist in the supporting bone of the maxilla. When this occurs, a higher than normal palatal vault accompanies the posterior crossbite. It is important to differentiate between lingually inclined maxillary teeth and a true transverse deficiency in the skeletal maxilla. Usually the mandibular molar teeth are situated properly over the supporting basal bone of the mandible. In patients who have a severe anteroposterior skeletal discrepancy, mandibular posterior teeth are inclined lingually. Any degree of asymmetry detected clinically should be confirmed by means of radiographs and with study casts mounted on a semi-adjustable articular. (See Chapter 9 for additional details.)

ANTEROPOSTERIOR RELATIONSHIPS

The most commonly cited feature of mandibular excess is the mesial relationship of the mandibular first molar to the maxillary first molar. Less discussed, but almost always accompanying the problem, is the mesial or Class III (Angle) relation of the mandibular canine to its maxillary counterpart. A reverse horizontal overlap in the incisor area is characteristic. Cephalometric and clinical studies are used to aid in assessing the degree of mandibular deformity relative to the face and the relationship of the dentition to the basal bone in the mandible and the maxilla. Vertical and horizontal relationships must be assessed. The true proportions of both the midface and the lower face should be determined clinically and confirmed with cephalometric studies.

VERTICAL RELATIONSHIPS

Facial height strongly influences the appearance of the lower third of the face. Most often a short posterior face is accompanied by an obtuse gonial angle and a steep mandibular plane as seen on the lateral cephalometric film. Anterior facial height may be increased, and an anterior open bite may accompany this condition if the teeth could not compensate by a differential eruption pattern. The anterior bite opening is often produced when the patient is in the final growth spurt and the teeth have compensated for the problem to their maximum before that time. It is this final manifestation of the condition of mandibular excess that alerts many patients to the fact that they have a problem.

ORTHODONTIC TREATMENT

Chin Cap Therapy

A "pressure bandage" applied to an excessively growing mandible was one of the earliest approaches to treatment of mandibular excess. The idea that force applied against the lower jaw during growth could improve a skeletal mandibular excess problem was developed and refined in the latter half of the 19th century, primarily by Norman Kingsley.[33] It was reasoned, then as now, that pressure against the chin would be transmitted to the growing areas of the mandible, and that growth would be impeded or at least redirected more favorably. Chin cap therapy, as this extraoral approach is known, has never been widely accepted in the United States. Two reasons for this lack of popularity are apparent:

1. Despite sporadic reports of success for many patients, the interceptive treatment did not work well enough to prevent a severe problem of mandibular excess in adult life.
2. Increasing emphasis on tooth movement as the preferred method for correcting dentofacial deformity led to virtual abandonment of extraoral appliances as a general approach.

From the 1930s on, if tooth position proved uncorrectable by full banded orthodontic appliances, surgery to reduce the size of the mandible was considered, and a relatively large amount of experience with combined orthodontic and surgical treatment was gained earlier with mandibular excess than with any of the other dentofacial deformity problems discussed in this book. As extraoral force in the treatment of maxillary excess (Class II) problems was reintroduced after World War II, interest in chin caps reappeared.

In today's context, there are two ways to use a chin cap for interceptive orthodontic treatment of skeletal mandibular excess. Both approaches have their advocates at present, and although the evidence is clear that the second approach is effective, it may be that true skeletal effects are achieved by the first mechanism as well. The first approach to correcting mandibular excess is based on impeding mandibular growth by applying heavy pressure in the vicinity of the growing condyle of the mandible.[18] These approaches are illustrated diagrammatically in Figure 11–2. Force is applied upward and backward, in approximate opposition to the vector of downward and forward mandibular growth. Such a force requires an extraoral attachment high on the head and relatively far forward. A modern appliance that uses precalibrated modules with coil springs to produce the force and a plastic frame to allow the prescribed direction is shown in Figure 11–3. It is now well established that sutures respond to externally applied forces, and that sutural responses to extraoral force delivered to

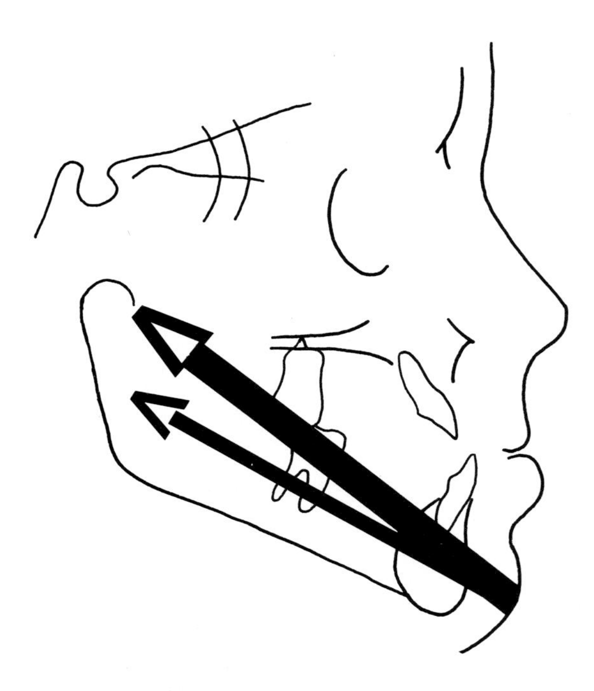

Figure 11–2. The two approaches to chin cap therapy differ in the direction and magnitude of force application. A higher direction of pull, with heavy force magnitude, is used to apply pressure directly against the condyle in an attempt to impede condylar growth (*upper arrow*). A lower direction of pull with lighter force is employed to rotate the mandible down and back, changing growth direction (*lower arrow*).

the maxilla via a facebow can be obtained (see Chapter 3). The situation with the mandibular condyle is not totally analagous, since instead of a suture there is a joint with a joint capsule and an articular disk. Cartilaginous growth as well as periosteal growth is involved. The extent to which growth at the condyle of the mandible is influenced by an impeding force remains controversial. Histologic studies tend to confirm a response in the pattern of bone deposition at the condyle when extraoral force is applied to the mandible.[29] The magnitude of the response is small and as such might not explain the clinical benefits. Similarly, clinical improvement can be achieved by various means besides directly impeding growth at the condyle.

The second theoretical possibility for influencing excess mandibular growth is to use extraoral force not to impede but to redirect growth of the mandible.[51] This approach takes advantage of the fact that when the mandible is rotated downward, it also rotates backward. Some patients appear to have horizontal mandibular excess when their problem is merely lack of posterior vertical development of the maxillary and mandibular alveolar processes, so that the mandible rotates closed more than it should. This same effect can be produced by loss of posterior teeth with resulting dental collapse and lack of posterior vertical dimension. Conversely, the impression of mandibular excess can be corrected in such patients by increasing the vertical dimension, thereby moving the chin backward as well as downward. If force is directed against the mandible during a period of rapid growth in such manner as to move the chin down and back, increased eruption of posterior teeth will "build in" this rotation, and the mandibular excess will be less prominent in the anteroposterior plane of space. This approach works exceptionally well in patients who have a deficit in vertical dimension. Obviously, the approach would be contraindicated if the vertical as well as horizontal dimensions of the mandible are too great. The trade-off between horizontal excess in the lower third of the face and vertical excess is satisfactory only when vertical development was deficient initially (see Chapter 9).

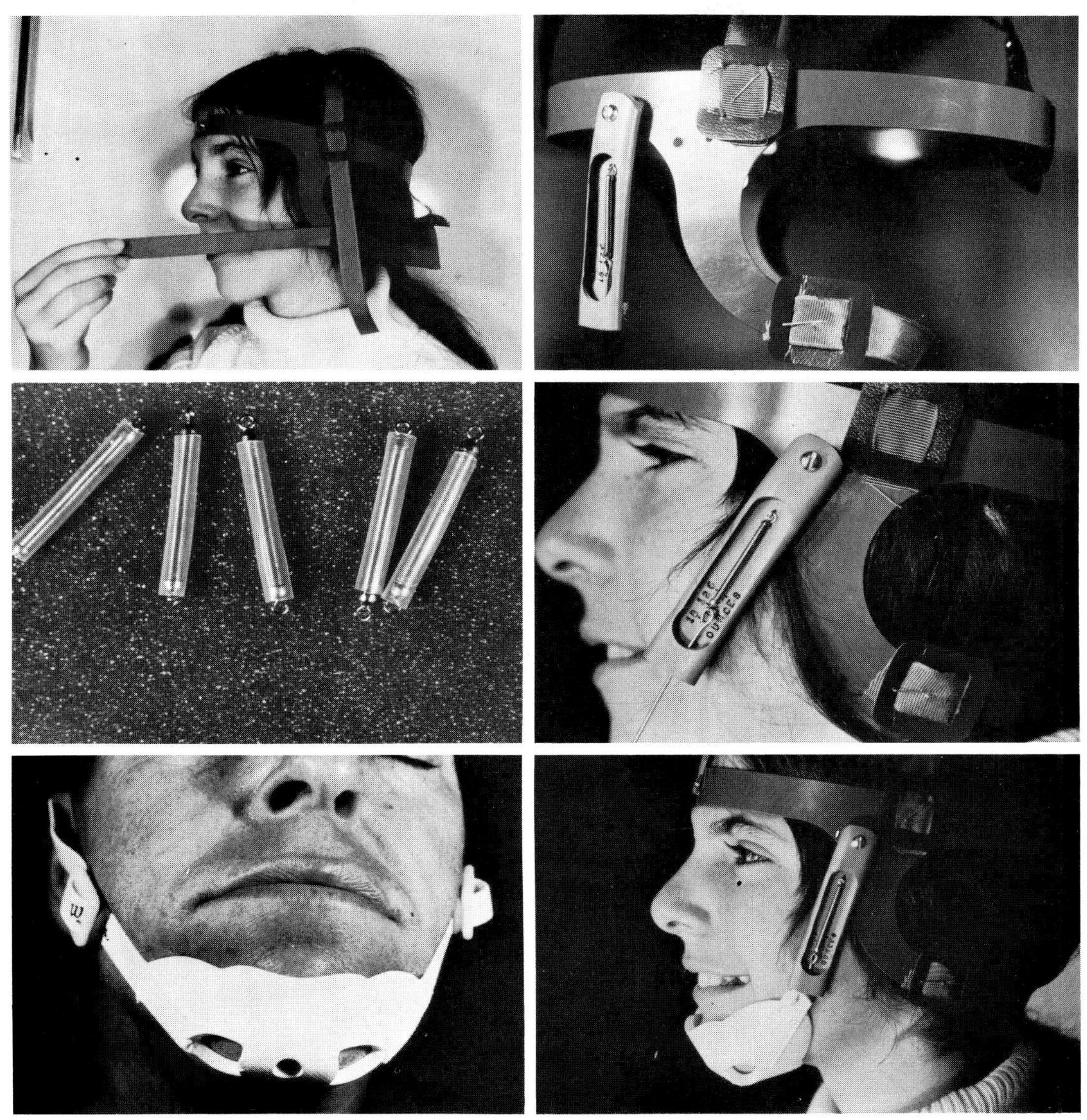

Figure 11–3. Semirigid calvarium cap specifically designed for forces within orthopedic range, although it may be used for conventional (lighter) tooth-moving applications. Force modules of calibrated coil springs are attached to a flexible plastic structure and are designed to measure the precise force delivered to the maxillary or mandibular region. The side members are sufficiently resistant to prevent impingement of wires on cheeks, which might dissipate the force and reduce its effectiveness. A popular foam rubber football helmet chin cap makes an excellent adjunct for Class III and open-bite cases (third row). (From Graber TM and Swain BF: Current Orthodontic Concepts and Techniques. 2nd edition. Philadelphia: W. B. Saunders Co., 1975. Courtesy of Unitek Corporation and Orthoband Corporation.)

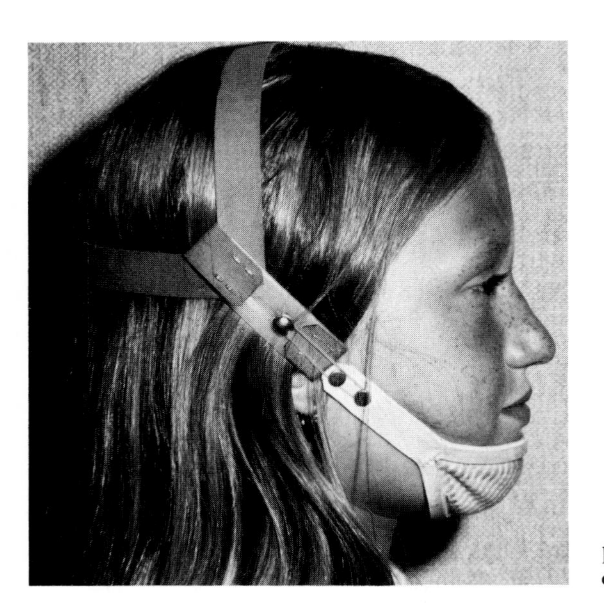

Figure 11–4. A chin cap with the direction of pull below the condyle tends to rotate the mandible downward and backward.

If the goal of extraoral chin cap therapy is to rotate the mandible rather than to impede its growth directly, both the direction and magnitude of force differ from therapy aimed at impeding growth. The direction of pull against the mandible would be lower in this instance, pulling on a line beneath the condyle rather than directly through it. Since the goal is redirecting rather than impeding growth, it would be logical also to utilize lower force levels. This approach, advocated particularly by Woodside in recent years, is presented diagrammatically in Figure 11–2. A head cap with a lower direction of pull is illustrated in Figure 11–4.

Downward and backward rotation of the mandible during growth tends to be a feature of all successful attempts to intercept mandibular excess, whether the clinician's orientation favored attempting to impede growth or rotation was the initial goal. There is no evidence that one or the other of the chin cap approaches is superior. In both instances, clinical success can be gained for some patients and improvement for others, while a third group do not respond favorably during the growth period and become candidates for surgical correction. Therapy employing the chin cap has been successful often enough to justify giving this therapeutic approach a trial in a growing individual with a developing mandibular excess problem. Deciding how long the chin cap should be worn calls for excellent clinical judgment. Prolonged treatment in the teens rarely produces a good esthetic result, so a good response prior to or at puberty is important. Because of the number of therapeutic failures, it is wise to anticipate something less than total success in many patients.

The alteration in position of the mandible that results from expansion of the maxillary dental arch has given rise to some misconceptions relative to the effect of this procedure. Many individuals with mandibular excess also have some maxillary deficiency. These patients benefit from treatment that expands the maxillary arch by opening the midpalatal suture during growth. When the suture is opened, clinical examination usually reveals that not only has the width discrepancy between the arches been decreased but any horizontal discrepancy related to mandibular excess has been minimized as well. Although it has been claimed that opening the suture displaces the maxilla forward, it is apparent that much of the anteroposterior improvement results, not from horizontal repositioning of the maxilla but from vertical repositioning of the mandible. When the posterior teeth are carried laterally, impingement of cusps and different interdigitation of the teeth always produces some downward and backward rotation of the mandible. The same can be true of intraoral elastic force such as cross-elastics: if molar teeth in either arch are moved laterally or extruded by elastic force so that mandibular rotation occurs, the chin will become less prominent.

Activator Appliances

The activator system of appliances can be effective in the treatment of Class III malocclusion despite the fact that in this instance there is no repositioning of the mandible so that muscles are stretched. During the fabrication of a Class III activator, the patient bites as far posteriorly as possible, but this position usually is little if any behind the habitual position of the mandible. Clinical success of the activator appliance in such a patient clearly depends on the same downward and backward rotation of the mandible. If the activator is trimmed to allow posterior teeth to erupt so that the increased vertical dimension is maintained, a diminution in the relative mandibular protrusion can be achieved.

Fully Banded Orthodontic Appliances

Fully banded orthodontic treatment for skeletal mandibular excess can be carried out satisfactorily without surgery only when the problem is minor, because it is very difficult to position mandibular teeth so as to camouflage the mandibular prominence. The teeth can be retracted, but the prominent chin remains. If teeth are severely crowded, it may be necessary to remove a tooth to gain space. This should be done only to maintain proper alignment of the teeth within their own arches. Marked displacement of the teeth relative to their supporting bone is not acceptable treatment for skeletal mandibular excess.

A patient with moderately severe Class III malocclusion in the preteen years can pose a difficult treatment planning decision. Interceptive treatment should be attempted. What if it almost but not quite succeeds in solving the occlusal and esthetic problems? The temptation is to place full-banded appliances for "final correction" of the problem. This should be avoided, simply because the correction may not be final. Late growth in patients with mandibular excess can and does occur. Orthodontic treatment should not involve severe retraction of mandibular incisors and protraction of maxillary incisors for two reasons: (1) the esthetic result is poor; and (2) if enough growth does occur to make surgery mandatory, such orthodontic treatment will have made surgical correction difficult or impossible.

SURGICAL TREATMENT

Considerations in Surgical Treatment Planning

The mandibular excess deformity typically involves the anterior dimension. Mandibular excess, however, must not be considered solely as a problem of excessive anterior growth; the vertical and horizontal dimensions are also frequently abnormal. If there is too much anterior growth alone, then surgical treatment may consist of retrusion by ramus osteotomy or body ostectomy. If vertical or horizontal abnormalities coexist, however, additional procedures are indicated. Indeed two or three mandibular procedures, sometimes in conjunction with a maxillary osteotomy, may be required for optimal surgical treatment of mandibular excess. The common growth disturbances in the vertical, horizontal, and anterior planes and the types of surgical procedures used for their correction are noted later.

Vertical abnormalities can involve either the chin, the vertical ramus, or the body of the mandible. Excessive chin height is correctable by genioplasty (see Chapter 14). Excessive height of the body and ramus, as can occur in condylar hyperplasia, is treatable by excision of the inferior border of the mandible (see mandibular asymmetry section of this chapter).

Horizontal growth abnormalities of the mandible are manifested by arch width anomalies. The mandibular arch may be too wide, or associated with transverse maxillary deficiency. In either case, when maxillary surgery is not indicated, a symphysis osteotomy or ostectomy in concert with vertical ramus osteotomies often corrects the wide arch. Asymmetry in body width and height, as occurs with condylar hyperplasia, can be corrected by mandibuloplasty (see Chapter 14 and mandibular asymmetry section) or an onlay of bone or alloplastic material.

Extraoral Approaches

Historical Development

Extraoral surgery to correct excess in the ramus of the mandible was described early in the 20th century. Although individual references to the approach can be found in both the American and European literature, the impetus for general acceptance of the procedure by American surgeons came from a paper published by Caldwell and Letterman in 1954.[11] These authors thoroughly reviewed the procedure itself and described in detail the diagnostic and technical aspects of surgery in the ramus of the mandible with access through a submandibular skin incision (Fig. 11–5). Further refinements in the procedure followed in the ensuing decade, and studies such as the one by Boyne on osseous healing confirmed the clinical impressions of surgeons who used the procedure routinely.[8] In 1968, Caldwell discussed the use of the procedure in correcting problems of extreme mandibular excess.[10] The importance of detaching the coronoid process at the time of surgery when the mandibular correction exceeds 10 mm was stressed as critical in preventing displacing forces from the temporalis muscle and relapse toward the pretreatment condition. Other minor

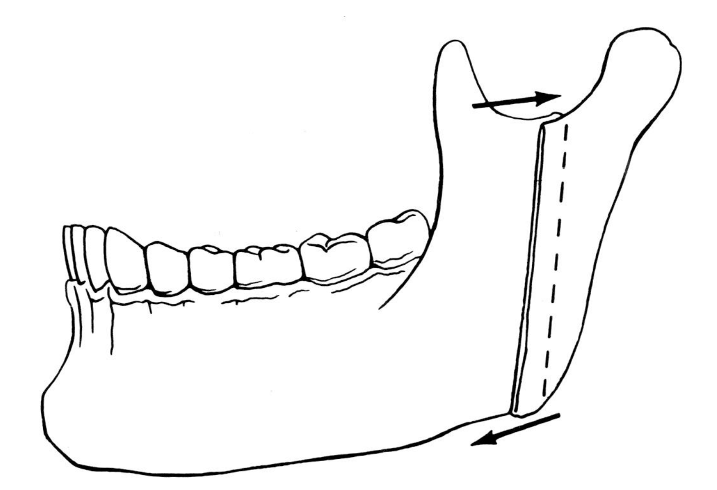

Figure 11–5. Following a bilateral bony cut in the mandibular ramus behind the mandibular foramen, the tooth-bearing segment is moved posteriorly and the condylar segments are positioned laterally, leaving the articular surface of the condyle as close as possible to its original position.

modifications such as the removal of bone in the area of the coronoid notch were advocated by Caldwell to facilitate good bony contact after repositioning of the proximal condylar segment and the tooth-bearing distal segment of the mandible. In 1967, Hinds and Girotti suggested that the skin incision for approaching the ramus of the mandible be made parallel to the posterior border of the mandible.[25] This incision, described as 2.5 cm in length or less, allows the surgeon to reach the posterior border of the mandible above its angle. It was suggested that through this approach the mandibular branch of the facial nerve could be avoided in the soft-tissue dissection. An extraoral approach to the mandible is used less frequently today by surgeons for the correction of mandibular excess.

Indications for Using the Extraoral Approach

Until recently, the extraoral approach to the ramus of the mandible was the most commonly preferred technique (Fig. 11–6). With recent refinements of intraoral osteotomies of the ramus, an extraoral approach is infrequently indicated. One relative indication for the extraoral approach is when wide exposure of the lateral aspect of the ramus is necessary. Such a situation occurs most often when the mandible is retruded more than 1.5 cm. When a large posterior movement is calculated preoperatively to have an inefficient biomechanical effect on the temporalis muscles or restrict the amount of posterior movement, an "inverted L" osteotomy technique is utilized to offset the decreased mechanical efficiency produced by altering the spatial relationship of the temporalis muscles. (See Chapters 13 and 24 for additional considerations.) When a large amount of retrusion or lengthening of the mandibular ramus is necessary, the periosteum along the inferior or posterior border, or both, of the mandible is incised to allow sufficient mobility of the distal segment. The splitting of the periosteum is an important adjunctive consideration and is achieved through an extraoral or intraoral approach. In clinical practice, however, the need for such large posterior movements is relatively rare; the distal segment is not frequently lengthened because of the propensity to relapse. Another uncommon indication exists when the mouth is very small and inelastic, or when visualization is restricted because of extreme bowing of the vertical rami. The extraoral vertical ramus osteotomy has also been recommended when severe asymmetry exists.[23] In this situation, the vertical ramus osteotomy is a better choice than the sagittal split osteotomy, because with the sagittal split osteotomy the large proximal segments may not be adapted well to the asymmetrically retruded mandible. However, the vertical ramus osteotomy can also be performed from an intraoral approach and, for reasons to be noted later, this approach is preferred to the extraoral approach. The extraoral approach also has been advocated because it permits reduction of a very obtuse gonial angle. Kelsey and Lash, in independent studies, however, demonstrated that the gonial angle remodels back to its former shape and may indeed be more obtuse than before surgery.[32, 35]

Surgical Technique

The extraoral approach to the ramus of the mandible is a clean surgical procedure, and the patient should be prepared and draped appropriately for such a procedure after the nasoendotracheal induction of gěneral anesthesia. The surgical procedure is facilitated by the use of an anesthetic technique that allows the surgeon to extend the patient's neck and tilt the head right or left as the bilateral surgical approaches are made. The skin incision may be made in a curvilinear fashion beneath the angle of the mandible or vertically parallel to the posterior border of the ramus of the mandible. The ramus of the mandible is approached by careful dissection through soft-tissue planes with care being taken not to damage the marginal mandibular branch of the facial nerve. Occasionally the facial vein and artery are encountered in the anterior aspect of the wound, and these vessels must be appropriately ligated. Additional detail regarding soft-tissue dissection may be found in Chapter 16.

Once the lateral aspect of the ramus of the mandible is reached, the masseter muscle and the anterior aspect of the medial pterygoid muscle are detached. After the lateral aspect of the ramus of the mandible is appropriately marked, a surgical bur or a reciprocating saw is used to make an osteotomy from the coronoid notch to a point anterior to the angle of the mandible (Fig. 11–6). Soft tissue should be reflected

Text continued on page 864.

Figure 11–6. Surgical technique for correction of mandibular excess by extraoral vertical ramus osteotomy. *A*, Typical dental, skeletal, and facial features of mandibular excess with mandible in centric relation and lips relaxed, prominent chin with procumbent and everted lower lip, and Class III malocclusion. Dental compensations have been removed by orthodontic treatment, which tipped lower incisors forward; upper incisors have been uprighted. Broken line indicates planned line of osteotomy. Position of masseter muscle. *B*, Position of medial pterygoid muscle and site for osteotomy. *C*, Relevant anatomical structures encountered in Risdon approach to vertical ramus or condylar region of mandible. *D*, The planned line of incision is inscribed on the neck with the blunt tip of a scalpel blade before the landmarks are obscured by the surgical drapes. Cross hatches are inscribed in the skin to provide a reference for accurate approximation of the skin edges at the time of closure. Local anesthetic solution containing 1:200,000 concentration of epinephrine is infiltrated into the skin and the subcutaneous and periosteal tissues for hemostasis and to facilitate the surgical dissection. A 3- to 4-cm incision is made in a natural flexion line of the neck or parallel to a skin fold in the submandibular area approximately one finger breadth below and behind the angle of the mandible. Digital pressure along the margins of the skin incision facilitates the dissection through the skin and subcutaneous tissue.

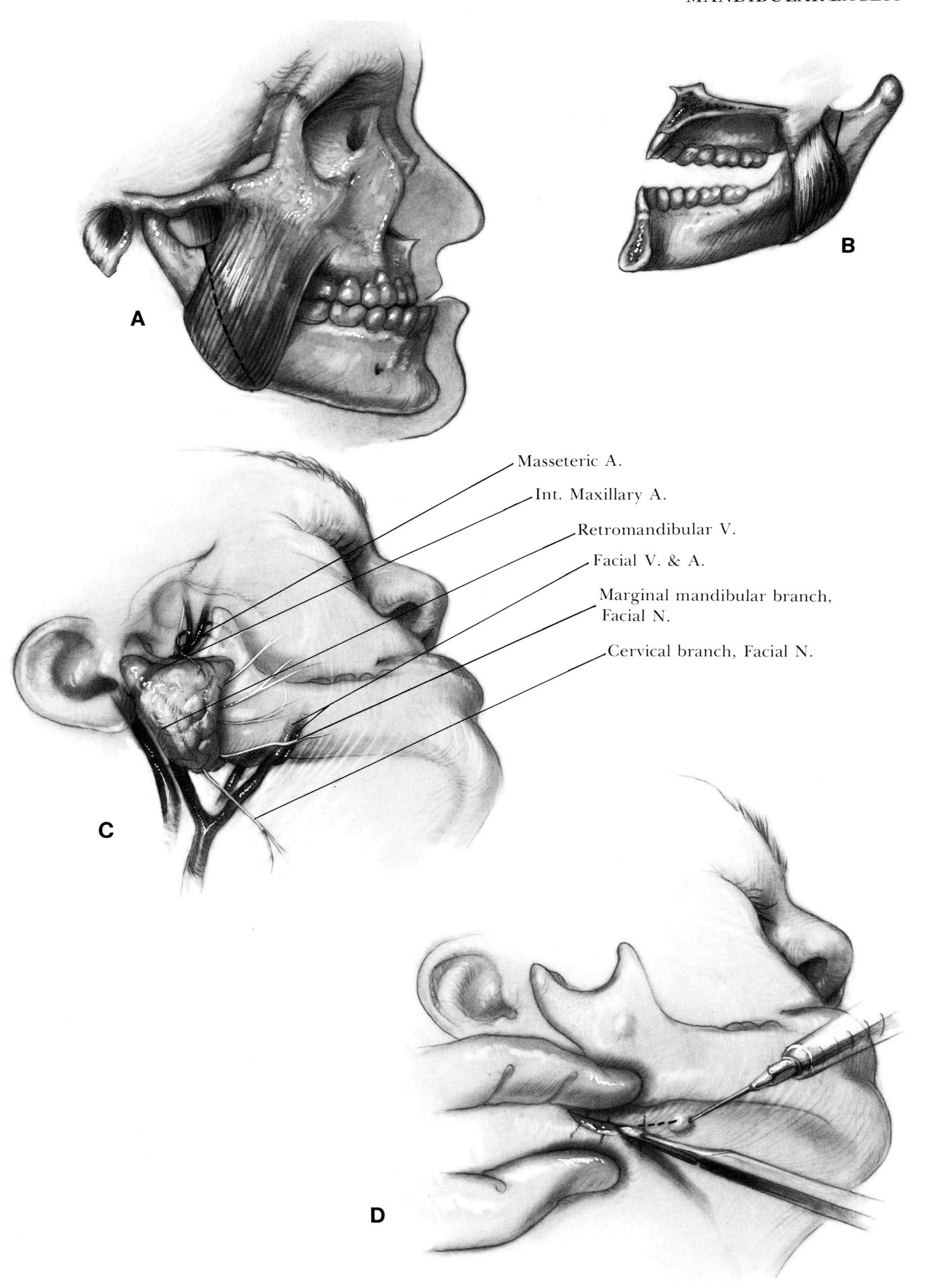

Figure 11–6. See legend on the opposite page.

Illustration continued on the following page

Figure 11–6 *Continued.* *E*, Sharp dissection is accomplished through the skin and subcutaneous fascia to deepen the surgical wound to the level of the platysma muscle. The platysma muscle is bluntly separated to facilitate cutting the muscle without injuring the underlying marginal mandibular branch of the facial nerve, which is located superficial to the superficial layer of the deep cervical fascia. *F*, If the marginal mandibular nerve is visualized, it is bluntly dissected free from the superficial layer of the deep cervical fascia and retracted superiorly along with the tissues along the superior margin of the incision. After identifying the insertion of the masseter muscle at the inferior border of the mandible, its fibers are incised at the inferior limits of their insertion along the inferior border, the angle, and the posterior border of the mandible. *G*, The masseter muscle insertion and periosteum are raised from the underlying ramus to expose the lateral aspect of the ramus. The dissection is continued superiorly to the sigmoid notch and the base of the condylar process, and anteriorly to the base of the coronoid process. The intimate attachments of the tendinous portion of the masseter and medial pterygoid muscles are not detached from the posterior and posteromedial aspects of the vertical rami. These muscle-tendon pedicles tend to maintain the preoperative spatial relationship of the condyles, thereby maintaining the condyles in the fossae, and usually eliminating the need for wiring the proximal segment. (Fibers of the masseter muscles insert directly into bone in the mandibular angle region.)

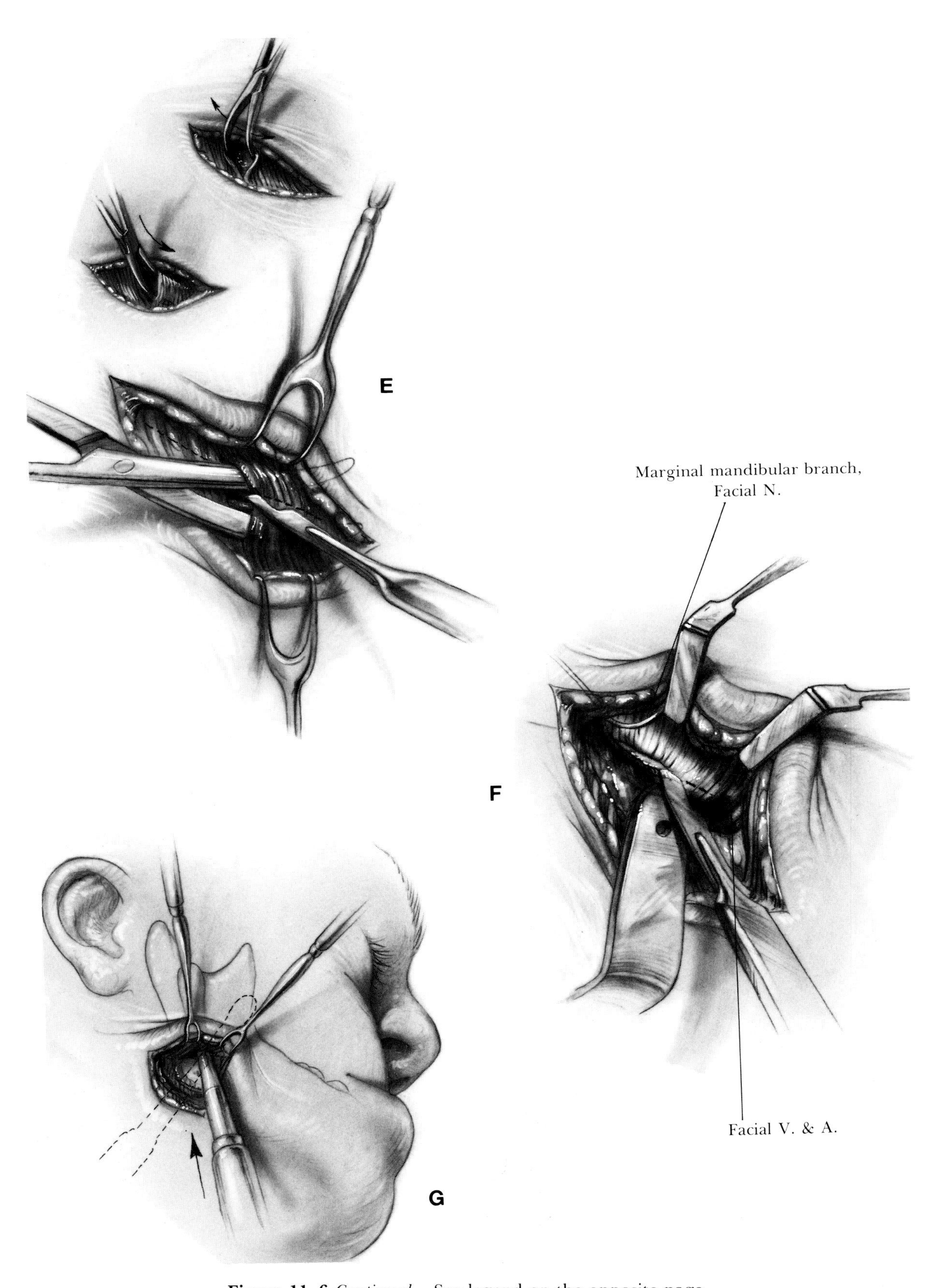

Figure 11-6 *Continued.* See legend on the opposite page.

Illustration continued on the following page.

Figure 11–6 *Continued.* *H*, With an appropriately angulated retractor hooked in the sigmoid notch to expose the lateral surface of the ramus, the bone is sectioned with a reciprocating saw blade or straight fissure bur. The line of section extends from the midsigmoid notch area inferiorly to a point immediately posterior to the mandibular foramen and then inferiorly to the antegonial notch. A radiograph of the ramus and four prime landmarks (sigmoid notch, posterior border, angle of the mandible, and antilingular prominence on lateral aspect of mandible) are used to determine where the osteotomy will be placed. The superior half of the osteotomy begins at a point immediately posterior to the antilingular prominence and curves slightly forward to the midpoint of the sigmoid notch. For most patients, an osteotomy 5 to 7 mm from the posterior border of the ramus is optimal and safe because the neurovascular bundle has not actually entered the mandibular foramen at this point. After the planned osteotomy between the sigmoid notch and the area opposite the mandibular foramen has been etched into the bone with a fissure bur, the bone is sectioned with a reciprocating saw blade. Next, the osteotomy is extended from the area immediately posterior to the antilingular prominence slightly forward to the antegonial notch. *I*, After the osteotomy is completed, the proximal segment is displaced laterally by inserting a periosteal elevator between the segment and the ramus. The elevator is used to move the segment laterally (1) and to stabilize it while a portion of the medial pterygoid muscle and the periosteum are stripped from the anterior medial surface (2). The amount of periosteum and muscle reflected from the proximal segment is largely a function of the degree of anticipated overlap and the width of the proximal segment. The mildly curved osteotomy maintains about a 1-cm wide bony segment at the angle. The goal is to obtain a broad, overlapping surface while maintaining an adequate pedicle of soft tissue. The proximal segment is usually placed lateral to the ramus; with minimal movements the proximal segment is occasionally not overlapped. *J*, Cross-hatched area indicates where the medial pterygoid muscle is detached; dotted area indicates where medial pterygoid muscle attachment is not detached. *K*, When a large posterior movement (1 to 1.5 cm) is calculated preoperatively to have an inefficient biomechanical effect on the temporalis muscles or restricts the amount of posterior movement, an "inverted L" osteotomy technique is utilized.

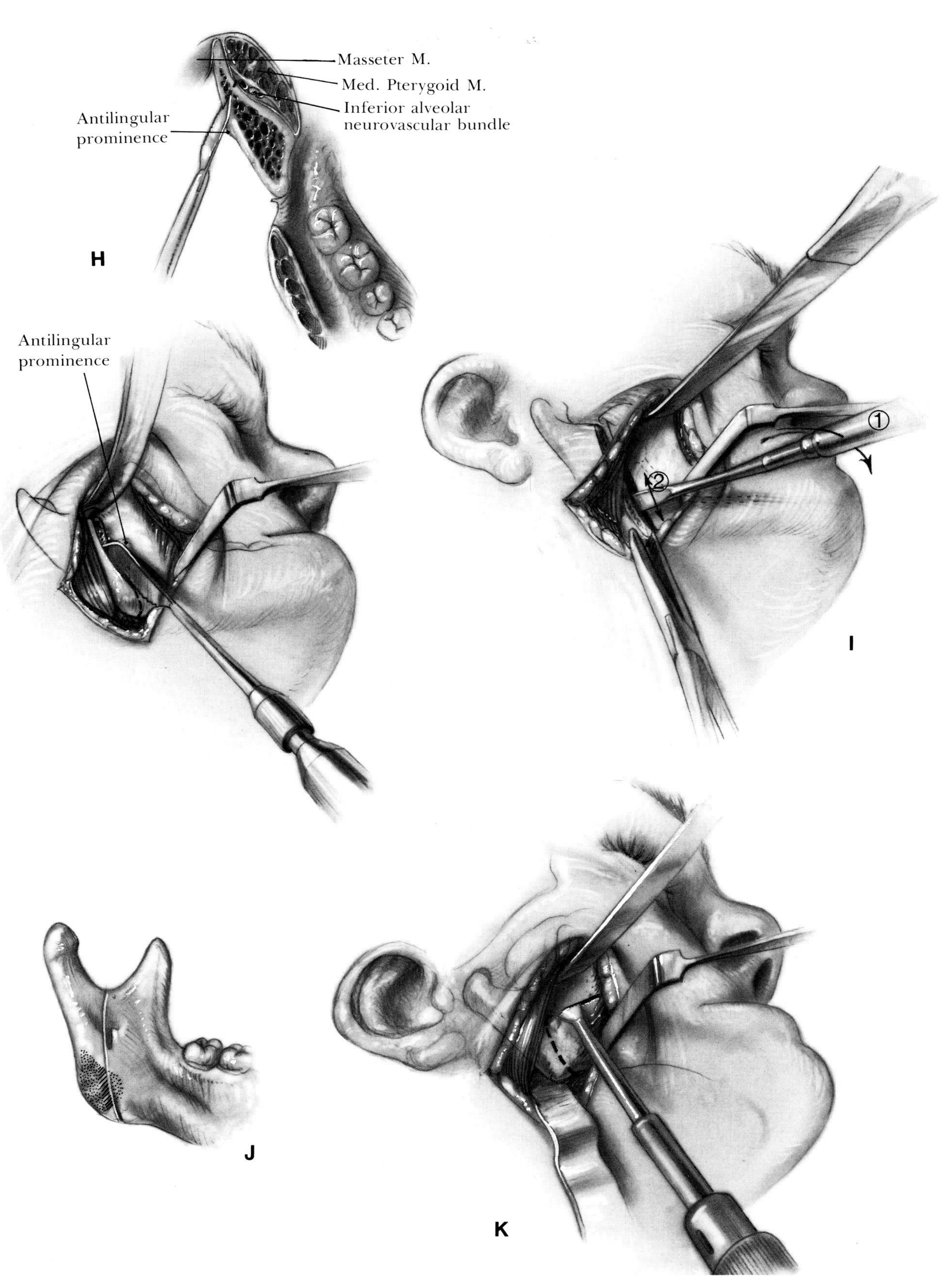

Figure 11–6 *Continued.* Techniques of Dr. William Bell, modified from Dr. Edward C. Hinds and Dr. H. D. Hall. See rest of legend on the opposite page.

Illustration continued on the following page.

Figure 11–6 *Continued.* *L*, Coronoidotomy is considered when unforeseen restriction to mandibular retrusion is encountered at the time of surgery. Sectioning the coronoid process not only alters the mechanical efficiency of the temporalis muscles but also may eliminate the function of these muscles completely, owing to excessive shortening. *M*, The line of action of the medial pterygoid and temporalis muscles, which remain attached to the proximal segment with the "inverted L" osteotomy, tend to maintain the same spatial relationship that exists prior to surgery and minimizes anatomical or functional change in the muscle and bone relationship of the proximal segment. *N*, After the contralateral ramus osteotomy is completed, the proximal segments are positioned laterally and anteriorly to the distal segments and the mandible is retracted until the teeth are in the planned occlusion. Intermaxillary fixation is accomplished with wire ligatures placed between vertical lugs soldered to the previously placed arch wires. *O*, After each proximal segment is manipulated to seat the condyles in the condylar fossae, the extraoral wound is closed in layers. the periosteum and the masseter and medial pterygoid muscles are approximated and sutured over the inferior edge of the osteotomy site. The platysma muscle is closed with interrupted plain catgut sutures. The margins of the skin and subcutaneous tissue are carefully aligned, approximated, and sutured to achieve slight eversion of the wound margins.

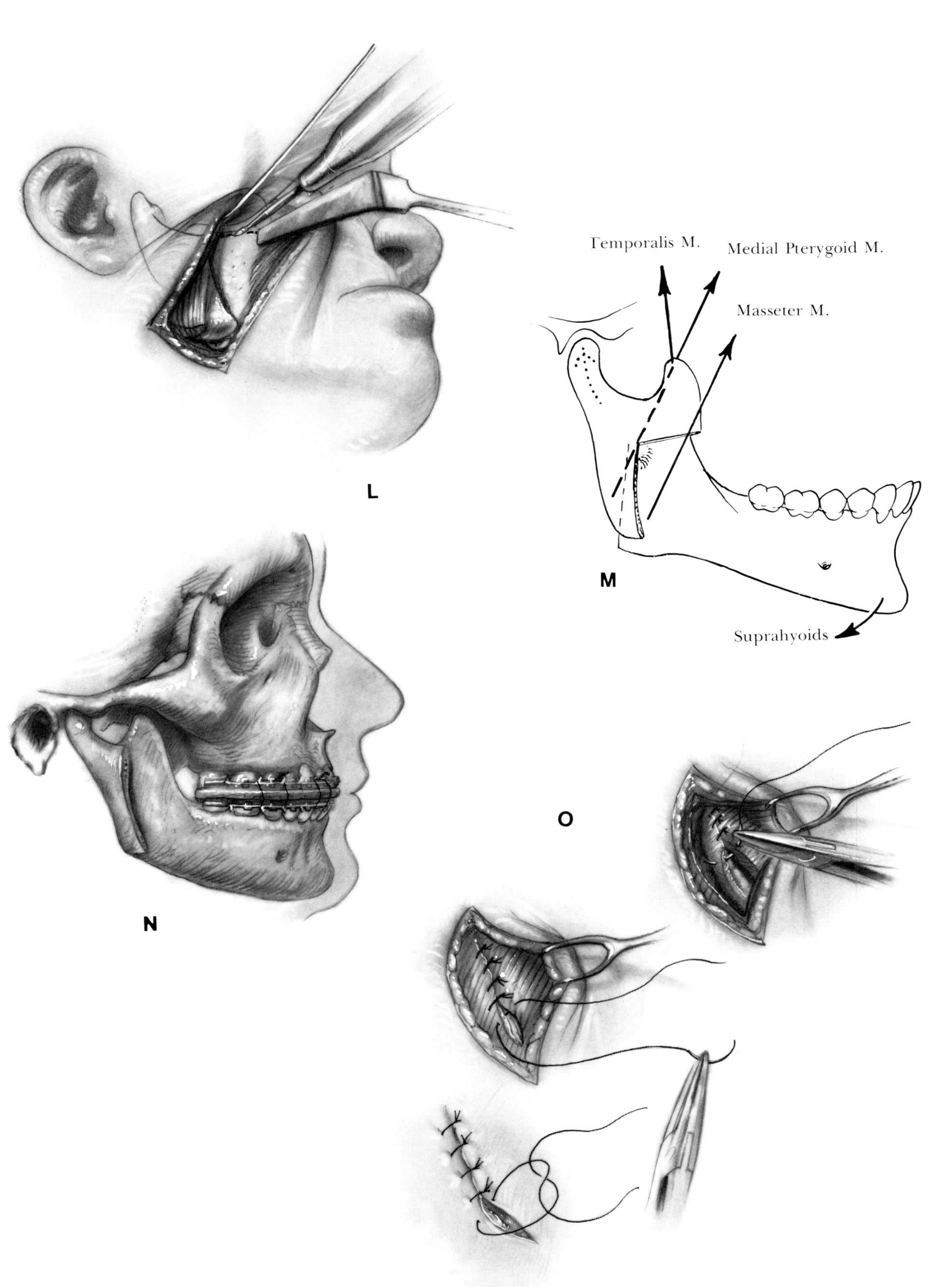

Figure 11–6 *Continued.* See legend on opposite page.

from the medial aspect of the proximal (condylar) segment only to the extent necessary to reposition the jaw after the bilateral cuts have been made.

After completing the procedure bilaterally, the surgeon or his assistant repositions the jaw to a predetermined position, and intermaxillary fixation is applied. At this point the proximal (condylar) segment should adapt laterally to the tooth-bearing distal segment. Segments are tied together with a wire suture or with a No. 2 catgut suture only when there is obvious condylar sag. It is important to be certain that the suture does not displace the condylar segment from its position in the mandibular articular fossa.

Once the surgeon is satisfied that the bony parts are in the preplanned position, the wound is thoroughly irrigated and closed in layers. Sterile dressings are applied to the surface of the skin incision, and appropriate dressings should cover the wound until healing is adequate to allow exposure to the air. Skin sutures should be removed before the fifth postoperative day, and the skin must be given care to minimize scarring. No matter which incision is used for the approach, the thin surgical scar can be cosmetic. Usually, it is very difficult to detect after only a few months have passed.

Nutrition and oral hygiene are most important in the postoperative period, as with any patient in intermaxillary fixation (see Chapter 7). The fixation usually is removed about 6 to 8 weeks following surgery, but some surgeons prefer to begin function in the mandible earlier than this. The patient's ability to cooperate may dictate how such a return to function is managed. Very close supervision of the patient's return to function is one of the most important phases of treatment, and this approach must be carried through the first 3 or 4 months following surgery. A clear understanding of this aspect is most important for the restorative dentist and/or orthodontist who might also be working with the patient.

Biologic Basis for Vertical Subcondylar Osteotomy

Even though the vertical ramus osteotomy is used to correct many different types of mandibular deformities, and numerous clinical successes have been achieved, the biologic rationale for using such surgical techniques has remained obscure until recently. To facilitate repositioning of the proximal (condylar) segments relative to the tooth-bearing anterior mandible — and to minimize relapse — many surgeons detach most of the muscles and periosteum from the mandibular vertical ramus. However, if the surgeon retains soft-tissue pedicles from the proximal segment only to a portion of the lateral pterygoid muscle and the articular capsule, circulation to the bone could be imperiled. Alteration of the circulation could reduce osseous viability, and affect the bone healing capacity of the osteomized segments.

The principal blood supply to the mandibular ramus and condyles is through perforating vessels emerging from the muscles that insert in the area.[12, 13, 14] The major arterial supply is a complex of branches that arise directly or indirectly from the maxillary branch of the external carotid artery and are named for the muscles they supply. The vessels that perfuse the mandibular condyle emerge from the superior belly of the lateral pterygoid muscle and from the joint capsule. The neck of the condyloid process receives its blood supply from the inferior belly of the lateral pterygoid muscle. The ramus receives the majority of its vessels from the medial pterygoid and masseter muscles.

It is hypothesized that success with the vertical ramus osteotomy is predicated on maintaining blood supply to the proximal condylar segment through a soft-tissue pedicle, the articular capsule, and the lateral pterygoid muscle. To test this hypothesis and to study the biologic aspects of pedicled and nonpedicled bone in vertical ramus osteotomies, experimental procedures were done in adult rhesus monkeys to elucidate the problem of vascular ischemia of the proximal segment and healing of the osteo-otomized bone (Figs. 11–7 through 11–13). The revascularization and bone healing associated with the operations have been studied by microangiographic and histologic techniques.[3, 39]

Microangiographic and histologic studies of vertical ramus osteotomies in which the proximal segment was not pedicled to soft tissue showed intraosseous necrosis, vascular ischemia, and delayed healing (Figs. 11–10 and 11–13). Similar studies of pedicled vertical ramus osteotomies showed early osseous union, minimal osteonecrosis, and transient vascular ischemia (Figs. 11–9, 11–11, and 11–12). The results of the studies indicate that continuous circulation to the proximal segment is necessary to retain osseous viability, and these results support the clinical practice of retaining a soft-tissue pedicle between the proximal condylar segment and the articular capsule and lateral pterygoid muscle and keeping the soft-tissue pedicle as large as possible.[4]

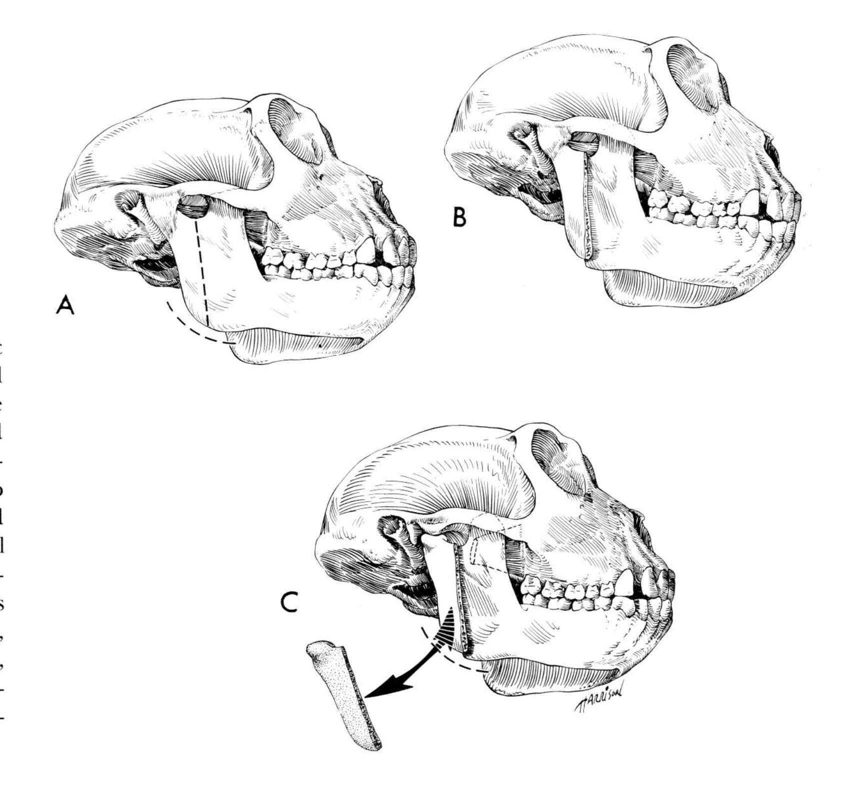

Figure 11–7. Schematic drawings of two experimental surgical techniques. Soft-tissue and bony incisions are illustrated by dotted lines (*A*); pedicled vertical ramus osteotomies (group A); proximal segment pedicled to capsular ligament and lateral pterygoid muscle (*B*); nonpedicled vertical ramus osteotomies (group B); proximal segment, devoid of soft tissue attachments, has been repositioned into glenoid fossa and placed lateral to distal segment (*C*).

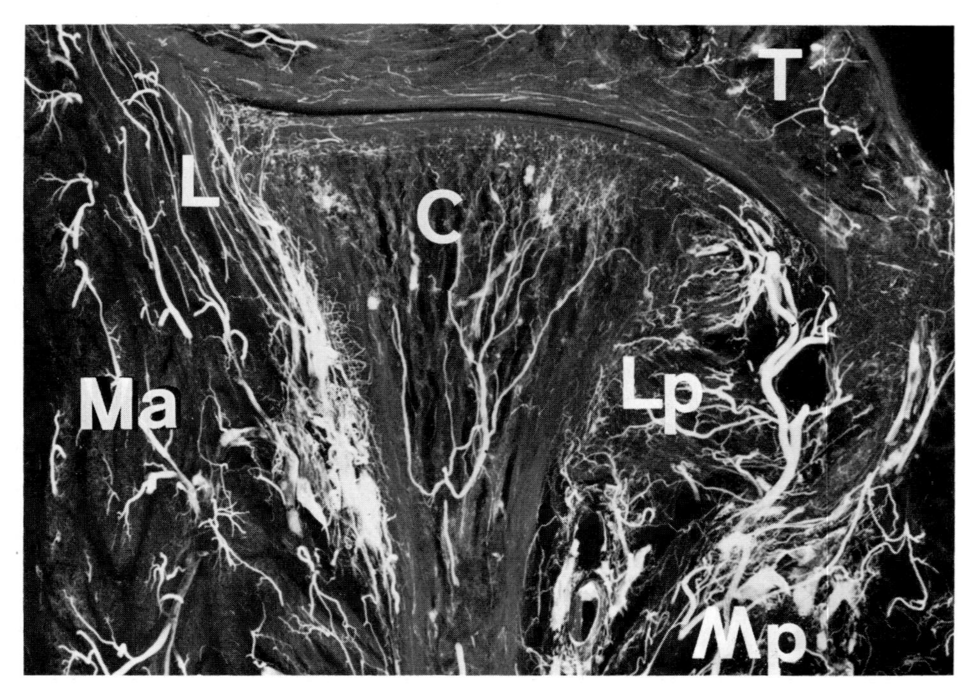

Figure 11–8. Microangiogram of transverse 1-mm section through condylar head and neck of control animal. C, condyle; T, temporal bone; L, capsular ligament; Ma, masseter muscle; Lp, lateral pterygoid muscle; Mp, medial pterygoid muscle. Penetration of cortices by numerous small vessels arising from lateral pterygoid muscle and capsular structure.

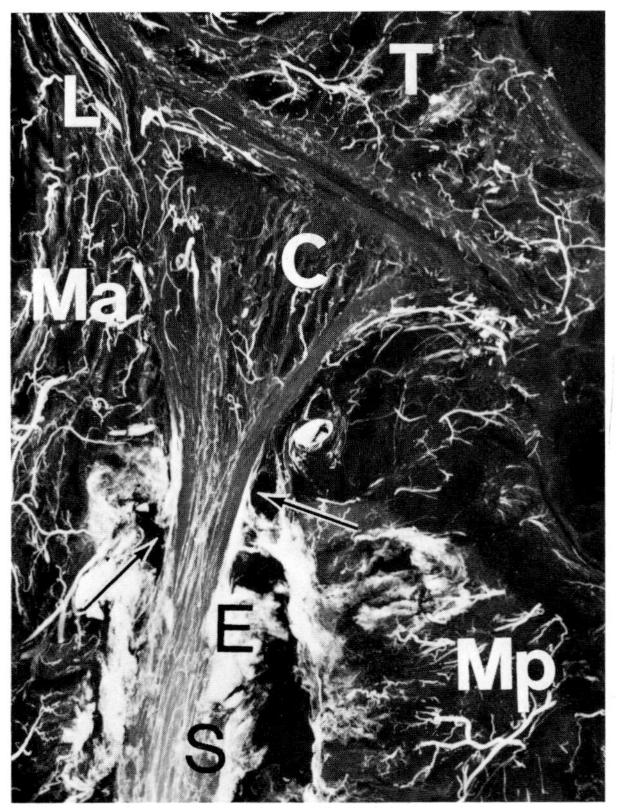

Figure 11–9. Microangiogram of immediate pedicled (group A) specimen. Arrows indicate avascular areas below detached soft tissues. Condylar area (C) is perfused with Micropaque. E, extravasated Micropaque; L, capsular ligament; Ma, masseter muscle; Mp, medial pterygoid muscle; S, distal segment; T, temporal bone.

Figure 11–10. Microangiogram of immediate nonpedicled (group B) specimen shows lack of perfusion of contrast medium into proximal segment. Arrows indicate avascular zone circumscribing proximal segment. Notice intraosseous vascular architecture of distal segment (S). C, condyle; E, extravasated Micropaque; Ma, masseter muscle; Mp, medial pterygoid muscle; T, temporal bone.

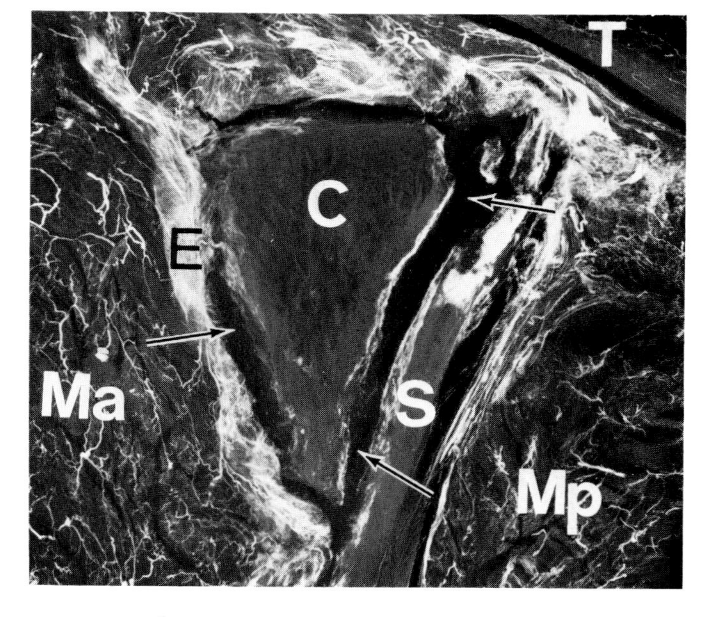

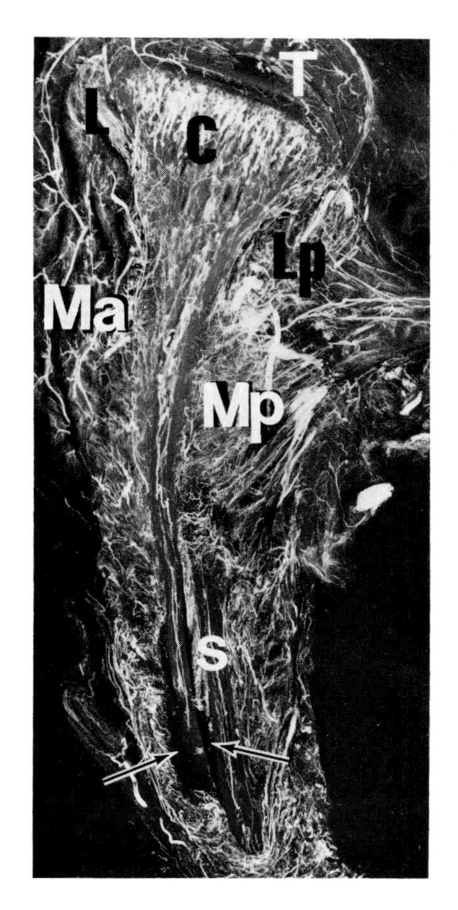

Figure 11–11. Microangiogram of section from the two-week pedicled (group A) specimen shows lack of reattachment of soft tissue (arrows) and avascular zone surrounding distal end of proximal bony segment; penetration of vessels arising from the hypervascular ligament (L) into the condylar area (C). Lp, lateral pterygoid muscle; Ma, masseter muscle; Mp, medial pterygoid muscle; S, distal segment; T, temporal bone.

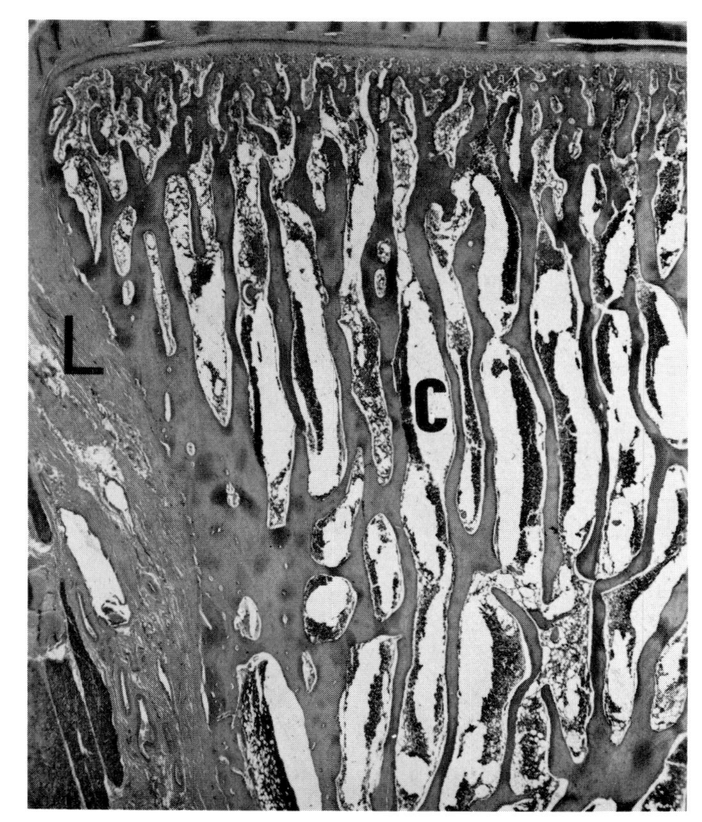

Figure 11–12. Photomicrograph of temporomandibular joint area of 12-week pedicled (group A) animal shows regular trabecular patterns running perpendicular to articular surface of condyle (C). L, capsular ligament. (Original magnification ×15.)

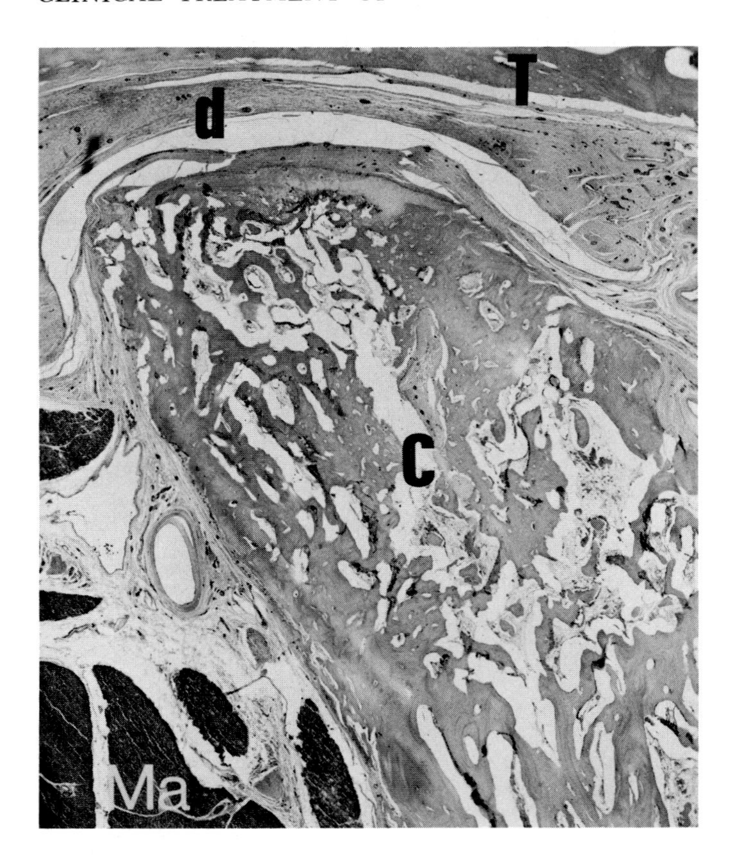

Figure 11–13. Photomicrograph of temporomandibular joint area of 12-week nonpedicled (group B) animal shows rounded irregular appearance of condyle (C) and random trabecular pattern; masseter muscle (Ma) has not reattached. T, temporal bone; d, articular disk. (Original magnification ×10.)

Intraoral Surgery

Historical Development

The chief appeal of intraoral surgical techniques is that the scar they produce is not ordinarily visible. Absence of a visible scar is especially important with surgical techniques involving the face. However, even with this decided advantage, intraoral surgical techniques were rarely used for treatment of the prognathic mandible until recent years. Apparently the fear that the wound would be contaminated by oral organisms deterred many surgeons. While the oral tissues have a good natural resistance to infection from oral microorganisms, infection may occur in a small percentage of cases. It is not surprising that the advent of the widespread use of antibiotics coincided with the development of intraoral surgical techniques. Moreover, surgical access formerly was more difficult with intraoral approaches than it was with extraoral approaches. The recent development of special instrumentation has facilitated greatly surgical access in intraoral procedures.

Curiously, the first recorded operation for treatment of a prognathic mandible utilized an intraoral approach. The procedure, a subapical osteotomy of the anterior mandible, was performed by Dr. S. P. Hullihen in 1848 (Fig. 11–14).[26] After this, only a few intraoral procedures of any kind were reported for almost one hundred years. Subsequently, Thoma,[42] Moose (Fig. 11–14),[36, 37] and others began to describe intraoral procedures they were using in treatment of mandibular excess.

The next significant step in development of intraoral procedures occurred with

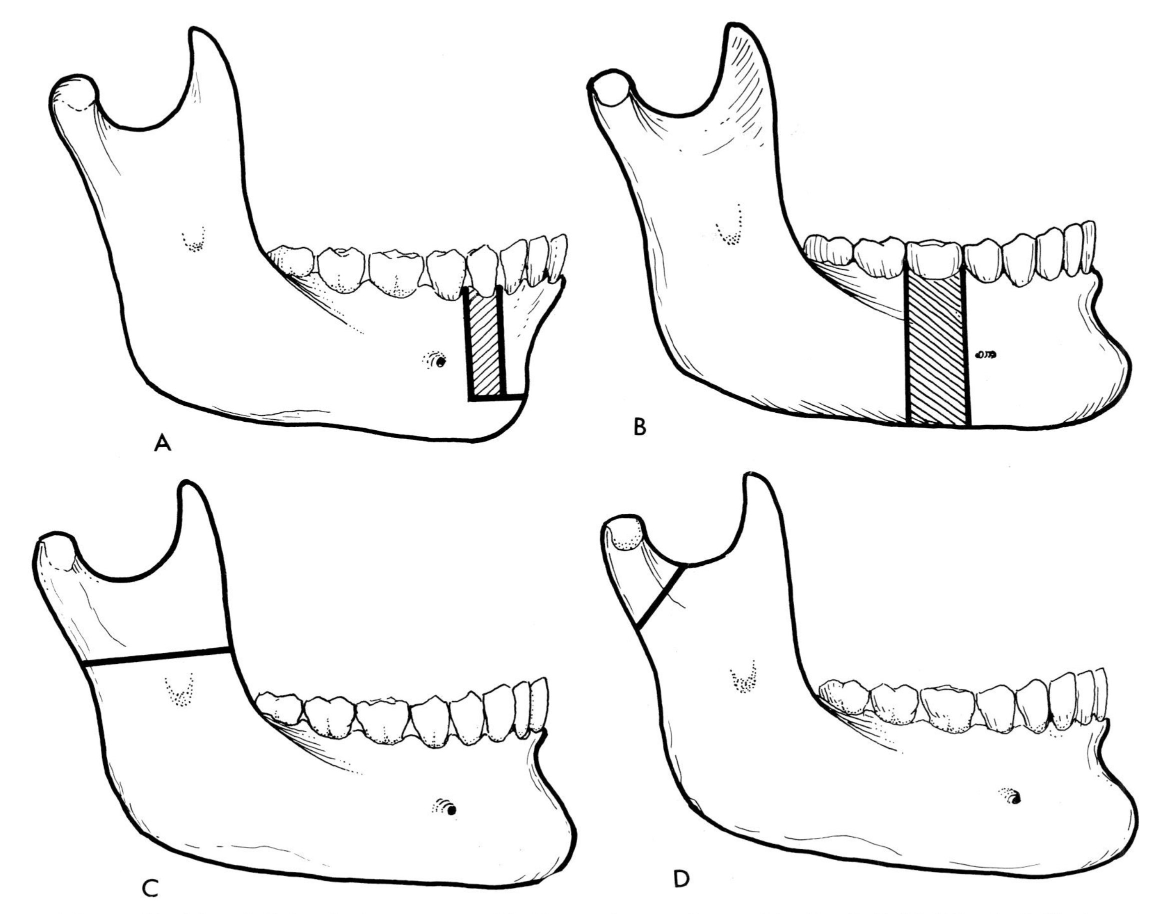

Figure 11–14. *A*, Subapical osteotomy (similar to that performed by Dr. S. P. Hullihen). *B*, Body osteotomy. *C*, Horizontal osteotomy. *D*, Subcondylar osteotomy.

the development of the sagittal split ramus osteotomy (SSRO), first reported in the English literature by Trauner and Obwegeser in 1957.[43] Refinements of this technique were subsequently reported by DalPont,[15] Hunsuck,[27] Epker,[17] and Bell.[6] In 1968, Winstanly reported the first intraoral vertical subcondylar osteotomy (IVSO), which he performed with a conventional dental drill.[49] A significant improvement in the intraoral vertical subcondylar technique was reported by Herbert, Kent, and Hinds in 1970.[24] Their osteotomy technique utilized a Stryker oscillating power unit. The technique has been further refined by Hall, Chase, and Payor[20] and by Walker,[44] as instrumentation has improved and greater surgical experience has been gained.

Of the various intraoral surgical techniques that have been advocated for reduction of the prognathic mandible, only four have merit today. The others were abandoned because of unsatisfactory results. For example, after horizontal osteotomy of the ramus, the bone tended to heal slowly, sometimes by fibrous union, and not infrequently an open bite resulted. Of the useful techniques, two (body ostectomy and subapical osteotomy) have occasional application; their use is described in this chapter. Both the sagittal split ramus osteotomy and the intraoral vertical ramus approach have much wider application and have become increasingly popular techniques as they are used today.

Advantages of Intraoral Surgical Procedures

Until recently, extraoral surgical techniques have been more commonly utilized than intraoral procedures for treatment of mandibular excess. Before the development of intraoral techniques that provided good stability and few complications, this choice was justified. The results obtained with intraoral techniques today appear not only to be comparable to those obtained with the extraoral techniques, but to surpass them in certain important ways. When extraoral techniques are used, a facial scar is invariably produced and, occasionally, the facial nerve (VII) is damaged. With the intraoral techniques, the major potential disadvantage is damage to the inferior alveolar nerve. When intraoral techniques are properly selected, this occurs in only a few patients and is almost always temporary. Intraoral techniques are perhaps more demanding of the surgeon and require special instrumentation, but neither of these factors should have much influence on the choice of technique. The advantages so far outweigh the disadvantages that the intraoral techniques are preferred for treatment of the prognathic mandible in almost all circumstances.

Surgical Techniques

BODY OSTECTOMY

William H. Bell

Blair (1907) was the first to describe the surgical correction of mandibular deformities by ostectomy in the body of the mandible, removing bone from the premolar and molar regions with a hand saw.[7] In 1912, Harsha accomplished a similar feat by excising a rhomboid section of bone from the third-molar region of a prognathic patient.[21] New and Erich reported on a one-stage intraoral-extraoral body ostectomy that preserved the mandibular neurovascular bundle.[38] They recognized that the mandibular body ostectomy was well suited for patients whose mandibular prognathism was associated with skeletal type anterior open bite. Thoma in 1943 described a Y-shaped ostectomy in the mandibular body for correction of mandibular prognathism associated with marked anterior open bite.[41] Dingman popularized the mandibular body ostectomy procedure by describing a two-stage technique that was designed to eliminate the compound intraoral and extraoral wound while preserving the integrity of the inferior alveolar nerve.[16] In 1961, Burch and associates reported a single-stage intraoral body ostectomy technique for correction of mandibular prognathism.[9]

Indications for Using Mandibular Body Ostectomy

A mandibular body ostectomy should be considered when the correction for mandibular excess is small — not more than the width of a tooth. If the procedure can be carried out bilaterally in the mandibular first premolar area, the surgical site is easily accessible and the inferior alveolar nerve and its mental branches need be disturbed only minimally. A body ostectomy may be accomplished at any point in the tooth-bearing area of the mandible, but the surgery must be precise so that there will be good bone-to-bone contact when bony segments are repositioned. Occlusion of teeth posterior to the ostectomy site should be carefully evaluated in the planning stages. The position of the posterior teeth (those posterior to the bone cuts) will not be changed at the time of surgery.

Radiographic examination of the potential ostectomy sites is very important to proper planning and execution of the surgery. Radiographs of the surgery sites provide information indispensable to evaluating tooth-root angulation in the areas that are contiguous to the planned osteotomies. These same radiographs reveal the position of the mental foramen and mandibular canal and demonstrate the architecture of the bone in the potential ostectomy sites. Adequate dental arch space and proper angulation of the tooth roots that are adjacent to the planned site of ostectomy can be gained by presurgical orthodontic treatment.

The body ostectomy is accomplished by a single-stage operation through a degloving-type incision under general endotracheal anesthesia. Animal studies using the adult rhesus monkey as an experimental model have demonstrated that intraosseous and intrapulpal circulation to the anterior mandibular segment is maintained by this technique (Fig. 11–15).[5] The proximal and distal segments healed by osseous union within 6 weeks without intermaxillary fixation.

When the inferior alveolar nerve traverses the planned ostectomy site, it must either be decorticated appropriately and repositioned or bypassed by a step osteotomy. After the nerve is carefully decorticated with thinly tapered osteotomes and rotary diamond burs, it is separated from its incisive branch and reflected posteriorly with the soft-tissue flap (Fig. 11–16). Great care must be exercised to preserve the integrity of the inferior alveolar neurovascular bundle. Careful retraction is paramount to execute a body ostectomy through the second premolar or molar regions. If the nerve should be trans-sected inadvertently, good apposition of the cut segments will facilitate postsurgical repair of the nerve.

Design of the Soft Tissue Incision

Proper design of the soft-tissue and bone incisions is important to ensure uncomplicated healing of the surgical wounds and prevent injury to the periodontium of the teeth contiguous to the planned ostectomy site. The soft-tissue incision is generally accomplished as shown in Figure 11–17. As depicted in Figures 11–16, 11–17, and 11–18, the design of the soft-tissue incision can be varied to provide accessibility, visualization, and an adequate soft-tissue pedicle for the individual patient without compromise to healing of the surgical wound.

A circumvestibular incision is extended from at least 1 cm distal to the planned posterior vertical osteotomy of one side to a similar area on the contralateral side. The lateral and mental symphysis regions of the mandible are degloved. With the margins of the superior flap retracted opposite the planned vertical ostectomy site, the vertical and horizontal bone cuts can be made under direct vision. Such an incision has the advantage of providing direct access to the planned ostectomy sites, exposure of the mental nerves, accessibility for geniohyoid and digastric myotomy, and exposure of the symphysis region for concomitant genioplasty or interdental osteotomy. Additionally, the design of the degloving incision provides an additional soft-tissue pedicle to the facial aspect of the mobilized segment and facilitates a tensionless closure of the soft-tissue incision in the lateral aspect of the facial sulcus away from the osteotomy sites. The attachment of the lingual mucoperiosteum is maximized —

Text continued on page 880

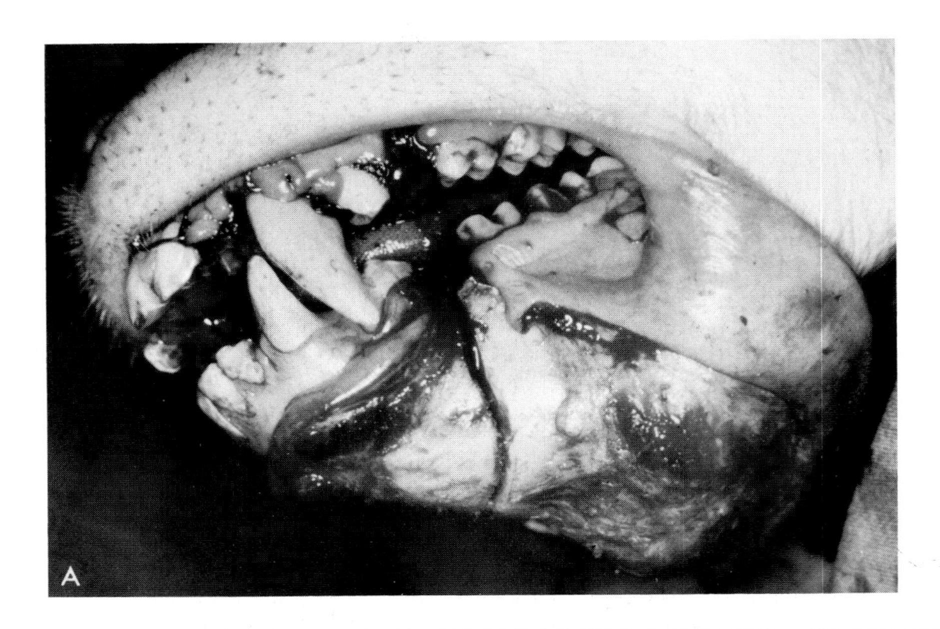

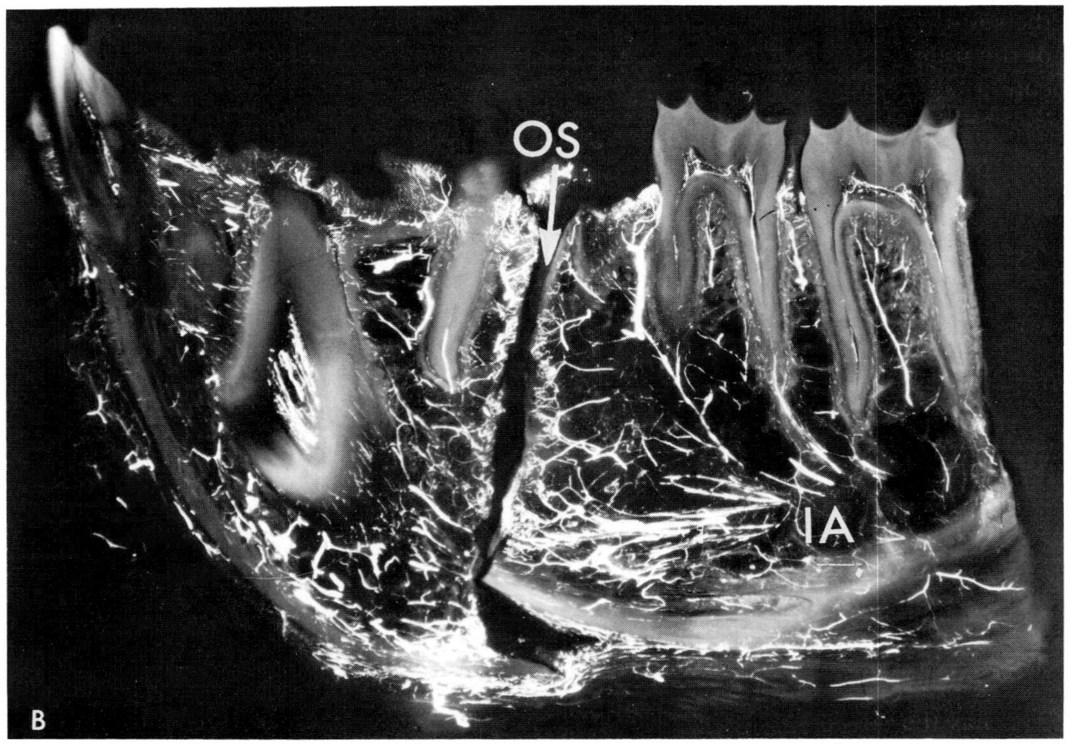

Figure 11–15. Wound healing associated with anterior mandibular osteotomy technique. *A*, Anterior mandibular osteotomy performed through a "degloving-type" incision. *B*, Microangiogram demonstrating intraosseous and intrapulpal distribution of injection medium one week after anterior mandibular osteotomy. Terminal branches of inferior alveolar artery (IA); increased number of blood vessels in bone approximating osteotomy site (OS). (Sagittal section.)

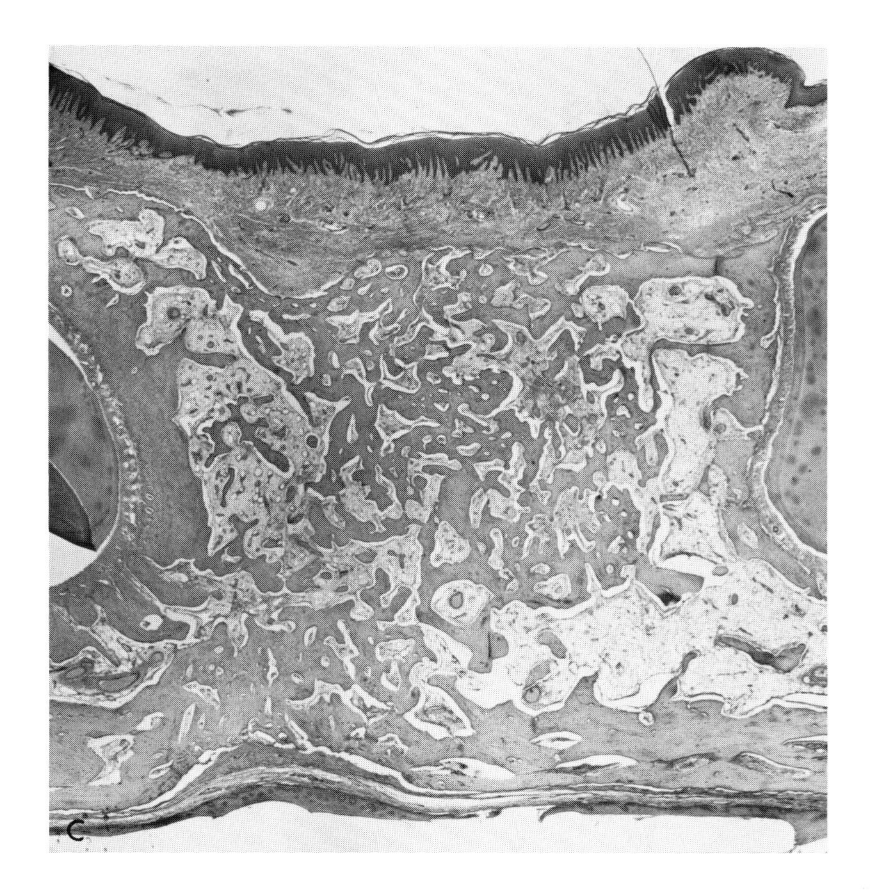

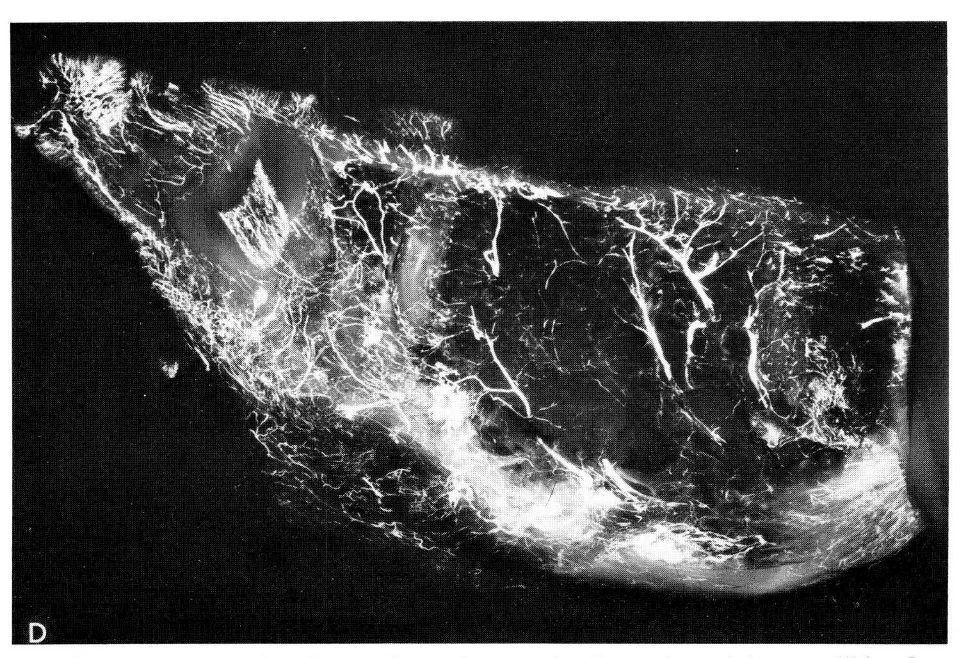

Figure 11–15 *Continued.* *C*, Photomicrograph of a section of the mandible of an animal six weeks following osteotomy. The osteotomy site is replaced by cancellous bone. Hematoxylin-eosin stain. (Original magnification × 10.) *D*, Microangiogram demonstrating generalized distribution of injection medium throughout the anterior mandibular bone fragment six months after anterior mandibular osteotomy. Reconstitution of normal vascular architecture. (Sagittal section.)

Figure 11–16. Method of decorticating bone overlying inferior alveolar nerve to facilitate mandibular body ostectomy when vertical osteotomy is made through area of the body of mandible traversed by inferior alveolar nerve. *A*, Planned ostectomy in 2nd premolar region; arrow indicates directional movement of anterior mandibular segment. *B*, Soft-tissue incision for exposure of the mental nerves. *C*, Intended line of osteotomy is etched into lateral cortical plate of mandible around the mental nerve and opposite the inferior alveolar nerve; holes are drilled through the cortical bone only along the intended line of osteotomy; the multiple bone incisions are connected with a tapered fissure bur. *D*, Buccal cortical plate circumscribing the mental nerves is chiseled away from its cancellous bony base with finely tapered osteotome. *E*, A rongeur is used to remove the bone circumscribing the mental nerve. *F*, Final removal of cancellous bone overlying inferior alveolar neurovascular bundle; separation of incisive branch from the inferior alveolar nerve. *G*, Nerve retracted from the surgical site with nerve hook to facilitate the planned vertical ostectomy in the body of the mandible. *H*, Apposition of proximal and distal segments fixed with interosseous wires; desired occlusion is maintained by rectangular arch wire ligated to orthodontic brackets.

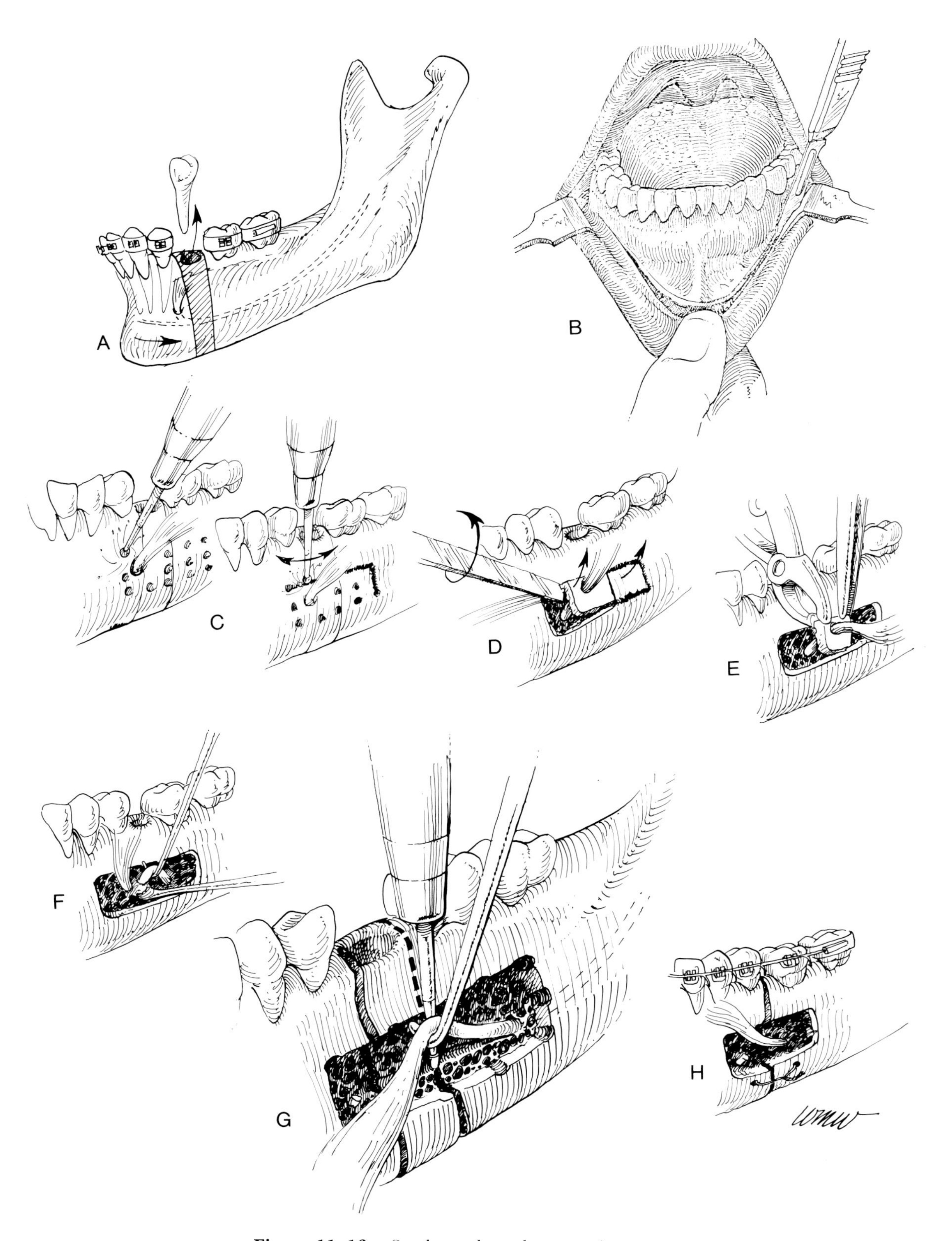

Figure 11–16. See legend on the opposite page.

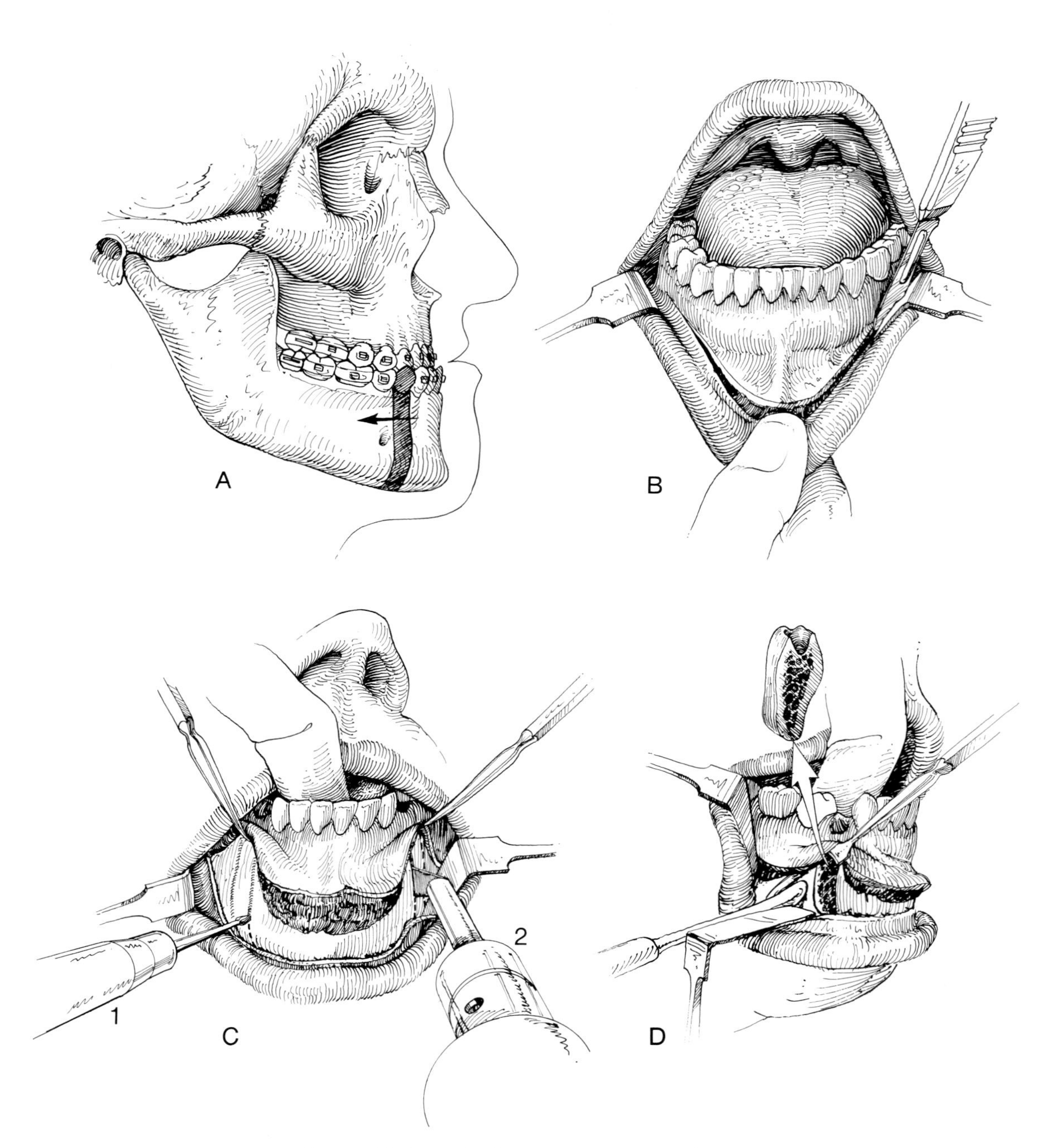

Figure 11–17. See legend on the opposite page.

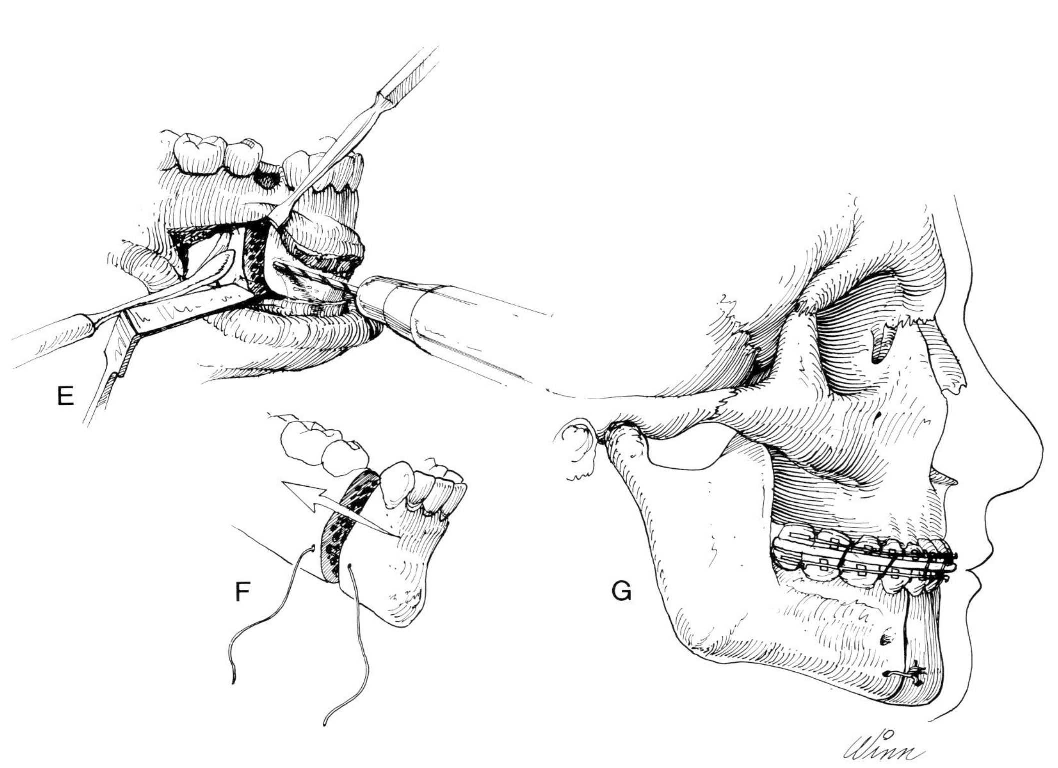

Figure 11–17. Mandibular body ostectomy in 1st premolar region accomplished through degloving incision. *A*, Typical dental, skeletal, and facial features associated with mandibular prognathism; planned ostectomy in 1st premolar region anterior to mental nerve; arrow indicates directional movement of anterior mandibular segment. *B*, Soft-tissue incision for exposure of mental symphysis and ostectomy site. *C* and *D*, Mental symphysis degloved to facilitate vertical ostectomies; planned ostectomies are etched into mandible with 701 fissure bur (1); with inferior margin of mucobuccal flap raised with skin hook or small retractor, vertical ostectomy is accomplished in extraction space with oscillating saw (2) or fissure bur. *E* and *F*, Interosseous wire placed through margins of osteotomized bone before body ostectomy is completed. *G*, Repositioned mandible fixed with interosseous wire and placed in intermaxillary fixation.

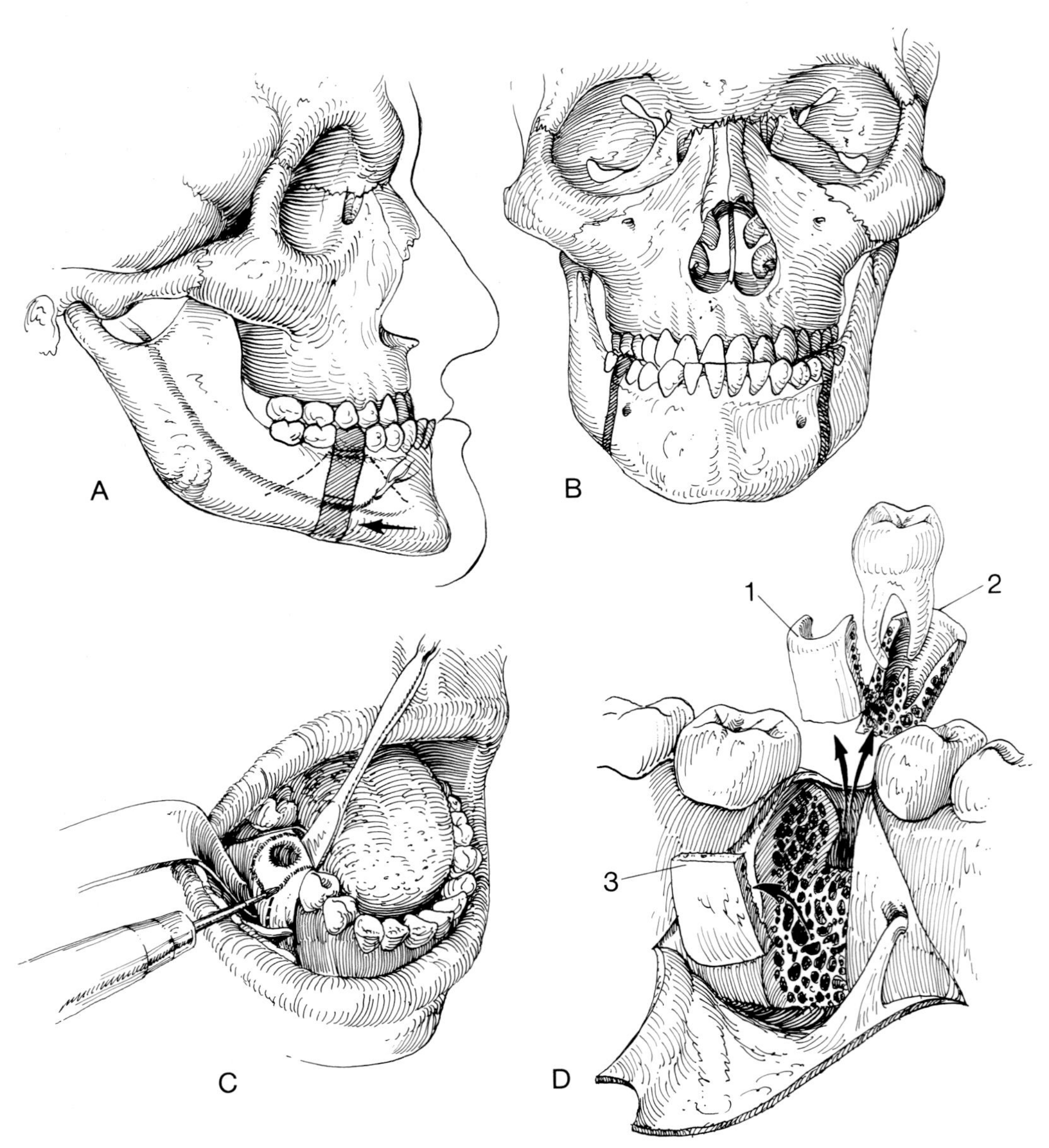

Figure 11–18. Preservation of integrity of inferior alveolar nerve when body ostectomy is used for correction of mandibular prognathism (technique of Dr. Robert V. Walker, Dallas, Texas). *A* and *B*, Planned ostectomies in 1st molar regions. *C*, Diverging vertical incisions in buccal vestibule adjacent to area of planned ostectomy; horizontal osteotomy is made superior to level of inferior alveolar nerve to intersect with vertical bone incisions. *D*, Sequential excision of buccal (1) and lingual (2) cortical plate above level of inferior alveolar nerve; excision of buccal inferior cortical plate (3). *E*, Exposure of inferior alveolar neurovascular bundle by careful excision of cancellous bone. *F* and *G*, Excision of residual inferior lingual cortical bone facilitated by retraction of inferior alveolar nerve; interosseous wire placed through margins of osteotomized bone before body ostectomy is completed. *H* and *I*, Removal of bone surrounding inferior alveolar nerve in margins of ostectomy site to facilitate apposition of proximal and distal segments without compressing nerve. *I* and *J*, Apposition of segments fixed with interosseous wires; mandible immobilized with intermaxillary wires between maxillary and mandibular orthodontic appliances.

Illustration continued on the opposite page.

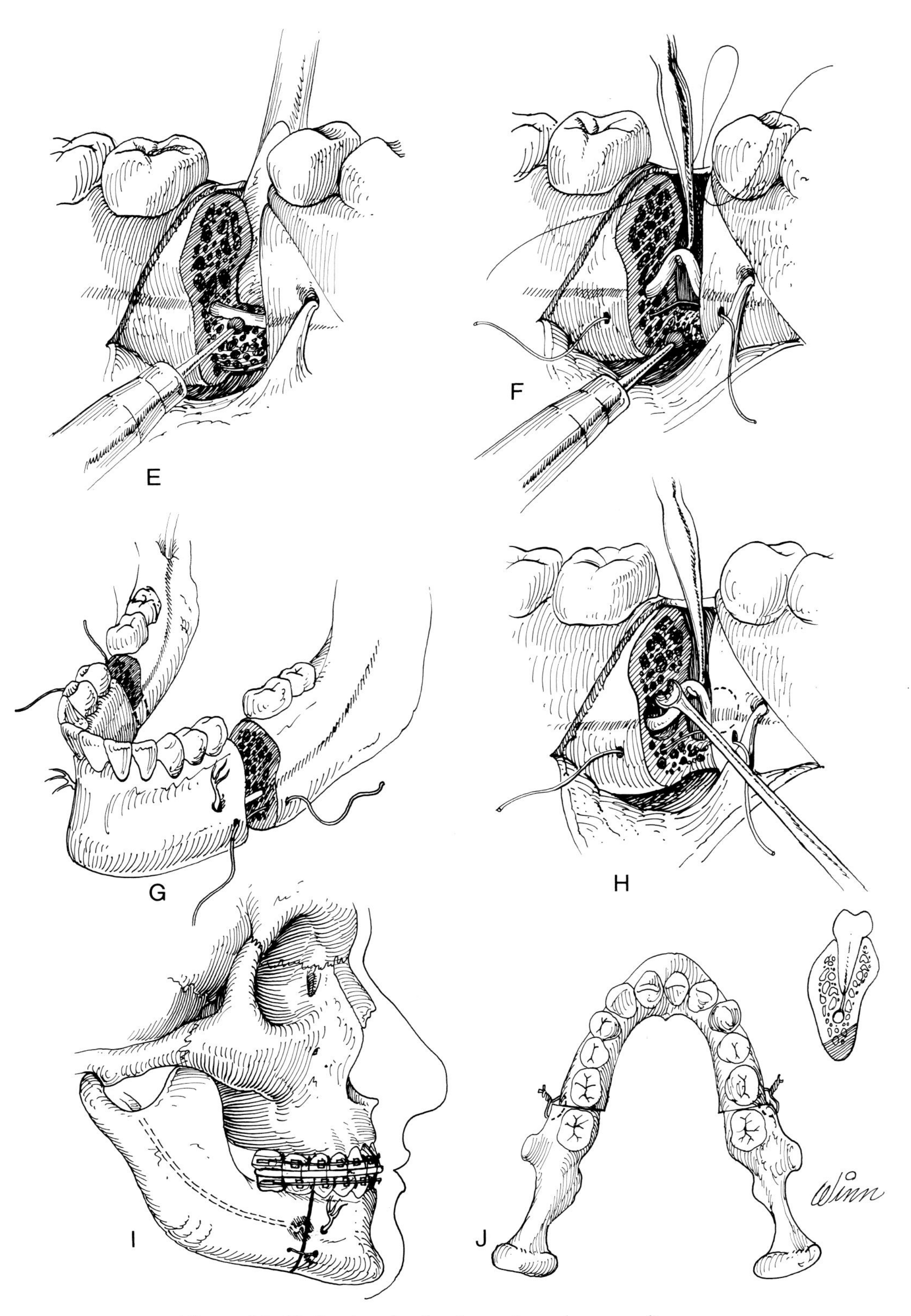

Figure 11–18 *Continued.* See legend on the opposite page.

only the lingual tissue at the alveolar level opposite the planned ostectomy site is detached. When vertical ostectomies are accomplished in the first premolar areas, they can be made very rapidly and with impunity when the mental nerve is inferior to the second premolar teeth. In cooperative individuals, such surgery can be executed on an outpatient basis with local anesthesia supplemented by sedation or with general anesthesia.

Arch wires and intraosseous wiring or a cast splint can be used to fix the mobilized segment without intermaxillary fixation. More frequently, the mandible is indexed into a wafer splint and immobilized with intermaxillary fixation for 4 to 6 weeks. The forces from the masseter, medial pterygoid, and temporalis muscles on the posterior segments and the suprahyoid muscles on the anterior segment make immobilization of the repositioned jaw parts a critical step. Without good contact of the bony parts at the completion of surgery and adequate fixation of the jaw parts, delayed union or non-union is predictable.

OPTIONAL SOFT-TISSUE INCISION. Diverging vertical incisions are made through the interdental papillae adjacent to the area of the planned ostectomy and extended obliquely, anteriorly and inferiorly, and posteroinferiorly into the buccal vestibule. A buccal mucoperiosteal flap is then elevated from the underlying bone inferiorly to the inferior border of the mandible. With a channel retractor positioned to protect the soft tissues from the rotating bur, the planned vertical and horizontal bone incisions are accomplished (Fig. 11–18). The incision, which affords excellent access to the ostectomy site, has distinct limitations by virtue of the fact that it does not provide access to the anterior part of the mandible for adjunctive genioplasty, myotomy, or interdental osteotomy.

Design of the Bone Incisions

MANDIBULAR BODY "V," "Y," OR "RECTANGULAR" OSTECTOMY. Mandibular prognathism with concomitant anterior open bite is the principal indication for "V," "Y," or "rectangular" ostectomies, which are accomplished in a single stage through intraoral degloving incisions (Fig. 11–19). A functional posterior occlusion associated with edentulous spaces also gives support to the use of the "V" body ostectomy when prognathism is associated with anterior open bite. Clinical and cephalometric studies of candidates for the "V" body ostectomy will typically reveal a reverse curve in the mandibular plane angle with associated open bite, high mandibular plane angle, adequate lower lip-to-tooth relationship, and satisfactory positioning of the lower anterior teeth with respect to their supporting basal bone. Some forward tipping of the mandibular anterior teeth by orthodontic forces may be necessary to upright mandibular anterior teeth over supporting bone. No attempt is made to level a severe reverse curve in the mandibular arch completely by orthodontics — such movement is accomplished by the body ostectomy, a subapical osteotomy, or both. When severe mandibular prognathism is associated with skeletal anterior open bite, maxillary surgery and mandibular ramus surgery may indeed be necessary to achieve occlusal balance and stability.

Despite the fact that mandibular body ostectomy reduces the volume of the oral cavity and the mandibular arch length, postoperative studies have demonstrated excellent stability with this procedure once healing takes place. This stability after healing has been attributed to the fact that the line of the osteotomies is anterior to major

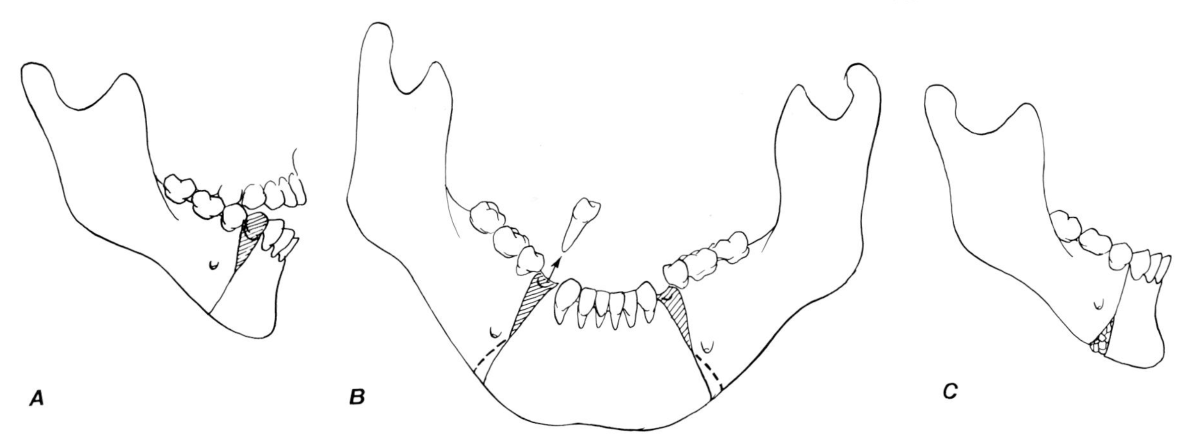

Figure 11–19. Mandibular body "Y" ostectomy. *A*, Mandibular prognathism associated with anterior open bite and reverse curvature of mandibular arch. *B*, Mandibular body "Y" ostectomy. *C*, Retropositioned mandible; bony gap at inferior border of mandible filled with autogenous particulate marrow bone graft.

muscles of mastication. The influence of the masseter, temporalis, and medial pterygoid muscles is thereby obviated.

The mandibular body "Y" ostectomy adds additional facility to treat cases of severe anterior open bite in which the dysplasia is manifest as a reverse curve in the mandibular arch (Fig. 11–19). Model surgery and cephalometric prediction studies using templates to determine the resultant interface of repositioned bone segments are essential to determine the feasibility of the procedure and the need for bone grafting of osseous defects at the inferior border of the mandible. The indications for the two procedures depend on a careful analysis of the individual case.

Mandibular Body "Step" Ostectomy. The mandibular body step ostectomy has been used most frequently to treat mandibular deficiency. The same principle is applicable to surgical management of selected patients with mandibular prognathism—it has particular application in treatment of patients with edentulous posterior mandibles. The design of the osteotomy and ostectomy provides a greater interference of bone and may obviate the need for cumbersome prosthetic splints. The surgery is accomplished in a single stage through an intraoral degloving incision (Fig. 11–20).

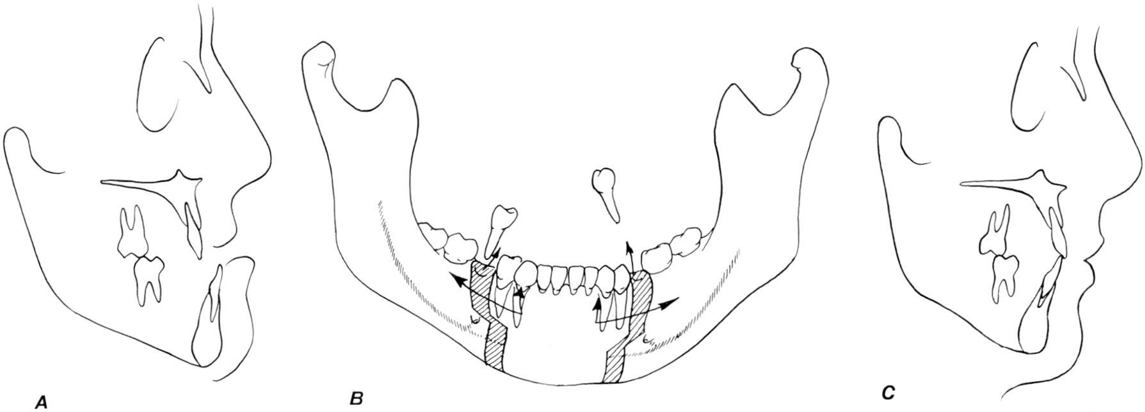

Figure 11–20. Mandibular body "step" ostectomy. *A*, Mandibular prognathism associated with anterior open bite; planned ostectomy in 2nd premolar region; arrow indicates directional movement of anterior portion of mandible. *B*, Mandibular body "step" ostectomy to circumvent inferior alveolar nerve. *C*, Repositioned mandible fixed with interosseous wire.

MANDIBULAR BODY "INVERTED-V" OR "INVERTED V–STEP" OSTECTOMY. Where there is extreme lingual tipping of the mandibular anterior teeth on the basal bone, the "inverted-V" or "inverted-V–step" ostectomy may be indicated. If the deformity is accentuated by premature loss of posterior teeth or imprudent extractions of premolars to facilitate orthodontic treatment, either of these two procedures may be indicated to allow uprighting of the mandibular incisors and posterior rotation of the bony chin (Fig. 11–21). Simultaneous sculpturing of the lateral and anterior aspects of the chin may be accomplished through the degloving exposure. In such patients the relationship between the upper and lower lips may be acceptable because of the dental

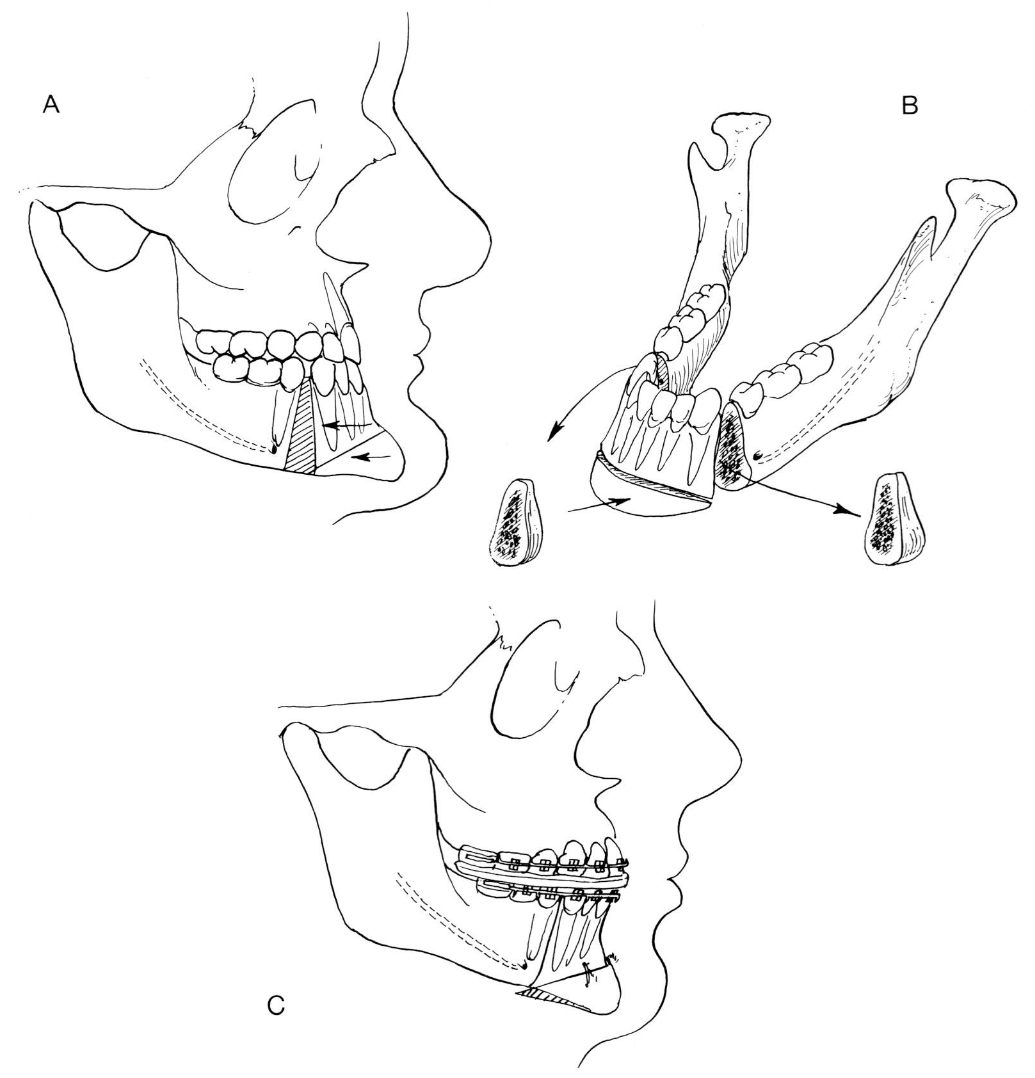

Figure 11–21. Mandibular body "inverted V" ostectomy and reduction genioplasty. *A*, Mandibular prognathism with end to end occlusion; severe retroinclination of mandibular anterior teeth as a consequence of dental compensations and premature loss of mandibular 1st premolar teeth. Imprudent extraction of maxillary and mandibular premolars to facilitate orthodontic treatment may create a "dished-in" facial profile, prominent chin, and relatively prominent nose. *B*, Mandibular "inverted V" ostectomies, reduction genioplasty, and rhinoplasty. *C*, Repositioned mandible and chin fixed with interosseous wire.

and osseous compensations. The end product is a patient with a concave facial-lip profile, prominent chin, and "relatively" prominent nose. As the anterior mandibular segment is advanced into a crossbite relationship, the maxilla may have to be advanced or the mandible retracted to achieve occlusal harmony.

The use of the "inverted-V–step" ostectomy may obviate the need to decorticate and uncover the neurovascular bundle in the mental foramen area and provides more extensive bony contact and increased stabilization of the osseous segments (Fig. 11–21).[20] The design of the "step" ostectomy when combined with the use of an orthodontic arch wire may obviate the need for intermaxillary fixation in selected patients.

Reduction in Transverse Width

When the mandibular intercanine width is greater than the maxillary intercanine width, a vertical interdental osteotomy or ostectomy may facilitate the attainment of occlusal harmony. If there is a concomitant posterior crossbite, ostectomy of the mandibular symphysis will allow narrowing of the mandible by medial rotation of its right and left halves, with rotation occurring around vertical axes in the mandibular condyles (Figs. 11–22, 11–23, and 11–24).[40] With such surgery there will be some concomitant shortening of the mandible. After the segments are fixed by interosseous wires, the chin can be sculptured to the planned dimensions before the wound is closed. Subapical osteotomy, symphyseal ostectomy or osteotomy, and chin remodeling may be combined with vertical ramus osteotomies to produce the desired anteroposterior and transverse changes in the mandible (Figs. 11–24 and 11–25).

Text continued on page 889.

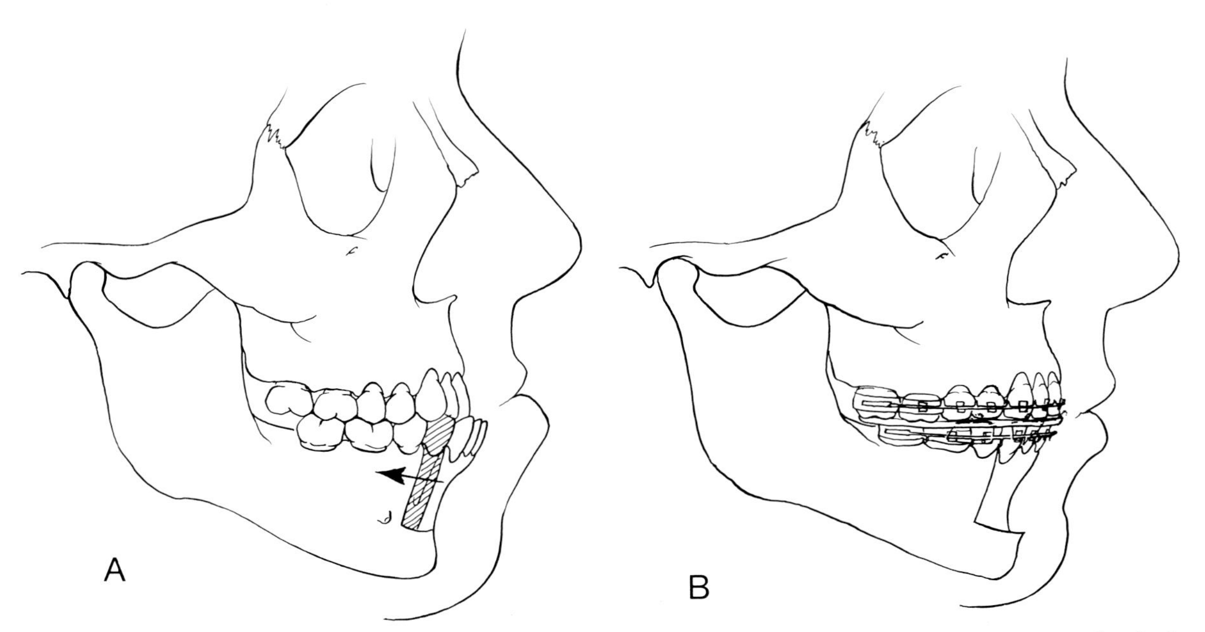

Figure 11–22. Subapical osteotomy (Kole) to correct anterior crossbite. *A*, Mandibular subapical osteotomy; stippled area indicates planned ostectomy; arrow indicates directional movement of anterior mandibular alveolar segment. *B*, Anterior mandibular alveolar segment retropositioned to achieve chin-lip-nose balance.

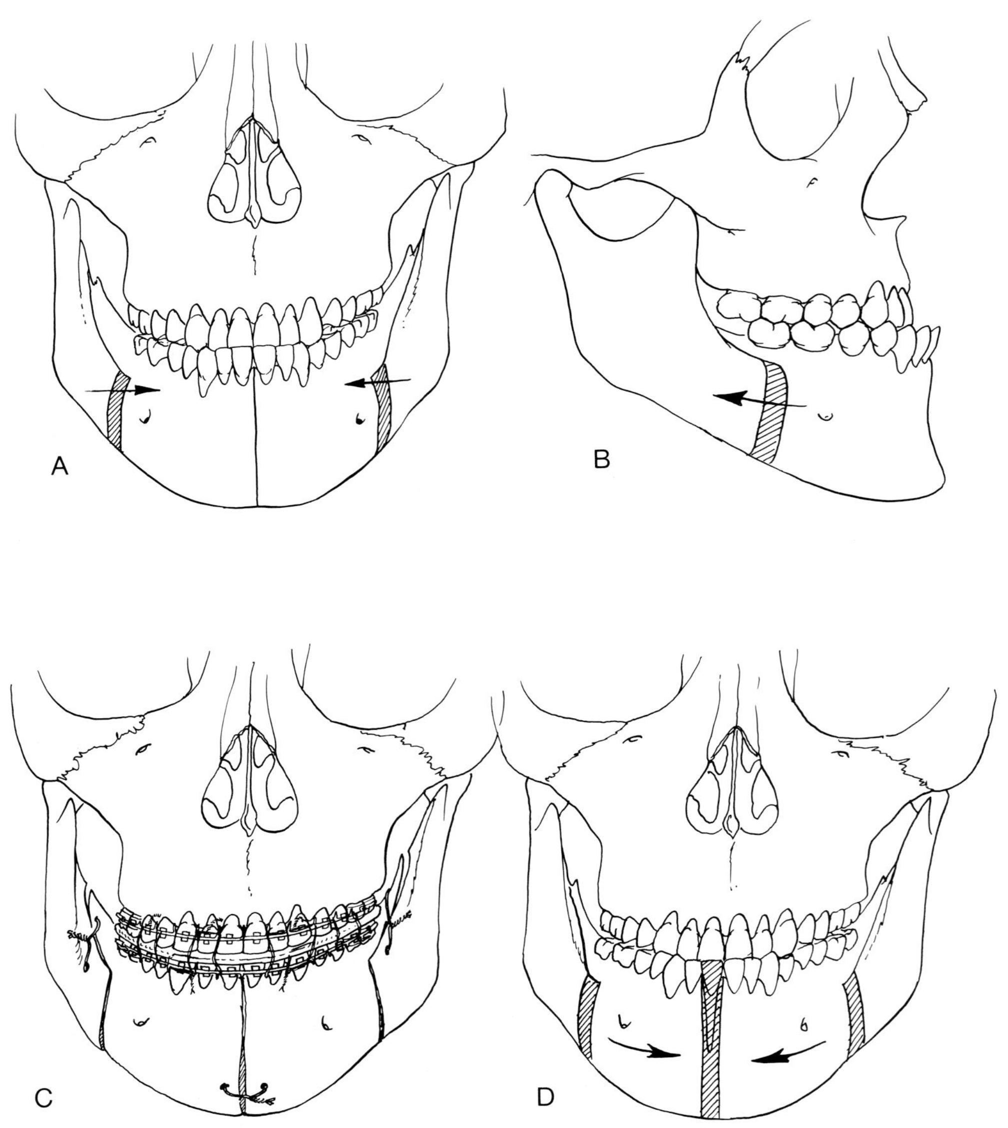

Figure 11–23. Adjunctive interdental osteotomy or ostectomy combined with sagittal split ramus osteotomies or intraoral vertical ramus osteotomies to correct crossbite associated with mandibular prognathism. *A* and *B*, Bilateral palatal crossbite and anterior crossbite; arrows indicate directional movement of mandible; stippled areas indicate planned ostectomies. *C*, Repositioned mandible fixed with interosseous wires. *D*, Optional technique for correction of crossbite; model surgery must indicate that three mandibular anterior teeth will harmonize with maxillary anterior teeth. *E*, Plan of surgery: interdental osteotomy in midsymphysis region combined with intraoral vertical ramus osteotomies. *F*, Degloving exposure of anterior aspect of mental symphysis. *G*, Planned interdental osteotomy is etched into midsymphysis region with 701 fissure bur.

Illustration continued on the opposite page.

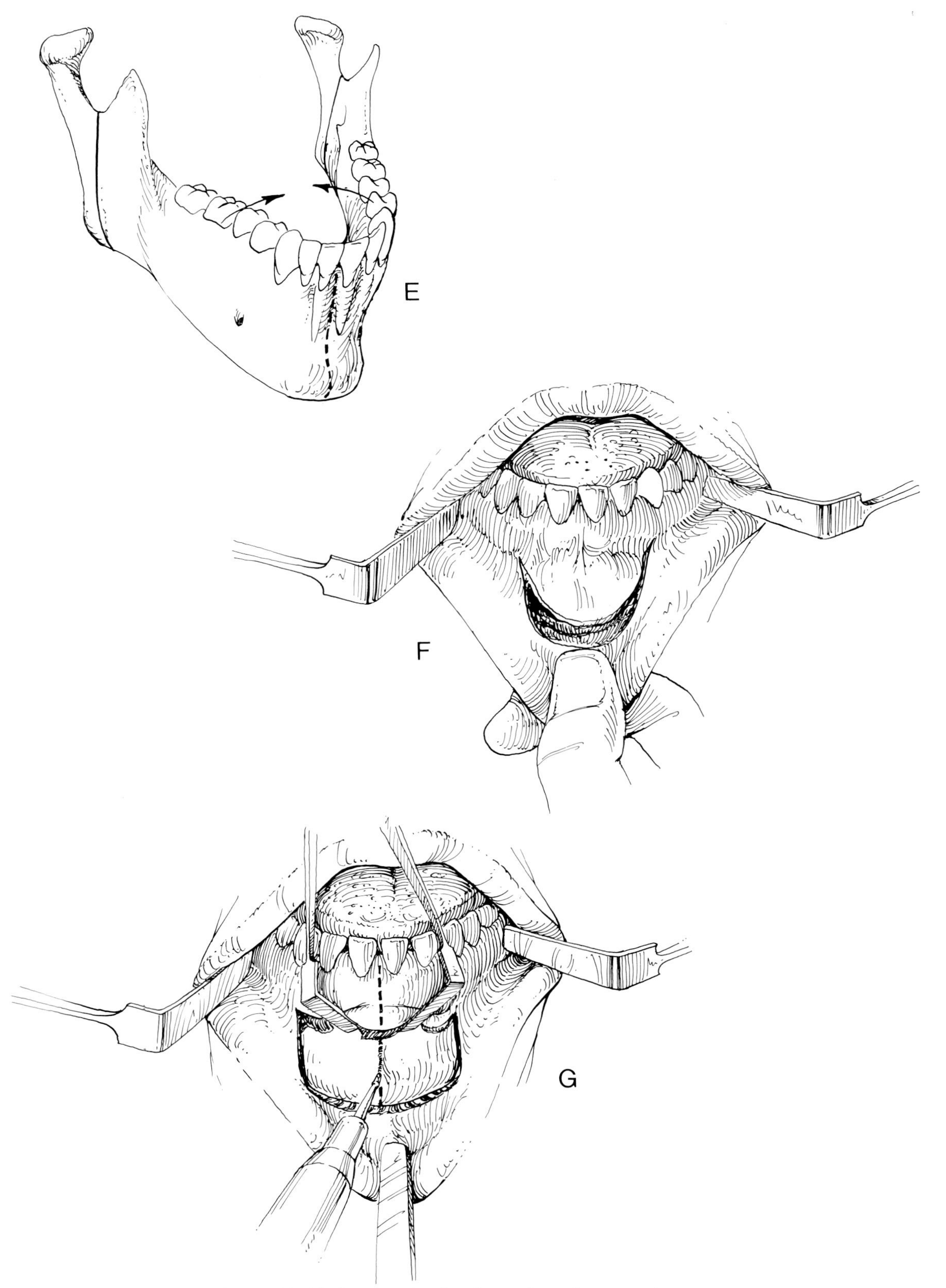

Figure 11–23 *Continued.* See legend on the opposite page.

Illustration continued on the following page.

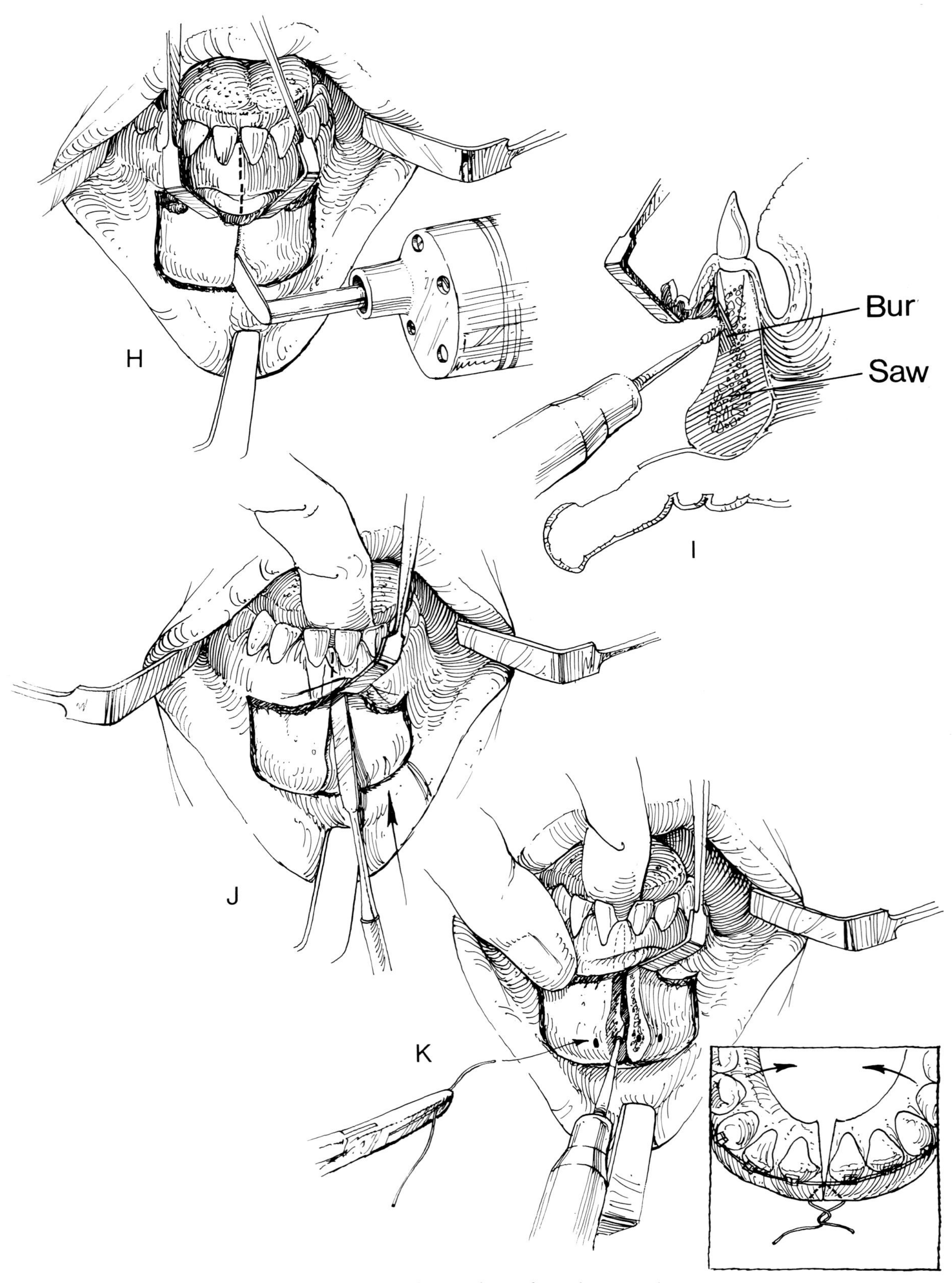

Figure 11–23 *Continued.* See legend on the opposite page.

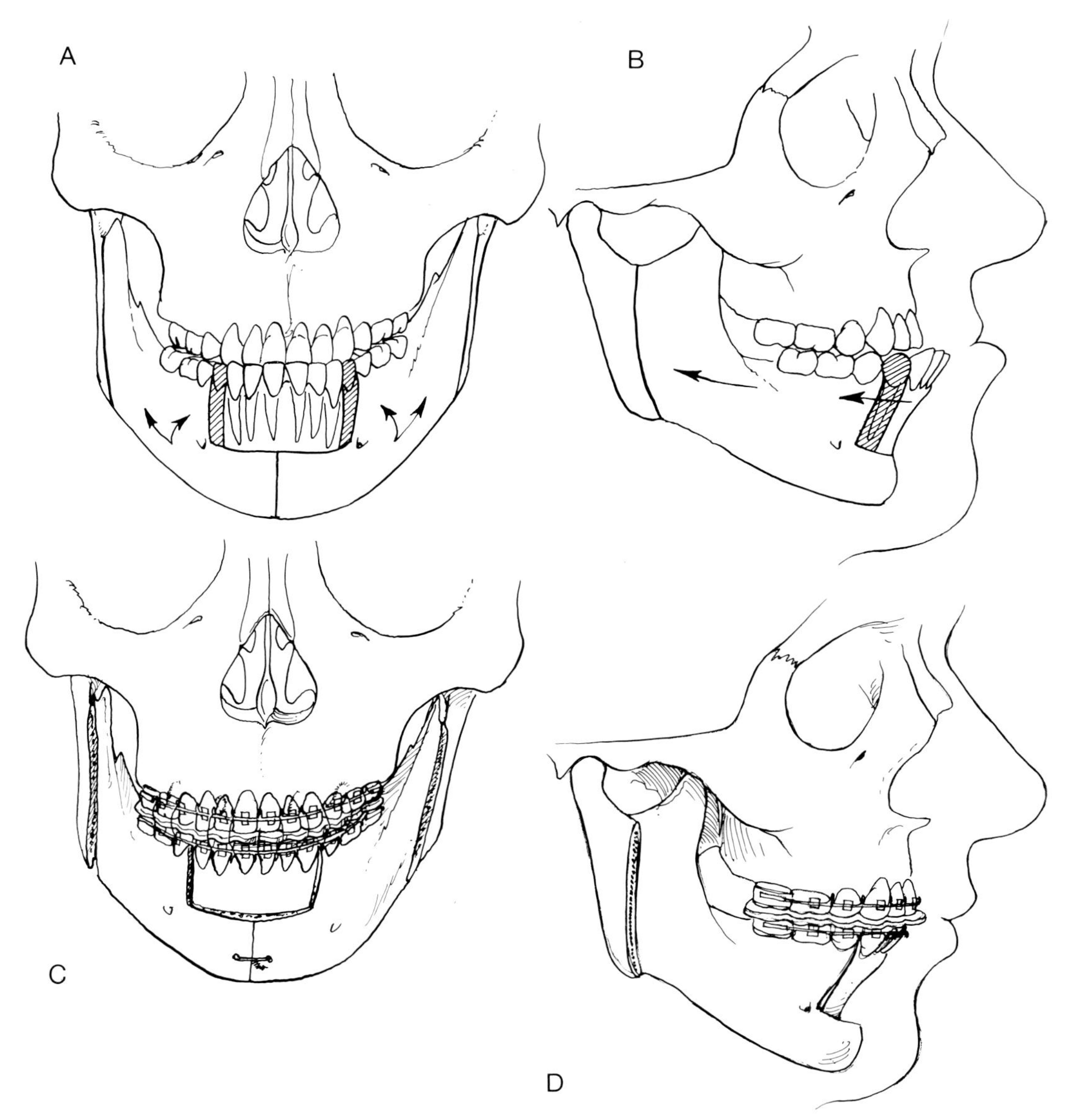

Figure 11–24. Technique for correction of mandibular prognathism with anterior and palatal crossbites by subapical osteotomy, symphyseal osteotomy, and intraoral vertical ramus osteotomies. Prominent lower lip, lack of labiomental fold, but adequate esthetic balance between the chin and nose give support to the surgical treatment plan in *A* and *B*. *A* and *B*, Stippled areas indicate planned ostectomies and premolar extractions; arrows indicate directional movements of segments; maxillary 1st premolars have been previously extracted to facilitate alignment of maxillary anterior teeth by orthodontics. *C* and *D*, Corrected crossbite and esthetic balance between nose, lips, and chin after surgery.

Figure 11–23 *Continued.* *H* and *I*, Inferior portion of mental symphysis, below level of incisors, is completely sectioned with oscillating saw blade (horizontal cross-hatched lines indicate where bone is sectioned by oscillating saw blade); with superior margin of soft tissue flap retracted, the labial cortical plate and alveolar bone immediately below the level of incisor apices are sectioned with a 701 fissure bur (vertically oriented cross-hatched lines indicate where bone is sectioned with fissure bur). *J*, The symphysis is sectioned into two halves by malleting a spatula osteotome into the partially sectioned interdental osteotomy site. *K*, Interosseous holes are drilled through the margins of the osteotomized bone at the inferior aspect of the mental symphysis. The lingual aspect of the margins of the sectioned bone are ostectomized to facilitate narrowing the mandible and apposition of the two segments, which are indexed into the planned relationship with an interocclusal splint and stabilized with an arch wire. Unless there is an alteration of the vertical dimension of the two segments, it is usually unnecessary to cut the arch wire in the planned osteotomy site.

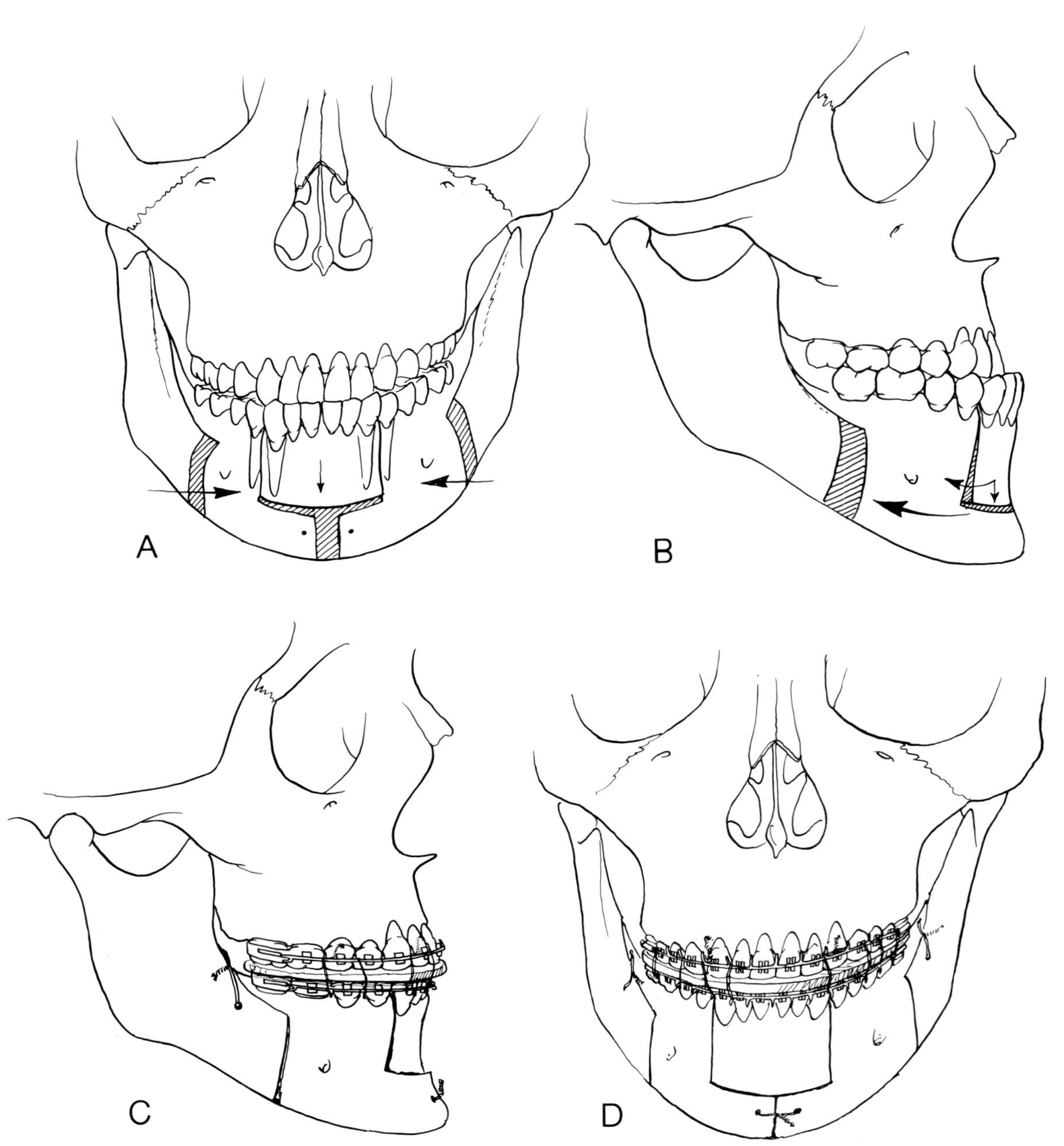

Figure 11–25. Combined subapical osteotomy, symphyseal ostectomy, and sagittal split osteotomies to correct various clinical manifestations of mandibular prognathism. *A* and *B*, Stippled areas indicate planned ostectomy sites. *C* and *D*, Postoperative relationship after surgery.

FOLLOW-UP STUDIES

The long-term results achieved with 21 body ostectomies (mean follow-up of 7 years, 4 months) were compared with similar follow-ups of 22 vertical ramus osteotomies (mean follow up 5 years, 2 months).[35] Each patient who had been surgically treated for severe mandibular prognathism was recalled for a long-term clinical, cephalometric, and model analysis.

The tongue and its associated pharyngeal musculature readapt to allow a patent and functional airway without causing flaring of the incisor teeth or significant anterior pogonial regression.[35] Although the space for the tongue significantly is reduced immediately after surgery, the space is eventually restored, possibly by a readjustment of the position of the hyoid bone. Insignificant labial proclination of the incisor teeth is observed in the cephalometric studies with either the body ostectomy or ramus osteotomy procedures.

Many clinicians have suggested surgical reduction in the size of the tongue to prevent relapse associated with body ostectomies. Wolk studied preoperative and postoperative cinefluorographic, electromyographic, and myometric data about six ramus osteotomy patients and concluded that the tongue and its associated musculature have a limited role, if any, in the anterior relapse seen in the mandible.[50] Wickwire and associates have similarly concluded that following surgery for mandibular excess in the ramus of the mandible, the hyoid, lingual, and cervical muscles adapt to their altered spatial and functional environment.[48]

Clinical studies indicate that there was no advantage of the ramus procedure over the body procedure in correcting crossbites.[35] The body ostectomy frequently was used to correct posterior crossbites by the medial rotation of the posterior segments, which was necessary to obtain apposition with the anterior segments. Despite the decrease in the size of the mandibular arch, there was no discernible relapse as a consequence of tongue pressure.

The majority of anterior open bites presently are corrected by maxillary surgery. When that approach is not feasible, the body ostectomy may eliminate the anterior open bite more predictably than ramus osteotomy. The vertical overlap of the anterior teeth following surgery is increased significantly more by the body ostectomy than by the ramus osteotomy. Clinical results from open bite patients support the hypothesis that the masticatory musculature in the vertical ramus can result in a lack of adequate control of the vertical dimension and the mandibular plane; these findings demonstrate the limitations of ramus osteotomy when this modality is used as the sole surgical procedure to manage vertical jaw dysplasias.

Subapical Osteotomy

When protrusion of the dentoalveolar portion of the mandible occurs alone, without lateral crossbite, the subapical osteotomy may achieve optimal esthetic appearance and correction of the anterior crossbite (see Figure 11–22).[34] Patients with such dentofacial deformities typically appear to have prominent chins. Because of the anterior position of the mandibular incisor teeth and their supporting bone, the contour of the lower anterior portion of the face appears flat, without a discrete labiomental fold. Masking off the lips and performing careful cephalometric prediction studies should reveal whether esthetic balance between the nose and chin is actually good. Surgical retraction of the lower incisors to correct the anterior crossbite will retroposition the lower lip, increase the relative prominence of the chin, and produce a discrete labiomental fold. Planning for such surgery is predicated on a knowledge of soft-tissue changes associated with retraction of the anterior mandibular dentoalveolar segment. The anteroposterior soft-tissue change is approximately two thirds of the change of the dento-osseous segment. The surgery is carried out through a standard degloving incision, which is described in Chapter 10, Mandibular Deficiency, and Chapter 12, Bimaxillary Protrusion.

In clinical practice, deformities amenable to this correction are relatively rare and usually defy correction by a single surgical procedure. Adjunctive osteotomies or ostectomies of the symphysis, body, or vertical rami frequently are necessary to correct the transverse, vertical, and anteroposterior manifestations of mandibular prognathism if the maxillomandibular disharmony is treated exclusively in the mandible (Figs. 11–23, 11–24, and 11–25).

INTRAORAL VERTICAL RAMUS OSTEOTOMY

H. David Hall

Indications for Using Intraoral Vertical Ramus Techniques

An intraoral ramus technique (intraoral vertical subcondylar or sagittal split osteotomy) is indicated when a good profile, arch, and dental relationship can be obtained by retruding the intact mandibular arch. Even in instances when the dental profile or arch relationship is not entirely satisfactory, this technique may be used in conjunction with midline ostectomy or osteotomy of the mandible, segmental osteotomies of the mandible or maxilla, or total maxillary osteotomy in order to provide better relationships. Ramus techniques have the advantage of not requiring removal of a tooth in the dental arch, as is usually the case with body ostectomy. A surgeon may choose between an intraoral and an extraoral approach on the basis of personal preference.

In most instances, the intraoral techniques are preferred to the older extraoral techniques. Although the vertical ramus and sagittal split techniques are comparable in many ways, there are minor differences. The intraoral vertical ramus osteotomy has a lower incidence of hypoesthesia of the inferior alveolar nerve; it is easier and faster, which are of special value in combined procedures, and it causes less rotational displacement of the proximal segment in asymmetric retrusions. Thus, everything being equal, we usually prefer the intraoral vertical ramus osteotomy to the sagittal split ramus osteotomy for correction of mandibular excess.

Biologic Considerations

Bell[21] has examined the blood flow in the proximal segment of the mandibular ramus after vertical subcondylar osteotomy in monkeys.[4] When the capsule and lateral pterygoid muscles served as pedicles, there was evidence of reduced blood flow in the proximal segment, especially in the distal tip, immediately after operation. There is also some indirect evidence that the blood flow in the distal portion of the proximal segment may be marginal under these circumstances. Necrosis and sequestration at the most distal tip of the proximal segment sometimes occur in man.[20] Thus, there is both experimental and clinical evidence that suggests that ischemia may occur in the distal portion of the proximal segment when only the capsule and lateral pterygoid muscle serve as pedicles. Ischemia may occur only infrequently and may not cause obvious difficulties, since there is rarely a problem in healing. Nonetheless, the intraoral vertical technique recently has been modified by maintaining attachment of a portion of the medial pterygoid muscle to the proximal segment.[44] This modification can be expected to improve blood flow, especially in the distal tip of the segment, and to minimize problems of avascular necrosis.

Evaluation of the Surgical Site

Visualization of the osteotomy site during the operation can be predicted from the radiographic configuration of the rami. The evaluation is made by using the submental-vertex view to show the rami. The more obtuse the angle formed where the lateral surface of the ramus meets the sagittal plane, the easier it will be to visualize the ramus. Since the osteotomy site is in the posterior third of the ramus, another factor affecting visualization is medial or lateral curvature of the posterior portion of the ramus. When there is a lateral curvature, visualization is enhanced. Conversely, when there is a medial curvature, the osteotomy site is more difficult to visualize. There is usually a difference between right and left rami; the side that provides the best view is cut first. Before the other side is cut, the mandible is rotated toward the side of the first osteotomy. This maneuver increases the angle formed by the ramus and the sagittal plane, enhancing visualization of the uncut ramus. It is quite rare for anticipated poor visualization of rami to contraindicate use of the intraoral vertical technique. Visualization also can be improved by sectioning the coronoid process before the ramus is sectioned.

Recent Modification and Advantages Thereof

Walker's recent modification in surgical technique for intraoral vertical ramus osteotomy represents a major improvement.[44] The key difference between this modification and the older technique used by Hall and associates[20] is that a pedicle of medial pterygoid muscle remains attached to the posterior and medial aspect of the proximal segment. This pedicle serves several useful purposes. First, it eliminates the need for wiring the proximal segment, thereby shortening and simplifying the procedure. Secondly, normal muscular tone will "seat" and maintain the condyles in the fossae. Not only does this constant muscle tone as well as active contraction during swallowing appear to maintain the condyles in the fossae, but the muscle tends to reestablish the position of the proximal segment in approximately the position existing before operation.[28]

With the older technique, in which a circumramus wire is used to stabilize the proximal segment, forward rotation of the segment almost always occurs when the circumramus wire is tightened (Fig. 11–26*A*). The wire moves the proximal segment forward until the posterior borders of the proximal and distal segments coincide where the wire passes around them. Only when the retrusion is great does the wired proximal segment retain an essentially normal angulation. It should be noted, however, that a circumramus wire does maintain the condyle in the fossa.

When the modified technique is used, the muscle pedicle tends to maintain a normal angulation (Fig. 11–26*B*). Extensive retrusions may produce some backward rotation of the proximal segment initially, but the segment subsequently assumes a more normal position. Finally, the pedicle of muscle and the periosteum provide a better blood supply to the proximal segment. This improved blood supply probably eliminates the necrosis of the distal tip of the proximal segment that occasionally occurs with the older technique, in which blood supply is less extensive. A better blood supply may also enhance rapid union of the bone segments.

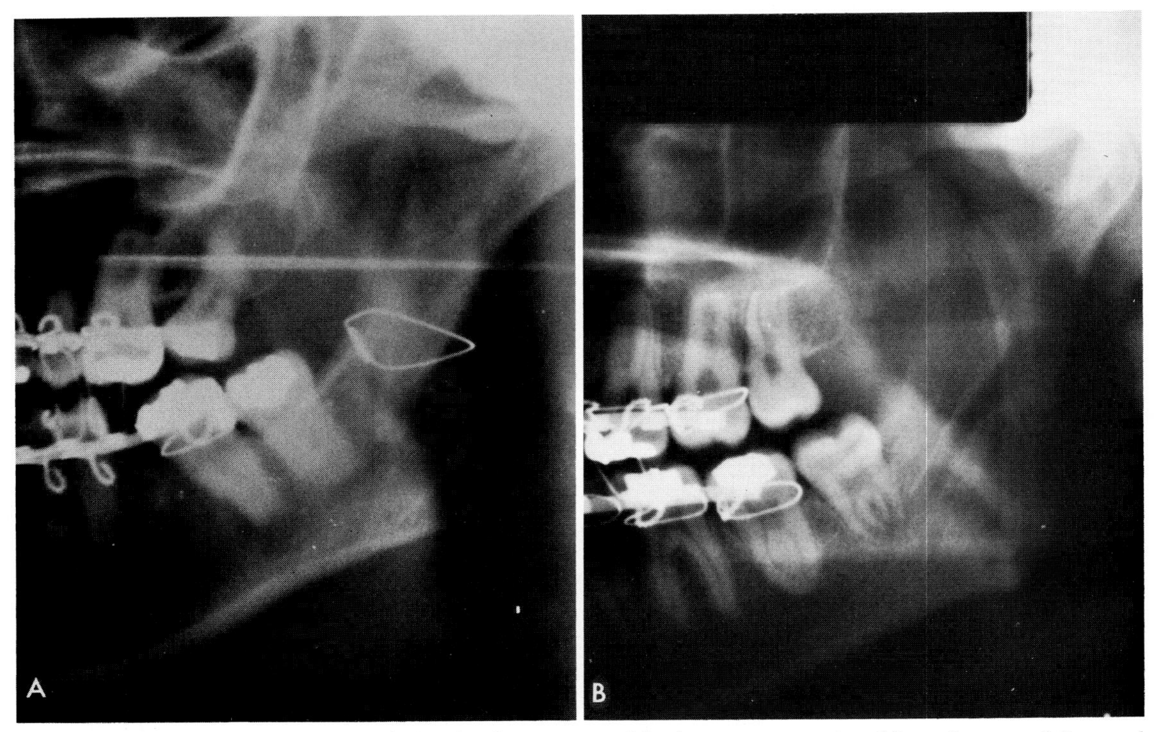

Figure 11–26. *A*, Position of proximal segment with circumramus wire. Note degree of forward rotation of proximal segment. Mandible retruded 7 mm. *B*, Position of proximal segment with attached pedicle of medial pterygoid muscle. Mandible retruded 6 mm.

Design of the Incision and Surgical Technique
(Fig. 11–27)

The mucosal incision is positioned over the external oblique line. The incision extends from the level of the occlusal plane anteriorly and inferiorly for about 3 cm. Beginning the incision low on the ascending ramus minimizes the possibility of cutting the buccal nerve and artery; moreover, it minimizes exposing the fat pad.

The periosteum is incised along the anterior border and is reflected from the lateral surface of the mandible but not from the posterior surface. The reflection extends from the sigmoid notch to the antegonial notch. A Bauer retractor is inserted into the sigmoid notch, and the opposite-handed Bauer retractor is inserted into the antegonial notch. The mandible should be in the closed position since this position minimizes tension of the soft tissues during retraction. Good lighting for the lateral surface of the ramus can be obtained by attaching a fiberoptic bundle to the retractor or by using a headlight.

The next step is to perform the osteotomy. This cut should extend in a mild curve from the sigmoid notch to the mandibular angle, immediately posterior to the mandibular foramen. A radiogram of the ramus and three prime landmarks (sigmoid notch, posterior border, and angle of the mandible) are used to determine where the osteotomy will be placed. The superior half of the osteotomy should begin at a point just posterior to the mandibular foramen and curve slightly forward to the midpoint of the sigmoid notch. Orientation for the angle of the cut is facilitated by relating the saw blade shaft to the occlusal plane. Measurements have shown that the mandibular groove just superior to the actual mandibular foramen is 5 to 7 mm from the posterior border in most patients.[22] Since the neurovascular bundle has not actually entered the foramen at this point, the inferior alveolar nerve should not be damaged by the oscillating saw blade, which only slightly protrudes through the medial cortex. Thus, for most patients, a cut 5 to 7 mm from the posterior border is optimal.

Sometimes, the posterior border may be difficult to visualize directly. One way to identify it in such instances is to feel it with a curved tip of a small instrument, such as a Freer elevator. For the osteotomy a Stryker saw with a rounded, angled blade that can make a 6-mm to 7-mm deep cut is preferred. A blade capable of making a deeper cut is more cumbersome, risks damage to the neurovascular bundle, and requires greater lateral retraction of tissues. The blade is placed in the detent on the shaft of the Stryker gas-powered oscillating unit, which provides the best visualization of the osteotomy site. After the location for the cut between the sigmoid notch and the area of the mandibular foramen has been established, the osteotomy is performed. Next, the osteotomy is extended from the area of the mandibular foramen slightly forward to the antegonial notch.

After the osteotomy has been completed, the proximal segment is displaced laterally. This can be accomplished by pulling the mandible forward and inserting a periosteal elevator between the segment and the ramus. The elevator is used to move the segment laterally and to stabilize it while portions of the medial pterygoid muscle and periosteum are stripped from the anterior, medial surface. The amount of periosteum and muscle reflected from the proximal segment is largely a function of the degree of anticipated overlap and of the width of the proximal segment. The goal is to obtain a broad, overlapping surface while maintaining an adequate pedicle of soft tissue. The mildly curved osteotomy maintains about a 1-cm wide bony segment at the angle. When necessary for larger retrusions, this permits stripping of all but the most posteroinferior pterygoid muscle fibers near the angle. Fortunately, these muscle fibers near the posteroinferior border are tenaciously attached and are less likely to be inadvertently stripped from the proximal segment. The proximal segment is placed lateral to the ramus. If a coronoidotomy is required, a periosteal elevator is passed to the sigmoid notch on the medial to the ramus. With the soft tissue thus protected by the elevator, the coronoid is easily sectioned with a drill or reciprocating saw and allowed to retract with the temporalis muscle.

The wound is packed with a moist gauze sponge, and a similar procedure is performed on the other side. After the second osteotomy is completed, the throat pack is removed and the mandible placed in its predetermined position. The teeth are fixed in occlusion with intermaxillary wires, and the extent of contact between the proximal and distal segments is assessed. A maximal area of contact of the proximal segments and the rami can be obtained by using a dental bur to decorticate any areas of premature contact. The proximal segments should be manipulated to ascertain that the condyles are not dislocated, even though the possibility of dislocation is remote when the medial pterygoid muscle attachment is retained. There is no need to wire these segments into position since the muscle pedicles will "seat" the condyles well in the fossae. Vacuum drains may be placed along the posterior and inferior borders of the ascending ramus, exiting through small punch incisions in the mucosa of the buccal sulcus or the skin anterior to the facial vessels. The proximal segments are examined again to assure that they are lateral to the rami. The wound is closed using a continuous horizontal mattress or similar suture.

The intraoral inverted L-osteotomy is an alternative technique to intraoral vertical ramus osteotomy and coronoidotomy for correction of extreme mandibular prognathism (Fig. 11–27 *L–O*). A theoretical advantage of this procedure relates to the fact that a good proportion of the temporalis and pterygoid muscles remain attached to the prox-

Text continued on page 898.

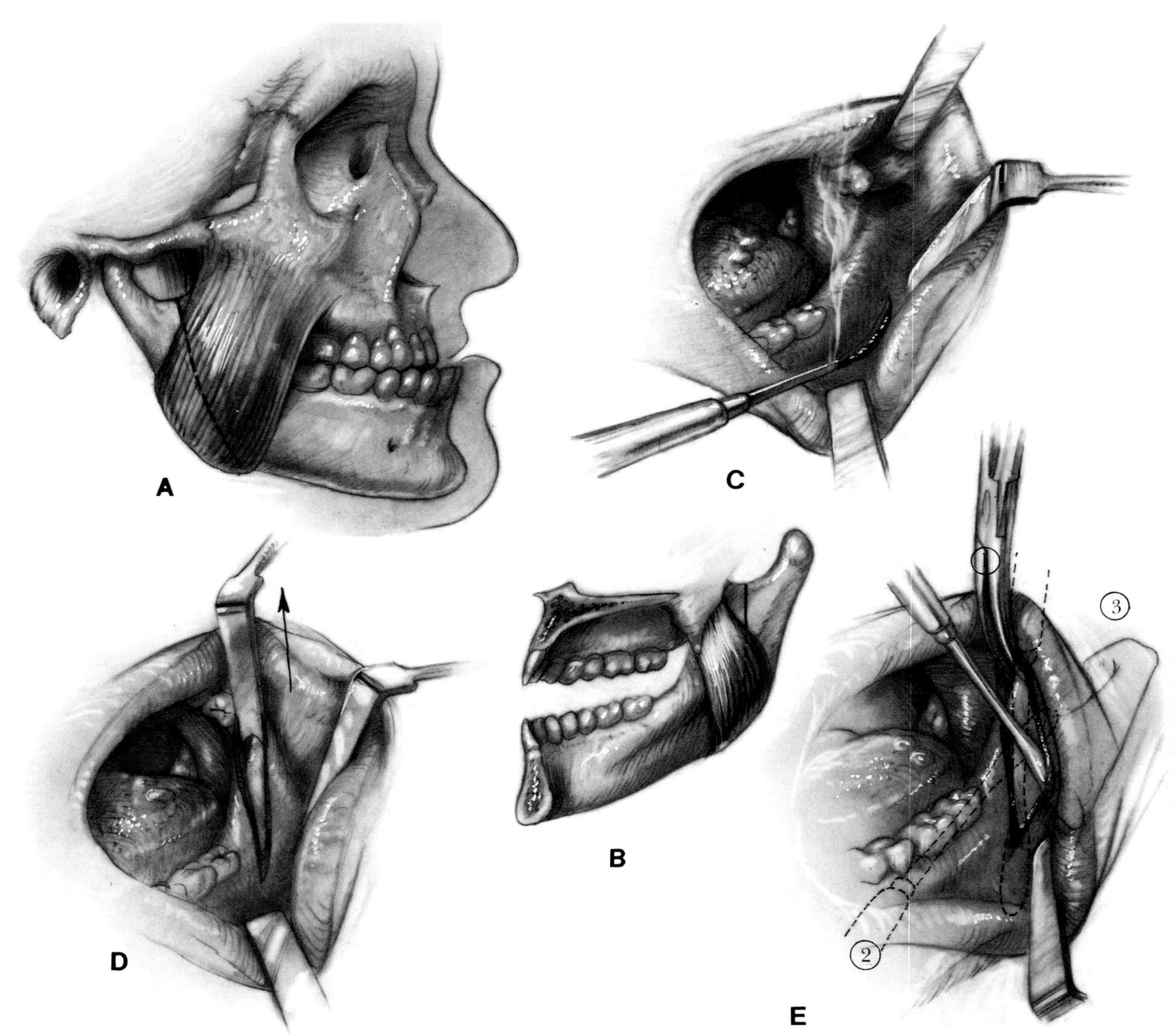

Figure 11–27. *A–K*, Surgical technique for correction of mandibular excess by intraoral vertical ramus osteotomy (IVRO). *A*, Position of masseter muscle and site for osteotomy. *B*, Position of medial pterygoid muscle and site for osteotomy. *C*, Location of mucosal incision for intraoral vertical ramus osteotomy. *D*, Exposure of coronoid process with a V-shaped right angle notch retractor positioned against the anterior and inferior aspects of the coronoid process. *E*, Subperiosteal reflection of lateral border of ramus: lateral and posterior aspects of the vertical ramus (1), sigmoid notch (2), and antegonial notch areas undermined (3). *F*, Bauer retractors are positioned in sigmoid notch and antegonial notch. The osteotomy is made with a rounded oscillating saw blade. The line of bone section extends from the midsigmoid notch area inferiorly to a point immediately posterior to the antilingular prominence and then inferiorly to the antigonial notch. *G*, A rounded angulated oscillating saw blade is used to section the ramus opposite the mandibular foramen 5 to 7 mm from the posterior border of the ramus; the osteotomy is extended inferiorly to the antegonial notch. *H*, After the osteotomy is completed, the proximal segment is displaced laterally by inserting a periosteal elevator between the segment and the ramus. With the proximal segment held laterally, a portion of the medial pterygoid muscle and periosteum are stripped from the anterior medial surface of proximal segment; the amount of periosteum and muscle reflected from the proximal segment is a function of the degree of anticipated overlap and the width of the proximal segment. *I*, Cross-hatched area indicates where the medial pterygoid muscle is detached; dotted area indicates where medial pterygoid muscle is not detached. *J*, After the contralateral ramus osteotomy is completed, the proximal segments are positioned laterally and anteriorly to the distal segments and the mandible is retracted until the teeth are in the planned occlusion. Intermaxillary fixation is accomplished with wire ligatures placed between vertical lugs soldered to the previously placed arch wires. The pedicle of medial pterygoid muscle stabilizes the segment in position.

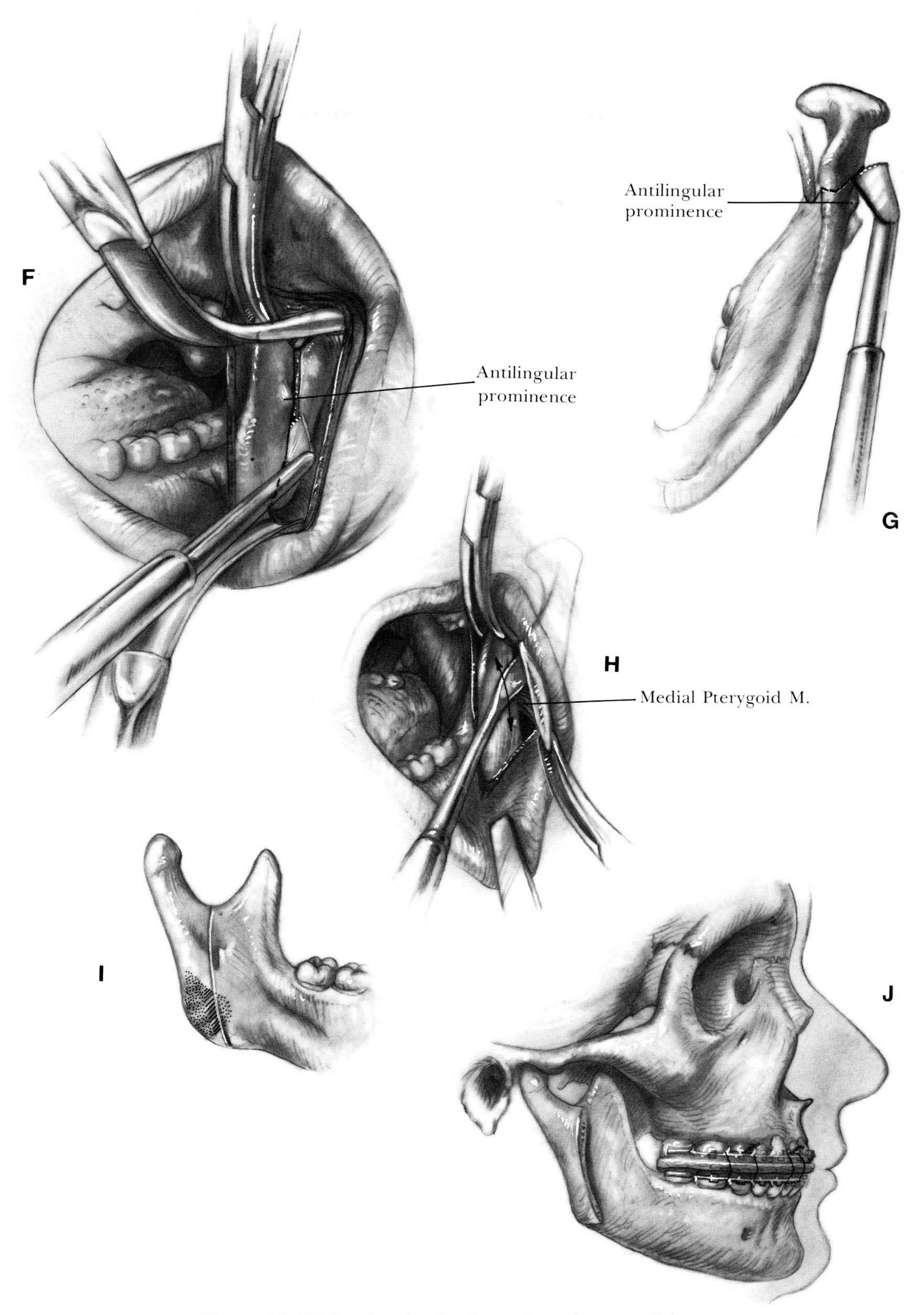

Figure 11–27 *Continued.* See legend on the opposite page.

Illustration continued on the following page.

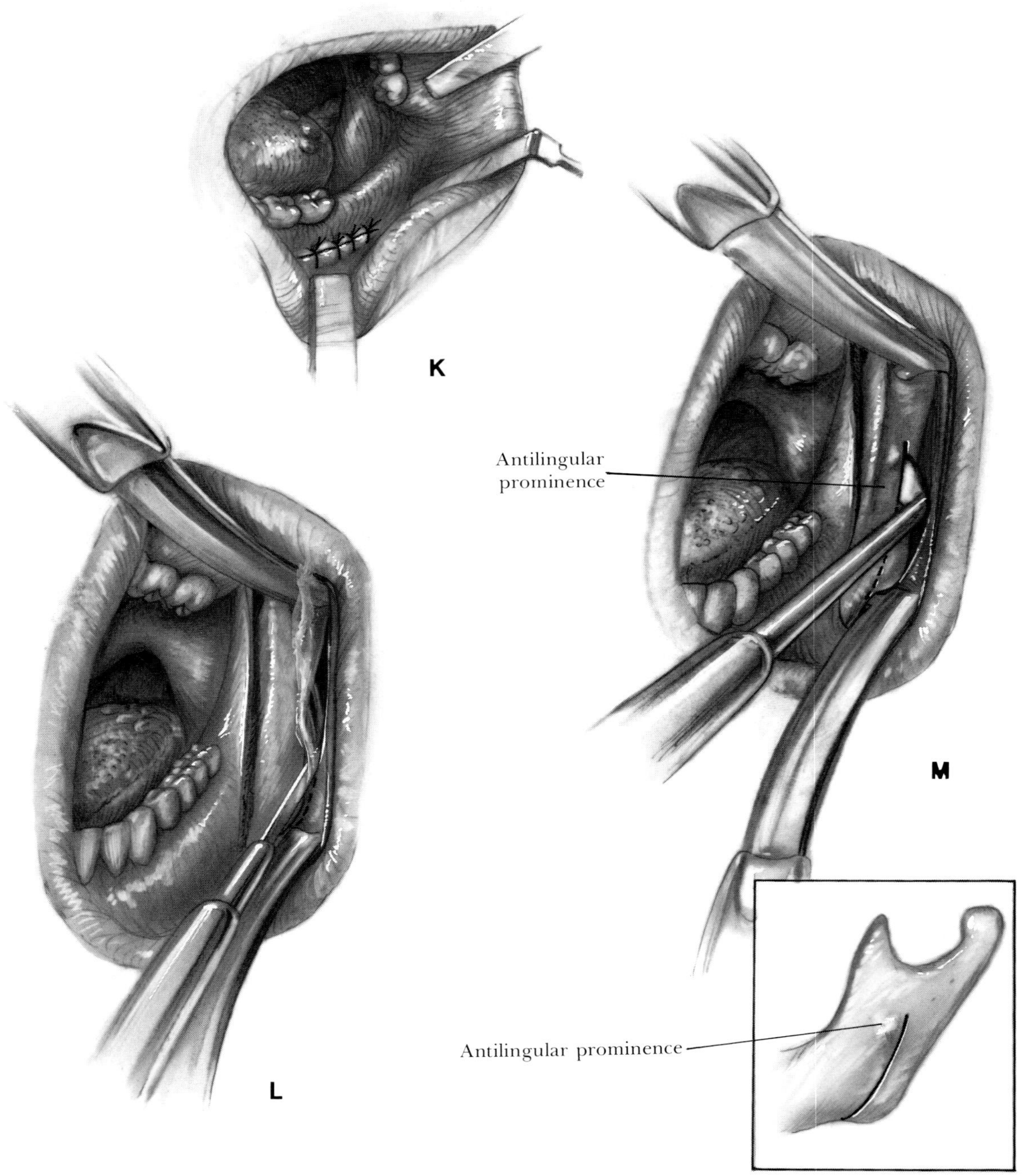

Figure 11–27 *Continued.* *K,* After each proximal segment is manipulated to be certain that the condyles are seated in the condylar fossae, the intraoral incisions are closed with continuous horizontal sutures. *L–O,* Surgical technique for correction of mandibular excess by intraoral "inverted L" osteotomy. *L,* After the lateral surface of the mandibular ramus is exposed, Bauer retractors are positioned in the sigmoid and antegonial notches. The periosteal sheath posterior to the vertical ramus is incised to expose the medial pterygoid-masseter muscle sling to facilitate subsequent retrusion of the distal segment. *M,* The vertical portion of the osteotomy is made with a rounded oscillating saw blade. The line of osteotomy extends from a point approximately 2 mm superior and immediately posterior to the antilingular prominence inferiorly to the antigonial notch.

Legend continued on the opposite page.

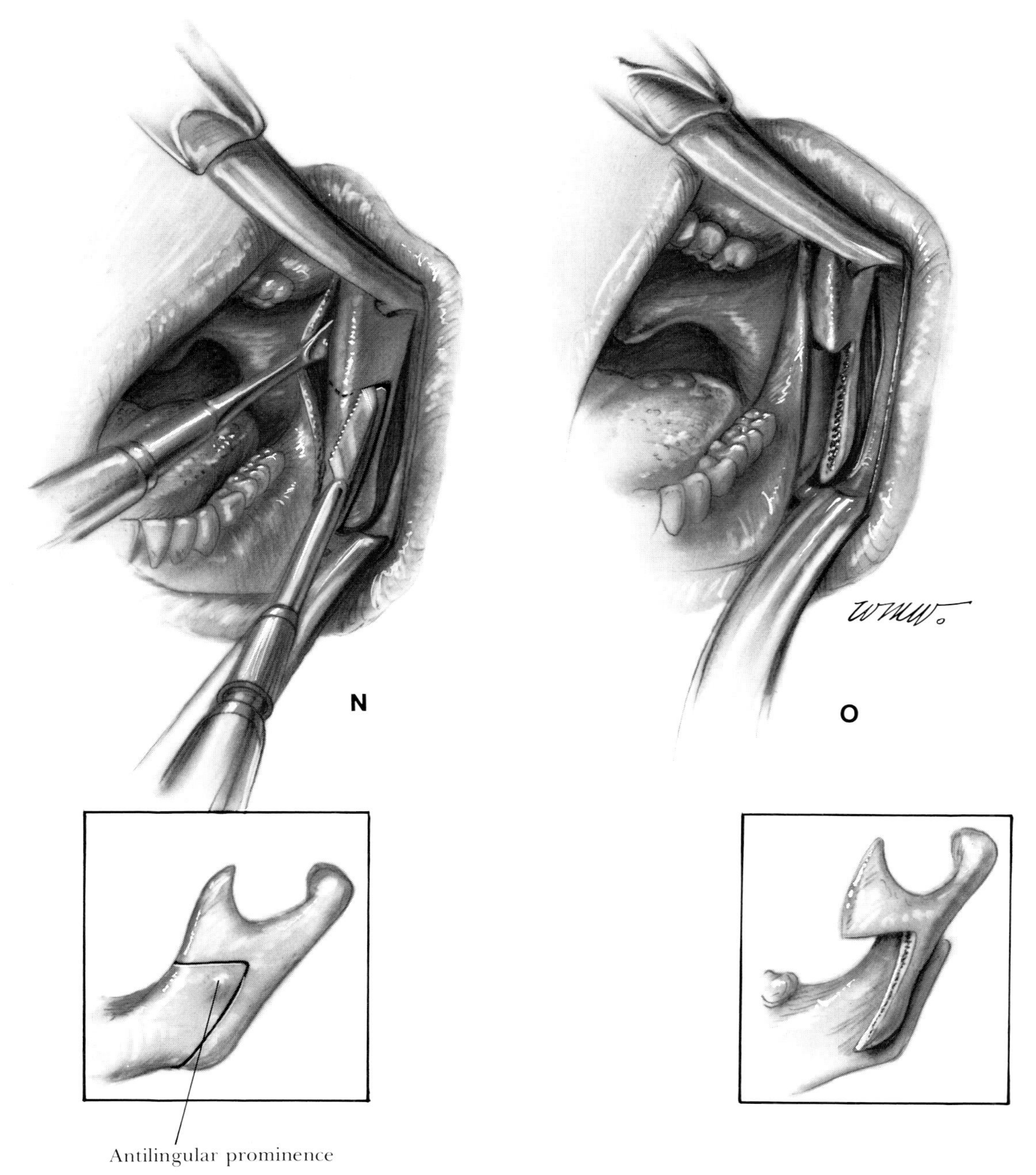

Figure 11–27 *Continued. N,* A periosteal elevator is positioned on the medial aspect of the ramus above the level of the lingula opposite the planned horizontal osteotomy to protect the neurovascular bundle and lingual soft tissues. A horizontal osteotomy is made from lateral to medial with either a reciprocating saw blade or a Lindemann bur to connect the posterior vertical osteotomy with the anterior aspect of the ascending ramus. Posteriorly, the horizontal osteotomy is made approximately 2 mm above the antilingular prominence. *O,* After the "inverted L" osteotomy is completed, the proximal segment is elevated laterally. The medial pterygoid muscle is detached as necessary from the medial aspect of the proximal and distal segments to facilitate retrusion of the distal segment. Posterior movement of the distal segment is facilitated by separation of the medial pterygoid and masseter muscles. Direct interosseous fixation of the repositioned segments is not routinely used.

imal segments. Consequently, the overall line of muscle action tends to maintain the preoperative spatial relationship of the proximal segment and hold the condyle in the condylar fossae. Carefully executed cephalometric prediction analyses and studies to simulate the planned movements with acetate overlay tracings are essential to determine that the margins of the horizontal osteotomies of the proximal and distal segments will be juxtaposed and overlap.

SAGITTAL SPLIT RAMUS OSTEOTOMY

Indications for Sagittal Split Procedures

Biologic considerations and evaluation of the surgical sites for sagittal split ramus osteotomy are discussed in Chapter 10, Mandibular Deficiency (see Fig. 10–22). The procedure is indicated specifically when two-dimensional changes are necessary to correct skeletal problems in the mandible. If a vertical change and an anteroposterior change are both anticipated, the sagittal split osteotomy provides a better bone contact than may be possible with the intraoral vertical subcondylar procedure. Occasionally, the sagittal split or the intraoral vertical approach may be equally appropriate and the decision as to procedure is largely the surgeon's choice.

Surgical Technique

The surgical technique for retruding the mandible by sagittal split ramus osteotomies is similar to that described in Chapter 10—through "splitting" of the rami (Fig. 11–28 *A–K*). The proximal segment is displaced laterally and the medial pterygoid muscle is stripped from this segment. The throat pack is removed and the teeth are wired into the desired occlusion. The proximal segments are seated firmly in the fossae. There will be some degree of overlap of the proximal segments with the most anterior osteotomy in the distal segments (Fig. 11–28*A*). This overlapping bone is removed by sectioning with a bone bur.

Figure 11–28. Surgical technique for correction of mandibular excess by sagittal split osteotomy of mandible. *A*, Typical dental, skeletal, and facial features of mandibular excess with mandible in centric relation and lips relaxed: prominent chin with procumbent and everted lower lip and Class III malocclusion. Dental compensations have been removed by orthodontic treatment, which tipped lower incisors forward; upper incisors have been uprighted. Cross-hatched area indicates planned ostectomy; broken line indicates osteotomy. *B*, Intraoral incision through the mucosa in the lateral aspect of the buccal vestibule opposite the 2nd and 3rd molar areas. *C*, Exposure of coronoid process with a V-shaped right angle notch retractor positioned against the anterior and inferior aspects of the coronoid process. *D*, Exposure of medial surface of the ramus by subperiosteal tunneling; tissue retraction by clamp positioned at the coronoid notch. A periosteal elevator is used to establish a periosteal tunnel on the medial aspect of the ramus of the mandible; the dissection is made superior to the mandibular foramen and carried to a point immediately posterior to the neurovascular bundle. *E*, Tip of modified lingual channel retractor is positioned immediately superior and posterior to neurovascular bundle to facilitate visualization of medial surface of the mandible. The medial retractor has been illustrated so that the reader can visualize the medial aspect of the ramus and neurovascular bundle. In clinical practice, however, the end of the retractor is positioned approximately parallel to the mandibular occlusal plane at about a 45° angle to the vertical ramus. Horizontal bone incision immediately above the mandibular foramen and inferior alveolar neurovascular bundle. The medial horizontal osteotomy is made with a Lindemann bur, taking care not to damage the inferior alveolar neurovascular bundle with the bur or by exaggerated retraction from the medial retractor. A lingual view is shown in the insert. The osteotomy shown here is made parallel to occlusal plane, from the area immediately posterior to the inferior alveolar neurovascular bundle to the anterior border of the mandible to a depth of one-half the mediolateral thickness of the ramus.

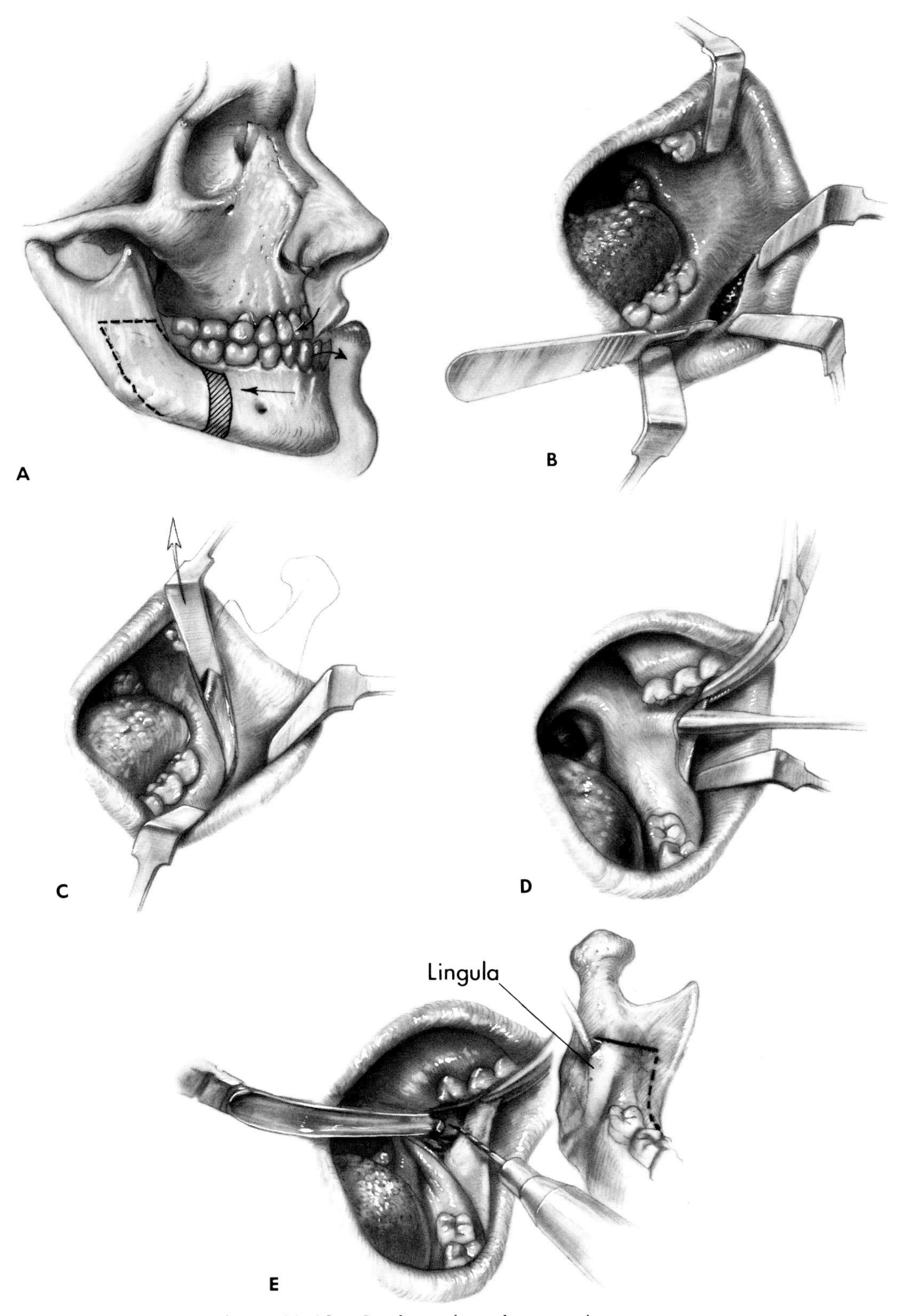

Figure 11–28. See legend on the opposite page.

Illustration continued on the following page

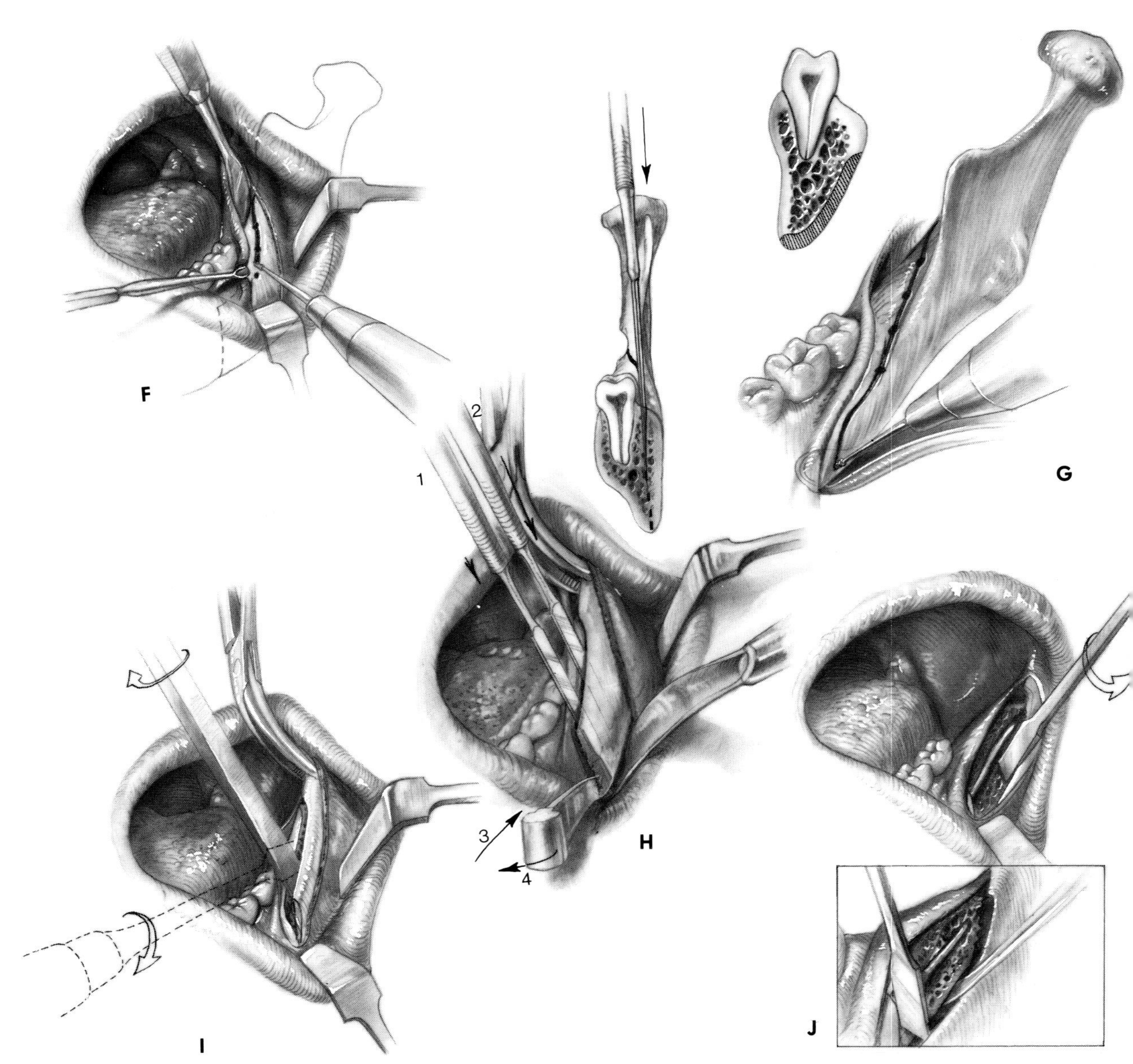

Figure 11–28 *Continued.* *F*, After multiple drill holes are made into the cancellous bone along the anterior border of the ramus, the sagittal osteotomy is continued along the anterior border of ascending ramus with a #703 tapered fissure bur; the masseter muscle is minimally retracted with a Henahan retractor. *G*, With the curved end of the channel retractor positioned in the area of the antegonial notch, a vertical osteotomy of the lateral aspect of the mandible is accomplished. The vertical cut is made through the buccal cortex with a fissure bur. In the insert, the cut is shown as the cross-hatched portion. Note that the cut penetrates only through the cortex. The cut extends completely through the cortex of the inferior aspect of the mandible. *H*, A thin sharp "spatula" osteotome is malleted to partially section the body of the mandible at the junction of the buccal cortical plate and the intramedullary bone. (1 and 2). The osteotome is then used to partially split the lateral and medial aspects of the ramus. Care should be taken to direct the osteotome against the internal surface of the lateral ramus so as not to damage or transect the inferior alveolar nerve and artery. A finely tapered sharp curved osteotome is malleted between the sectioned bony margins at the inferior border of the body of the mandible at the junction of the proximal and distal bone fragments; the osteotome is then levered against the distal segment to apply force against the inner surface of the proximal segment. *I* and *J*, An orthopedic osteotome is inserted in the split and twisted to separate the ramus fragments; the inferior alveolar nerve should be visualized as it passes into the medial or distal fragment. When the nerve is in the proximal segment, the enveloping cancellous bone must be carefully removed with small curettes to allow medial repositioning of the nerve. Detachment of residual attachment of medial pterygoid muscle.

Legend continued on the opposite page.

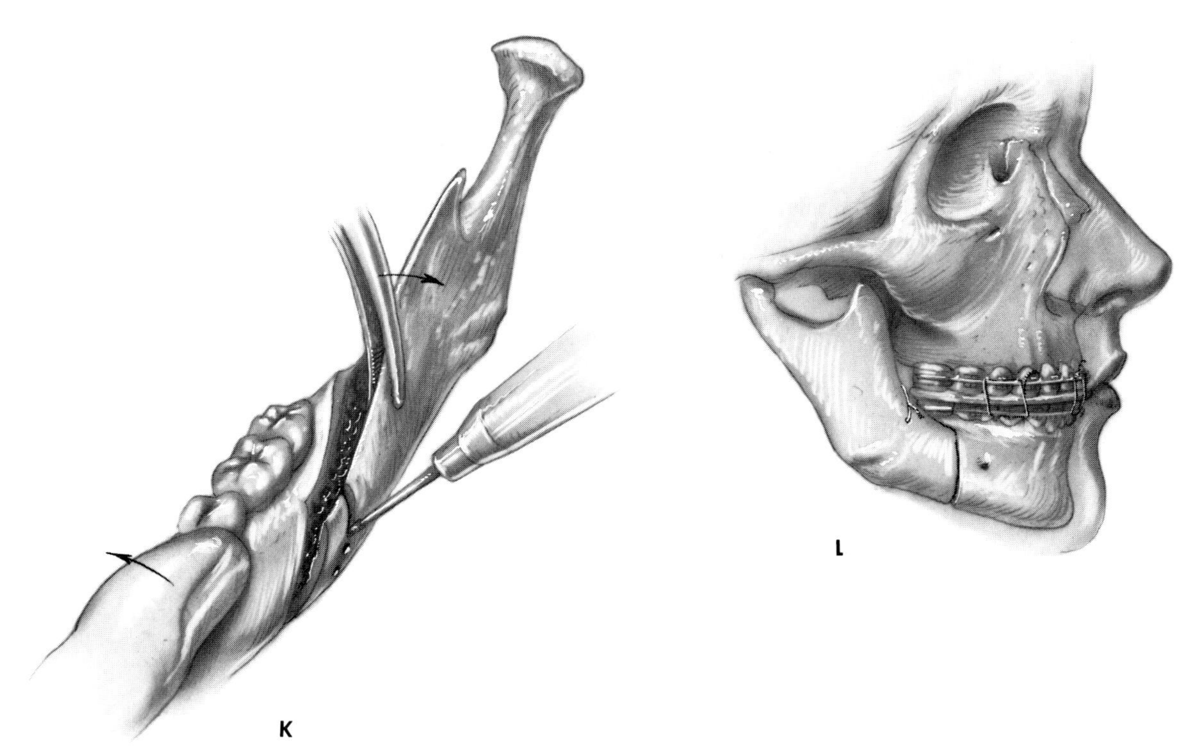

Figure 11–28 *Continued.* *K*, The proximal and distal segments are held apart by repositioning the distal segment to the contralateral side. With the proximal segment stabilized with a Kocher clamp, the anterior aspect of the proximal segment is shortened the amount calculated to juxtapose the margins of the proximal and distal fragments. This procedure is usually accomplished after the splits are accomplished bilaterally and the mandible is fixed into the planned intermaxillary relationship. *L*, The repositioned distal part of mandible is fixed with interosseous wire, which tends to reposition the condyle in the glenoid fossa. After the mandible is retracted and immobilized, the proximal fragments should be fixed with wire ligatures to insure an active direct force seating the condylar head positively in the glenoid fossa. Lateral view of completed osteotomy, showing interosseous wire in solid cortical bone securing the proximal and distal segments together along the anterior aspect of the ramus.

INTERMAXILLARY FIXATION AFTER INTRAORAL RAMUS OSTEOTOMY

The mandible has a strong tendency to rotate backward during intermaxillary fixation following surgical procedures in which the ramus is cut. The rotation is apparently secondary to force exerted by muscles of mastication. With the ramus no longer intact, the molar teeth become a fulcrum. This produces superior movement of the angle of the mandible and inferior movement of the chin. The force causing inferior movement of the chin is sufficiently strong to induce skeletal relapse in most instances. The force is also strong enough to cause supraeruption of the mandibular and even the maxillary incisor teeth when the force is transferred to the incisors during fixation. Conversely, if the force is applied only to the posterior teeth and the canines, as is the case when an arch bar is ligated to these teeth only, supraeruption occurs in the posterior and canine teeth, creating a mild open bite between the incisors. It is important to take this force into account when designing appliances for intermaxillary fixation. One simple way to counteract this force is to stabilize the mandibular arch bar with a circum-mandibular wire placed in the symphysis area. A piriform aperture wire attached to the maxillary arch bar serves the same purpose, i.e., transferring this force to bone through wire rather than through teeth. Whatever means of fixation is employed, it is important to understand this tendency for inferior movement of the chin and to make appropriate adjustments in the fixation appliances.

The majority of relapse during intermaxillary fixation appears to occur when the mandible is moved posteriorly in a counterclockwise direction after ramus osteotomies. These relapse tendencies are best minimized by proper planning and execution of surgery, careful preoperative cephalometric prediction studies and programming of maxillary surgery when indicated.

It is frequently wise to construct a thin occlusal splint to guide the mandible into the desired occlusion at the time of surgery. This is especially true if there are any occlusal interferences or if intercuspation of teeth is not good.

Usually the splint is ligated to the maxillary appliances with fine wires passed through holes in the slightly thickened lateral aspect of the splint. If a good intercuspation of teeth is possible, the splint is removed at four to six weeks and intermaxillary fixation immediately reapplied for the remainder of the period of fixation. If elastic traction is used, the teeth can be "settled" into a better occlusion before removal of the intermaxillary fixation. If, however, the occlusion is such that the mandible cannot be guided easily into the desired occlusion, the occlusal splint should be maintained for the entire period of intermaxillary fixation. In addition, it can be used during the first week of intermittent mobilization to assure proper positioning of the mandible. Whenever the splint is removed, if there are interferences or an unstable occlusion, the orthodontist should take over the management of the occusion.

COMBINED SURGICAL AND ORTHODONTIC TREATMENT

Timing of Treatment

The timing of combined surgical and orthodontic treatment of mandibular excess problems can pose real difficulties for both the surgeon and the orthodontist. Difficulties arise both in deciding whether to attempt interceptive orthodontic treatment or to wait for definitive surgical correction and in timing the surgery once the necessity for surgery has been determined.

As has been pointed out previously in this chapter, the prognosis for success using orthodontic treatment alone for true mandibular excess problems is relatively poor if the skeletal jaw discrepancy is large. In children who have moderate jaw discrepancies, orthodontic treatment during growth can succeed in producing a satisfactory occlusion and satisfactory facial esthetics. If there is any doubt as to whether surgical treatment is necessary, an attempt at interceptive orthodontics during the elementary school years is warranted. The goal of this orthodontic treatment should be to influence the growth of the jaws without producing exaggerated protrusion of maxillary incisors and retrusion of mandibular incisors. In the long term, "masking" of the skeletal discrepancy by tooth movement is unsatisfactory because of the compromise in facial esthetics that this treatment can produce. Even more significantly, displacement of incisors produced by vigorous orthodontic treatment may have to be reversed in order to achieve a satisfactory surgical correction later. Early orthodontic treatment, then, should be attempted whenever there is a chance of success, but should not be overdone.

Once it has been decided that surgical correction of the mandibular excess will be required, timing of the surgery and of any preparatory orthodontic treatment must be considered carefully. Here, there are two opposing influences. For psychologic reasons, early surgical intervention to correct the deformity frequently is desired by the patient and his or her family. For maximum long-term stability and predictability of result, surgical correction should be delayed until mandibular growth is essentially complete. If for psychologic reasons surgical correction of an extremely severe mandibular excess is done in the early teens, it is highly likely that a second operation will be needed in the late teens because of continued disproportionate mandibular growth, and the patient and the parents should be informed of this likelihood. In most instances, it is better to delay surgery until growth is completed and to meet the patient's psychologic need for positive action in some other way.

When orthodontic preparation for surgery is required, beginning the orthodontic treatment a year or so in advance of any possible surgery date can have psychologic benefits. The visible orthodontic appliance is a symbol to the patient's contemporaries that this problem has been recognized and that effective treatment is under way. Occasionally, it may be necessary to place bands on incisor teeth at a time when no real tooth movement is required in order to give the patient psychologic support during the final phase of disproportionate mandibular growth. The orthodontic treatment, however, should be aimed at eliminating or preventing dental compensation for the skeletal discrepancy, not accentuating it as the teeth are brought into occlusion.

Several methods have been proposed for determining when mandibular growth is complete or so nearly complete that there is no longer a major risk that continuing growth will cause postsurgical relapse. By far the most effective method is careful comparison of serial cephalometric radiographs (Fig. 11–29). Ideally, a determination that mandibular growth has ceased should be made from three serial films taken at six-month intervals. Three films at four-month intervals are adequate if there is real pressure for speed in making the decision. A decision made on the basis of only two films is more subject to tracing error or other inaccuracies in the comparison itself.

At one time it was hoped that measuring the blood levels of growth hormone or other hormones associated with the adolescent growth spurt would provide an accurate biochemical indication of mandibular growth status. This hope has not been borne out — at present no reliable biochemical methods for evaluating facial growth state have been discovered. Despite the correlations between the stage of ossification of the hand and wrist bones and mandibular growth, individual variation makes wrist films unreliable for determining whether mandibular growth has ceased in any given patient; there is no substitute for direct observation, especially because patients with disproportionate mandibular growth are likely to be at the extremes of normal variation and, therefore, may not follow correlation patterns established by observing individuals who are growing normally.

Presurgical Orthodontic Treatment

The general rules for combining surgical and orthodontic treatment have been presented in Chapter 6. With mandibular excess, as with other types of problems, it is desirable to carry out the surgery as early in the combined treatment phase as is feasible, leaving the detailed orthodontic finishing until after jaw movement has been accomplished. Nevertheless, in many instances, considerable orthodontic preparation is re-

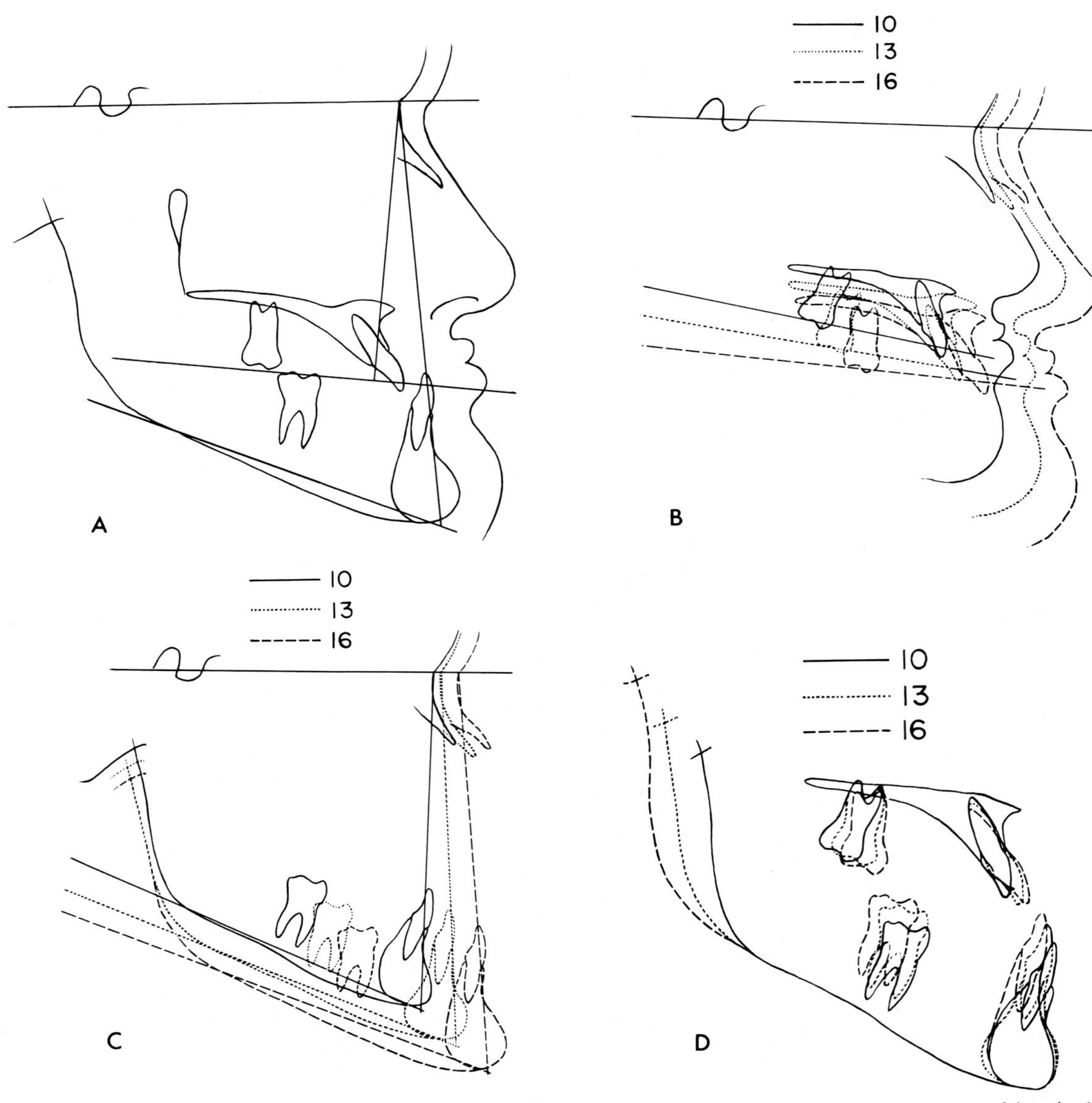

Figure 11–29. *A*, Typical dental, facial, and skeletal characteristics of mandibular prognathism in 16-year-old boy. *B–D*, Six-year growth study of mandibular prognathism between ages 10 and 16. Growth and development caused labial migration of maxillary teeth (*B and D*) and lingual migration of mandibular teeth (*C* and *D*). Patient had no orthodontic treatment during this period of time.

quired. The "surgery early" approach simply means that it is better to defer some finishing orthodontics until after surgery, while completing the necessary preparatory tooth movements before surgery.

The three major goals in orthodontic preparation before surgical correction of mandibular excess are:

1. *Eliminating or reducing dental compensation for the skeletal deformity.* Typically, when mandibular growth has been excessive, the mandibular incisors are upright and positioned lingually, whereas maxillary incisors are severely protruded (Fig. 11–30). In this circumstance, the goal in preparatory orthodontic treatment is to relate the teeth of each

arch to their own jaw, without regard to the dental occlusion at that time. This almost always requires making the occlusion worse, retracting maxillary teeth while mandibular teeth are being proclined.[7] Sometimes it is difficult for the orthodontist to appreciate that correct treatment in preparation for surgery requires moving the teeth in just the opposite direction to that needed to bring them into occlusion with orthodontics alone, but this is the case.

2. *Obtaining alignment of teeth and establishing anteroposterior incisor position.* When the dental arches are crowded, it is necessary to decide whether appropriate alignment can be obtained without extraction of teeth. If the maxillary and mandibular arches are mildly crowded but the mandibular incisors are quite upright while the maxillary incisors protrude forward off their bony base, it may be desirable to extract premolars in the maxillary arch while treating the mandibular arch by expansion. In such a case, the eventual molar relationship could be Class II, but this approach to treatment often is necessary in order to position the incisors in good alignment and in good relationship to their supporting bone. If extraction is necessary, the extraction sites should be closed orthodontically prior to surgery (although it is not necessary to complete root paralleling and other finishing tooth movements at that stage).

Before a decision to advance the mandibular incisors is made, it is important to evaluate the periodontium around these teeth carefully. Frequently the labial plate of bone is thin, and the gingivae already show signs of recession. In this instance, it is unwise to bring the incisors further forward, because increased loss of supporting tissue around the teeth is highly likely. In a patient with this problem, genioplasty to reduce the prominence of the bony chin may have to be considered as an alternative.

Alignment of the teeth in the vertical plane of space also is needed — if there is an exaggerated curve of Spee a decision must be made as to whether the necessary leveling of the arch would be done best by intrusion of incisors or extrusion of premolars. Leveling by

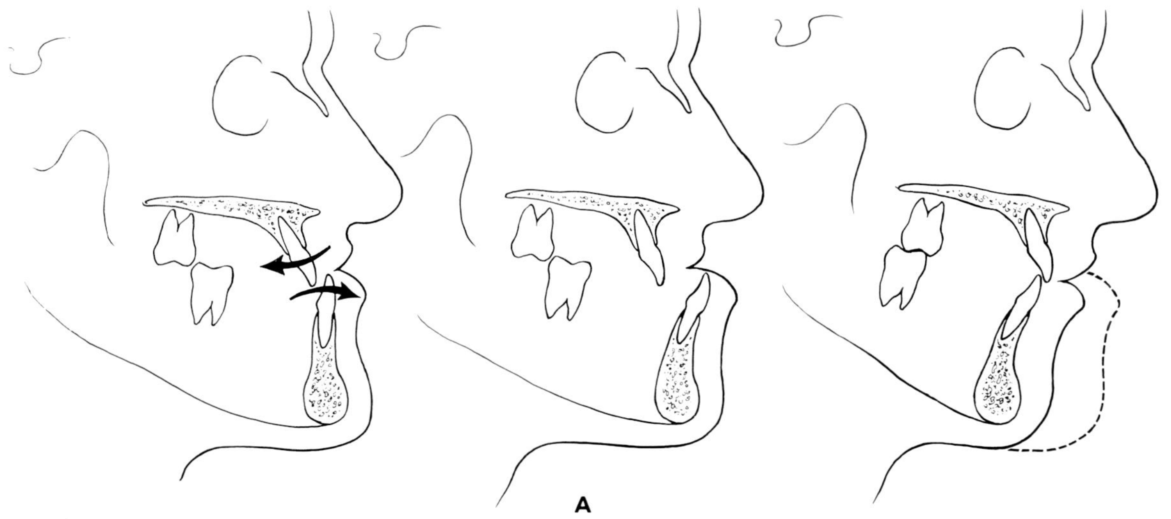

Figure 11–30. *A*, The maxillary incisor teeth, which clinically appear to be retrusive, are usually protrusive and labially inclined when compared to their ideal position. The lower incisors are usually retrusive and lingually inclined when compared to their ideal position. The objective of orthodontic treatment is to position the malaligned teeth in the best possible position on the individual jaw. The jaws are aligned surgically to produce the best occlusal relationship. If the teeth were positioned properly, this restores facial balance.

intrusion can be done using the appropriate orthodontic mechanics for incisor intrusion (which requires a segmented arch approach rather than continuous arch wires) or by an alveolar segmental surgical procedure. The orthodontic intrusion should be accomplished as part of pre-surgical preparation, whereas the segmental surgery to establish incisor position can be done at the same time the ramus osteotomy to reposition the jaw is carried out. If leveling would be carried out best by extrusion of premolars, this may be done orthodontically following the correction of jaw position.

Missing maxillary lateral incisors and a tendency toward skeletal maxillary deficiency as well as mandibular excess frequently are found in patients whose major problem is in the size of the mandible. If maxillary lateral incisors are missing, it may be quite feasible to place the canines in the lateral position, in essence using the lateral incisor space to allow proper positioning of the central incisors. The canine teeth can be reshaped by a combination of strategic grinding and the addition of composite restorative materials. Occasionally esthetic considerations related to unusual shape of the canines may make it desirable to extract first premolars and retract the canines into the first premolar space, opening space for a bridge pontic replacing the lateral incisor. Reshaping the canine and using it as a lateral incisor is generally preferable.

3. *Obtaining reasonable arch compatibility.* The form of the maxillary and mandibular dental arches may be quite different in patients who have mandibular excess. Often the mandibular arch is wide and rounded, whereas the maxillary arch is relatively constricted, particularly in the canine and premolar area, producing a V-shaped arch. It is imperative that proper diagnosis of any absolute transverse discrepancy be made. Proper treatment should be designed to correct problems such as skeletal aberrations either prior to or at the time of surgery for correction of mandibular excess. (See Chapter 9) (Fig. 11–30*B*). This correction may be facilitated by concomitant segmentalized maxillary surgery or, in mild cases, by sectioning the mandible at the midline of the symphysis to constrict the mandibular arch. Extreme care should be taken to avoid excessive use of crossbite elastics or expanded arch wires to obtain correction of transverse discrepancies through dental tipping.

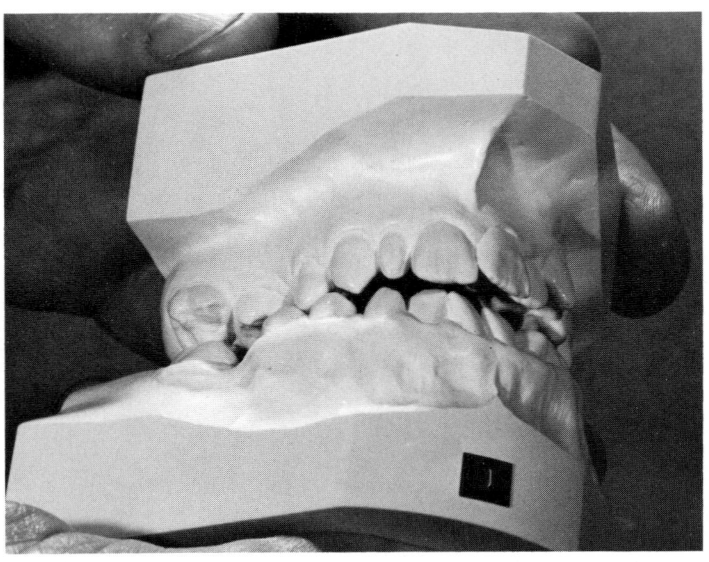

B

Figure 11–30 *Continued. B,* Discrepancies in lateral widths between maxillary and mandibular arches can be determined by placing the models into their postoperative occlusal relationship. The maxilla originally in crossbite may actually be too wide when the mandible is moved back. Minor dental width discrepancies are usually corrected with orthodontic arch wires postoperatively. When the maxilla is excessively narrow, maxillary osteotomy, presurgical orthodontic treatment, or rapid maxillary expansion with lateral maxillary osteotomies may be needed. Excessive maxillary width usually requires maxillary surgery.

Orthodontic and Surgical Interaction at Surgery

If any postsurgical orthodontic correction is planned, it is much better to have the orthodontic appliance in place presurgically than to perform the surgery and then refer the patient for placement of the orthodontic appliance and movement of the teeth. Any presurgical orthodontic movement obviously will require that the appliance be in place. But even if it is planned that all orthodontic tooth movement will be done after mandibular surgery, the orthodontic appliance should be in place at the time of surgery and should be used as part of the postoperative fixation.

Full-dimension rectangular orthodontic arch wires, fitting precisely in rectangular (edgewise) brackets, provide excellent intermaxillary fixation following ramus osteotomy. There are three ways in which the necessary hooks for maxillary fixation can be provided:

1. Small loops may be bent in the arch wire in interproximal spaces.
2. Short spurs of brass wire may be soldered to the arch wire, also in the interproximal spaces.
3. Hooks may be tied to the brackets when the stabilizing arch wire is placed (Kobayashi hooks).

Bent-in loops make it easy to change the vertical level of the arch wire or to change the amount of twist in the arch wire between adjacent teeth. This can be quite helpful in fitting a large rectangular arch wire to teeth that still are relatively irregular; therefore, this approach is particularly helpful for patients who have had minimal preliminary orthodontic correction. With the .022-inch slot edgewise appliance, the stabilizing arch wire should be .021 × .025 or .0215 × .028. Blue Elgiloy is an excellent material for these large arch wires, because it can be fabricated more easily and then heat-hardened. Satisfactory fixation also can be obtained with the .018-inch slot edgewise appliance, in which case .018 × .025 arch wires are used for stabilization. Bending in hooks in the .018 × .025 arch wires is not satisfactory, because the loop decreases the rigidity of the small wire. Soldered hooks are preferred for stabilizing arch wires in the .018 slot system. Placing hooks for fixation on the brackets rather than on the arch wires is easier for the orthodontist and seems to have no important contraindications. In this case, a plain stabilizing arch wire with neither soldered nor bent-in hooks is used. This does have the effect of placing greater stress on the band or the bonded attachment and so may increase the risk of losing an attachment during the fixation period.

The stabilizing arch wires should be placed at least 48 hours prior to surgery. They should be made to fit as passively as possible and should not incorporate any provision for tooth movement, but it is impossible to make such a wire perfectly passive. Therefore, the stabilizing arch wires should be placed first; then, after they have been tied in for at least 24 hours, the impressions for making the interocclusal wafer splints should be taken. This will ensure a precise fit of the wafers at time of operation, which is important to ensuring that the planned result is achieved.

If an ostectomy in the body of the mandible or an alveolar segmental surgical procedure is planned, intermaxillary fixation may not be necessary. When cuts are to be made within the dental arches, it is not possible to place stabilizing arch wires prior to surgery. In this instance, a stabilizing arch wire is made to fit the casts that were sectioned in planning the surgery, and this arch wire is tied into the brackets in the operating room. A full-dimension rectangular arch wire offers surprisingly good intra-arch fixation and is satisfactory as the only fixation for anterior segmental procedures. If intermaxillary fixation is not planned following a body ostectomy procedure to reduce mandibular excess, it may be wise to supplement the orthodontic arch wire with a cast splint or other device to obtain greater rigidity in the vertical plane of space.

Postsurgical Orthodontic Treatment

Excellent coordination between surgeon and orthodontist is critical as the patient begins to resume jaw function following intermaxillary fixation. If the occlusion has not been perfected presurgically (which is the situation for most patients), active tooth movement should begin under the control of light arch wires and interarch elastics as soon as the wafer splint is removed. It is permissible, and frequently desirable, to allow the patient to begin jaw function before the surgical stabilizing arch wires are removed, but it is critically important that the patient function into the wafer splint at this time. There should be no opportunity for the patient to encounter occlusal interferences while the teeth are held rigidly by the stabilizing arch wires, because he will begin shifting the mandible to one side or anteriorly in search of better occlusion. This can lead quickly to relapse tendencies and distortion in arch form. To repeat: if the surgeon wishes the patient to begin jaw function before turning him back over to the orthodontist for completion of the orthodontic treatment, the wafer splint should be tied to the maxillary or mandibular arch, so that the patient can function into the splint. This can be done easily by drilling small holes through the edge of the wafer splint and ligating it to the orthodontic stabilizing arch wire.

When the surgeon is satisfied that good bony union has occurred, the patient is ready to resume orthodontic treatment. Following a ramus osteotomy to correct mandibular excess, this usually is 6 to 8 weeks after surgery. At this time, the surgical stabilizing arch wires are removed and the wafer splint is discarded. The stabilizing arch wire should be replaced with light round ideal arches (usually .016-inch). Small omega loops can be bent into these arch wires as points for attachment of light elastics. The amount of traction on the elastics is vastly different from what the surgeon uses for intermaxillary fixation. Now the elastic pull is designed to produce rapid tooth movement, and this means that only a few ounces of force produced by light latex elastics are needed or desirable. The patient should have anterior and posterior vertical box elastics in conjunction with any needed cross-elastics. With such an arrangement, the teeth move quickly into an ideal occlusion. As the occlusion is perfected, heavier rectangular arch wires are placed if needed and the importance of the vertical elastics is lessened. This phase of postsurgical orthodontic treatment should take no more than a few months.

Orthodontic retention following correction of mandibular excess differs only slightly from retention after other forms of orthodontic treatment. If the patient has been treated surgically at a relatively early age, so that there is some probability of renewed growth, a retainer that ties the arches together is helpful, and a positioner can serve this purpose reasonably well.

In an older patient, renewed growth leading to forward positioning of the mandible is highly unlikely, and retention should concentrate on problems that are likely to recur, such as crowding of incisors if there was severe crowding initially or return of crossbite if a great deal of maxillary expansion was necessary. Achieving a good occlusion in the immediate postoperative period and not allowing the patient to function without guiding elastics until a good occlusion has been achieved are the keys to post-treatment stability in nongrowing patients. Relapse due to continued mandibular growth is almost impossible to control; such relapse is a silent indictment of failure to anticipate further growth when planning treatment timing.

MINIMIZING COMPLICATIONS

Intraoral Vertical Ramus and Sagittal Split Ramus Osteotomies

The only apparent difference in complication rates between sagittal split and vertical ramus techniques is the incidence of altered sensation of the inferior alveolar nerve. With the sagittal split osteotomy, the incidence of immediate hypoesthesia or anesthesia is greater[19, 45, 47] than experienced with the intraoral vertical ramus technique.[1, 20] Additional surgical experience with the intraoral vertical ramus technique has reduced the incidence of inferior alveolar nerve hypesthesia to 1 to 2 per cent. Moreover, physical damage to the nerve with intraoral vertical ramus procedures appears to be less severe than with the sagittal split, although recent technical refinements have also reduced nerve damage after sagittal split ramus procedures. Normal lower lip sensation usually returns within a few weeks or months when the inferior alveolar nerve is traumatized during the intraoral vertical ramus osteotomy. The most important question that remains to be answered relates to stability after the two different techniques. Valid comparative stability studies are needed to elucidate the differences, if indeed there are such differences.

The principal causes of nerve trauma with intraoral vertical surgery are (1) cutting too close to the mandibular foramen and (2) letting the proximal segment become "trapped" medial to the ramus where it can impinge on the mandibular nerve. Cutting too close to the mandibular foramen can usually be avoided by using the posterior border of the ramus as a landmark for the cut. The mandibular foramen is rarely less than 5 mm from the posterior border.[22] A radiograph of the rami provides additional help in relating the foramen to the border. By using the posterior border of the mandible as a landmark, the cut can be placed so as to provide for a maximal width of the proximal segment with minimal risk of damage to the inferior alveolar nerve. The risk can be further diminished by use of a saw blade that cuts only deep enough to pass through the medial cortex of the ramus. Even if the neurovascular bundle is near the osteotomy, an oscillating blade would likely cause at most only transitory neuropathy. The other major cause of inferior alveolar nerve trauma, "trapping" of the proximal segment, can be prevented by maintaining better control of the segment while positioning it laterally.

Although the incidence of nerve damage with sagittal split ramus osteotomy cannot be modified greatly by good surgical technique, the severity of the damage can be minimized. Details of the surgical technique that will reduce neural trauma have been described by Epker[17] and also are discussed in Chapter 10, Mandibular Deficiency.

Necrosis and sequestration of the distal portions of the proximal segment occur in a small number of patients treated with either technique. Whichever technique is used, retention of larger soft-tissue pedicles increases blood flow to the proximal segments. Although these innovations should eliminate ischemic necrosis, presently available data are insufficient for absolute certainty on this point.

Skeletal relapse tends to occur with the sagittal split ramus osteotomy and the intraoral vertical ramus osteotomy, regardless of whether the approach is intraoral or extraoral. Certain factors that seem particularly important in reducing these skeletal changes are (1) the effects of altering the resting length of the closing muscles of the mandible, (2) the integrity and healing of the ramus of the mandible, (3) the position of the condyle in the glenoid fossa during the period of intermaxillary fixation, and (4) biomechanical considerations in the surgical correction of mandibular excess.

Both the area of bone overlap and the closeness of adaptation of the segments will affect ramus integrity and consolidation of the osteotomized segments. The sagittal split osteotomy provides a broad area of bone contact. There is also an adequate area of contact with the vertical ramus osteotomy technique when the cut is designed to maximize overlap. One method of maximizing bone contact is to extend the osteotomy to the angle rather than terminating the cut at the posterior border. Sometimes with the vertical ramus osteotomy there is poor adaptation between the proximal segment and the ramus after the teeth are fixed in occlusion. In these instances, a good adaptation of the two segments can be obtained by decorticating the ramus or the proximal segment, or both, in the areas of premature contact. A broad area of overlap with close adaptation of the proximal and distal segments enhances the chance for an early solid union.

Close apposition of bony segments, early union after ramus osteotomies, and indeed long-term immobilization (8 to 12 weeks) do not necessarily produce skeletal stability, however. Significant relapse occurring during intermaxillary fixation is most commonly the result of improper planning and failing to recognize and treat associated vertical maxillary dysplasias. Short- and long-term stability after mandibular ramus surgery to shorten the mandible relates strongly to the vertical component of mandibular retraction. If the mandible is retruded and repositioned in a counterclockwise direction, dental and skeletal changes may continue during intermaxillary fixation and for a long time after release from intermaxillary fixation. The biomechanics of mandibular ramus surgery that involves rotation around a fulcrum at the molar teeth is inefficient and may generate large forces that tend to displace the proximal and distal segments.

The biomechanical consequences of surgical procedures designed to alter facial morphology must be appreciated. Many of the noted undesirable occurrences subsequent to mandibular ramus surgery may have underlying biomechanical explanations. These results partially explain the noted problems associated with orthodontically and surgically corrected high angle class III open bites. Biomechanical influences are important considerations for the surgeon as he plans any technical procedure designed to correct facial disharmonies. With a knowledge of relapse propensities and careful simulation of the planned surgical change by cephalometric prediction studies a surgical procedure can be designed to maximize esthetics, function, and stability. Maxillary surgery in concert with mandibular ramus surgery is frequently necessary to achieve these objectives in treating the spectrum of problems associated with mandibular prognathism. (See Chapters 10, 13, and 24 for further details.)

The position of the proximal segment during intermaxillary fixation may contribute to skeletal relapse. The condyle should be "seated" well in the glenoid fossa. Occasional difficulty in achieving this may constitute the biggest disadvantage of the intraoral vertical ramus procedure. When the condyle is found to be poorly "seated" in the postoperative radiographs, re-operation should be seriously considered. If the condyle remains poorly "seated," the closing muscles may "seat" it after release of intermaxillary fixation and cause an immediate anterior open bite. In addition to the position of the condyle in the fossa, the position of the proximal segment should approximate its spatial position before operation. If the proximal and distal segments are fixed to each other by wire or other means, the proximal segment must be positioned carefully in its preoperative position. Only when there is obvious condylar lag at the time of surgery is the proximal segment fixed directly to the distal segment with an interosseous wire. Isaacson and associates have presented data suggesting that wiring the proximal segment in a new position may cause a shift in mandibular position after release of occlusal fixation.[28] By retaining muscle attachment to the proximal segment, a self-repositioning of the condylar segment may occur to approximately that which existed before surgery.

Postsurgical Occlusal Problems

In addition to complications or problems related to the surgical intervention itself, three types of occlusal problems are noted in patients who have had combined surgical and orthodontic treatment of mandibular excess. These are:

1. *Appearance of Class II malocclusion or mandibular asymmetry soon after function has resumed.* In a few instances, it has been noted that soon after patients begin to function following removal of the wafer and stabilizing arch wires, the mandible dropped back farther unilaterally or bilaterally. This complication results if the surgeon fails to ascertain that the condyle was seated in the temporal fossa after completion of the osteotomy. If the condyle is forward on the eminence when it is wired into position, healing will occur with an extensively shortened ramus and the mandible will drop posteriorly at the first opportunity. To avoid this possibility, muscles should be left attached to the proximal segment. Evidence published to date suggests that with both intraoral vertical subcondylar and sagittal split ramus osteotomy techniques, a muscle pedicle may "seat" the condyle well in the fossa. Occasionally, the condyle may not appear well "seated" on the radiograph taken immediately after the operation, but a repeat radiograph taken during the next day or two will usually show the condyle to be well positioned in the fossa. Increased muscle tone is a likely explanation for this change. If the proximal segment is to be wired, great care should be taken to assure that the condyle is well "seated" before tightening the wire. The position of the condyle also should be checked with a radiograph immediately after operation. If it is not well "seated," an operation to reposition the condyle is indicated. Thus the problem of a poorly "seated" condyle is related entirely to surgical technique.

2. *Relapse toward renewed mandibular excess.* This complication can be brought about in two ways: first, by renewed mandibular growth after the operation, and second, by change in mandibular position or change in relative position of the jaw segments. As indicated previously, the surgical procedures to correct mandibular excess have little or no effect on growth potential of the mandible. The earlier the surgical procedure is done, the greater the chance of difficulties due to renewed growth. Tooth position can be controlled to an extent with Class III elastics used postsurgically, but continuing skeletal growth inevitably results in return of anterior crossbite and chin prominence. If the patient begins to function too soon or is allowed to begin function without removing occlusal interferences, new postural adaptive positions of the mandible may be seen; these initially simulate skeletal relapse and can lead to frank skeletal changes in the short term. When the wafer splint is removed after intermaxillary fixation, it is important that the patient have a solid

place to bite in centric relation, or that active orthodontic treatment including interarch elastics be in progress.

3. *Lateral open bite developing several months after surgery, frequently occurring in the early stages of retention following removal of orthodontic appliances.* It is not uncommon to observe in patients whose mandibular excess was treated 6 to 12 months previously that incisor and molar teeth occlude in centric relation, whereas premolars do not. Occasionally, a posterior open bite including the molars will develop, so that only the incisors are in function. The cause of this is obscure. It may be related to a tendency for premolar teeth that have been extruded in the final stages of orthodontic treatment to re-intrude slightly. It also may be influenced by resting posture of the tongue — if the tongue is carried between the teeth at rest, an open bite is likely to be observed. If a total posterior open bite develops (a complication that occurs rarely), lateral spreading of the tongue between the teeth is the most likely cause, and further treatment including surgical reduction of the tongue may be needed. An open bite affecting only the premolars is of less clinical consequence and can be corrected with bonded orthodontic brackets and extrusion of the teeth with light elastics. If such retreatment is needed, the brackets should be left in place and light elastics continued at night for 2 to 3 months after the teeth have been brought back into occlusion.

NERVE COMPLICATIONS AND THEIR MANAGEMENT

Douglas P. Sinn
Stephen C. Hill

When mandibular surgery involves the mandibular body, ramus, lateral symphysis, or temporomandibular joint, the possibility of injury to neural structures exists.[1] Behrman reported injury to both the inferior alveolar and the lingual nerves after sagittal split osteotomies.[2]

Injury may occur when completing osteotomies or mobilizing the bone segments or by improper soft-tissue retraction. Similarly, an improperly positioned intraoral vertical ramus osteotomy may traumatize the inferior alveolar nerve. During body osteotomy or ostectomy the neurovascular bundle may be inadvertently stretched, torn during manipulation of the mandibular segments, or sectioned at the time of the actual osteotomy. In certain cases the nerve may require repositioning to accomplish a segmental osteotomy that places the cutting instrument in close proximity to the nerve, thereby increasing the chance for nerve trauma. When performing genioplasty, the mental nerve is particularly vulnerable to injury as a result of poorly designed soft-tissue incisions, improper osteotomy level, and excessive tissue retraction. Regardless of special precautions and best intentions, the integrity of the inferior alveolar nerve is in jeopardy with most mandibular surgical procedures. In addition to the inferior alveolar nerve, the facial nerve may be injured when approaching the mandibular ramus extraorally and in preauricular dissections for temporomandibular joint surgery. Inadvertent transection of head and neck neural structures is an emergent surgical complication that can benefit from primary management.

Neuropraxia, axonotmesis, and neurotmesis are terms introduced by Seddon to classify and describe increasing degrees of nerve injury.[3] Neuropraxia refers to a transient period of complete interruption of nerve impulse conduction without distal degeneration of the nerve axons. Nerve conduction is normal proximal and distal to the lesion, and recovery is rapid, usually days or weeks. Function is usually completely restored. For example, this type of injury frequently occurs after an orthognathic surgical procedure secondary to moderate traction upon the mental nerve producing a transient paresthesia or anesthesia. Axonotmesis results when there is a separation of nerve fibers but continuity of the endoneurial tube and connective tissue structure of the nerve remains intact. Wallerian degeneration occurs distal to the lesion and recovery is dependent on axonal regeneration along the intact endoneurial tube. Clinically this situation occurs when vigorous retraction is applied to the mental nerve. This results in significant compression of nerve tissue and secondarily in anesthesia for a period of some weeks to months after injury. The potential for reinnervation is good, however, and the delay between injury and recovery is dependent on the distance from the site of reinnervation to the site of injury. Neurotmesis is the term applied to injured nerves that exhibit total disruption of nerve fibers and endoneurial architecture usually secondary to a severe crushing type of trauma or to complete severance of the nerve itself. This injury occurs when the mental nerve is inadvertently transected during an osteotomy, resulting in anesthesia of its peripheral sensory distribution. Recovery of nerve function is imperfect and unpredictable after this type of injury, although results are best after skilled microsurgical repair of the injured nerve.[4]

Management of Nerve Injuries

Partially separated nerves will benefit by careful repositioning of the partly torn nerve in a tension-free position. If complete tension-free repositioning is not possible, however, which is the usual situation, microsurgical repair of the nerve is indicated to provide the optimal conditions for nerve regeneration.

Complete transections of the lingual, inferior alveolar, or mental nerve or of the facial nerve will benefit from primary microsurgical repair. The objective of treatment, as described by Hausamen and others, is to suture the nerves together microscopically in an end-to-end tension-free adaptation.[5, 6] When this is not possible, nerve graft transplantation is indicated to create a tension-free repair. Small nerve segment donor grafts are readily obtained from the great auricular nerve, whereas the sural nerve is better suited for nerve grafts greater than 10 to 12 cm.

Prior to attempting microsurgical nerve repair it is essential that one should have a thorough knowledge of neural microanatomy and develop good microsurgical techniques (Fig. 11–31*A*). The most important factor in the prognosis of a nerve repair is the skill of the surgeon in handling and suturing the injured nerve tissue.[7] The microsurgical technique involves careful dissection of the epineurium away from the nerve fascicles, leaving only the perineurium over the fascicles (Fig. 11–31*B*). The axons are trimmed back to the perineural tube and a suture is placed through the perineurium to approximate the ends (Fig. 11–31*C*). Wound plasma will assist in the coaptation as it has a certain adhesive quality that aids in positioning the nerve ends. Tension-free adaptation is difficult without grafting since the nerve contracts when cut, and trimming

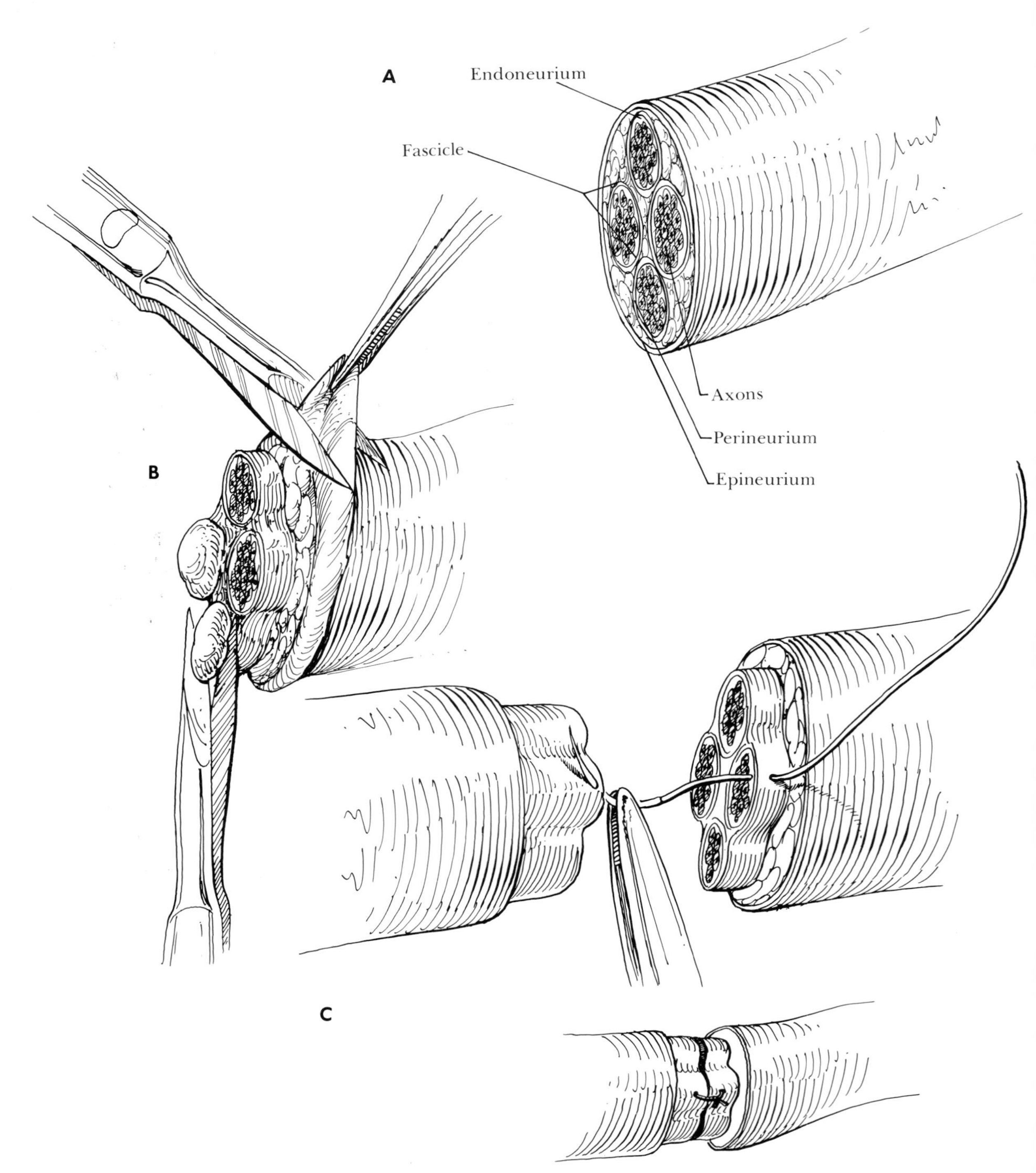

Figure 11–31. *A*, Cross section of a peripheral nerve showing the microanatomy that can be visualized through the operating microscope. A thorough working knowledge of the architectural arrangement of the axons and their supporting connective tissue structures is essential for a successful nerve repair. *B*, The epineurium is trimmed away from the nerve end to prevent proliferation of epineurium into the repair site and resultant interference with axonal regeneration. The epineurium is lifted with fine forceps and excised away from the suture site for a short distance with microscissors. As the axoplasm extrudes from the nerve fascicles, microscissors are used to remove the excess and straighten the perineural sheath in preparation of suturing. *C*, To reapproximate the nerve ends an 11–0 suture is placed through the perineural sheath at the microscopic level and carefully tied to avoid a tight suture that could damage the perineurium or tear through the nerve sheath.

Legend continued on the opposite page.

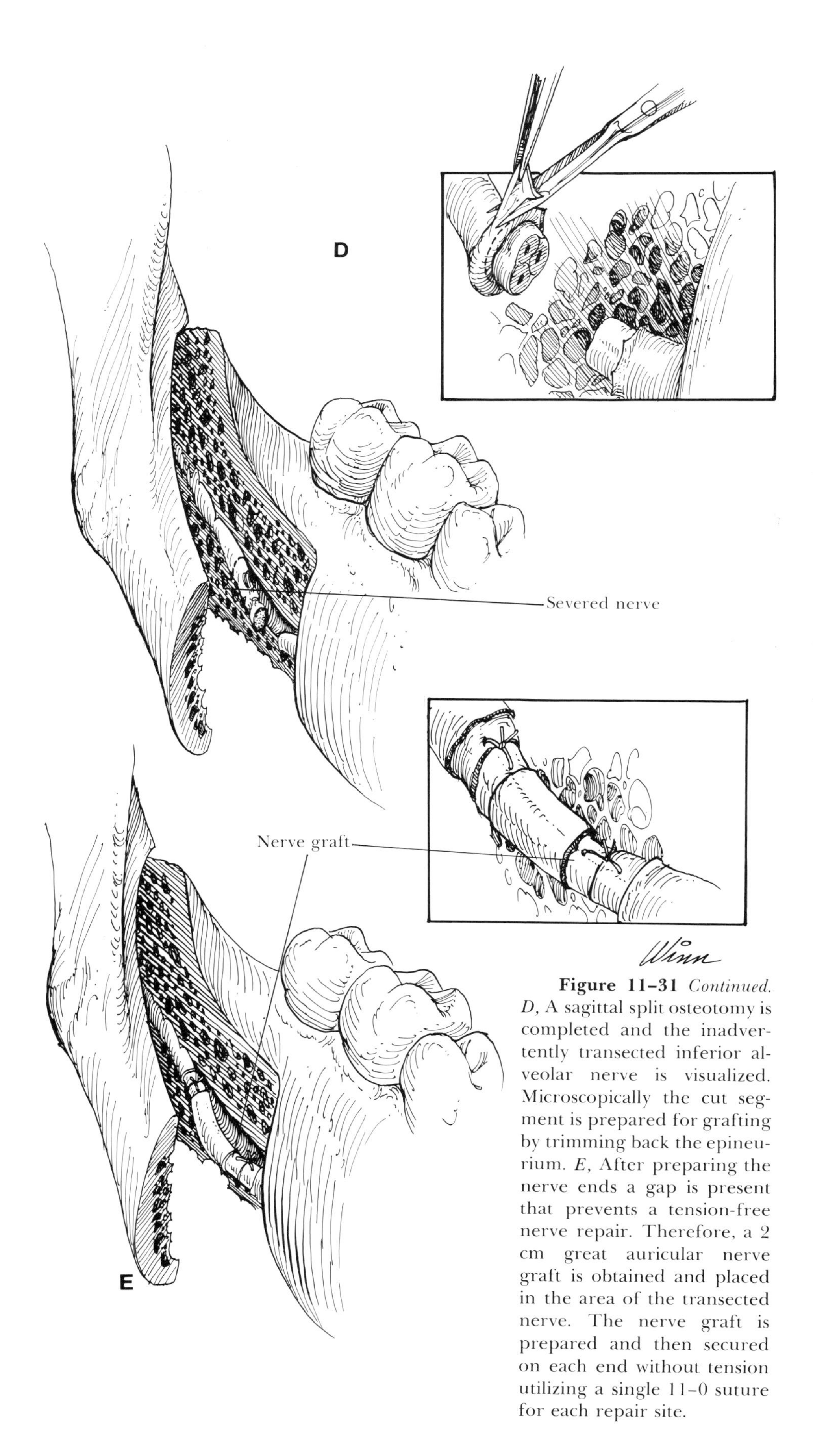

Figure 11–31 *Continued.* *D,* A sagittal split osteotomy is completed and the inadvertently transected inferior alveolar nerve is visualized. Microscopically the cut segment is prepared for grafting by trimming back the epineurium. *E,* After preparing the nerve ends a gap is present that prevents a tension-free nerve repair. Therefore, a 2 cm great auricular nerve graft is obtained and placed in the area of the transected nerve. The nerve graft is prepared and then secured on each end without tension utilizing a single 11–0 suture for each repair site.

of the axons will further reduce the tissue available for reapproximation (Fig. 11–31*D* and *E*). If the repair would finish under tension, a nerve transplantation from the great auricular nerve, just below the ear and superficial to the sternocleidomastoid muscle, is indicated. This is accomplished by taking a 1- to 2-cm length of nerve from the donor site and interposing it between the cut segments. One suture is then placed through the perineurium at each end to hold the nerve graft passively in position.

The repair of a nerve is a delicate procedure that is best done as late as possible in the procedure, thereby minimizing trauma to the suture site by subsequent manipulation. These repairs are performed utilizing an operating microscope and require experience, skill, and patience to be completed successfully.

CASE STUDIES

CASE 11–1 (Fig. 11–32)

D. S., a 15-year-old student, was seen initially in consultation with her orthodontist. Study parameters showed the typical dentofacial features of mandibular prognathism and were the basis for developing the following problem list.

PROBLEM LIST

Esthetics (Fig. 11–32*A, B,* and *C*)

FRONTAL. Long face with prominent narrow chin.
PROFILE. Excessive prominence of chin; protruding lower lip; oblique gonial angle.

Cephalometric Analysis (Fig. 11–32G)

1. Increased vertical dimension of lower third of face; excessive mental prominence.
2. Mandibular incisors tipped backward $\bar{1}$ to NB 2.5 mm.
3. Skeletal type Class III malocclusion; ANB difference −3°.

Occlusal Analysis (Fig. 11–32*K* through *O*)

DENTAL ARCH FORM. V-shaped maxillary and mandibular arches in basic harmony with one another when models placed into a simulated postoperative occlusal relationship.
DENTAL ALIGNMENT. Palatally impacted maxillary right canine; remaining maxillary anterior teeth shifted 2 mm to the right, crowded, and slightly proclined; mild anterior crossbite from canine to canine; lingual inclination of mandibular incisors, one of which was congenitally missing, contributed to 5 mm crowding in the lower arch.

TREATMENT PLAN

Presurgical Orthodontic Treatment

1. Extract maxillary 2nd premolar teeth to allow correction of maxillary anterior asymmetry and to provide space for eruption of the palatally impacted canine.
2. Treat lower arch by tipping lower anterior teeth labially over their supporting alveolar bone without extraction of teeth.
3. Narrow maxillary arch to correct the lateral width discrepancy produced by retracting mandible surgically; diagnostic set-up indicated that the three mandibular incisors would harmonize with the four maxillary incisors.

Surgical Treatment

1. Reposition mandible posteriorly by bilateral ramus osteotomies to achieve the desired overbite and overjet and reduce chin prominence.
2. Genioplasty to reduce height and prominence of chin.

Postsurgical Orthodontic Treatment

1. Obtain final interdigitation and positioning of teeth.

ACTIVE TREATMENT

The maxillary and mandibular teeth were aligned and the rotations were corrected within 10 months with edgewise orthodontic appliances. After osteotomies of the vertical rami, the mandible was repositioned distally 12 mm; 7 mm of chin height and 4 mm of chin prominence were removed concomitantly through an intraoral degloving incision. Final space closure and alignment of the arches were completed in another 5 months by orthodontic treatment. Post-treatment dental symmetry, normal overbite, and overjet attained by 15 months of combined surgical and orthodontic treatment have remained stable during 60-month postoperative follow-up period (Figs. 11–32*P* through *T*). There was a marked change in lip posture and soft-tissue profile after treatment (Fig 11–32*D, E,* and *F*). Upward and forward movement of the mandible in the post-treatment period was observed in progress cephalometric tracings (Fig. 11–32*I* through *J*).

COMMENT

Even though skeletal changes took place postoperatively, the occlusion remained stable. Clinical assessment of the occlusion only may be misleading. Although the occlusal interrelationships appeared stable, the jaw position was changing minimally as shown in the sequential cephalometric radiographs.

Oral Surgeon: William H. Bell, Dallas, Texas. *Orthodontist:* Thomas Creekmore, Houston, Texas.

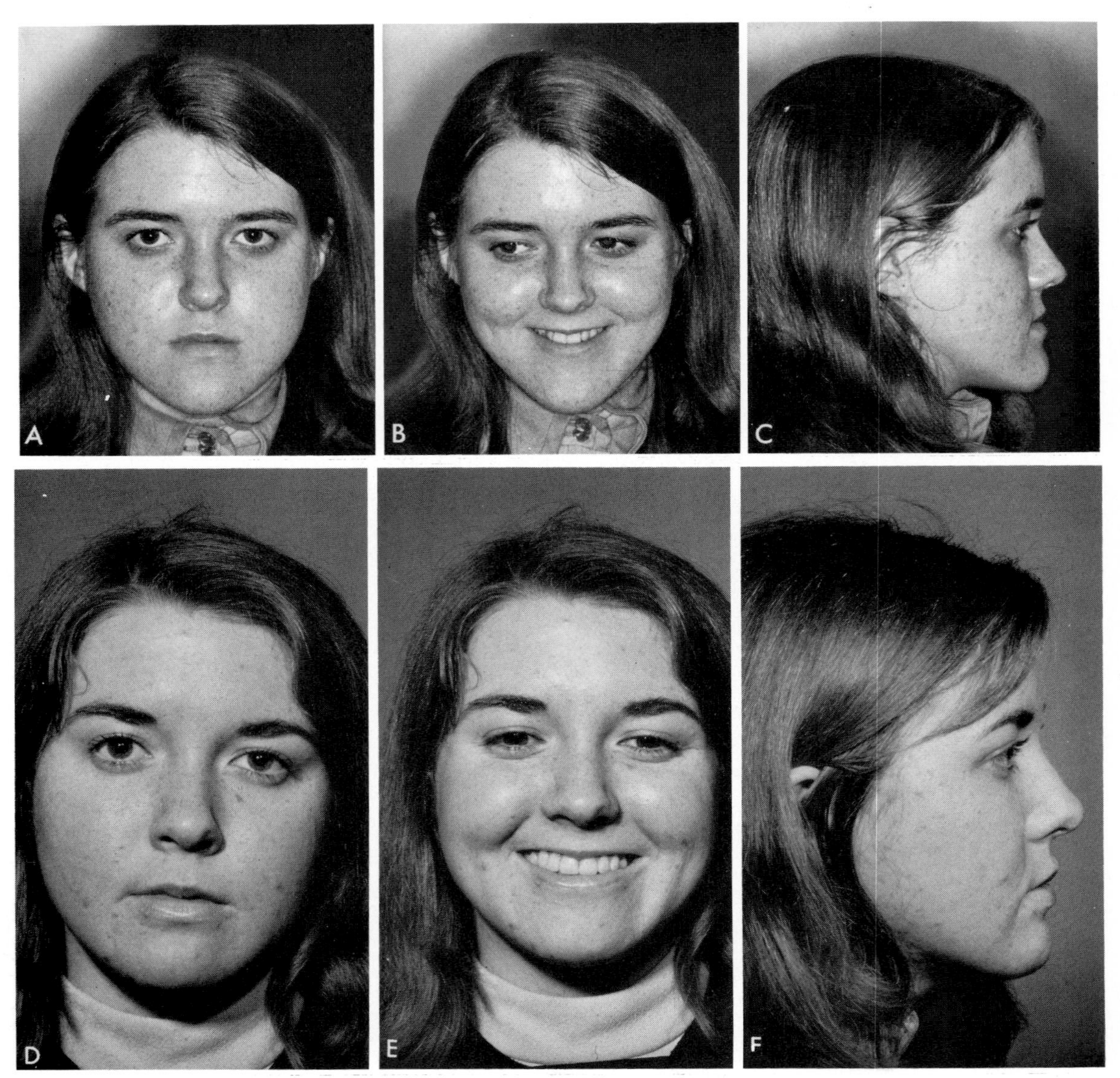

Figure 11–32 (Case 11–1). 15-year-old patient with mandibular prognathism before (*A–C*) and after (*D–F*) treatment.

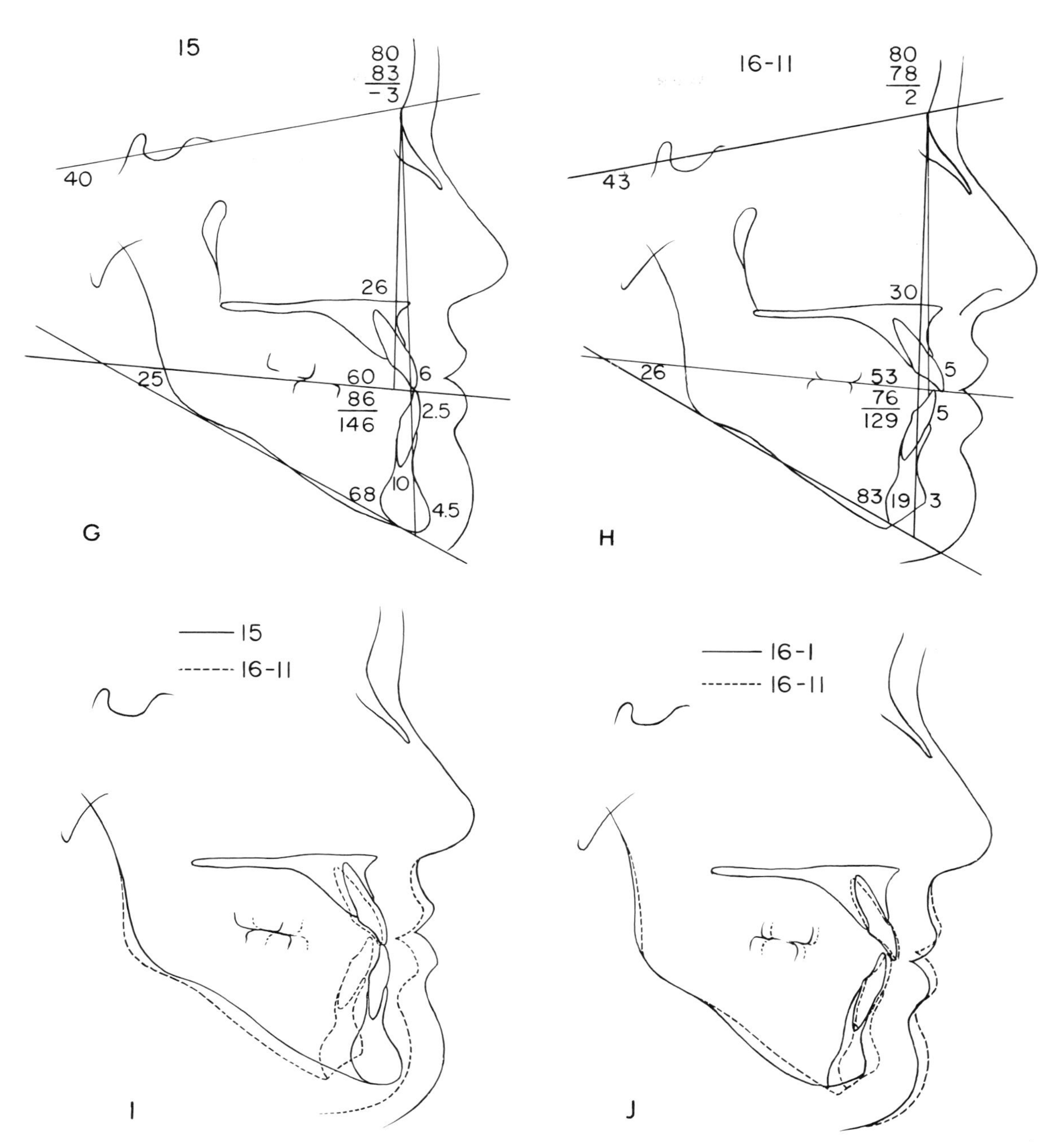

Figure 11–32 *Continued.* *G,* Cephalometric tracing at age 15, before treatment, showing increased vertical dimension of lower third of face, excessive mental prominence, and mandibular prognathism. *H,* Cephalometric tracing six months after orthodontic bands were removed (age 16 years, 11 months). *I,* Cephalometric tracings before treatment (*solid line,* age 15 years) and six months after orthodontic bands were removed (*broken line,* age 16 years, 11 months) showing short-term results of treatment. *J,* Cephalometric tracings showing dental and skeletal adjustments 11 months after operation. Immediately after operation (*solid line,* age 16 years, 1 month) and six months after orthodontic bands were removed (*broken line,* age 16 years, 11 months). *Illustration continued on the following page.*

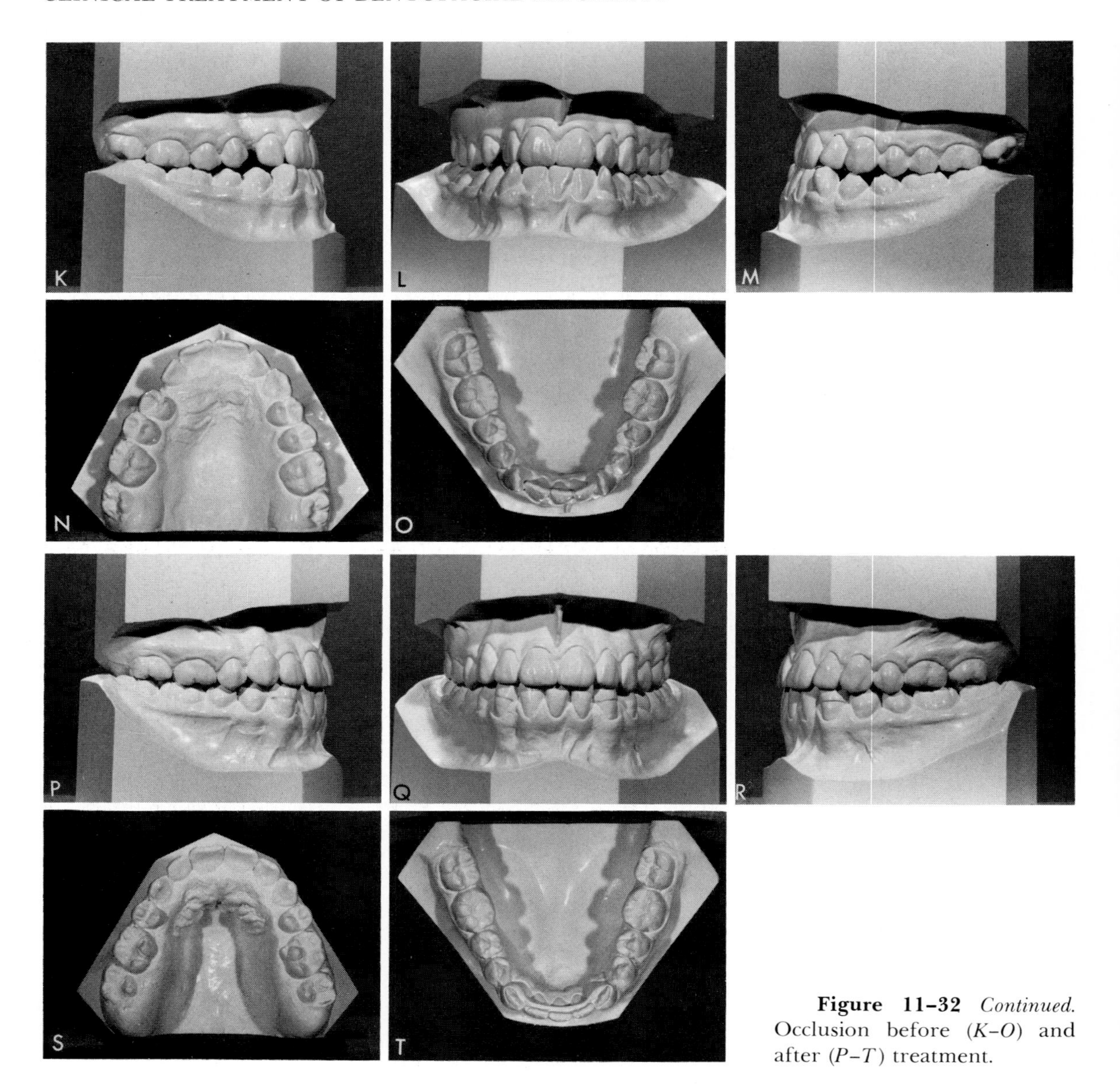

Figure 11–32 *Continued.* Occlusion before (*K–O*) and after (*P–T*) treatment.

CASE 11–2 (Fig. 11–33)

J. B., a 24-year-old teacher, exhibited the typical dentofacial characteristics of mandibular prognathism when she was initially seen. She sought treatment to improve the function of her teeth and the appearance of her face.

PROBLEM LIST

Esthetics (Fig. 11–33*A, B,* and *C*)

FRONTAL. Narrow nose with mild paranasal deficiency; dental disharmony revealed when patient smiled; maxillary incisors deviated from midline of face.

PROFILE. Prominent nose; poor balance between nose, upper lip, and chin; prominent chin and protruding lower lip; recessive upper lip.

Cephalometric Analysis (Fig. 11–33*G*)

1. Excessive prominence of chin; oblique gonial angle; maxillary deficiency.
2. Maxillary incisors inclined forward, $\overline{1}$ to NB 12 mm.
3. Mandibular incisors tipped backward, $\overline{1}$ to NB 2 mm.
4. Class III molar and canine relationship; ANB difference −10°.

Occlusal Analysis (Fig. 11–33*K* through *O*)

DENTAL ARCH FORM. V-shaped maxillary and mandibular arches; reverse curve of mandibular occlusal plane. Study of the lateral widths of both arches showed that maxillary second molars were too wide — only the first molars were constricted (Fig. 11–33*U*).

DENTAL ALIGNMENT. Constricted first molars; palatal premolar; peg-shaped lateral incisor; 4 mm of crowding in the canine-lateral incisor area; missing lower first molars; approximately 7 mm of crowding in lingually inclined lower anterior teeth.

DENTAL OCCLUSION. Class III canine and molar relationship; entire lower dentition positioned in front of upper dentition.

TREATMENT PLAN

Presurgical Orthodontic Treatment

1. Extract maxillary right second premolar and left first premolar teeth to allow some retraction of the protruding maxillary incisors and correction of the midline; space would be opened to allow restoration of the peg-shaped maxillary lateral incisor.
2. Correct crowding of lower anterior teeth by tipping lower incisors forward into more favorable position without closing the first molar spaces.
3. Correct posterior lateral width discrepancy.

Surgical Treatment

1. Perform bilateral osteotomies of mandibular rami to retract mandible surgically into Class I anterior relationship.

Postoperative Orthodontic Treatment

1. Obtain final interdigitation and positioning of teeth.

Restorative Dentistry

1. Restore pegged lateral incisor and replace missing lower first molar tooth.

ACTIVE TREATMENT

The preoperative phase of orthodontic correction was accomplished within a period of 8 months with an edgewise orthodontic appliance (Fig. 11–33*V*). After the arches were properly coordinated, the mandible was retracted 16 mm by bilateral osteotomies of the mandibular rami. Postoperative orthodontic treatment was completed in 11 months. The restoration of the patient's previously mutilated occlusion was completed by the general dentist, who restored the peg-shaped maxillary lateral incisor and replaced missing lower first molar teeth. The preoperative malalignment of teeth was in sharp contrast to their postoperative position (Fig. 11–33*K* through *T*). Sequential cephalometric tracings showed the immediate and long-term skeletal, dental, and soft-tissue changes (Fig. 11–33*G* through *J*). Despite the apparent stability of the occlusion, there was a marked change in the position of the mandible as evidenced by the anterior superior movement of pogonion (Fig. 11–33*J*).

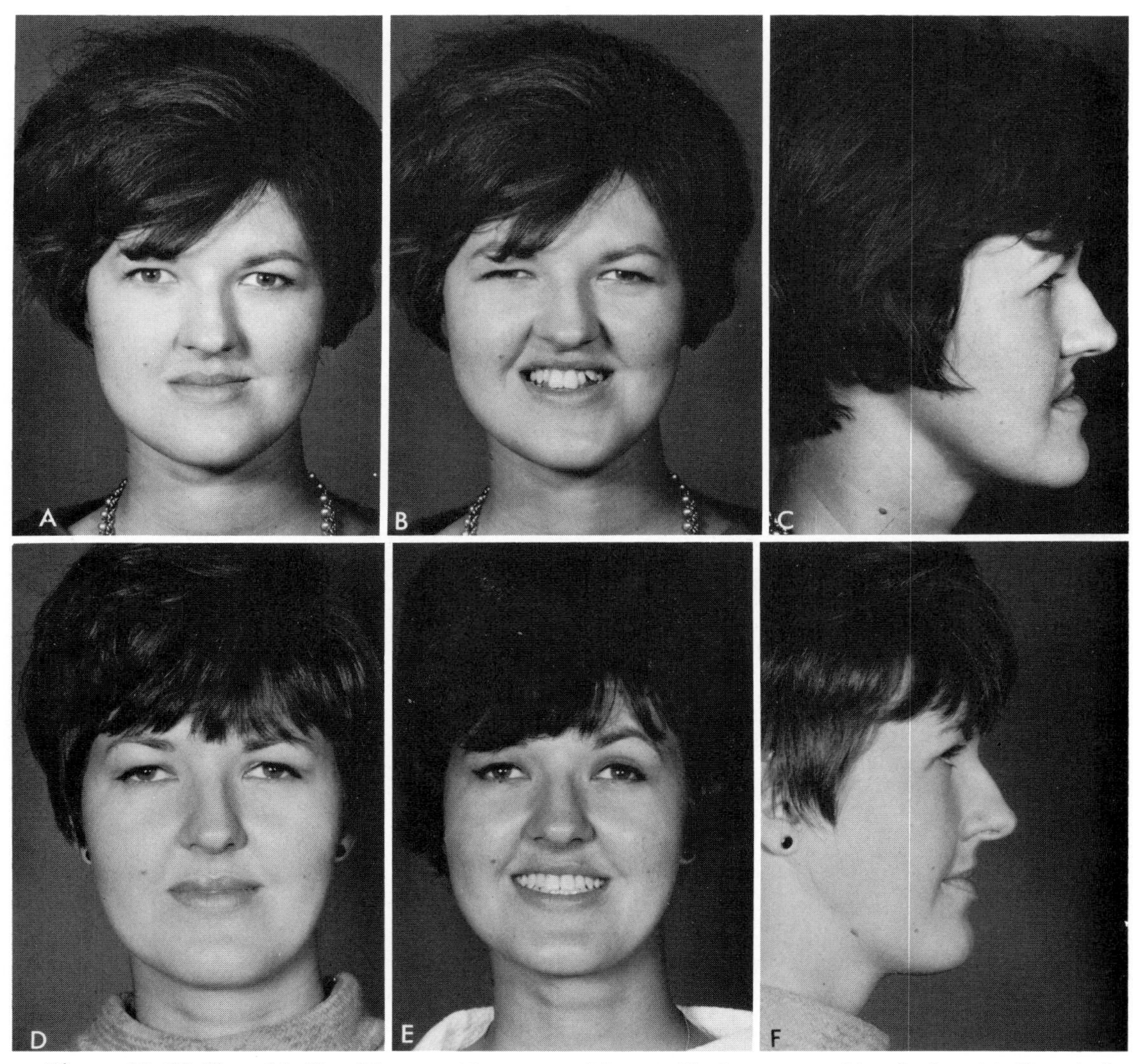

Figure 11–33 (Case 11–2). 25-year-old woman with mandibular prognathism before (*A–C*) and after (*D–F*) treatment.

Legend continued on the opposite page.

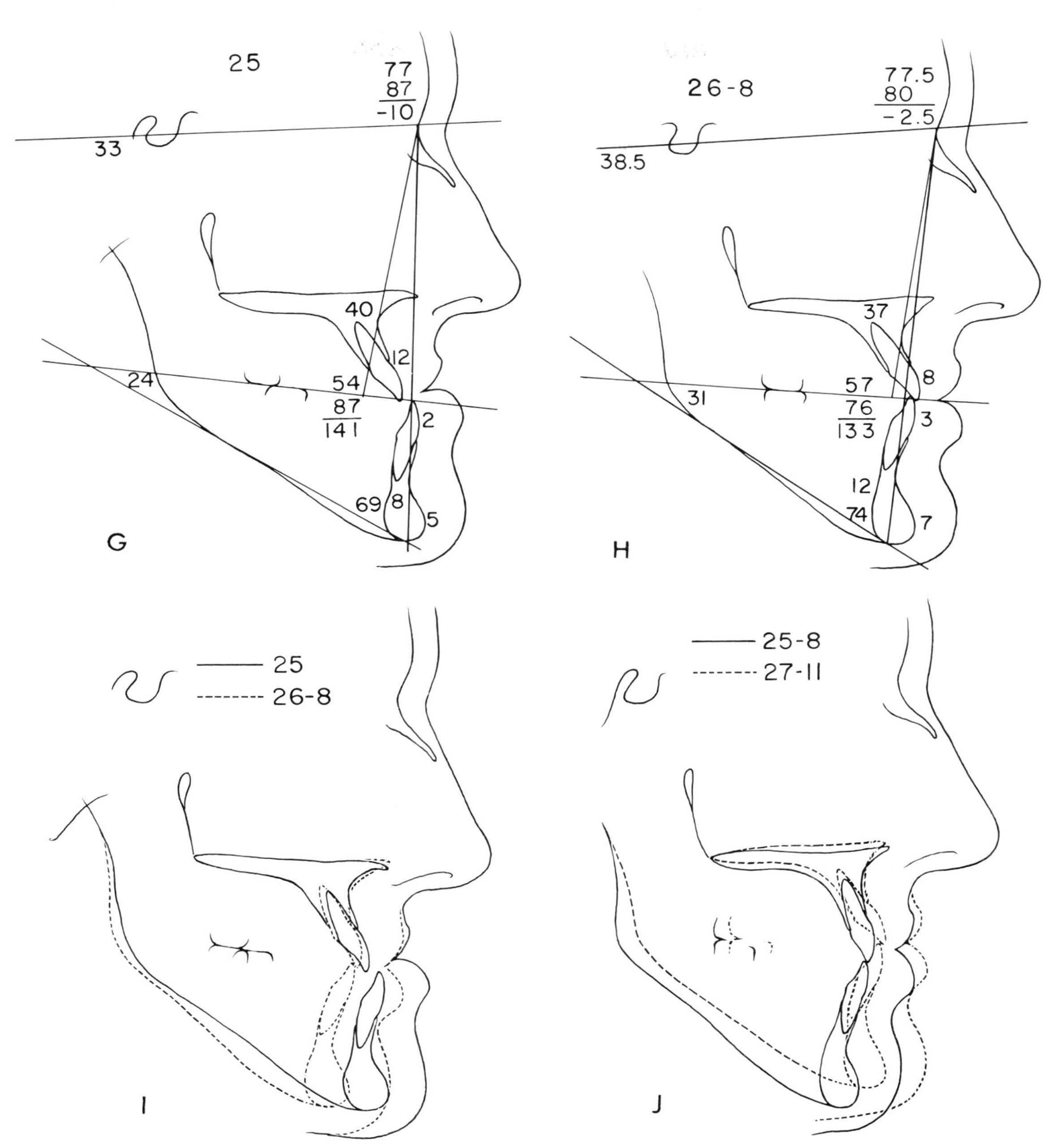

Figure 11–33 *Continued. G,* Cephalometric tracing (age 25) before treatment showing excessive prominence of chin, protruding lower lip, oblique gonial angle, and Class III occlusal relationship. *H,* Cephalometric tracing after orthodontic bands were removed (age 26 years, 8 months). *I,* Cephalometric tracings before treatment (*solid line,* age 25) and after orthodontic bands were removed (*broken line,* age 26 years, 8 months). *J,* Cephalometric tracings immediately after operation (*solid line,* age 25 years, 8 months) and 18 months after band removal (*broken line,* age 27 years, 11 months) showing postoperative dental and skeletal changes.

Illustration continued on the following page.

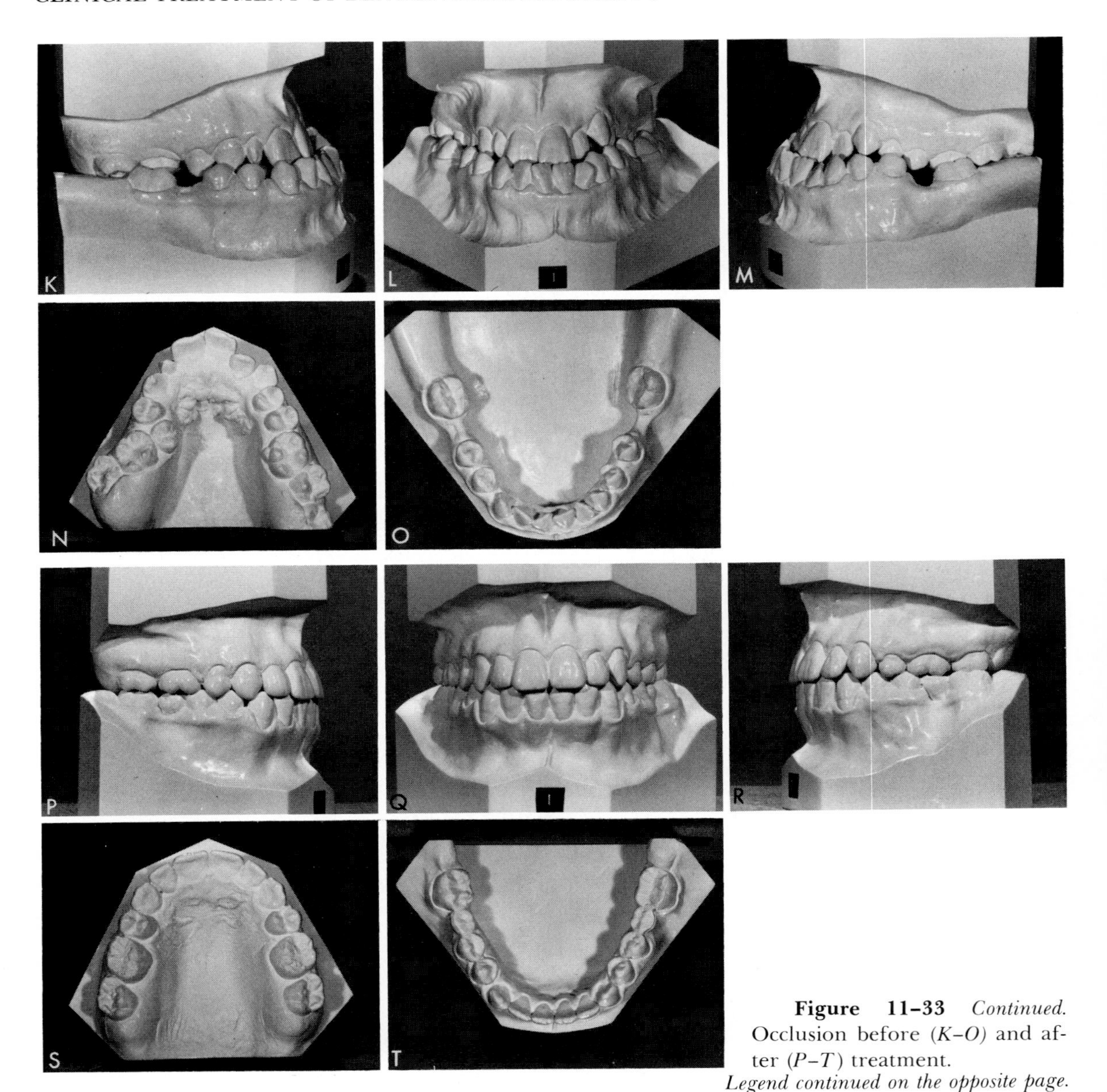

Figure 11-33 *Continued.* Occlusion before (*K–O*) and after (*P–T*) treatment.

Legend continued on the opposite page.

COMMENT

Functional and esthetic changes were achieved by mandibular surgery and orthodontic treatment. In retrospect, however, it appears that maxillary advancement or a combination of maxillary advancement and mandibular retraction might have achieved even more — increased stability, decrease of the nasolabial angle, increased nasal width, and increased prominence of the paranasal deficient areas could have been anticipated with this plan of treatment. The advantages of surgical treatment in both maxilla and mandible must be carefully weighed against the anticipated results gained from surgery in the mandible or maxilla alone.

Oral Surgeon: William H. Bell, Dallas, Texas. *Orthodontist:* Thomas Creekmore, Houston, Texas.

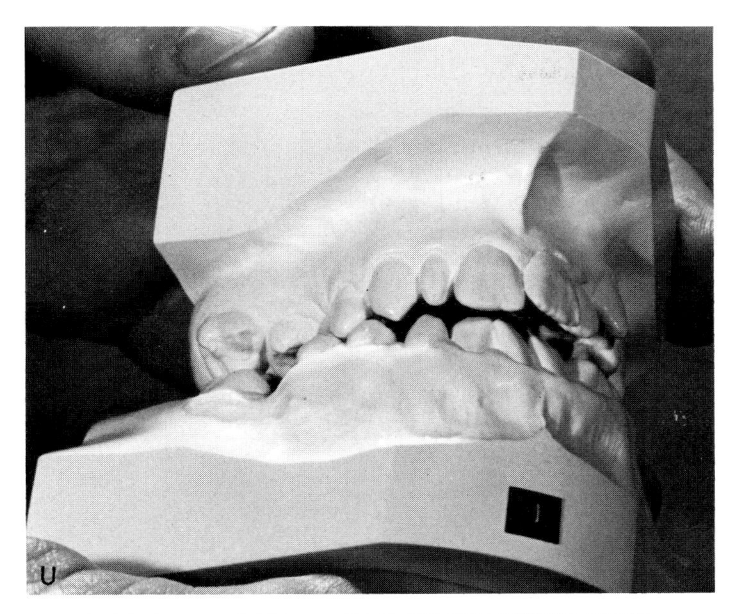

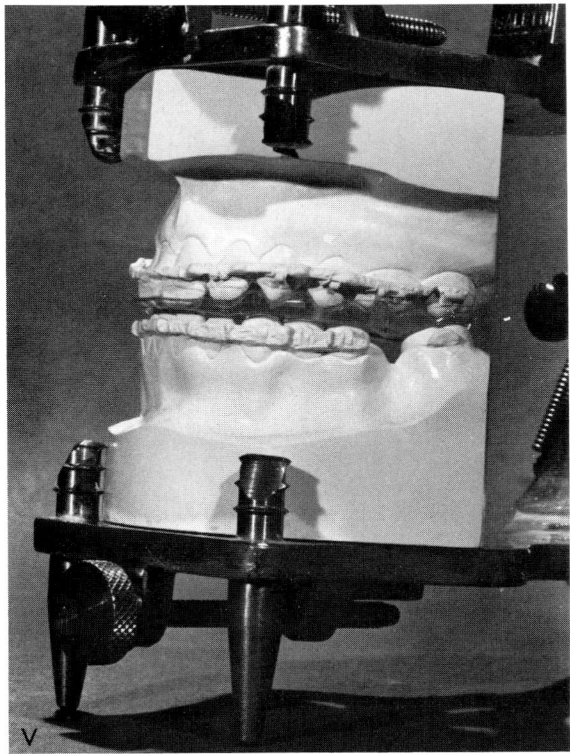

Figure 11–33 *Continued.* *U*, Model of lower arch placed into planned Class I canine relationship to simulate surgical repositioning of mandible and analyze the transverse maxillo-mandibular relationship. *V*, Repositioned study casts after eight months of orthodontic treatment keyed into place with wafer-type interocclusal acrylic resin splint.

CASE 11–3 (Figure 11–34)

J. M., a 46-year-old man, was seen in consultation with his orthodontist and periodontist regarding treatment to improve his occlusion and preserve his mutilated dentition. The patient related that several other family members had jaw deformities similar to his own. From time to time he was affected by allergies and asthma. The following problem list was evolved after appropriate clinical and laboratory examination and consultation with the patient's general dentist, periodontist, and orthodontist.

PROBLEM LIST

Esthetics (Fig. 11–34*A, B,* and *C*)

FRONTAL. Prominent chin and lower lip.
PROFILE. Prominent chin and everted lower lip; nasolabial angle acceptable esthetically.

Cephalometric Analysis (Fig. 11–34*J*)

1. Mandibular excess with typical Class III skeletal pattern; −6 ANB difference.
2. Protrusive maxillary incisors.
3. Mandibular incisors fairly well related to large bony chin.

Occlusal Analysis (Fig. 11–34*O* through *R*)

DENTAL ARCH FORM. Maxillary arch narrow and constricted; wide mandibular arch compared with the maxillary denture. The analysis was based upon the occlusal relationship that was achieved when the models were hand articulated into a simulated corrected Class I canine and molar relationship.
DENTAL ALIGNMENT. Mutilated malocclusion; missing posterior teeth including the maxillary right second premolar and all second and third molars with the exception of the lower left third molar; extensive periodontal bone loss and bifurcation involvement of the lower right first molar.
DENTAL OCCLUSION. Class III molar and canine relationship with upper dentition in total lingual crossbite to the mandibular dentition; reverse horizontal overlap, 7 mm; vertical overlap 7 mm.

TREATMENT PLAN

Presurgical Orthodontic Treatment

1. Treat without extractions with exception of lower third molar, which exhibited pulpitis.
2. Expand lateral maxilla with fixed palatal orthopedic appliance to widen maxilla.
3. Align all maxillary and mandibular teeth.
4. Open the space of the missing maxillary right second premolar for a fixed partial denture.

Surgical Treatment

1. Retract mandible by bilateral osteotomies of mandibular rami to achieve desired horizontal and vertical overlap of the teeth and Class I canine relationship and to reduce chin prominence.

Postsurgical Orthodontic Treatment

1. Completely align and interdigitate the teeth.

Adjunctive Treatment

1. Restorative procedures to replace missing teeth.
2. Periodontal treatment.

ACTIVE TREATMENT

All lower teeth were banded with an .018 × .025 Lewis rotation edgewise appliance. A fixed palatal expander was placed in the maxilla on the first molars, the right canine, and the left first premolar; the maxilla was expanded 7 mm over a period of 17 days. The upper incisors were banded and an .016 multiloop placed. The palatal expander remained in position for 2 months, then all maxillary teeth were banded in .018 × .025 Lewis rotation edgewise appliance and a lingual arch were placed with a facial root torque on the first molars together with posterior cross-elastics to maintain the expansion. The lower arch wire progression was from .016 to .018 × .025 stabilizing and finishing arch wire. The upper arch wire progression was from .016 multiloop to .017 × .022 opening loop arch wire to open the second premolar space. From this point, posterior cross-elastics were worn to help maintain the expansion achieved. An upper retainer was also worn for 4 months to aid as a fulcrum for torque and to prevent relapse of the upper expansion (Fig. 11–34*S*). After the upper teeth were aligned and the premolar space was opened, an .018 × .025 maxillary facial root torque in the posterior teeth was placed (Fig. 11–34*T*, *U*, and *V*).

Bilateral osteotomies of the mandible rami to retract the mandible 8 mm were uncomplicated, and the patient experienced minimal discomfort. His intermaxillary fixation was discontinued after 6 weeks (Fig. 11–34*W*, *X*, and *Y*). Bands were removed 4 months later after minimal Class II elastic wear (Fig. 11–34*Z* through *CC*).

COMMENT

Overall facial balance was gained by the surgical and orthodontic treatment (Fig. 11–34*D*, *E*, and *F*). Pogonion was repositioned 12 mm and the lower incisor 8 mm. The ANB difference was increased from −6° to 0.5°. The overbite and overjet were fully corrected (Fig. 11–34*Z* through *FF*). The transverse maxillary arch deficiency was widened considerably to achieve Class I interdigitation.

Periodontal pocket depth had been reduced — the general good condition of the periodontium was in sharp contrast to its pretreatment appearance. There was minimal and clinically insignificant root resorption (Fig. 11–34*II*). Very little periodontal bone loss resulted from the orthodontic-surgical correction. Occlusal adjustment was completed shortly after band removal. Upper and lower removable Hawley retainers were worn for 10 months.

Records taken 2 years, 3 months out of treatment (17 months out of retention) showed that the occlusal and functional relationships had been very stable (Fig. 11–

Text continued on page 933.

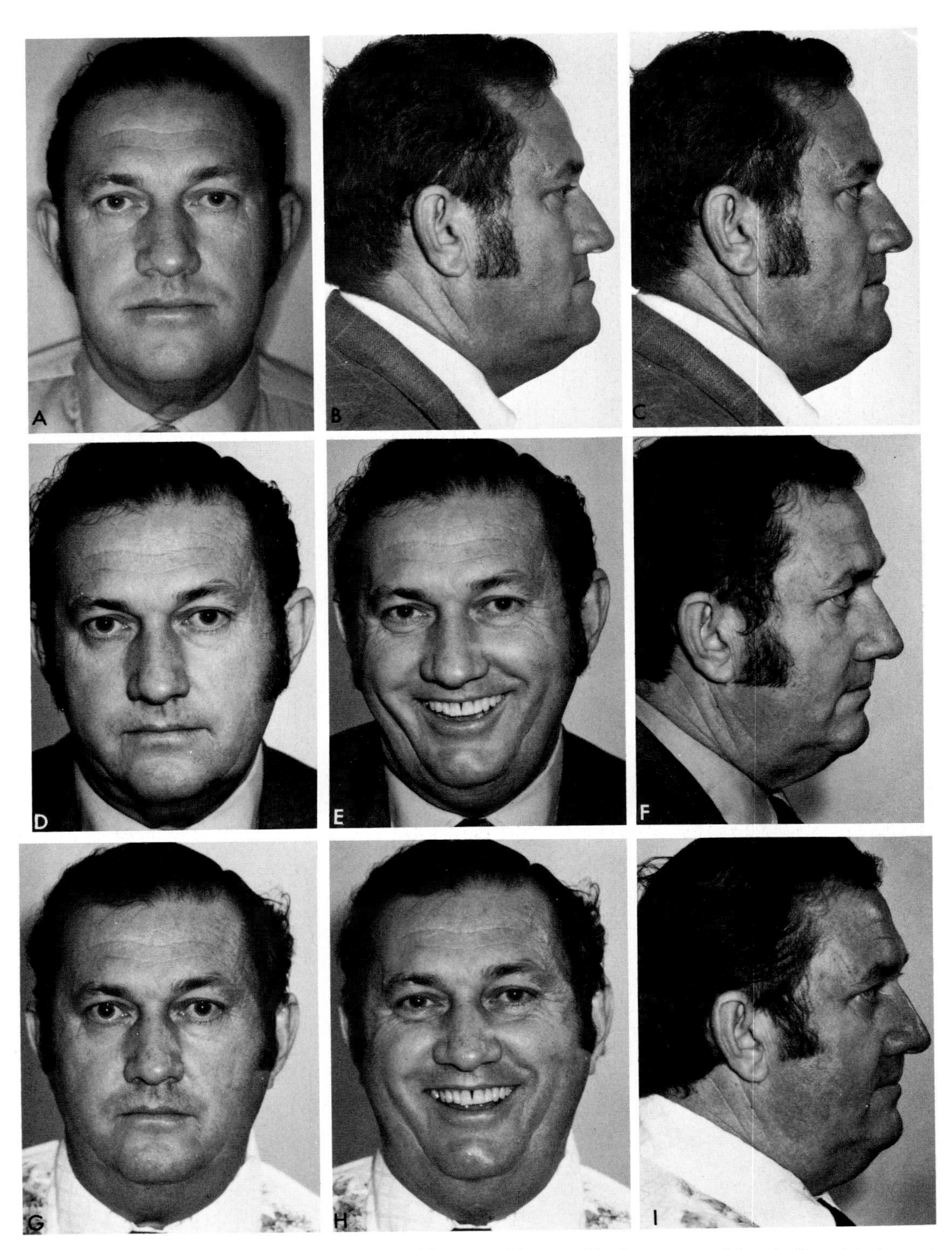

Figure 11–34 (Case 11–3). 46-year-old man with mandibular prognathism before (*A*, frontal view; *B*, centric occlusion; *C*, centric relation) and after (*D–F*) treatment. *G–I*, Five years after treatment.

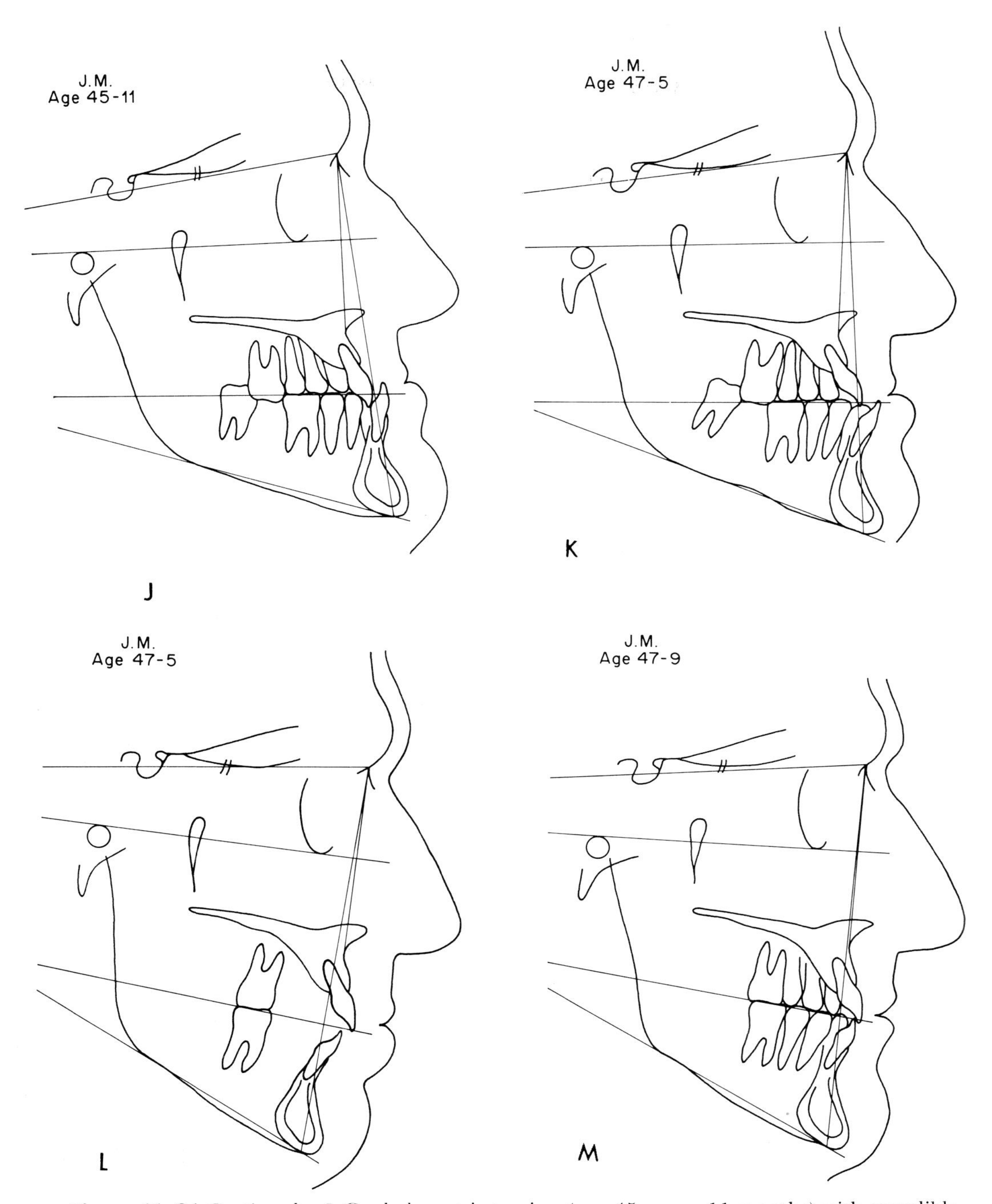

Figure 11–34 *Continued.* *J*, Cephalometric tracing (age 45 years, 11 months) with mandible in centric occlusion. *K*, Cephalometric tracing (age 47 years, 5 months) after presurgical orthodontics. *L*, Cephalometric tracing (age 47 years, 5 months) during intermaxillary fixation. *M*, Cephalometric tracing after orthodontic bands were removed (age 47 years, 9 months).

Illustration continued on the following page.

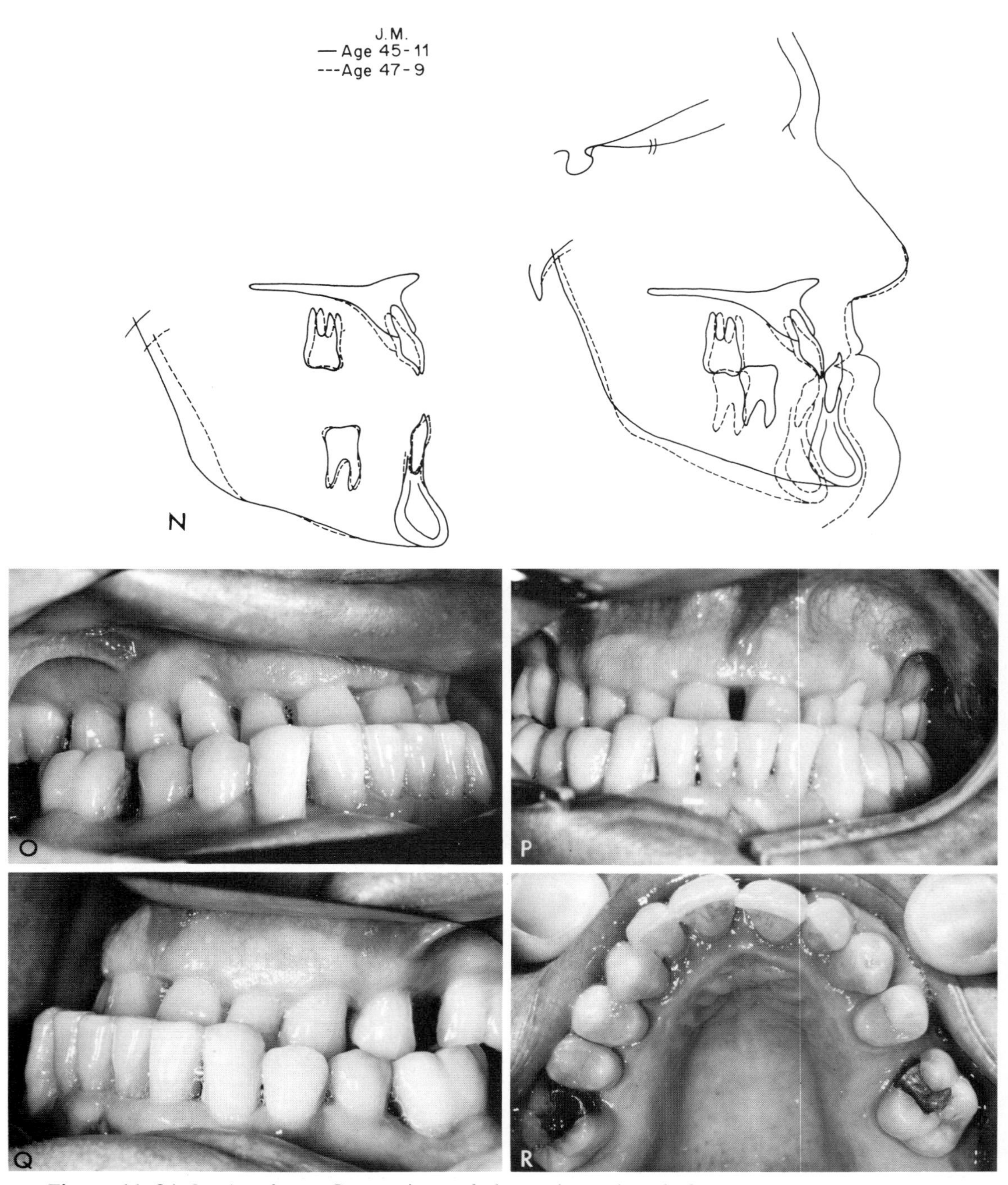

Figure 11–34 *Continued.* *N*, Composite cephalometric tracings before treatment (*solid line*, age 45 years, 11 months) and after orthodontic bands were removed (*broken line*, age 47 years, 9 months). *O–R*, Occlusion before treatment.

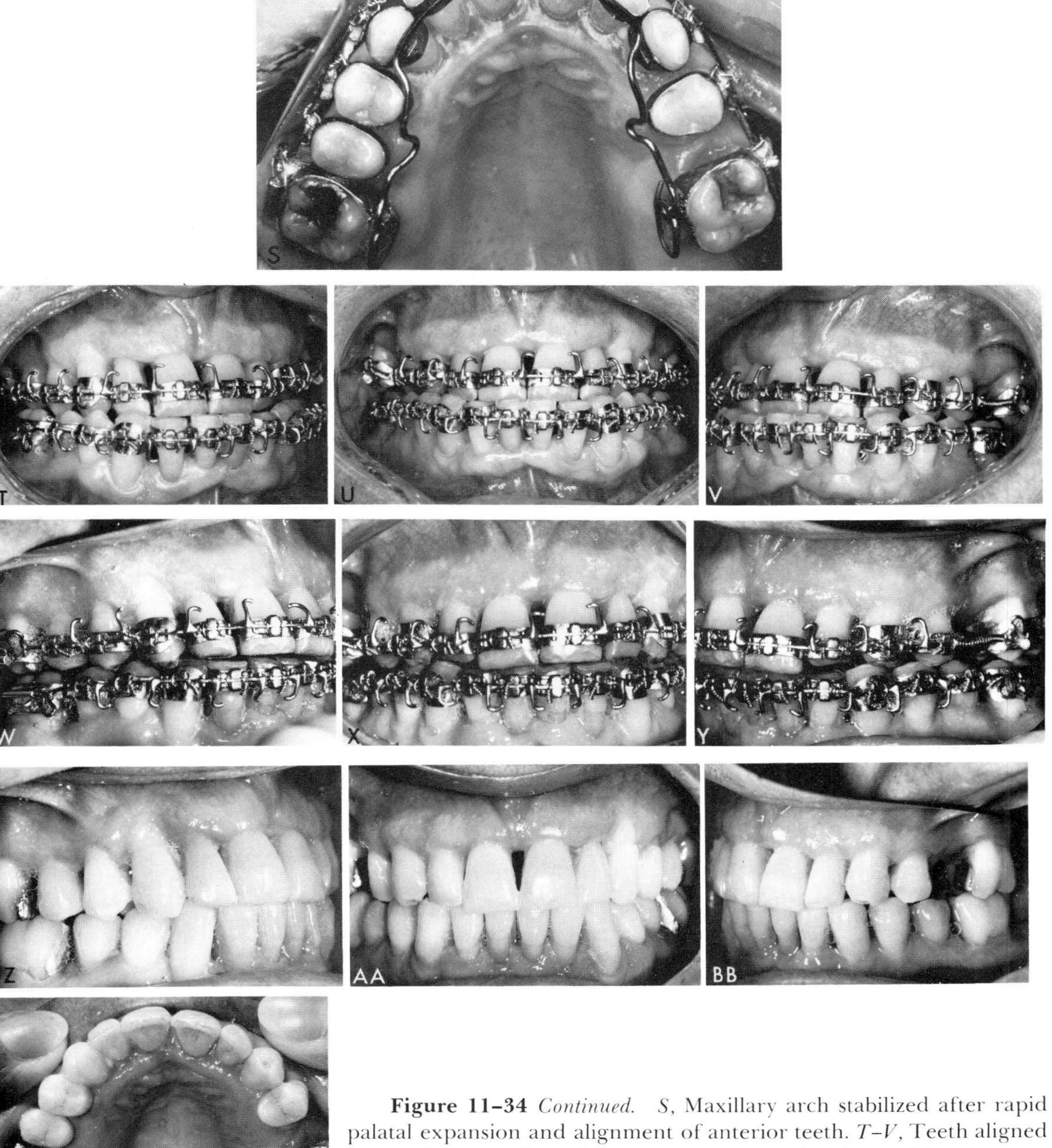

Figure 11–34 *Continued.* *S,* Maxillary arch stabilized after rapid palatal expansion and alignment of anterior teeth. *T–V,* Teeth aligned and arches coordinated before surgery; vertical lugs soldered to rectangular arch wire that is ligated to orthodontic brackets. *W–Y,* Occlusion after surgery and release from intermaxillary fixation. *Z–CC,* Occlusion after removal of orthodontic appliances.

Illustration continued on the following page.

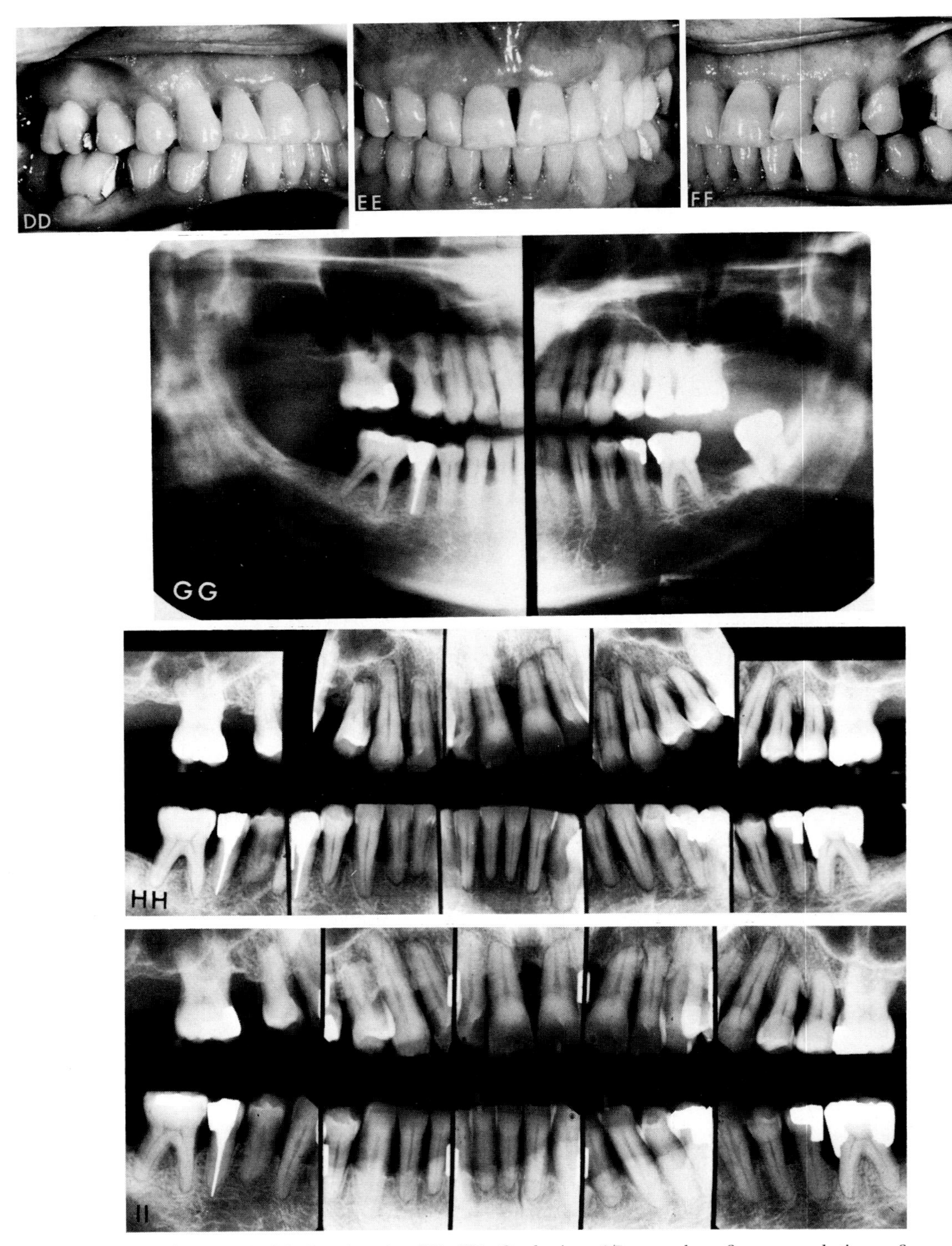

Figure 11–34 *Continued. DD–FF,* Occlusion 27 months after completion of orthodontic treatment (17 months out of retention). *GG,* Panographic view before treatment (periapical radiographs were lost). *HH,* Periapical survey accomplished immediately after orthodontic appliances were removed. *II,* Periapical survey two years after treatment, showing virtually the same radiographic appearance of the teeth and their supporting alveolar bone that was present when orthodontic treatment was completed.

34*DD, EE,* and *FF*). There was slight recrowding in the lower arch and left canine lateral incisor area, spacing distal to the right canine and a very slight settling and deepening of the anterior bite.

In cephalometric terms, the anterior facial height was decreased 1 mm by the upward and forward movement of the mandible concomitant with 1 mm lingual and incisal bodily positioning of the lower incisor. The face was improved by changes in the upper lip, which was altered between the beginning of treatment and the time when post-treatment records were taken. At follow-up, the upper lip had assumed a fuller, more balanced anteroposterior relation to the lower lip and the soft-tissue chin.

There was very little discernible radiographic change in the osseous architecture of the supporting bone as well as the gingival height (Fig. 11–34*GG, HH,* and *II*). Considering the amount of supporting bone, the teeth were very stable with minimal mobility.

Periodontal therapy was resumed shortly after debanding. All the post-treatment study parameters have remained virtually unchanged and stable over a postoperative period in excess of 6 years.

The retention of this adult's teeth was dependent on a number of factors — periodontal care, occlusal stability, surgery to reposition the mandible into an acceptable relationship to the maxilla, proper tooth-to-bone relationship, restoration of the mutilated dentition, and patient motivation. Post-treatment views in Figure 11–34 show that treatment to date has been successful as evidenced by the stable, functional, and esthetic result achieved.

Oral Surgeon: William H. Bell, Dallas, Texas. *Orthodontist:* Kermit Welch, Houston, Texas. *Periodontist:* Lawrence A. Friedman, Houston, Texas.

CASE 11–4 (Fig. 11–35)

C. P., a 19-year-old student, initially seen for treatment of her dentofacial deformity after undergoing 3 years of orthodontic therapy during adolescence. Four first premolar teeth had been extracted to facilitate alignment of the crowded anterior teeth. A retrospective study of sequential cephalometric radiographs taken before, during, and after orthodontic treatment revealed continued mandibular growth during the period of treatment and the typical dentofacial-skeletal characteristics of mild mandibular prognathism. Clinical and radiographic examination yielded the following information.

PROBLEM LIST

Esthetics (Fig. 11–35, *A, B, C*)

FRONTAL. Symmetric long face; narrow nasal alar bases; deficiency in nasolabial areas.

PROFILE. Deficient nasolabial and nasomaxillary areas and prominent nose; prominent chin; protrusive lower lip.

Cephalometric Analysis (Fig. 11–35*H*)

1. Moderate increase in chin prominence and height; oblique gonial angle.
2. Mandibular incisors tipped backward, $\overline{1}$ to NB 2.5 mm.
3. Class III canine and molar relationship: ANB difference –3°.

Occlusal Analysis (Fig. 11–35*J, K,* and *L*)

DENTAL ARCH FORM. Normally tapered and shaped maxillary and mandibular arches. A study of the lateral widths of the two arches showed that the maxillary arch was a little too wide.

DENTAL ALIGNMENT. Satisfactory.

DENTAL OCCLUSION. Class III canine and molar relationships; missing maxillary and mandibular first premolars as a result of previous treatment.

TREATMENT PLAN

Surgical Treatment (Fig. 11–35*P*)

1. Bilateral intraoral vertical subcondylar osteotomies of mandibular rami to surgically retroposition mandible into a Class I canine and molar relationship and reduce prominence of chin; interdental osteotomy between the lower central incisors to facilitate widening of the mandibular arch.
2. Genioplasty to reduce height and prominence of chin.
3. Augmentation of nasolabial and nasomaxillary areas with an alloplastic material (Proplast).

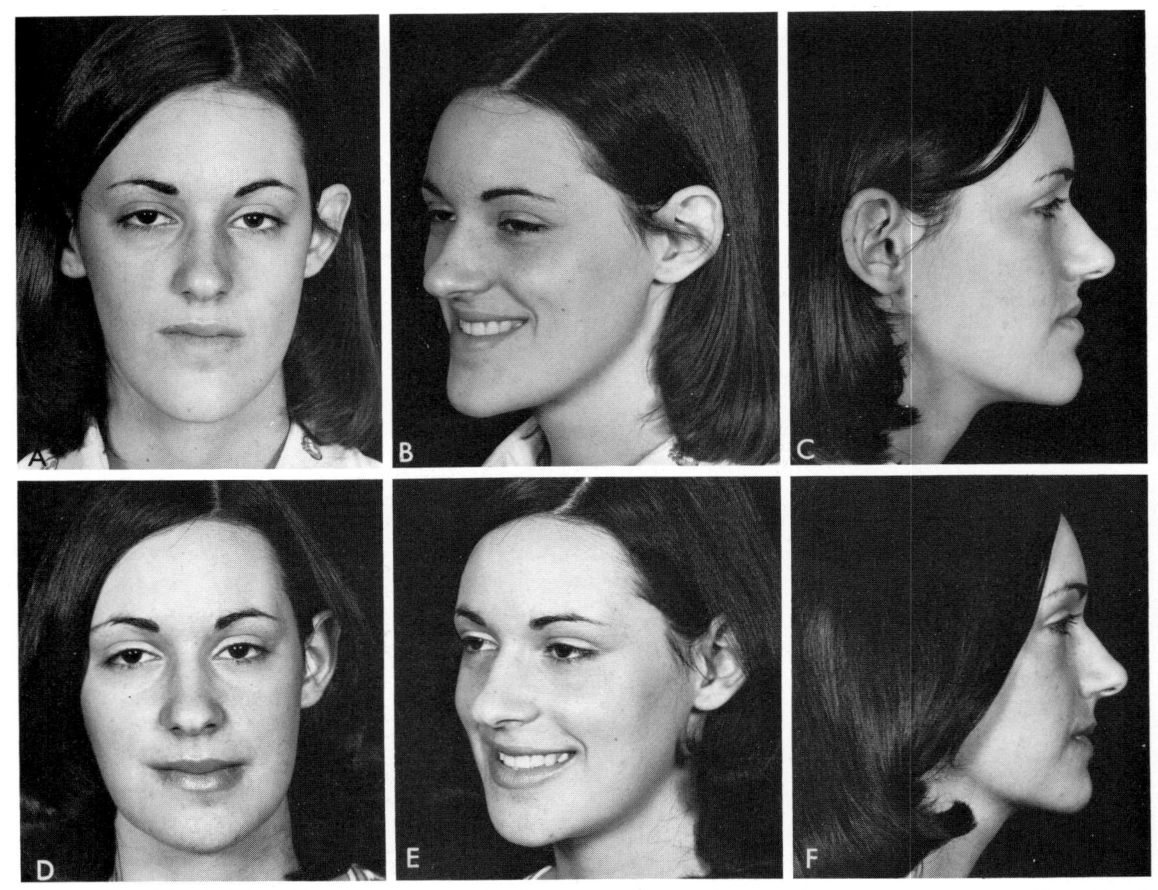

Figure 11–35 (Case 11–4). 19-year-old female patient with mandibular prognathism before (*A–C*) and after (*D–F*) surgical intervention.

Legend continued on the opposite page.

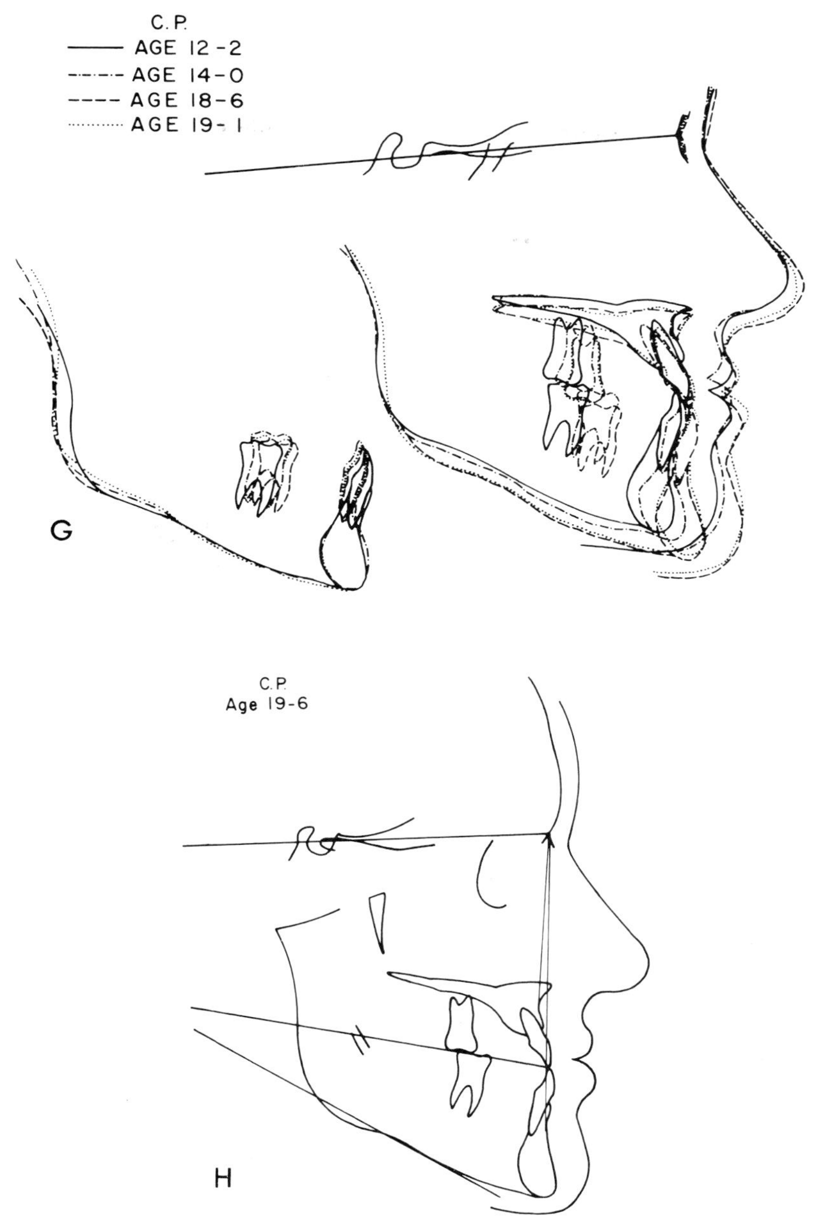

Figure 11–35 *Continued.* *G*, Composite cephalometric tracings showing seven-year growth of mandibular prognathism between ages 12 and 19. *H*, Cephalometric tracing (age 19 years, 6 months) before surgical treatment.

Illustration continued on the following page.

ACTIVE TREATMENT

After bilateral intraoral vertical subcondylar osteotomies of the vertical rami, the mandible was repositioned distally approximately 3 mm. A 5-mm horizontal wedge of bone was excised from the mental symphysis through a degloving incision. With the pedicled mental symphysis segment positioned inferiorly, the line of the proposed

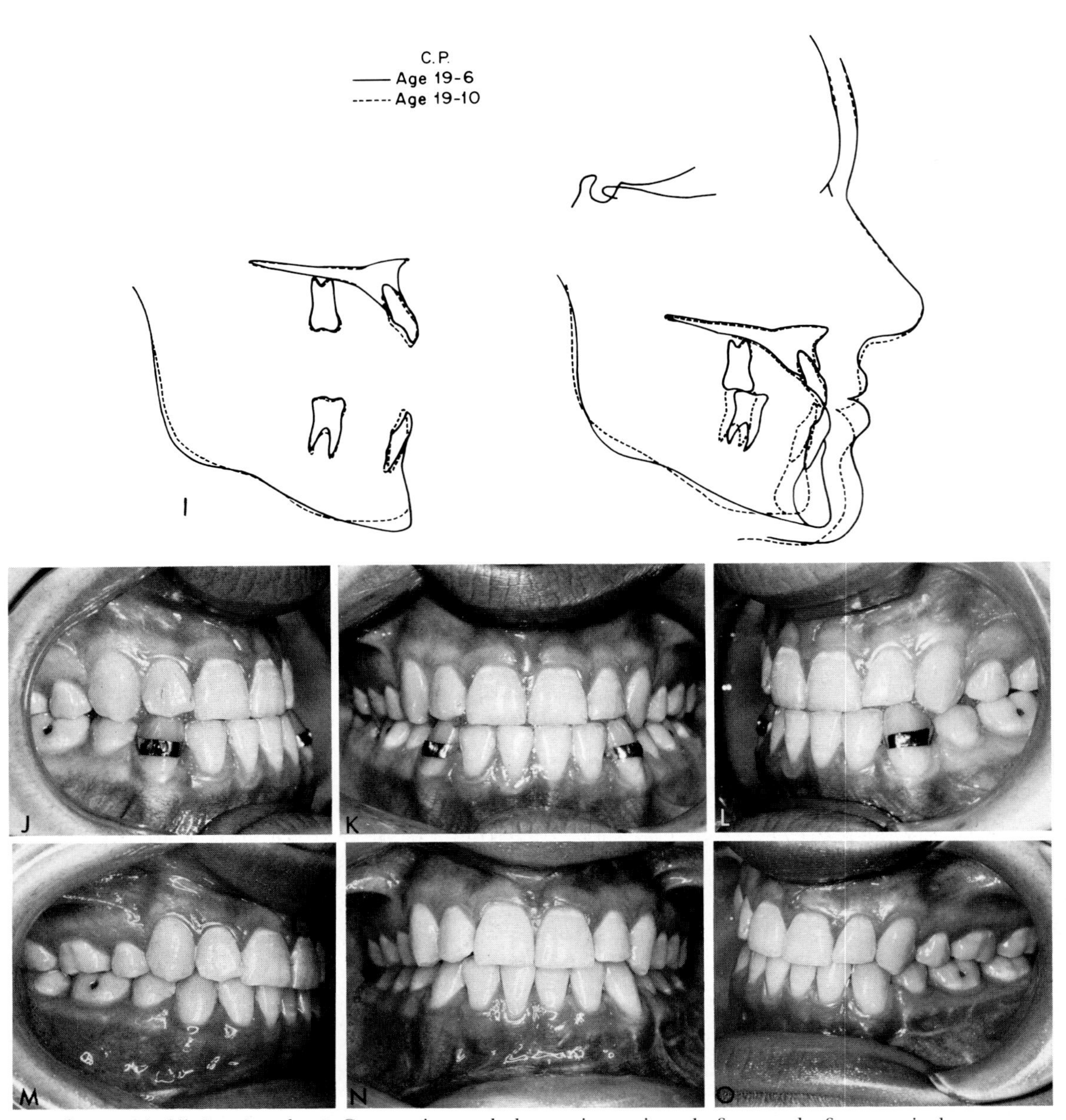

Figure 11–35 *Continued.* *I,* Composite cephalometric tracings before and after surgical treatment showing subtle changes in soft-tissue drape. Occlusion before (*J–L*) and after (*M–O*) surgical intervention.

Legend continued on the opposite page.

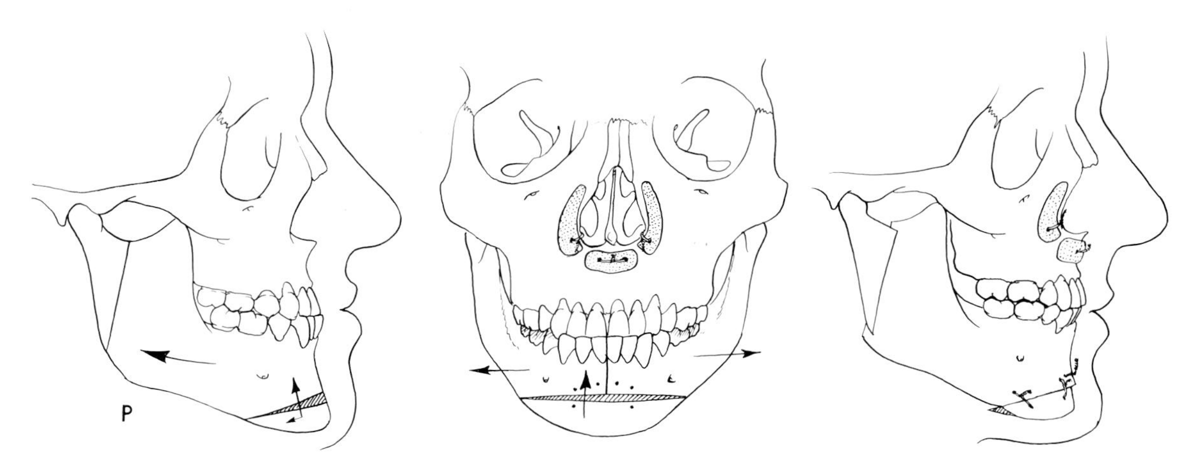

Figure 11–35 *Continued.* *P*, Schematic view of maxillary and mandibular surgical procedures used to correct patient's dentofacial deformity; bilateral intraoral vertical oblique osteotomies of the vertical rami; interincisal osteotomy to widen mandibular arch; genioplasty to reduce the height and prominence of chin; augmentation of nasolabial and paranasal areas with Proplast.

interdental osteotomy was etched into interproximal bone with a fissure bur. This line extended from the crestal alveolar bone to the previously made horizontal bone incision, and the bone cut was completed with an oscillating saw. The surgeon's forefinger was positioned on the lingual side of the mandible to feel the oscillating saw blade as it trans-sected the thicker portion of the mandible below the apices of the incisors. Finally, the two segments were separated by malleting a thin osteotome into the interseptal and interradicular areas. The inferior chin segment was re-retracted approximately 3 mm and ligated to the proximal segments. Implants of Proplast, 5 mm thick, were simultaneously placed in the nasolabial and nasomaxillary areas (Fig. 11–35*P*). The mandible was immobilized for approximately 6 weeks.

Dental symmetry and normal overbite and overjet have remained stable during a 4 year postoperative follow-up period. Facial balance was achieved by a number of subtle changes in the drape of soft tissues (Fig. 11–35*D, E,* and *F*). The nasal prominence was deaccentuated by augmentation of the nasolabial and nasomaxillary areas. Lower lip and jaw prominence was reduced by retropositioning of the mandible. Genioplasty reduced the height and prominence of the chin slightly.

COMMENT

Recognition of the typical dentofacial-skeletal characteristics and growth monitoring with sequential cephalometric radiographs are essential for proper treatment planning of mandibular prognathism. A "functional end-to-end occlusion" with severely retroclined lower anterior teeth is too often a practical compromise when mandibular prognathism is treated orthodontically in adolescence without surgical intervention. Postadolescent growth is not uncommon and further complicates the esthetic and occlusal problem. Despite late jaw growth, tooth alignment achieved by orthodontic correction usually remains satisfactory. To achieve both facial balance and occlusal harmony, however, carefully planned and executed surgery in the maxilla, the mandible, or both, coordinated with orthodontic treatment, is mandatory.

Oral Surgeon: William H. Bell, Dallas, Texas. *Orthodontist:* Thomas Byrne, St. Louis, Missouri.

CASE 11–5 (Fig. 11–36)

Patient M. B., a young woman aged 16 years, was referred by her orthodontist for assistance in the treatment of her prognathic mandible. Her father also has a prognathic mandible.

PROBLEM LIST

Esthetics (Fig. 11–36 *A* and *B*)

FRONTAL. Satisfactory.
PROFILE. Mildly prominent chin. Protruding lower lip.

Occlusal Analysis (Fig. 11–36*G*)

1. DENTAL ARCH FORM. Satisfactory.
2. DENTAL ALIGNMENT. Minor crowding and malalignment of maxillary and mandibular teeth. Teeth Nos. 1, 16, 17, and 32 were found to be impacted.
3. DENTAL OCCLUSION. Class III molar and canine relationships; 7-mm reverse horizontal overlap; 2-mm vertical overlap.

TREATMENT PLAN

Surgical Treatment

1. Perform bilateral intraoral vertical subcondylar osteotomy with 7-mm posterior repositioning of the mandible.

Postsurgical Orthodontic Treatment

1. Final orthodontic alignment of teeth after surgery.
2. Remove teeth Nos. 1, 16, 17, and 32.

COMMENT

The patient experienced mild pain the first few days after operation. The intermaxillary fixation was also mildy annoying. No hypoesthesia or anesthesia of the lip and chin occurred. The patient was well pleased with the results.

The mandible was immobilized for 6 weeks after the operation. A normal range of motion was re-established within a few weeks after release of intermaxillary fixation. The patient had a satisfactory improvement of appearance. (Figs. 11–36*C* and *D*). Cephalometric analysis 1 year after operation is contrasted with that before operation in Fig. 11–36*F*. Orthodontic treatment was completed 1 year after the operation, and at that time the teeth were well-aligned and the patient had a Class I molar and canine occlusion (Fig. 11–36*J*).

Surgeon: H. David Hall, Nashville, Tenessee. *Orthodontist:* William E. Beaumont Jr., Clarksville, Tennessee.

Text continued on page 942.

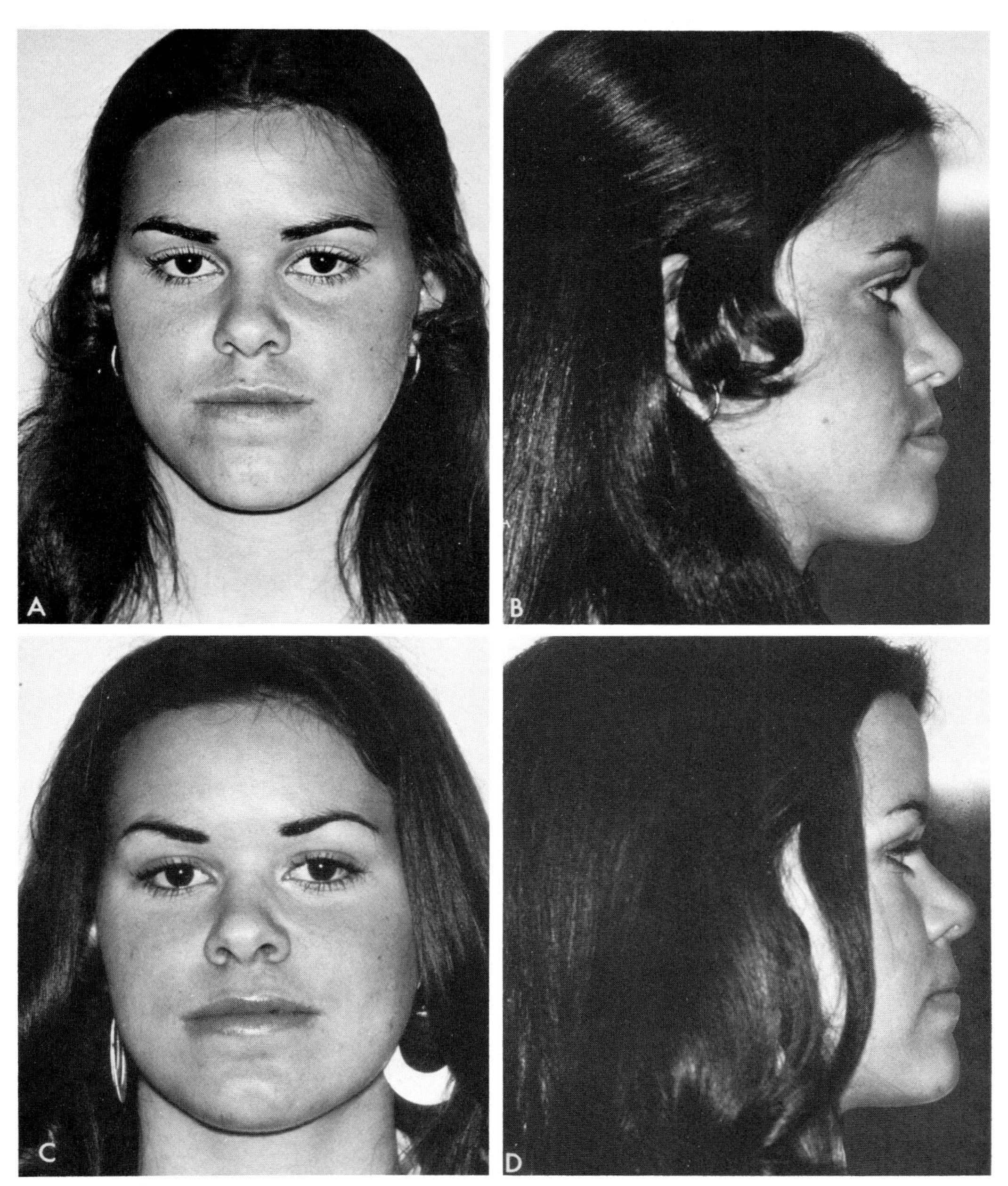

Figure 11–36 (Case 11–5). *A* and *B*, Appearance of patient before operation (IVRO): frontal view (*A*) and profile (*B*). *C* and *D*, Appearance of patient two years after surgery: frontal view (*C*) and profile (*D*).

Illustration continued on the following page.

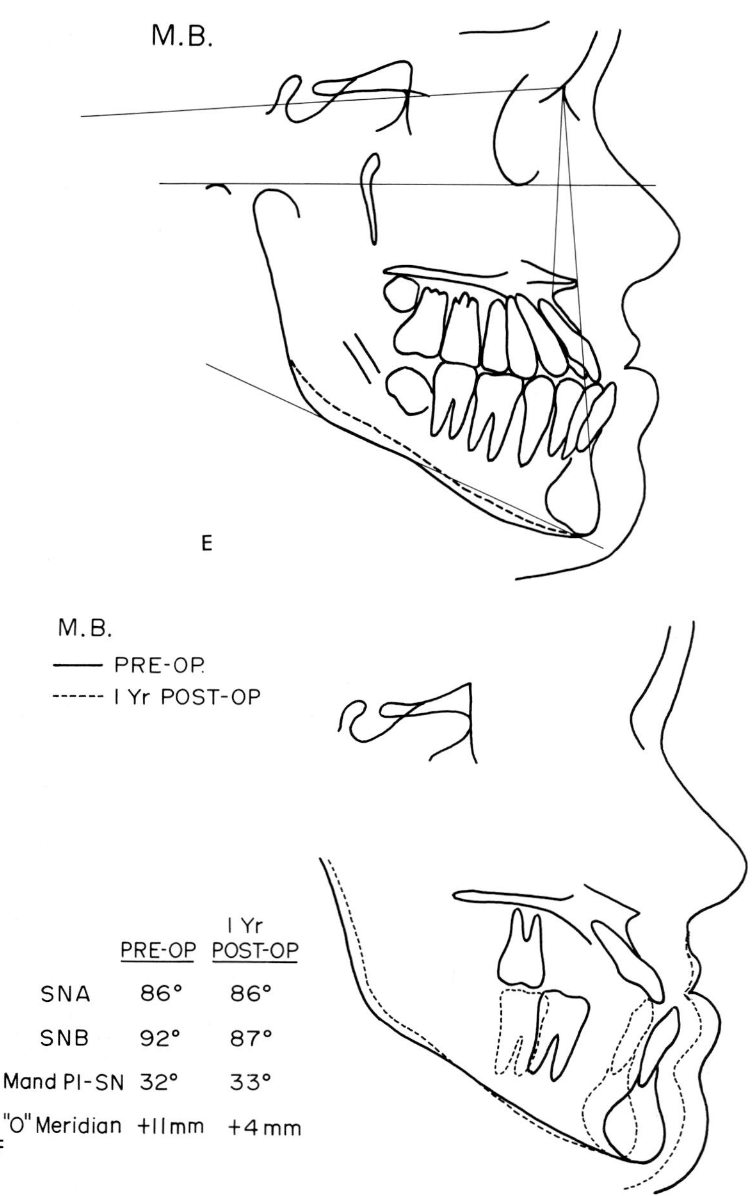

Figure 11–36 *Continued.* *E*, Cephalometric tracing before operation. *F*, Comparison of cephalometric tracing before operation and one year after operation.

Legend continued on the opposite page.

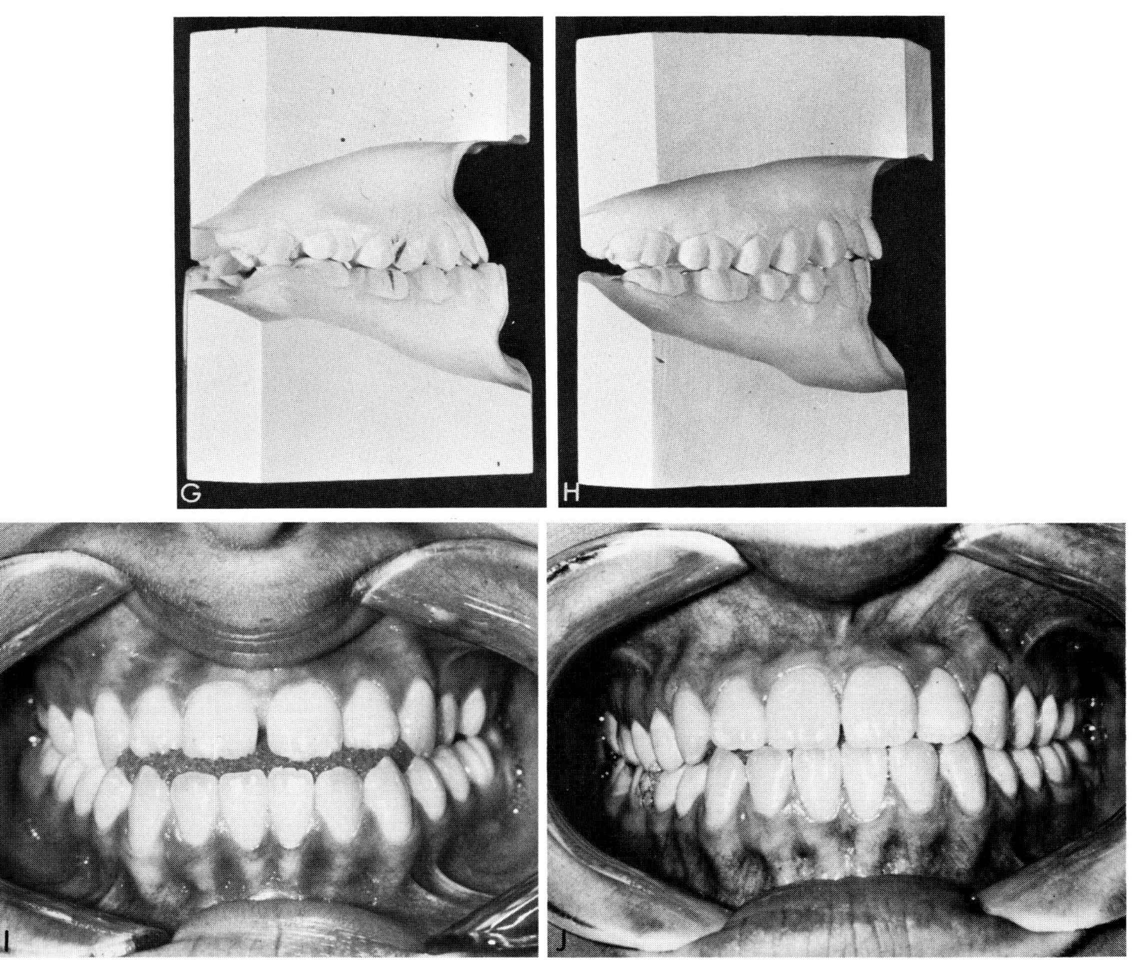

Figure 11–36 *Continued.* *G*, Occlusion cast before operation: lateral view. *H*, Occlusion cast one year after completion of orthodontic treatment: lateral view. *I*, Occlusion before operation: intraoral frontal view. *J*, Dentition and occlusion one year after completion of orthodontic treatment: intraoral frontal view.

CASE 11-6 (Fig. 11-37)

D. S., a young woman aged 17 years, was referred by her orthodontist for correction of a prominent chin and Class III occlusion.

PROBLEM LIST

Esthetics (Fig. 11–37)

FRONTAL. Excessive chin prominence.
PROFILE. Mandibular excess and prominent chin.

Cephalometric Analysis (Fig. 11–37*E)*

1. Mandibular excess; SNB 87°; ANB –7°
2. Prominent chin.
3. Recumbent mandibular incisors, $\bar{1}$ to NB, 1 mm.

Occlusal Analysis (Fig. 11–37*G, H,* and *I)*

DENTAL ARCH FORM. Satisfactory.
DENTAL ALIGNMENT. Mild crowding and malalignment of maxillary and mandibular teeth; tooth No. 25 missing.
DENTAL OCCLUSION. Class III molar and canine relationship; 3-mm reverse horizontal overlap; left posterior crossbite; mandibular dental midline 2 mm to left of maxillary dental midline (Figs. 11–37*G* and *I*).

TREATMENT PLAN

Surgical Treatment

1. Perform bilateral sagittal split ramus osteotomy with posterior repositioning of mandible 10 mm on left and 8 mm on right.
2. Perform reduction genioplasty with posterior movement of 6 mm.

Postsurgical Orthodontic Treatment

1. Align teeth and correct left posterior crossbite after sagittal split procedure.

COMMENT

The patient had moderate discomfort for several days after the operation. Right and left mental nerve hypoesthesia returned to normal in 6 months. The patient was well pleased with the result.

The mandible was mobilized about 6 weeks after the surgical procedure, and a normal range of motion was rapidly reestablished. The profile was satisfactory (Fig.

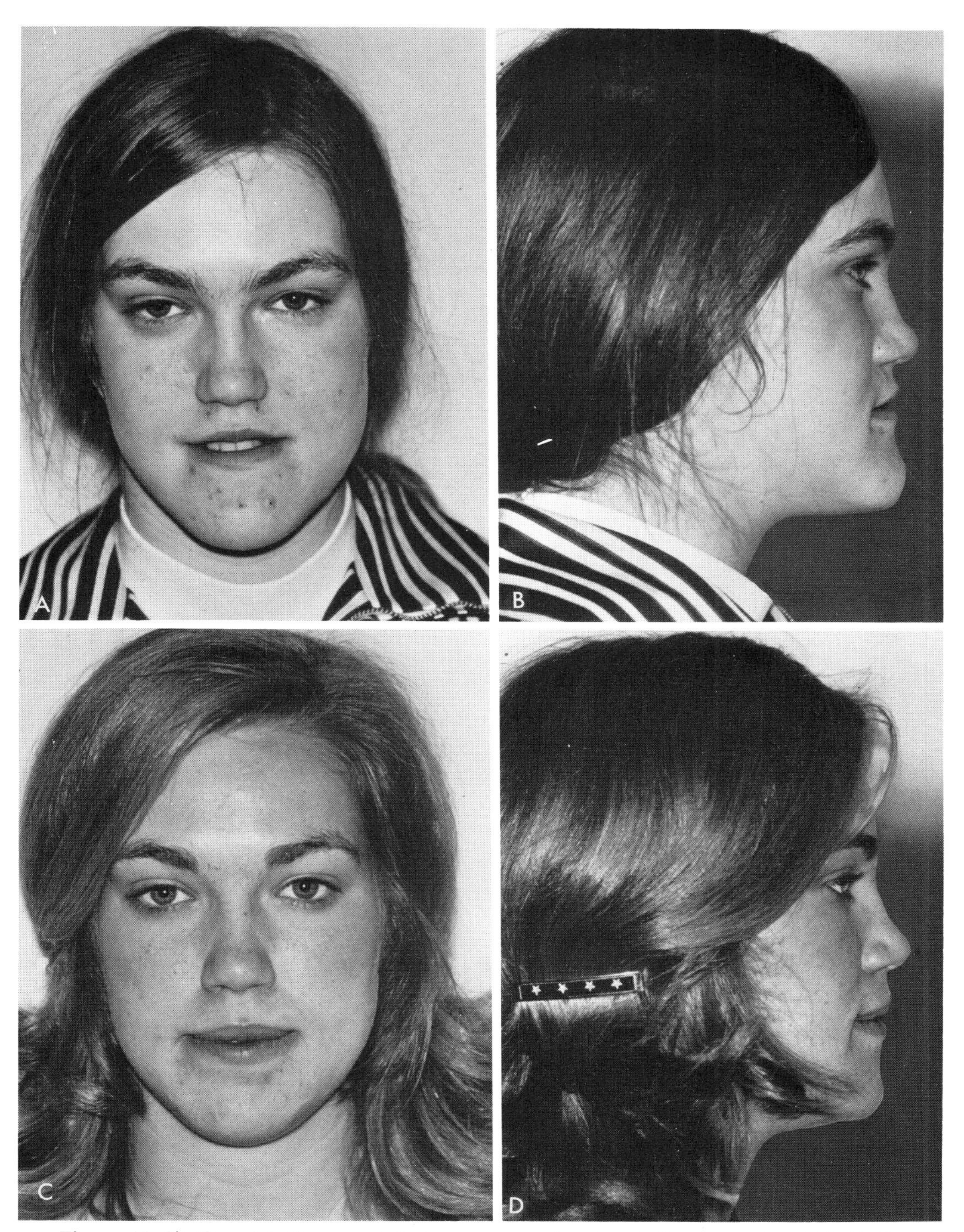

Figure 11–37 (Case 11–6). *A* and *B*, Appearance of patient before operation (SSRO). Frontal view (*A*) and profile (*B*). *C* and *D*, Appearance of patient 2 years after operation. Frontal view (*C*) and profile (*D*).

Illustration continued on the following page.

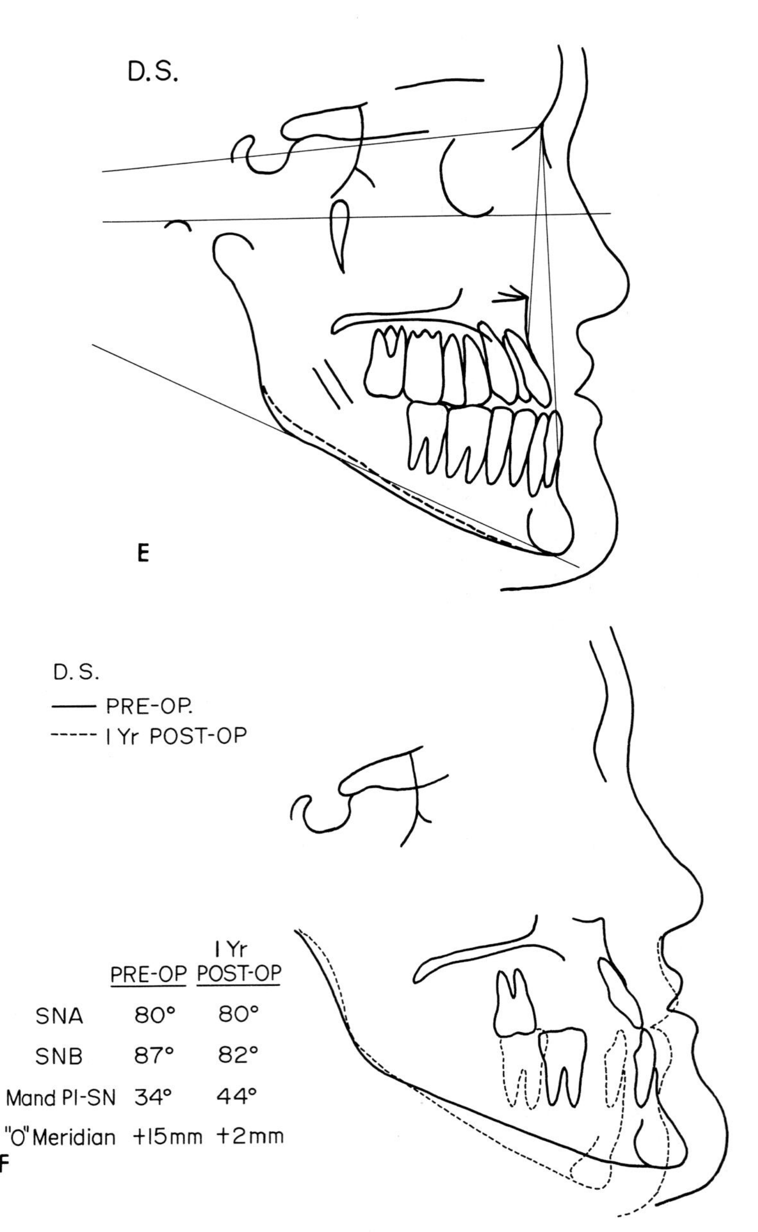

Figure 11–37 *Continued. E,* Cephalometric tracing before operation. *F,* Comparison of cephalometric tracings before and 1 year after operation.

Legend continued on the opposite page.

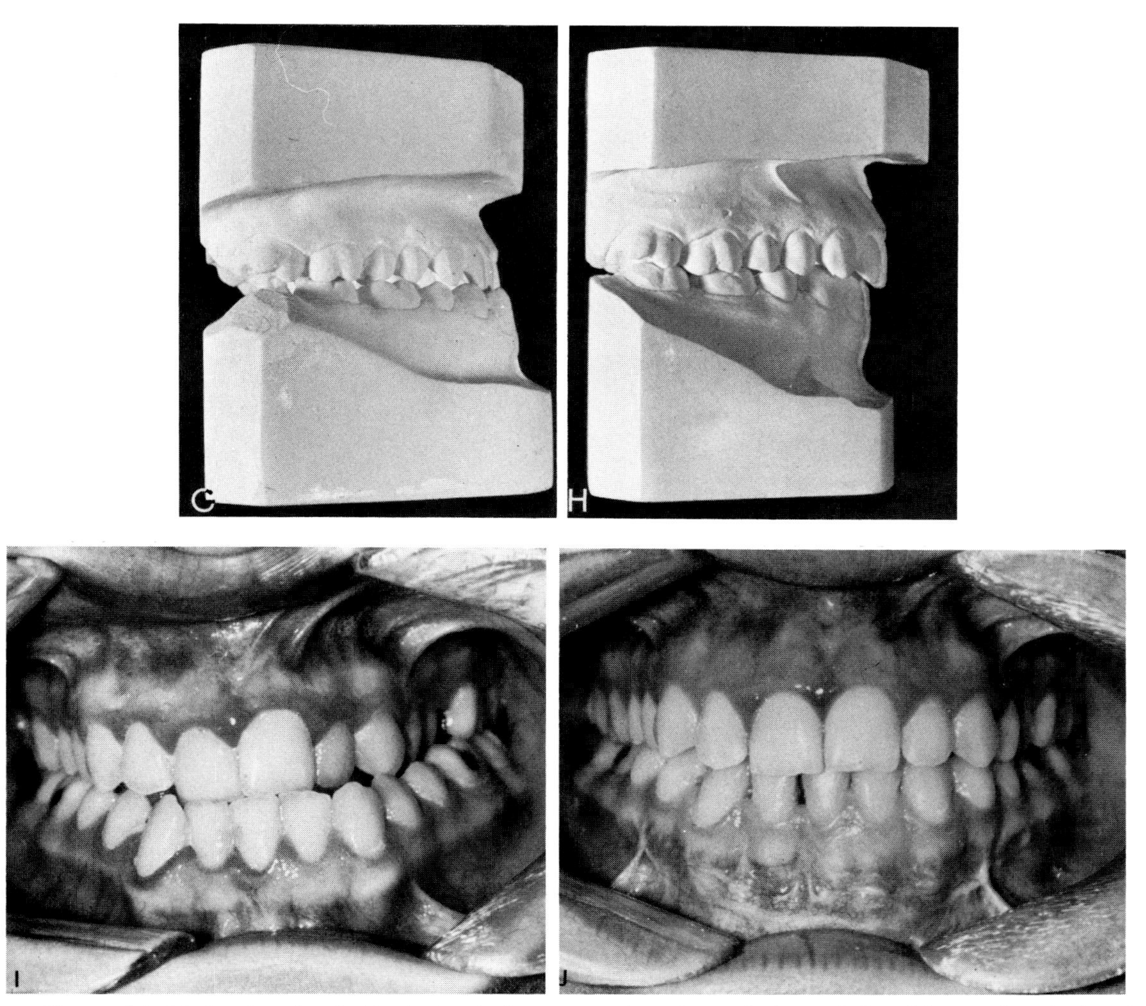

Figure 11–37 *Continued.* *G*, Occlusion before operation. Lateral view. *H*, Dentition and occlusion 1 year after completion of orthodontic treatment. Lateral view. *I*, Occlusion before operation. Intraoral view. *J*, Dentition and occlusion 1 year after completion of orthodontic treatment. Intraoral view.

11–37*D*). Cephalometric analysis 1 year after the operation showed mild backward rotation of the mandible (Fig. 11–37*F*). The teeth were well aligned, and a class I molar and canine occlusion was achieved after completion of the orthodontic treatment (Figs. 11–37*I* and *J*).

The mild backward rotation of the mandible that occurred after operation was typical of the tendency to develop an open bite that sometimes appears with both sagittal split ramus osteotomy and the intraoral vertical subcondylar osteotomy. It was corrected by orthodontic means while crowding and alignment were also being corrected.

Surgeon: H. David Hall, Nashville, Tennessee. *Orthodontist:* William B. Thetford, Nashville, Tennessee.

REFERENCES

1. Akin RK, Walters PJ: Experience with the intraoral vertical subcondylar osteotomy. J Oral Surg *33*:343, 1975.
2. Angle EH: Double resection for the treatment of mandibular protrusion. Dental Cosmos *45*:268–274 1903.
3. Bell WH: Revascularization and bone healing after anterior maxillary osteotomy: a study using adult rhesus monkeys. J Oral Surg *27*:249 1969.
4. Bell WH, Kennedy JW: Biological basis for vertical ramus osteotomies — a study of bone healing and revascularization in adult rhesus monkeys. J Oral Surg *34*:215 1976.
5. Bell WH, Levy BM: Revascularization and bone healing after anterior mandibular osteotomy. J. Oral Surg *28*:196–203, 1970.
6. Bell WH, Schendel SA: Biologic basis for modification of the sagittal ramus split operation. J Oral Surg *35*:362, 1977.
7. Bell WH, Creekmore TD: Surgical-orthodontic correction of mandibular prognathism. Am J Orthodontics *63*:256, 1973.
8. Boyne PJ: Osseous healing after oblique osteotomy of the mandibular ramus. J Oral Surg *24*:125, 1966.
9. Burch RJ, Bowden GW, Woodward HW: Intraoral one-stage ostectomy for correction of mandibular prognathism: report of case. J Oral Surg *19*:72–76, 1961.
10. Caldwell JB: Surgical correction of extreme mandibular prognathism. J Oral Surg *26*:253, 1968.
11. Caldwell, JB, Letterman GS: Vertical osteotomy in the mandibular rami for correction of prognathism. J Oral Surg *12*:185, 1954.
12. Castelli W: Vascular architecture of the human adult mandible. J Dent Res *42*:786, 1963.
13. Castelli WA, Huelke DF: The arterial system of the head and neck of the rhesus monkey with emphasis on the external carotid system. Am J Anat *116*:149, 1965.
14. Cohen L: Further studies into the vascular architecture of the mandible. J Dent Res *39*:936, 1960.
15. Dalpont G: Retromolar osteotomy for correction of prognathism. J Oral Surg *19*:42, 1961.
16. Dingman RO: Surgical correction of mandibular prognathism, an improved method. Am J Ortho Oral Surg *30*:683–692, 1944.
17. Epker BN: Modifications in the sagittal osteotomy of the mandible. J Oral Surg *35*:157, 1977.
18. Graber TM: Dentofacial orthopedics. *In* Graber TM, Swain BF (Eds). Current Orthodontic Concepts and Techniques, ed. 2. Philadelphia: WB Saunders Co, 1975.
19. Guernsey LH, DeChamplain RW: Sequelae and complications of intraoral sagittal osteotomy in the mandibular rami. Oral Surg *32*:176, 1971.
20. Hall HD, Chase DC, Payor LG: Evaluation and refinement of the intraoral vertical subcondylar osteotomy. J Oral Surg *33*:333, 1975.
21. Harsha WM: Bilateral resection of the jaw for prognathism. Surg Gynecol Obstet *15*:51–53, 1912.
22. Hayward J, Richardson ER, Malhotra SK: The mandibular foramen: its anteroposterior position. Oral Surg *44*:837, 1977.
23. Hayward JR, Walker RV: Personal communication. 1979.
24. Herbert JM, Kent JN, Hinds ED: Correction of prognathism by an intraoral vertical subcondylar osteotomy. J Oral Surg *28*:651, 1970.
25. Hinds EC, Girotti WJ: Vertical subcondylar osteotomy: a reappraisal. Oral Surg *24*:164, 1967.
26. Hullihen SP: Case of elongation of the under jaw and distortion of the face and neck, caused by a burn, successfully treated. Am J Dent Sci *9*:157, 1849.
27. Hunsuck EE: Modified intraoral splitting technique for correction of mandibular prognathism. J Oral Surg *26*:250, 1968.
28. Isaacson RJ, Kopytov OS, Bevis RR, Waite DE: Movement of the proximal and distal segments after mandibular ramus osteotomies. J Oral Surg *36*:263, 1978.
29. Janzen EK, Bluher JA: The cephalometric, anatomic, and histologic changes in *Macaca mulatta* after the application of a continuous acting retraction force on the mandible. Am J Orthod *51*:823, 1965.
30. Keller EE, Hill AJ, Sather AH: Orthognathic surgery, review of mandibular body procedures. Mayo Clin Proc *51*:117–133, 1976.
31. Kelly JE: An assessment of the occlusion of the teeth of youths 12–17 years, United States. Vital & Health Staitstics: Series II, Data from the National Health Survey. (DHEW Publication No. [HRA] 77–1644). Washington DC: Government Printing Office. 1973.
32. Kelsey CC: Radiographic cephalometric study of surgically corrected mandibular prognathism. J Oral Surg *26*:283, 1968.
33. Kingsley NW: Oral Deformities. New York: Appleton, 1908.
34. Kole H: Results, experience, and problems in the operative treatment of anomalies with reverse overbite (mandibular protrusion). J Oral Surg *19*:427–450, 1965.
35. Lash SM: Comprehensive evaluation of long term results of two types of surgical correction of mandibular prognathism. (Master's Thesis, The University of Michigan, July 1972).
36. Moose SM: Correction of abnormal mandibu-

lar protrusion by intraoral operation. J Oral Surg *3*:304, 1945.
37. Moose SM: Surgical correction of mandibular prognathism by intraoral subcondylar osteotomy. J Oral Surg *22*:197, 1964.
38. New GB, Erich JB: The surgical correction of mandibular prognathism. Am J Surg *53*:2–12, 1941.
39. Rhinelander FW, et al: Microangiography in bone healing. Displaced closed fractures. J Bone Joint Surg *50*:643, 1968.
40. Sowray JH, Haskell R: Ostectomy at the mandibular symphysis. Br J Oral Surg *5–6*:97–102, 1967–1969.
41. Thoma KH: Y-Shaped osteotomy for correction of open bite in adults. Surg Gynecol Obstet *77*:40–50, 1943.
42. Thoma KH: Oral Surgery. St. Louis: CV Mosby Co, 1948.
43. Trauner R, Obwegeser H: The surgical correction of mandibular prognathism and retrognathia with consideration of genioplasty. Part I. Surgical procedures to correct mandibular prognathism and reshaping of the chin. Oral Surg *10*:677, 1957.
44. Walker DG: Personal communication, 1978.
45. Wang JH, Waite DE: Evaluation of the surgical procedure of sagittal split osteotomy of the mandibular ramus. Oral Surg *38*:167, 1974.
46. Whipple JW: Double resection of the inferior maxilla for protruding lower jaw. Dental Cosmos *40*:552–557, 1898.
47. White RP Jr, Peters PB, Costich ER, Page HL: Evaluation of sagittal split ramus osteotomy in 17 patients. J Oral Surg *27*:851, 1969.
48. Wickwire NA, White RP, Proffit WR: The effect of mandibular osteotomy on tongue position. J Oral Surg *30*:184, 1972.
49. Winstanly RP: Subcondylar osteotomy of the mandible and the intraoral approach. Br J Oral Surg *6*:134, 1968.
50. Wolk RS: Cinefluorographic, electromyographic and myometric study of muscular activity during swallowing in patients with mandibular resections. (Master's Thesis, Loyola University, Chicago, 1969).
51. Woodside DW: Some aspects of present and future control of mandibular, alveolar, and midface growth. Symposium on Control Mechanisms in Craniofacial Growth. University of Michigan, 1974.

Nerve Complications and Their Management

1. Walter JM, and Gregg JM: Analysis of postsurgical neurological alteration in the trigeminal nerve. J Oral Surg *37*:410, 1979.
2. Behrman S: Complications of sagittal osteotomy of the mandibular ramus. J Oral Surg *30*: 554, 1972.
3. Seddon HJ: Three types of nerve injury. Brain *66*:237, 1943.
4. Terzis J, and Williams HB: Functional evaluation of free nerve grafts. *In* Symposium on Microsurgery. St. Louis: CV Mosby Co, *14*:144, 1976.
5. Hausamen JE, and Schmidseder MS: Repair of the mandibular nerve by means of autologous nerve grafting after resection of the lower jaw. J Maxillofac Surg *1*:74, 1973.
6. Hausamen JE, Samii M, and Schmidseder R: Indication and technique for the reconstruction of nerve defects in head and neck. J Maxillofac Surg *2*:159, 1974.
7. Daniel RK, and Terzis JK (Eds.): Reconstructive Microsurgery. New York: Little, Brown, and Co, 1977.

Part B: Asymmetric Mandibular Excess

J. D. Hayward, R. V. Walker, D. G. Poulton, and W. H. Bell

Asymmetric mandibular excess presents a special set of problems related to both diagnosis and treatment. The growth patterns of the mandible that produce facial asymmetry may be the result of a localized oddity in growth or they may reflect a generalized growth problem affecting the entire face. Facial enlargements that produce asymmetry may occur at many sites, but those associated with the mandible are usually the most striking. The masseter muscles may become hypertrophied and their enlargement causes a distinctive facial imbalance, to which exostoses of the mandible occasionally contribute. Enlargement of the facial soft tissues associated with enlargement of all the facial bones on the affected side is seen in facial hemihypertrophy, a rare congenital disorder characterized by generalized or total hemifacial enlargement involving soft tissues, jaws, and teeth.

In this section, discussion will center on problems that are related directly to the mandible and the lower face and result from excessive growth in an uncommon pattern. Asymmetry resulting from excessive and unusual growth patterns in the lower face is classified into three types: laterognathism or asymmetric prognathism, condylar hyperplasia, and unilateral macrognathia (Fig. 11–38). These terms are discussed in detail later in this section.

Recognizing the difference between a skeletal asymmetry and a localized excessive growth is difficult. A fundamental diagnostic problem is the differentiation of a real from a relative excess in the asymmetric condition. For example, arrested growth of the mandible as a result of injury in childhood may produce an asymmetry in which the unaffected side of the mandible appears to be enlarged when it is actually normal. The process of diagnosis must identify that such a problem is the result of inhibited or arrested growth on the smaller side of the face rather than excessive growth on the opposite normal side.

The adjustments that are caused by remodeling of bone or by a pathologic condition complicate the issue. For example, permanent asymmetry of the mandible does not result from infantile cortical hyperostosis, although this is a disease that generally involves only one side of the mandible. This bony enlargement, which occurs during infancy, disappears as growth proceeds in later childhood and the mandible remodels to a normal contour. Unilateral fibrous dysplasia will produce asymmetry of the mandible. Characteristics of the bone in these and other forms of unilateral expanding pathologic conditions of the mandible must be differentiated clinically and radiographically. Identifying specific bone characteristics associated with a pathologic process may be the only way such conditions can be distinguished from an asymmetric growth pattern.

Minor asymmetry of the face is entirely normal, and it is only when the degree of asymmetry becomes obvious that patients desire its correction.

HISTORY

Asymmetric conditions attributed to condylar hyperplasia have been reported extensively in the literature. Condylar hyperplasia was first reported and described in 1836 by Adams, who associated hyperplasia of a mandibular condyle with a variety of rheumatoid arthritis.[10] Since that time, many causes have been reported in the literature. An outstanding early review article on condylar hyperplasia by Gruca and Meisels considered 17 cases reported up to 1926, including 3 of their own; they emphasized the importance of an early operation to correct the condition.[12] Rushton described the histologic features of the hyperplastic condyle in 1944.[20] Cernea added 8 cases to the literature in 1948,[5] and Gottlieb reported on the correction of the deformity in 12 patients and thoroughly described the gross morphology of the hyperplastic condylar head.[10] Blomquist and Hogeman chronologically listed the cases reported in the literature up to 1963.[2] Bruce and Hayward in 1968[13] and Tarsitano and Wooten in 1970[26] reviewed the subject as well.

Most of the early reports of condylar hyperplasia originated in Europe, and the condition was considered to be relatively common there. American authors, reporting on a limited number of cases, considered the condition to be rare in the United States until Gottlieb's report reviewing 62 cases appeared in 1951. Gottlieb recognized that his own large series of 12 cases did not reflect an increasing incidence but rather an increased awareness of the problem by patients who demanded its correction. The increased demand for surgical correction of asymmetric deformities was substantiated in an article by Hinds, Reid, and Burch[15] in 1960. These authors' 15 cases of mandibular asymmetry associated with unilateral condylar hyperplasia were seen within a four-year period. An extensive study of reports in the literature of condylar hyperplasia by Blomquist and Hogeman showed that in 102 cases reviewed, there was an almost equal sex distribution.[2] Included in the literature are several reports of unilateral condylar hyperplasia and macrognathia with asymmetry that were not reported by Blomquist and Hogeman, and there are many cases reported since 1963.* It is now obvious that unilateral condylar hyperplasia and the associated types of mandibular asymmetry are relatively common conditions for which patients readily seek surgical attention.

CLASSIFICATION

The complexities of etiology and the characteristics of mandibular hyperplasia and associated asymmetry have resulted in a variety of classifications. Rushton related the type of mandibular laterognathia to the time-span of abnormal condylar growth.[20] He stated that any unilateral condylar overgrowth occurring in childhood would be compensated for by secondary alveolar growth of both the mandible and maxilla. He also suggested that the affected side of the mandible would be larger and longer than normal, but the condyle ramus and body of the mandible would remain in proportion (as seen in unilateral macrognathia). If the condylar growth continued beyond or resumed after a normal cessation of growth, remodeling of the mandible and downward growth of the maxilla could not occur. Accordingly, the deformity would be primarily evident in the condyle (condylar hyperplasia).

In discussing mandibular prognathism, Waldron, Peterson, and Waldron also described patients with mandibular laterognathism.[29] They classified patients with this deformity into two types: those with molar infraocclusion and incisive supraocclusion and those with molar contact and incisive infraocclusion. In both instances, the patients did not have unilaterally enlarged condyles. Instead, they had crossbite with a prognathic mandibular relationship, an asymmetric prognathism. Many conditions described in the literature as unilateral condylar hyperplasia are probably examples of asymmetric mandibular prognathism, which is termed *laterognathism.* With these deformities, the patient generally has lateral facial asymmetry with a Class III malocclusion in addition to a crossbite relationship. These types of asymmetry are quite distinct morphologically from the types (condylar hyperplasias) described by Rushton.

Gottlieb[10] classified condylar hyperplasia as an osteoma resulting from a unilateral condylar deformity and prognathic deviation consequential to a bilateral disproportion in size of the condyles. Hinds and his coworkers classified mandibular asymmetry involving condylar overgrowth into two categories: unilateral condylar hyperplasia and deviation prognathism (with the condyles being approximately the same size).[15]

*See references 1, 3, 4, 7–9, 11, 15–18, 20, 21, 23, 25, and 27 for further information.

In two thorough articles on mandibular deformities, Rowe classified asymmetric protrusion into three groups: unilateral condylar hyperplasia, unilateral macrognathia confined to the skeletal element only, and unilateral macrognathia of both osseous and muscular components.[23] He characterized unilateral condylar hyperplasia as being associated with elongation of the condylar neck, bowing of the inferior body of the mandible, lateral crossbite, and concavity of the lateral aspect of the ramus.

Rowe's second classification, unilateral skeletal macrognathia, was characterized by elongation of the bone alone "since ramus growth is restricted by the pterygomasseteric sling." A crossbite is apparent, but there is no twisting of the vertical axis of the chin and no bowing of the lower border of the mandible.

Rowe's third classification, involving the osseous and muscular tissues, is characterized by downward displacement of the mandibular gonial angle, no crossbite (since the abnormal muscle component did not limit downward growth), increase in the size of the entire side of the mandible, slanting of the apices of the teeth toward the unaffected side, and unilateral masseter muscle hypertrophy. Rowe did not classify the laterognathic malformation that is the result of an enlarged condyle with normal proportions of the ramus and body of the mandible.

In an evaluation of unilateral condylar hyperplasia, Cernea proposed four classes of asymmetry and occlusal disturbances: laterodeviation with prognathism and open bite in the posterior region on one or both sides; laterodeviation with posterior open bite without prognathism; laterodeviation with prognathism without open bite; and facial asymmetry without prognathism.[6]

Of the several classifications presented in the literature, those of Rushton[20] and Rowe[23] are perhaps the most inclusive. Rushton's classification is based primarily on a time period, and it suggests that, ultimately, mandibular morphology is related to the length of time that the excessive unilateral growth was active in the pattern of morphogenesis. Subtle variations in configuration such as the increase in body height and maxillary alveolar growth occur as compensatory mechanisms to maintain dental occlusion. Rowe's ideas relate to genetic predisposition of bone growth or muscle growth or an interrelationship between the two that ultimately controls the mandibular morphology.

The etiology of asymmetric mandibular excess is not well understood. It is often suggested that a congenital imbalance is related to some chromosomal aberrance. Efforts to relate unilateral condylar hyperplasia to trauma, infection, neoplasia, or an inheritable trait have not been successful. In describing the histologic characteristics of specimens of hyperplastic condyles that were surgically removed, Oberg and others suggest that increased vascularization in the condyles could have led to excessive growth.[20] Walker also noted increased vascularity in three condylar specimens that were characterized as hyperplastic.[30] Excessive proliferation in repair after injury to the condyle remains a suspected cause of condylar hyperplasia.

For simplicity, the problems caused by a unilateral growth excess can be sorted into three general groups of mandibular asymmetry: asymmetric prognathism, condylar hyperplasia, and unilateral macrognathism.

Asymmetric Prognathism

Asymmetric prognathism comprises the largest group of asymmetry problems caused by growth excess. This particular term suggests that the growth potential of the mandible at the right and left condyles is unequal, with one side having the greater tendency to become prognathic, although the condyles themselves are of equal size and within normal size limits. There is often a degree of anterior open bite as well as crossbite relationship. There may be no significant maxillary compensatory change (Fig. 11–38*A*).

Condylar Hyperplasia

In patients with condylar hyperplasia, the mandibular arch form remains approximately symmetric with the maxillary arch, and there is no major compensatory alveolar modification. The condyles are decidedly unequal in size. The uninvolved side has a normal contour and dimension and the hyperplastic side is significantly enlarged (Fig. 11–38*B*). Except for the condylar enlargement and increased length of the condylar neck, which causes deviation of the mandible to the opposite side, the general contour of the displaced mandible is symmetric. It appears that mandibular growth has been completed and that hyperplasia of the condyle occurred after maturation of the skeleton.

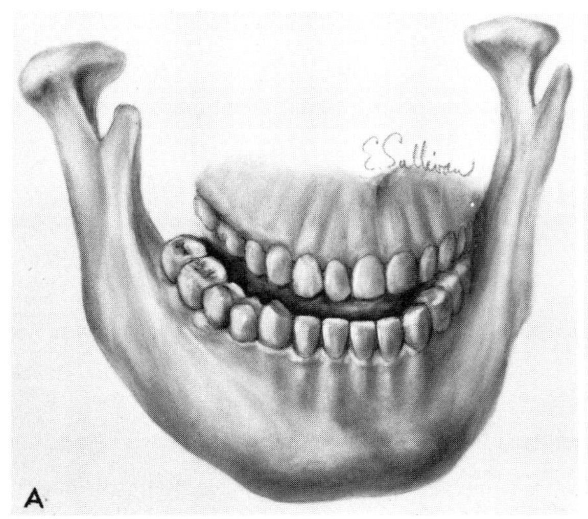

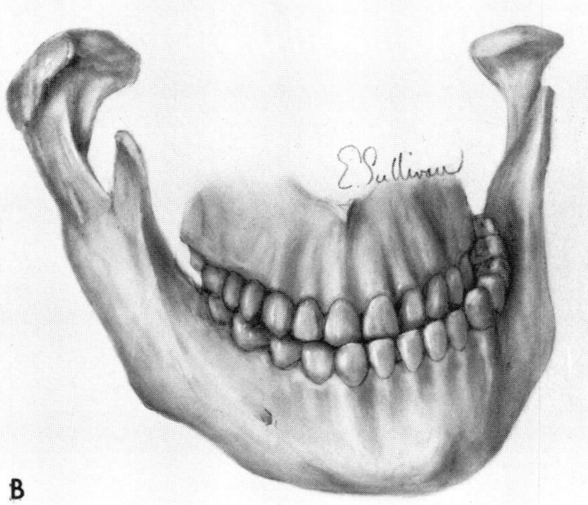

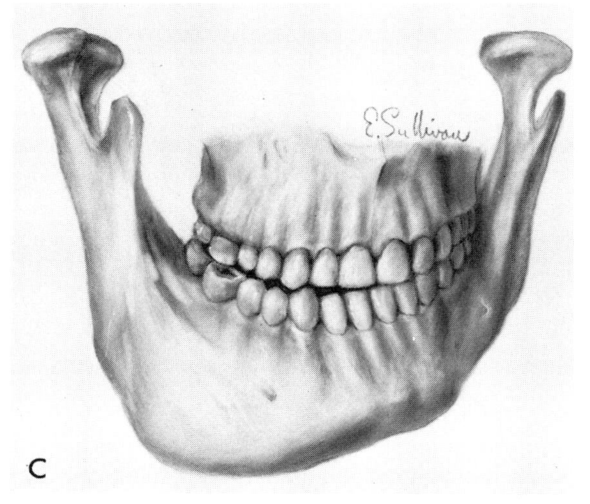

Figure 11–38. *A*, Deviation prognathism with a generalized proportionate increase in the size of the mandible and an increased unilateral growth component. *B*, Unilateral condylar hyperplasia manifested by an enlarged condylar head resulting in a crossbite and laterognathia. *C*, Unilateral macrognathia with a generalized increase in half of the mandible, "bowing" of the inferior mandibular body, open bite, compensatory maxillary growth, and deviation of the teeth from the affected side of the mandible. (*A–C* from Bruce RA, and Hayward JR: Condylar hyperplasia and mandibular asymmetry: a review. J Oral Surg *26*:281–290.

Illustration continued on the following page.

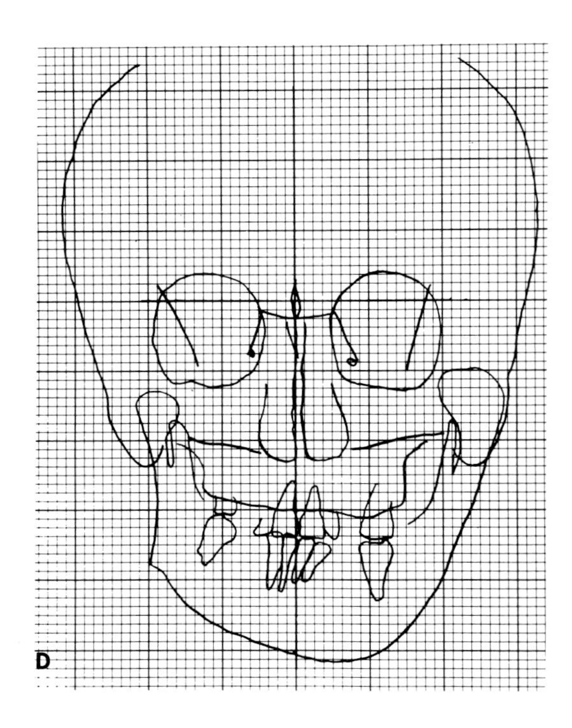

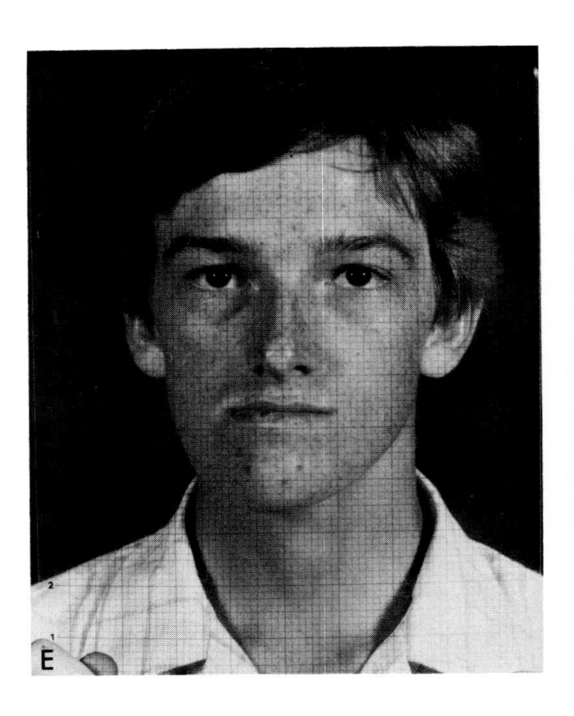

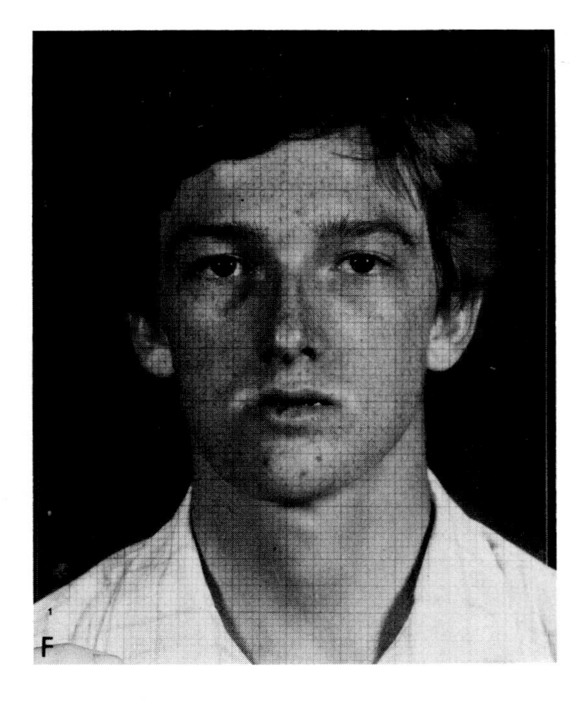

Figure 11–38 *Continued.* *D,* P–A cephalogram with horizontal plane axis through right and left zygomaticofrontal sutures and vertical axis perpendicular to this plane on a line passing through the crista galli. Measurements from these axes permit the quantitation of asymmetry. *E,* Use of computagrid to evaluate and quantitate facial asymmetry. The computagrid consists of a grid of horizontal and vertical lines scribed on an 11- × 9-inch clear plastic sheet. It provides a series of coordinates to aid in evaluating frontal and profile facial esthetics. A clear plastic grid is held in front of patient, the horizontal line on the grid is oriented to the natural horizontal passing through orbital rims or interpupillary line, the balance and symmetry of facial structures are evaluated in relation to vertical lines, and the vertical relations are evaluated in relation to horizontal lines. (See also Figure 14–3.) *F,* The patient has been instructed to move his mandible laterally until his mandibular dental midline coincides with the midsagittal plane of the face and skull. Residual facial and chin asymmetry can then be evaluated with computagrid, which is oriented to a natural horizontal.

Unilateral Macrognathism

In unilateral macrognathism, the entire involved side of the mandible, including the condyle, is enlarged (Fig. 11–38*C*). The vertical ramus is long, the inferior border bows excessively downward, the horizontal body of the mandible has excessive bony height, and the mandibular contour is flat in the region of the mental foramen on the involved side. The incisors are tipped toward the involved side, and the occlusal plane is dropped to a lower level. The degree of open bite on this side varies in accordance with whether the alveolar growth in both the mandible and the maxilla has been able to compensate to maintain a functional occlusion.

SYSTEMATIC DESCRIPTION OF THE DEFORMITY

Asymmetric mandibular excess is characterized by deviation of the chin to one side of the facial midline. One must look beyond the most prominent feature to completely define the patient's deformity. The exact position of the dental midline in both mandible and maxilla must be noted in relation to the jaws themselves and to the general facial midline. Mercier suggests that the facial photographs are helpful in precisely defining the location of the deformity.[19] The profile view will identify a prominent lower face. Specific relationships for mandibular excess will be the same as those discussed earlier in this chapter. Alterations in facial height must be assessed as well. The use of a clear plastic grid with horizontal and vertical reference lines provides a means of clinically evaluating asymmetric mandibular excess (Fig. 11–38*E* and *F*).

Discrepancies in the dental occlusion may be seen unilaterally or bilaterally. Dental arch form in both the mandible and the maxilla must be studied. The maxilla may have made an adjustment to the mandibular arch, and deviations of tooth position must be assessed with this in mind. Both anterior and posterior dental crossbites may be found. Deviations from the correct retruded contact position of the teeth may be difficult to determine. For ease of analysis, dental casts must be mounted on an anatomic, semi-adjustable articulator. Because vertical jaw discrepancies almost always accompany the transverse and anteroposterior deviations, three planes of space must be assessed in defining the problem for patients with the deformity. (See Chapters 9 and 21.)

The maxillary cast is mounted on an anatomic articulator to duplicate the position in which the arch is oriented in the skull. A face-bow is used to accomplish the transfer from the patient to the articulator. The point of reference on the hyperplastic side may be arbitrary if there is an aberrant position of the temporomandibular joint. The pretragal points overlying the lateral poles of the condyles are used for this purpose. The face-bow is oriented so that the arms are parallel and equidistant from the midsagittal plane of the skull. The mounting is used to simulate the spatial relationship of the maxillary and mandibular arches to the skull (see Chapter 21 for details of mounting casts.)

Various clinical measurements are useful in planning corrective surgery (see case reports at end of this chapter). The maxillary tooth-to-lip measurements (mm), symmetry of the smile, and the relationship of the maxillary midline to the midsagittal plane of the skull are all critical for proper planning of maxillary surgery. If the orbits are symmetric, the interpupillary plane is useful for orientation.

The mandibular cast is temporarily luted to the mounted maxillary cast in the desired surgical position. Treatment is planned so that the midline of the maxilla approximates the midsagittal plane of the skull. After simulating correction of the cant of the maxillary occlusal plane, proper tooth-to-lip relationship and correction of the maxillary dental midline with the midsagittal plane of the skull, the mandibular occlusal plane can be corrected by repositioning the mandible to coincide with the *corrected maxillary midline and occlusal plane.* Correction of the mandibular occlusal plane and dental midline is therefore predicated upon correction of the maxillary occlusal plane and dental midline or on a preexisting normal position of the maxilla in all three planes of space. Successful treatment of asymmetric mandibular excess is predicated and based upon proper and systematic three-dimensional diagnosis and treatment of concomitant maxillary dysplasias. Once this is accomplished, three dimensional analysis and treatment of the asymmetric mandibular excess is not complicated.

In a radiographic assessment of facial skeletal asymmetry, a posteroanterior radiograph that has been oriented with grid lines is a common tool for helping to localize the degrees of asymmetry (Fig. 11–38). One patient with condylar hyperplasia described in this chapter was studied by this method (Fig. 11–46). A horizontal axis between the zygomaticofrontal sutures on the orbital rims is used for orientation of that plane. The midline is dropped perpendicular to the horizontal and intersects the crista galli of the cranial base. Lack of specific cephalometric data prevents giving the posteroanterior radiograph the same detailed evaluation that is possible for assessing anteroposterior and vertical facial deformities on the lateral cephalogram.

There are perhaps several ways of using posteroanterior cephalograms to assist in an analysis of facial skeletal asymmetry. A variation in the above technique is to drop perpendicular lines from the Frankfort plane on a posteroanterior cephalogram through gonion on each side (see Figure 11–46). By direct measurement in millimeters, the difference in distance of gonion from the Frankfort plane on each side can be immediately appreciated. When such radiographs and measurements are done in a serial manner over whatever period of time is deemed appropriate, an assessment of the progressive nature of an asymmetry can be documented. Reliability of the technique is dependent upon a relatively valid Frankfort plane without a skeletal deformity existing in the upper middle face. The technique is not suggested as being absolutely accurate, but it serves as a reasonable guide in appraising a deformity and planning for the timing of a surgical correction.

ORTHODONTIC TREATMENT

The planning for orthodontic correction depends upon the degree to which the maxillary teeth and alveolar process have compensated for the asymmetric position of the mandible. In cases where there has been deviation of the maxillary structures, it may be necessary to employ maxillary surgery as well as orthodontic correction in addition to mandibular surgery. In other situations, presurgical orthodontic treatment alone may be indicated to bring the individual teeth into symmetric relationship with their respective jaw while keeping them on basal bone. Tooth movement can be accomplished with a fully banded orthodontic appliance capable of axial control of teeth in all dimensions, e.g., the edgewise appliance.

Orthodontic treatment prior to surgery usually increases the severity of the apparent malocclusion. Posteroanterior radiographs of the head are used to determine the degree of maxillary dental asymmetry as it relates to the overall cranial midline. The orthodontic goal prior to surgery generally is to bring the maxillary teeth into harmony with this midline. This approach will entail full banding of the teeth and the use of rubber bands from the upper to the lower teeth as well as full labial and lingual archwires. Determination of progress during this phase of treatment cannot be made by clinical examination alone but will require progress dental casts to determine the developing conformity of the arches to the final goal.

It is possible to do the surgical correction first and the orthodontic treatment later, and it is easier to visualize the necessary tooth movement in this way. The problem is that complete surgical correction of the jaw position will severely overcorrect the malocclusion, and the orthodontic forces that are needed to move teeth into good position will tend to cause relapse of the surgical result. Lack of occlusal fit may contribute toward instability of a surgical correction.

At the completion of active treatment, when orthodontic appliances are removed, there will be a marked tendency for relapse. To offset this, completion and ultimate firm stabilization of the orthodontic correction is best achieved with an orthodontic tooth positioner. This appliance has interarch control as well as tooth control and can be worn for a long time to assure stability of the treatment result.

Basic Follow-up Physiotherapy: Use of Night Elastics

When correction of the asymmetric mandible requires a condylectomy or an osteotomy of the vertical ramus or body to shift the mandible, the occlusion is markedly affected. The instruction to reposition the mandible to the midline as well as possible does not mean that the teeth need immediately intercuspate satisfactorily, even though good upper and lower arch alignment be obtained. When preoperative and follow-up orthodontic care is available and can be a part of the overall treatment plan, adjustments to obtain optimum occlusion may confidently be produced in this manner. Even if orthodontic care is not available, good occlusion and intercuspation of teeth can still be obtained. After intermaxillary fixation for postoperative jaw immobilization is removed, a program of careful follow-up physiotherapy is initiated. This consists of allowing the patient's jaw to function as normally as possible during the day and then holding the teeth in optimal occlusion with two or three small elastics while the patient sleeps at night. The small elastics are attached to the hooks of upper and lower arch bars secured to the teeth by wiring. A small elastic placed at the cuspid area bilaterally will usually suffice (see Figures 11–43 and 11–45). If slightly heavier pull seems desirable, an additional small elastic may be placed at the central incisor area (see Figure 11–42). Rarely will more than three small elastics be needed for this nocturnal up-and-down traction.

The elastics are hooked into position before the patient retires for the night. Immediately upon awakening in the morning, the patient removes the elastics. The whole ritual must be repeated devotedly every day for a *minimum* of 3 months while the teeth slowly move into good intercuspation. The various processes that occur during this regimen are almost impossible to measure. Posterior teeth are intruded slightly, anterior teeth are extruded slightly, and the mandible settles to its best functional position while bony modeling and healing of the sectioned areas and muscle retraining and adaptation subtly take place simultaneously. It is desirable that the therapist appreciate these subtle changes and express confidence that they *are* happening while the patient's progress is being closely monitored.

SURGICAL TREATMENT

The surgical correction of *asymmetric mandibular prognathism* or *condylar hyperplasia* is planned to adjust the length of the ramus with the condyle, modify the occlusal plane to function, and contour the inferior and lateral borders of the mandible to produce facial balance (see Figures 11–39 and 11–41). The surgery may be done intraorally or extraorally and must be designed to solve the chief presenting problems.

Surgical correction is done through standard approaches for an osteotomy to correct prognathism, and the only difference is in the extent to which the correction is made on each side. When an anterior open bite is associated with the prognathism, additional surgery or orthodontic treatment must be planned to correct the added problem (see Chapters 11 and 14). Long-standing mandibular asymmetry is frequently associated with some degree of secondary or incidental maxillary asymmetry. With careful and systematic diagnosis and treatment planning for the individual's three-dimensional problems, maxillary and mandibular surgery are frequently indicated to achieve optimum function, esthetics, and stability.

In Figure 11–39 are presented various methods for surgical correction of actively growing unilateral condylar hyperplasia and asymmetric mandibular prognathism. The plan of surgery in Figure 11–39*B* and *C* is a technique intended to arrest the continued excessive condylar growth and to correct the clinical manifestations of unilateral condylar hyperplasia. This plan includes the following: a Le Fort I osteotomy to level the maxillary occlusal plane, a condylectomy to arrest the continued condylar growth or to excise the neoplastic condyle, bilateral vertical ramus osteotomies to allow horizontal rotation of the mandible without significantly altering the temporomandibular articulations, an arthroplasty by superior repositioning of the pedicled stump of the proximal condylar segment into the condylar fossa, and a mandibuloplasty to restore the facial symmetry by differential excision of the bone from the inferior aspect of the mandible. (See Figures 11–44 to 11–46 for details of mandibuloplasty technique.) Arrows indicate the directional movement of the segments and cross-hatched areas indicate ostectomy sites (Fig. 11–39*B* and *C*).

The vertical ramus osteotomy is accomplished through the extraoral retromandibular approach, which affords excellent access to the entire ramus and decreases the potential trauma to the inferior branches of the facial nerve; the contralateral ramus is sectioned by intraoral vertical ramus osteotomy (Fig. 11–39*D*). In Figure 11–39*E*, subperiosteal exposure of the condylar neck and the enlarged condyle is seen with minimal detachment of the medial pterygoid muscles from the proximal segment. The muscle attachments serve as a vascular pedicle for the proximal segment after the condylectomy. The neck of the condylar process is sectioned with a fissure bur below the level of the tumor (Fig. 11–39*F*).

In an optional technique to remove the condyle, the proximal segment is completely freed from its soft tissue attachments and removed from the surgical site after the extraoral vertical ramus osteotomy in order to facilitate reshaping of the segment to the desired dimensions (Fig. 11–39*G* and *H*). The completely detached segment is used as a free bone graft that consolidates with the host bone, and remodels and maintains the normal condylar form. This procedure is technically easier to accomplish than pedicling the proximal segment to periosteum and muscle. Because the proximal segment is a free bone graft, however, the segment is slower to remodel and may be associated with more resorption and a higher incidence of infection. The wound is carefully closed to eliminate dead space and facilitate early revascularization of the segment. After sculpturing the distal portion of the residual "stump" of the proximal segment to simulate the form of the mandibular condyle, the segment is repositioned superiorly into the condylar fossa (Fig. 11–39*I*).

With the repositioned mandible and maxilla in intermaxillary fixation, the proximal condylar segment is fixed to the distal segment with interosseous wires (Fig. 11–39*J*). An interocclusal splint is used as a template for mandibular positioning at surgery and during fixation. A costochondral graft may be used to restore temporomandibular articulation when the residual proximal segment is too small to replace the excised condyle or if the condyle is congenitally missing (Fig. 11–39*K*).

Figure 11–39*L* shows the maxillomandibular relationship after surgery. The maxilla, mandible, and chin have been repositioned into line with the midsagittal plane of the face.

In Figure 11–39*M–S*, condylectomy and modified sagittal split ramus osteotomy are used for the surgical correction of actively growing unilateral condylar hyperplasia or condylar neoplasm. (This is the technique of Dr. Frank Pavel of San Diego, California.) The plan of surgery includes a Le Fort I osteotomy to level the maxillary occlusal plane, a condylectomy accomplished through preauricular incision to arrest continued mandibular growth or to resect a condylar neoplasm (Fig. 11–39*O*); bilateral sagittal split ramus osteotomies to allow horizontal rotation and posterior retrusion of mandible without significantly altering the temporomandibular articulations; and, after the condylectomy and sagittal split ramus osteotomy, a reshaping of the condylar stump of the proximal segment to simulate the form and size of the contralateral mandibular condyle (Fig. 11–39*P*). A portion of the sigmoid notch may be excised to increase the relative length of the newly created condylar neck; the proximal segment is then repositioned superiorly into the condylar fossa and fixed to the distal segment (Fig. 11–39*Q* and *R*).

Nongrowing unilateral condylar hyperplasia or asymmetric mandibular prognathism is treated by intraoral vertical ramus osteotomies and other jaw surgery. Condylectomy in such individuals is indicated only when intolerable functional problems are present as a consequence of the enlarged condyle (Fig. 11–39*S*).

The correction of asymmetric mandibular prognathism is shown in Figure 11–39*U* and *V*. The plan of surgery includes the following: bilateral intraoral vertical ramus osteotomies to allow horizontal rotation of mandible into Class I canine occlusion without significantly altering temporomandibular articulations, genioplasty to reposition chin into line with midsagittal plane of the skull and face (for additional details, see Chapter 14); and maxillary surgery, if indicated, for correction of canting of the occlusal plane and any other associated maxillary vertical dysplasia. Canting of the maxillary occlusal plane is not a dominant feature of asymmetric mandibular prognathism. The maxillomandibular relationship after surgery can be seen in Figure 11–39*W* and *X*. The mandible and chin have been repositioned into line with the midsagittal plane of the face and skull.

Text continued on page 969.

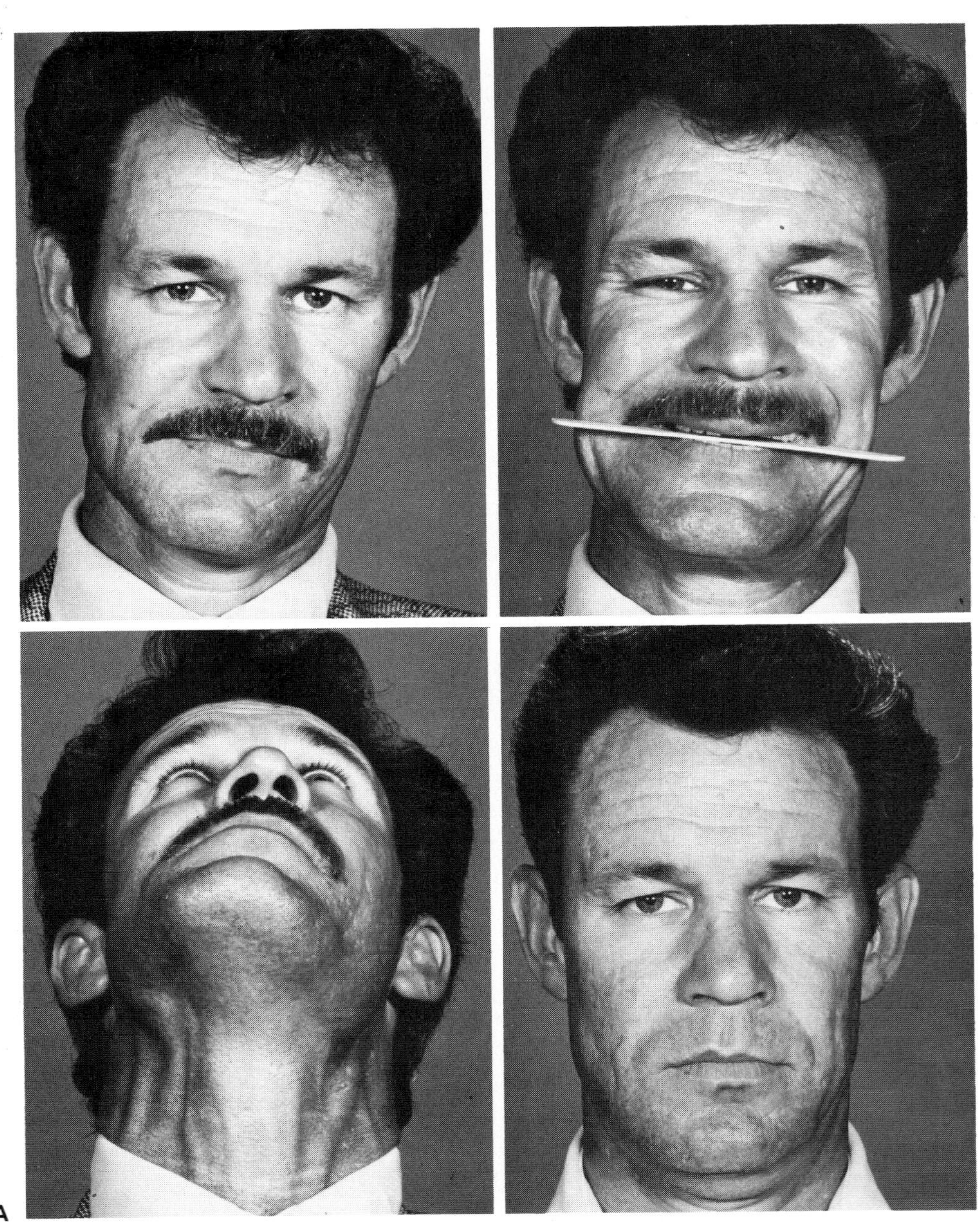

Figure 11–39. *A*, Typical facial appearance of patient with unilateral condylar hyperplasia who manifests facial asymmetry in all three planes of space and aberrant natural head posture. Upper left and right and lower left before surgery; lower right after surgery. (*Surgeon:* William H. Bell.)

Legend continued on the opposite page.

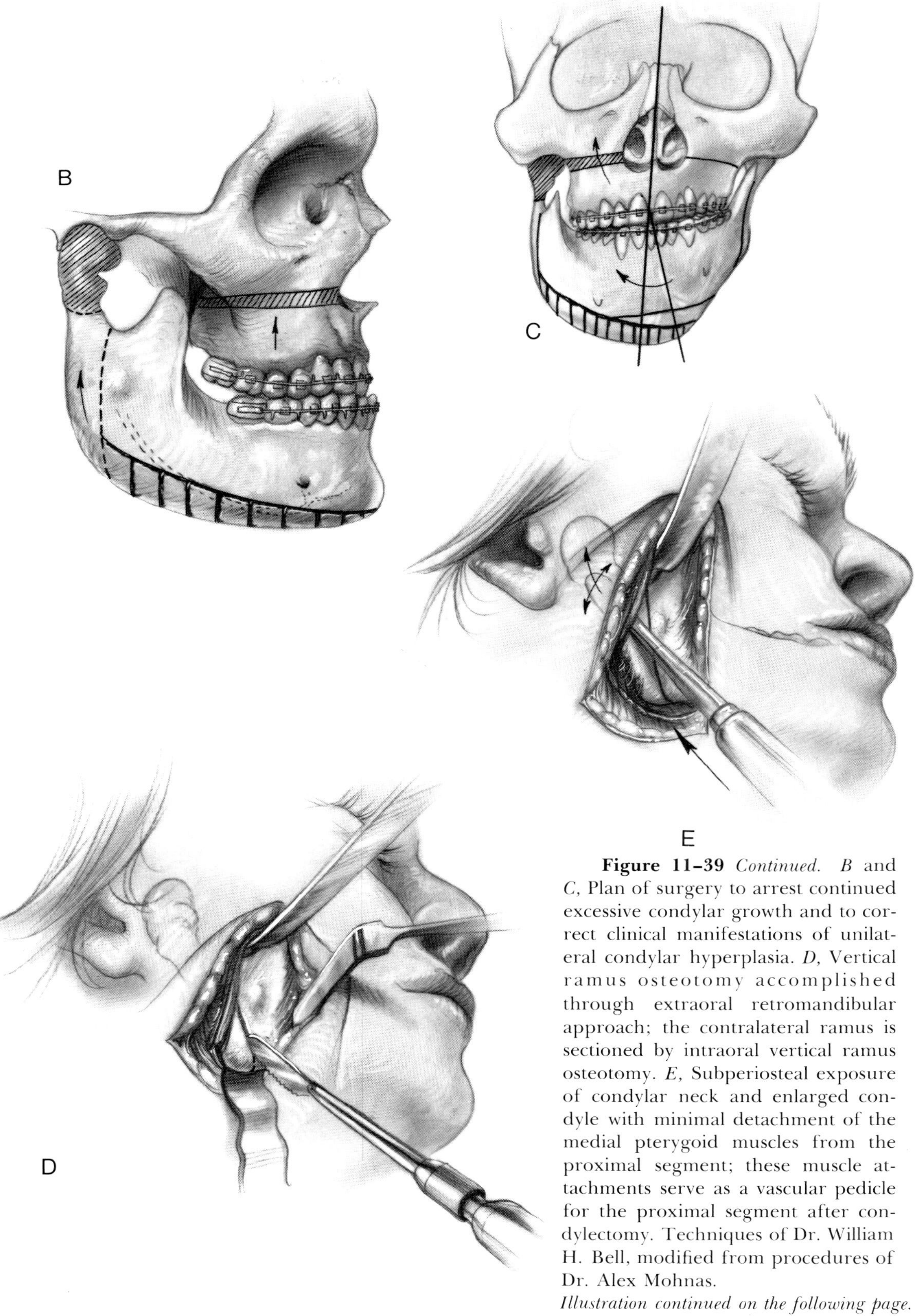

Figure 11–39 *Continued.* *B* and *C,* Plan of surgery to arrest continued excessive condylar growth and to correct clinical manifestations of unilateral condylar hyperplasia. *D,* Vertical ramus osteotomy accomplished through extraoral retromandibular approach; the contralateral ramus is sectioned by intraoral vertical ramus osteotomy. *E,* Subperiosteal exposure of condylar neck and enlarged condyle with minimal detachment of the medial pterygoid muscles from the proximal segment; these muscle attachments serve as a vascular pedicle for the proximal segment after condylectomy. Techniques of Dr. William H. Bell, modified from procedures of Dr. Alex Mohnas.

Illustration continued on the following page.

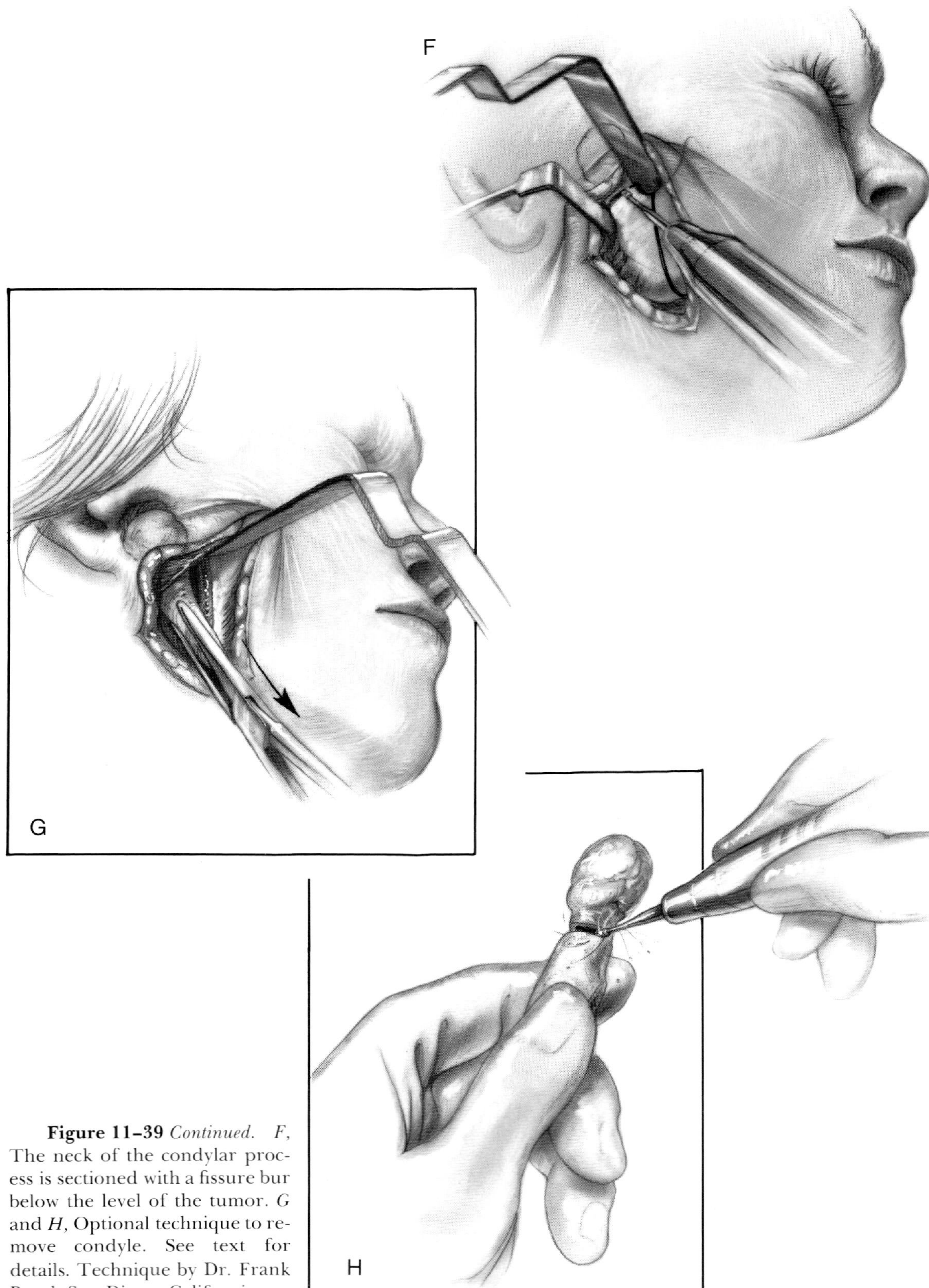

Figure 11–39 *Continued.* *F*, The neck of the condylar process is sectioned with a fissure bur below the level of the tumor. *G* and *H*, Optional technique to remove condyle. See text for details. Technique by Dr. Frank Pavel, San Diego, California.

Legend continued on the opposite page.

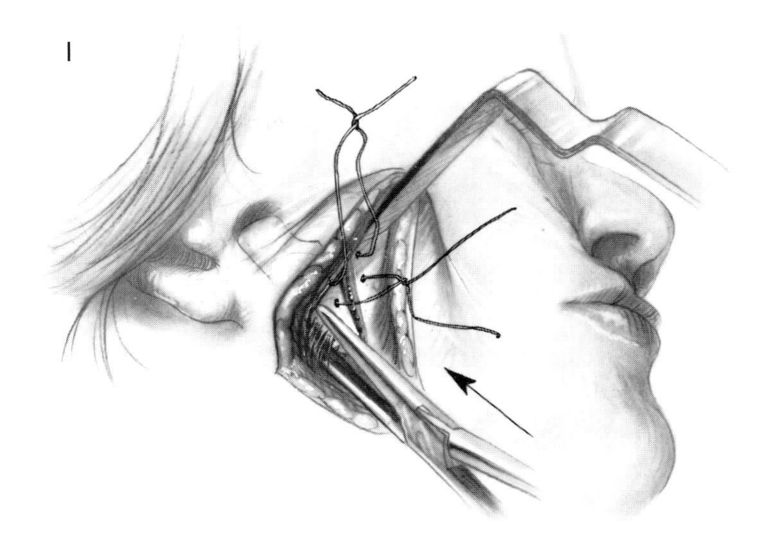

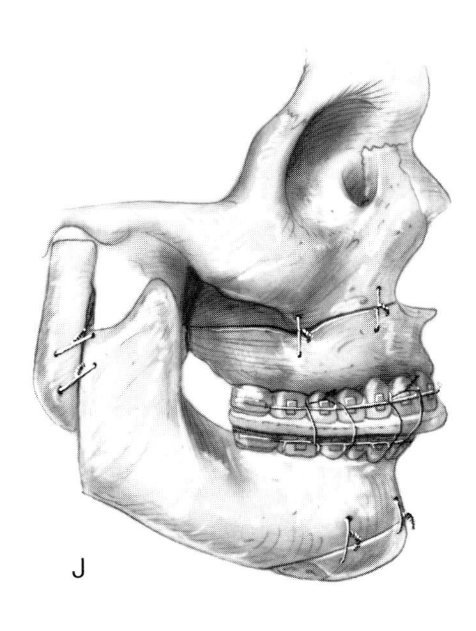

Figure 11–39 *Continued.* *I,* The segment is repositioned superiorly into the condylar fossa. *J,* The proximal condylar segment is fixed to the distal segment with interosseous wires. An interocclusal splint is used as a template for mandibular positioning at surgery and during fixation. *K,* A costochondral graft may be used to restore temporomandibular articulation when the residual proximal segment is too small to replace the excised condyle or if the condyle is congenitally missing.

Illustration continued on the following page.

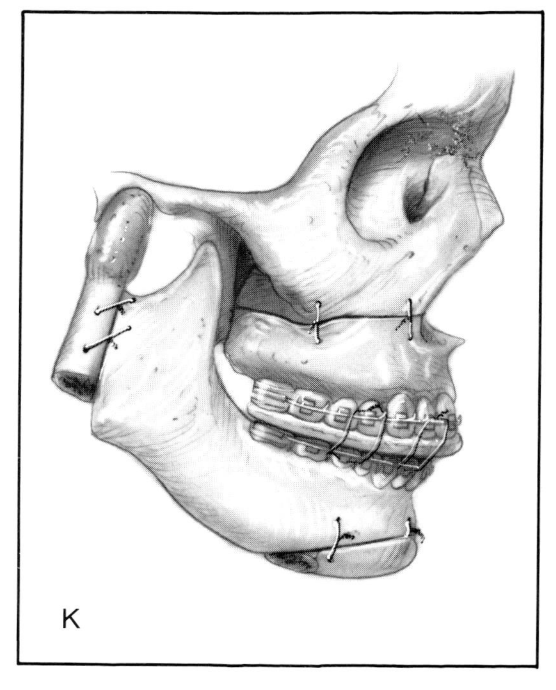

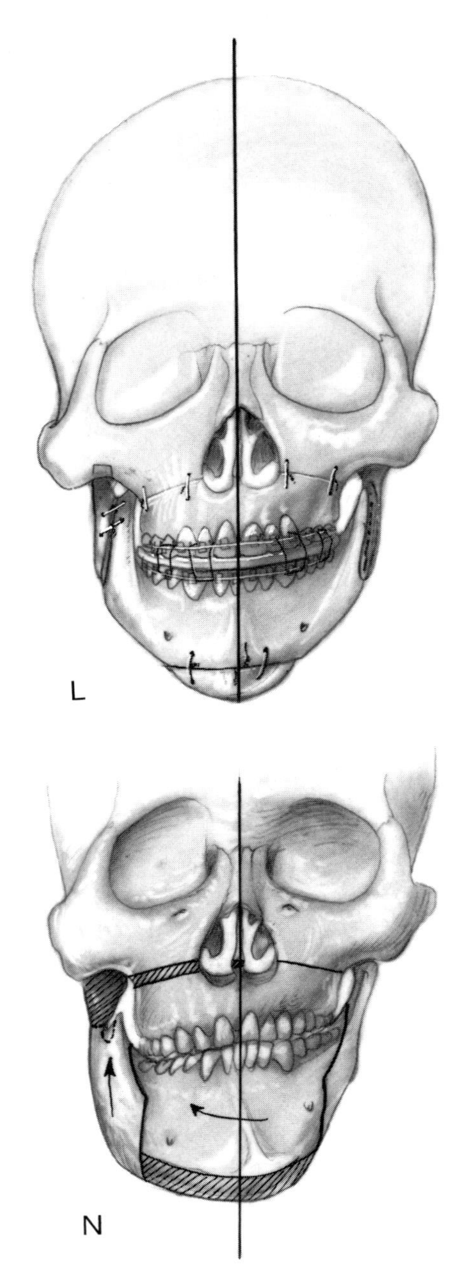

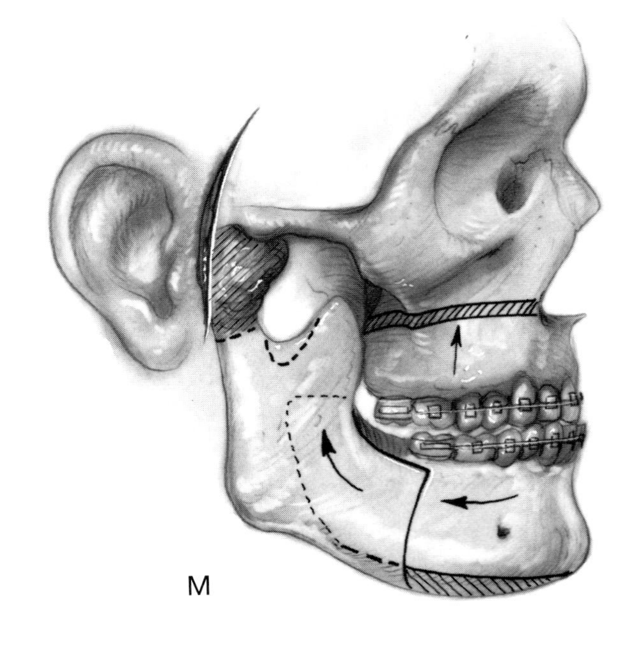

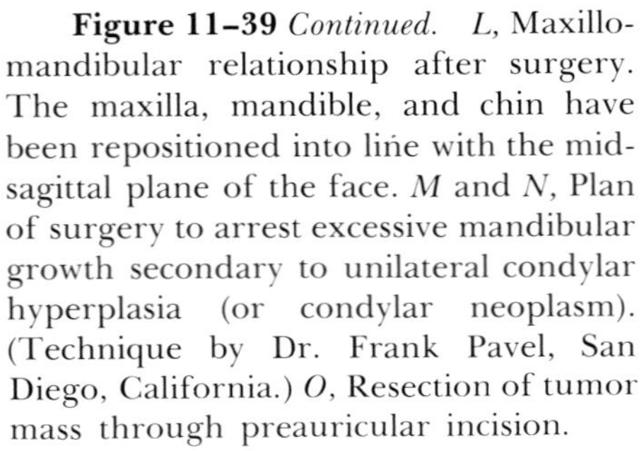

Figure 11–39 *Continued.* *L,* Maxillomandibular relationship after surgery. The maxilla, mandible, and chin have been repositioned into line with the midsagittal plane of the face. *M* and *N,* Plan of surgery to arrest excessive mandibular growth secondary to unilateral condylar hyperplasia (or condylar neoplasm). (Technique by Dr. Frank Pavel, San Diego, California.) *O,* Resection of tumor mass through preauricular incision.

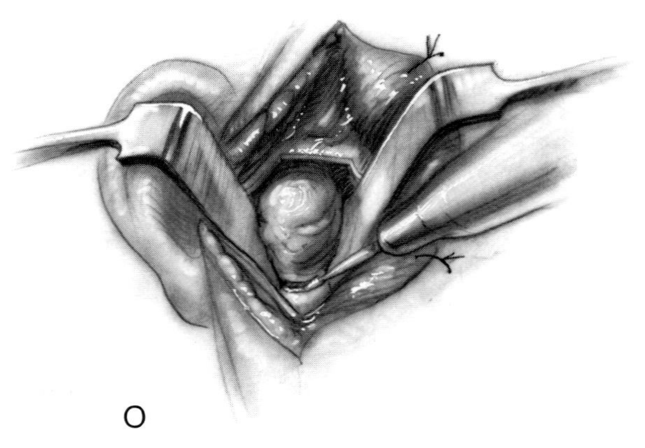

Legend continued on the opposite page.

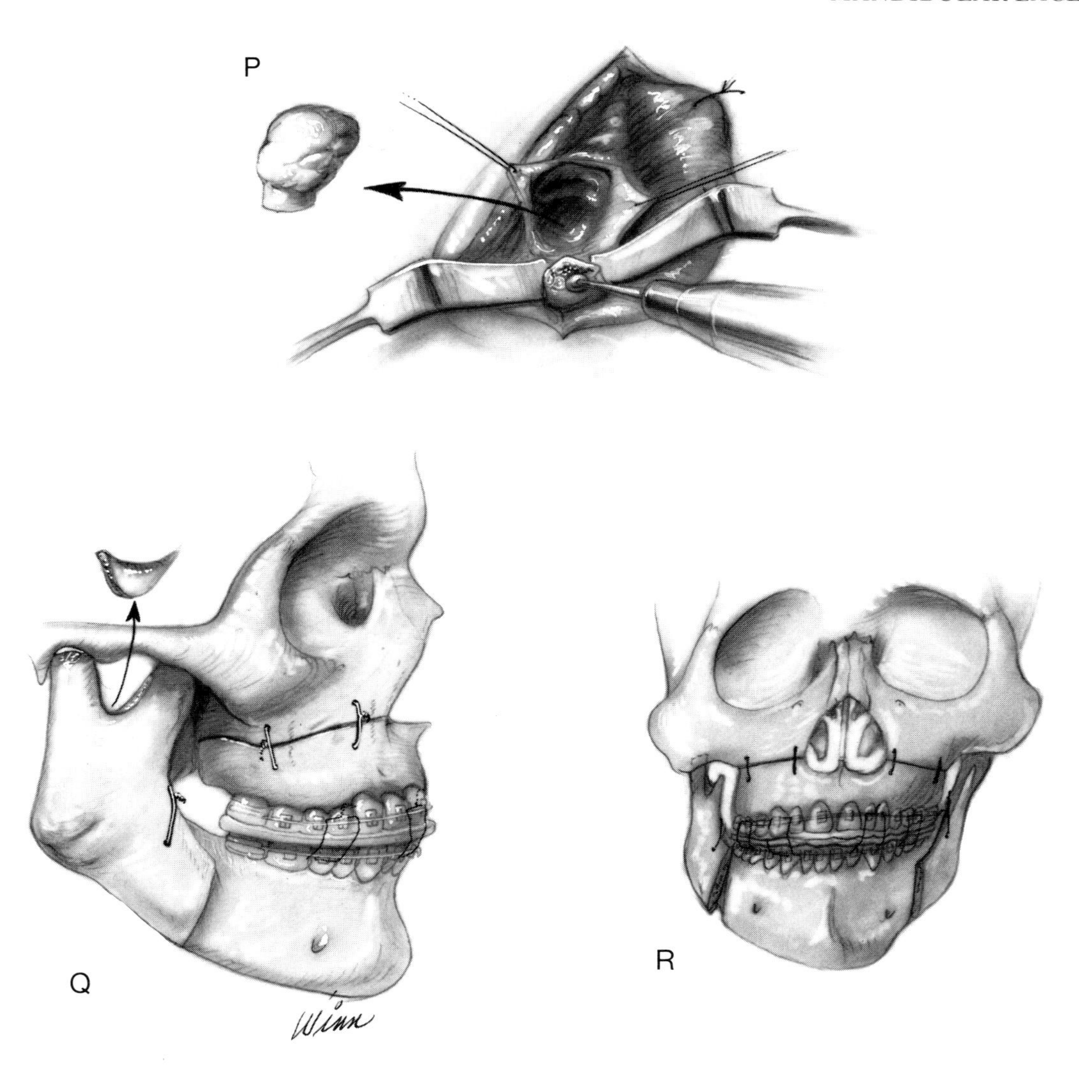

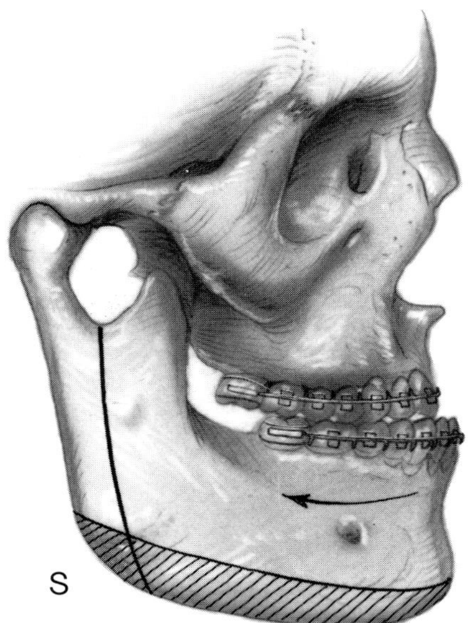

Figure 11–39 *Continued. P,* The condylar neck "stump" is reshaped to simulate the form and size of the contralateral mandibular condyle. *Q* and *R,* A portion of the sigmoid notch may be excised to increase the relative length of the newly created condylar neck; the proximal segment is then repositioned superiorly into the condylar fossa and fixed to the distal segment. *S,* Nongrowing individuals with unilateral condylar hyperplasia or asymmetric mandibular prognathism are treated by intraoral vertical ramus osteotomies and other jaw surgery.

Illustration continued on the following page.

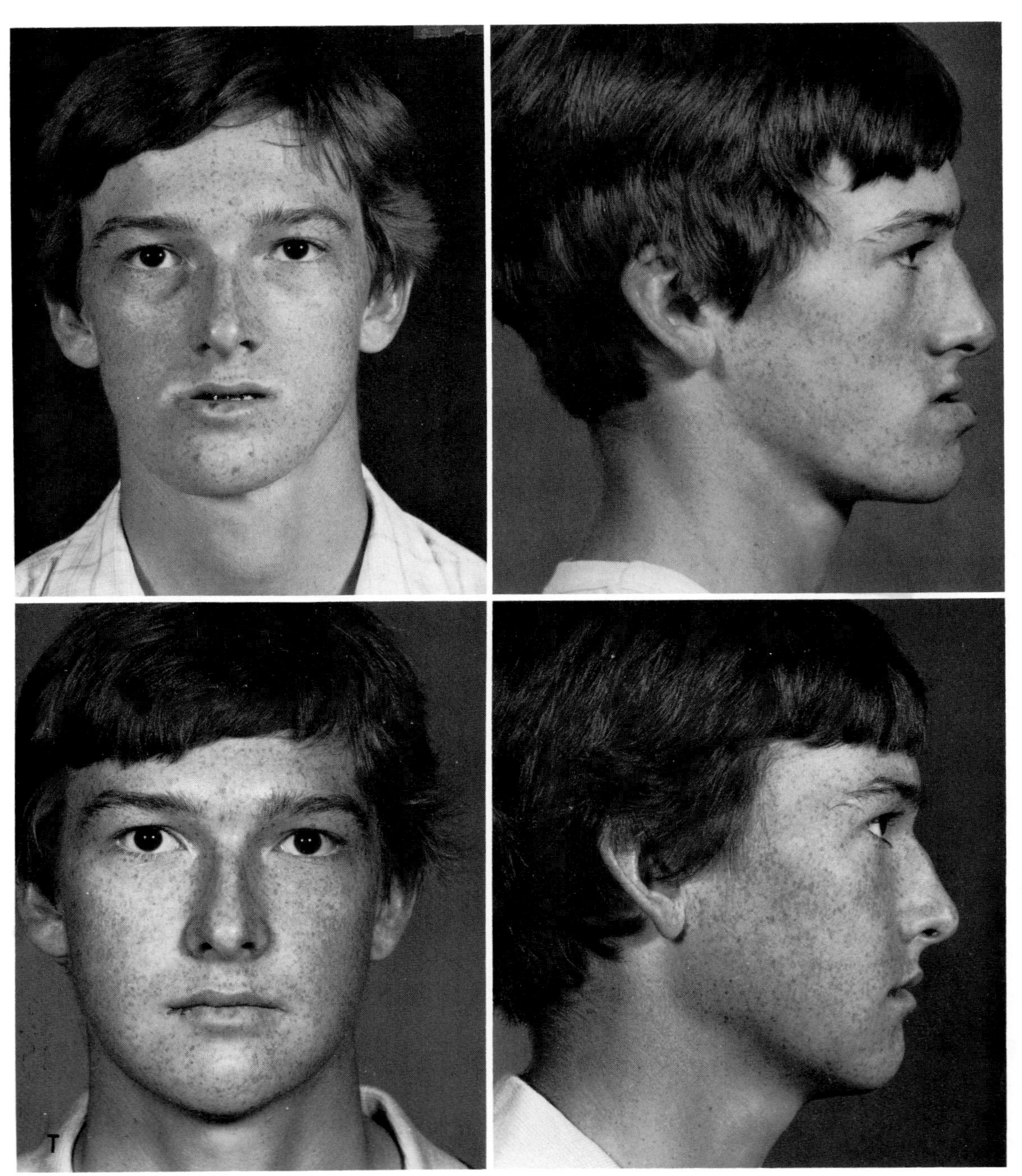

Figure 11–39 *Continued.* *T*, Typical facial appearance of patient with asymmetric mandibular prognathism. (Before and after surgery illustrated in *U* to *X*). (*Surgeon:* William H. Bell.)

Legend continued on the opposite page.

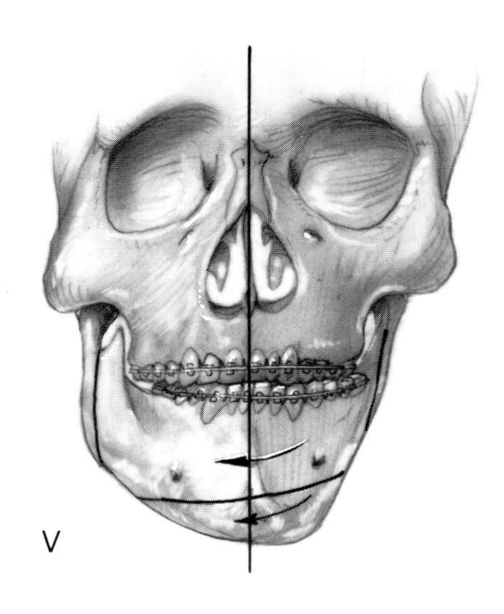

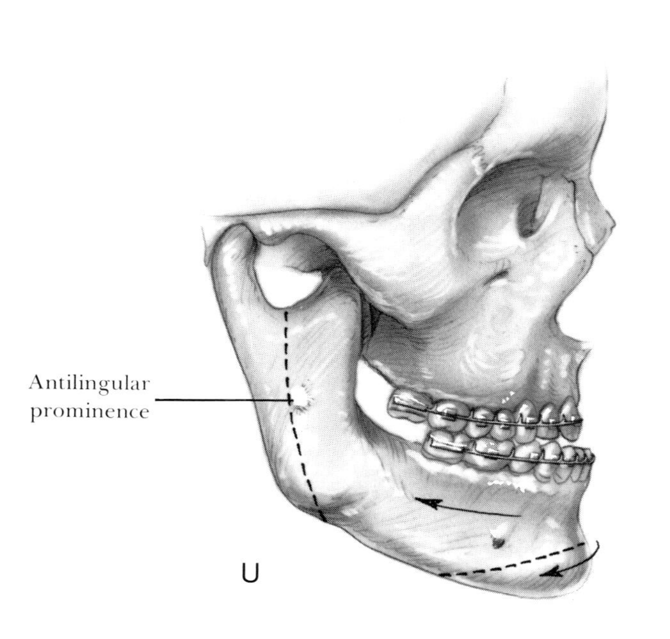

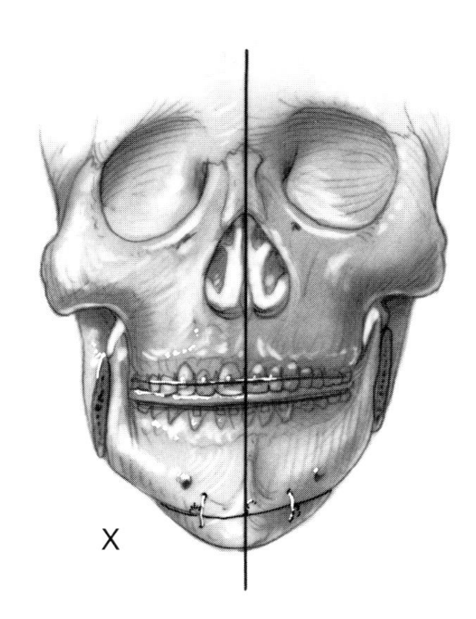

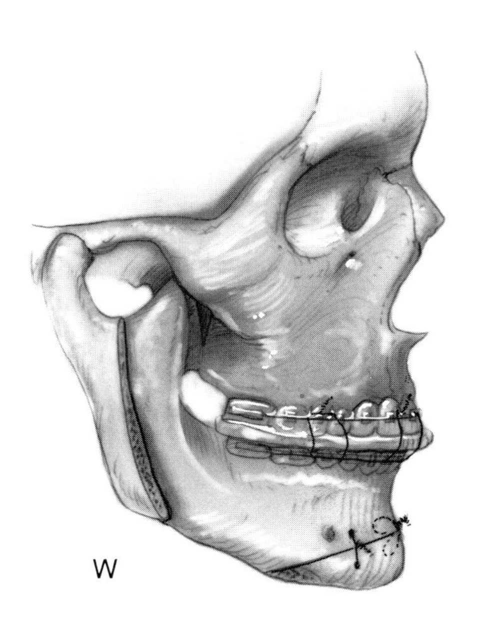

Figure 11–39 *Continued.* *U* and *V*, Plan of surgery to correct clinical manifestations of asymmetric mandibular prognathism. *W* and *X*. Maxillomandibular relationship after surgery. The mandible and chin have been repositioned into line with the midsagittal plane of the face and skull.

Illustration continued on the following page.

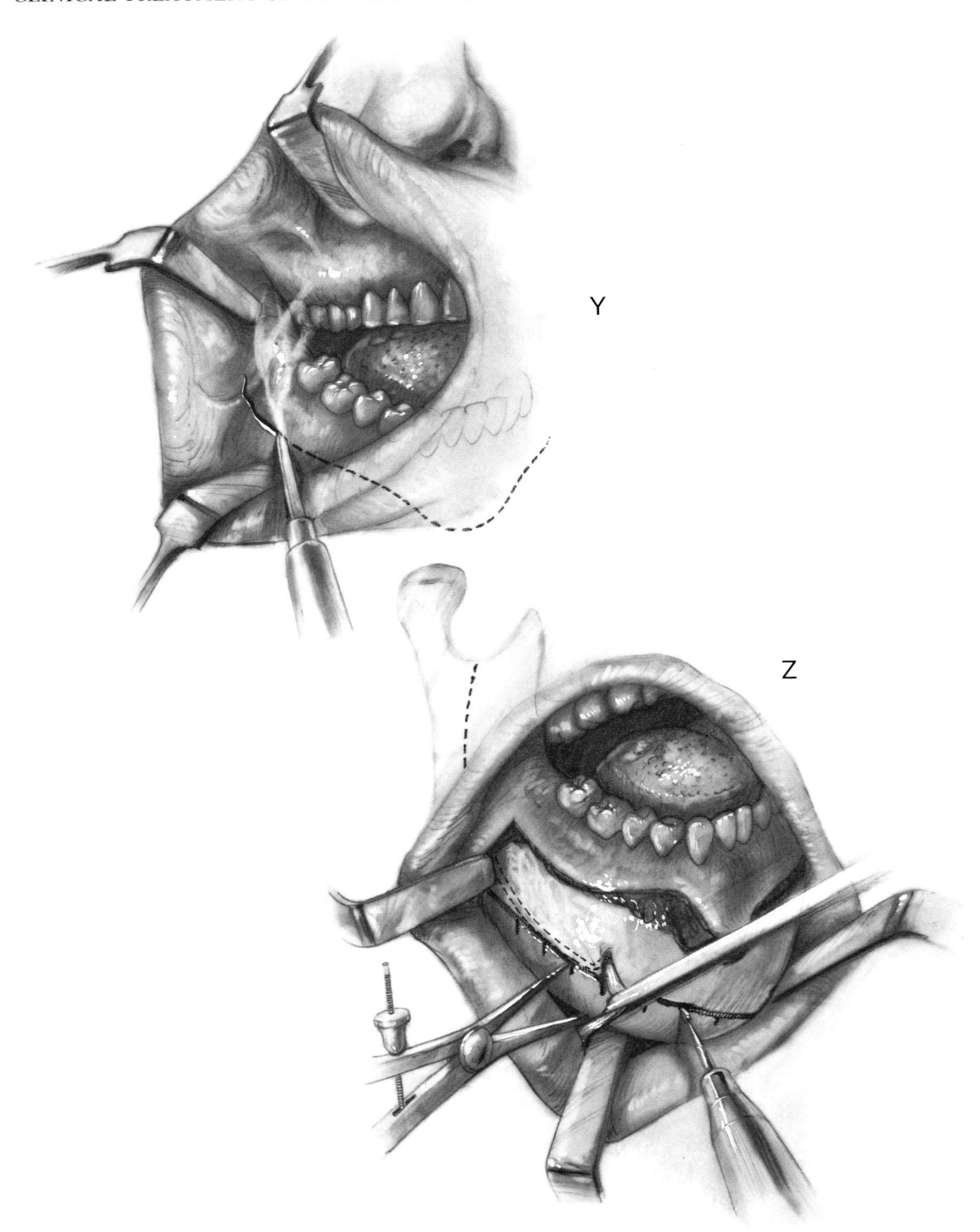

Figure 11–39 *Continued.* *Y–HH,* Intraoral removal of bowing of angle, body, and symphysis of mandible associated with either condylar hyperplasia or unilateral macrognathism. *Y,* The entire lateral surface of the mandible and mental symphysis is exposed through a circumvestibular incision. *Z,* Direct measurements are made with calipers and marked with a bur. Seven or eight marks are inscribed along the bowed mandible.

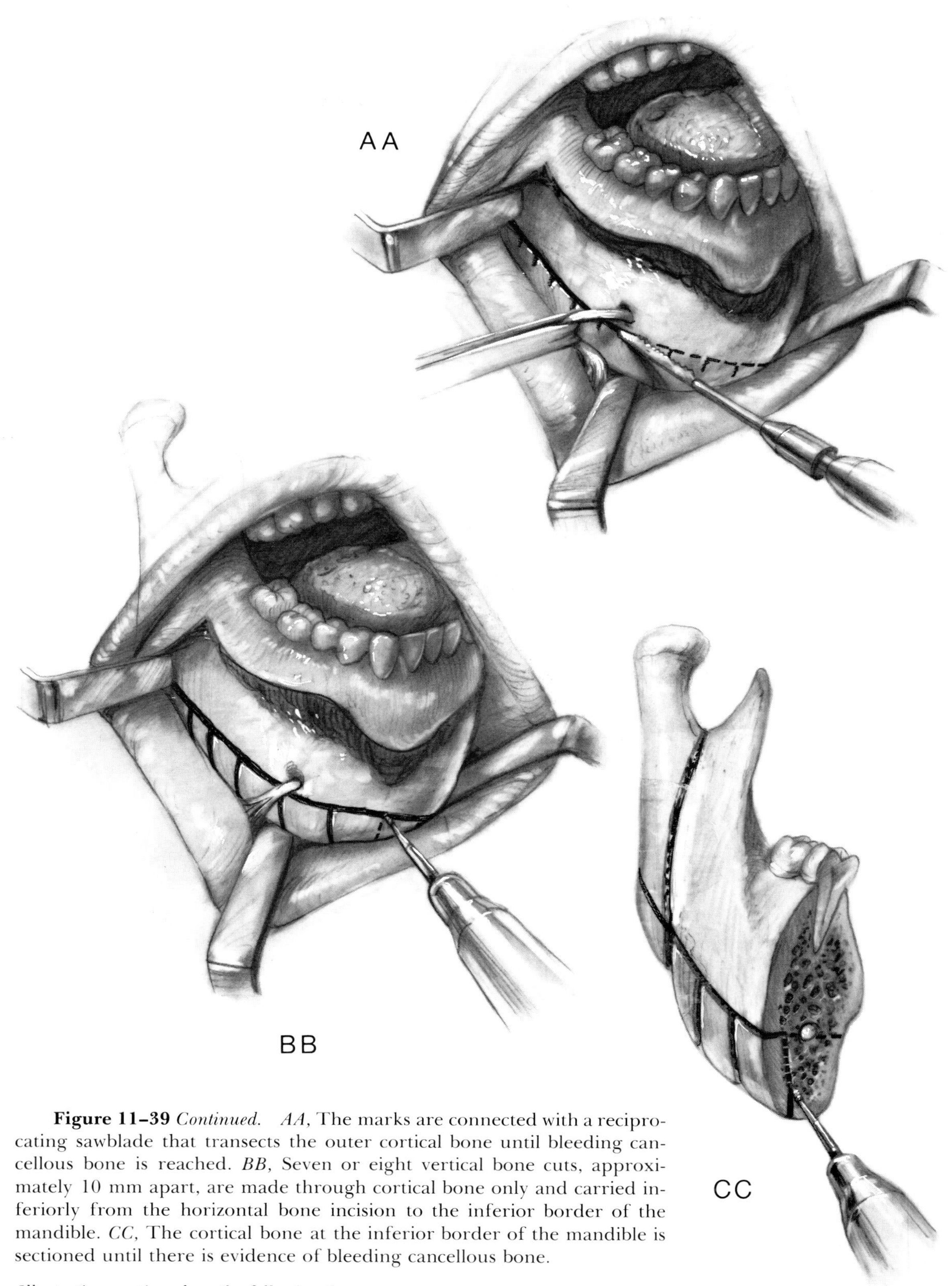

Figure 11–39 *Continued.* *AA,* The marks are connected with a reciprocating sawblade that transects the outer cortical bone until bleeding cancellous bone is reached. *BB,* Seven or eight vertical bone cuts, approximately 10 mm apart, are made through cortical bone only and carried inferiorly from the horizontal bone incision to the inferior border of the mandible. *CC,* The cortical bone at the inferior border of the mandible is sectioned until there is evidence of bleeding cancellous bone.

Illustration continued on the following page.

Figure 11–39 *Continued. DD,* A spatula osteotome is malleted into the corticocancellous junction (1) and manipulated (2) to pry the squares of cortical bone away from the underlying cancellous bone. *EE,* A curette is used to lift away cancellous bone overlying the thin bony lamina. The neurovascular bundle is exposed by lifting away the thin overlying bony lamina with a curette. *FF,* The entire length of the lingual cortical plate of bone is removed with a reciprocating saw blade or #703 fissure bur. *GG,* Postoperative result. Technique of Dr. Robert V. Walker, Dallas, Texas.

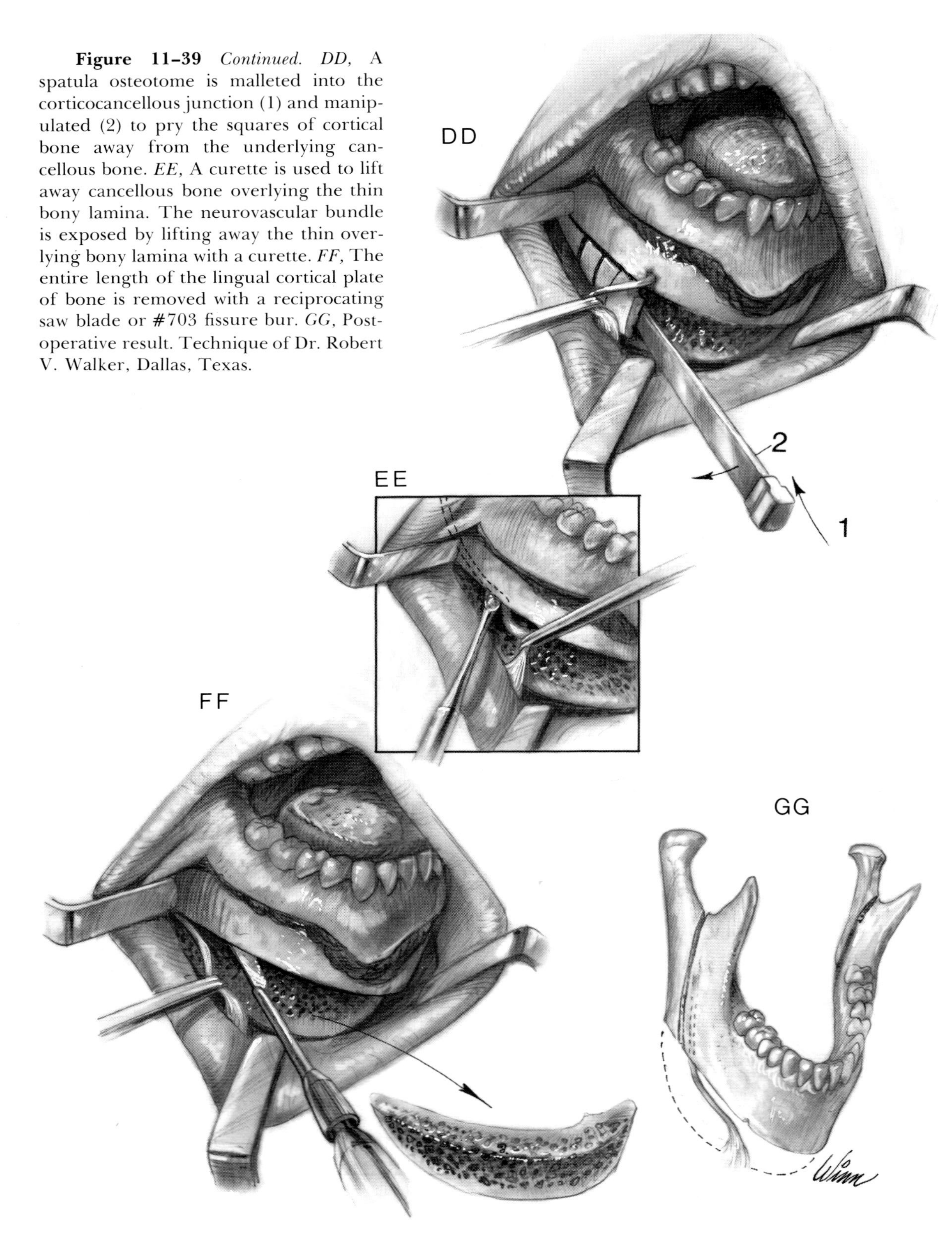

The procedure for the intraoral removal of bowing of the angle, body, and symphysis of the mandible associated with either condylar hyperplasia or unilateral macrognathism is shown in Figure 11–39*Y–GG*. The entire lateral surface of the mandible and the mental symphysis is exposed through a circumvestibular incision extending from the 2nd molar region of one side to the contralateral premolar region. Care is taken to protect the mental nerve emerging from its foramen.

The amount and location of bone to be excised from the bowed mandible is determined from a panoramic radiograph. Based upon these preoperative calculations, the projected horizontal bone cut is inscribed into the lateral aspect of the mandible. Direct measurements are made with calipers from the inferior margin of the mandible to the appropriate places along the lateral surface of the mandible and marked with a bur (Fig. 11–39*Z*). The mental nerve and foramen serve as landmarks from whence to begin marking the lateral surface of the mandible. Seven or eight marks are inscribed along the bowed mandible at the various heights derived from the measurements on the preoperative tracing.

The marks are connected with a reciprocating sawblade that transects the outer cortical bone until bleeding cancellous bone is reached (Fig. 11–39*AA*). Seven or eight vertical bone cuts, approximately 10 mm apart, are made through cortical bone only and carried inferiorly from the horizontal bone incision to the inferior border of the mandible (Fig. 11–39*BB*). The cortical bone at the inferior border of the mandible is sectioned until there is evidence of bleeding cancellous bone (Fig. 11–39*CC*).

As seen in Figure 11–39*DD*, a spatula osteotome is malleted into the corticocancellous junction and manipulated to pry the squares of cortical bone away from the underlying cancellous bone. After all of the cortical bony squares are removed, a curette is used to lift away the cancellous bone overlying the thin bony lamina that makes up the neurovascular canal (Fig. 11–39*EE*). The neurovascular bundle is exposed by carefully lifting away the thin overlying bony lamina with a curette. With the neurovascular bundle retracted with a Penrose drain, the entire length of the lingual cortical plate of bone is removed with a reciprocating saw blade or a #703 fissure bur. The superoinferior height of the excised lingual cortical bone should approximately equal the amount of bone removed laterally (Fig. 11–39*FF*). In Figure 11–39*GG*, the postoperative result is shown.

Condylar Hyperplasia

Robert V. Walker

Isolated condylar hyperplasia that occurs unilaterally after maturation of the bony skeleton causes a distinct shift in the midline and produces a crossbite malocclusion on the opposite side. The contour of the mandibular arch generally still matches that of the maxilla; the mandible and teeth are simply displaced bodily by a late or delayed condylar enlargement.

In deciding whether to perform a condylectomy or to retain the condyle and shorten the ramus by osteotomy, the clinician must consider the following factors: (1) the duration of the condition and adjustments that have taken place in the dentition to compensate for it; (2) evidence of active change in the hyperplastic condyle; (3) radiographic or clinical suggestions of chondroma, osteoma, or other neoplastic conditions. If a condyle is mature and stable, has a normal functional excursion within the joint, and shows an unequivocal cessation of its progressive increase in size, an osteotomy to shorten the ramus is indicated. Thus, the enlarged condyle that functions normally within the temporomandibular joint is left intact. If serial radiographs indicate progression in size of the condyle or if a patient notices rather early that the jaw is shifting and causing an asymmetry, the condition can reasonably be diagnosed as condylar hyperplasia. Excision of the rapidly growing condyle is the treatment of choice. The active lesion should be removed.

No one knows what triggers a condyle suddenly to start growing and become hyperplastic, and no one knows how long such active growth continues. From an accurate history given by the patient, the study of recent photographs, and conferences with the patient's dentist, one can gain a reasonable idea of the duration of the condition. It is believed that the rapid growth process lasts at least 4 years and perhaps as long as 6 or 7 years. When the jaw has moved rapidly in adulthood, the compensations of tooth movement and alveolar growth are not a major, immediate part of the problem.

Lengthening of the condylar neck or overall increase in size of the condyle are the usual causes for the mandible's being moved to the opposite side, resulting in a crossbite, deflected chin, tilting, and similar associated conditions. Accordingly, if the lengthening of the involved condyle that caused the jaw shift has been accurately measured, that amount can be cut from the top of the condyle to allow the mandible to move back to its normal position. By removing the top of the condyle, the actively growing site is removed and the whole process is stopped without producing a greater deformity. The amount of bone to be removed from a condyle is determined from transpharyngeal radiographs made of both temporomandibular joints in the closed and open positions of the mandible.[28] The x-ray head should not be angulated more than 2 or 3 degrees upward from the horizontal in making the views of the two sides. Exactly the same angulation should be used on both sides. By tracing the condyle, sigmoid notch, coronoid process, and ramus areas of both sides, a straight anteroposterior line can be drawn that touches the very top of the condyle. By drawing a similar line paralleling the upper one and touching the very lowest swing of the sigmoid notch, the overall length of the condyle and its neck on each side can then be measured in millimeters between the parallel lines (see Figures 11–43 and 11–45). By subtracting the lesser figure on the normal side from the greater figure on the hyperplastic side, an acceptable determination of the increased length of the condyle and condylar neck on the involved side can easily be made. This figure can be used at surgery as a reliable guide to the amount of the condylar top to be removed. Calipers are used at surgery to measure from the top of the condyle downward to the predetermined level for the bone cut. Occasionally, removal of the condyle alone will not allow the mandible to move back to its original posture. In such an instance, an intraoral vertical ramus osteotomy of the opposite ramus will permit an easier positioning of the mandible even though an accurate length of condyle and condylar neck has been excised on the involved side. Judgment at surgery dictates whether or not this relief will be needed on the side opposite the condylectomy.

EXCISION OF THE CONDYLE

Removal of the condyle is best done from a preauricular approach (Figs. 11–39 and 11–40). Direct vertical measurements from the top of the condyle downward are much easier to make and more accurate than measurements made from a submandibular ap-

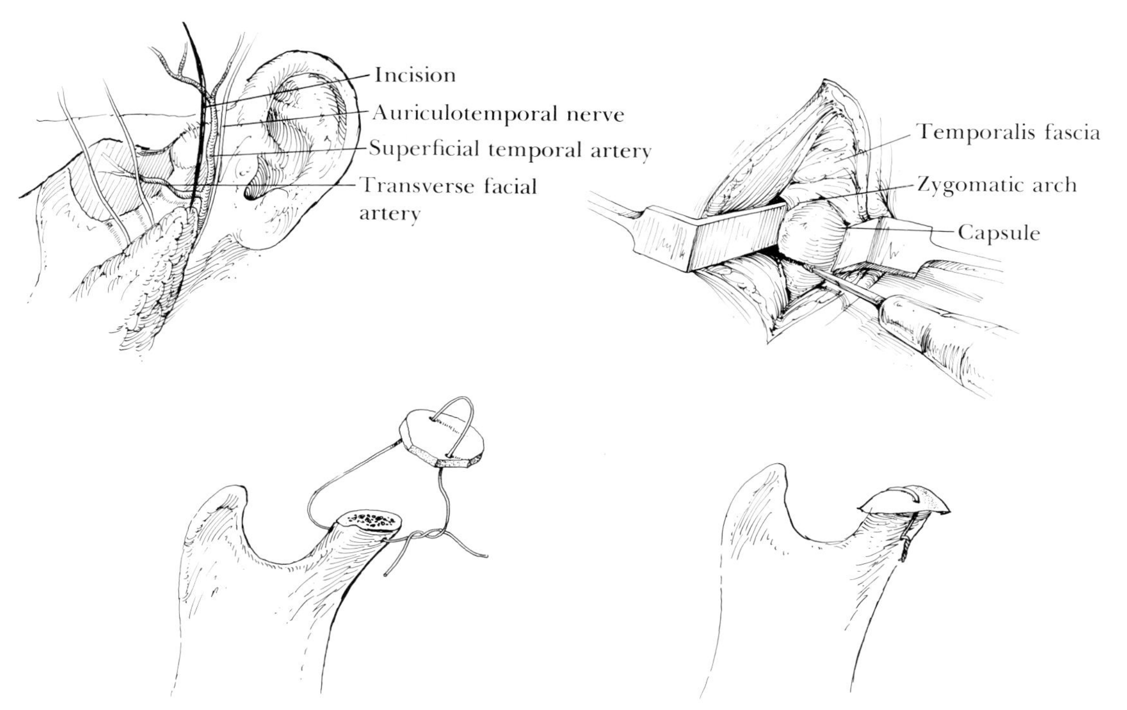

Figure 11–40. Diagrams depicting the preauricular incision for excision of a condylar head; the subperiosteal, subcapsular placement of narrow, right-angled retractors while cutting through the condylar neck; the fitting and scheme for wiring in a posteroanterior direction of a Silastic disk atop the condylar neck; and the firm cinching down of the Silastic disk atop the condylar neck.

proach. There will hardly ever be reason for removing only a 5-mm superior-inferior portion of the condyle, but a section of this size is sufficient to include the actively growing epiphyseal-like cartilage that is the cause of the deformity and asymmetry. Removing this cartilage stops the process of growth, and if the entire cartilage is included in the specimen and removed, the lesion will not recur.

Rehabilitation of the joint and jaw to normal use is done in exactly the same manner as described for habilitating or restoring incuspation of occlusion after moving the jaw back to its usual position. The patient is *required* to increase the incisal opening of the jaw progressively during the postoperative period. If the patient is reluctant, positive jaw levering maneuvers are instituted. Jaw opening has to be regained early and maintained through the minimum three-month period of physiotherapy. Happily, this is not difficult to achieve following removal of a normally moving condyle and is not comparable to the difficult period of physiotherapy that must follow an arthroplasty for relief of ankylosis. Night elastics are used as described earlier. The cut end of the condylar stump covers with cortical bone and remodels itself to the demands of jaw movement and the contours of the articular fossa and eminence. If the cut end of the condylar stump is covered with a Silastic disk or other alloplastic material, remodeling often occurs beneath the replacement part and also within the articular fossa. This remodeling, again, takes place according to the demands of jaw movement and the articular parts. Radiographs taken serially over a few years show redone joints to be constantly changing even though symptoms are seldom experienced by the patient.

Unilateral Macrognathism

The classic features of unilateral macrognathism include enlargement of the entire side of the mandible. There is a downward bending of the long inferior border of the mandible and a loss of lateral convexity in the premolar area of the mandible on the same side. The occlusal plane is dropped downward, and the vertical dimension of bone in the body of the mandible is excessive, reflecting the compensatory mechanisms of the erupting mandibular posterior teeth and the supporting alveolar process. The anterior teeth are tipped so that their long axes are directed toward the involved side. The overall downward contour of the concave occlusal plane of the mandible is matched by the convexity of the dropped maxillary occlusal plane, where the teeth have continually erupted downward in an effort to maintain their functional position.

Whether or not an osteotomy of the ramus is needed to shift the position of the mandible will depend in part upon the degree to which occlusal compensation has been successful through the years of growth disparity. If the arches are fully functional and the only malformation is a disparity of the occlusal plane, contouring of the inferior border of the mandible may be the only surgery that is necessary. Such an osteotomy-ostectomy would reduce the extreme downward contour of the body of the mandible. If necessary, the bone removed can be added at another site to improve contour. If an open bite is present and there is lack of posterior function, an osteotomy of the mandibular ramus may be required. This osteotomy may be either unilateral or bilateral, depending upon the degree of shift in the mandibular muscular suspension that is required to restore symmetry. Small adjustments may require only a unilateral procedure, whereas major shifts will require bilateral ramus osteotomies. The condyle that is not operated upon will tolerate rotations of 10 to 15 degrees as the mandible is swung toward the opposite side by a unilateral osteotomy in the ramus.

If the condyle is especially large and functions poorly, a condylectomy may be required along with an osteotomy of the contralateral ramus. In such a case, the matter of adjusting the occlusal plane by intruding the maxilla may also be considered. The question of contouring the inferior and lateral borders of the mandible depends entirely upon the esthetic goals of surgery and the correction that has been obtained by a shift of the suspended mandible via the ramus changes. Combinations of horizontal and vertical osteotomies for this correction have been reported. The correction of the vertical ramus and of the inferior border may be done entirely from either an intraoral approach (see Figure 11–45) or an extraoral approach (see Figures 11–39, 11–44 and 11–46). Surgical access from an intraoral approach provides excellent visualization of the surgical site, obviates a long extraoral incision, and is our preferred method.

The technical duties of calculating the amount of bone to be removed from a downward bow of the mandible and then excising that amount of excess bone are crucial. Panoramic radiographs, which produce the least distortion of mandible and tooth size, have proved adequate to determine the location and amount of bone to be excised from the bowed mandible.

A direct tracing is made of the entire mandible, the teeth, and the neurovascular canal (Figs. 11–45*E* and 11–46*K*). Vertical lines are drawn from the crest of alveolar bone (assuming there is no abnormal resorption present) between teeth to the inferior margin of the mandible at five or six places on each side. Direct measurement in millimeters of the lengths of these lines will obviously vary from an area on the bowed side to the same comparable area on the opposite or normal side. By continuing the measuring of vertical lines at comparable areas on both sides and subtracting the lesser number marked off on the normal size from the greater number marked off on the bowed side, the exact amount of bone to be excised all along the inferior portion of the bowed mandible can be determined in millimeters. As illustrated, the amount will vary at different areas.

Next, a line depicting the projected line of the bone cut on the bowed side of the mandible can be drawn by measuring upward from the inferior border of the mandible using the already determined millimeter differences at the various areas. Making a dot at each of these points on the tracing and then connecting them with a linear line in an anteroposterior direction provides an adequate depiction of the bone to be removed along the inferior border of the mandible. Almost always, the neurovascular canal will be found to swing downward into the bowed area of bone projected for removal. The relationship of the projected cut to the apices of the teeth is easily discerned.

The measurements are used at surgery, and whether the entire lateral surface of the mandible is bared extraorally or intraorally, direct measurements are made with calipers from the inferior margin of the mandible to the appropriate places along the lateral surface of the mandible and marked with a bur (see Figures 11–44*F* and 11–45*F*). In reflecting the periosteum upward or downward depending upon the extraoral or intraoral approach, care is given to protect the mental nerve emerging from its foramen. If the mandible is approached extraorally, the mental nerve and foramen serve as excellent landmarks from whence to begin marking the lateral surface of the mandible. After seven or eight marks are inscribed along the bowed mandible at the various heights derived from the measurements on the preoperative tracing, the marks are connected with a No. 6 round bur or a No. 703 crosscut fissure bur. These cuts are made through the *outer cortical bone only*. When bleeding cancellous bone is reached, the deepening of the bone cut must be stopped. Vertical cuts approximately 10 mm apart are then made downward from this long anteroposterior bone cut to the inferior border of the mandible. There will be seven or eight of these vertical cuts, which are also made through cortical bone only (see Figures 11–44*F* and 11–46*M*). When these cuts are completed, the several squares of cortical bone separated by cuts to the cancellous layer give a "waffled" appearance to the area. A chisel or other heavy, narrow-bladed instrument is used to pry these squares of cortical bone and lever them away from the underlying cancellous bone. (See Fig. 11–39*Y–GG*.)

After removal of all cortical bony squares, a curette is then used to discreetly lift away the cancellous bone overlying the thin bony lamina that makes up the neurovascular canal. This thin lamina can be carefully picked and lifted away from the neurovascular bundle without damage to the bundle using small double-ended curettes and a thin-bladed periosteal elevator. The connective tissue that makes up the covering wall of the neurovascular bundle has great elasticity. After the bony lamina covering the bundle is removed, the bundle's inherent elasticity draws it upward to lie at the highest point of the bony operative wound (see Figure 11–44*H* and 11–46*N*). While the neurovascular bundle is protected with a retractor, the lingual cortical plate of bone can be easily removed along its entire length with burs. The superior-inferior height of lingual cortical bone removed should equal the amount of bone removed laterally.

Seemingly, the neurovascular bundle is left unprotected at the completion of surgery, but the abundant soft tissue covers it after a layered closure of the operative wound. The periosteum that is its immediate covering tissue quickly lays down a vesture of new bone over the cut surfaces of the inferior border of the mandible. Within a year, a prominent new neurovascular canal is evident on follow-up radiographs (see Figure 11–46*J*).

Straightening of the Chin

Often, the chin is obviously deflected toward the normal side as a part of macrognathia. Even though basic management of the deformity consists of trimming away the mandible's deeply bowed inferior margin, osteotomies of some sort are needed to straighten the chin. Bilateral vertical cuts may be made between appropriate teeth anteriorly (usually at the cuspid-premolar area) and extended downward through the inferior border to tilt the chin back to a straight position (see Figure 11–44*D*). This maneuver is dependent upon the allowances of the occlusion. If this procedure is not possible because of the limitations of the occlusion, a horizontal osteotomy of the inferior border of the mandible, done in much the same manner as for a bone advancement genioplasty, will aid in shifting the chin to the midline for straightening. Careful planning is necessary for making an angled cut that will allow straightening of the chin during a slide of the chin along the bony cut to the midline. (See Chapter 14 for details.)

DISCUSSION

Unilateral macrognathism is perhaps the most puzzling of the asymmetric mandibular deformities. The etiology of unilateral mandibular macrognathism is not known. Genetic etiology is discounted on the basis of examinations of siblings or other relatives of patients, none of whom has been found to have tendencies for this problem. A major genetic role can be discounted also by the finding of this deformity in one of two monozygotic twins.[14] The combination of genetic and environmental factors may play a role in the deformity, and one cannot rule out genetic vulnerabilities when this asymmetric response to growth stimulation occurs. The development of the deformity parallels the general skeletal growth period, and the condition seems to be stable after final mandibular growth has been completed. In contrast, the change in condylar hyperplasia is progressive after skeletal growth has been completed; there are no late or delayed compensatory changes after skeletal maturity has been obtained.

As pointed out by Tarsitano, the extent to which the matured mandible is asymmetric depends upon the time when the excessive growth takes place and the rate at which it occurs.[26] For example, if onset is early and excessive unilateral mandibular growth progresses relatively slowly from childhood to adulthood, there is ample opportunity for compensations in the elaboration of alveolar process to maintain a functional dental occlusion. When development of this compensatory bone is followed by progressive eruption of the teeth, the height of the body region of the mandible is greatly increased where the inferior border of the mandible has been displaced downward. The maxillary teeth in this situation drop down in an attempt to establish the occlusal plane and bring alveolar bone with them to sustain posterior occlusal function at a much lower level than on the opposite side.

If, on the other hand, the excessive condylar growth response that is excessive occurs rapidly during the late teens or in adulthood, there will be an absence of posterior occlusion with an open bite where the compensation has not been possible. The vertical bone height in the body region of the mandible will not be increased in the same degree.

CASE 11–7 (Fig. 11–41)

The mandible of B. L., a 21-year-old woman with pronounced dental and facial asymmetry of the mandible, deviated to the left. She was diagnosed as having hyperplasia of the right mandibular condyle.

PROBLEM LIST

Esthetics (Fig. 11–41*A*)

FRONTAL. Upper face and nose in good balance but mandible and lower face markedly shifted to the left side. Facial contour is concave in the mandibular area on the right and convex on the left.

PROFILE. General appearance good with some protrusion in the dentolabial area.

Cephalometric Analysis (Fig. 11–41 *C* and *D*)

1. In the lateral view, skeletal features within normal range, except for steep mandibular plane angle (38°).
2. Upper and lower teeth prominent.
3. In the frontal view, asymmetry of the mandible apparent, with overgrowth of the right condyle.

Occlusal Analysis (Fig. 11–41 *I*, *J* and *K*)

DENTAL ARCH FORM. Marked asymmetry of maxillary and mandibular arches, with the maxillary left posterior teeth deviated and tipped buccally. Mandible flattened in the cuspid area.

DENTAL ALIGNMENT. Upper and lower incisors crowded; upper right first premolar missing and space closed.

DENTAL OCCLUSION. Mandibular teeth in buccal crossbite from left central incisor to the second premolar. Molar relationship Class I on right and Class II on left.

TREATMENT PLAN

Presurgical Orthodontic Treatment

1. Align upper and lower dental arches after extracting lower first premolar tooth.
2. Shift maxillary posterior teeth to right side to make them symmetric with the maxilla.
3. Retract upper and lower incisors moderately.

Surgical Treatment

1. Correct mandibular asymmetry by performing bilateral oblique osteotomy of the rami, advancing the mandible on the left side and retruding it on the right.

Postsurgical Orthodontic Treatment

1. Refine occlusion and stabilize it with a tooth positioner.

ACTIVE TREATMENT

A full edgewise appliance with .022" slot brackets and lingual arch sheaths on the first molar was placed (Fig. 8–41*L, M,* and *N*). The remaining three first premolar teeth were extracted and the spaces were closed with pull coil springs. An acrylic palatal plate was placed to relieve the occlusion and allow the necessary shifting of the posterior teeth. Cross-elastics were used extensively, being attached from the lingual side of the upper right posterior teeth to the buccal side of the lower right and from the buccal of the upper left posterior teeth to the lingual of the lower left. After 16 months of active treatment, the arches were adequately aligned and ready for surgical correction. A frontal tracing was done to show the shift of the molars and the increased severity of the crossbite (Fig. 8–41*E*).

Surgical correction was by a bilateral oblique section of the vertical rami followed by advancement of the mandible on the left side and retrusion on the right side. Intermaxillary fixation was maintained for 8 weeks and followed by elastic traction employing Class II elastics on the left side and Class III elastics on the right. Initially, there was some loss of the advancement on the left side, but the correction was regained, stabilized, and maintained. The fixed appliances were removed 8 months after surgery. Active treatment time totaled 25 months.

FOLLOW-UP

The occlusion was stabilized with an orthodontic tooth positioner that controlled individual tooth position and interarch relationship (Fig. 11–41*H*). It was worn at night for 12 months and then discontinued. The facial appearance was pleasing and symmetric (Fig. 11–41*B*), and the occlusion was satisfactory and stable (Fig. 11–41*O, P,* and *Q*). Frontal headfilm tracings showed corrected symmetry (Fig. 11–41*F*), and the lateral headfilm tracings demonstrated reduction of the protrusion (11–41*G*).

Surgeon: William H. Ware, San Francisco, California. *Orthodontist:* Donald G. Poulton, Alameda, California.

CASE 11–8 (Fig. 11–42)

V. T., a 23-year-old college student, was referred by her dentist for correction of mandibular asymmetry and malocclusion. The condition was eventually diagnosed as asymmetric prognathism.

PROBLEM LIST

Esthetics (Fig. 11–42*A*)

FRONTAL AND PROFILE. Good facial balance except for deviation of the chin to the left.

Cephalometric and Panoramic Radiographic Analysis (Fig. 11–42*C* and *D*)

1. Modest prominence of mandible in profile projection.
2. Significant deviation of mandibular midline to the left (Fig. 11–42*C*).
3. Relatively normal condylar neck length on both sides.

Text continued on page 980.

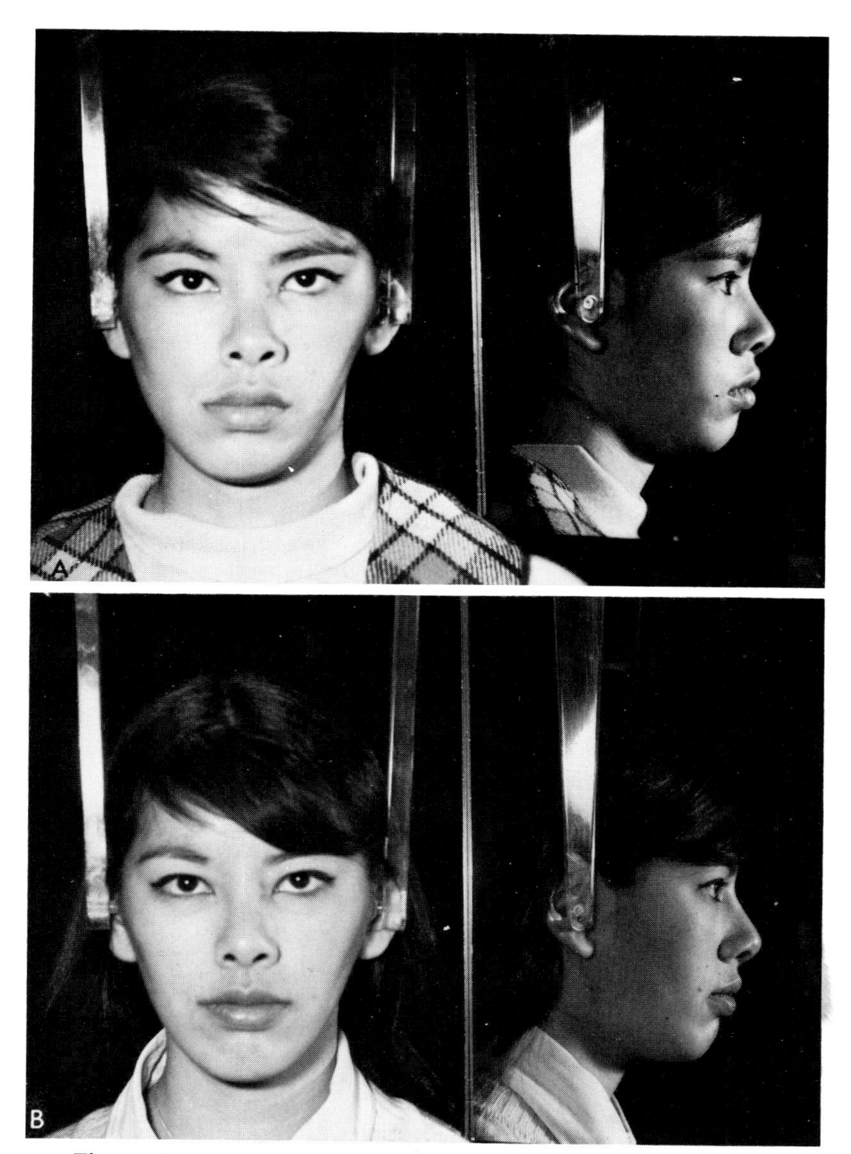

Figure 11–41 (Case 11–7). *A,* Frontal and lateral facial appearances before correction. *B,* Frontal and lateral facial appearances after correction.

Illustration continued on the following page.

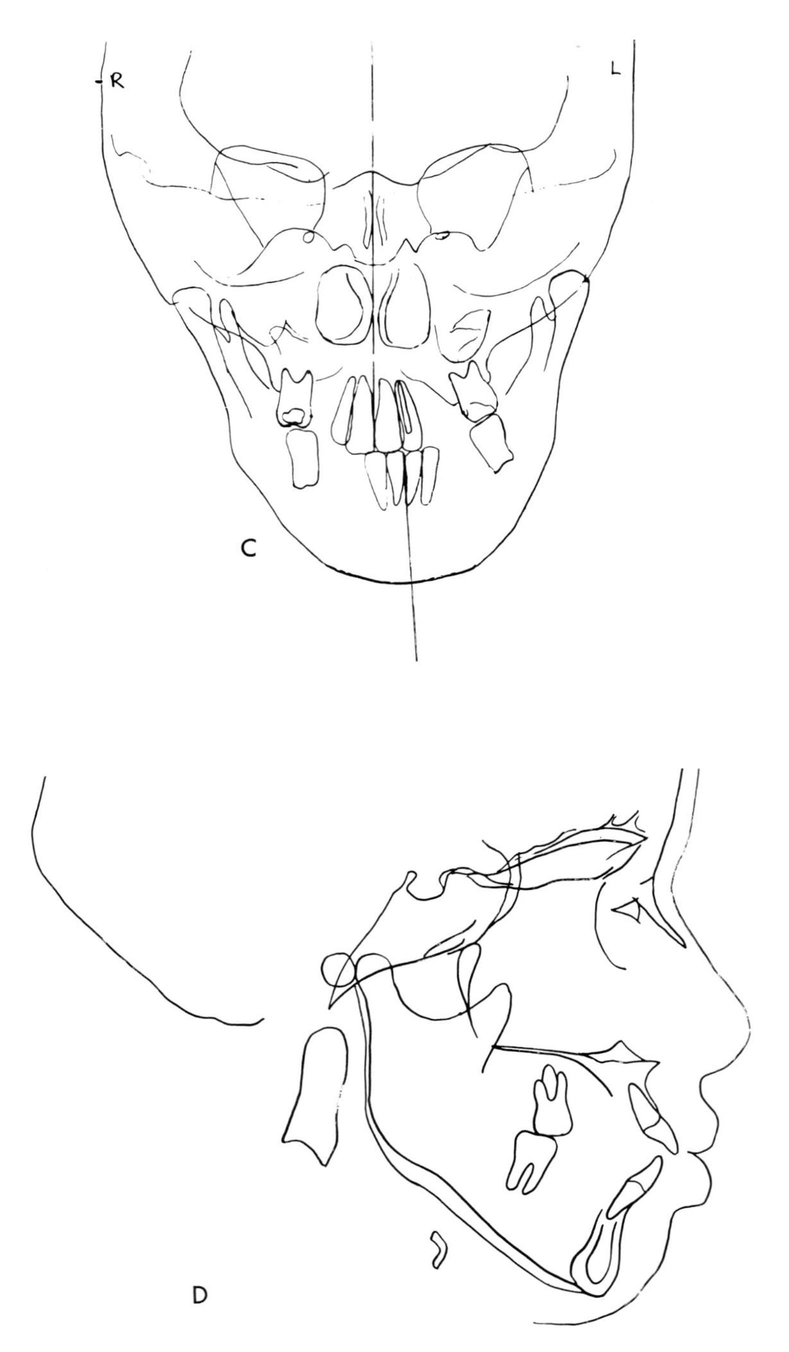

Figure 11–41 *Continued.* *C* and *D*, Pretreatment cephalometric tracings, frontal (*C*) and lateral (*D*).

Legend continued on the opposite page.

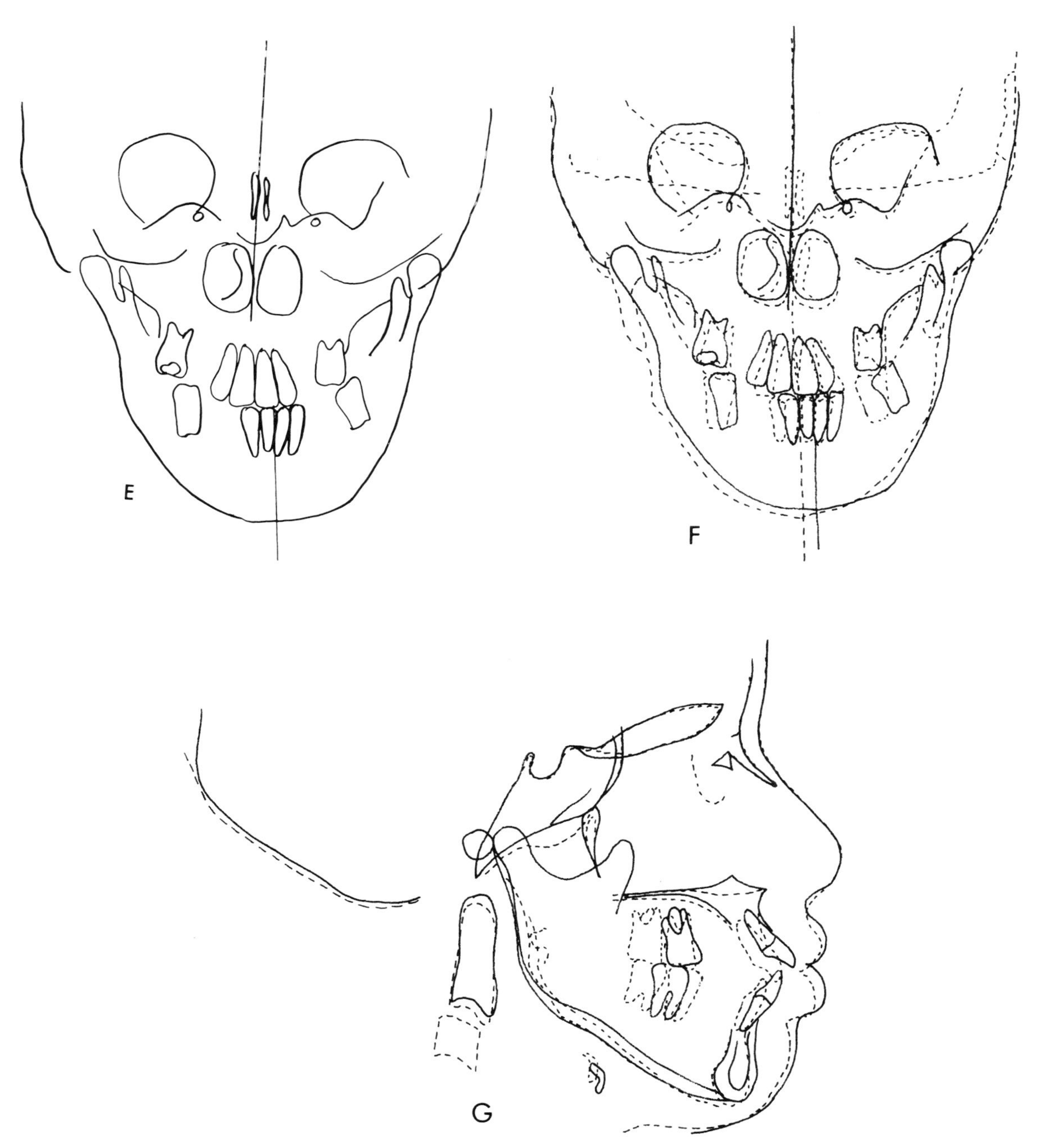

Figure 11–41 *Continued.* *E,* Frontal tracing, teeth ready for surgery; note change in molar relation. *F,* Composite frontal head film tracings before (*solid line,* age 21 years, 5 months) and after (*broken line,* 23 years, 6 months) treatment. Maxillary change is orthodontic; mandibular change is surgical. *G,* Lateral head film tracings before (*solid line,* age 21 years, 5 months) and after (*broken line,* age 23 years, 6 months) correction.

Illustration continued on the following page.

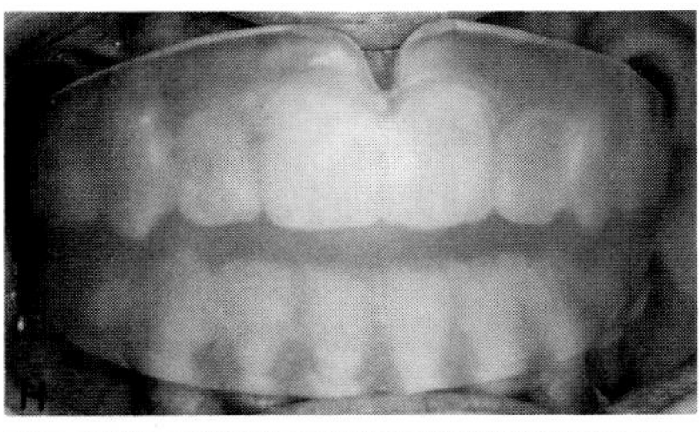

Figure 11–41 *Continued.* *H*, Orthodontic tooth positioner. *I–K*, Intraoral views of dental occlusion before correction. *L–N*, Intraoral views of teeth prepared for surgery; note change in buccal overjet. *O–Q*, Intraoral views of dental occlusion after correction.

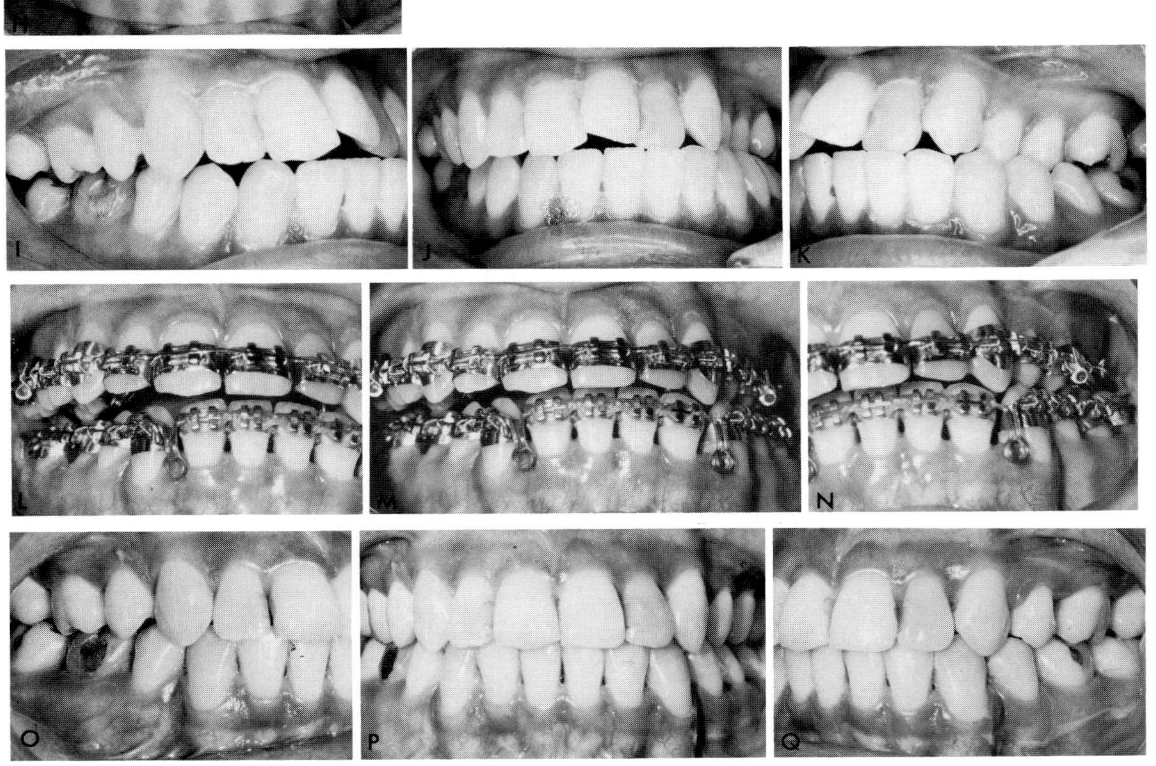

Occlusal Analysis (Fig. 11–42*E*)

DENTAL ARCH FORM. Arch forms surprisingly symmetric although mandible was displaced to the left by the skeletal abnormality.

DENTAL ALIGNMENT. No excessive crowding except for slight outward flaring of the maxillary left lateral incisor and moderate rotation of maxillary left cuspid (Fig. 11–42*E*).

DENTAL OCCLUSION. The only functional occlusal contact was between the maxillary and mandibular posterior molars. The mandibular anterior teeth were positioned in front of the maxillary anterior teeth. A prominent open bite existed at the maxillary and mandibular left cuspid–premolar areas, and open bite of lesser degree extended around the midline to the maxillary and mandibular right cuspid–premolar areas. The tongue was interposed in the open bite spaces when the mandible was in rest position. The mandibular central incisors were approximately a half tooth off the midline to the left of the maxillary central incisors (Fig. 11–42*E*).

TREATMENT PLAN

Assessment of the study models showed a potentially satisfactory posturing of the mandibular teeth relative to the maxillary teeth by a unit shift of the mandible to the right and posteriorly. Occlusion was far from perfect, but it was planned to institute elastic traction at night after intermaxillary fixation was removed. Bilateral vertical osteotomies of the mandibular rami to be done via an intraoral approach were planned.

ACTIVE TREATMENT

During hospitalization and under general anesthesia delivered via a nasoendotracheal route, bilateral vertical osteotomies of the mandibular rami were performed via an intraoral approach. The mandible was then shifted from left to right in aligning the symphysis to the midline (Fig. 11–42*D*). The mandible was immobilized in this position for 3 weeks by arch bars and multiple intermaxillary wires. After the jaw was mobilized by removal of the intermaxillary wires, an active regimen of daytime use of the jaws and night-time use of elastic traction was followed for 3 months (Fig. 11–42*F* and *G*). The marked disocclusion that was present on removal of the intermaxillary wires slowly and firmly resolved during the follow-up regimen of physiotherapy (Fig. 11–42*H*).

FOLLOW-UP

Restoration of normal facial proportion, symmetry, and midlines was achieved, as well as a tight full-arch occlusion that functioned well (Fig. 11–42*B*). Follow-up assessment of the occlusion 2 years after surgery showed the result to be completely stable (Fig. 11–42*H*). Radiographically, the mandibular midline was confirmed to be correctly related to the maxilla and the open bite was well closed (Fig. 11–42*D*).

Surgeon: Robert V. Walker, Dallas, Texas.

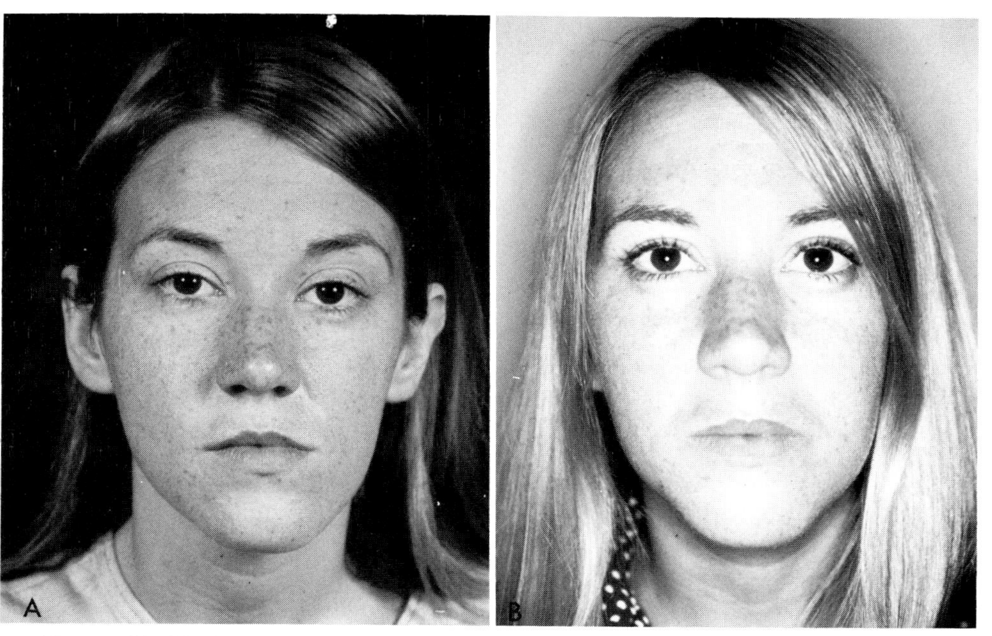

Figure 11–42 (Case 11–8). *A*, Preoperative facial view; asymmetric prognathism. *B*, Postoperative facial view.

Illustration continued on the following page.

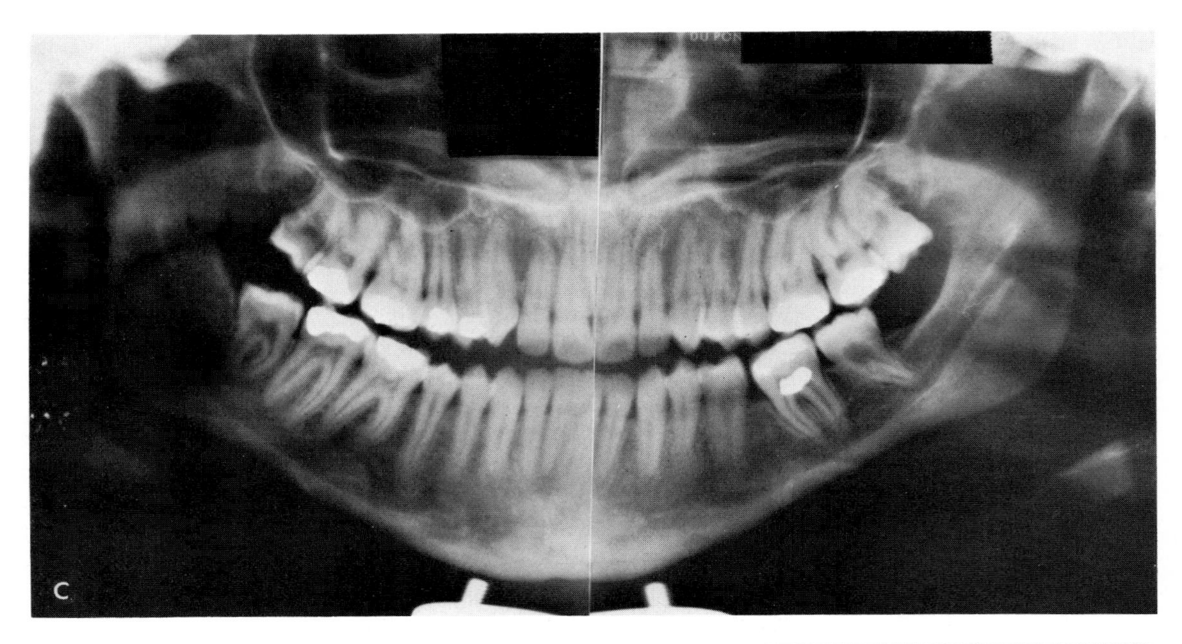

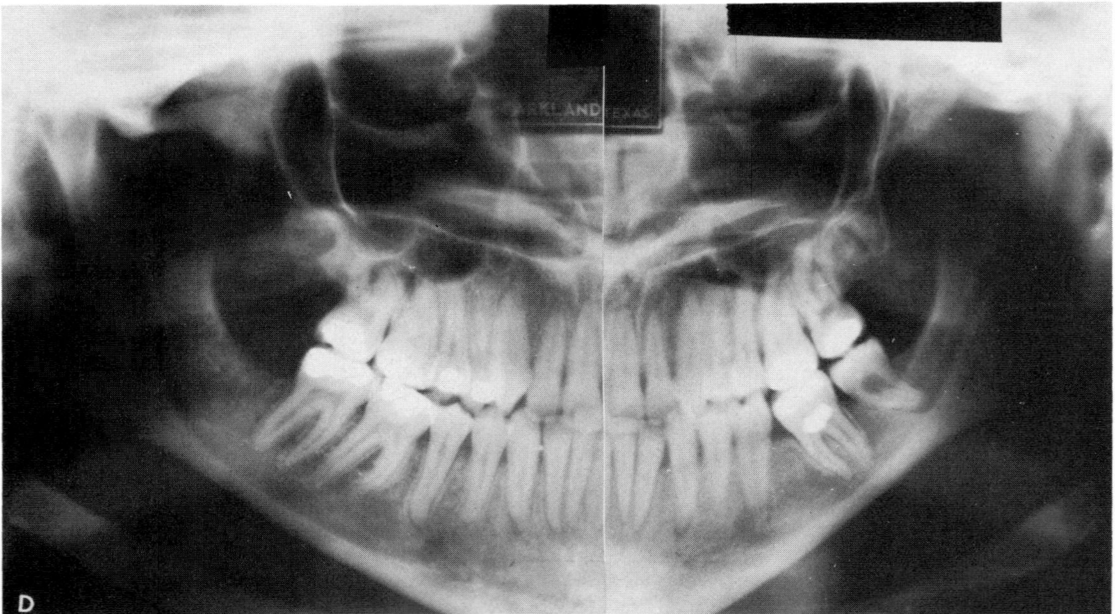

Figure 11–42 *Continued.* *C,* Preoperative panoramic radiograph. *D,* Follow-up panoramic radiograph after physiotherapy was completed.

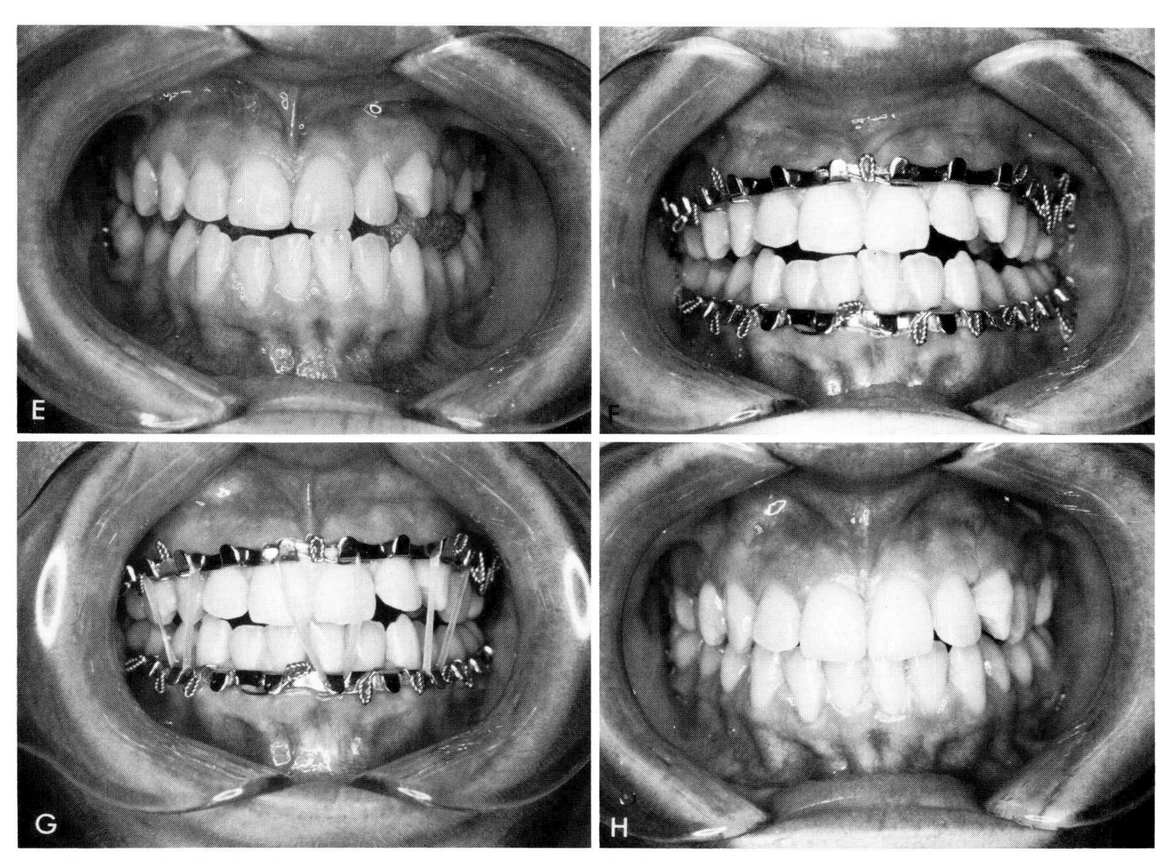

Figure 11–42 *Continued.* *E*, Preoperative malocclusion with open bite. *F*, Occlusion (disocclusion) three weeks after surgery and intermaxillary wiring was removed. *G*, Three small elastics in place for nighttime traction. *H*, Final occlusion. *I*, Diagrammatic representation of surgical procedures done: bilateral vertical osteotomies of the right and left mandibular ascending rami done via an intraoral approach; mandible shifted from the left to the right side for correction of the asymmetry.

CASE 11–9 (Fig. 11–43)

W. W., a 19-year-old college student, noticed a rapidly developing shift of his chin and jaw to the right. He was also aware of a change in his occlusion with a crossbite on the right. Photographs taken 18 months previously while he was a senior in high school confirmed that the face and jaw had previously been symmetric. He first sought assistance from his dentist and was then referred for consultation with an oral surgeon. His condition was diagnosed as left mandibular condylar hyperplasia. The case of W. W. represents early detection of the condition by the patient himself.

PROBLEM LIST

Esthetics (Fig. 11–43*A*)

1. The patient's chin was deviated to the right. Facial proportions were otherwise very well balanced.

Radiographic Analysis (Fig. 11–43*C*, *D*, and *E*)

1. A panoramic radiograph demonstrated a shift of the midline to the right and an elongated left condylar neck (Fig. 11–43*C*).

2. Transpharyngeal radiographs of the right and left temporomandibular joints in the closed and open positions of the mandible showed a markedly enlarged left condyle and an elongated condylar neck (Fig. 11–43*D*).

Occlusal Analysis (Fig. 11–43*G* and *H*)

DENTAL ARCH FORM. Maxillary and mandibular arches symmetric.

DENTAL ALIGNMENT. Modest diastema between the maxillary central incisors (Fig. 11–43*G*).

TREATMENT PLAN

Assessment and manipulation of study models showed a potentially functional occlusion provided the mandible was shifted back to the left side.

Tracings of the right and left condyles and condylar necks made from the transpharyngeal radiographs demonstrated an enormous difference in length of the left condylar neck as compared with the shorter right condylar neck (Fig. 11–43*E*). Because of the relatively rapid progression of the jaw asymmetry, it was planned to excise the left condyle, which seemed to be still growing, thus allowing the mandible to shift back to the left side.

ACTIVE TREATMENT

After hospitalization and under general anesthesia delivered via a nasoendotracheal route, a left condylectomy was performed through a preauricular approach (Fig. 11–43*F*). The condylar neck was cut 17 mm below the top of the condyle, the difference in length between the left condylar neck and the right having been determined on the preoperative tracings of the transpharyngeal radiographs. After excision of the condyle, the jaw was shifted from right to left in aligning the occlusion and symphysis in the midline (Fig. 11–43*J*). The jaw was maintained in a slight state of disocclusion in this correct alignment via intermaxillary fixation for 5 days. The jaw was then mobilized, and an active regimen of daytime use of the jaws and night-time use of elastic traction was begun and maintained for 4 months. The disocclusion slowly and firmly resolved during the period of physiotherapy (Fig. 11–43*H*, *I*, and *J*).

FOLLOW-UP

Restoration of normal facial proportion, symmetry, and midlines was achieved, as well as a tight, full-arch occlusion that functioned well. A follow-up assessment of facial symmetry (Fig. 11–43*B*) and the occlusion 4 years after surgery (Fig. 11–43*K*) showed the result to be completely stable. Temporomandibular joint function was normal.

Surgeon: Robert V. Walker, Dallas, Texas.

Text continued on page 989.

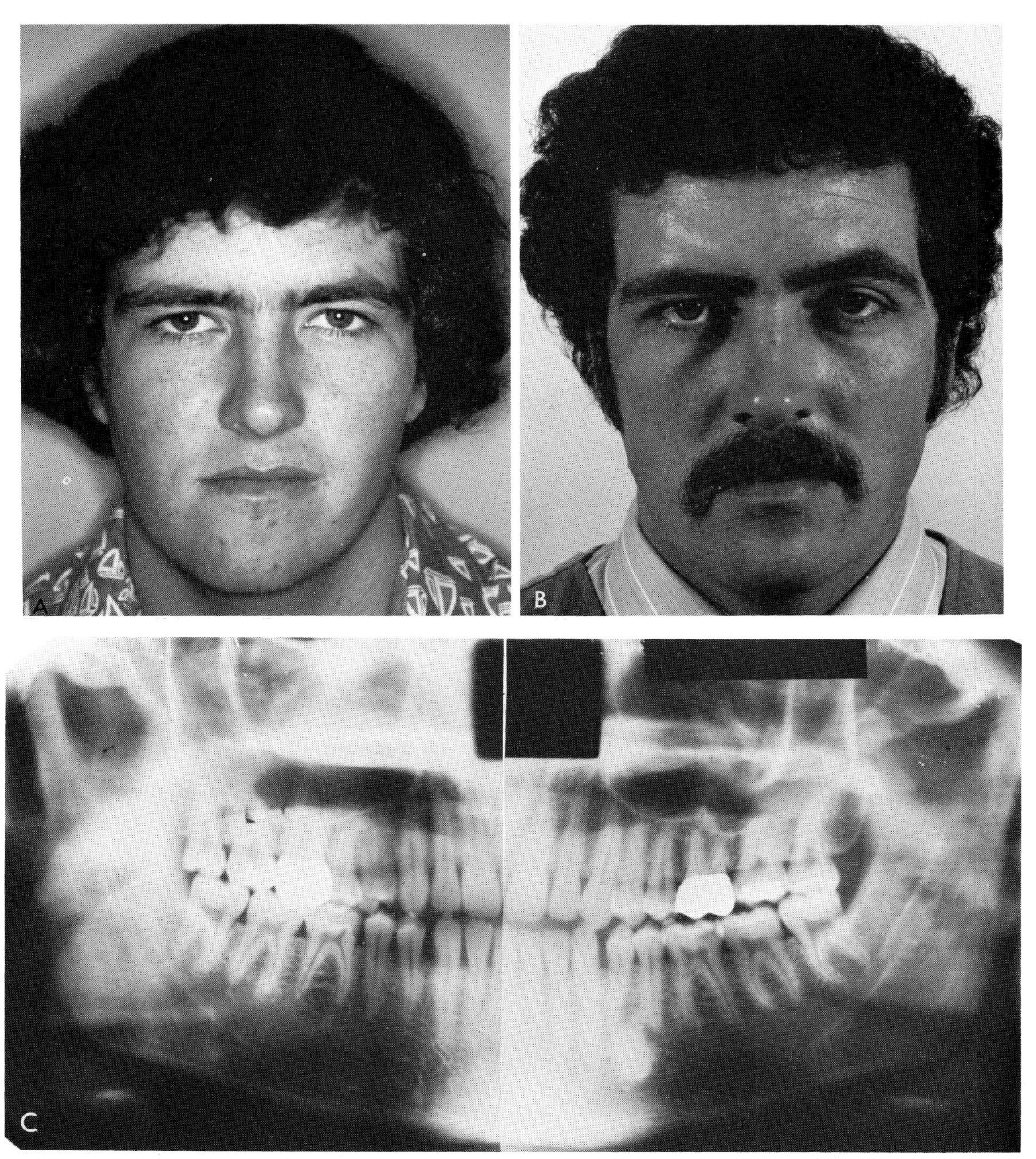

Figure 11–43 (Case 11–9). *A*, Preoperative facial view; left mandibular condylar hyperplasia. *B*, Facial view four years after surgery. *C*, Preoperative panoramic radiograph.

Illustration continued on the following page.

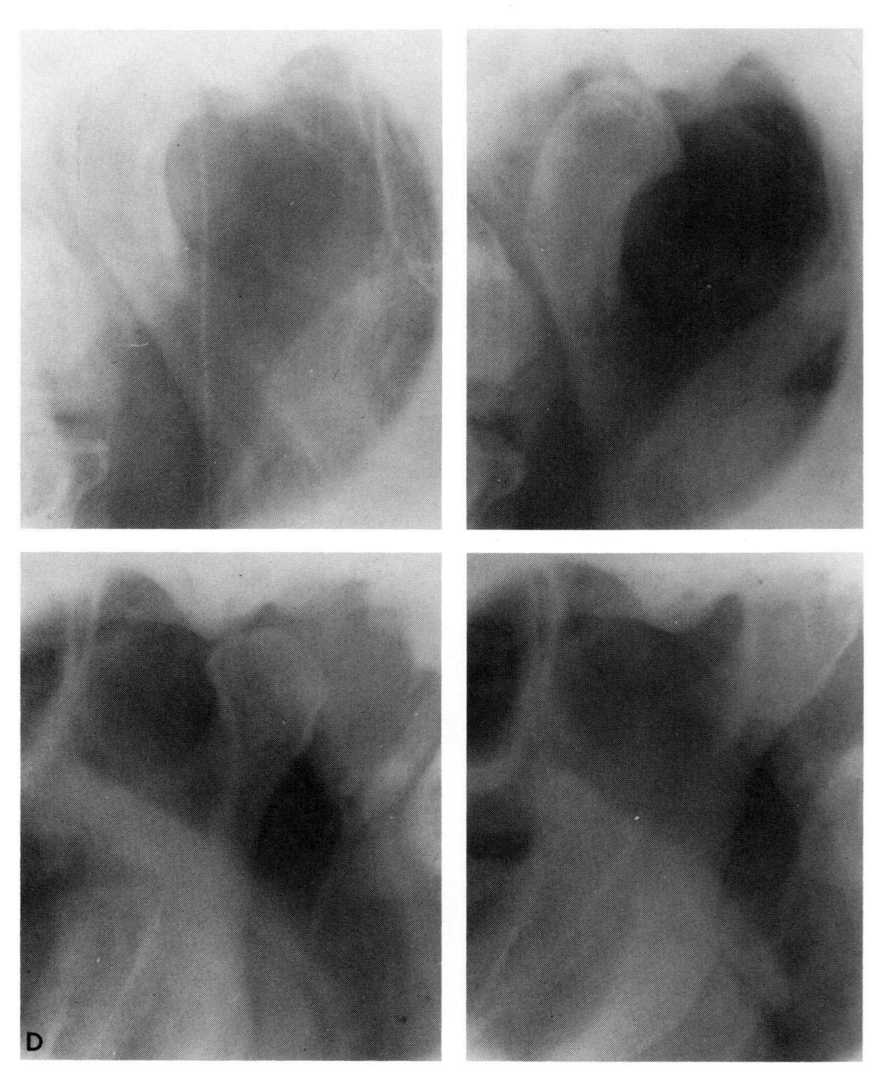

Figure 11–43 *Continued. D,* Preoperative transpharyngeal radiographs of left and right temporomandibular joints in closed and open positions of mandible.

Legend continued on the opposite page.

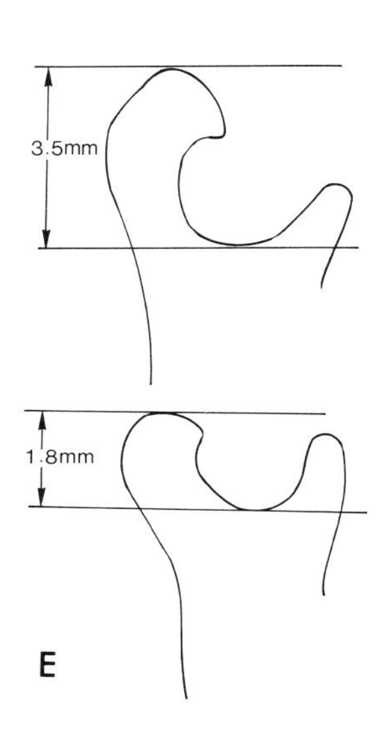

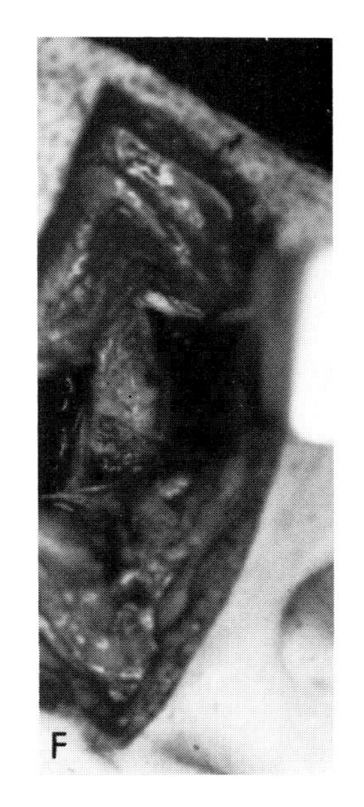

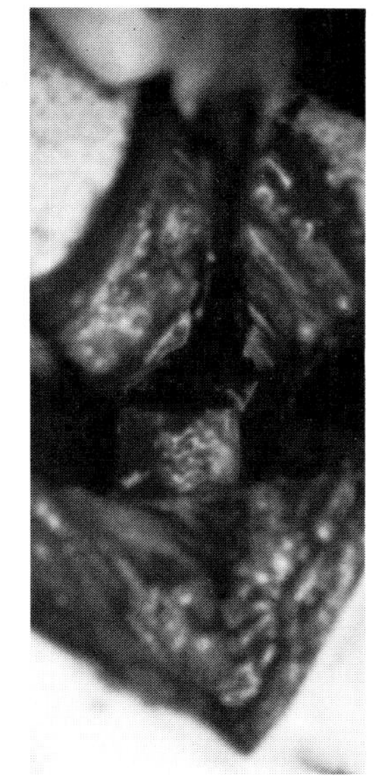

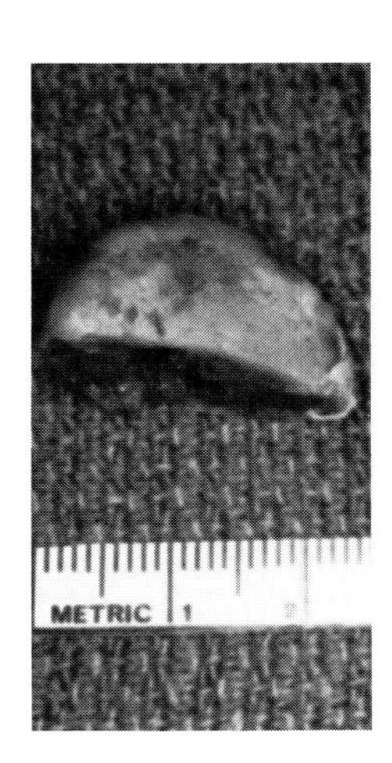

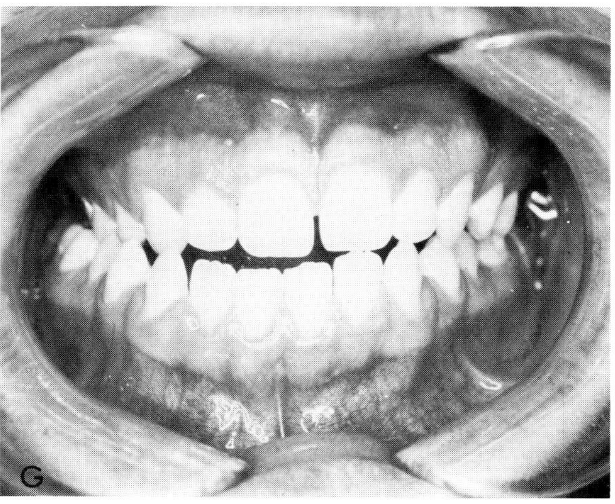

Figure 11–43 *Continued.* *E*, Tracings of left and right transpharyngeal radiographs in open position of mandible; right radiograph reversed prior to tracing for easier comparison of the two condyles. *F*, Surgery: excision of the mandibular left condyle via preauricular approach. *G*, Preoperative malocclusion with crossbite.

Illustration continued on the following page.

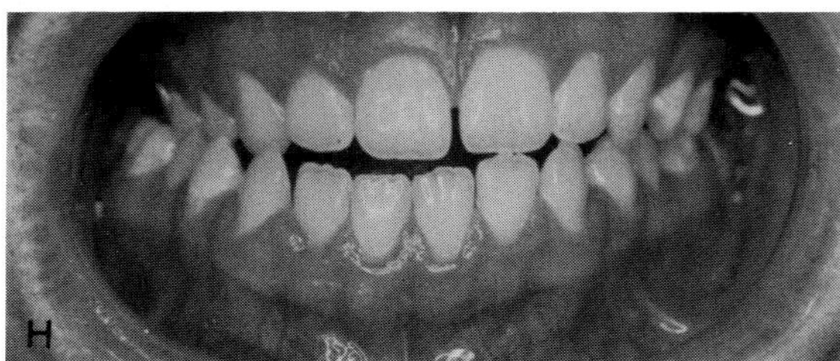

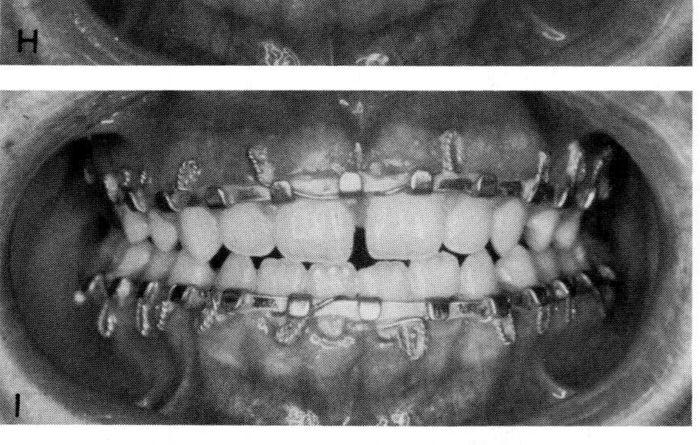

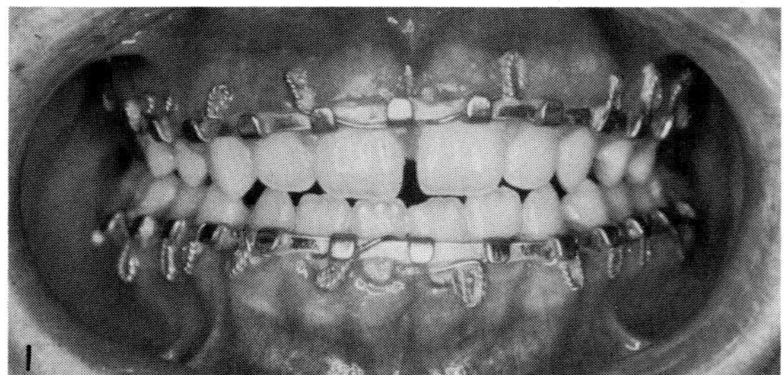

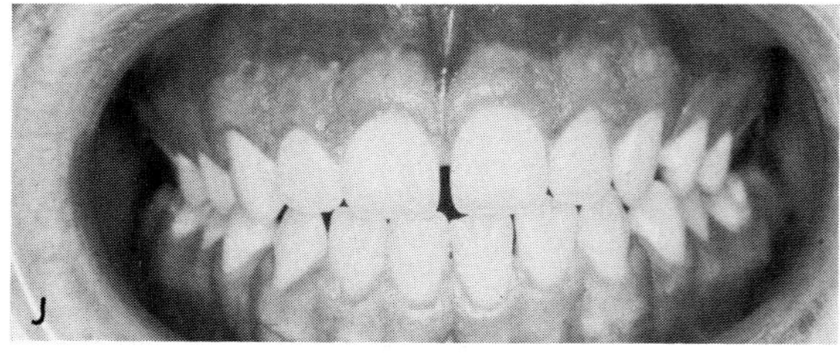

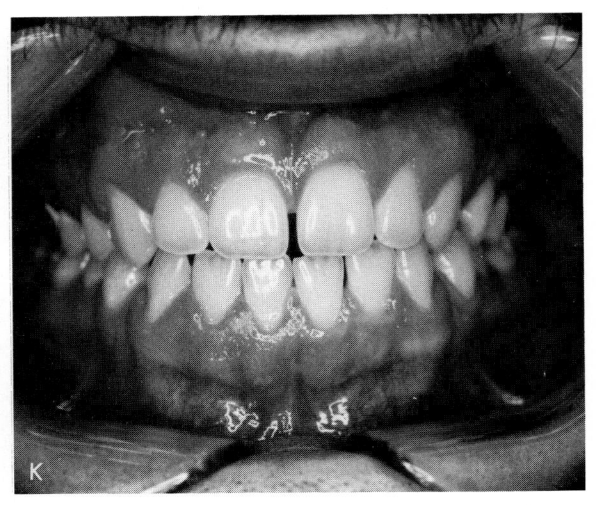

Figure 11–43 *Continued. H–J,* Occlusion prior to surgery (*H*), during physiotherapy (*I*), and at completion of physiotherapy (*J*). *K,* Final occlusion stable; four years after surgery.

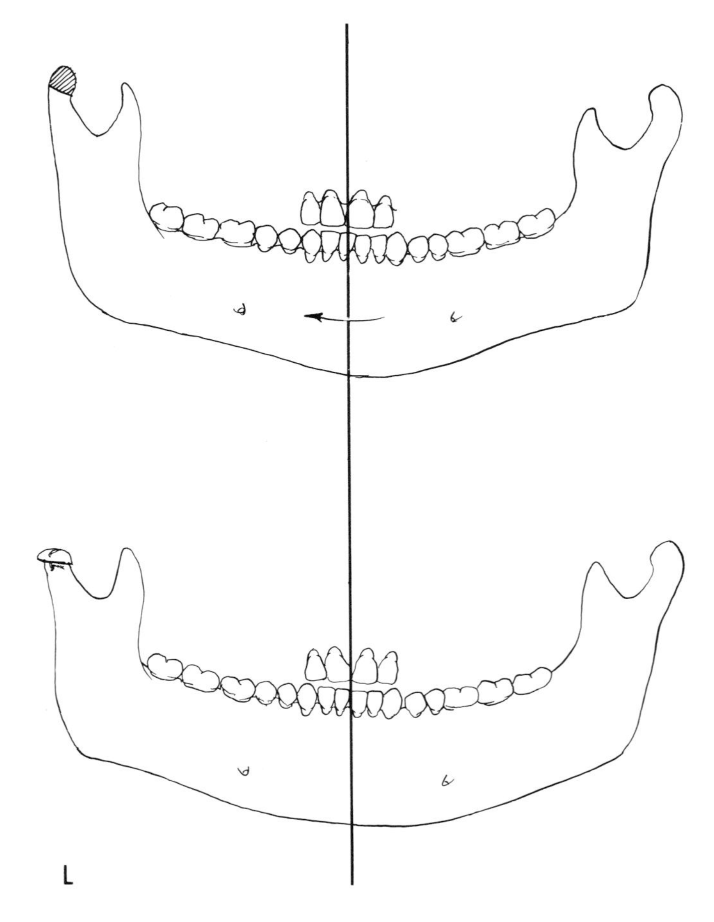

Figure 11–43 *Continued. L,* Diagrammatic representation of surgical procedures done: mandibular left condyle excised via a preauricular approach with wiring of a Silastic disk atop the remaining condylar stump; mandible shifted from the right to the left side for correction of the asymmetry.

CASE 11–10 (Fig. 11–44)

L. F., a 29-year-old woman, was concerned about her facial and jaw asymmetry, of which she had been aware for 15 years. Photographs taken during her early high-school years confirmed the presence of a slight asymmetry at that time. She was diagnosed as having unilateral macrognathism of long duration.

PROBLEM LIST

Esthetics (Fig. 11–44*A*)

Asymmetry appeared chiefly as downward displacement of the entire right mandible with a deep bowing effect of the body and a significant deviation of the chin to the left.

Radiographic Evaluation (Fig. 11–44*C*)

1. Downward overgrowth of the mandibular condyle.
2. Elongation of the condylar neck.
3. Long mandibular ramus.
4. Deep bowed effect of the mandibular body area.
5. Downward extension of the neurovascular canal through the bowed area.

Occlusal Analysis (Fig. 11–44*I*)

DENTAL ARCH FORM. Maxillary and mandibular arch forms relatively symmetric.

DENTAL ALIGNMENT. Modest compensation for the awkward jaw growth by slight downward eruption of the maxillary right posterior teeth with alveolar bone growth accommodating the eruption of the teeth.

DENTAL OCCLUSION. The mandibular midline was deviated slightly to the left, and all mandibular anterior teeth from cuspid to cuspid were slanted with the incisal edges angled to the right and the roots angled in the opposite direction, to the left. The mandibular left cuspid was in a deeper overbite positon than mandibular right cuspid. The mandibular right first premolar was missing, but its space was closed by tilting of the second premolar into the space. The mandibular left first molar was missing and its space was still present.

Temporomandibular Joint Analysis

Both the right and left temporomandibular joints opened and closed and moved normally in a complete excursive range. There was no pain or discomfort during joint use. There was a slight bulge overlying the right temporomandibular joint.

TREATMENT PLAN

In deference to the normal working of the temporomandibular joints, the obviously burned-out condition of the mandibular right condyle's hyperplastic process, and the minimal downward compensation of the maxillary right teeth and alveolar process, attention was directed to planning correction of the downward bow of the right mandible and the chin deviation. A tracing of the panoramic radiography was made and the amount of the downward bowed part to be removed was calculated. The chin was to be straightened by means of bilateral vertical osteotomies at the cuspid-premolar areas.

ACTIVE TREATMENT

By an extraoral approach, the entire right mandible was exposed from the posterior border of the vertical ramus to the symphysis area. A series of holes was drilled through the cortical plate of bone at the predetermined height above the inferior border of the mandible (Fig. 11–44*F*). The holes were connected with a linear cut through the outer cortex of bone in an anteroposterior direction, and this marked the amount of bone to be removed from the inferior border. A series of vertical cuts were then made downward from the anteroposterior cut to the inferior border of the mandible (Fig. 11–44*G*). This allowed flipping away the outer cortex of bone and careful dissecting free of the neurovascular bundle. The lingual cortex was then cut away (Fig. 11–44*H*). Through-and-through vertical cuts were made between the cuspid and first premolar on the left and the cuspid and second premolar on the right (Fig. 11–44*D*). This allowed the chin to be tilted to a straightened position. Removal of the downward-bowing part of the right mandible and the vertical cuts at the cuspid-premolar area on both sides for straightening the chin are depicted by diagram (Fig. 11–44*K*). The mandible was then immobilized for 6 weeks by means of arch bars and intermaxillary fixation. This was followed by an additional 2 months of jaw physiotherapy (daytime use of the jaw and night-time use of intermaxillary elastic traction). A lower Hawley type appliance was used for an additional three months to firmly stabilize the anterior osteotomy sites while bony union became solid at these areas (Fig. 11–44*E*).

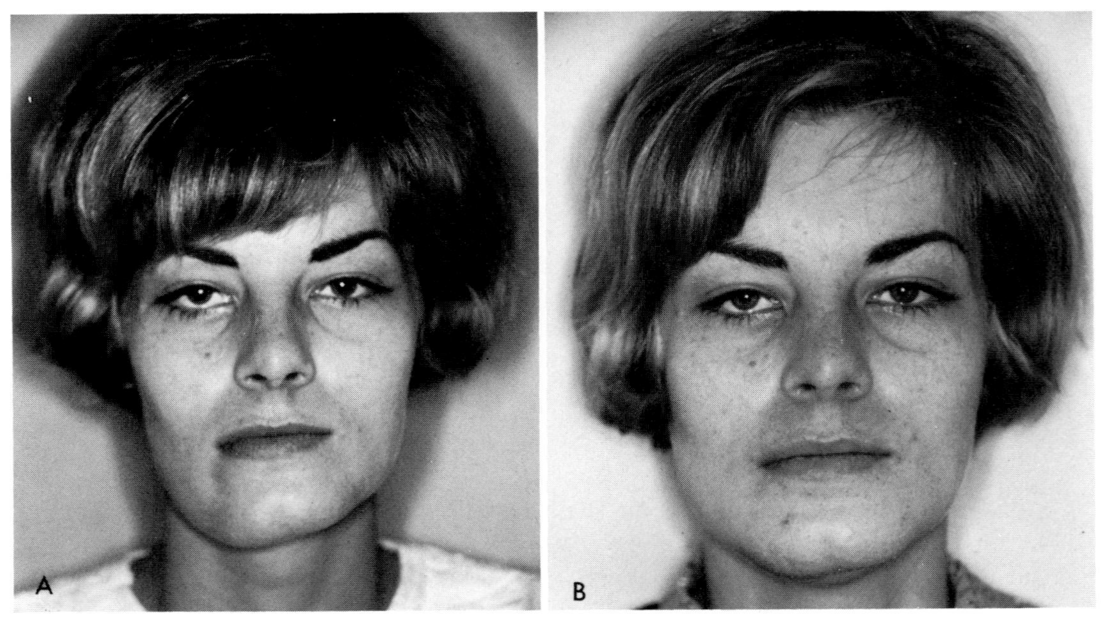

Figure 11–44 (Case 11–10). *A*, Preoperative facial view; unilateral macrognathism. *B*, Postoperative facial view.

Legend continued on the opposite page.

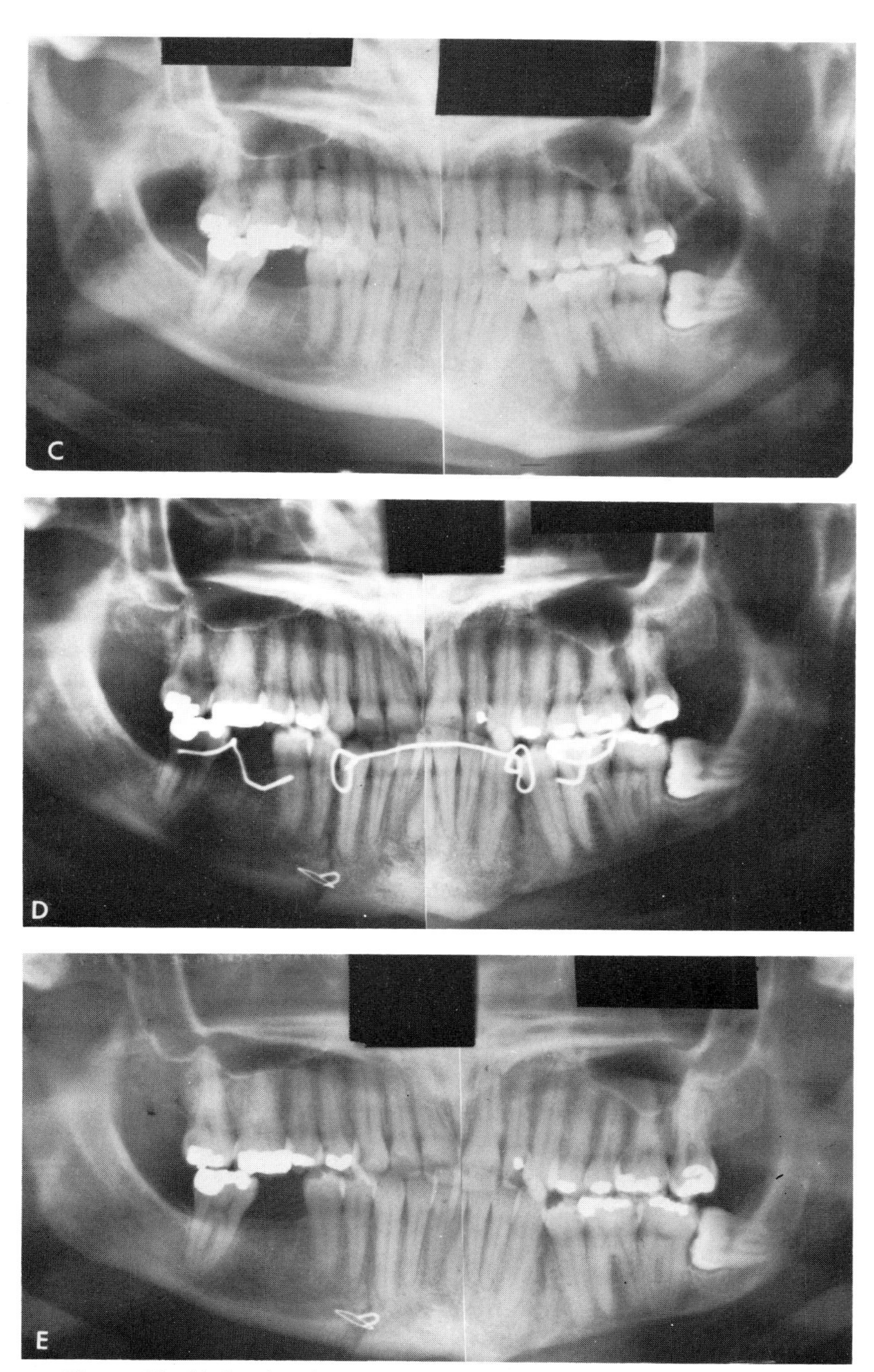

Figure 11–44 *Continued.* *C*, Preoperative panoramic radiograph. *D*, Postoperative panoramic radiograph showing areas of vertical osteotomies between cuspid and bicuspid teeth that allowed straightening of chin; Hawley type of appliance in place. *E*, Panoramic radiograph one year after surgery.

Illustration continued on the following page.

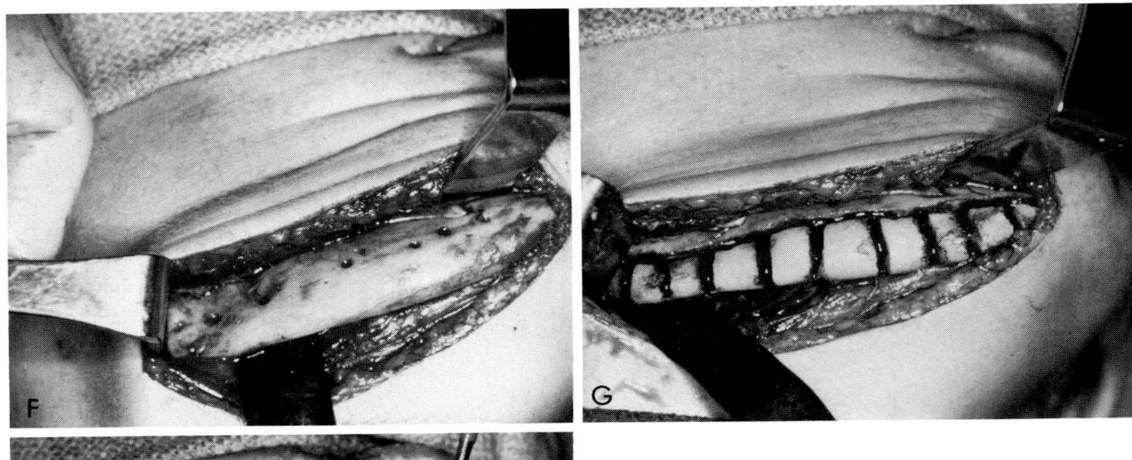

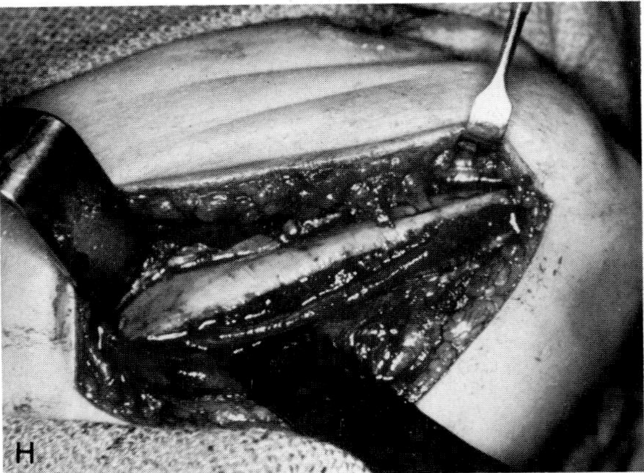

Figure 11–44 *Continued. F–H,* Operative procedure. *F,* Exposure of right mandible from posterior border of the ramus to the symphysis; holes drilled through outer cortex of bone to mark upper level of bone to be removed. *G,* Anteroposterior cut through outer cortex of bone at level of previously drilled holes; vertical cuts extended from anteroposterior cut to inferior border of mandible. *H,* Neurovascular bundle dissected free; lingual cortex of bone removed. *I,* Preoperative occlusion. *J,* Final occlusion.

Legend continued on the opposite page.

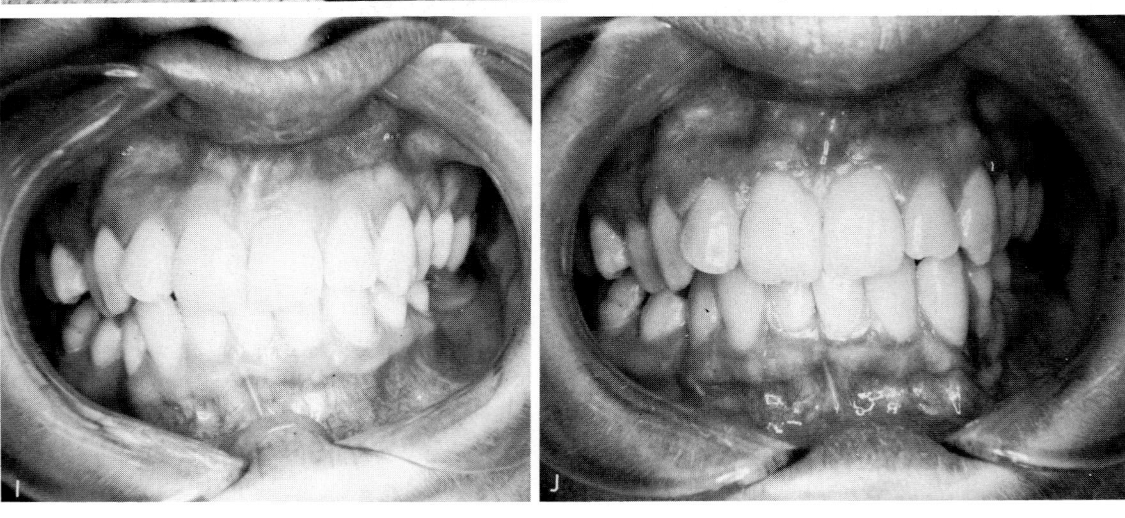

FOLLOW-UP

Satisfactory symmetry was restored to the mandible and face (Fig. 11–44*B*). Though not appreciably changed by the procedures, the occlusion has remained functional and stable through a two-year follow-up (Fig. 11–44*J*).

Surgeon: Robert V. Walker, Dallas, Texas.

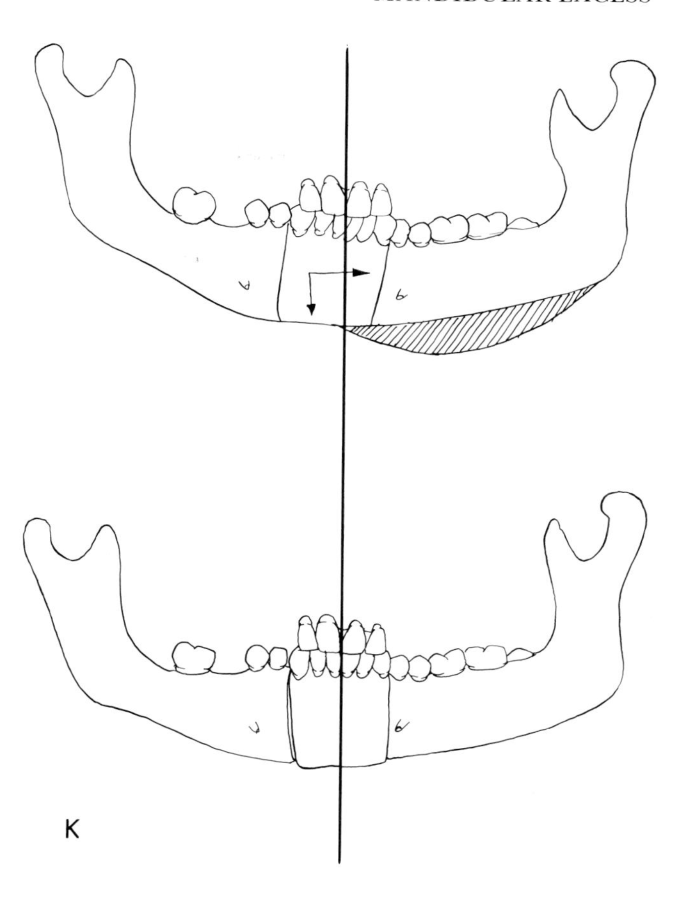

Figure 11–44 *Continued. K,* Diagrammatic representation of surgical procedures done: mandibular excess trimmed from inferior portion of right mandible via submandibular approach; vertical osteotomies of the mandibular body done between the left cuspid and 1st bicuspid tooth and between the right cuspid and 2nd bicuspid tooth (1st bicuspid tooth missing) to allow straightening of the chin by slight shifting of the chin from the left to the right side; direct interosseous wiring of bone done on the left side only.

CASE 11–11 (Fig. 11–45)

D. H., a 17-year-old high-school student, had a marked mandibular asymmetry that had been present for at least 6 years, and she had repeatedly sought a diagnosis and management of the condition. She appeared for consultation on referral from an orthodontist loaded with a few years' accumulation of radiographs. The patient and her parents felt that the deformity was continuing to progress. The final diagnosis was unilateral macrognathism.

PROBLEM LIST

Esthetics (Fig. 11–45*A*)

1. The patient had an acceptable upper facial balance despite a lowered right eyebrow. The total mandible was markedly deflected to the right, with chin deviation in the same direction. The left cuspid–premolar area of the mandibular body was flattened. The lower lip was procumbent to the upper lip.

Panoramic Radiographic Evaluation (Fig. 11–45*C*)

1. Elongated mandibular left condylar neck.
2. Significant deviation of the mandibular midline to the right.
3. Marked bowing of mandibular left body in a downward direction.
4. Downward extension of the left neurovascular canal into the bowed portion of bone.

Occlusal Analysis (Fig. 11–45*G, H,* and *I*)

DENTAL OCCLUSION. Class III malocclusion and mandibular buccal crossbite on the right. Marked Class III malocclusion on the left with an open bite from the mandibular left second molar forward to the left lateral incisor.

DENTAL ARCH FORM. Mandibular anterior teeth forward to the maxillary anterior teeth and off the midline to the right by the width of the left central incisor; mandibular anterior teeth angled slightly to the left.

TREATMENT PLAN

An excision of the mandibular left condyle via a preauricular approach was planned to stop the progression of the condition. On the basis of tracings of transpharyngeal radiographs of the right and left temporomandibular joints, it was planned to remove a 13-mm superior-inferior section of the condyle (Fig. 11–45*E*). A vertical osteotomy of the mandibular right ramus was planned to allow a substantial swing of the mandible back to the left side. The downward-bowed portion of the left mandible was then to be trimmed via an intraoral approach. A tracing of the preoperative panoramic radiograph was also used to calculate the amount of bone to be removed from the lower part of the left mandible. Bone removal and dissecting free of the neurovascular bundle was to be in the same manner as if done extraorally.

ACTIVE TREATMENT

During hospitalization and under general anesthesia delivered via a nasoendotracheal route, the three planned surgical maneuvers of left condylectomy, intraoral vertical osteotomy of the right ramus, and intraoral excision of the bowed part of the

Text continued on page 999.

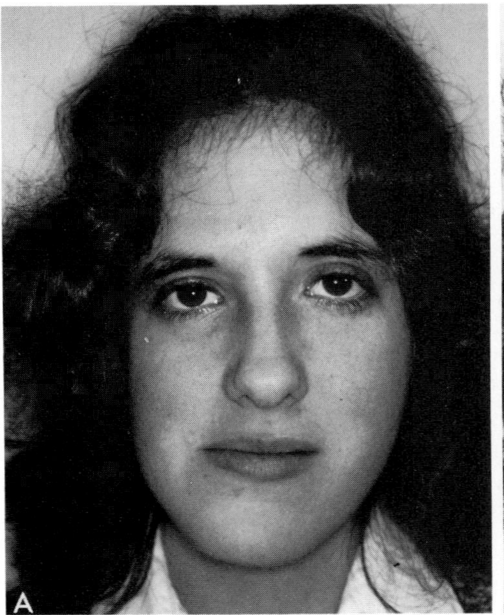

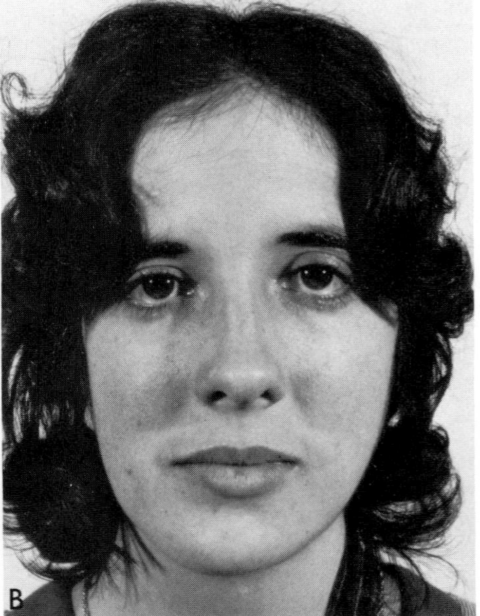

Figure 11–45 (Case 11–11). *A*, Preoperative facial view; condylar hyperplasia and unilateral macrognathia. *B*, Postoperative facial view.

Legend continued on the opposite page.

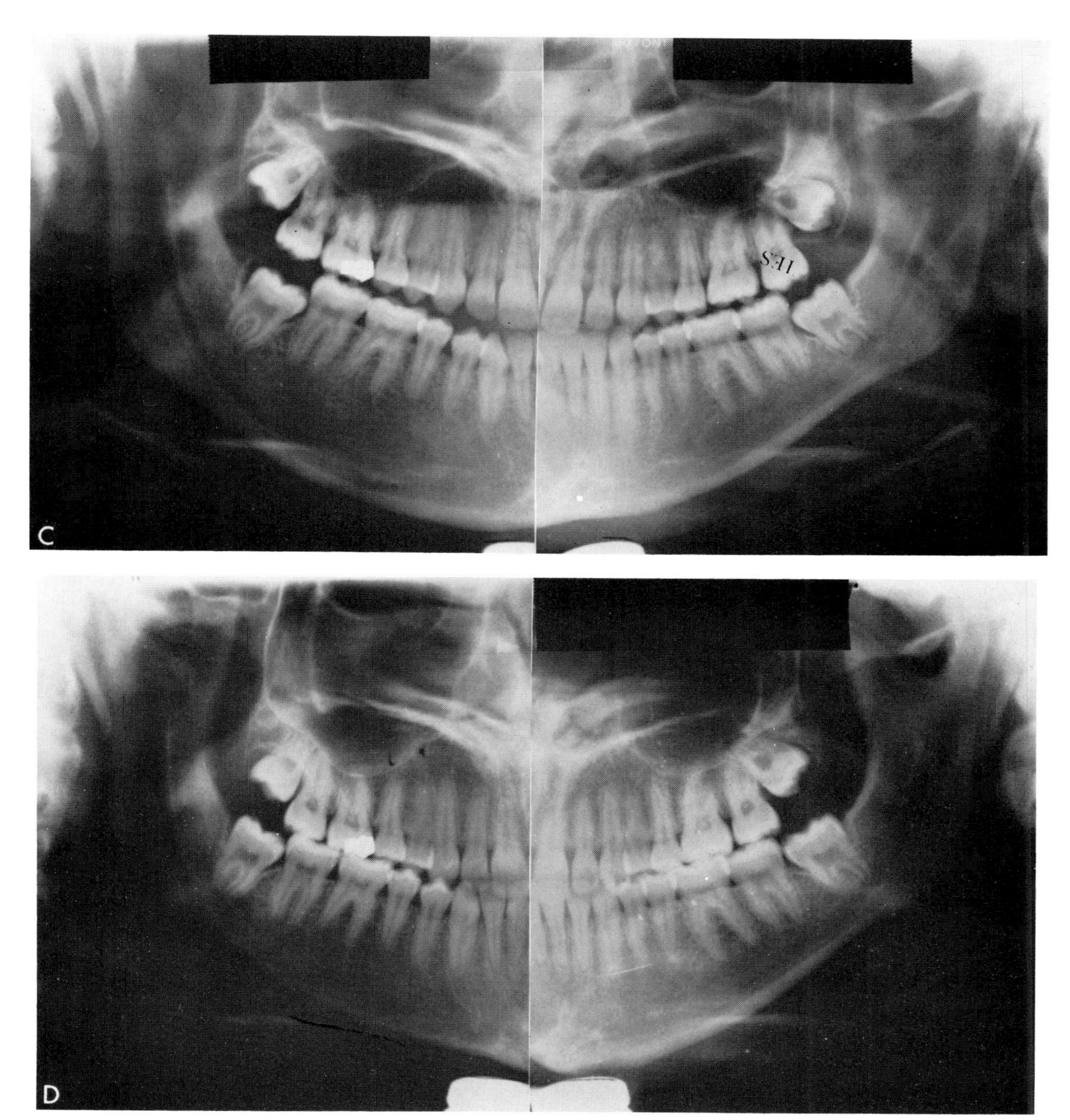

Figure 11–45 *Continued.* *C*, Preoperative panoramic radiograph. *D*, Follow-up panoramic radiograph.

Illustration continued on the following page.

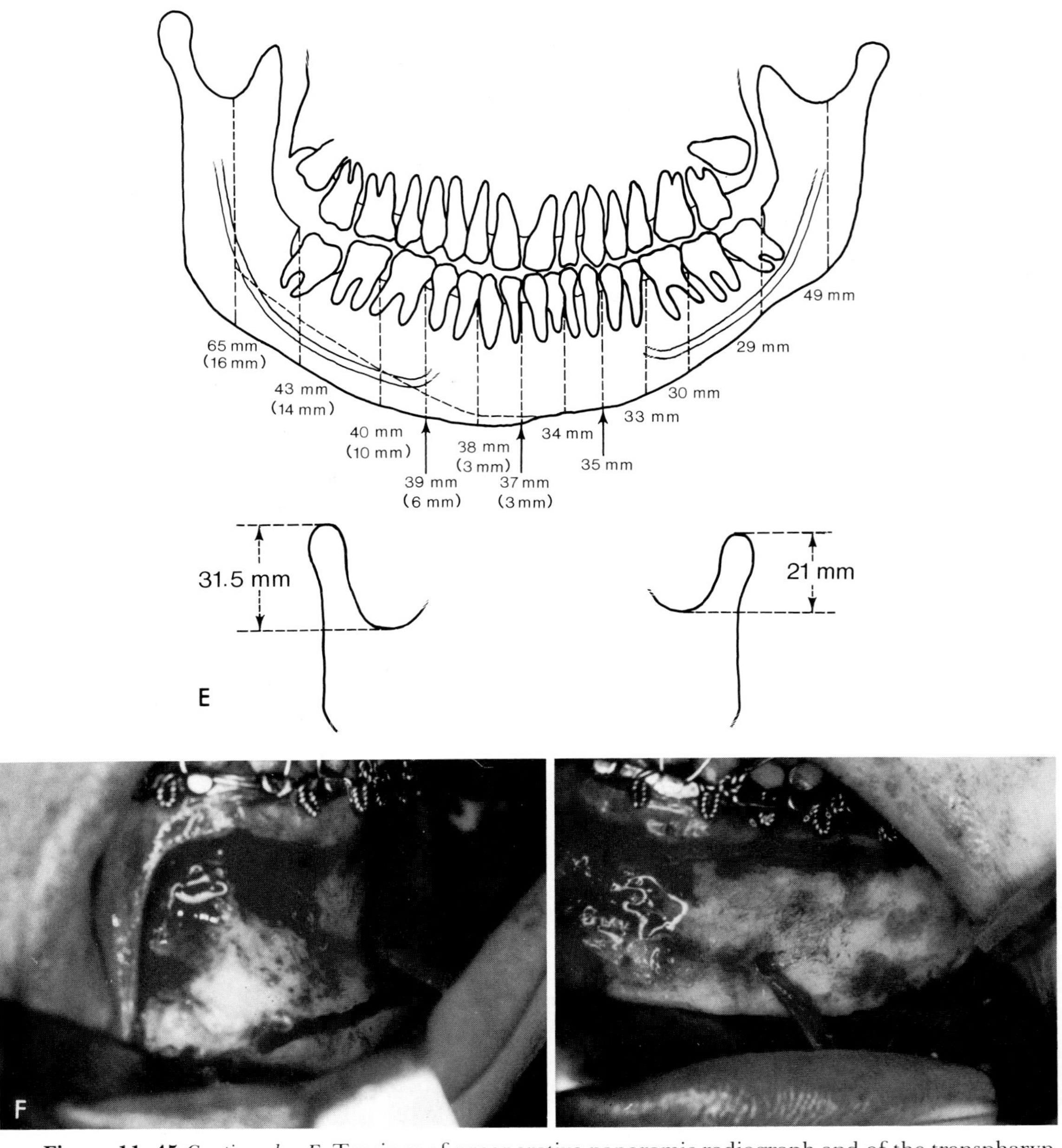

Figure 11–45 *Continued.* *E,* Tracings of preoperative panoramic radiograph and of the transpharyngeal radiographs of the left and right temporomandibular joints in the open position of the mandible. *F,* Intraoral view showing the beginning of the excision of the bowed lower portion of the left mandible.

Legend continued on the opposite page.

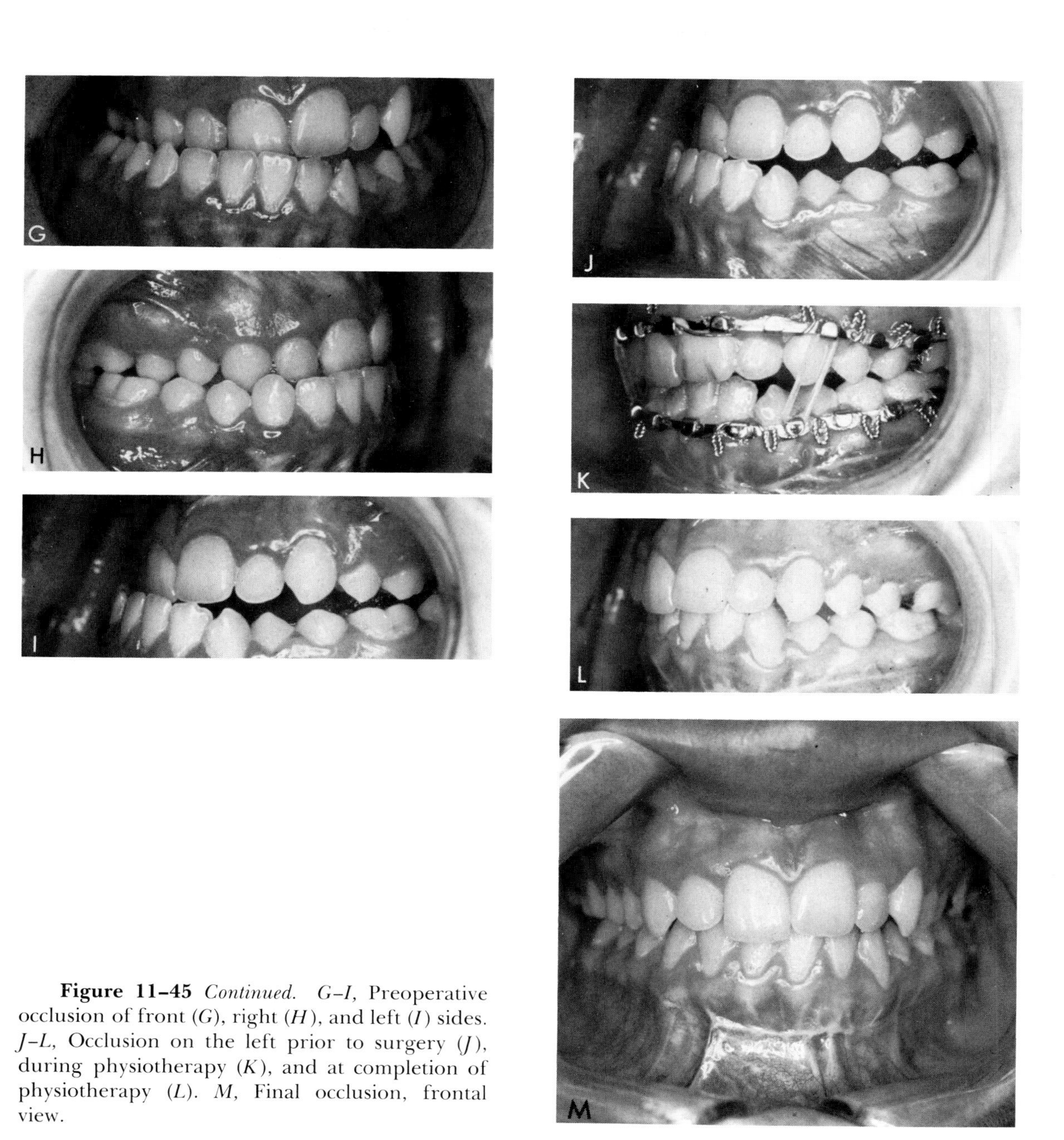

Figure 11–45 *Continued. G–I,* Preoperative occlusion of front (*G*), right (*H*), and left (*I*) sides. *J–L,* Occlusion on the left prior to surgery (*J*), during physiotherapy (*K*), and at completion of physiotherapy (*L*). *M,* Final occlusion, frontal view.

Illustration continued on the following page.

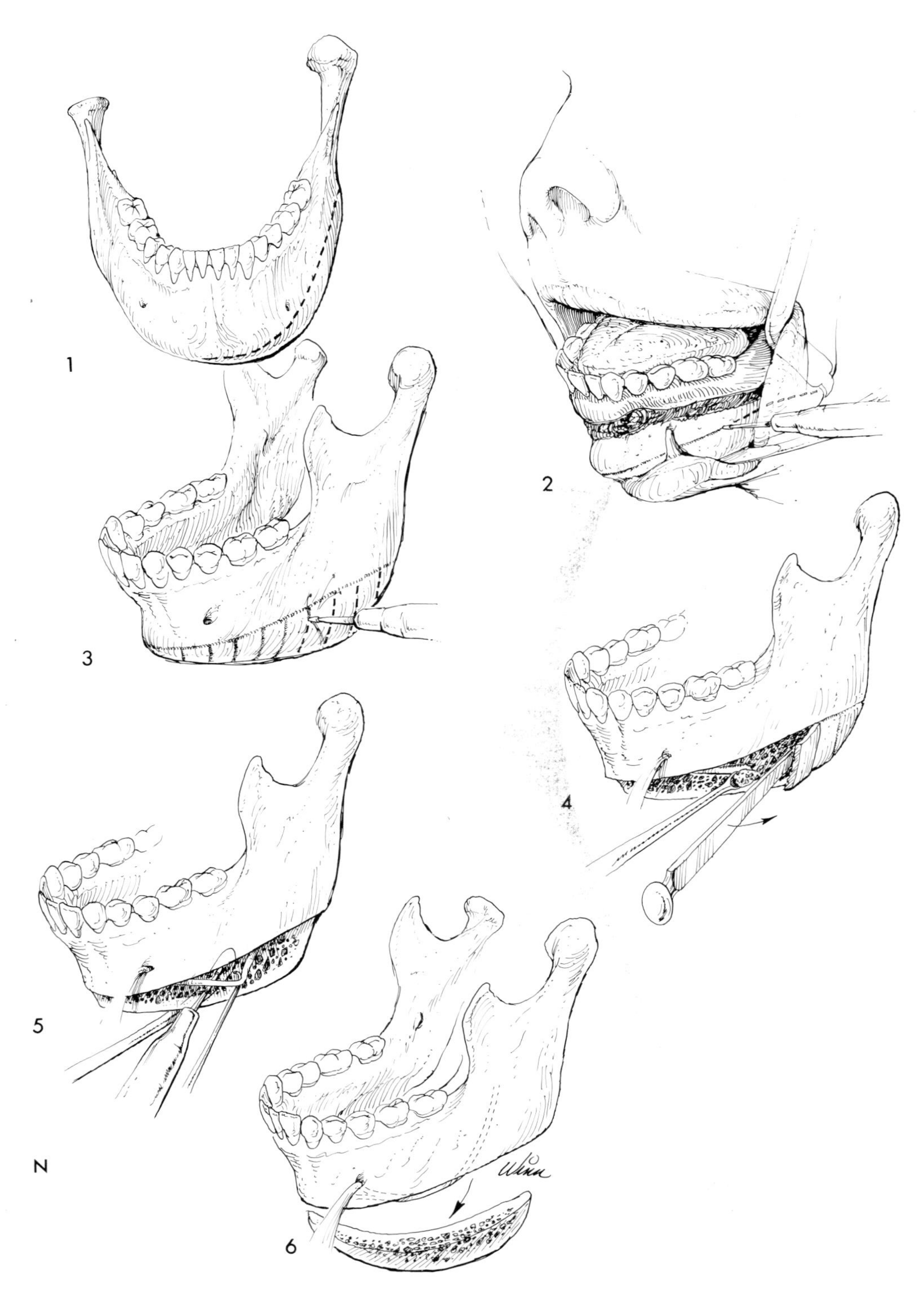

Figure 11–45 *Continued.* *N,* Diagram of surgical procedure. *1,* Line of osteotomy. *2,* Retraction of soft tissue. *3,* Marking and scoring of bone to be removed. *4,* Excision of the outer cortex of bone. *5,* Dissecting free of the neurovascular bundle. *6,* Final excision of the lingual cortical bone with protection of the neurovascular bundle. Technique is same as that used in extraoral approach except that the exposure is more limited. (See Fig. 11–39*Y–GG* for further details.)

left mandible were done (Fig. 11–45*N*). The mandible was immobilized for 3 weeks by arch bars and intermaxillary wiring. After mobilization of the mandible, the physiotherapy of daytime use of the jaw and night-time use of elastic traction was continued for 4 months. The open bite on the left closed during this therapy (Fig. 11–45*J, K,* and *L*).

FOLLOW-UP

Facial proportion and symmetry were brought to an acceptable state (Fig. 11–45*B*). The patient still plans to have the chin shifted a bit more to the left at a later date via an osteotomy of the inferior portion of the anterior mandible. The occlusion has been brought to a good Class I position and has remained stable and functional for two years (Fig. 11–45*M*). The incisal opening is wide and the jaw moves in all excursions without difficulty. A follow-up panoramic radiograph documents the shift of the mandible to the midline and the amount of bone excised from the lower part of the left mandible (Fig. 11–45*D*).

Surgeon: Robert V. Walker, Dallas, Texas.

CASE 11–12 (Fig. 11–46)

W. W., an 11-year-old boy, was being followed by his orthodontist for minimal malocclusion and a significant jaw asymmetry. He was referred for oral surgery consultation. It was determined that the boy had a mandibular right condylar hyperplasia as well as a deep bowing of the right angle and body of the mandible (Fig. 11–46*A*). It was not known at that time (1968) whether or not it was prudent to excise the mandibular right condyle in view of the boy's remaining years of growth. It was jointly decided by parents, orthodontist, and oral surgeon to follow the youngster an additional two years to see whether the condition was progressive. Accordingly, a posteroanterior cephalogram was made, with measurements being made from the Frankfort plane to gonion on each side (Fig. 11–46*E*). Two years later, the posteroanterior cephalogram and comparable measurements from the Frankfort plane to gonion on each side were repeated (Fig. 11–46*F*). It was immediately apparent that no favor was provided the boy by waiting 2 years for a repeat study of his deformity. The asymmetry became a great deal worse during the 2-year wait (Fig. 11–46*B*).

PROBLEM LIST

Esthetics (Fig. 11–46*B*)

1. Good middle and upper facial balance and proportion.
2. Marked right mandibular asymmetry with downward bowing of the inferior border.
3. Tilting of the chin slightly to the left.

Cephalometric and Panoramic Radiographic Evaulation

1. Good anteroposterior position of mandible and maxilla.
2. Excessively long mandibular right condyle, condylar neck, and ramus as measured from the Frankfort plane to gonion on a posteroanterior cephalogram (Fig. 11–46*F*).

3. Deep bowing of the mandibular right body and angle as reflected on the panoramic radiograph (Fig. 11–46*H*).

4. Downward extension of the neurovascular canal through the bowed portion of the right mandible.

Occlusal Analysis

DENTAL ARCH FORM. Symmetric and correctly related.

DENTAL ALIGNMENT. Good.

DENTAL OCCLUSION. Class I occlusion on the left and slight Class II occlusion on the right; good intercuspation of teeth.

TREATMENT PLAN

The treatment plan included trimming away the excess bowing of the right mandible, excising the mandibular right condyle, and attaching a Silastic disk atop the remaining condylar neck stump.

ACTIVE TREATMENT

The excessive bowing on the right mandible, as determined on a tracing of a preoperative panoramic radiograph (Fig. 11–46*K*), was removed (Fig. 11–46*L* through *N*); the mandibular right condyle was excised, a Silastic disk was secured by wiring atop the right condylar neck stump (Fig. 11–46*P*; see also Fig. 11–40). The condyle specimen was soft and appeared to have a deep cartilaginous covering (Fig. 11–46*Q*). This clinical observation was confirmed through study of the histopathologic section, which showed an abundantly growing cartilaginous top of the condyle (Fig. 11–46*R*). No shift of the mandible to the right or left was needed for this patient. After these procedures, the jaw was immobilized for 5 days in the occlusal position by means of an orthodontic labial arch wire and intermaxillary wiring. After 5 days the jaw was mobilized, and a follow-up physiotherapy regimen of daytime use of the jaw and night-time elastic traction with the teeth in occlusion was followed for 2 months.

FOLLOW-UP

Satisfactory mandibular symmetry was achieved (Fig. 11–46*B*). The occlusion remained very good and stable after a 2-year follow-up (Fig. 11–46*S*). Follow-up panoramic radiographs showed new bone covering the neurovascular canal within a year after surgery. A posteroanterior cephalogram with measurements made from the Frankfort plane to gonion on both sides showed satisfactory symmetry of the mandible (Fig. 11–46*G*). A 7-year follow-up facial view of the patient showed the clinical result to be stable with no further progression of the asymmetry (Fig. 11–46*D*).

Surgeon: Robert V. Walker, Dallas, Texas

Text continued on page 1006.

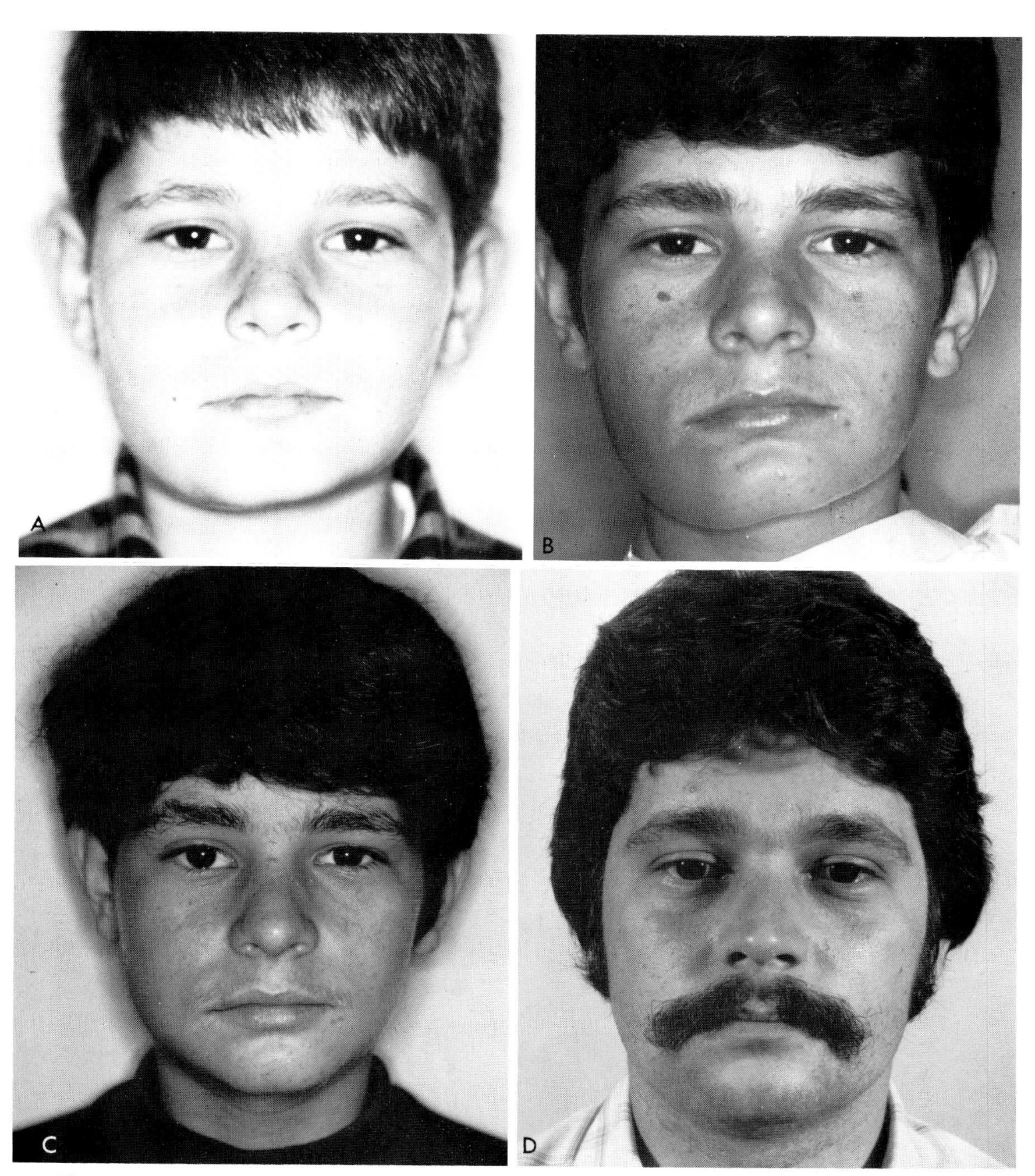

Figure 11–46 (Case 11–12). *A*, Original facial view of patient at age 11. *B*, Preoperative facial view of patient two years later, age 13. *C*, Facial view one year after surgery. *D*, Facial view seven years after surgery.

Illustration continued on the following page.

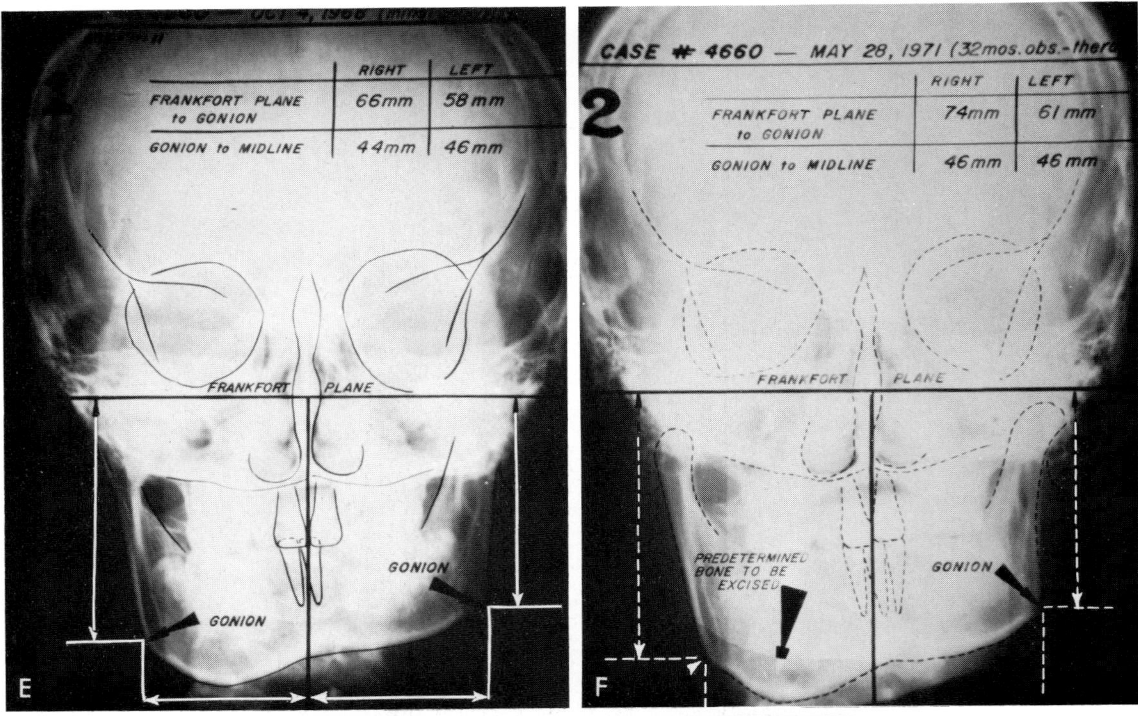

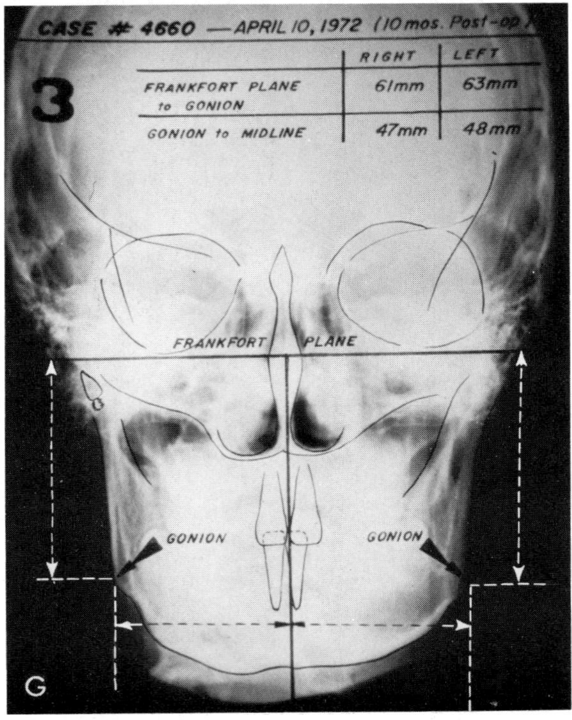

Figure 11–46 *Continued. E,* Original P–A cephalogram with measurements of distance from the Frankfort plane to right and left gonion. *F,* Follow-up P–A cephalogram with repeat measurements of distance from the Frankfort plane to right and left gonion documenting the significant increase on the right side. *G,* Follow-up P–A cephalogram showing gonion on the right and left sides to be at the same level as determined by measurements from the Frankfort plane.

Legend continued on the opposite page.

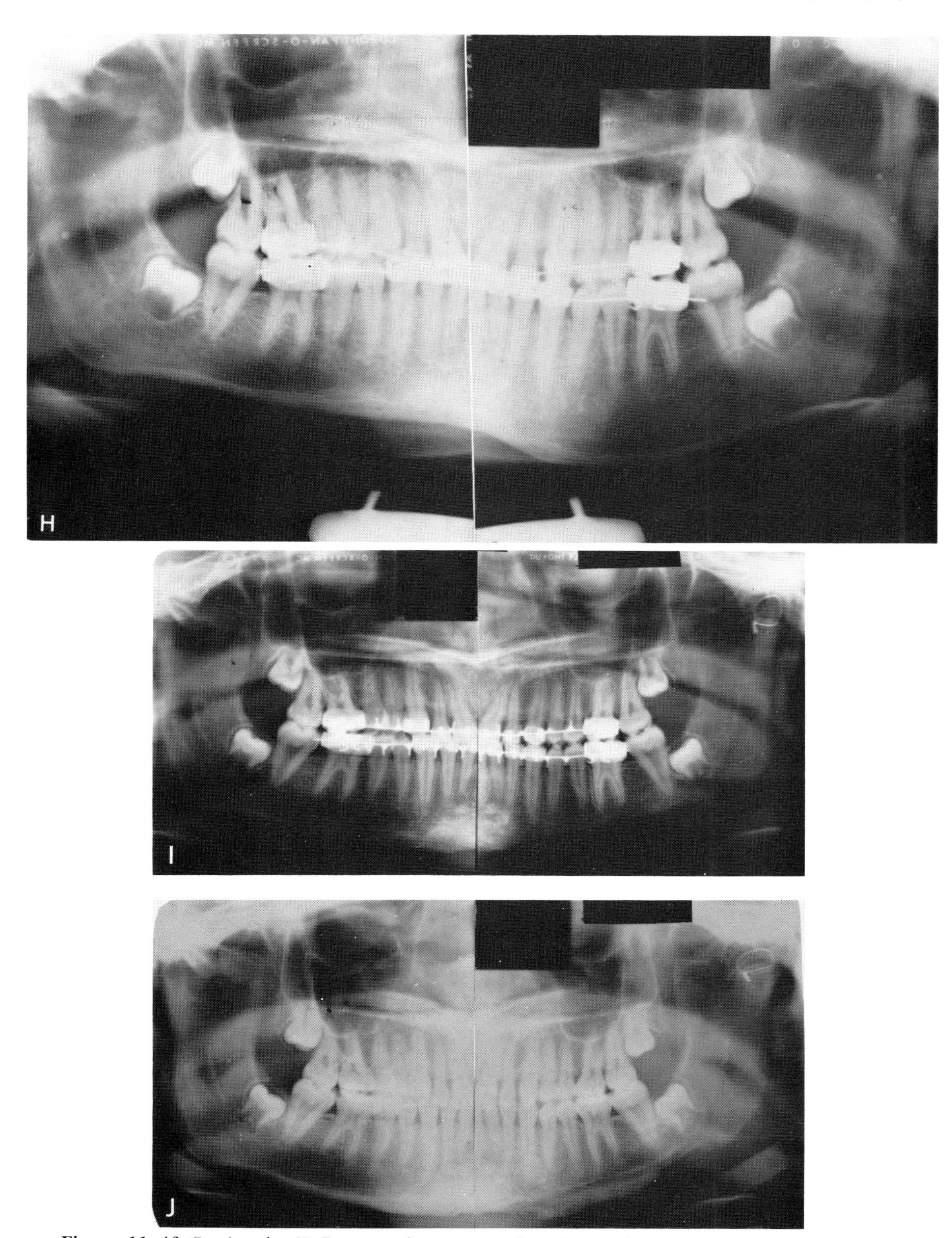

Figure 11–46 *Continued.* *H*, Preoperative panoramic radiograph. *I*, Immediate postoperative panoramic radiograph and (*J*) one year follow-up panogram showing subperiosteal bone now covering neurovascular bundle.

Illustration continued on the following page.

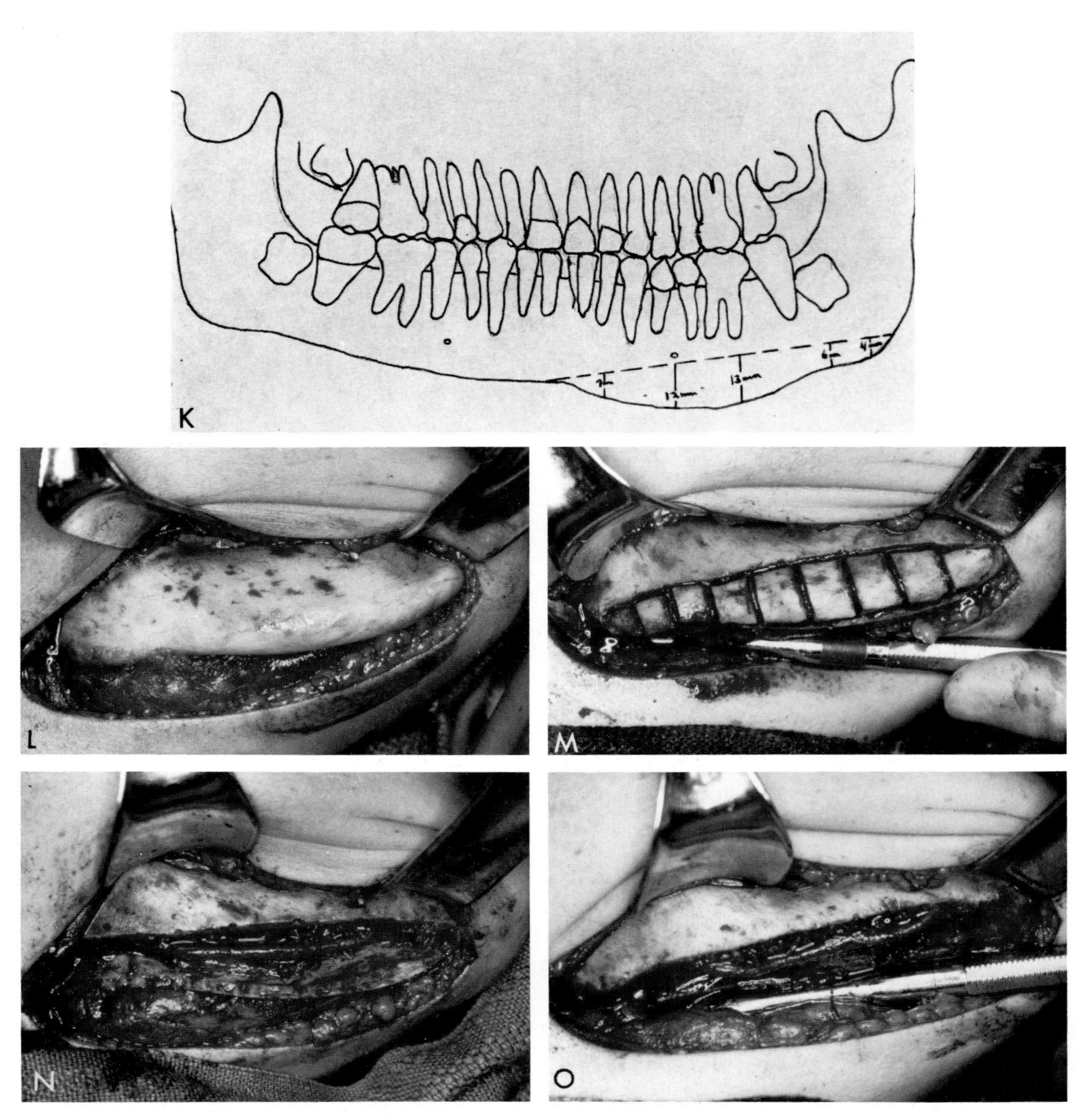

Figure 11–46 *Continued.* *K*, Tracing of preoperative panoramic radiograph for determination of bone to be removed from inferior border of the right mandible. *L–P*, Operative procedure. *L*, Right mandible exposed from submandibular approach; *M*, lateral cortical bone marked and cut prior to removal for dissection of neurovascular bundle. *N*, Neurovascular bundle dissected free, and *O*, lingual cortical bone then removed.

Legend continued on the opposite page.

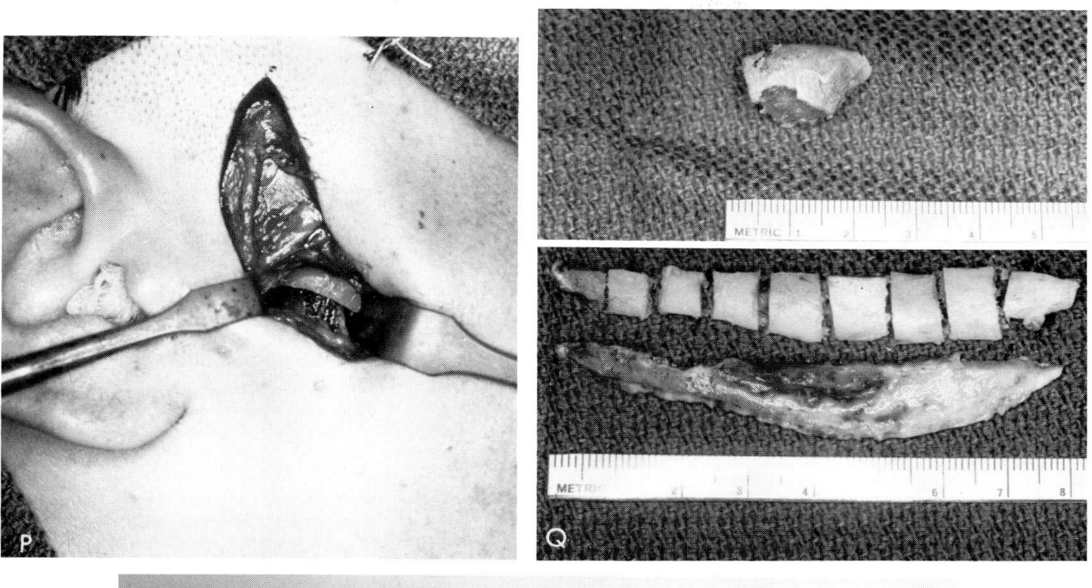

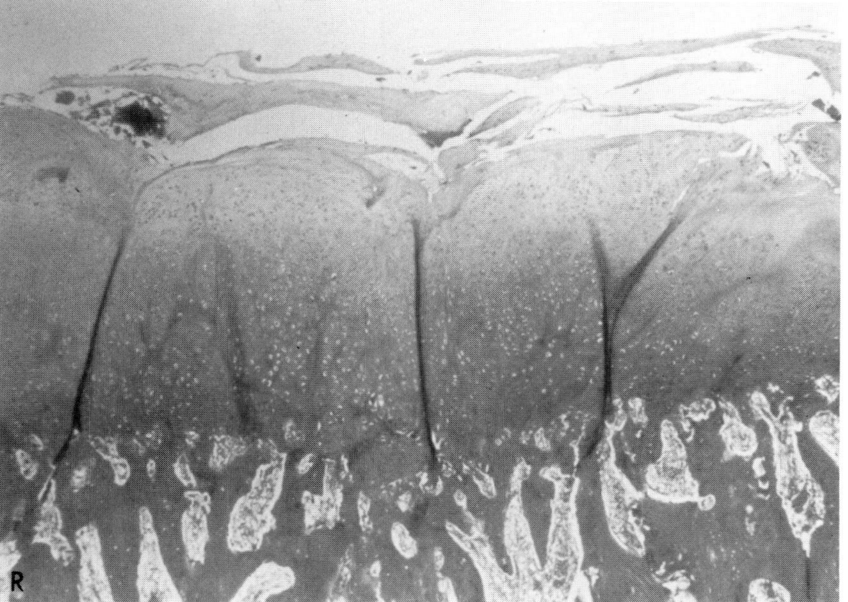

Figure 11–46 *Continued.* *P*, Preauricular approach for removal of right condyle and attachment of Silastic disk atop the condylar stump. *Q*, Condyle specimen and bone excised from lower part of right mandible. *R*, Photomicrograph of section from right condyle showing abundant growth arising in the cartilage covering.

Illustration continued on the following page.

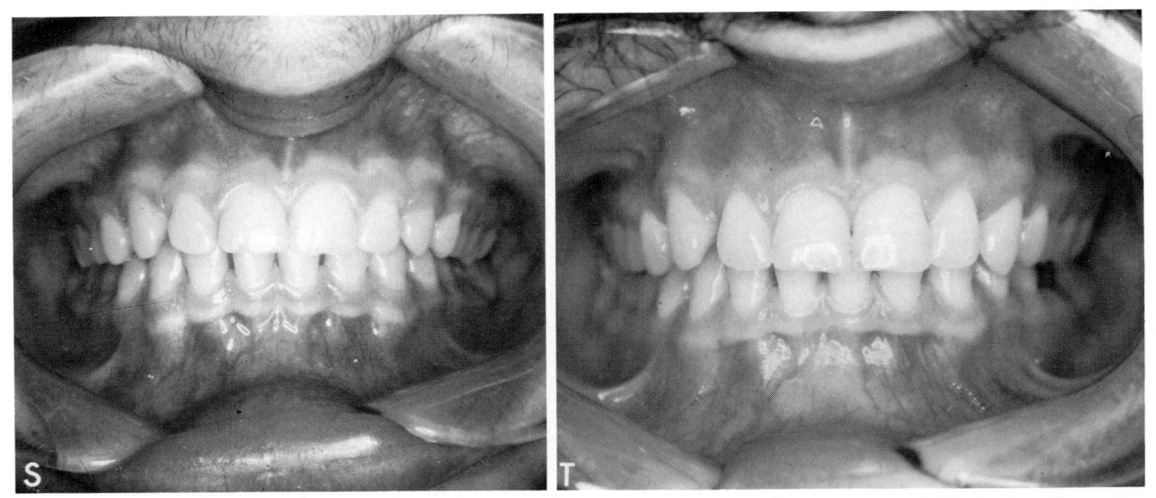

Figure 11–46 *Continued.* *S,* Occlusion from the front two years after surgery. *T,* Occlusion from the front seven years after surgery; no change.

CASE 11–13 (Fig. 11–47)

A 25-year-old man desired treatment to correct his facial asymmetry and malocclusion. At age 11 years the patient's "crossbite" had been treated by orthodontics, facilitated by extraction of four 1st premolar teeth.

PROBLEM LIST

Esthetics (Fig. 11–47*A* and *B*)

FRONTAL. Facial asymmetry: Right side of lower face was angular and flattened anteriorly, the left side was plump and rounded, the chin deviated 6 mm to the left, and the lip-line and occlusal plane tilted upwards toward the right. Examination of repose upper lip: The maxillary incisor relationship revealed a lack of tooth exposure. Asymmetric smile line: There was less tooth exposure on the left side than on the right when smiling. Asymmetric maxillary dental midline: The dental midline deviated 2 mm to the right of the facial midline.

PROFILE. Contour deficient–chin with protruding lower lip.

Cephalometric Analysis (Fig. 11–47*E*)

1. ANB ∠ = 2°
2. Mandibular plane angle = 41°
3. Right mandibular ramus and condylar neck were 5 mm longer than the left mandibular ramus and condylar neck.
4. Maxillary and mandibular anterior teeth tipped forward slightly: T to Na = 31°, T to NB = 32°

Occlusal Analysis (Fig. 11–47*F*)

DENTAL ARCH FORM. Asymmetric in all three planes of space; canting of maxillary occlusal plane; maxillary left incisors positioned 2 mm superior to maxillary right incisor teeth; maxillary posterior teeth positioned 5 mm superior to maxillary right posterior teeth.

DENTAL ALIGNMENT. Minimal crowding of maxillary and mandibular arches.

DENTAL OCCLUSION. Class III molar and canine relationship; midline of mandibular incisors positioned 6 mm to left of maxillary incisors.

TREATMENT PLAN

Presurgical Orthodontic Treatment (Fig. 11–47*G*)

1. Align maxillary and mandibular teeth without extractions; correct dental rotations; align lower anterior teeth without opening bite, facilitated by the use of direct bonded appliances (Fig. 11–47*G*).
2. Stripping of maxillary and mandibular anterior teeth as needed to harmonize arches; orthodontic diagnostic set-up (Fig. 11–47*H*).

Surgical Treatment (Fig. 11–47*J*)

1. Two-piece Le Fort I osteotomy to level maxillary occlusal plane, correct dental midline, widen maxilla 4 mm to achieve transverse harmony with mandible, achieve esthetic tooth to lip relationship and esthetic smile line. The vertical changes would be accomplished by raising the right maxillary molar-premolar region 5 mm; rotating the maxilla to left side 2 mm; lowering the maxillary right incisor region 3 mm and left maxillary incisor region 5 mm to increase amount of maxillary incisor tooth exposure and produce an esthetic and symmetric smile line.
2. Posterior repositioning of mandible with rotation by bilateral intraoral vertical ramus osteotomies to correct midline and produce Class I canine and molar relationship.
3. Seven-mm advancement genioplasty to increase prominence of chin and offset the effect of surgically retracting the mandible; inferior aspect of mental symphysis would be repositioned laterally to achieve chin symmetry (see Chapter 14 for details of surgery technique).
4. Augmentation of right mandibular body with 6 mm thick Proplast implant.

Postsurgical Orthodontic Treatment (Fig. 11–47*I*)

1. Detailing of occlusion with fixed orthodontic appliances.
2. Final detailing of occlusion and retention with positioner and orthodontic retention appliances.

TREATMENT AND FOLLOW-UP

This case illustrates how a good occlusal and esthetic result was achieved by numerous subtle three-dimensional changes. The therapy was effective despite the

Text continued on page 1011.

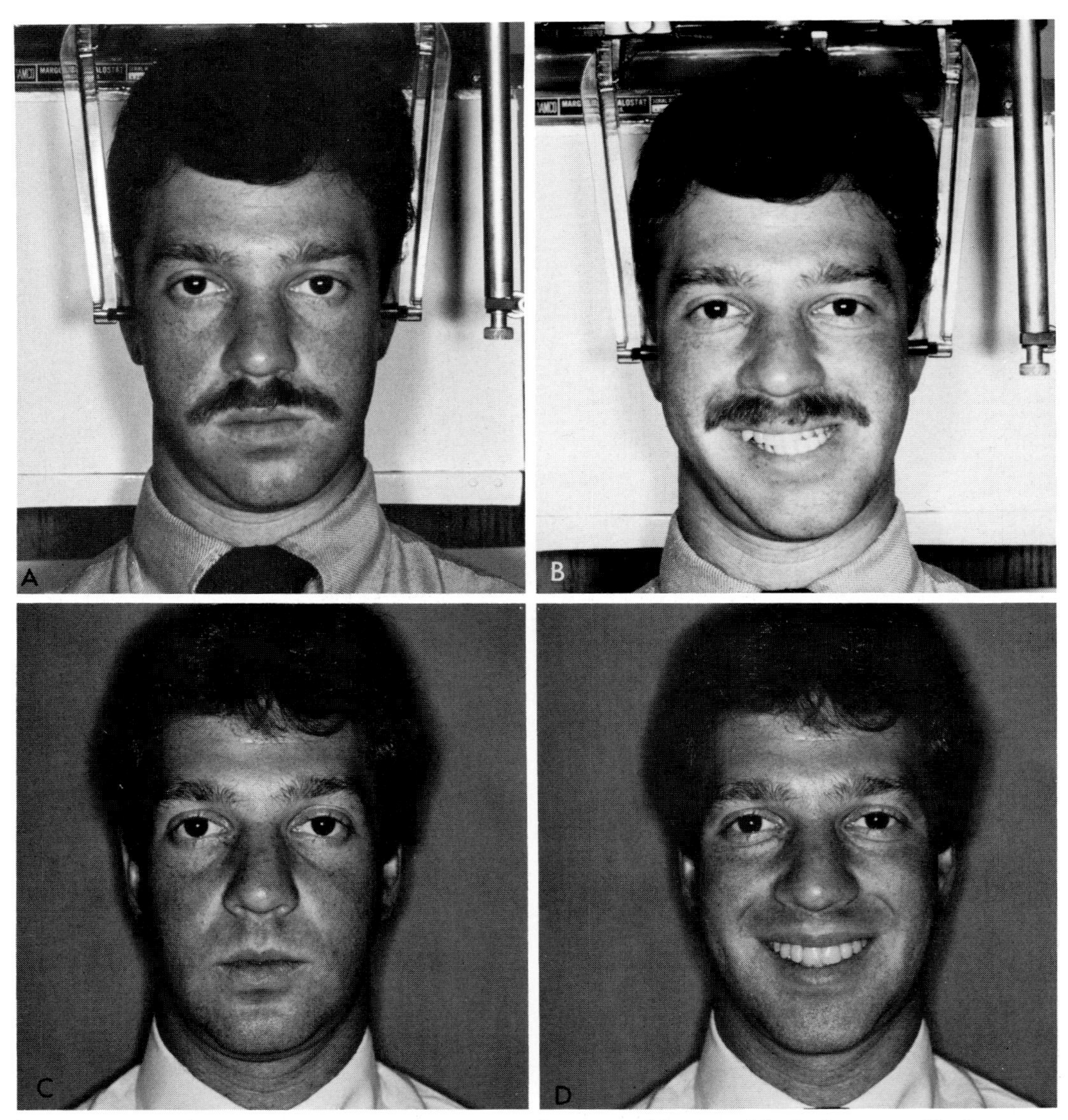

Figure 11–47 (Case 11–13). *A to D,* Twenty-five year-old man with deviate mandibular prognathism and facial asymmetry before (*A* and *B*) and after treatment (*C* and *D*). Note the asymmetric smile and relative lack of tooth exposure before treatment.

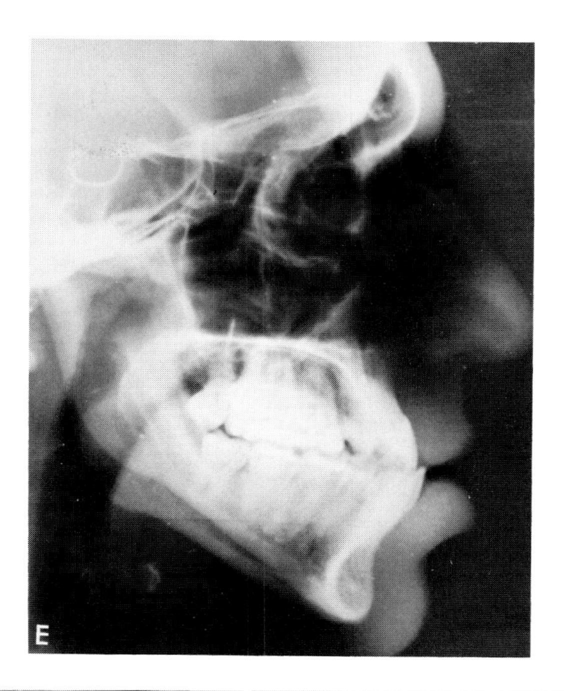

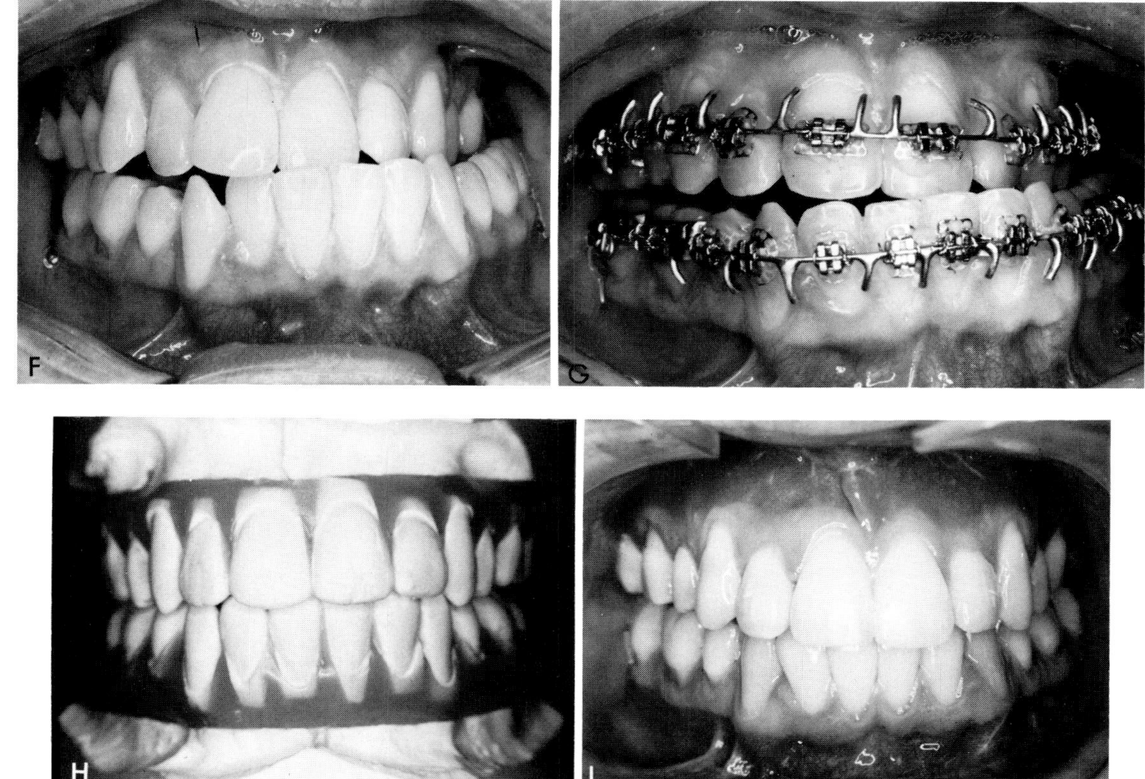

Figure 11–47 *Continued.* *E,* Pretreatment cephalogram. *F,* Occlusion before treatment. *G,* Teeth aligned and arches levelled and coordinated before surgery. *H,* Orthodontic diagnostic setup which indicated the feasibility of treatment without extractions. *I,* Occlusion immediately after removal of orthodontic appliances.

Illustration continued on the following page.

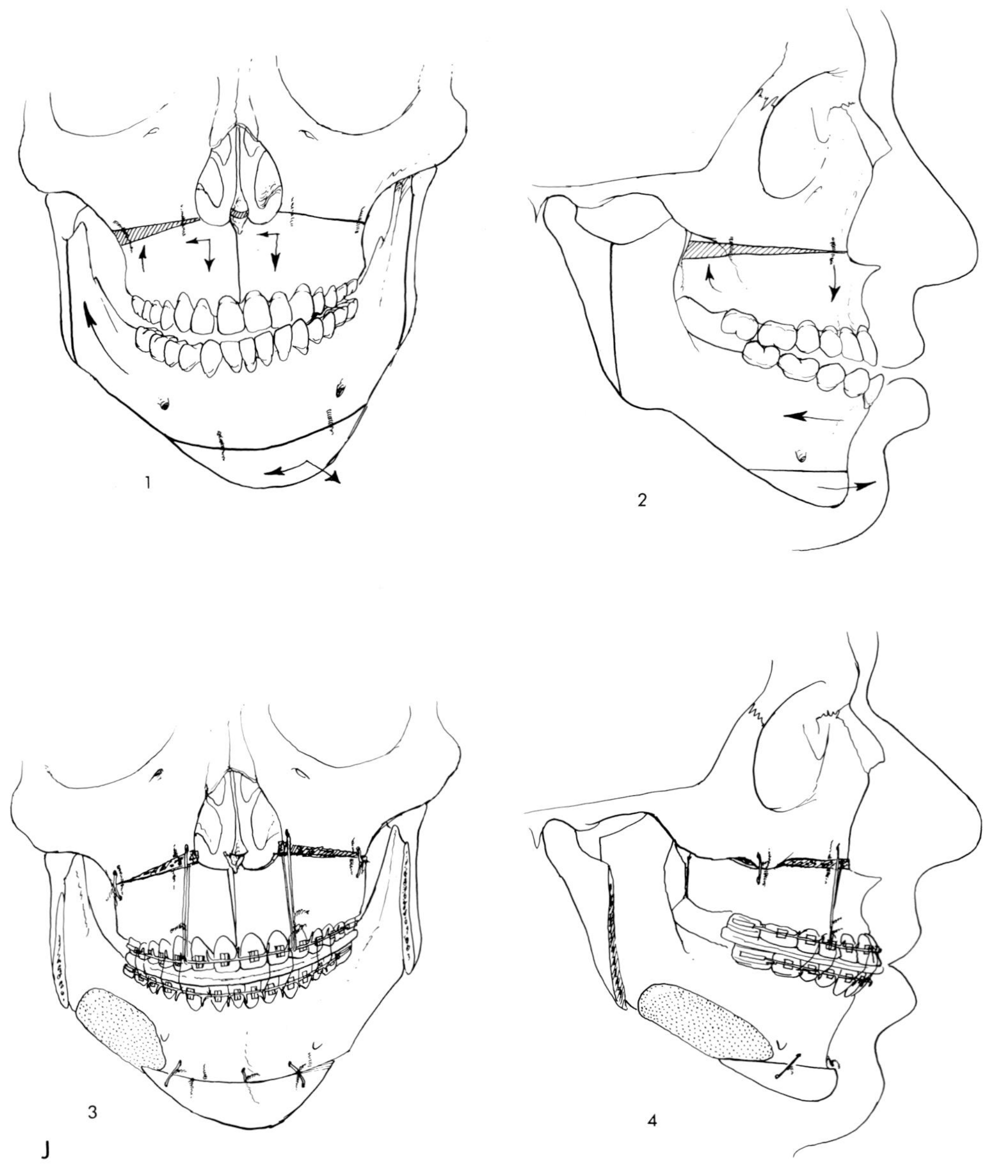

Figure 11–47 *Continued.* *J,* Plan of surgery: 1) Two-piece Le Fort I osteotomy to level maxillary occlusal plane, rotate maxilla to center dental midline; widen maxilla; differentially lower right and left anterior maxilla by interpositional bone grafts to increase tooth exposure and achieve symmetric smile. 2) Bilateral intraoral vertical ramus osteotomies to reposition mandible posteriorly and rotate mandible to correct dental midline and achieve Class I canine and molar relationship. 3) Genioplasty to reposition chin anteriorly and laterally to increase chin prominence and achieve chin symmetry. 4) Augmentation of right mandibular body with 6 mm thick proplast implant.

fact that the initial orthodontic plan of treatment was accomplished when the patient was 12 years old, without plans to surgically correct the facial asymmetry. At age 26, three-dimensional occlusal and facial esthetic balance was achieved by orthodontic and surgical treatments over a period of 12 months.

An orthodontic diagnostic set-up, model surgery, and cephalometric prediction studies of both PA and lateral head radiographs indicated the feasibility of the surgical plan. A three-dimensional assessment of the maxillary spatial relationship and planned changes was made by model surgery of dental casts mounted on an anatomic articulator with the aid of a face-bow mounting. The indication for and size of bone grafts was calculated from a study of the lateral head cephalograms, tooth-to-lip measurements and three-dimensional measurements of the repositioned sectioned study casts. (See Chapters 9, 18, and 21 for additional details.)

Proper planning and execution of maxillary surgery is the key to correcting facial asymmetry. The maxilla is repositioned to achieve three-dimensional facial balance. The plan to level the maxillary occlusal plane and correct the canted occlusal plane is based upon multiple factors. In the anterior, the lip-to-tooth relationship and asymmetric smile line are the principal diagnostic parameters used to plan for differentially raising or lowering the anterior maxilla. In the posterior region, the smile line, mandibular plane angle, and occlusal plane angle in an anteroposterior direction are all considered to determine whether the posterior occlusion will be leveled by raising one side of the maxilla or lowering the contralateral "short" side of the maxilla by interpositional bone grafting. In this particular case the decision was made to raise the right posterior maxilla because of the relatively high mandibular plane angle and the propensity for relapse after mandibular surgery. Consequently, from a biomechanical point of view, greater stability was "built" into the treatment plan. (See Relapse Considerations in Chapter 13.)

After treatment is planned to correct maxillary asymmetry in all three planes of space, the asymmetric mandible is repositioned to achieve the best possible occlusal and esthetic result. Genioplasty is usually indicated to achieve adequate prominence and symmetry of the chin. (See Figure 11–47*J*.)

Presurgical orthodontic treatment was accomplished within a period of 7 months. The alignment of the anterior teeth was achieved with minimal bite opening by judicious stripping of the anterior dentition. All of the planned surgery was accomplished simultaneously. The maxilla and mandible were immobilized 6 weeks by intermaxillary fixation between the vertical lugs that were soldered to the orthodontic arch wires. This was followed by an additional 6 weeks of jaw physiotherapy (daytime use of the jaw and nighttime use of intermaxillary elastic traction). Final detailing of the occlusion was achieved by an additional 3 months of orthodontic treatment through the use of a positioner and finally with orthodontic retention appliances.

Surgeon: William H. Bell, Dallas, Texas. *Orthodontist:* I. D. Buchin, Forest Hills, New York.

REFERENCES

1. Berry DC: Mandibular condyle hyperplasia. Oral Surg *11*:420, 1958.
2. Blomquist J, Hogeman KE: Benign unilateral hyperplasia of the mandibular condyle: report of eight cases. Acta Chir Scand *126*:414, 1963.

3. Broadway RT: Two cases of unilateral hyperplasia of the mandibular condyle. Proc Roy Soc Med *51*:691, 1958.
4. Burch RJ, Shuttee TS: Unilateral hyperplasia of the left mandibular condyle and hypoplasia of body of right side of mandible: report of case. J Oral Surg Anesth Hosp Dent Serv *18*:255, 1960.
5. Cernea P: Les deviations mandibulares d'origine epiphysaire. Rev Stomat *49*:388, 1948.
6. Cernea P: Unilateral hypertrophy of the mandibular condyle. *In* Husted E, Hjorting-Hansen E (Eds): Oral Surgery, First International Conference. Copenhagen: Munksgaard, 1967, pp 255–257.
7. Cowan A: Case of unilateral condylar hyperplasia. Br Dent J *93*:118, 1952.
8. Dingman RO, Grabb WC: Mandibular laterognathism. Plast Reconstr Surg *31*:563, 1963.
9. Engel MB, Brodie AG: Condylar growth and mandibular deformities. Surgery *22*:976, 1947.
10. Gottlieb, O: Hyperplasia of the mandibular condyle. J Oral Surg *9*:118, 1951.
11. Grellet M, Scheffer P: Traitements chirugicaux des latérognathies mandibulaires. Rev Stomat *67*:85, 1966.
12. Gruca A, Meisels E: Asymmetry of the mandible from bilateral hypertrophy. Ann Surg *83*:755, 1926.
13. Hayward JR, Bruce RA: Condylar hyperplasia and mandibular asymmetries: a review. J Oral Surg, April 1968.
14. Hayward JR, Kahn SP: Skeletal differences in identical twins. J Oral Surg, Feb. 1974.
15. Hinds EC, Reid LC, Burch RJ: Classification and management of mandibular asymmetry. Am J Surg *100*:825, 1960.
16. Hovell JH: Condylar hyperplasia. Br J Oral Surg *1*:105, 1963.
17. Levignac J: Laprognathie et la laterognathie mandibulaire dans les formes avec beance d'articule et exces vertical de l'étage inferieru de la face. A propos de son traitement. Ann otolaryng (Paris) *82*:941, 1965.
18. Litzlow TJ, et al.: Surgical correction of deformities of the mandible. Surg Clin North Am *43*:979, 1963.
19. Mercier P: Asymmetries of the mandible. Proposed classification and analysis. J Can Dent Assoc *35*:146, 1969.
20. Oberg T, et al: Unilateral hyperplasia of the mandibular condylar process. A histological, microradiographic, and autoradiographic examination of one case. Acta Odontol Scand *20*:485, 1962.
21. Peyrus J: Apropos of the treatment of a unilateral mandibular hypertrophy. Lyon Med *93*:1265, 1961.
22. Plumpton S: The surgical correction of mandibular deformities. J Roy Col Surg Edinb *9*:279, 1964.
23. Rowe NL: Aetiology, clinical features, and treatment of mandibular deformity. Br Dent J *108*:41, 1960.
24. Rushton MA: Growth at the mandibular condyle in relation to some deformities. Br Dent J *76*:57, 1944.
25. Sung RY: Facial asymmetry and malocclusion from unilateral hyperplasia of the mandibular condyle; report of five cases. Chinese Med J *76*:59, 1958.
26. Tarsitano JJ, Wooten JW: The asymmetrical mandible. J Oral Surg *28*:832, 1970.
27. Taylor RS, Cook HP: Surgical correction of skeletal deformities of the mandible. Br Dent J *105*:349, 1958.
28. Toller PA: The transpharyngeal radiography for arthritis of the mandibular condyle. Br J Oral Surg *7*:47, 1969.
29. Waldron CW, Peterson AG, Waldron CA: Surgical treatment of mandibular prognathism. J Oral Surg *4*:61, 1946.
30. Walker RV: Condylar abnormalities. *In* Husted E, Hjorting-Hansen E (Eds) Oral Surgery, First International Conference. Copenhagen: Munksgaard, 1967, pp 81–96.

Suggested Reading

Avis V: The significance of the angle of the mandible; an experimental and comparative study. Am J Phys Anthrop *19*:55, 1961.
Bell WE: Temporomandibular joint disease: etiology, diagnosis, principles of treatment. Dallas, Texas: Etan Co, 1960.
Converse JM, Shapiro HH: Treatment of developmental malformations of jaws. Plast Reconstr Surg *10*:473, 1952.
Deady JJ, Silagi JL, Hutton CE: Hemihypertrophies of the face and mandible. Oral Surg *27*:577, 1969.
Dufourmentel L: Deviation irreductible de la Machoire inferieure traiteé par la resection orthopedique du condyle. Rev Odont *48*:162, 1927.
Fickling BW, Fordyce GL: Mandibular osteotomy for facial asymmetry. Proc Roy Soc Med *48*:989, 1955.
Gorski M, Tarczuska IH: Surgical treatment of mandibular asymmetry. Br J Plast Surg *22*:370, 1969.
Ivy RH: Benign bony enlargement of the condyloid process of the mandible. Ann Surg *85*:27, 1927.
Jacobs FJ, Rafel SS, Weiss B: Correction of asymmetric prognathism by unilateral ostectomy. J Oral Surg *11*:42, 1953.
McNichols JW, Roger AT: Original method of correction of hyperplastic asymmetry of mandible. Plast Reconstr Surg *1*:288, 1946.
Mavaddat I: Intraoral correction of mandibular asymmetry. J Oral Surg *29*:422, 1971.
Moyers RE: Handbook of Orthodontics; for the Student and General Practicioner, ed 2. Chi-

cago: Year Book Medical Publishers, 1963, p 3.

Prasad U: Congenital true hemihypertrophy of the face. J Laryngol Otolarngol *85*:607, 1971.

Reichenbach E., et al: Chirurgische Kieferothopadie. Leipzig: Johann Ambrosius Barth, 1965, p 154.

Sercer A, Bock J: Angeborene einseitige Hypertrophie des Unterkiefers. Deutsch Zahn Mund Kieferheik 7:404, 1940.

Thoma KH: Tumors of the condyle and temporomandibular joint. Oral Surg *7*:1091, 1954.

Weis RS, Thompson JL: Infantile cortical hyperostosis: A study to determine if residual deformities exist in mandibles. J Dent Child *36*:441, 1969.

Chapter 12

BIMAXILLARY PROTRUSION

William R. Proffit and William H. Bell

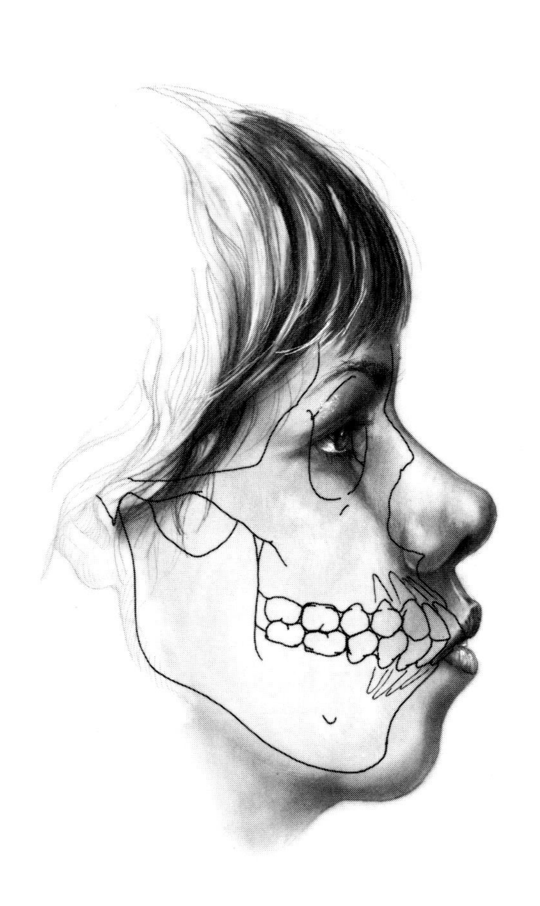

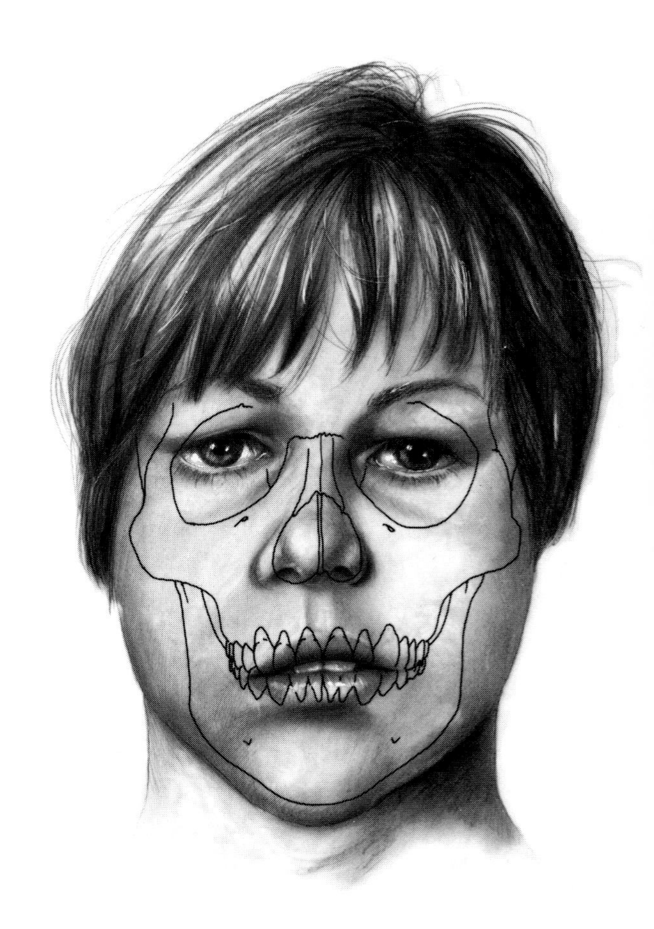

The term *bimaxillary dentoalveolar protrusion* refers to a condition in which the maxillary and mandibular incisor teeth are so severely protruded that the lips cannot be closed without strain. The condition may or may not accompany relative protrusion of the jaws themselves. Lip incompetence (i.e., failure of the lips to meet at rest) and lip strain on closure are important diagnostic features. The primary indication that the incisors are too far forward is that the lips cannot be brought into proper function because of the protruding teeth.

There is a great deal of racial variation in the degree of protrusion of the teeth as well as the jaws. In general, the faces of blacks and orientals are more prominent than those of caucasoids; that is, their maxillae and mandibles are farther forward in relation to the cranium. In addition, these racial groups also have a greater degree of dental protrusion (protrusion of incisor teeth relative to their supporting bone). Moreover, variations occur within each of the major racial groups. In white populations, dental protrusion is more common in individuals of Mediterranean background than in those from more northern areas. The Australian aborigines, who are classified as caucasoid on the basis of blood groups, have a great deal of facial as well as dental protrusion. A possible explanation for interracial differences in dental protrusion is that the soft-tissue contours related to greater prominence of the cheekbones allow more dental protrusion in some groups than others.[11] At any rate, the variance in dental protrusion seems to be related to both racial and soft-tissue differences.

Whatever the racial group, lip strain and lip incompetence are the hallmarks of excessive dental protrusion. Since bimaxillary protrusion is compatible with excellent occlusal relationships of the teeth, the patient's problems are primarily esthetic. Some protrusion of incisors is found in many patients with dental crowding, but extremely protrusive teeth usually are well aligned.

SYSTEMATIC DESCRIPTION OF THE DEFORMITY

Esthetic Features

Four related esthetic problems occur in patients with bimaxillary protrusion:

1. Extreme protrusion of maxillary and mandibular incisor teeth so that either the teeth are prominent and visible in the full-face and profile views, or lip strain is evident in both views if the teeth are covered.
2. Lip incompetence such that the lips remain apart most of the time rather than covering the protruding teeth.
3. Thick-looking lips, with an everted vermilion border and a "rolled" appearance. Lips actually are not thicker than normal in most instances; they are merely more prominent.
4. Apparent chin deficiency. The patient invariably has a very "toothy" appearance. The maxillary teeth may protrude more than the mandibular teeth; therefore, the differential diagnosis often is between bimaxillary dentoalveolar protrusion and maxillary dental or skeletal protrusion. True deficiency in chin contour often adds to the convexity of the face, exaggerating the appearance of skeletal mandibular underdevelopment.

Cephalometric and Dental Cast Relationships

Patients with bimaxillary protrusion may have mild crowding or spacing of teeth within the dental arches but usually have good alignment. (Occasionally, a single tooth may be significantly malpositioned.) In most of these patients, however, the potential crowding has expressed itself as protrusion instead, and so alignment problems have taken care of themselves.

Occlusal relationships in the transverse plane of space also are likely to be good. There may be mild vertical discrepancies, ranging from open bite to deep bite. If the maxillary incisors protrude more than the mandibular incisors, some mandibular incisor crowding, an accentuated curve of Spee, and an accompanying dental deep bite may be found. The major problem lies in the anteroposterior plane of space. The incisor teeth can be seen to be positioned forward relative to any cephalometric vertical reference line. The N-A, N-B, A-Pog, and N-Pog lines are most often used for this purpose. When the lips are strained to closure, the various soft-tissue cephalometric measurements, such as the Ricketts or Holdaway lines, also reveal lip protrusion. The prominence of the mandibular incisor teeth in relation to the chin is particularly well revealed by comparing the prominence of the incisor to the N-B line with the prominence of the bony chin to the same line. The ratio of these numbers, the "Holdaway ratio," should be about 1:1 plus 2 mm for the lower incisors (i.e., 3:1, 4:2, 5:3).

ORTHODONTIC TREATMENT

Historical Background

Orthodontic treatment for bimaxillary protrusion was first attempted in the late 19th century and was carried out quite successfully in the early 1900s. The technique involved removing the first premolars and retracting the protruding incisors orthodontically. Successful treatment required development of full-banded appliances so that roots could be positioned properly. This was done concurrently by Edward Angle and Calvin Case in the early 1900s.

Angle was an uncompromising opponent of the extraction of teeth for orthodontic purposes, and so he never discussed the use of his appliances to manage premolar extraction sites, although they were well suited for that purpose. In his later years, Angle refused to admit that there was such a thing as bimaxillary protrusion. He used full-banded appliances to expand the arches to bring the teeth into ideal alignment, whatever the amount of protrusion created by doing so.

Case, on the other hand, disagreed sharply with Angle on this point. In 1921, he wrote, "One of the most dangerous features of the Angle classification is the universally applied teaching that when the dentures are placed in normal occlusion, the facial outlines will take care of themselves."[6] By the time of World War I, Case had worked out most of the mechanical principles that are required for successful management of orthodontic extraction sites with full-banded appliances. In many ways, his work presages that done by other investigators 40 years later. Nevertheless, it was not until after Angle's death that orthodontists who had been trained by Angle began to use his full-banded appliances for extraction treatment. The modern techniques for orthodontic management of bimaxillary protrusion were worked out independently by two of Angle's students, Charles Tweed in the United States and Raymond Begg in Australia. Tweed reintroduced extraction treatment into American orthodontics after Case's early work had been all but forgotten. Improvements in the full-banded orthodontic appliances necessary for good management of extraction sites have continued over the intervening 40 years.

Treatment Approach

Whatever the orthodontic treatment approach, the challenge in successful management of bimaxillary protrusion is to close the extraction space by retraction of the incisors, maintaining the posterior teeth in their original position and thus "protecting the posterior anchorage." Tweed developed a detailed mechanical approach for this purpose in the 1940s. This consisted of establishing the maxillary arch as an anchorage unit, setting up the mandibular posterior teeth in a position that he believed gave maximum resistance to mesial movement, and then retracting the mandibular incisors. At this stage of treatment, a considerable overjet of the maxillary incisors was produced. The mandibular arch was then stabilized, and the maxillary incisors were retracted, leading to an ultimate correction of the protrusion in both arches. Extraoral force was exerted upon both arches to help support the posterior teeth. Treatment time in nongrowing individuals was 24 to 30 months, and as many as sixteen separate sets of arch wires were required. Although the technique has been somewhat simplified now, the basic approach is still valid: all teeth in the opposite arch, and posterior teeth in the arch where incisors are being retracted, are pitted against the six incisors to be retracted, while the posterior anchorage is augmented by extraoral force.[13] If this approach is carried out carefully, excellent orthodontic retraction can be achieved.

One of the advantages of this orthodontic treatment approach is that any necessary leveling of the mandibular arch is automatically taken care of as part of the overall procedure. Many patients with bimaxillary protrusion have an accentuated curve of Spee in the mandibular arch; this requires correction. In growing children, it is not necessary to intrude mandibular incisors in order to correct a deep curve of Spee. All that is required is to maintain the vertical level of the incisors while premolars and molars erupt concomitantly with continued vertical growth. In nongrowing individuals, some intrusion of elongated mandibular incisors usually is needed.

Orthodontic correction of bimaxillary protrusion can be carried out quite successfully in both growing children and nongrowing adults. The more the incisors must be retracted, the more carefully the retraction must be done in order to keep from "losing anchorage" and slipping posterior teeth forward. For this reason and because incisor intrusion is needed, patients who are not growing often require relatively long periods of treatment and must cooperate well in the use of extraoral force and interarch elastics.

SURGICAL TREATMENT

In its simplest form, surgical treatment of bimaxillary protrusion involves maxillary and mandibular alveolar segmental osteotomies following extraction of first or second premolars, to retract and frequently to intrude the protruding maxillary and mandibular incisors. In many instances, even after retraction of mandibular incisors, an augmentation genioplasty is needed in order to achieve good facial appearance (Fig. 12–1).

Historical Background

Although anterior segmental surgical procedures in both arches were described in the 1920s, it was not until after World War II, in Europe, that these procedures came into common use. Significant contributions to the anterior maxillary segmental surgery were made by Wassmund,[14] Cupar,[7] and Wunderer[15] — with variations, the surgical techniques advocated by these men remain in use. The anterior mandibular segmental osteotomies were evaluated in detail by Köle.[9] (The variation for correcting anterior open bite that is now commonly known as the Köle procedure rarely is indicated in bimaxillary protrusion.) These surgical procedures were not introduced in the United States until the late 1950s and 1960s, by which time they were in common use in Europe. Correlated surgical and orthodontic treatment has been emphasized in American papers during the 1970s.[2, 3, 10]

Treatment Approach

The surgical history of and detailed surgical technique for anterior maxillary osteotomy to retract maxillary incisors is described in Chapter 8. The downfracture method, which is usually indicated for superior movement of the total maxilla, also is described in Chapter 8. Use of the downfracture technique may be indicated if significant open bite accompanies bimaxillary protrusion. Anterior mandibular osteotomy is described in Chapter 10 and genioplasty in Chapter 14. In this chapter, we comment on application of these surgical techniques specifically to bimaxillary protrusion.

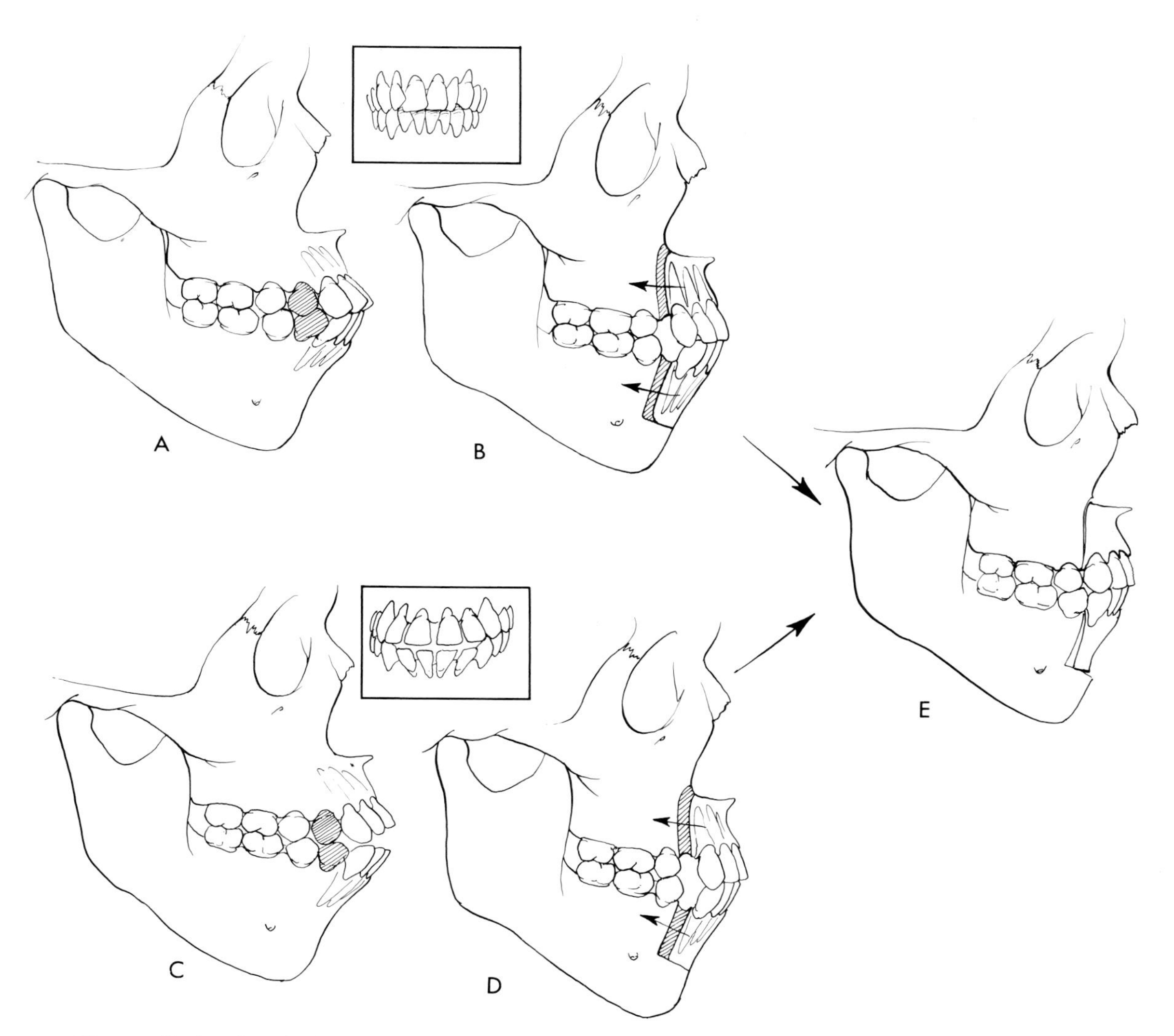

Figure 12–1. Surgical and orthodontic correction of bimaxillary protrusion associated with closed bite and crowded anterior teeth (*A* and *B*) and with anterior open bite and spaced teeth (*C* and *D*). After extraction of 1st premolars, the anterior teeth are aligned by orthodontic treatment. The anterior maxilla and anterior mandible are then surgically repositioned by anterior subapical ostectomy (*E*).

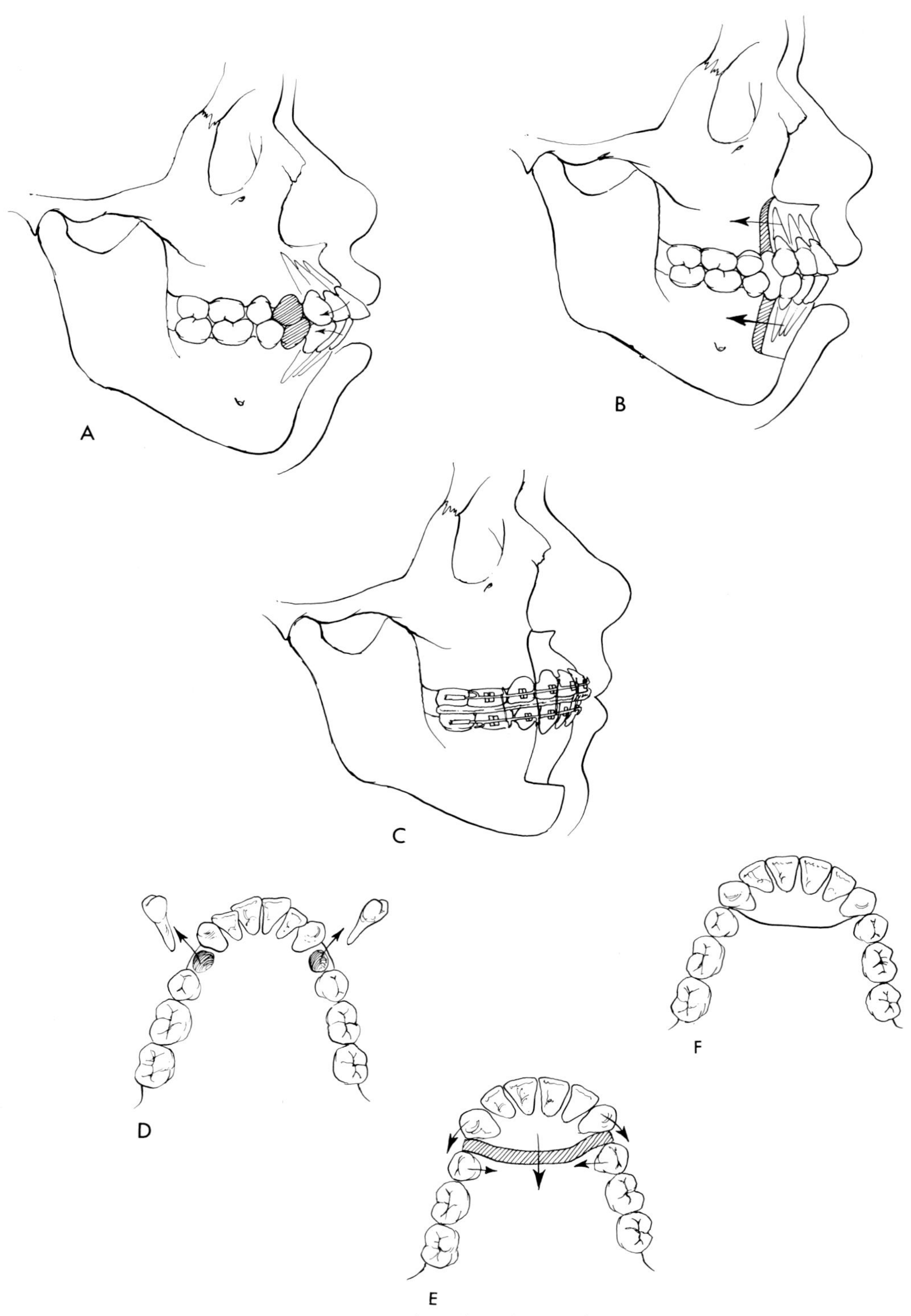

Figure 12–2. *See legend on the opposite page.*

When surgery is accomplished without preliminary orthodontic treatment, the procumbent anterior maxillary and mandibular teeth are easily retracted and raised or lowered by anterior maxillary and mandibular subapical ostectomy in the first or second premolar regions (Fig. 12–2). Bodily retraction of a tapered anterior maxilla or mandible by anterior subapical ostectomy produces a step defect in the interface between the proximal and distal segments (Fig. 12–3). This malalignment problem can be obviated surgically by one of several methods. The anterior maxillary or mandibular dentoalveolar segments can be split by interincisal osteotomies to allow lateral transposition of the two halves of the maxilla, the mandible, or both. Alternatively (or simultaneously), maxillary or mandibular ostectomies may be accomplished in the second premolar or first molar regions when model surgery indicates that improved alignment can be achieved by operating at these sites.

Simultaneous tipping and retraction of proclined maxillary or mandibular canines by dentoalveolar surgery frequently tends to raise the canine teeth off the occlusal plane and to tip the canine roots forward. The same effect is seen in more severe form when first premolars are included in the anterior segment. This must be foreseen by studying the preoperative cephalometric predictions and by performing model surgery. The elevated canines can be brought down into occlusion by postsurgical orthodontic treatment. Alternatively, proper axial inclination of the anterior teeth can usually be achieved by presurgical orthodontic correction after extracting first premolar teeth, thus avoiding the need to tip the segment at the time of surgery (see Fig. 12–2).

When severe bimaxillary protrusion is treated by surgery alone, however, segmentalization of the maxilla or mandible may be necessary to achieve proper anteroposterior and axial inclination of the maxillary and mandibular anterior teeth (Fig. 12–4).[1,3] Similar surgical techniques can also be used as adjuncts to orthodontic treatment if the anterior teeth are excessively proclined. Interdental osteotomies can usually be made in the canine–lateral incisor interspaces with relatively little risk to the contiguous teeth. When osteotomies are accomplished in these areas, vertical ostectomies are usually accomplished in the second premolar sites. Multiple small dento-osseous segments are mobilized and repositioned to accomplish the desired three-dimensional changes (Figs. 12–4 and 12–5). The feasibility of such interdental bone cuts must be determined on the

Text continued on page 1025.

Figure 12–2. *A–C,* Surgical and orthodontic techniques for correction of Class I bimaxillary protrusion. *A,* Preoperative deformity with mandible in centric relation and lips relaxed: prominent lips, acute nasolabial angle, mild degree of lip incompetence, contour deficient–chin, Class I malocclusion, and procumbent and slightly crowded maxillary and mandibular anterior teeth. First premolar teeth are extracted to facilitate alignment and uprighting of anterior teeth by orthodontic treatment. *B,* Plan of surgery: anterior maxillary and mandibular subapical ostectomies to retract anterior teeth, reduce prominence of lips and facial convexity, partially level mandibular occlusal plane, and produce relative increase in prominence of chin. Cross-hatched areas indicate planned vertical and horizontal ostectomy sites. Arrows indicate planned directional movements of anterior part of maxilla and mandible. Amount of bone to be excised is determined from cephalometric prediction studies and mock sectioning of study casts after presurgical orthodontic treatment. *C,* Repositioned anterior portion of maxilla and mandible indexed into interocclusal wafer splint and fixed to posterior teeth with an arch wire ligated to the posterior teeth; mandible is immobilized with intermaxillary wire ligatures. *D–F,* Orthodontic and surgical treatment of Class I bimaxillary protrusion. *D,* Retraction of anterior teeth by orthodontic treatment after extraction of 1st premolar teeth. *E,* Movement of teeth is accomplished by posterior and lateral movements of the anterior teeth into extraction spaces, medial movement of the anterior teeth into extraction spaces, and medial movement of the posterior teeth. *F,* Closure of residual extraction space by anterior subapical ostectomy.

See illustration on the opposite page.

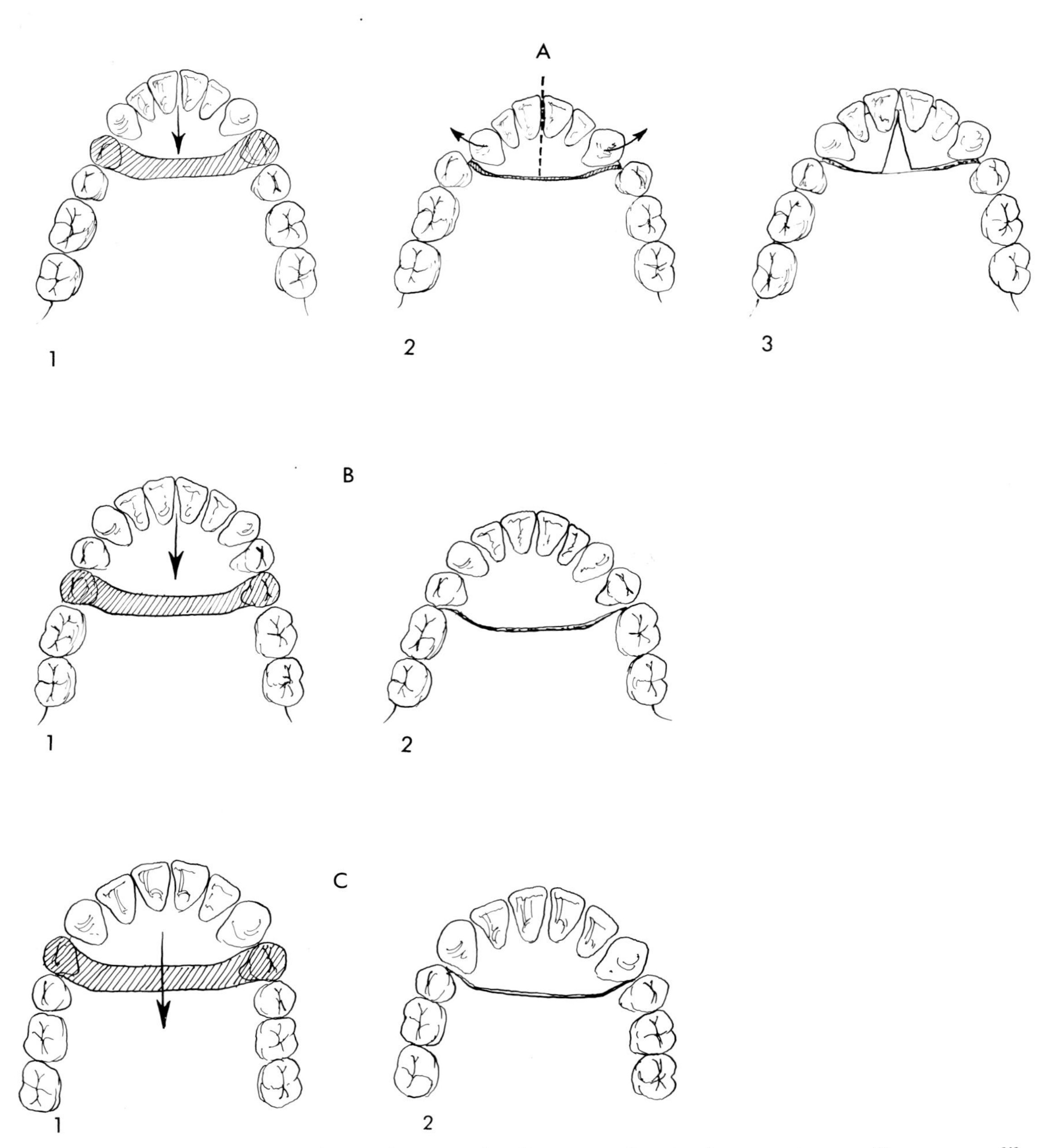

Figure 12–3. Surgical options to improve the alignment of teeth after anterior maxillary or mandibular subapical ostectomies. Careful occlusal analysis and model surgery will indicate which surgical technique, or combination of procedures, is feasible and will produce the best alignment. *A: 1,* Retraction of anterior maxilla or mandible by subapical ostectomy in 1st premolar region of V-shaped maxilla or mandible results in malalignment of canine and 2nd premolar teeth. *2,* Interincisal osteotomy to increase intercanine width. *3,* Improved alignment between canine and 2nd premolar teeth. *B: 1,* Subapical ostectomy in *2nd premolar regions* of same tapered arch illustrated in *A 1. 2,* Improved alignment between 1st premolars and molar teeth. *C: 1,* Retraction of anterior maxilla or mandible by anterior subapical ostectomy in 1st premolar region of U-shaped maxilla or mandible. *2,* Postoperative: satisfactory alignment of the canine and 2nd premolar teeth.

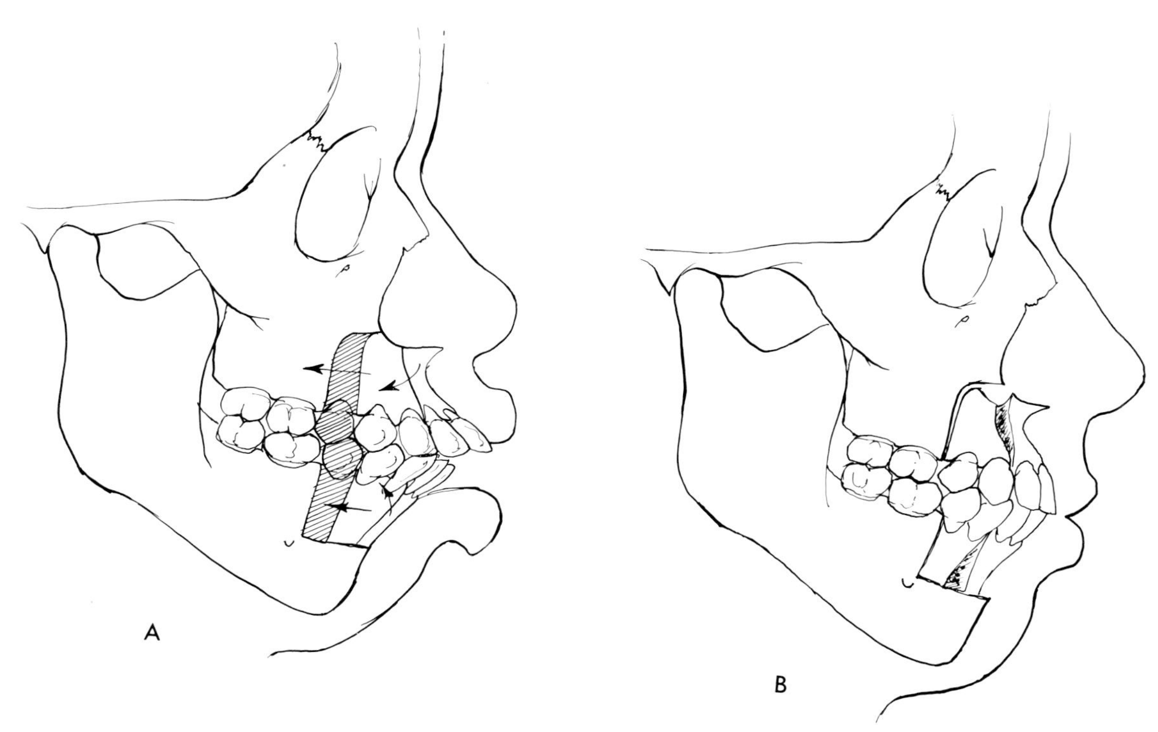

Figure 12–4. Severe bimaxillary protrusion corrected by simultaneous retraction and uprighting of anterior teeth. *A*, Plan of surgery: vertical ostectomies in 2nd premolar regions and vertical interdental osteotomies in lateral incisor-canine interspaces are connected by horizontal subapical osteotomy. Surgery is designed to retract anterior teeth, upright incisors, reduce prominence of lips and facial convexity, and produce relative increase in prominence of chin. *B*, Repositioned dentoalveolar segments indexed into interocclusal wafer splint and fixed to posterior teeth with an arch wire ligated to the posterior teeth. The mandible is immobilized with intermaxillary wire ligatures. Cross-hatched areas indicate planned vertical and horizontal ostectomy sites. Arrows indicate planned directional movements of maxillary and mandibular segments.

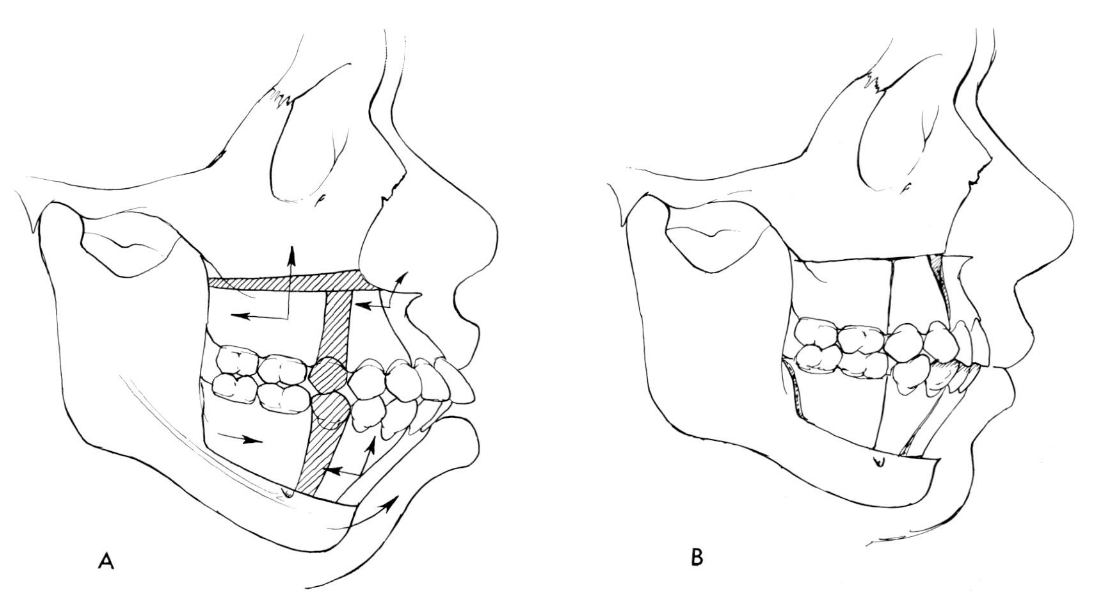

Figure 12–5. Preoperative deformity: severe bimaxillary protrusion associated with vertical maxillary excess, excessive exposure of teeth, lip incompetence, prominent lips, acute nasolabial angle, contour deficient–chin, malaligned teeth, and maxillomandibular disharmony. Multiple maxillary and mandibular osteotomies are made to achieve the desired vertical, horizontal, and anteroposterior dimensional changes. *A*, Plan of surgery. Maxilla: Le Fort I osteotomy to raise and segmentalize the maxilla. Mandible: Vertical ostectomy in 2nd premolar region, vertical interdental osteotomy in canine-lateral incisor interspace and total subapical osteotomy. Planned osteotomies and ostectomies are shown by cross-hatched areas; arrows indicate planned directional movements of anterior and posterior parts of jaws. *B*, Postoperative.

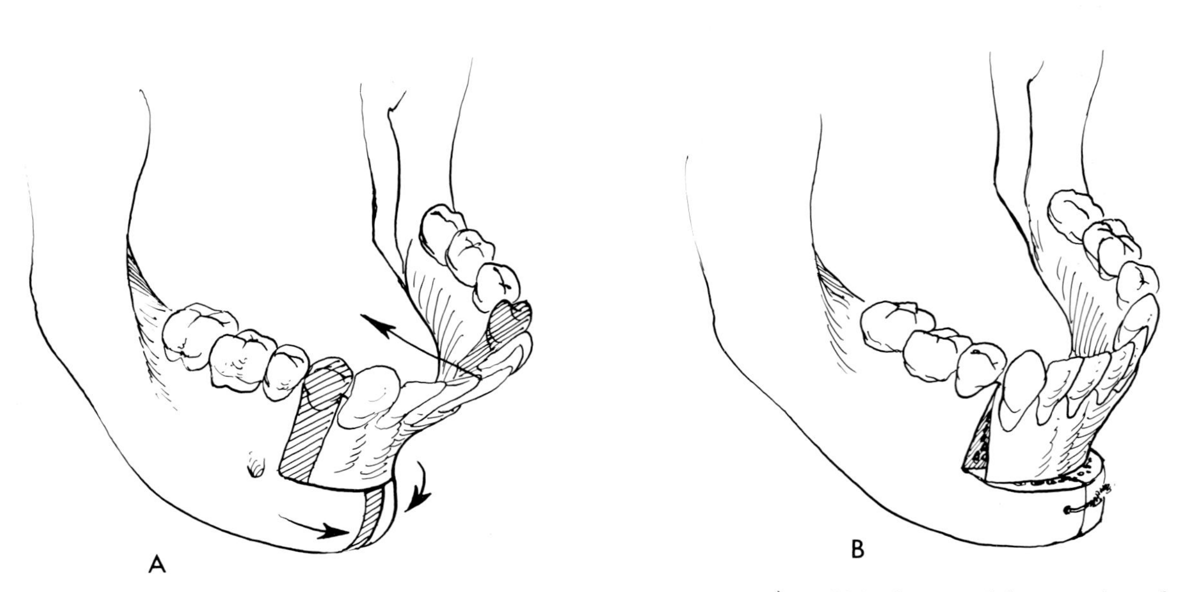

Figure 12–6. *A* and *B*, Mandibular intercanine and intermolar width decreased by symphyseal ostectomy and mandibular subapical osteotomy. Cross-hatched areas indicate planned vertical ostectomies in 1st premolar areas and symphyseal ostectomy.

basis of careful clinical and radiographic study of the potential interdental osteotomy sites.

Total maxillary osteotomy, involving simultaneous movement of the anterior and posterior dento-osseous segments, affords even greater versatility (Fig. 12–5).[4] Any of the three methods—total maxillary osteotomy, anterior or posterior segmental osteotomy, small segment osteotomy—or combinations may be used to improve the canine-premolar relationship and simultaneously to alter the axial inclination of the anterior teeth.

Midsymphyseal ostectomy (Fig. 12–6) may also be combined with subapical osteotomy or ostectomy to narrow the posterior part of the mandible.[12] (Technical details may be found in Chapter 11.) This narrowing will improve canine-premolar alignment and may partially correct a palatal crossbite. When a tooth mass problem is present in the mandibular arch, an ostectomy in an incisor tooth extraction site may be combined with the subapical osteotomy or ostectomy.

Importance of Treatment Planning

Ultimately, the feasibility of the planned movements must be demonstrated by cephalometric prediction studies and model surgery. A prediction of the postoperative results of the treatment is made by simulating the surgical and orthodontic movements on a lateral cephalogram. The anterior maxillary and mandibular dentoalveolar segments to be repositioned are registered onto a second piece of overlay tracing paper. Templates of the segments to be moved are cut out and positioned over the previous cephalometric tracing to simulate the desired positional changes of the anterior portions of the maxilla and mandible. After the templates are repositioned according to the amount of correction desired, a third tracing is made of the new soft-tissue profile on the basis of the ratios between bone and soft-tissue changes presented in Chapter 6. The new soft-tissue profile in turn serves as the basis for simulating additional changes by genioplasty, cheiloplasty, or rhinoplasty. (A detailed discussion of treatment planning by cephalometric prediction studies appears in Chapters 6 and 8.)

Adjunctive Procedures

Genioplasty

Analysis of patients with bimaxillary protrusion will frequently demonstrate a need for genioplasty, which usually can be accomplished simultaneously with anterior maxillary or mandibular osteotomies. In selected cases, however, when the amount of chin augmentation required is marginal and there is a question about the actual need for genioplasty, the procedure is best deferred until several months after definitive jaw surgery. When the amount of mental symphysis is marginal and precludes simultaneous horizontal osteotomy of the chin, the genioplasty is accomplished several months later as a secondary procedure or an alloplastic material is used.

A variety of nonbiologic (alloplastic) materials has been used for augmentation genioplasty. It has been observed over time that silicone materials (Silastic or equivalent) tend to be absorbed gradually into the bone and have a distressing tendency to migrate (Fig. 12–7). At present, Proplast is the preferred alloplastic material. The most stable results are obtained from a sliding osteotomy along the lower border of the chin. This

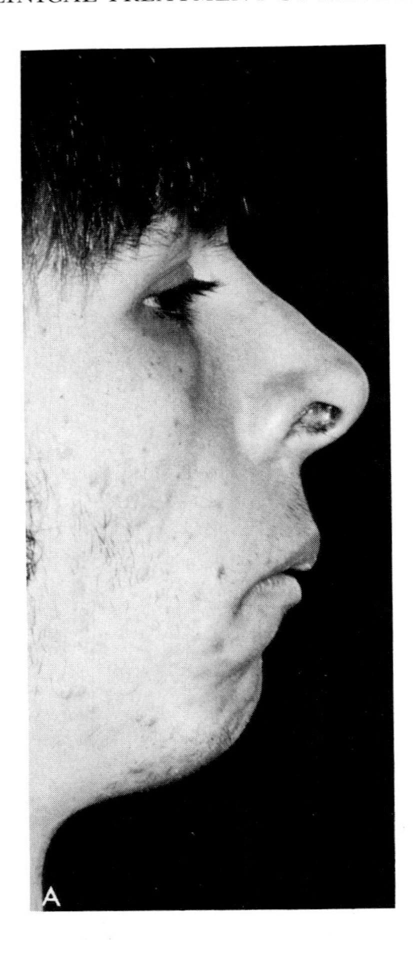

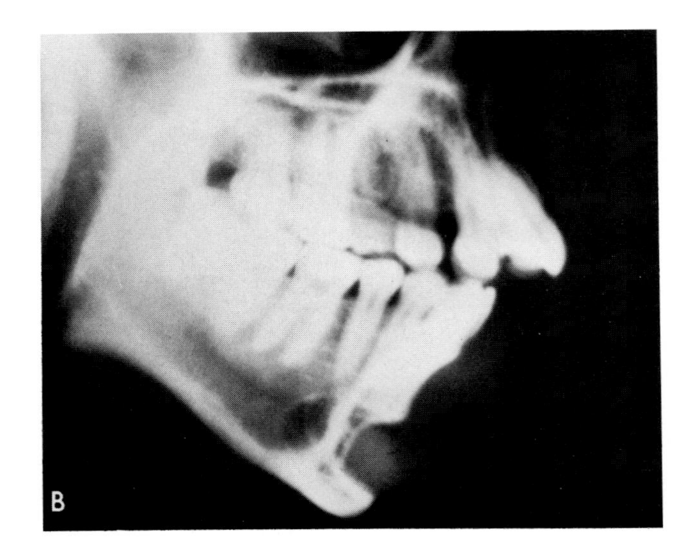

Figure 12-7. Silicone implant at the chin was placed 10 years prior to cephalometric film at age 21. Note the extreme resorption beneath the implant. (Courtesy of Dr. R. Justus.)

allows the surgeon to move the lower border forward while maintaining a soft-tissue pedicle.[3]

In planning for augmentation genioplasty, the clinician should keep in mind that when an alloplastic material like Proplast is inserted, the soft tissue will be increased in about the same amount as the size of the alloplastic insert (1:1 augmentation). When the patient's own bone is used via a sliding osteotomy at the chin, augmentation of the soft tissue is only 60 to 70 per cent of the amount the bone is moved forward.[3] The soft-tissue effect of both kinds of augmentation is highly predictable. For bimaxillary protrusion patients, the sliding osteotomy is preferred when it can be done. If alveolar osteotomies are done in both arches, however, there may not be enough bone to allow a lower border osteotomy. In this case, augmentation with Proplast is employed.

Cheiloplasty

After correction of the anteroposterior jaw and tooth disharmony, the upper and lower lips may yet appear too prominent because of excessive tissue in the lips themselves. In such cases a portion of the upper and lower lips is easily excised by secondary cheiloplasty to reduce the prominence of the lips and amount of vermilion border exposure (see Chapter 16). The original treatment must be carefully planned so that lip competency is achieved by jaw surgery. A tendency toward skeletal open bite, which contributes to lip incompetence, should not be overlooked. If this is the problem, a segmentalized Le Fort I osteotomy may be needed to reduce the interlabial gap by allowing the mandible to rotate closed.

Rhinoplasty

Rhinoplasty, if needed for complete treatment of a patient with bimaxillary protrusion, should be deferred until the protrusion has been corrected and postoperative soft-tissue contours of the lower face have been well established. This will allow the best planning for optimum contour of the nose (see Chapter 15).

COMBINED SURGICAL AND ORTHODONTIC TREATMENT

Surgical correction of bimaxillary protrusion rarely is indicated for children, but combined surgical and orthodontic management can make the overall treatment considerably easier and provide a better result for adults. There are three major advantages to surgical repositioning of alveolar segments:

1. *The incisor segment can be repositioned vertically as well as horizontally once it is freed surgically.* This is particularly advantageous when intrusion of incisors to correct an anterior deep bite is required.
2. *The requirements for patient cooperation in treatment are lessened.* Particularly, it is not necessary to utilize extraoral force to control posterior anchorage, and there is no danger of losing anchorage as posterior segments slip forward. Because the most difficult and time-consuming part of treatment, the incisor retraction, is eliminated, treatment time can be shortened considerably.
3. *Augmentation genioplasty can be performed at the same time as the retraction.* If the patient will have to be admitted to the hospital for surgery on the chin in any event, it may be desirable to have the surgeon retract the incisors while the patient is anesthetized instead of retracting them orthodontically.

Bimaxillary protrusion can be handled by combined surgical and orthodontic treatment in two ways:

1. Using maxillary and mandibular segmental osteotomies to retract the teeth and finishing the case by establishing proper occlusal relationships with an orthodontic appliance.
2. Using orthodontic forces to align and retract the mandibular arch and then performing an osteotomy to retract the maxillary teeth.

In both circumstances, a genioplasty frequently is needed at the time of surgery. The two types of treatment are discussed separately.

Combined Treatment Using Maxillary and Mandibular Segmental Osteotomies

If the maxillary and mandibular incisors are well aligned initially, and if there is no severe curve of Spee in the mandibular arch, it may be possible to retract the teeth surgically in both arches and achieve good postoperative occlusion. The osteotomies in both arches provide a certainty of maximal retraction. Both maxillary and mandibular segments can be intruded as they are moved posteriorly if this is needed, without producing any strain on anchorage by this tooth movement. Occasionally finishing orthodontic treatment is not necessary, but in most instances some postsurgical orthodontic treatment is required. For example, if the surgeon places the anterior segment so that incisor inclination is correct, the canine position usually is poor. When the mandibular segment is intruded, differences in vertical level between central incisors and canines remain. It is unlikely that extraction sites can be totally closed by surgery alone, and patients usually require some root paralleling.

It is better to carry out orthodontic tooth movement to correct these discrepancies after surgery. Accordingly, the best way to manage patients who will have surgical retraction of maxillary and mandibular incisors is as follows:

1. Band (or bond) maxillary and mandibular teeth except the first (or second) premolars, which will be extracted at surgery. The edgewise appliance, which is uniquely adapted to stabilization as well as tooth movement, should be used. Other fixed appliances are not as successful in handling both stabilization following surgery and the tooth movement that is necessary later.

2. Proceed with maxillary and mandibular osteotomies. Postsurgical stabilization is achieved by placing full-dimension rectangular orthodontic arch wires into the appliance at the time of surgery. An acrylic interocclusal splint should be made on the casts after model surgery. Orthodontic arch wires also are made to fit the casts following model surgery. In the operating room, the mobilized segment is placed firmly in the splint and held there while the arch wires are tied in and tied back tightly against the last molar to be sure that the extraction site remains closed. After both arches have been stabilized, the splint can be left in place during intermaxillary fixation, or it may be discarded and the patient allowed to continue jaw function, at the discretion of the surgeon. With both anterior segments mobile, intermaxillary fixation may be needed postoperatively.

An alternative method to placing an arch wire at the time of surgery is to fix the repositioned segments into the planned relationship with an interocclusal acrylic splint. After the arch wires are sectioned in the planned osteotomy sites, the repositioned segments are indexed and fixed into the splint with wire ligatures passed through the splint and around vertical lugs on the arch wire. In some instances, circumandibular wires should be used for adjunctive stabilization. With either method, intermaxillary fixation is usually not necessary. When vertical ramus or total maxillary osteotomy surgery is accomplished simultaneously, however, intermaxillary fixation is routinely used.

3. After approximately 6 weeks for healing, remove the surgical stabilizing arches and replace them with lighter working arch wires (typically 0.016-inch round arch wires) for final positioning of incisors and canines. A heavier rectangular wire may be needed 4 to 6 weeks later to complete tooth positioning. This includes extrusion of canines (which may have been tipped up off the occlusal plane), root paralleling at the extraction sites, and general perfection of the occlusal relationships.

With this approach, little presurgical preparation is needed. It should be possible to complete treatment in a few months postoperatively. Using the orthodontic appliance for stabilization at the time of surgery and proceeding with final tooth movement as soon as healing allows makes the treatment efficient and produces an immensely better occlusal result than that typically obtained by surgery alone.

Combined Treatment Using Orthodontic Leveling and Alignment of the Mandibular Arch Followed by Surgical Retraction of Maxillary Incisors

The major indication for this treatment plan is a requirement for orthodontic alignment and leveling of the mandibular arch prior to surgery, combined with a need for maxillary intrusion, genioplasty, or both. If the mandibular teeth are irregular, they should be aligned prior to retraction, and it is almost always necessary to have the mandibular arch reasonably level before maxillary retraction can begin. A decision must be made as to whether surgical or orthodontic retraction of mandibular incisor segment will be the more advantageous. In many instances, if surgical retraction were done, considerable orthodontic alignment of teeth would still be required postsurgically. It would take no longer to achieve the desired retraction along with leveling if all the tooth movement were done orthodontically. Sometimes it is necessary to align maxillary teeth in preparation for retraction, and this can be done while the mandibular arch is being prepared.

From an orthodontic point of view, cases handled in this fashion very much resemble cases treated with the Tweed-oriented approach to bimaxillary protrusion. Mandibular but not maxillary first premolars are extracted in the initial phase of treatment, the maxillary arch is banded except for the first premolars and is stabilized, and the mandibular arch is leveled and aligned using Class III elastics from the stabilized maxillary arch. Usually, high-pull headgear to the maxillary molars is indicated to prevent their extrusion by the Class III elastics. (If the maxillary molars are elongated initially, a total maxillary osteotomy for intrusion will be needed. Then vertical stabilization with headgear is not needed, since posterior intrusion can be done at the time of surgery.) In clinical practice, total maxillary osteotomy (segmentalized in two, three, or four pieces) is usually accomplished to achieve three-dimensional occlusal and esthetic balance. To achieve maxillomandibular harmony, all of the lower teeth may have to be repositioned by either mandibular ramus surgery or total mandibular subapical osteotomy (see Chapter 10 for technique).

Since this treatment approach creates a transient appearance of maxillary protrusion as the mandibular teeth are retracted, the patient must understand that he or she will look temporarily worse. Leveling of the lower arch, however, can be accomplished as the retraction proceeds, and there is no problem in producing differential vertical movement of mandibular canines and lateral and central incisors. Orthodontic preparation of the mandibular arch typically requires 6 to 8 months.

The difference in treatment comes when the orthodontist would be ready to "reverse mechanics" in typical Tweed orthodontic treatment. At that stage, new impressions are made, model surgery and cephalometric prediction are carried out, and a rectangular stabilizing arch wire for the maxilla is prepared on the sectioned cast representing the postsurgical maxillary dental arch. An interocclusal splint is made on the casts, and this is used to stabilize the anterior maxillary segment in the operating room while the stabilizing arch wire is tied in and tied back. Since surgery is confined to the maxillary alveolar segment, intermaxillary fixation is not required. The full-dimension rectangular arch wire provides excellent stabilization, and the patient can continue jaw function (on a restricted diet) while healing occurs. Orthodontic treatment can proceed in the mandibular arch during the 6 weeks or so following surgery. The mandibular extraction spaces should have been closed before surgery, but if some tipping of canines has occurred, root paralleling in the mandible can proceed unhindered by the maxillary surgery.

A significant advantage of the maxillary surgical procedure is that not only can the maxillary segment be retracted, but it can also be intruded. Usually, at least 2 to 3 mm of intrusion is needed along with the retraction. A sliding osteotomy for chin augmentation also can be done in the operating room at the same time as the maxillary retraction.

Often the maxillary anterior segment is rotated somewhat as it is retracted surgically. This allows the central incisors to be placed at about their correct axial inclination but pulls the canines up off the occlusal plane. If the correct axial inclination of the maxillary incisors is obtained prior to surgery, the segment can be retracted without rotation, and the canines will not be lifted off the occlusal plane. This can be accomplished by removing the maxillary premolars earlier and tipping the incisors back orthodontically. If this method of presurgical treatment is used, posterior anchorage must be protected (with headgear or Class II elastics).

Six weeks following the maxillary surgery, the rectangular stabilizing arch wire is removed and lighter working arch wires are placed to achieve detailed interdigitation. Postoperative orthodontic treatment will consist largely of vertical positioning of teeth, especially maxillary canines, and any necessary root positioning. Typically, the postsurgical orthodontic phase of treatment requires 3 to 5 months.

There is a definite time advantage in handling the maxillary retraction surgically as opposed to orthodontically. The total orthodontic treatment time for a typical adult bimaxillary protrusion case is 24 to 27 months. If the mandibular arch is handled orthodontically but the maxillary arch is retracted surgically, treatment time is reduced to about 15 months.

COMPLICATIONS

Complications related to treatment of bimaxillary protrusion fall into two categories: problems related to the surgery itself and problems related to relapse.

Complications Related to Anterior Segmental Osteotomy

Interruption of Blood Supply with Consequent Necrotic Changes

In any segmental surgical procedure, it is important to maintain an adequate soft-tissue pedicle to the mobilized segment so that its blood supply is maintained. Flap designs for segmental surgery have been worked out so that complications due to loss of blood supply almost never occur. Clinical experience as well as experimental evidence from work with monkeys by Bell has demonstrated that if a soft-tissue flap is maintained either buccally or lingually, perfusion of the bone segment is adequate to maintain its vitality.[5]

Devitalization of Teeth in the Anterior Segments

Although the neurovascular bundle that supplies the incisor teeth is sectioned during anterior segmental osteotomy, collateral circulation provides a blood supply adequate to maintain pulp vitality. Immediately after surgery, this results in a situation unusual in dentistry: although the teeth have been denervated and do not respond to electrical or other pulp stimulators, they are vital. Only if the osteotomy cuts pass through the apices of the teeth is the blood supply to the pulp interrupted so that pulp vitality is lost. Since canines have the longest roots, the canine teeth are most likely to be at risk of this complication. One or 2 per cent of teeth in the osteotomized alveolar segments can be expected to require endodontic treatment following surgical mobilization. About 80 per cent of the teeth will respond to an electrical pulp tester within 6 months of the surgical procedure, demonstrating successful re-innervation.[8] The remaining 18 or 19 per cent are vital despite having been denervated by the osteotomy.

Ankylosis of Canine Teeth

If an osteotomy cut passes too close to a canine tooth, penetrating into the periodontal ligament, ankylosis can result. This can be a significant complication if the canine was depressed during the osteotomy and part of the postsurgical orthodontic plan is to elongate it. If a canine, or any other tooth, that requires extrusion does not respond to orthodontic forces postsurgically, it is likely that there are small areas of ankylosis. Any necessary tooth movement usually can be accomplished by anesthetizing the tooth, luxating it lightly, and immediately reapplying the orthodontic force. If this method is unsuccessful, surgical repositioning of the ankylosed tooth by alveolar surgery is another treatment option. (See Chapter 22 for details of surgery).

Complications Related to Relapse

Many clinicians worry that tongue pressure will push the maxillary and mandibular teeth forward again after they have been retracted. This rarely happens. Physiologic adaptation to an altered position of the teeth can be demonstrated, and this helps to explain the stability that almost always is observed following surgical or orthodontic retraction. Although tongue function adapts to the new position of the teeth, tongue pressures do not become abnormally high after the surgery. Usually, tongue pressures had been low when the teeth were protrusive and became normal when tooth position was corrected.[10]

Probably the most important single factor in determining whether the teeth will be stable in the new position is attainment of proper lip function postoperatively. Lip pressure against the teeth is important in maintaining them in the retracted position. It is important diagnostically to evaluate whether pretreatment lip incompetence is due to horizontal protrusion of the teeth or whether there is a vertical component as well. If lip incompetence is due to vertical excess as well as horizontal protrusion, anterior maxillary and mandibular surgery may not be enough to create sufficient lip competence to maintain stability after treatment. When vertical dimension is excessive, total maxillary osteotomy to obtain posterior intrusion along with incisor retraction may be necessary to obtain a stable result.

In comparison with orthodontic treatment alone, combined surgical and orthodontic treatment of bimaxillary protrusion offers advantages in control of anchorage, in ease and duration of treatment, and in the degree of facial change possible. From the patient's point of view, surgery carries greater risk, but the chance of significant complications is very small, so that such risk usually is not a serious contraindication. The greatest disadvantage to the patient is the higher cost of combined surgical and orthodontic treatment. Since the involvement of the orthodontist in treatment planning, appliance fabrication, surgical stabilization, and retention is nearly as great as for orthodontic treatment alone, the orthodontist's fee typically is 75 to 80 per cent of the fee the patient would have paid for orthodontic treatment alone, whereas the surgeon's fee and hospital costs combine to make the total cost considerably higher. This higher cost and the slightly greater risk must be balanced against the greater ease of treatment and the greater potential benefit. Careful integration of orthodontic and surgical treatment is required to obtain the best result, but with cooperation between the specialists, better patient care can be provided.

CASE STUDIES

CASE 12–1 (Fig. 12–8)

N. F., a 27-year-old woman, originally sought surgical correction for her deficient chin and was referred for further orthodontic consultation when her bimaxillary protrusion was recognized.

PROBLEM LIST

Esthetics (Fig. 12–8*A, B,* and *C*)

FRONTAL. Good facial contour and symmetry; dimpling and strain evident in the lips and chin with lips together.

PROFILE. Extreme lip protrusion and chin deficiency.

Cephalometric Analysis (Fig. 12–8*D*)

1. Extreme incisor protrusion: $\underline{1}$ to NA 5 mm; $\overline{1}$ to NB 12 mm.
2. Chin deficiency: Holdaway ratio $\left(\frac{\overline{1}-NB}{Pog-NB}\right)$ 12:1
3. Mild skeletal open bite pattern.

Occlusal Analysis (Fig. 12–8*E* through *I*)

1. Mild maxillary and mandibular incisor crowding.
2. Mild anterior open bite.

TREATMENT PLAN

Presurgical Orthodontic Treatment

1. Band posterior and anterior teeth.
2. Align teeth minimally.

Surgical Treatment

1. Maxillary anterior osteotomy for retraction.
2. Mandibular anterior osteotomy for retraction and slight elevation.
3. Augmentation genioplasty using Proplast.

Postsurgical Orthodontic Treatment

1. Complete detailed alignment.

ACTIVE TREATMENT

Bonded plastic brackets (.018 slot edgewise) were placed on maxillary and mandibular incisors, posterior teeth were banded, and .016 arches were placed for 4 weeks to improve incisor alignment before the impressions for final surgical planning were taken.

At surgery, maxillary and mandibular osteotomies plus genioplasty were carried out as planned. Stabilizing arch wires (.018 × .025) were tied into place in the operating room, and the patient was put into intermaxillary fixation for 2 weeks. A dramatic facial improvement was achieved immediately. Six weeks postoperatively light round arches were placed; then .017 × .022 closing loops were used for space closure and final alignment. Orthodontic appliances were removed 6 months after surgery, and maxillary and mandibular removable retainers were worn full time for 4 months and at night for 12 months before being discarded. Two years after treatment, the occlusal result seems stable, and facial esthetics are pleasing.

COMMENT

Bonded plastic brackets can be used quite successfully for surgical stabilization, but the ligature ties must be made carefully. Augmentation of the chin with Proplast was used in this case because bone support was insufficient for the osteotomized alveolar segment and for advancement of the lower border by means of osteotomy.

Surgeon: Timothy A. Turvey, Chapel Hill, North Carolina. *Orthodontist:* William R. Proffit, Chapel Hill, North Carolina.

Text continued on page 1039.

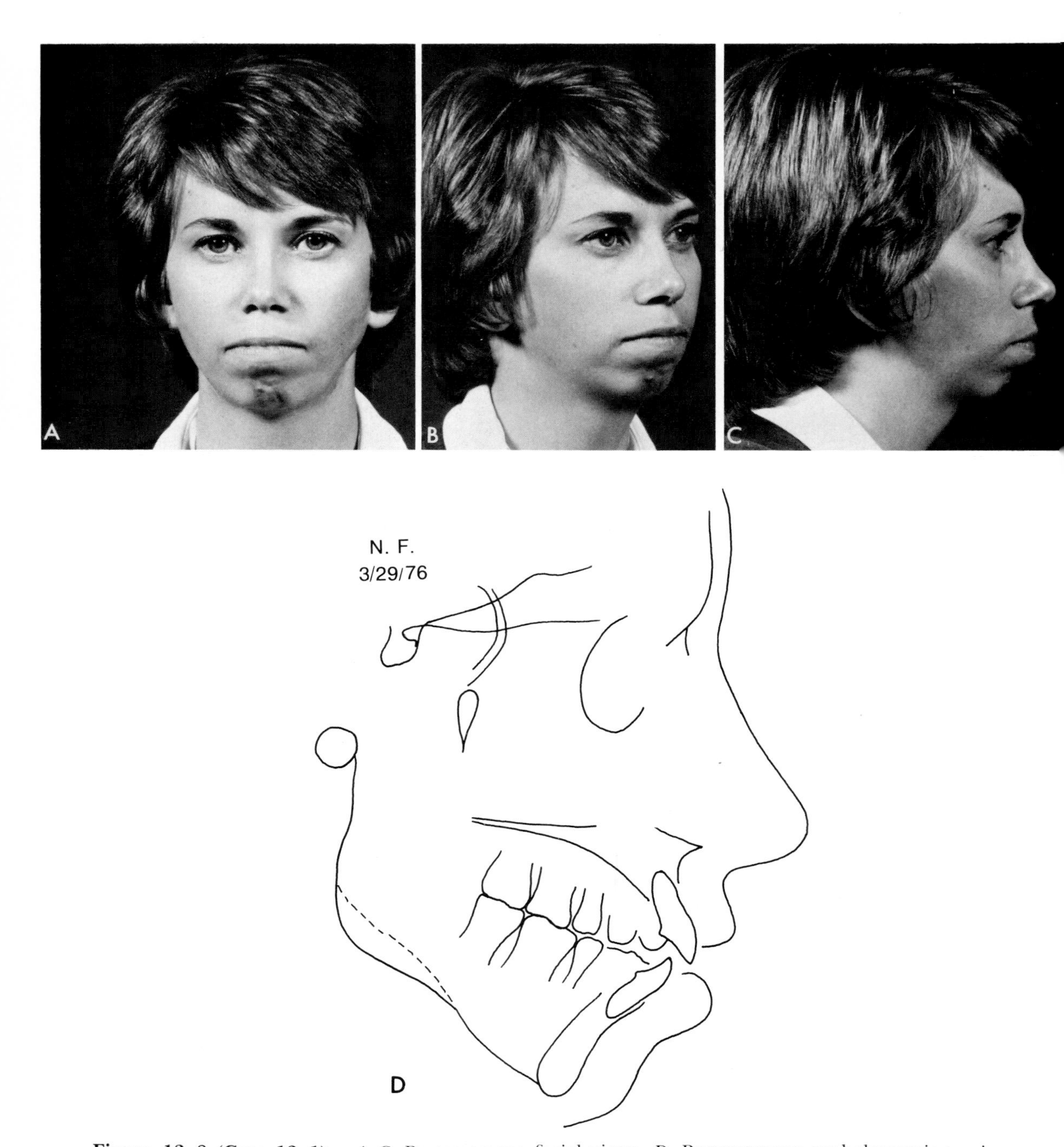

Figure 12–8 (Case 12–1). *A–C,* Pretreatment facial views. *D,* Pretreatment cephalometric tracing.
Legend continued on the opposite page.

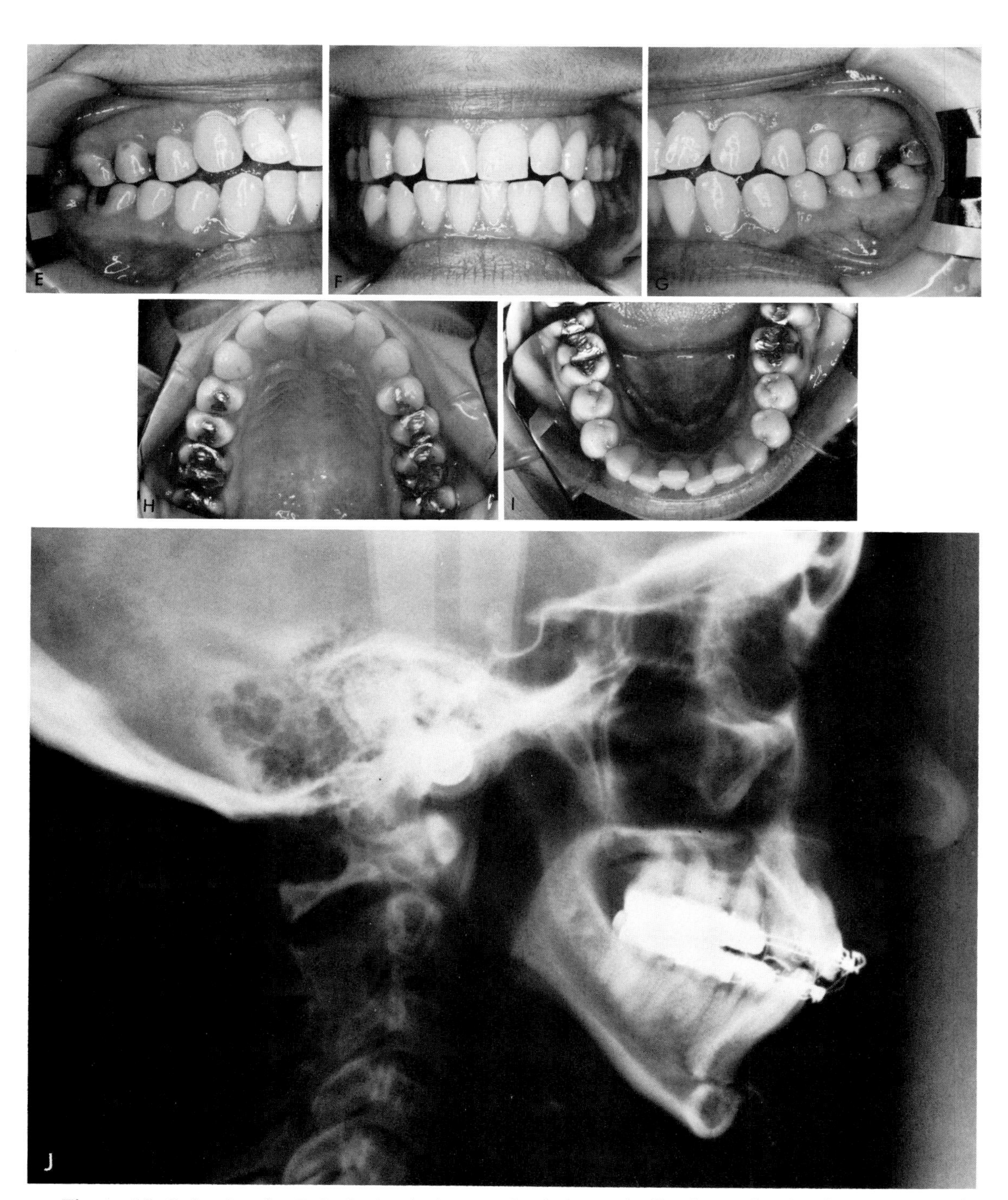

Figure 12–8 *Continued.* *E–I,* Occlusal views. *J,* Cephalometric film immediately after surgery. The Proplast chin insert cannot be seen radiographically.

Illustration continued on the following page.

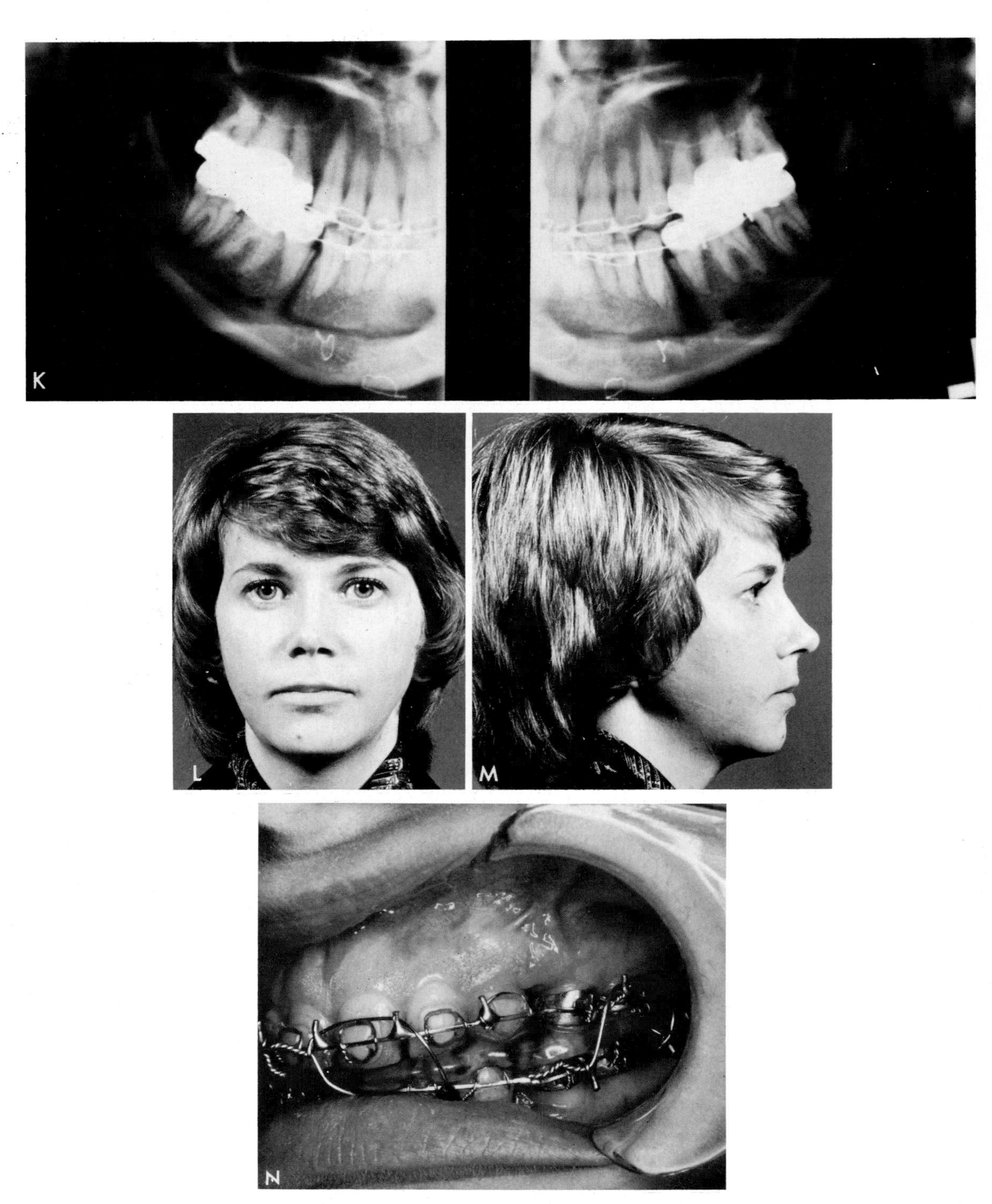

Figure 12–8 *Continued.* *K,* Panoramic film immediately after surgery. *L* and *M,* Facial views 2 weeks after surgery. *N,* Stabilizing wires with wafer splint during intermaxillary fixation.

Legend continued on the opposite page.

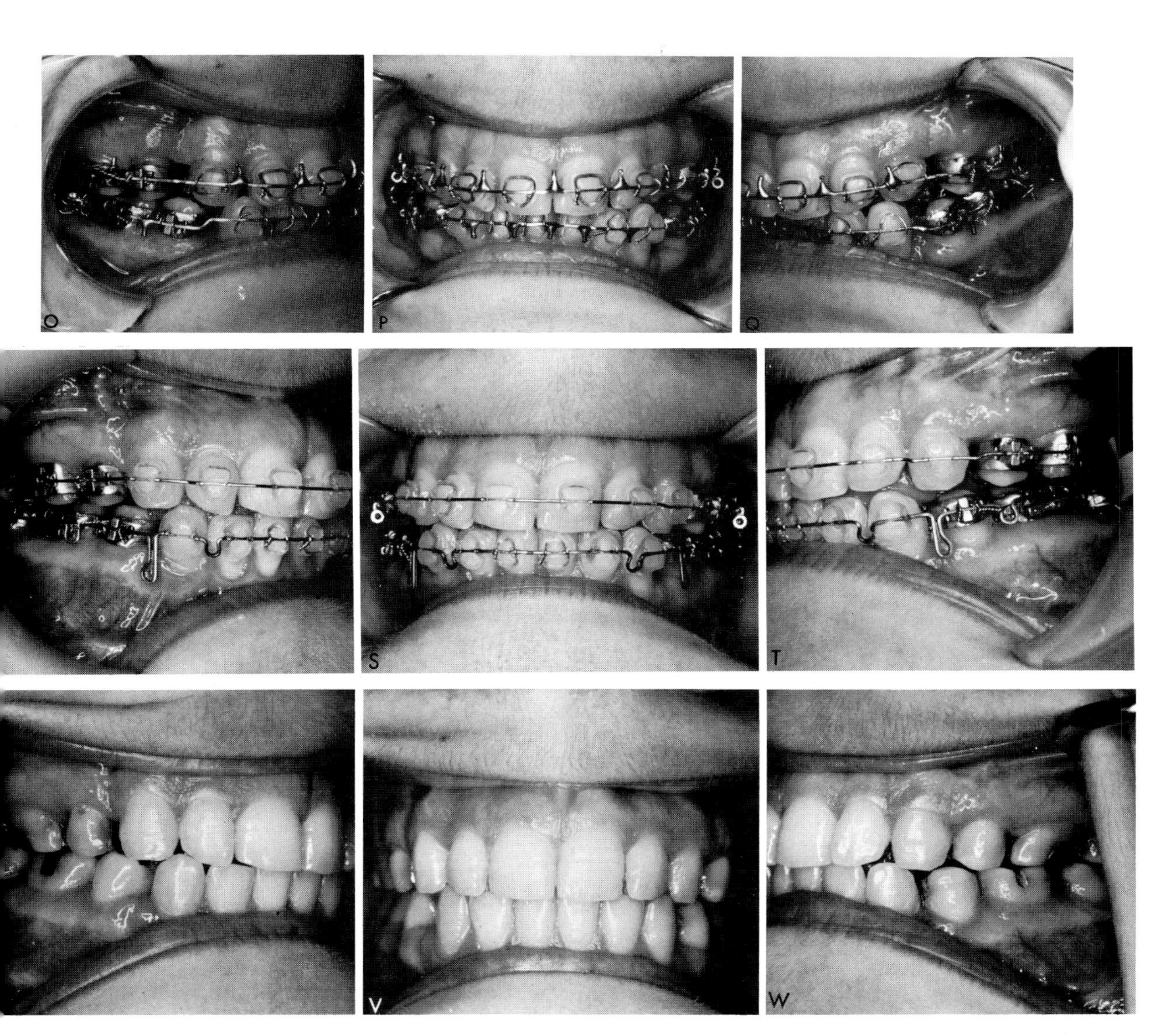

Figure 12–8 *Continued.* *O–Q*, Occlusion just prior to removing stabilizing arch wires. *R–T*, Postsurgical orthodontic treatment: space closure and final alignment. *U–W*, Post-treatment occlusion.

Illustration continued on the following page.

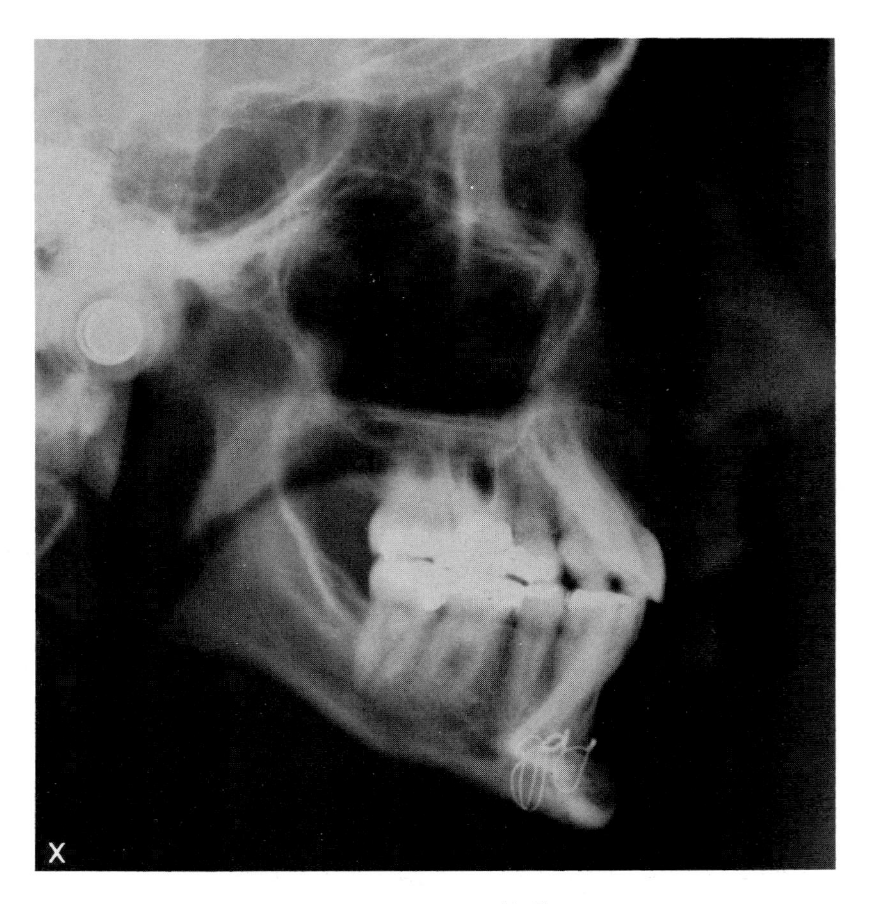

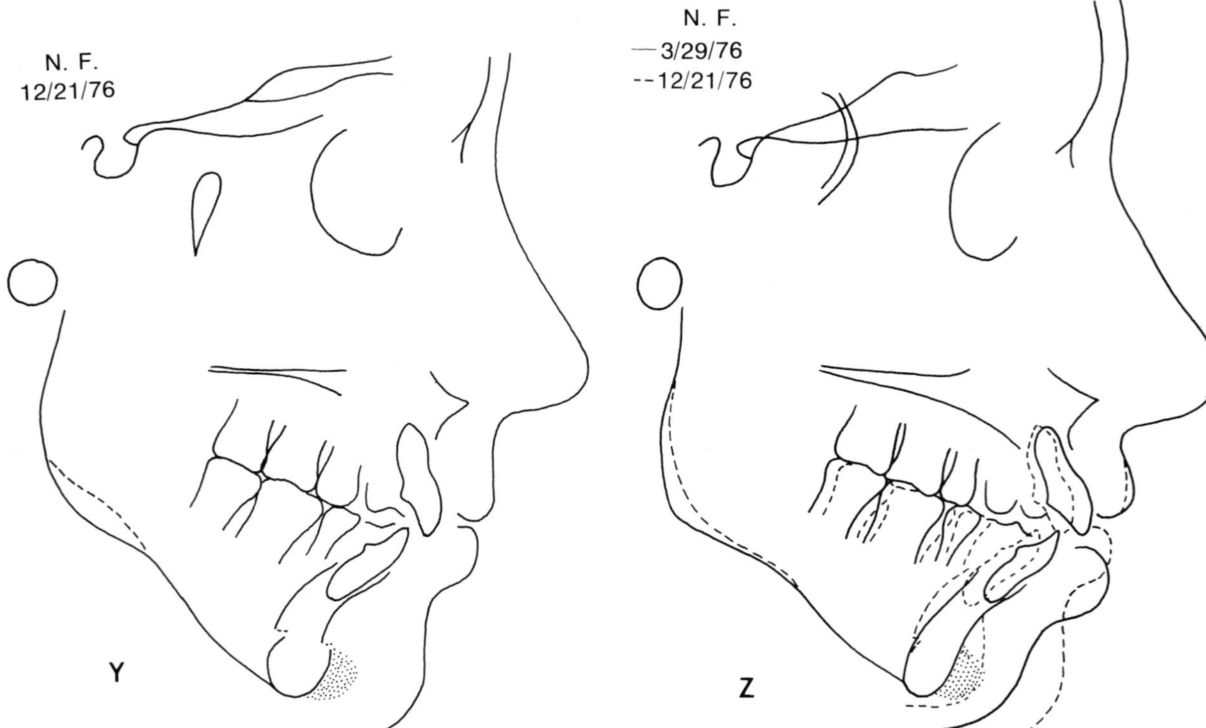

Figure 12–8 *Continued.* *X* and *Y*, Cephalometric film and tracing 1 year after surgery. *Z*, Cephalometric superimposition before (*solid line*) and after (*broken line*) surgery.

Legend continued on the opposite page

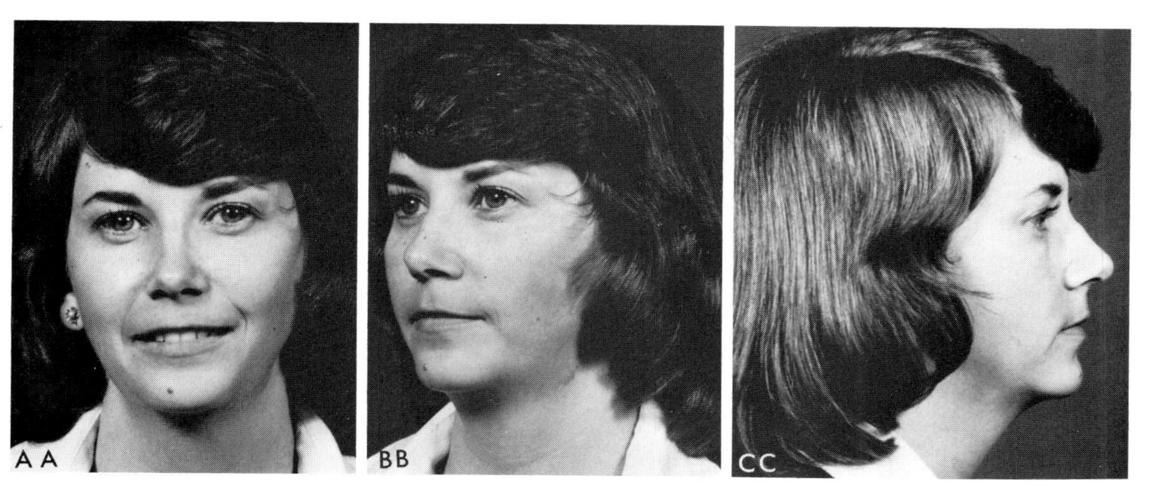

Figure 12–8 *Continued.* *AA–CC,* Facial views 2 years after treatment.

CASE 12–2 (Fig. 12–9)

D. W., a 23-year-old woman, sought treatment for her chief complaint of protruding front teeth.

PROBLEM LIST

Esthetics (Fig. 12–9*A, B,* and *C*)

FRONTAL. Good facial contour and symmetry, with prominent everted lips.
PROFILE. Extreme facial convexity: midface prominence; protruding lips; deficient chin.

Cephalometric Analysis (Fig. 12–9*D*)

1. Extreme protrusion of maxillary and mandibular incisors: $\underline{1}$ to NA 9mm; $\overline{1}$ to NB 12 mm.

Chin deficiency: Holdaway ratio 12:0.

Occlusal Analysis (Fig. 12–9*E* through *H*)

1. Excellent posterior interdigitation and Class I relationship.
2. Mild mandibular incisor crowding.

TREATMENT PLAN

Maximum retraction of maxillary and mandibular incisor teeth; chin augmentation.

Presurgical Orthodontic Treatment

1. Extraction of mandibular first premolar teeth.
2. Orthodontic stabilization of maxillary arch, supported by extraoral force to first molars.
3. Alignment and retraction of mandibular incisors.

Surgical Treatment

1. Retraction and intrusion of maxillary anterior alveolar segment, with removal of maxillary first premolars.
2. Augmentation genioplasty by sliding osteotomy.

Postsurgical Orthodontic Treatment

1. Extrusion and root positioning of maxillary canines.
2. Final space closure and detailing of occlusion.

ACTIVE TREATMENT

At the beginning of treatment, mandibular first premolar teeth were extracted but maxillary first premolars were not in order to help maintain maxillary posterior anchorage. Initially, only maxillary first molars and the mandibular arch were banded. High-pull headgear to the upper molars was used when Class III elastics were employed during mandibular alignment and retraction. Later, bonded brackets were placed on maxillary incisors. The .018 slot edgewise appliance was used. Alignment and retraction of mandibular incisor teeth in preparation for surgery required 9 months.

Surgical rather than orthodontic retraction of the maxillary anterior teeth was decided upon for two reasons:

1. Since genioplasty was needed to obtain good facial balance, a surgical procedure would be carried out anyway.
2. Segmental alveolar surgery would allow easier intrusion of the maxillary anterior segment.

Cast predictions revealed that canines would be rotated up out of occlusion at surgery if the correct inclination of central incisors was obtained, which frequently is the case. A .018 × .025 arch wire was prepared to fit the prediction cast. After the anterior segment had been placed in the wafer splint in the operating room, the arch wire was tied in and tied back. With the arch wire in place, the splint was discarded. After the maxillary osteotomy was completed, an osteotomy on the lower border of the chin was performed through an incision in the labial vestibule, and the chin was advanced.

Six weeks postsurgically, the stabilizing arch wire was removed and an ideal .014 arch wire was tied into the maxillary arch. As the canines moved down into position, a .016 arch wire was placed; then the residual space was closed with a .017 × .022 closing loop arch. The fixed appliance was removed and retainers (mandibular, fixed 3–3; maxillary, Hawley) were placed 6 months after treatment was begun.

Follow-up studies showed excellent stability of the occlusal and facial results 2 years following completion of treatment. At that time, the maxillary retainer still was being worn on occasional nights.

Text continued on page 1048.

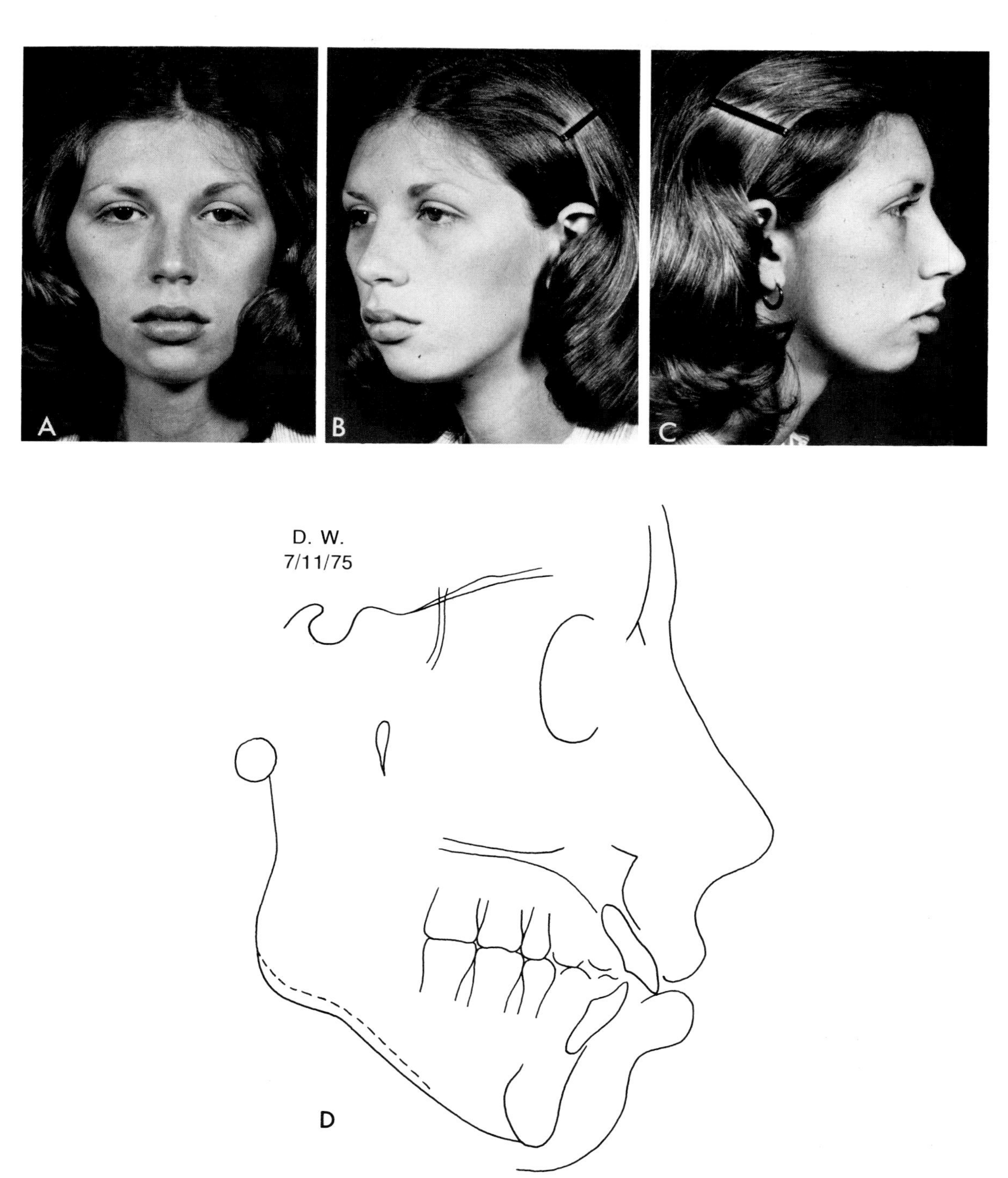

Figure 12-9 (Case 12-2). *A–C,* Pretreatment facial views. *D,* Pretreatment cephalometric tracing.

Illustration continued on the following page.

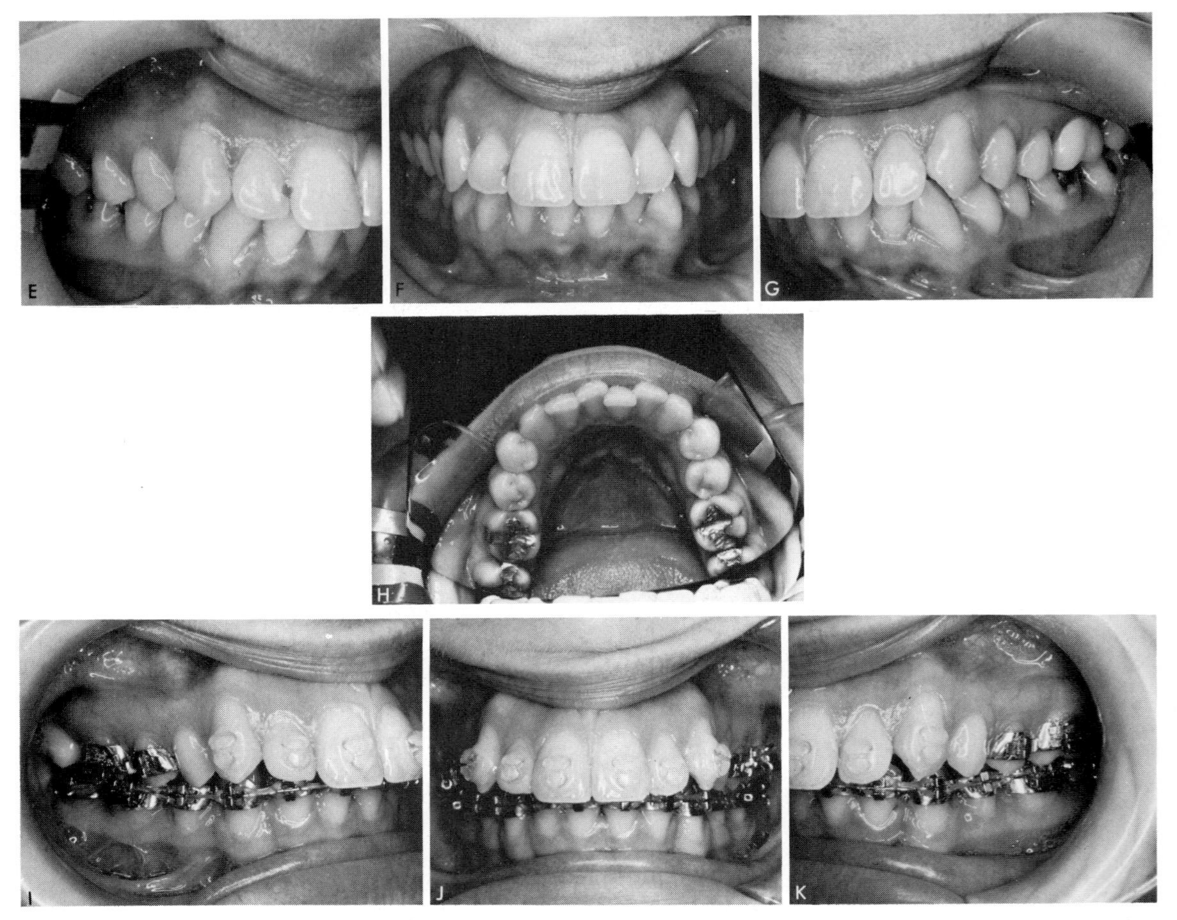

Figure 12–9 *Continued.* *E–H,* Pretreatment occlusal views. *I–K,* Occlusion after surgical preparation of mandibular arch.

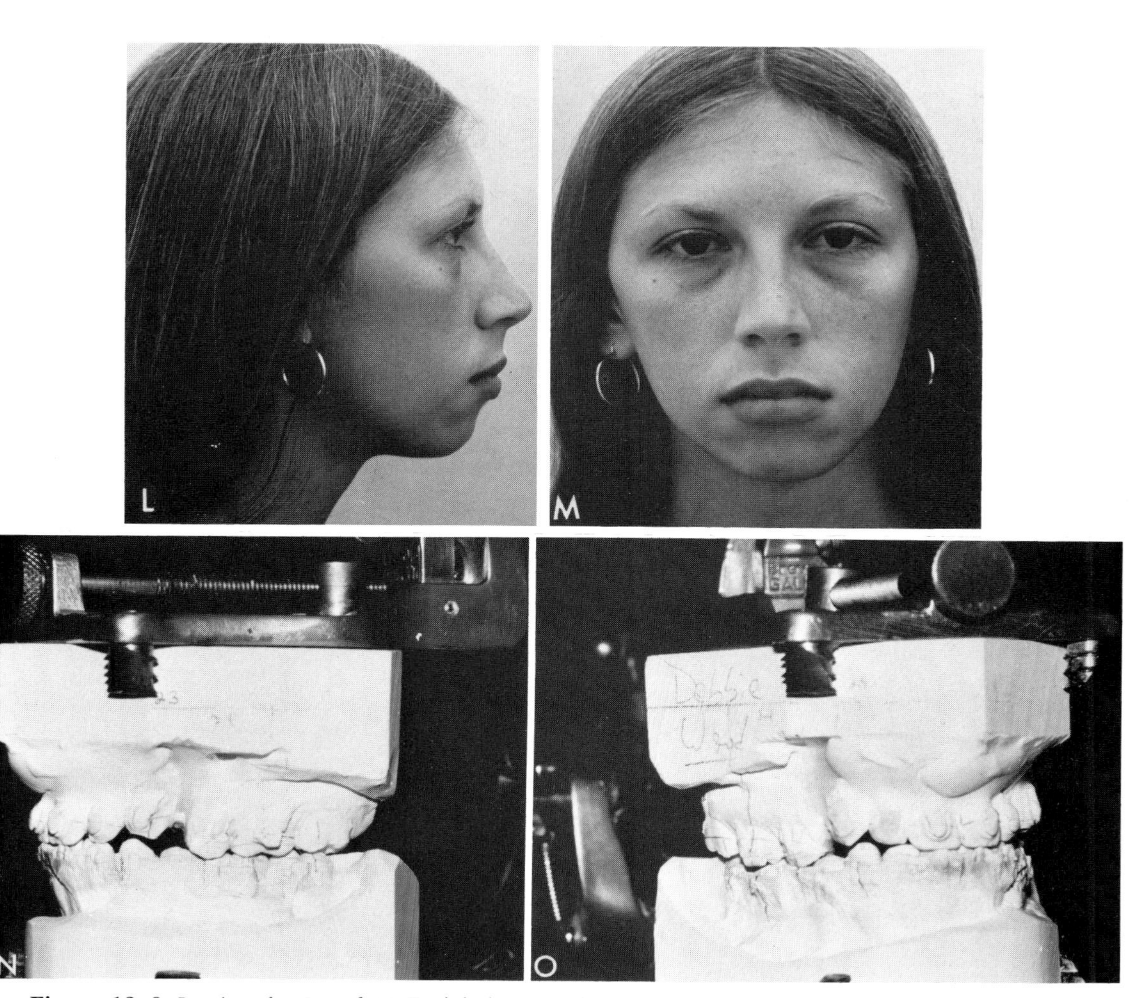

Figure 12–9 *Continued.* *L* and *M*, Facial views, patient ready for surgery. *N* and *O*, Model surgery on casts.

Illustration continued on the following page.

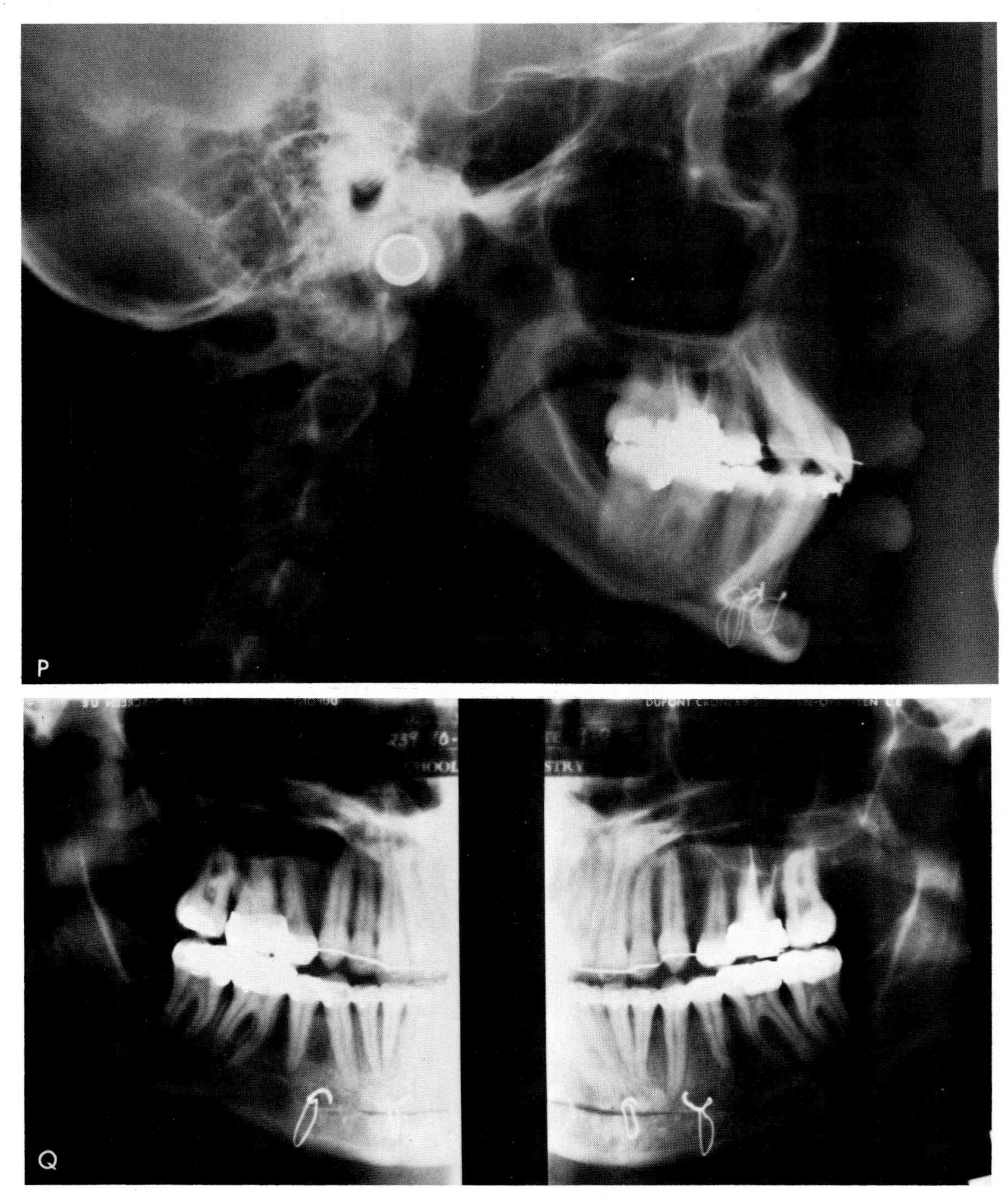

Figure 12–9 *Continued.* *P,* Postoperative cephalometric film. *Q,* Postoperative panoramic film.

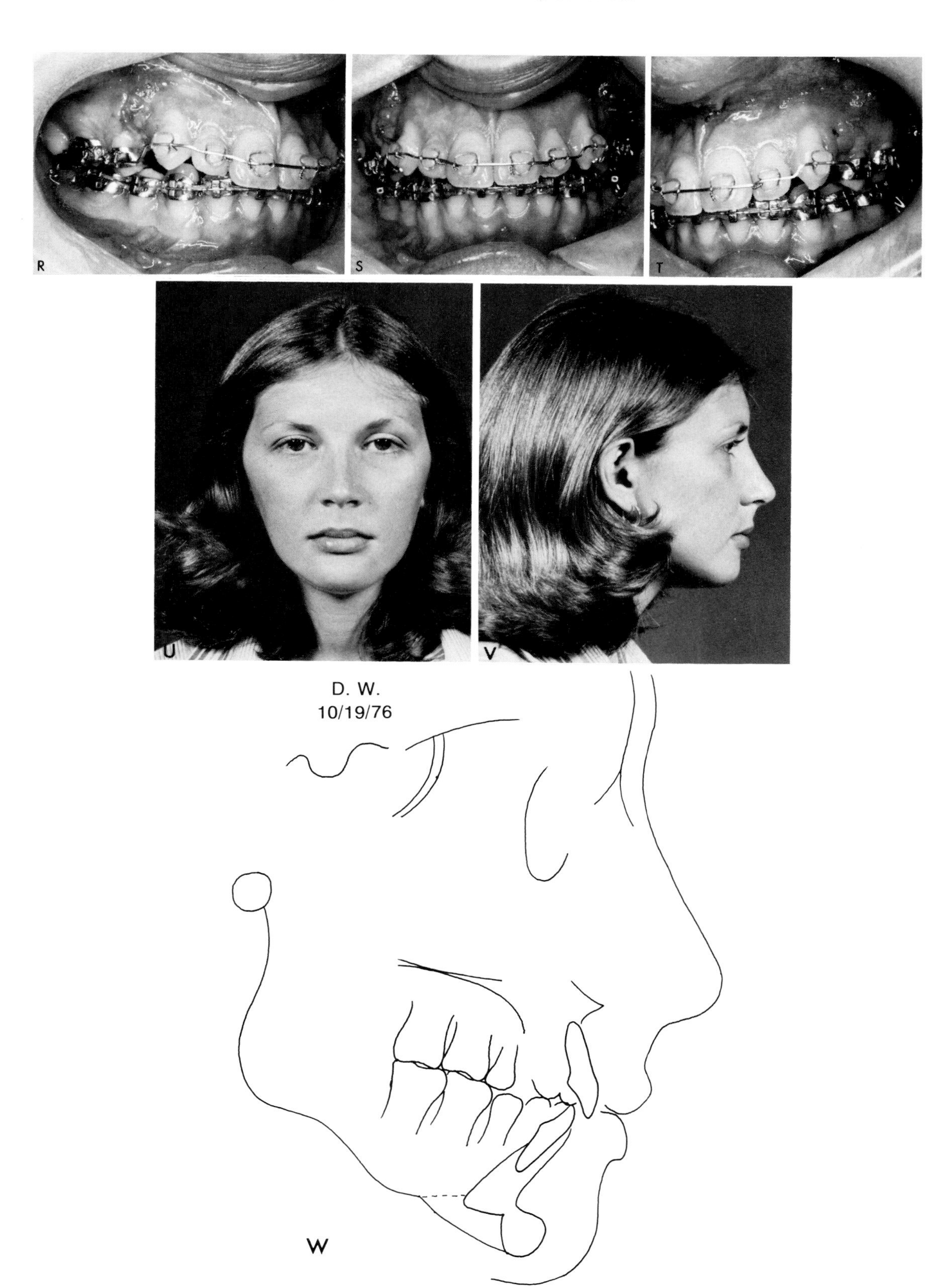

Figure 12–9 *Continued.* *R–T*, Occlusion 1 week after surgery. *U* and *V*, Facial appearance 4 weeks after surgery. *W*, Cephalometric tracing after surgery.

Illustration continued on the following page.

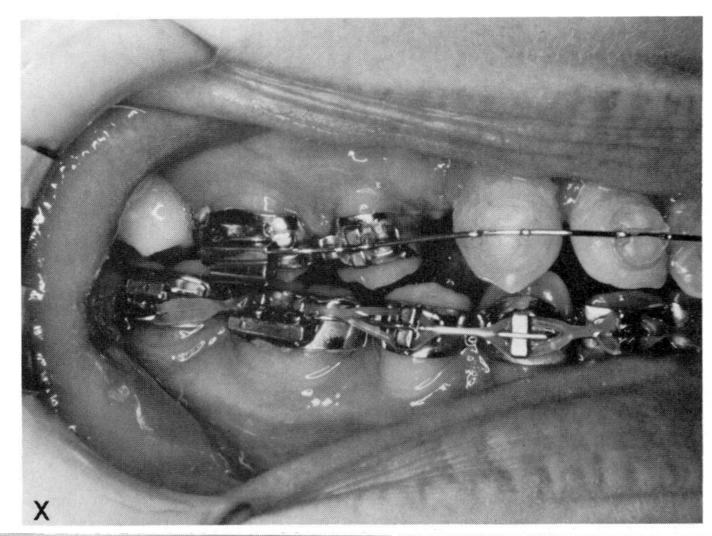

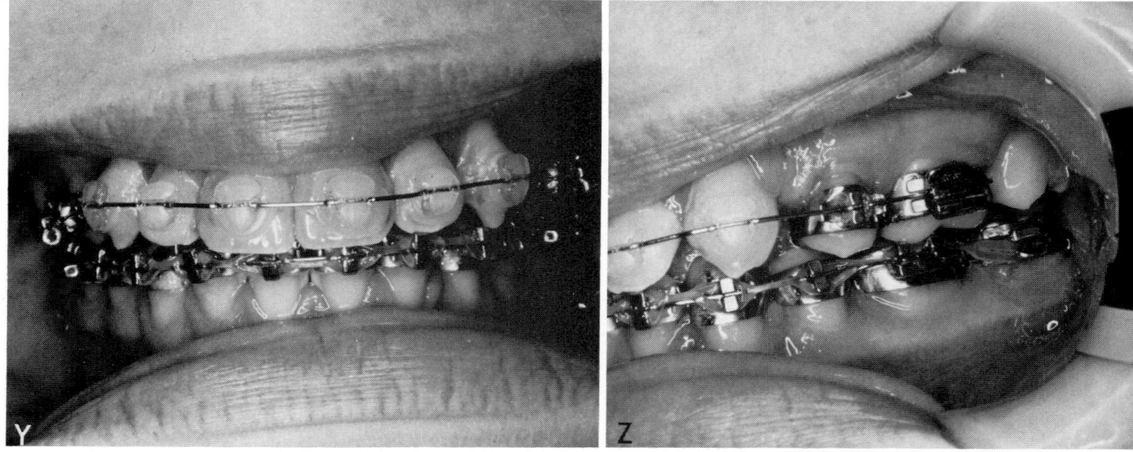

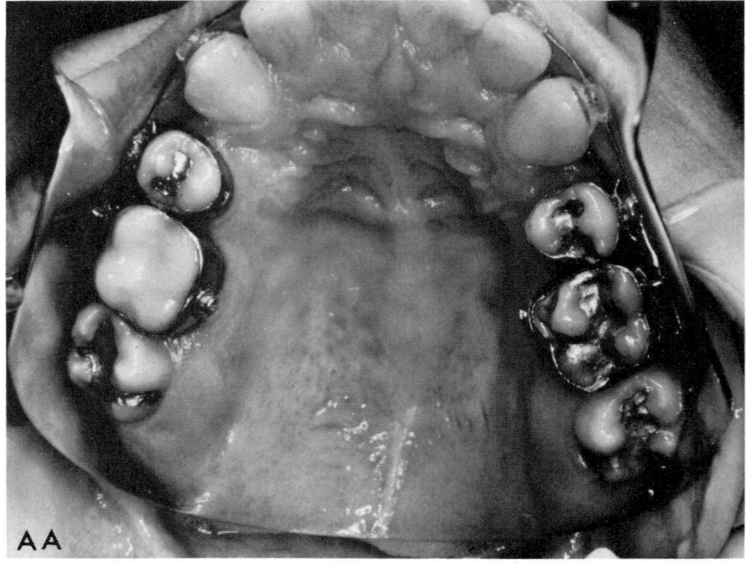

Figure 12–9 *Continued.* *X*, .014 arch wire placed when stabilizing arch was removed. *Y* and *Z*, Canine position 4 weeks later. *AA*, Occlusal view of maxillary arch prior to final space closure.

Legend continued on the opposite page.

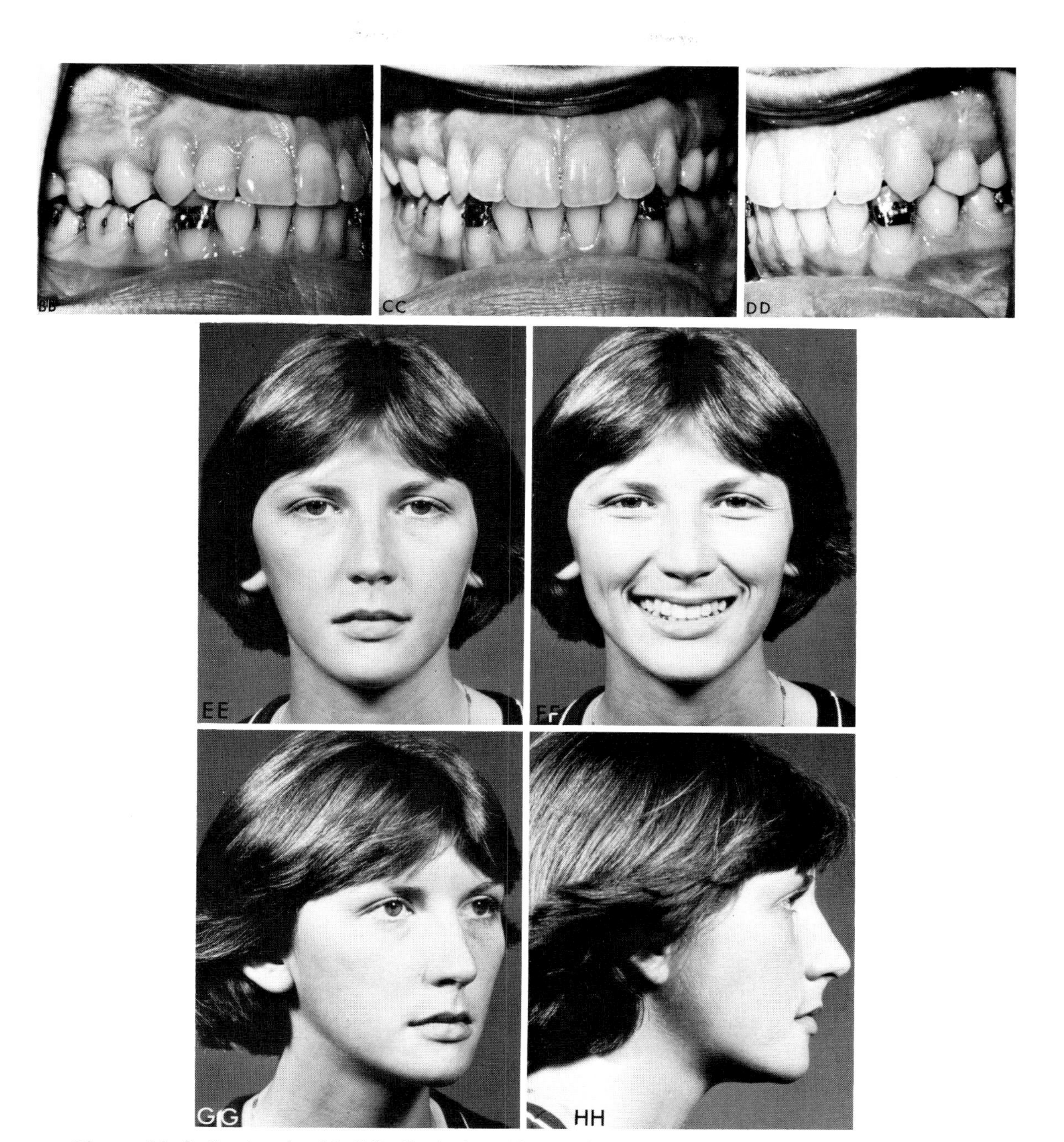

Figure 12–9 *Continued. BB–DD,* Occlusion 12 months after treatment. *EE–HH,* Facial views 18 months after treatment.

Illustration continued on the following page.

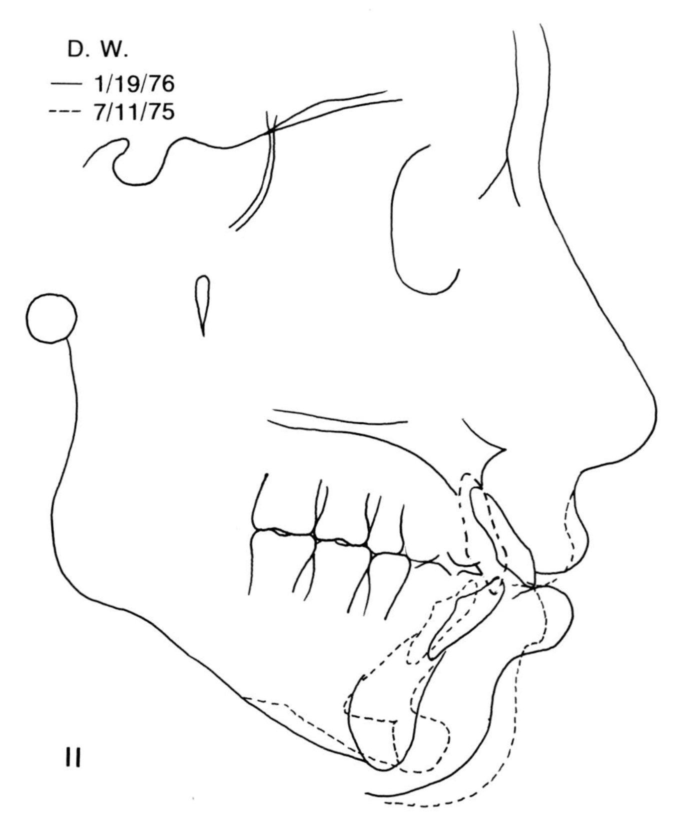

Figure 12–9 *Continued. II,* Cephalometric superimposition before (*solid line*) and after (*broken line*) treatment.

COMMENT

This treatment approach, utilizing orthodontic retraction of the mandibular segment with surgical retraction of the maxillary segment and genioplasty to correct profile convexity, can be very helpful in treatment of bimaxillary protrusion. Orthodontic treatment of the mandibular arch was required to correct the crowding, so there was no advantage to surgical retraction of the mandibular segment. Orthodontic retraction of the maxillary segment could have been done, but it would have required greater patient cooperation and longer treatment time, and genioplasty was required for the optimum facial improvement.

Surgeon: Timothy A. Turvey, Chapel Hill, North Carolina. *Orthodontist:* William R. Proffit, Chapel Hill, North Carolina.

CASE 12–3 (Fig. 12–10)

K. M., a 25-year-old woman, had the facial, dental, and skeletal characteristics commonly associated with bimaxillary protrusion. She spoke with a slight lisp. When she swallowed, her tongue was thrust through a small anterior open bite. Clinical and cephalometric examination revealed Class I bimaxillary dental protrusion.

PROBLEM LIST

TREATMENT PLAN

Esthetics (Fig. 12–10*A, B,* and *C*)

FRONTAL. Procumbent upper and lower lips. (Fig. 10, *A* and *B*)

PROFILE. Stretching of the perioral and mentalis musculature with the lips sealed; contour-deficient chin; prominent lips; mild lip incompetence.

Cephalometric Analysis (Fig. 12–10*G*)

1. Procumbent maxillary and mandibular anterior teeth: $\underline{1}$ to NA 27°; $\overline{1}$ to NB 40°.
2. ANB angle 6°.

Occlusal Analysis (Fig. 12–10 *I* through *L*)

DENTAL ARCH FORM. Maxilla and mandible ovoid and symmetric.

DENTAL ALIGNMENT. Minimal crowding in anterior part of maxilla and mandible; minimally rotated canines.

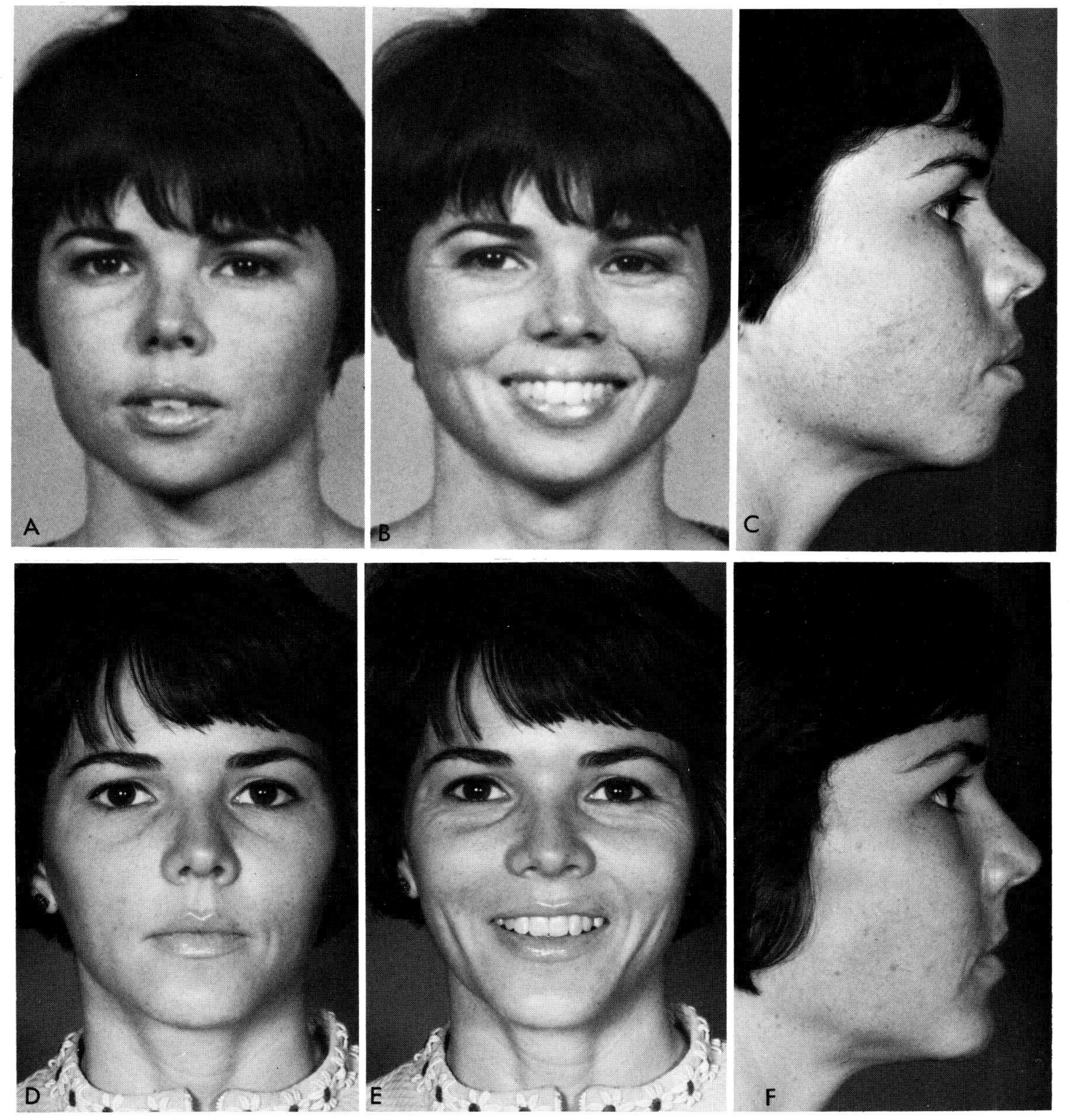

Figure 12–10 (Case 12–3). *A–F*, Photographs of a 25-year-old woman with bimaxillary dental protrusion before (*A–C*) and after (*D–F*) treatment.

Illustration continued on the following page.

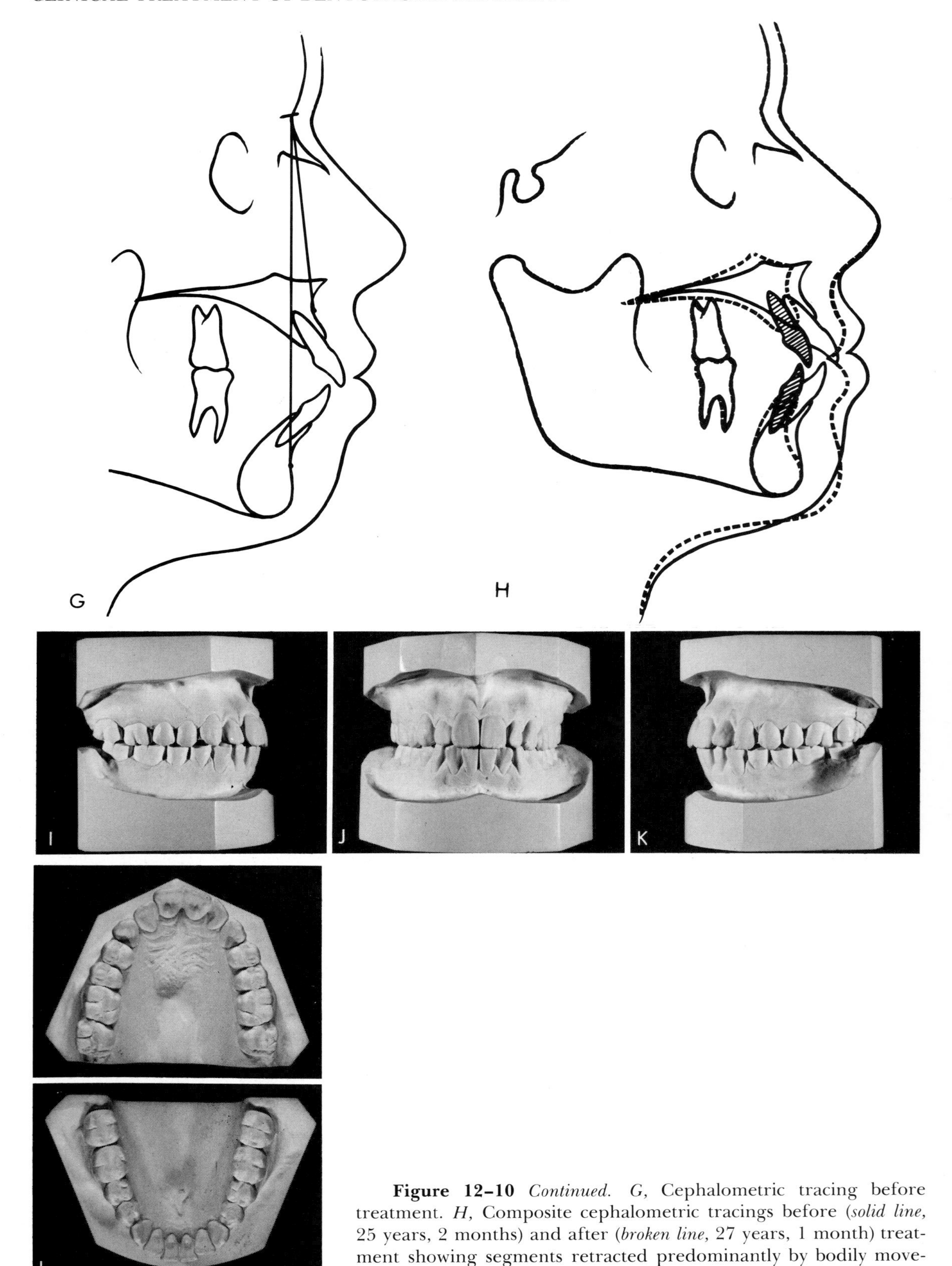

Figure 12–10 *Continued. G,* Cephalometric tracing before treatment. *H,* Composite cephalometric tracings before (*solid line,* 25 years, 2 months) and after (*broken line,* 27 years, 1 month) treatment showing segments retracted predominantly by bodily movement. *I–P,* Occlusion before (*I–L*) and after (*M–P*) treatment.

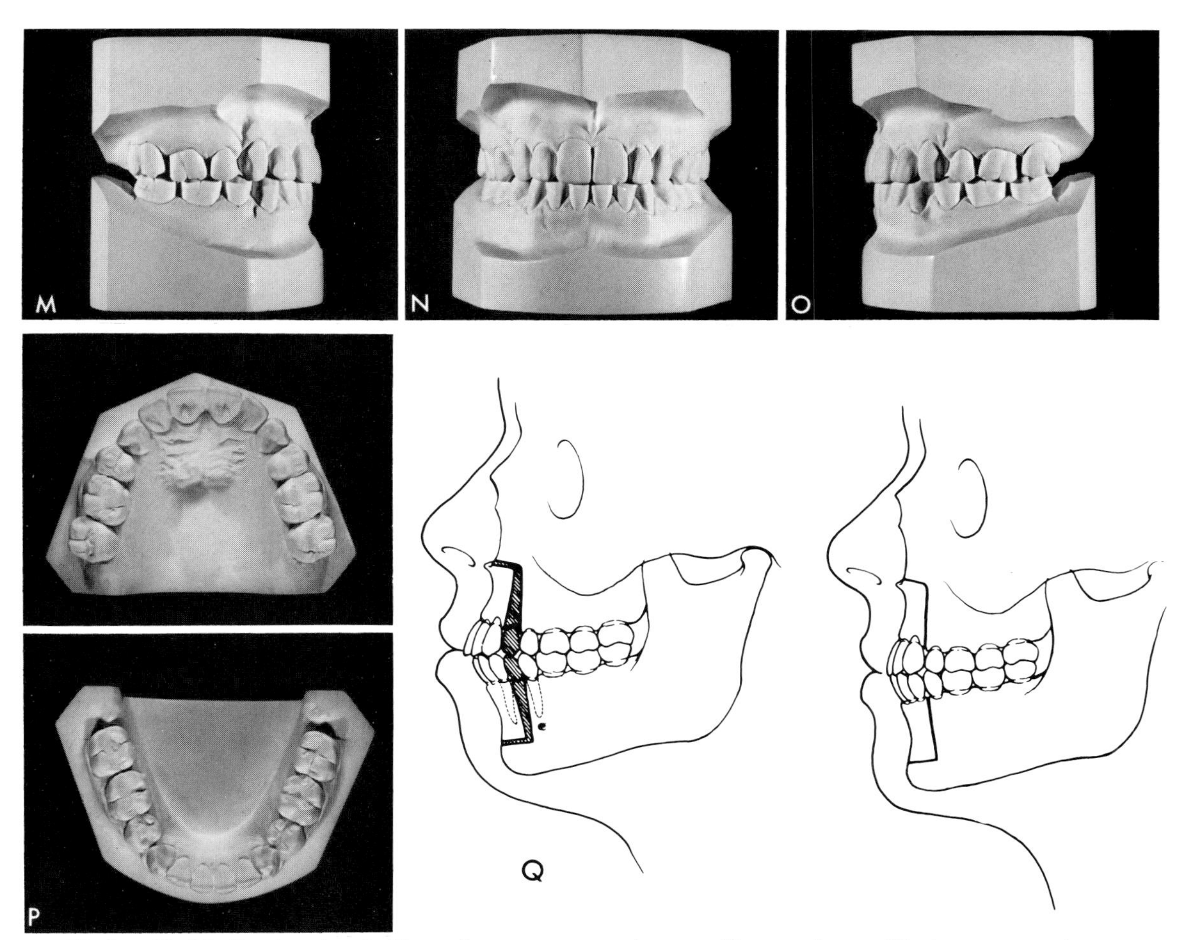

Figure 12–10 *Continued.* *Q*, Plan of surgery: anterior maxillary and mandibular ostectomies to retract anterior teeth, reduce prominence of lips and facial convexity, and produce relative increase in prominence of chin.

See also legend on the opposite page.

DENTAL OCCLUSION. Class I bimaxillary protrusion with minimal anterior open bite.

TREATMENT PLAN

Presurgical Orthodontic Treatment

1. Extract maxillary and mandibular first premolars to facilitate alignment of anterior teeth and position incisors in good relationship to bony bases.
2. Full-band with edgewise orthodontic appliance.
3. Align maxillary and mandibular teeth.
4. Correct rotation of canines.
5. Widen arches in canine region slightly to improve the second premolar to canine approximation at the time of surgery.

Surgical Treatment (Fig. 12–10*Q*)

1. Anterior maxillary ostectomy to retract anterior maxillary teeth and close residual extraction spaces; raise anterior maxilla slightly to improve the upper lip line to incisor relationship.
2. Anterior mandibular ostectomy to close residual extraction space by retraction and canting and raise anterior mandibular dentoalveolar segment to close anterior open bite.

Postsurgical Orthodontic Treatment

1. Final space closure and alignment of dental arches.

ACTIVE TREATMENT

A mock correction of the articulated study casts was made by extracting four first premolars and moving the anterior segments distally 5 mm until the spaces were closed. Satisfactory alignment of the teeth indicated the feasibility of the treatment plan.

After presurgical orthodontic treatment was accomplished, the arch wires were removed and study casts were made for final surgical planning and preparation of the occlusal splints. Following surgery, the mobilized segments were fixed into the desired position for approximately 6 weeks. Healing of the surgical sites was uneventful. Final space closure and alignment were completed in another 4 months. At that time all appliances were removed, and upper and lower Hawley retainers were placed and worn night and day for 6 months and at night only for another 6 months.

FOLLOW-UP AND COMMENT

The occlusion has remained stable during a postoperative follow-up period of 7 years. The slight lisp and anterior tongue thrust are no longer noticeable. Postoperative cephalometric tracings show the degree of retraction and uprighting of the maxillary and mandibular incisors. The amount of bony chin increased from 0.5 to 4.0 mm as a result of moving the mandibular anterior dentoalveolar segment distally 6 mm. The maxillary segment was moved distally 4.5 mm. A balanced facial profile with a pleasing smile line was produced by orthodontic treatment coordinated with segmental surgery.

Surgeon: William H. Bell, Dallas, Texas. *Orthodontist:* Clifford L. Condit, Houston, Texas.

CASE 12–4 (Fig. 12–11)

T. B., a 17-year-old black male, desired treatment to reduce the prominence of his lips. Clinical and cephalometric analysis revealed bimaxillary protrusion.

PROBLEM LIST

Esthetics (Fig. 12–11 *A* and B)

FRONTAL. Face symmetric with prominent upper and lower lips; esthetic smile line.

PROFILE. Prominent but competent upper and lower lips; acute nasolabial angle; moderate facial convexity with relatively good balance between the chin and nose.

Cephalometric Analysis (Fig. 12–11*E*)

1. Bimaxillary dental protrusion, moderate severity.
2. Procumbent maxillary and mandibular teeth.
3. Good lip-to-tooth relationship.
4. Anterior and posterior facial height within normal limits.

Occlusal Analysis (Fig. 12–11*G*)

DENTAL ARCH FORM. Maxilla and mandible ovoid and symmetric.

DENTAL ALIGNMENT. Minimal crowding and malalignment of teeth.

DENTAL OCCLUSION. Class I bimaxillary dental protrusion with satisfactory overbite and overjet.

TREATMENT PLAN

1. Anterior maxillary and mandibular ostectomies in second premolar sites to bodily retract the maxillary and mandibular dentoalveolar segments in order to:
   a. Decrease prominence of upper and lower lips.
   b. Increase the nasolabial angle.
   c. Produce relative increase in prominence of chin.

ACTIVE TREATMENT

A cephalometric prediction analysis indicated that facial convexity could be adequately reduced by anterior maxillary and mandibular subapical ostectomies in the

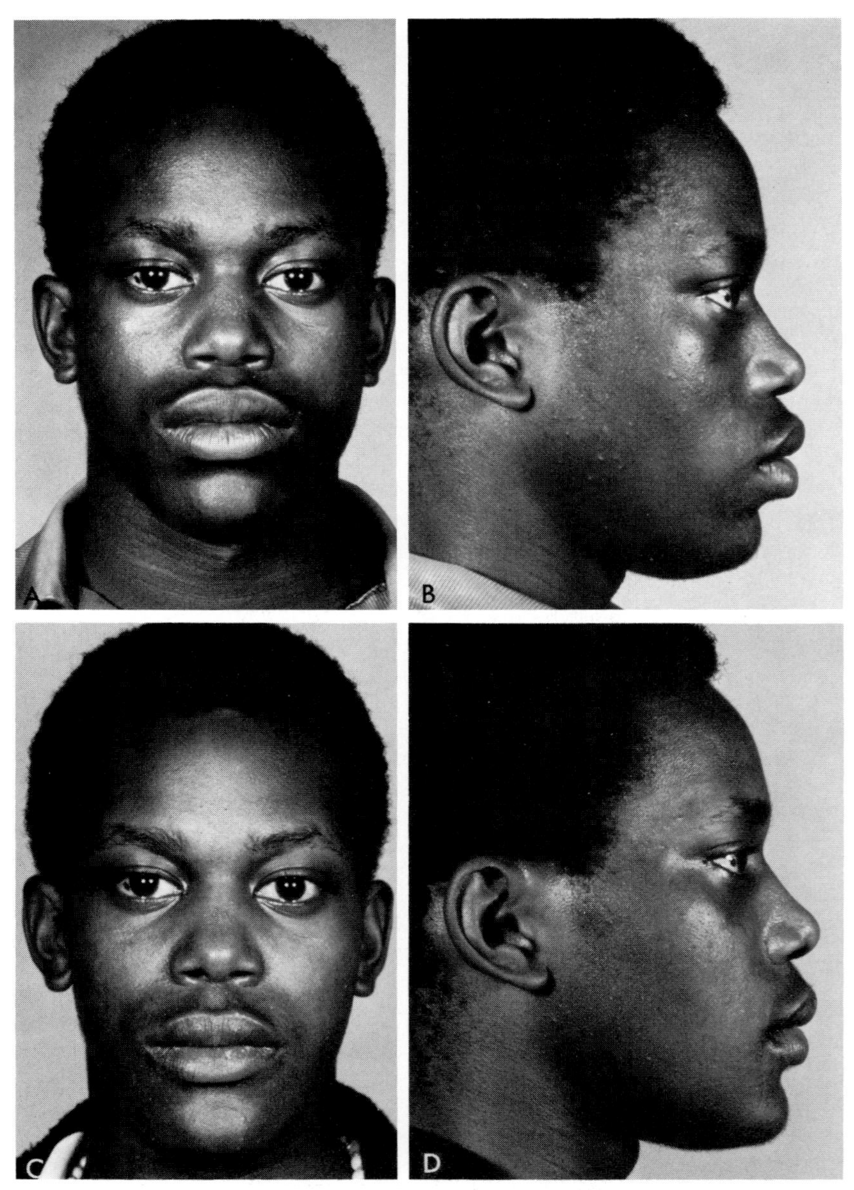

Figure 12–11 (Case 12–4). *A–D,* Photographs of 17-year-old male with bimaxillary dental protrusion before (*A* and *B*) and after (*C* and *D*) treatment.

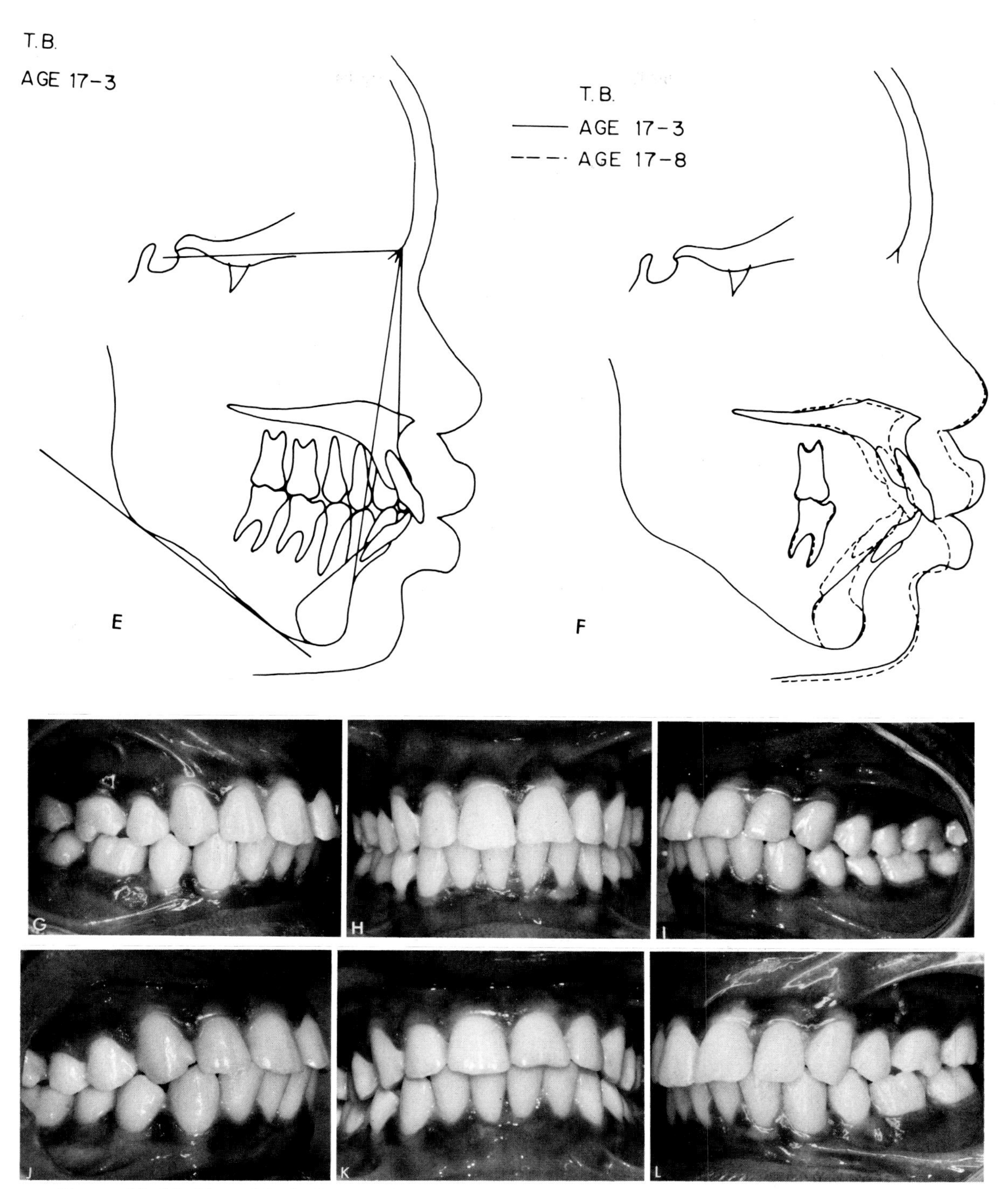

Figure 12–11 (Case 12–4) *Continued.* *E*, Cephalometric tracing before treatment (age 17 years, 3 months). *F*, Composite cephalometric tracings before (*solid line*, 17 years, 3 months) and after (*broken line*, 17 years, 8 months) treatment. *G–I*, Occlusion before treatment. *J–L*, Occlusion after treatment.

second premolar regions. Model surgery demonstrated a satisfactory relationship between the first premolars and first molars when the anterior dentoalveolar segments were retracted the full dimension of the second premolar extraction spaces (7 mm). An interocclusal splint was fabricated from the sectioned models.

The jaw surgery was accomplished under general anesthesia according to the preoperative plan. The Wunderer technique of anterior maxillary osteotomy was used because of the need for bodily retraction. After the mobilized segments were indexed into the previously prepared interocclusal splint, the mandible was immobilized with intermaxillary elastics placed between Erich arch bars that had been previously ligated to the upper and lower teeth.

Approximately 2 weeks after surgery the interocclusal splint was removed. Vertical intermaxillary elastics were worn continuously for another 4 weeks to improve the interdigitation of the teeth and allow the osteotomized segments to stabilize. When the intermaxillary fixation was removed 6 weeks after surgery the segments were firm. Light nighttime elastics were worn for another 2 weeks, after which time the arch bars were removed.

FOLLOW-UP

Bodily retraction of the anterior maxillary dentoalveolor segments reduced the facial convexity and the prominence of the upper and lower lips (Fig. 12–11 *C, D,* and *F*). As a consequence, there was good balance between the nose, lips, and chin. The postoperative occlusal relationship, which was functional and similar to the preoperative occlusion, has remained stable during a 2-year postoperative follow-up period (Fig. 12–11 *G–L*).

When good interdigitation is achieved by subapical surgical procedures and maintained until there is adequate union of the osteotomized segments, the need for postoperative retention appliances is usually precluded. Excellent esthetic and functional results can be achieved by properly planned and executed segmental surgical procedures when treatment is not complicated by malaligned teeth, or anterior teeth that are severely proclined. Despite the fact that the resulting incisal inclination of the maxillary and mandibular anterior teeth is frequently not ideal, occlusal and skeletal stability is usually achieved and the tongue adapts to its new environment. Post-treatment lip competence and proper interdigitation of the teeth are keys to attaining occlusal stability.

Surgeons: Philip Freeman, Campbellsville, Kentucky. William H. Bell, Dallas, Texas.

REFERENCES

1. Bell W: Correction of maxillary excess by anterior maxillary osteotomy. Oral Surg Med Pathol *43*:323, 1977.
2. Bell W, Condit C: Surgical-orthodontic correction of adult bimaxillary protrusion. J Oral Surg *28*:578, 1970.
3. Bell WH, Dann JJ: Correction of dento-facial deformities by surgery in the anterior part of the jaws. Am J Orthod *64*:162, 1973.
4. Bell W, McBride K: Correction of the long face syndrome by Le Fort I osteotomy. A report on some new technical modifications and treatment results. Oral Surg Med Pathol *44*:493, 1977.
5. Bell WH, *et al*: Bone healing and revascularization after total maxillary osteotomy. J Oral Surg *33*:253, 1975.
6. Case CC: Dental Orthopedia and Correction of Cleft Palate. New York: Leo L. Bruder, reprinted 1963.
7. Cupar I: Die chirurgische behandlung der Form und Stellungsveranderungen des Oberkiefers. Ost Z Stomotol *51*:565, 1954.
8. Kohn MW, White RP Jr: Evaluation of sensa-

tion after segmental alveolar ostectomy in 22 patients. J Am Dent Assn *89*:154, 1974.

9. Köle M: Surgical operations on the alveolar ridge to correct occlusal abnormalities. Oral Surg *12*:277, 1959.
10. Proffit WR, Knight JM: Tongue pressures and tooth stability after anterior maxillary osteotomy. J Oral Surg *35*:798, 1977.
11. Proffit WR, McGlone RE, Barrett MJ: Lip and tongue pressures related to dental arch and oral cavity size in Australian aborigines. J Dent Res *54*:1161, 1975.
12. Sowray J, Haskell R: Ostectomy at the mandibular symphysis. Br J Oral Surg *5*:97, 1967.
13. Tweed CH: Clinical Orthodontics. St Louis: C V Mosby Co, 1966.
14. Wassmund M: Lehrbuch der praktischen Chirurgie des Mundes und der Kiefer. Vol I. Leipzig: H Meusser, 1935.
15. Wunderer S: Erfahrungen mit der operativen behändlung hochgradiger Prognathien. Dtsch Zahn-Mund-Kieferheilkd *39*:451, 1963.

Chapter 13

OPEN BITE

William R. Proffit and William H. Bell

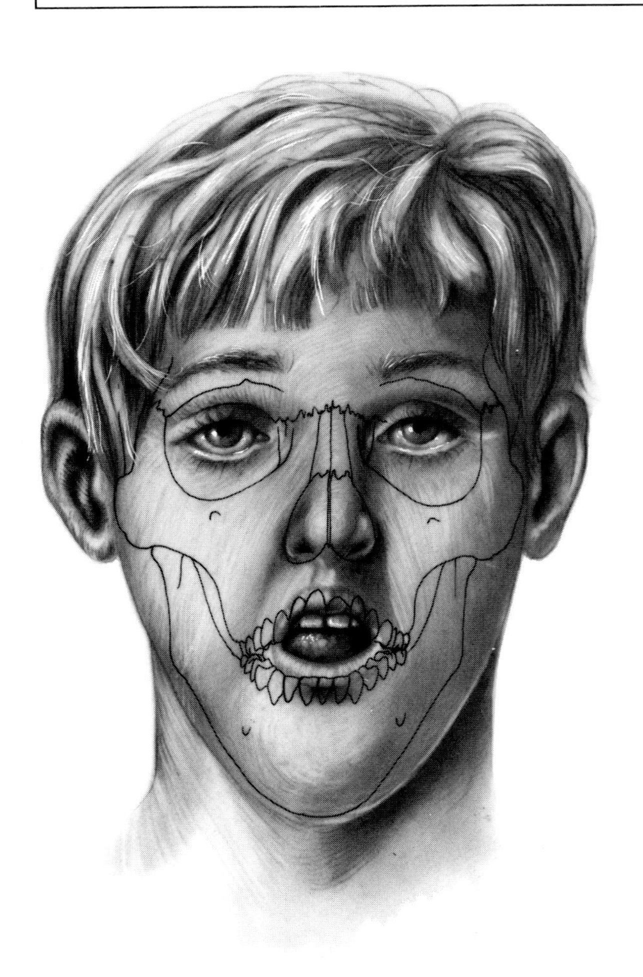

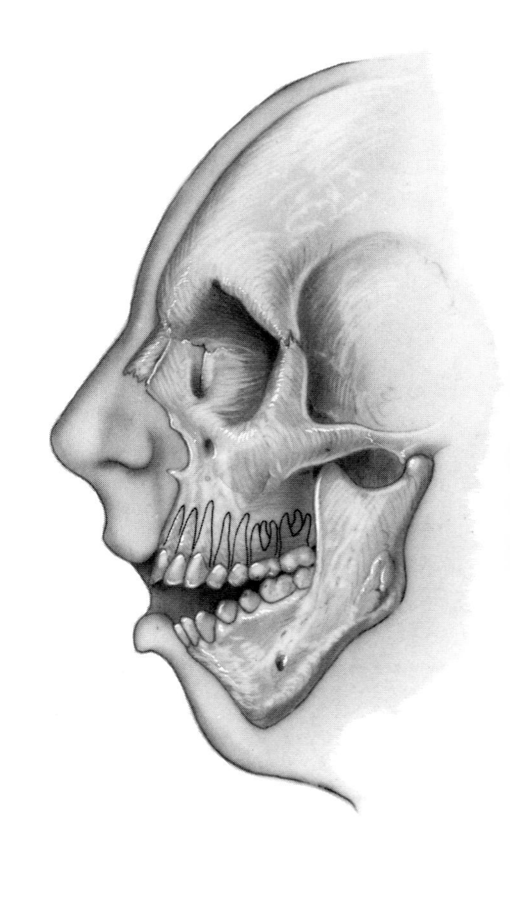

To a greater extent than most other dentofacial syndromes, open bite is a neuromuscular rather than solely an anatomic problem. Development of severe open bite is related to positioning of the mandible relative to the maxilla — a purely muscular phenomenon, and to differential eruption of the teeth — usually associated with differential growth of the anterior and posterior portions of the maxilla. The differential dentoalveolar development may be related to muscular or environmental influences as well. This does not preclude the importance of genetic influences and overall skeletal proportions in the development of open bite as in other types of dentofacial deformity. Both neuromuscular and genetic influences operate while the patient is growing. Although much remains to be learned, it has now been established that surgical intervention in severe open bite problems can improve anatomic relationships caused by aberrant growth. Improvement in physiologic adaptation follows surgery by means of altered neuromuscular function. The deformity can be treated in nongrowing patients by approaching the anatomic problem directly, and the prospects for long-term stability of the corrections are no different from those for other types of deformities in which neuromuscular influences may be less important etiologic factors.

In any discussion concerning the etiology of open bite, three general influences are usually considered. Two of these are environmental: (1) sucking habits in childhood and (2) tongue posture, tongue position in swallowing, or both. The third factor, the proportions of the facial skeleton, is primarily determined genetically. Data regarding the incidence rate of open bite in the United States population at various ages provide considerable insight into the operation of these three causative factors. For this as for other aspects of dentofacial deformity, the best data are from the U.S. Public Health Service surveys of incidence of malocclusion in American children aged 6 to 11 and youths aged 12 to 17. Both were large-scale surveys, utilizing 8000 and 7000 subjects respectively at numerous locations in the United States.

ETIOLOGIC FACTORS

Thumb Sucking and Other Sucking Habits

Most infants engage in some kind of "non-nutritive sucking." This behavior is entirely normal. The frequency of non-nutritive sucking decreases with age, but the U.S.

TABLE 13–1. Percentage of United States Children with Thumb-Sucking Habit[24]

Age	*Percentage*	
	Boys	Girls
6	11.8	15.4
7	11.5	14.4
8	5.7	11.8
9	8.6	13.1
10	6.3	8.7
11	8.3	6.2

Public Health Service data reveal that approximately 11 per cent of boys and 15 per cent of girls still suck their thumbs at least occasionally when they begin school at age 6 (Table 13–1). Even at age 11, a surprisingly large percentage of children still reportedly engage in sucking behavior. An examination of the data reveals that approximately 80 per cent of the children who still suck their thumbs at ages 6 to 11 have an anterior open bite, and 60 per cent have noticeable incisor protrusion. Both figures are highly significant statistically. There is no question but that there is a strong relationship between thumb sucking in the elementary school years and open bite malocclusion.

Data for incidence of anterior open bite in the 6 to 11 age group are displayed in Table 13–2. Two factors are immediately apparent:

1. There is a wide racial variation in the incidence of anterior open bite. Looking at all cases of failure of the incisors to overlap vertically, one finds that open bite occurs four times as often in the Black population as in the White. If only open bites of 2 mm or more are considered, the racial difference is even more striking, the incidence in the Black population then being seven times as high as that in Whites.

TABLE 13–2. Incidence of Open Bite in United States Children and Youths

	Percentage	
	Age 6 to 11[24]	Age 12 to 17[23]
Any open bite (no vertical overlap)		
Total	5.7	5.2
White	4.0	3.5
Black	16.3	16.3
Open more than 2 mm		
Total	1.4	1.1
White	0.6	0.5
Black	6.4	5.7

2. The statistics for incidence of open bite in this age group, when compared with the statistics for thumb sucking, suggest that the great majority of patients who have open bite at this age do in fact continue to suck their thumbs.

By the time a child reaches the school years, the sucking habit is likely to have become an empty one, often stopping spontaneously or being corrected by some kind of intervention. (Treatment of sucking habits is discussed briefly in the section on orthodontic treatment.) Almost all children in this age group wish to stop sucking their thumbs because of peer pressure, and it is rare that the dentist needs to do more than encourage the child. Spontaneous correction of the open bite after thumb sucking stops is a common observation. In a cross-sectional study of Navajo Indian children, Worms and associates found that the number of anterior open bites decreased tremendously, with the greatest improvement occurring between the ages of 10 and 12.[45] Cross-sectional data from the two U.S. Public Health Service epidemiologic studies also indicate a decrease in open bite with age, but a much smaller decrease than was reported in the Navajo children (see Table 13–2). Correction or improvement in open bite is much more likely to occur in children with good skeletal jaw relationships — skeletal open bites improve spontaneously only rarely and may become worse with age.

Tongue Pressure or Posture

Although there is no doubt that the position of the teeth depends upon a balance between opposing forces applied to them, equilibrium is not defined solely by the opposing pressures of tongue and lips. This has been extensively investigated in recent years by Proffit and others.[28, 36] It is now apparent that there is no balance of pressures between tongue and lips during swallowing, when all activities including resting pressures are summed up, or at rest. The concept that tongue pressure from an incorrect swallow pushes the teeth into open bite or protrusion is incorrect. The tongue thrust swallow that is commonly seen in children and occurs in 15 per cent of otherwise normal adults appears to be an adaptation to the open bite, rather than cause.

This does not mean that tongue and lips have no influence. Indeed, animal experiments strongly suggest that resting posture of tongue and lips is an important etiologic factor in open bite, and that the resting posture is determined largely by respiratory requirements.[16, 30] For instance, severe open bite malocclusion has been produced in primates merely by creating obstruction to nasal breathing. In order to breathe through the mouth, the animal alters the resting posture of the mandible and carries the tongue lower and more forward. The development of a severe open bite follows, often accompanied by mandibular protrusion. Similar effects can be achieved by placing an obstruction in the roof of the mouth which requires the animal to carry the tongue low in the floor of the mouth. Accommodation to the obstruction includes an altered resting posture of the mandible in addition to repositioning of the tongue. The association of mouth breathing with elongation of the face and a tendency toward anterior open bite has long been recognized in patients. In the English literature the "adenoid facies" has been discussed frequently. Resting posture of both tongue and lips contributes in a major way to the etiology of open bite.

As previously noted, open bite incidence decreases around the time of puberty. There are two reasons for an alteration in respiratory needs and a consequent alteration

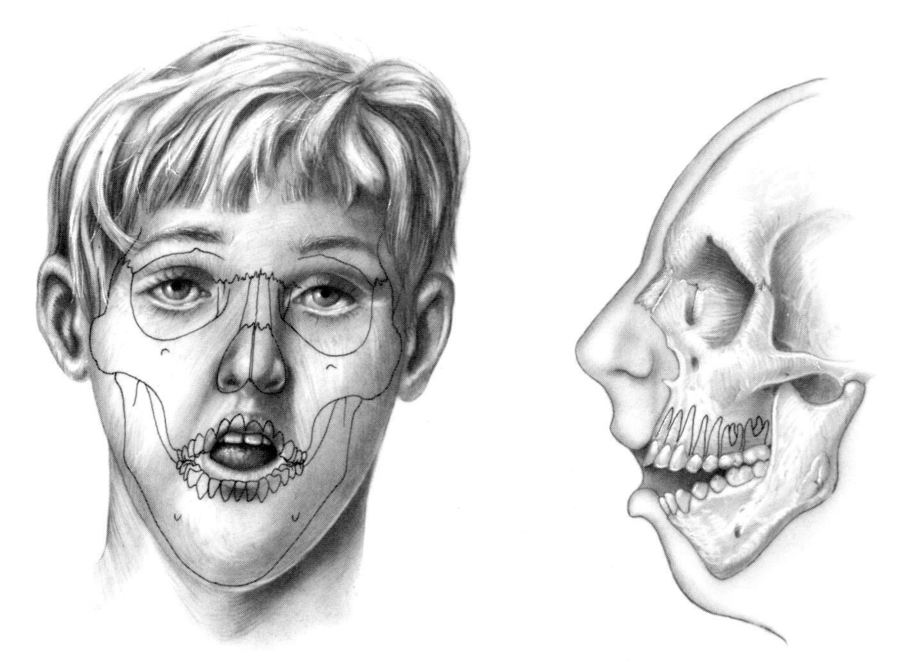

Figure 13–1. Anatomic characteristics of skeletal open bite deformity.

in tongue posture at this time: (1) the tendency for adenoids and tonsils to shrink rather than grow at puberty, and (2) the vertical growth of the jaws that occurs at the same time. These anatomic changes provide more room for the tongue, allowing it to be carried higher and more posteriorly without interfering with respiratory requirements. Tongue thrust swallow tends to disappear as this change in resting posture occurs.

The combination of a decrease in sucking habits and a change in resting posture seems to account for the decrease in open bite prior to and during adolescence. In children who do not have skeletal dysplasias, open bite is a transient phenomenon.

Skeletal Influences

Neuromuscular interaction makes it difficult to separate primary skeletal influences on open bite from those arising from alterations in resting posture and dictated by respiratory needs. Nevertheless, it is true that anterior open bite is more likely in individuals with certain anatomic characteristics (Fig. 13–1):

1. An obtuse "saddle angle" between the middle and anterior cranial fossae.
2. A normal or short mandibular ramus.
3. A tipped palatal plane, higher in front than in back.
4. A steep mandibular plane angle.
5. Increased anterior facial height.

The "saddle angle" is determined very early in life and does not change thereafter. The other characteristics are influenced by growth and may be altered by the facial environment, but all have a strong familial tendency.

The strongest evidence for a genetic influence on the development of vertical problems of the face and jaws derives from an examination of the data for incidence of open bite versus deep bite in Caucasian and Black races. The much higher incidence of anterior open bite in the Black population has been pointed out already. The reverse is true for deep bites. The incidence of overbite of more than 6 mm is seven times as high in Whites, just as open bite of more than 2 mm is seven times as common in Blacks. It is highly unlikely that this great a difference can be explained on environmental grounds alone. The slightly different facial proportions of the two racial groups affect dental and skeletal relationships in the vertical plane of space.

Putting the whole etiologic picture in perspective is difficult. Patients who have severe anterior open bite as part of an overall dentofacial deformity are likely to have skeletal relationships that predispose them to vertical problems. Almost always, neuromuscular imbalances are superimposed on the pre-existing skeletal pattern, further complicating the situation and contributing to the deformity as it develops.

Classification of Severity

The severity of the open bite influences the decision as to when and how it should be treated. Differentiations are commonly made on the basis of the degree of (1) skeletal involvement, i.e., distortion of facial proportions; (2) dental involvement, i.e., vertical displacement of teeth; and (3) neuromuscular involvement. Moyers, making the reasonable assumption that increasing neuromuscular involvement would be reflected in the dentition, classifies open bite as simple, compound, or infantile (skeletal), depending on how far posteriorly the open bite extends.[33] Such a classification into various types based upon specific occlusal characteristics may be very misleading to the clinician, however. For example, an individual may have a relatively small vertical spacing between his anterior teeth—which can be classified as simple open bite—and yet have the skeletal and facial features of a severe skeletal open bite deformity. Treatment of such a patient would be anything but as simple as implied by the definition; moreover, skeletal open bite is not self-correcting. A more clinically meaningful and practical method involves looking at the open bite deformity as a syndrome: a constellation of facial, cephalometric, and occlusal characteristics. By systematically describing the esthetic, cephalometric, and occlusal characteristics of the individual patient, a more meaningful plan of treatment based upon the individual's specific needs can be evolved.

Only limited data are available concerning the effect of growth on severe open bite problems, in which both skeletal malrelationships and neuromuscular imbalances are present. It is clear that the very severe open bites are not likely to be self-correcting. Self-correction of dental open bites is a phenomenon of the mixed dentition and the preadolescent growth spurt. Such *dental* open bites are *not* the central concern of this chapter. If a severe open bite is still present at the end of puberty (age 12 to 15), therapeutic intervention including surgery should be considered.

Physiologic Response to Alteration in Vertical Position of Teeth: Does Rest Position Change?

One conceptual difficulty with treatment of open bite by intrusion of posterior teeth is in visualizing the effect this has on the musculature. Would intrusion of the teeth merely lead to an increase in the freeway space? Or would the rest position of the mandible somehow change, so that it would rotate closed at rest as well as in occlusion, maintaining approximately the same freeway space as existed prior to the surgery? Prosthodontic experience indicates that rest position is not altered by changing the vertical level of prosthetic teeth. Patients with dentures do not tolerate significant changes in the vertical dimension of occlusion. But it is not logical to anticipate that patients with natural teeth would react in exactly the same way. Since the periodontal membrane has important sensory connections to the medullary centers that control the postural position of the facial muscles, it would be physiologically possible for patients with natural teeth to adapt differently from patients with artificial teeth. Indeed, this appears to be the case.

When surgical intrusion of maxillary teeth is carried out, the mandible rotates closed at rest as well as in function. For most patients, a new resting position is "programmed" by the surgery, in a way which as yet is not completely understood. In planning and carrying out surgery for correction of open bite, however, it is important to comprehend the principle of physiologic adaptation in resting jaw position. Adaptation to changes in vertical dimension occurs only in patients with natural teeth, not in patients with artificial teeth. It seems, furthermore that the key element of change in altering the rest position of the mandible is a change in the position of the teeth relative to their supporting jaw. Physiologic adaptation is observed commonly in patients who have maxillary intrusion. In this instance, the mandible rotates closed at rest, and a new resting position is observed. When the mandibular rotation that closes an open bite is achieved by mandibular osteotomy, however, so that the rotation is around the posterior teeth rather than at the condyle, physiologic adaptation does not seem to occur in the same way. In this instance, the relationship of maxillary and mandibular teeth to their supporting bone is unchanged. It is also significant that in patients who undergo rotation around the posterior teeth, the surgery lengthens the ramus and moves the chin away from the hyoid bone, thus stretching both the elevator muscles of the mandible and the suprahyoid musculature. If the rotation would tend to obliterate previously existing freeway space and increase posterior vertical dimension, the periodontal proprioceptive mechanisms serve to protect the natural teeth from occlusal interferences that might occur in patients with dentures. No one has natural teeth that click during speech, for instance. Despite this degree of physiologic adaptation, rerotation of the mandible may occur after rotation produced by ramus surgery.

SYSTEMATIC DESCRIPTION OF THE DEFORMITY

As with other dentofacial deformities, a spectrum of characteristics are associated with open bite. Only by systematically describing each individual with an open bite deformity can the specific characteristics of that patient be seen and a rational treatment evolved. The format for diagnosis in Chapter 6 is followed here with emphasis on findings pertinent to open bite.

History and General Physical Findings

Dental open bite is considered to be a condition created within the facial environment rather than an inherited or innate problem. True skeletal type open bite deformities, however, are more closely related to genetic factors and do not tend to regress spontaneously at age 11 to 12. The recognition and treatment of this type dentofacial deformity is the central theme of this chapter. In all severe facial deformities, there are complex interactions between environmental and inherent factors, and open bite differs only in the extent of neuromuscular involvement. In documenting the history, it is especially important to inquire about breathing problems. Since stability after correction of open bite may relate to the patient's ability to breathe through his nose, allergies and chronic nasal blockage should be investigated. If these are severe, an otolaryngologic consultation may be needed. Sucking habits must be identified. Invariably, a "tongue thrust" swallow is found to be present in patients with open bite, since an anterior tongue position is necessary to obtain an oral seal for swallowing. This finding must not lead the examiner to conclude that the tongue thrust is the cause of the open bite.

Esthetic Features

Considerable variation exists in esthetics when individuals with open bite deformity are seen in front or profile view (Fig. 13–2). Most patients with open bite do not have right–left asymmetries, and the upper and middle thirds of the face are generally well-balanced. The lower third of the face is almost always elongated. Ideally, the upper-, middle-, and lower-third facial heights should be approximately equal. The distance from the base of the nose to the inferior aspect of the upper lip should be approximately one third of the lower-third facial height. Typically, the individual with an open bite deformity has narrow nasal alar bases — ideally the alar base width should be about one fifth of the total width of the face as measured along a line through the pupils of the eyes.

Two aspects of lip posture should be studied carefully: (1) lip competence and (2) the relation of the upper lip to the underlying teeth and gingiva. Lip competence exists when lip closure can be achieved easily without hyperfunction of the perioral musculature. Separation of the lips at rest by more than 3 to 4 mm makes this impossible. In individuals with severe open bite, the lip separation may be as great as 10 to 12 mm. Lip incompetence must be considered carefully in the treatment approach. The vertical relation between the upper lip and the maxillary incisors is equally important. Although considerable variability exists in this relation, pleasing appearance usually requires that about one quarter (2 to 4 mm) of each upper anterior tooth be exposed when the upper lip is at rest. Patients with open bite deformity usually have considerably more exposure than this. The amount of lip incompetence (if any) and the amount of upper anterior teeth and gingiva exposed beneath the upper lip at rest must be measured accurately and recorded (see Chapter 8, Maxillary Excess, for details of case analysis). The amount of superior repositioning of the anterior maxilla is based upon the relationship between the maxillary incisors and the upper lip. The smile line frequently helps to substantiate the need for superior movement of the maxilla, but it is *not* the basis for planning the

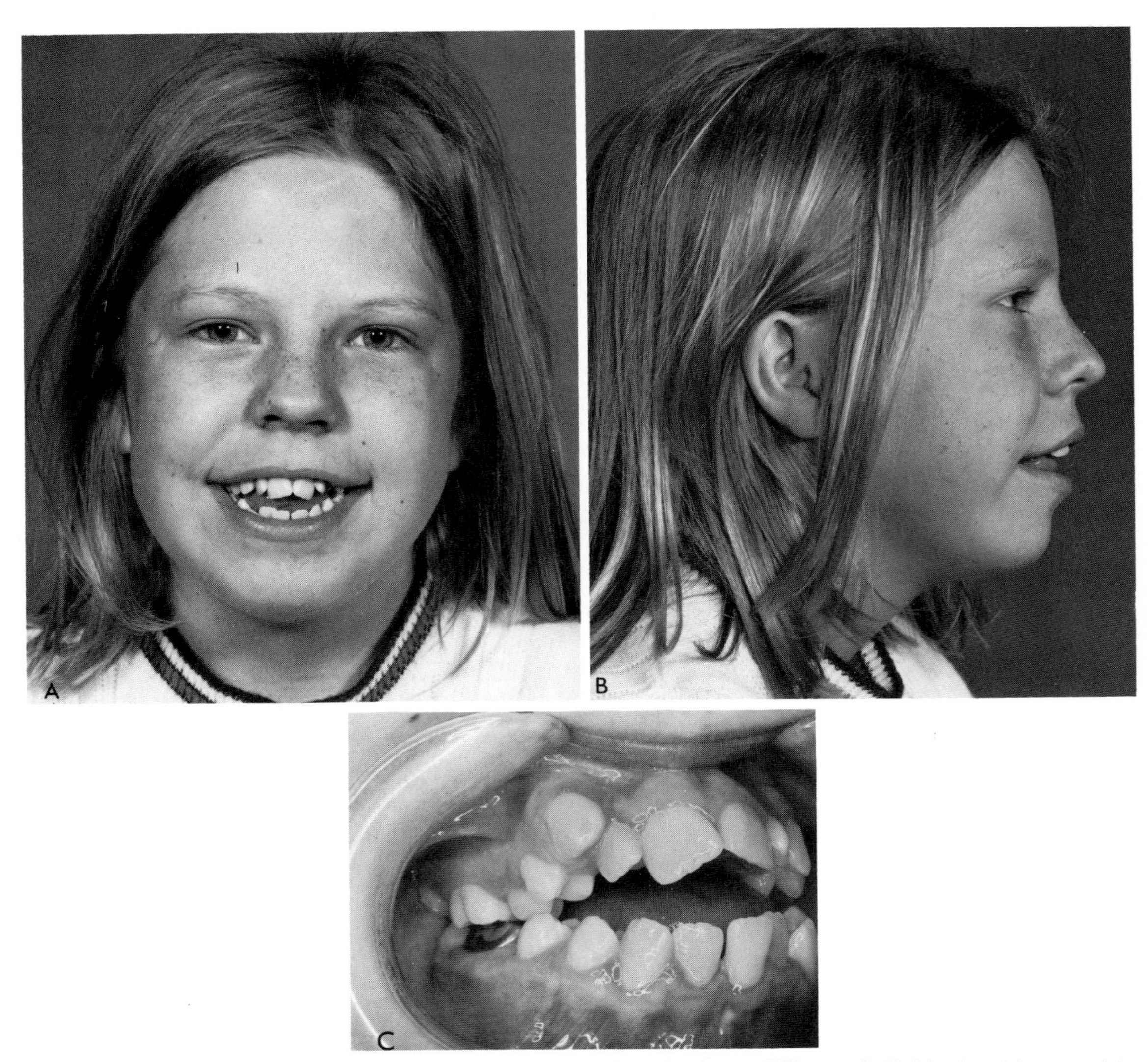

Figure 13–2. Variable facial esthetics and smile lines in three different individuals with open bite deformities. *A–C,* 11-year-old female with Class I occlusion.

Legend continued on the opposite page

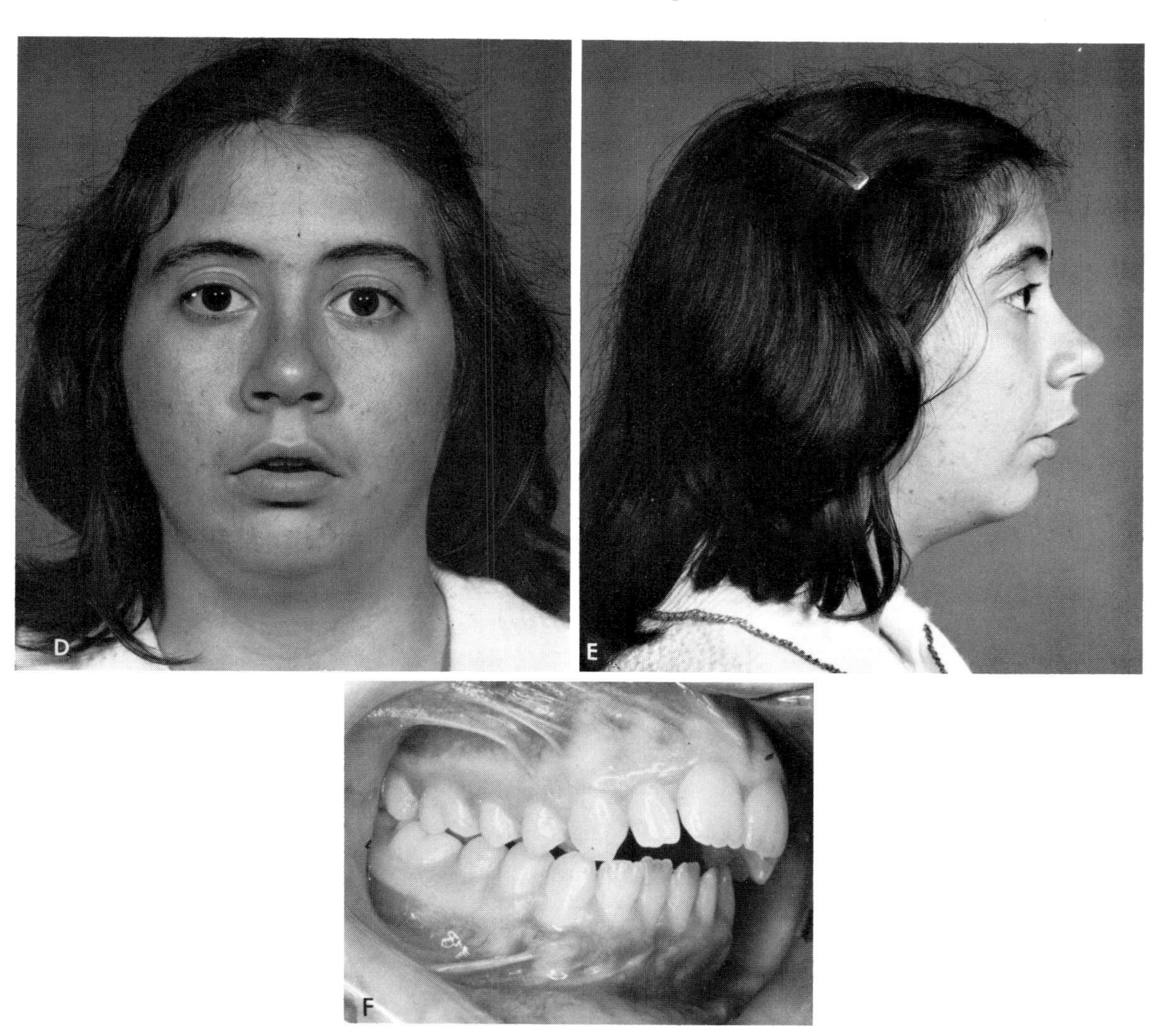

Figure 13–2 *Continued.* *D–F,* 17-year-old female with Class II occlusion.

Illustration continued on the following page

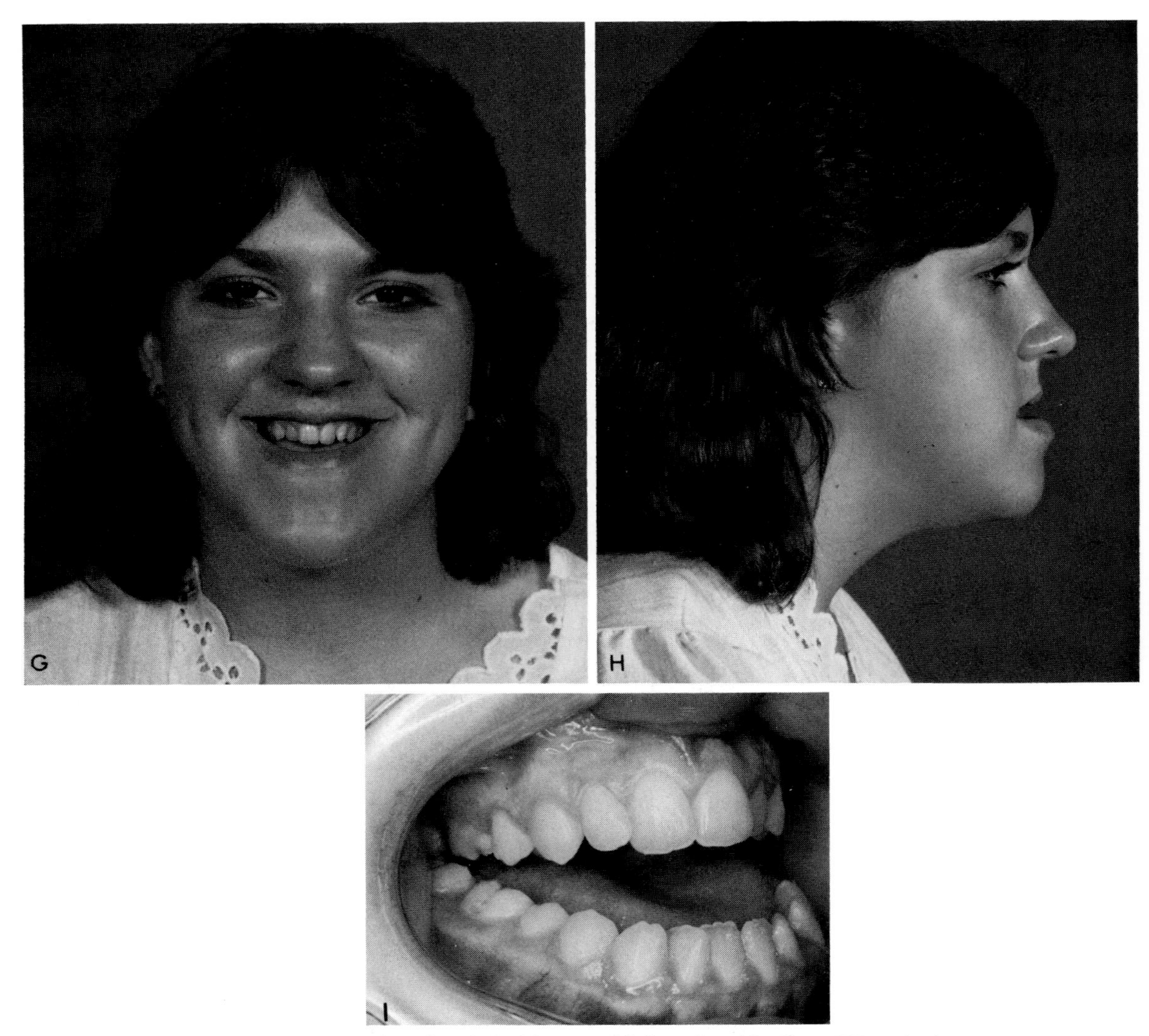

Figure 13–2 *Continued.* *G–I,* 16-year-old female with Class III occlusion.

exact amount of movement. Individual variation in the smile line produced by variation in the anatomy of a smile (i.e., variable activity of perioral muscles) precludes specific treatment planning based upon the amount of gingival exposure when smiling.

When the profile is evaluated, the esthetic disharmony is most often found to exist in the nasolabial area and the lower third of the face. The relation of the nose to the remainder of the face and the nasolabial angle must be considered carefully. A nasolabial angle between 90° and 110° is considered esthetic. Such measurements are predicated upon a normal columella-nose relationship. A "hanging" columella may, however, alter the esthetic priorities and necessitate modification of the surgical plan of treatment. (See Chapter 15, Nasal Deformities, for further diagnostic considerations.) When the angle is acute, the anterior maxillary dento-osseous segment can be retracted and appearance will be improved. When the angle is obtuse, frequently the case in open bite deformity, retraction of the anterior maxillary dento-osseous segment will worsen the appearance. Lip competence and the relation of the upper lip to upper teeth should be checked again. Lip incompetence, the interlabial gap, and the relationship between the upper lip and the maxillary incisors are measured with the lips in relaxed position. These clinical measurements are compared with comparable measurements made from a lateral cephalometric radiograph exposed with the lips in repose. It is extremely important to do this evaluation with the lips at complete rest. For some patients this evaluation is time-consuming, difficult, and frustrating, but an accurate record is mandatory.

The second principal area of esthetic consideration is the lower third of the face. An elongated lower face with a retrusive chin is a frequent finding. This indicates that the mandible has rotated down and backward. A well-balanced chin indicates less skeletal involvement.

Thus, the clinical evaluation of facial esthetics in individuals with open bite deformity concentrates on the following:

1. Lip competence.
2. Relation of the upper teeth to upper lip.
3. Nasolabial angle.
4. Length of the lower face.
5. Anteroposterior position of the chin.
6. Balance between chin, lips, and nose.

Additionally, the cephalometric films and models must be analyzed to decide upon a specific therapeutic approach to the problem.

Analysis of Dental Casts, Radiographs, and Other Records

Intra-arch Alignment and Symmetry

Crowding may be present, but alignment of the teeth usually is good in patients with open bite. Protrusion of incisors is likely. Arch form usually is satisfactory and symmetric, although constriction of the maxillary arch may exist.

Transverse Relationship of Teeth and Jaws

A difference in arch form between the maxilla and mandible is a common finding in an open bite deformity. The maxillary arch tends to be somewhat narrow and V-shaped, whereas the mandibular arch tends to be wide and ovoid or U-shaped. This situation creates a width discrepancy, which may be exhibited as a crossbite in all areas but is greatest in the premolar and canine areas. Rapid maxillary expansion facilitated by lateral maxillary osteotomies to round out the canine–premolar region may be required (see Chapter 9).

Anteroposterior Relationships

Although open bite may be associated with all types of malocclusion, relative or absolute mandibular deficiency and Class II malocclusion are most common. This situation arises from the downward and backward rotation of the mandible accompanying bite opening. Downward positioning can convert a Class I relationship to Class II, or Class III to Class I. The impression of a normal mandibular body length with a short ramus is confirmed cephalometrically. The length of the posterior cranial base (S–Ba distance) may be decreased.

Flatness of the midfacial region secondary to anteroposterior maxillary deficiency is occasionally associated with anterior open bite deformity. The affected area may extend from the base of the maxillary alveolar process to the infraorbital foramen and is variably manifest in the paranasal and canine fossae areas.

Vertical Relationships

Open bite is primarily a vertical problem, the common denominator of all such cases being failure of the anterior teeth to occlude. The teeth may be 2 to 14 or more mm apart anteriorly with the open bite extending posteriorly to the canines, or in the most severe instances, back to the third molars. Cephalometric analysis almost always reveals increased vertical facial height, an obtuse gonial angle, and a steep mandibular plane angle. The palatal plane is likely to be tipped up anteriorly and down posteriorly. The angle between the palatal and mandibular planes is excessive. Overall anterior facial height is increased, but middle-third facial height usually is normal or even decreased. The bulk of the increase in facial height is found in the lower third.

The common but variable cephalometric findings of the skeletal type anterior open bite deformity are as follows (Fig. 13–3):

1. Increased anterior facial height.
2. Steep mandibular plane angle.
3. Normal mandibular body length.
4. Normal or decreased ascending ramus height.
5. Increased distance from nasal floor to maxillary teeth apices.
6. Tipped palatal plane, higher anteriorly than posteriorly.
7. Low position of mental foramen.
8. Decreased posterior cranial base (S–basion).
9. Flat or reverse curve of mandibular occlusal plane.

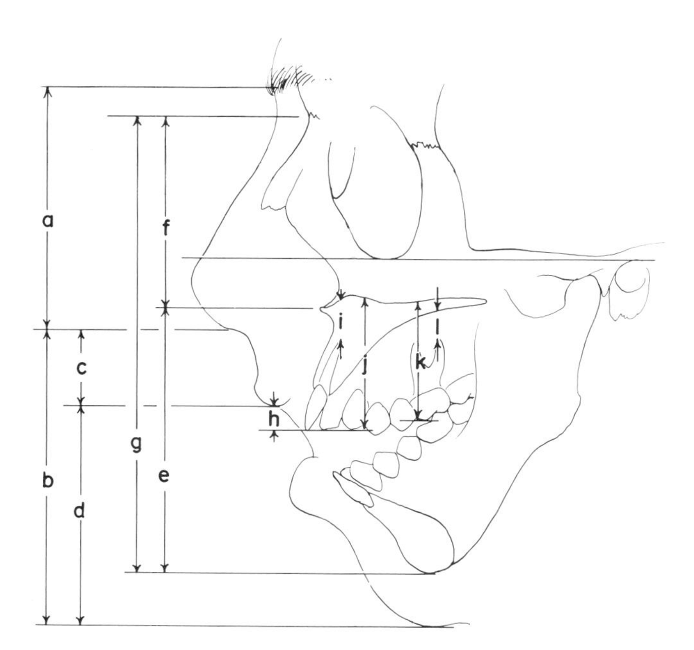

Figure 13–3. Common vertical cephalometric measurements of open bite deformity.

	soft tissue facial height mm.				skeletal facial height mm.			tooth lip mm.	tooth to alveolus mm.			
Measurement	a	b	c	d	e	f	g	h	i	j	k	l
Example	68	81	20.5	60	73	52	125	6.4	10.1	36.5	32.5	7.5
Normal	66	66	22	44	63	53	116	2.3	0	28.7	19.6	0

To analyze the dental component of the open bite, four dentoskeletal relationships must be evaluated. The open bite may affect any one of these or a combination. The vertical relationships are: (1) maxillary incisor to nasal floor, (2) maxillary molar to nasal floor, (3) mandibular incisor to lower border of the mandible, and (4) mandibular molar to the lower border of the mandible. If the molars are extruded while the incisors are normally positioned, there will be an open bite. If the molars are normally positioned but the incisors are under-erupted, there will be an open bite also, but of course the treatment would be different because the underlying problem is different.

In many deformities, the vertical position of teeth is symmetric; that is, maxillary and mandibular teeth will be found to have divided the vertical space between the jaws evenly. This often is not the case in open bite. If molar super-eruption has occurred, it will be exhibited mostly in the maxilla (usually) or mostly in the mandible (relatively rare). Superior repositioning of the maxilla by surgery is indicated when the extrusion is primarily a maxillary problem. Cephalometric data for vertical positioning of maxillary and mandibular teeth are given in Chapter 6. Relative mandibular deficiency is frequently correctable by superior repositioning of the maxilla; absolute mandibular deficiency associated with vertical maxillary excess will, however, require maxillary surgery in addition to mandibular advancement.

Vertical skeletal dysplasias show up cephalometrically as distortions of overall vertical symmetry. Projecting the cranial base and the palatal, occlusal and mandibular planes (method of Sassouni) is particularly helpful in detecting which jaw or area is most at fault. A palatal plane that tips down in back and up in front is an indication of skeletal maxillary involvement and may relate to failure of the anterior palate to descend properly during growth.

ORTHODONTIC TREATMENT

Correction of severe open bite deformity has been among the least successful of all forms of orthodontic treatment. Some cases defy any and all forms of orthodontic therapy. Others are corrected only to relapse due to late vertical growth when therapy is discontinued in the late teens. In some cases, facial appearance is compromised by conventional orthodontic therapy to the extent that the patient appears worse following treatment. Because of such failures and the complexity of the problems, the orthodontic literature abounds with treatment methods. Though the suggestions are diverse, all orthodontic treatment methods can be placed in one or more of the following general categories: (1) redirection of growth, (2) habit control, and (3) tooth movement.

Redirection of Growth

Even severe dental open bite problems in growing children tend to improve or even to correct spontaneously. If redirection of growth can be accomplished, orthodontic correction can be achieved. Redirection of growth is the initial treatment of choice in growing patients with moderate open bite. The objective of treatment in open bite is to prevent further eruption of posterior teeth while allowing normal eruption of incisors, and thereby to achieve a counterclockwise rotation of the mandible during its growth, decreasing the mandibular plane angle.

Three appliance systems are used currently for this type of growth redirection therapy: (1) high-pull headgear directed to the posterior maxilla, (2) chin cup with high-pull forces, and (3) functional appliance systems (activator types or, most promising of all, the Frankel appliance). High-pull headgear prevents eruption of maxillary molars and vertical growth of the maxillary posterior alveolar process. It may lead to intrusion of the maxillary molars. Vertical pull chin cups impede molar eruption in both arches, and in theory could produce intrusion. Intrusion has been observed to occur with the Milwaukee brace appliance used to correct scoliosis.[1] Intrusion of molar teeth rarely happens with the chin cup, probably because it is difficult to obtain near-constant use of the appliance. The functional appliance systems aim at impeding molar eruption while facilitating incisor eruption.

Since all these methods aim at reducing excess posterior vertical dimension, this should be a major component of the problem when they are used. Therapeutic success will be influenced by the amount and direction of growth and also by patient cooperation.

Tooth Movement

Vertical tooth movement in open bite correction may be divided into two types: (1) intrusion of teeth that are in occlusion and (2) extrusion of teeth at the site of the open bite.

Direct intrusion of posterior teeth has been discussed as a type of growth redirection. Of the appliances discussed, high-pull headgear to maxillary molars seems most likely to produce true intrusion and functional appliances least likely. In addition, reduction of posterior vertical height and bite closure may be obtained by extraction of posterior teeth. Typically, when bite closure through this effect is desired, first molars are extracted, and space is closed largely by moving the second and third molars mesially. If the posterior teeth are kept at their original vertical level relative to their supporting jaw as the extraction space is closed, anterior open bite will be reduced.

In an open bite case in which surgery is not planned, one should consider treating mild arch-length problems that otherwise would be treated by extraction of first premolars by extracting the first molars instead. Molar extraction may help with correction of mild open bites, but the extent of intrusion obtained by this method alone is not enough to correct the majority of open bite deformities. In these, direct intrusion is needed. If it is believed that maxillary surgery may be necessary, it may be wise to avoid using high-pull headgear. Because patients with skeletal open bite usually have excessive anterior facial height, superior movement of the anterior and posterior maxilla is usually indicated and should be programmed when the treatment plan is initially evolved.

Extrusion of teeth at the open bite site can be accomplished readily by orthodontic forces. Anterior vertical or "box" elastics are used in most instances. Continuous arch wires impede open bite correction when extrusion of some but not all teeth is needed. Segmental arch wires or continuous wires that have been cut at the point where the open bite ends should be used instead. If alveolar development is indeed insufficient, extruding the teeth may produce desirable and stable results. In the more usual instance when the problem is excessive anterior and posterior maxillary dentoalveolar height, extruding the anterior teeth to match is likely to produce results that are unstable and detrimental to facial appearance as well. Vertical elastics should not be used to elongate incisors when the basic problem is not infraeruption of incisors but supraeruption of molars.

Habit Control

An association between sucking habits, tongue thrusting, and anterior open bite has been recognized by generations of clinicians. What is cause and what is effect in these situations remains controversial. Although thumb or finger sucking in the preschool years may create an anterior open bite, rapid spontaneous correction normally follows abandonment of the habit when the open bite is dental and not skeletal. Treatment to stop thumb sucking prior to age 5 rarely is indicated. As sucking habits continue past this age, especially if a skeletal pattern favoring open bite is present, increasing deformity can be created by the habit. Current research indicates that behavior modification techniques to stop sucking habits can be used in school-age children without fear of psychologic side effects.[17, 18]

Appliances such as the crib, elbow retraints, or other direct approaches to breaking sucking habits should be used in conjunction with psychologic support for the child; i.e., the child should be given to understand what is being done and why. It is important that, once undertaken, the treatment approach not fail. Otherwise, the habit may be reinforced rather than extinguished.

The approach to "tongue thrusting" is not so clear-cut, simply because cause and effect relative to the tongue is not so simple. More and more modern research data indicate that tooth and jaw relationships are not sensitive to pressures of tongue contacts during swallowing, speaking, and other activities.[35, 38] Speech and swallowing therapy for open bite therefore has little rational underpinning. Resting positions of lips and tongue are the crucial environmental factors in determining tooth position, and one should keep in mind that the resting posture of the entire orofacial musculature (particularly the muscles of mastication, but also the suprahyoid and infrahyoid musculature and the deep muscles of the neck) relates to this. Excessive posterior vertical development can occur only if the muscles of mastication allow it. Tongue posture is but a small part of the overall picture.

Current recommendations regarding speech and swallowing exercises as part of open bite treatment are:[31, 37]

1. Exercises are not indicated for children with a tongue thrust who do not at present have malocclusion. There is no evidence that a child who has a tongue thrust but no open bite is at any risk of developing one. For this reason, swallowing therapy has no place in the armamentarium of preventive dentistry.
2. If open bite is present, swallowing exercises are not indicated prior to the approach of puberty. Prominent anterior tongue position is a normal developmental stage, and a high percentage of mild and moderate open bites in children aged 5 to 9 spontaneously correct themselves during puberty.
3. Swallowing exercises are most helpful for older children when this therapy is combined with orthodontic appliance therapy, rather than preceding it. The clinical rule should be, "Treat the open bite, not just the tongue thrust."
4. Swallowing exercises are of no additional help when speech articulation therapy is being employed. In order for treatment to be effective, the resting posture of the tongue and other orofacial muscles must be altered, not just what the tongue tip does during swallowing. It appears that articulation therapy is at least as effective as swallowing therapy in accomplishing this.

SURGICAL TREATMENT

Hullihen in 1849 apparently was the first to surgically correct an open bite.[21] The procedure he used to correct the deformity acquired as a result of scar contracture was an operation in the anterior part of the mandible (Fig. 13–4). Since that time the operation has been termed *anterior mandibular subapical osteotomy,* and has been modified and popularized by Trauner, Hofer,[19] and Köle.[25] In the Köle procedure, the mandibular incisor segment is freed and elevated to close an open bite, with the defect beneath the segment grafted with bone from the chin. This procedure is ideal for problems of infraeruption of the lower incisors.

In the late 1950s, numerous variations of the open subcondylar osteotomy in the ascending ramus of the mandible were introduced. Although these procedures were a modification of the much older closed subcondylar and open oblique osteotomy introduced by Limberg in 1925 (Fig. 13–5), it was believed that dissecting free several of the muscles of mastication during surgery would prevent the high incidence of relapse noted with the closed procedure. Despite early claims that the procedures were successful in correcting open bite deformity, follow-up observation of individuals treated with these procedures has shown a high incidence of relapse (see Case 13–9, page 1187). If counterclockwise rotation of the mandible with ramus surgery must be used to close anterior open bite, it should be undertaken with full knowledge of the tendency to relapse.

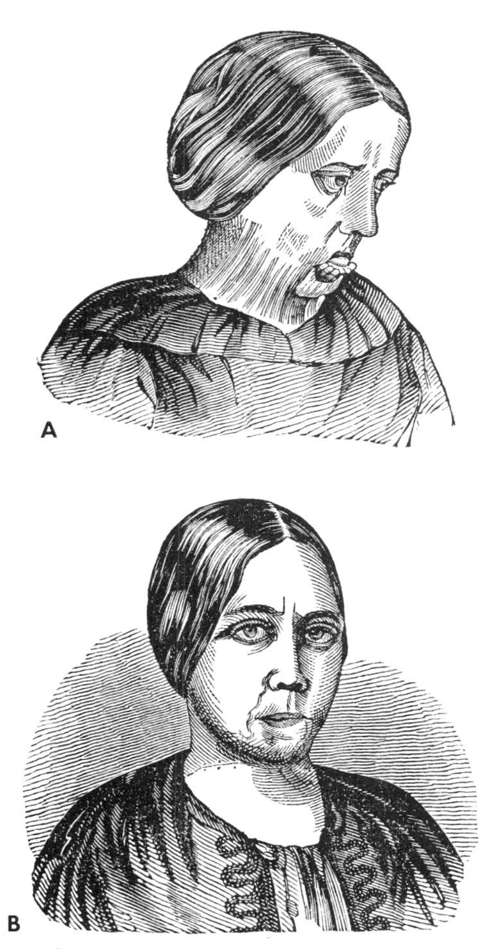

Figure 13–4. Case report of patient who was operated on in 1848 by Simon Hullihan of Wheeling, West Virginia.[21] *A*, The result of contraction of burns of the face and neck. *B*, Postoperative appearance.

Illustration continued on the following page

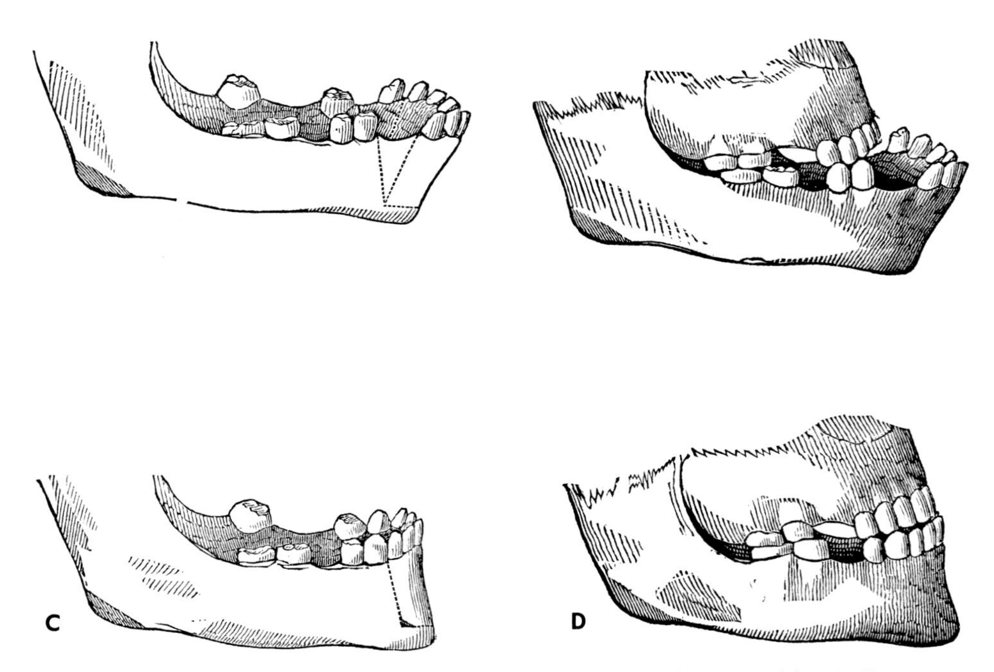

Figure 13–4 *Continued.* *C,* Surgical procedure used to close open bite. *D,* Postoperative result.

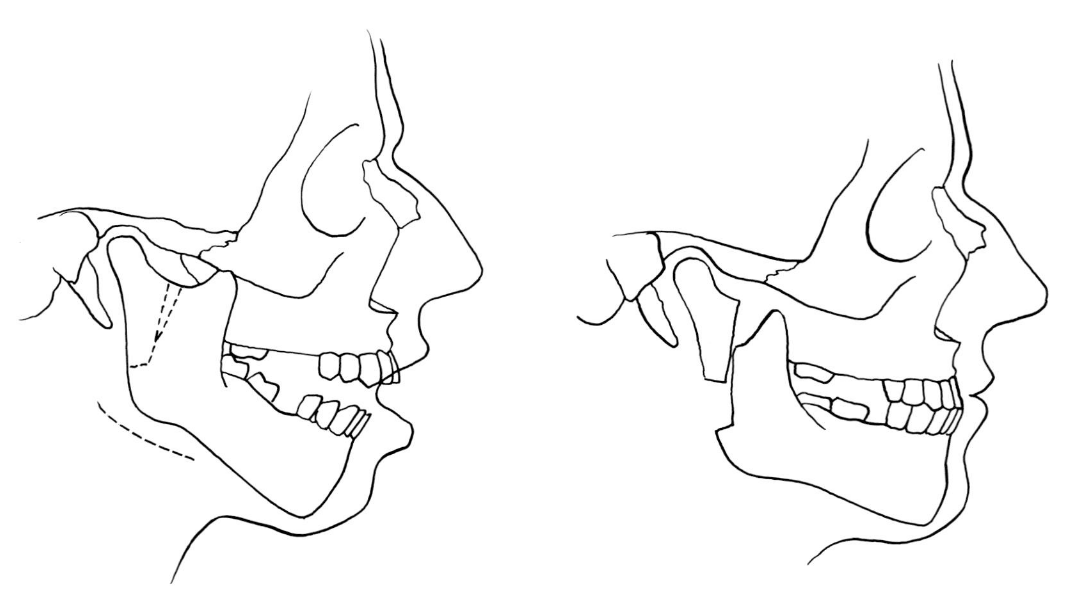

Figure 13–5. The first reported surgical technique for treatment of anterior open bite in vertical rami by Limberg in 1925.[29]

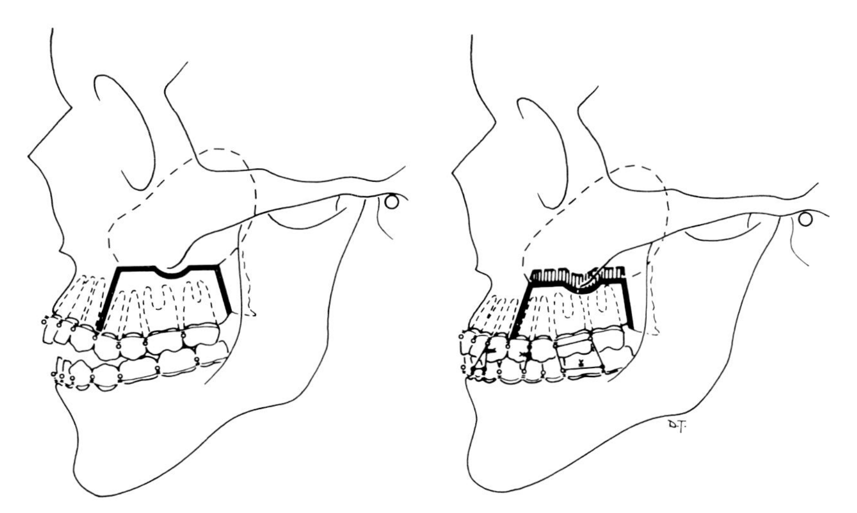

Figure 13–6. The first successful technique to close skeletal type open bite by posterior maxillary osteotomy (Schuchardt, 1959). The posterior maxillary dentoalveolar segments were repositioned superiorly in two stages. (From Mustardé, J. C.: Plastic Surgery in Infancy and Childhood. Philadelphia, W. B. Saunders, 1971.)

The first maxillary procedure used to correct open bite was the *anterior maxillary osteotomy,* which was introduced by Cohn-Stock in 1921[11] and modified by Wassmund,[42] Wunderer,[46] and Cupar.[12] When extrusion of the maxillary anterior segment is necessary, this procedure does result in a stable occlusion, but intrusion of the anterior and posterior teeth is more frequently required. A *posterior maxillary osteotomy* designed to produce intrusion of the posterior teeth was first described as a two-stage procedure by Schuchardt (Fig. 13–6).[40] Early relapses with Schuchardt's technique seem to have been related to failure to free the posterior segment adequately before intrusion. Posterior maxillary osteotomy is now usually performed as a single-stage procedure as described by Kufner.[26] Recently, good stability of posterior maxillary intrusion has been reported by several authors.

Modern techniques for maxillary surgery are based on the Le Fort I downfracture technique to free the entire maxilla. Our present-day surgical technique has evolved over more than 50 years and is the result of many technical modifications by surgeons throughout the world (Fig. 13–7).[4, 5, 9, 20, 34] After the entire maxilla has been cut free, it is frequently sectioned into anterior and posterior segments to obtain the differential movement necessary for optimum correction of the open bite deformity. This maxillary surgery allows the surgeon to approach the most common anatomic sites of open bite deformity directly.[9]

At present, surgical treatment for anterior open bite involves maxillary surgery for combinations of anterior and posterior intrusion and mandibular alveolar surgery to elevate the incisor segment. Surgical procedures in the ramus or body of the mandible are sometimes necessary because of special characteristics of the patient. Choice of the appropriate surgical technique requires a careful diagnostic evaluation.

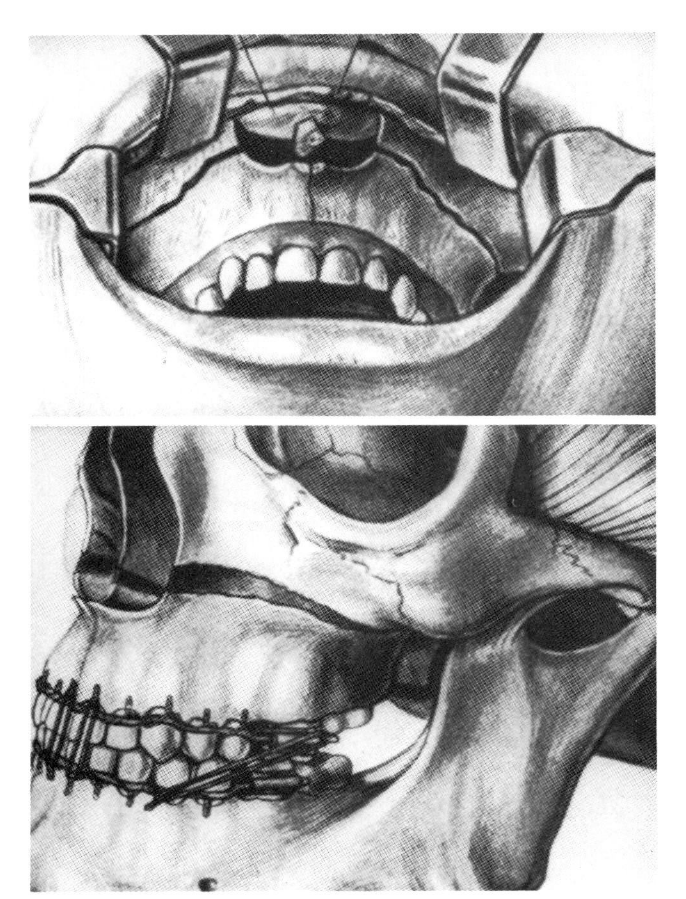

Figure 13–7. The first attempt to reposition the entire maxilla to close an anterior open bite by Wassmund in 1927 (as illustrated in "Handbook of Practical Surgery of the Mouth and Jaw," Martin Wassmund).[42] Osteotomies of the lateral maxilla were made without any attempt to mobilize and reposition the maxilla immediately after surgery.

Planning for Surgical Closure of Open Bite

The extent and direction of surgical repositioning of the maxilla or mandible and the feasibility of the tentative plan of treatment are determined from a coordinated study of the patient, including clinical examination, analysis of lateral cephalometric tracings, and model analysis. The cephalometric prediction of postoperative changes and the model surgery are accomplished in the manner described in Chapter 8, Maxillary Excess, pages 271–278. Trial repositioning of the maxillary and mandibular acetate tracing templates is continued until a satisfactory overbite-overjet and interincisal relationship is achieved and is consistent with the planned esthetic objectives.

The desired movements of the maxilla and mandible determined from clinical and cephalometric studies are then simulated on dental study casts. Extreme care must be used to mount the casts properly in centric relationship with the correct vertical and anteroposterior interarch relationship. The model and the cephalometric measurements serve as references when the planned maxillary and/or mandibular movements are executed during surgery and are used to sculpture the jaws to the dimensions that will effect the desired esthetic and functional changes. The principal difference between maxillary surgery for treatment of open bite and maxillary surgery for treatment of vertical maxillary excess deformity without open bite concerns the more extensive superior movement of the posterior maxilla necessary to close the anterior open bite. This greater movement has the additional advantage of allowing more autorotation superiorly and anteriorly. Excessive extrusion of maxillary anterior teeth by preoperative orthodontics may increase the possibility of postoperative relapse.

The most commonly used surgical procedures for correction of the anterior open bite deformity are described below in the following sections.

Anterior Maxillary Subapical Osteotomy for Extrusion

When consideration is given to planning treatment in all three dimensions of space, relatively few patients with open bite will be treated by isolated anterior maxillary osteotomies. Excessive tooth exposure and lip incompetence are important clinical manifestations of the skeletal type open bite problem, and closing the open bite by anterior maxillary osteotomy alone will increase the amount of tooth exposure and does not address itself to the problem of lip incompetence. A small open bite associated with minimal tooth exposure or none, lip competence, a good nasolabial angle, and adequate lower anterior facial height, may be an indication for anterior subapical osteotomy or for orthodontic extrusion of maxillary incisors.

Occasionally, the maxillary incisors are positioned too high and concealed behind the upper lip. The relationship between the upper lip and the concealed maxillary incisors in rest, speech, and smiling produces an unesthetic edentulous appearance. In such cases, lowering the anterior maxilla to close the open bite will actually improve the facial appearance and the smile line. Thus, when nonskeletal open bite is associated with sufficient upper lip length or a "long" upper lip, consideration may be given to closing the open bite by lowering the anterior maxilla. When there is esthetic balance between the nose and upper lip, excessive chin height, lack of chin contour, or excessive chin prominence can be managed by concomitant genioplasty (see Chapter 14). The basic surgical techniques for respositioning the anterior part of the maxilla by anterior maxillary subapical osteotomy, and the criteria for selection, are reviewed in Chapter 8.

SURGICAL TECHNIQUE FOR ANTERIOR MAXILLARY AND MANDIBULAR SUBAPICAL OSTECTOMY FOR EXTRUSION (Fig. 13–8)

The indications for and advantages of raising the anterior portion of the mandible by subapical osteotomy are similar to many of the indications for and advantages of mandibular body ostectomy. If the open bite manifests in the anterior part of the mandible as a reverse curve in the mandibular arch and there is transverse maxillomandibular harmony with good esthetic balance between the upper lip and the maxillary anterior teeth, the occlusal deformity can be corrected by elevating the mandibular

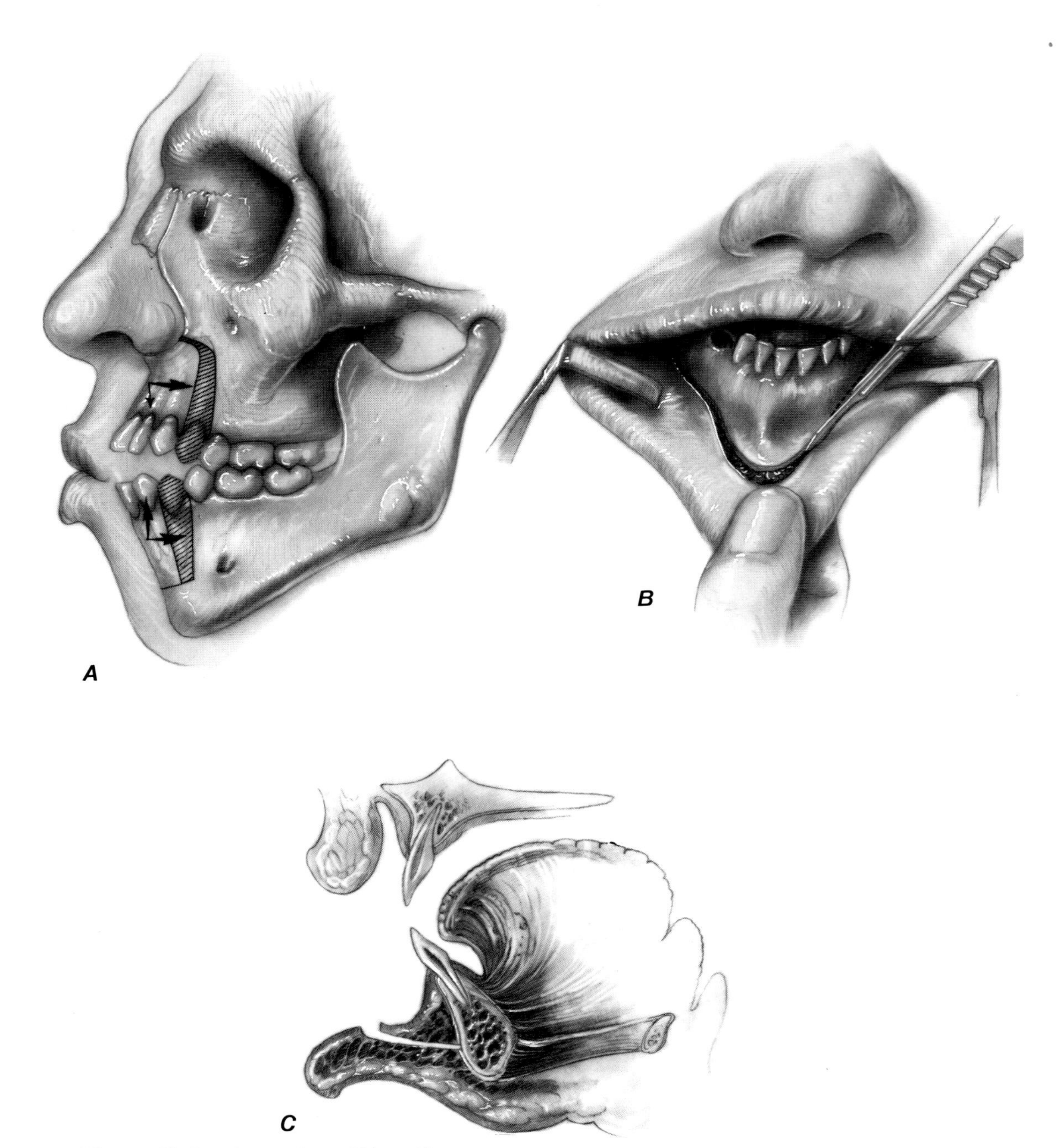

Figure 13–8. Correction of bimaxillary protrusion and anterior open bite by anterior maxillary and mandibular subapical ostectomies. *A,* Dental, skeletal, and facial features associated with bimaxillary protrusion and anterior open bite. Arrows indicate planned directional movements of maxillary and mandibular dentoalveolar segments to close anterior open bite and reduce facial convexity. *B,* Soft-tissue incision for exposure of mandible. *C,* Incision through orbicularis oris and mentalis muscles.

Legend continued on the opposite page

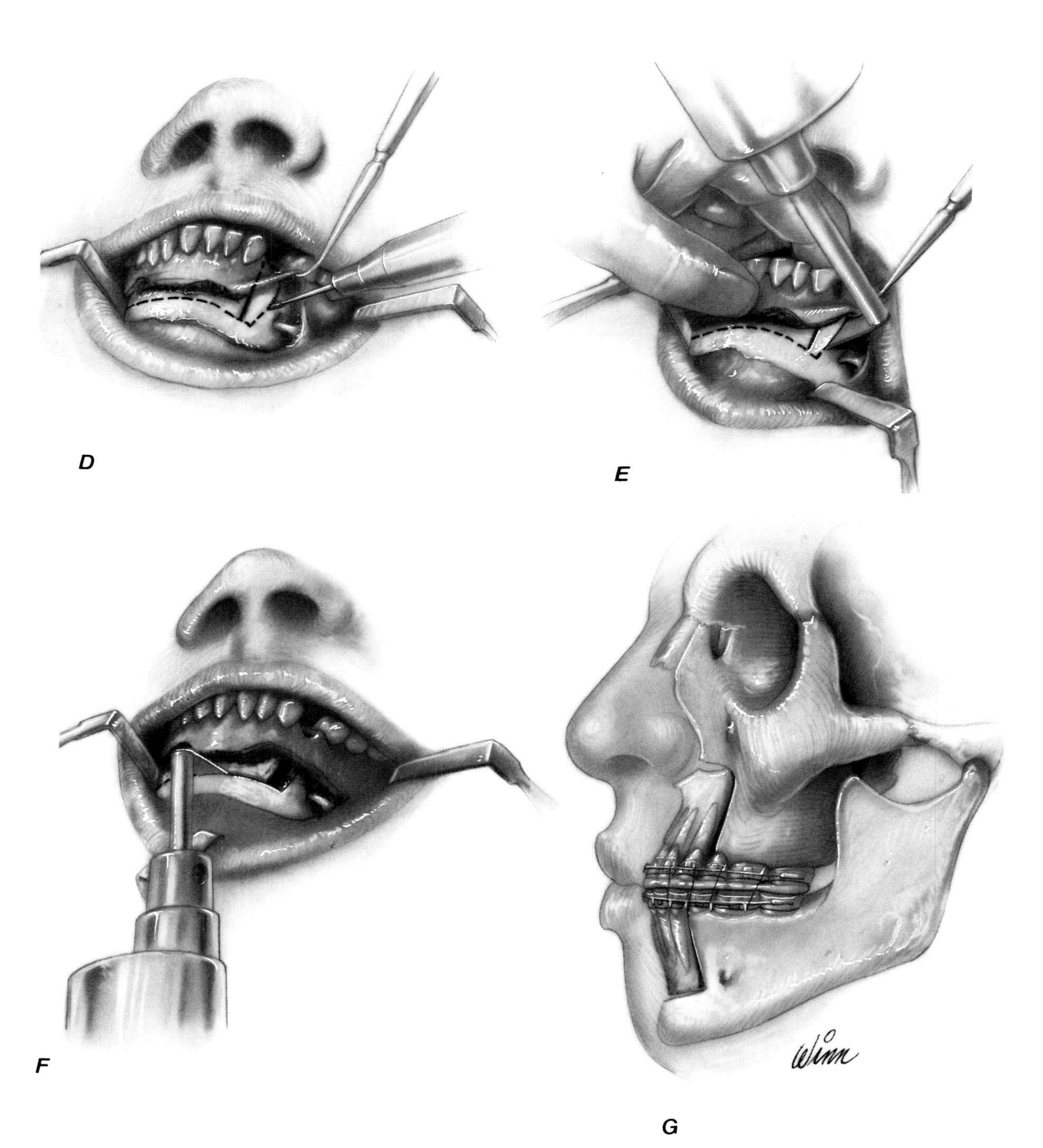

Figure 13–8 *Continued.* *D,* With inferior margin of mucobuccal flap raised with skin hook, the planned vertical ostectomy and horizontal osteotomy are etched into mandible with fissure bur. *E,* Vertical ostectomy is accomplished in residual extraction space with oscillating saw blade. *F,* Subapical osteotomy accomplished with oscillating saw. *G,* Intermaxillary fixation with repositioned dentoalveolar segments indexed into interocclusal splint.

anterior dentoalveolar segment into the desired occlusal relationship. The subapical osteotomy is a biologically sound surgical technique that is easily executed through an intraoral degloving type incision. Because the entire mandible is not sectioned, the mobilized and repositioned dentoalveolar segment can be fixed for a relatively short period of time (5 to 6 weeks) without the use of intermaxillary fixation. The details of the basic surgical technique for anterior mandibular subapical osteotomy are described in Chapter 10. Some of the essential steps are depicted in Figure 13–8. The procedure is most frequently used in concert with LeFort I osteotomy or anterior maxillary osteotomy.

Relapse potential of the repositioned dentoalveolar segment is minimal because the segment is usually moved in the same direction as the pull exerted on it by the attached genioglossus and geniohyoid muscles. Relapse may occasionally be caused by chronic posturing of the tongue against the lingual and occlusal surfaces of the mandibular anterior teeth. Clinically this kind of relapse can be identified by interdental spacing, proclination of the anterior teeth, and recurrence of the open bite. When and if this occurs after surgery, strong consideration should be given to the need for partial glossectomy.

KÖLE MODIFICATION OF MANDIBULAR SUBAPICAL OSTEOTOMY (Figs. 13–9 and 13–10)

When mandibular prognathism is associated with anterior open bite, occlusal and cephalometric studies typically reveal a reverse curve in the mandibular occlusal plane. If the reverse curve in the mandibular arch is severe and is associated with anterior open bite and excessive chin height, the Köle modification of the standard mandibular subapical osteotomy[19] may be used to effect simultaneous correction of the occlusal and esthetic problems (Figs. 13–9 and 13–10). Additionally, the technique makes it unnecessary to procure bone from a secondary surgical site for grafting purposes. Bone from the inferior aspect of the mental symphysis is transposed into the horizontal bony defect created by raising the mandibular dentoalveolar segment to close the open bite — if the chin is deficient, the excised bone may also be used to augment its contour. If this procedure used alone is to be successful, the patient must have a functional posterior occlusion without a significant transverse deficiency problem in the maxillary arch, as well as a satisfactory lip-to-tooth relationship in the anterior maxilla. In severe cases of open bite, however, combined maxillary and mandibular surgical procedures are usually necessary to accomplish the desired occlusal and esthetic result.

When excessive lower anterior facial height is associated with anterior open bite, the Köle procedure may be used to raise the mandibular anterior teeth and decrease the height of the chin. Clinical studies have shown the results of this procedure to be very stable; it is a predictable means of closing an open bite and leveling the mandibular plane of occlusion.

Vertical ostectomies in the premolar or molar extraction sites are usually combined with a horizontal subapical bone incision. The choice of extraction site depends on the magnitude of the anterior crossbite and open bite and the location of the reverse curve in the mandibular occlusal plane. After a horseshoe-shaped segment of bone is excised from the mental symphysis to reduce lower anterior facial height, a portion of the excised bone is placed into the horizontal bony defect created by raising the mandibular dentoalveolar segment. Because the integrity of the mandible is maintained, the reposi-

Text continued on page 1087

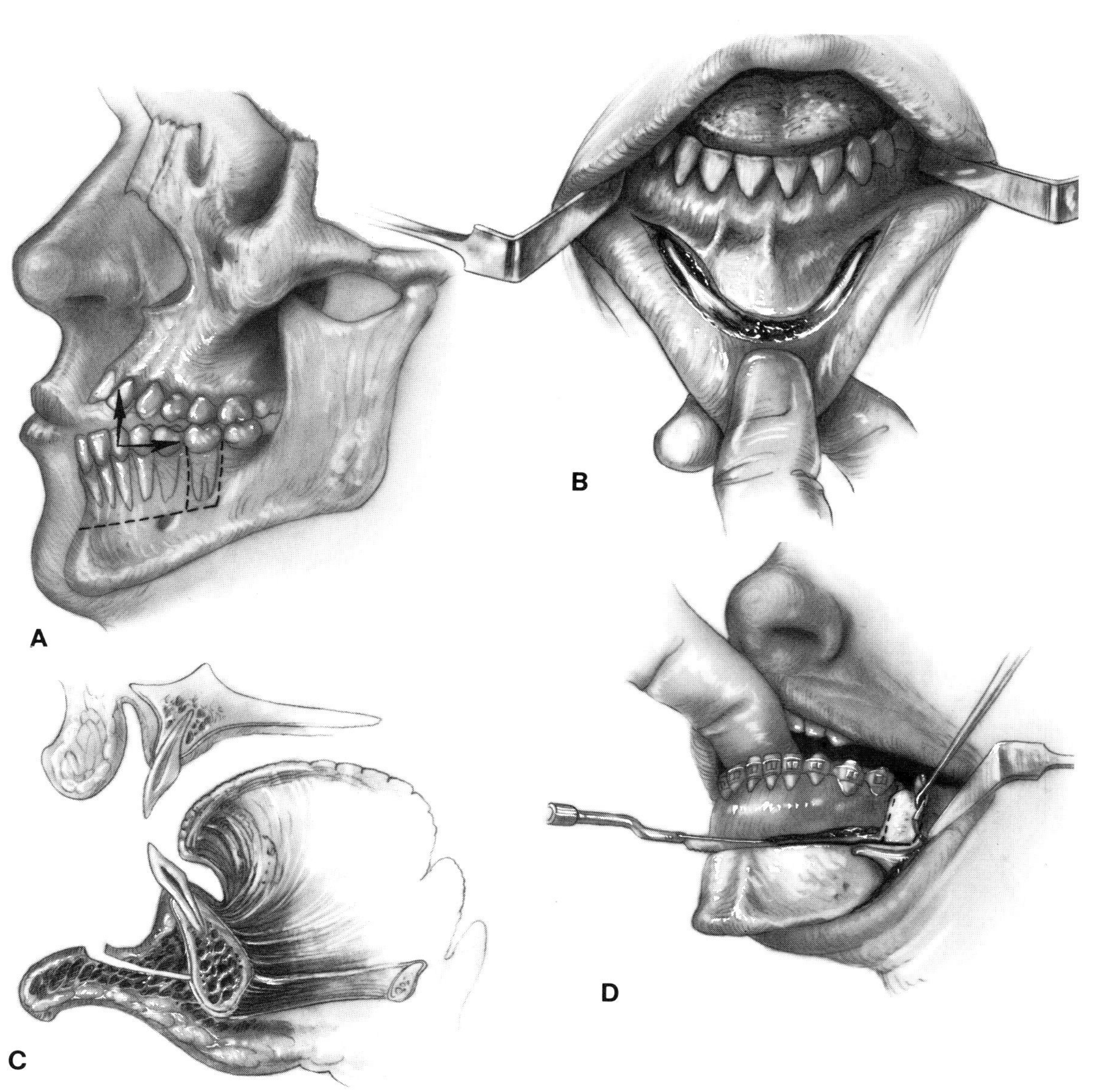

Figure 13–9. Correction of anterior open bite associated with mandibular prognathism by Köle modification of mandibular subapical osteotomy with extraction of 1st molar teeth. *A,* Dental, skeletal, and facial features associated with mandibular prognathism and anterior open bite with mandible in centric relation. Arrows indicate planned directional movements of mandibular dentoalveolar segment to close anterior open bite and achieve a satisfactory overjet. *B,* Soft-tissue incision for exposure of mandible. *C,* Incision through orbicularis oris and mentalis muscles. *D,* Subapical osteotomy accomplished with oscillating saw through degloving incision; vertical osteotomy made after margin of soft tissue flap is retracted posteriorly.

Illustration continued on the following page

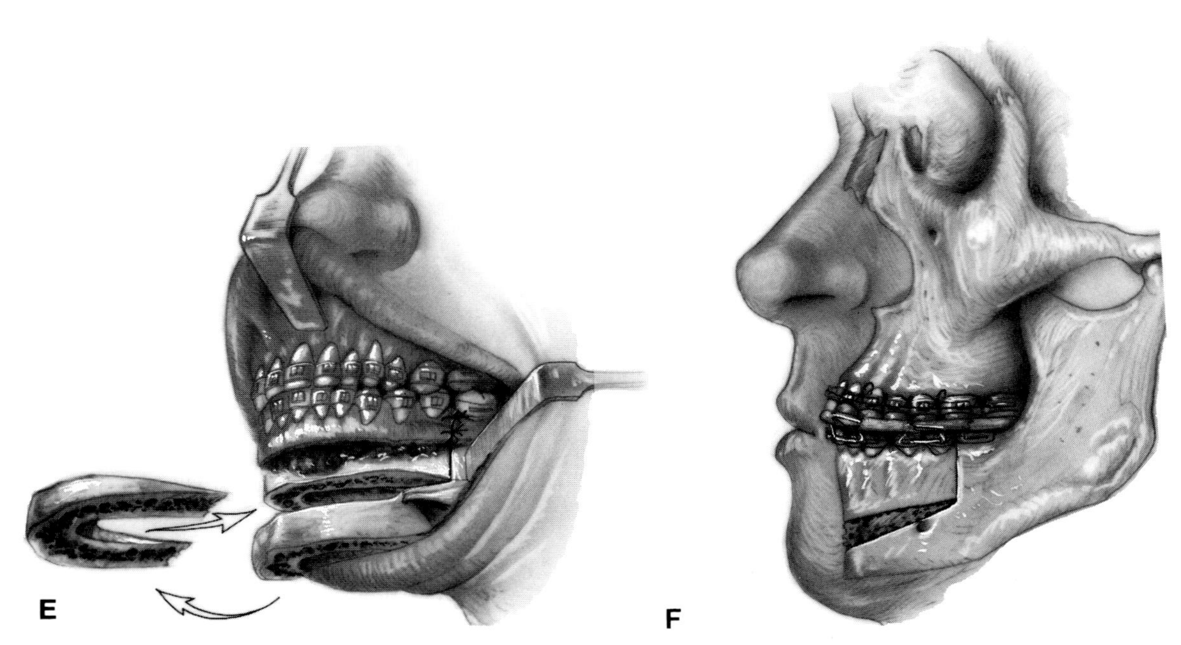

Figure 13–9 *Continued.* *E,* Excised bone is sculptured to proper dimensions and interposed into bony gap created by repositioning mandibular dentoalveolar segment to close anterior open bite and correct underjet. *F,* Anterior mandibular segment fixed with wire ligatures that extend between the interocclusal splint and the mandibular arch wire.

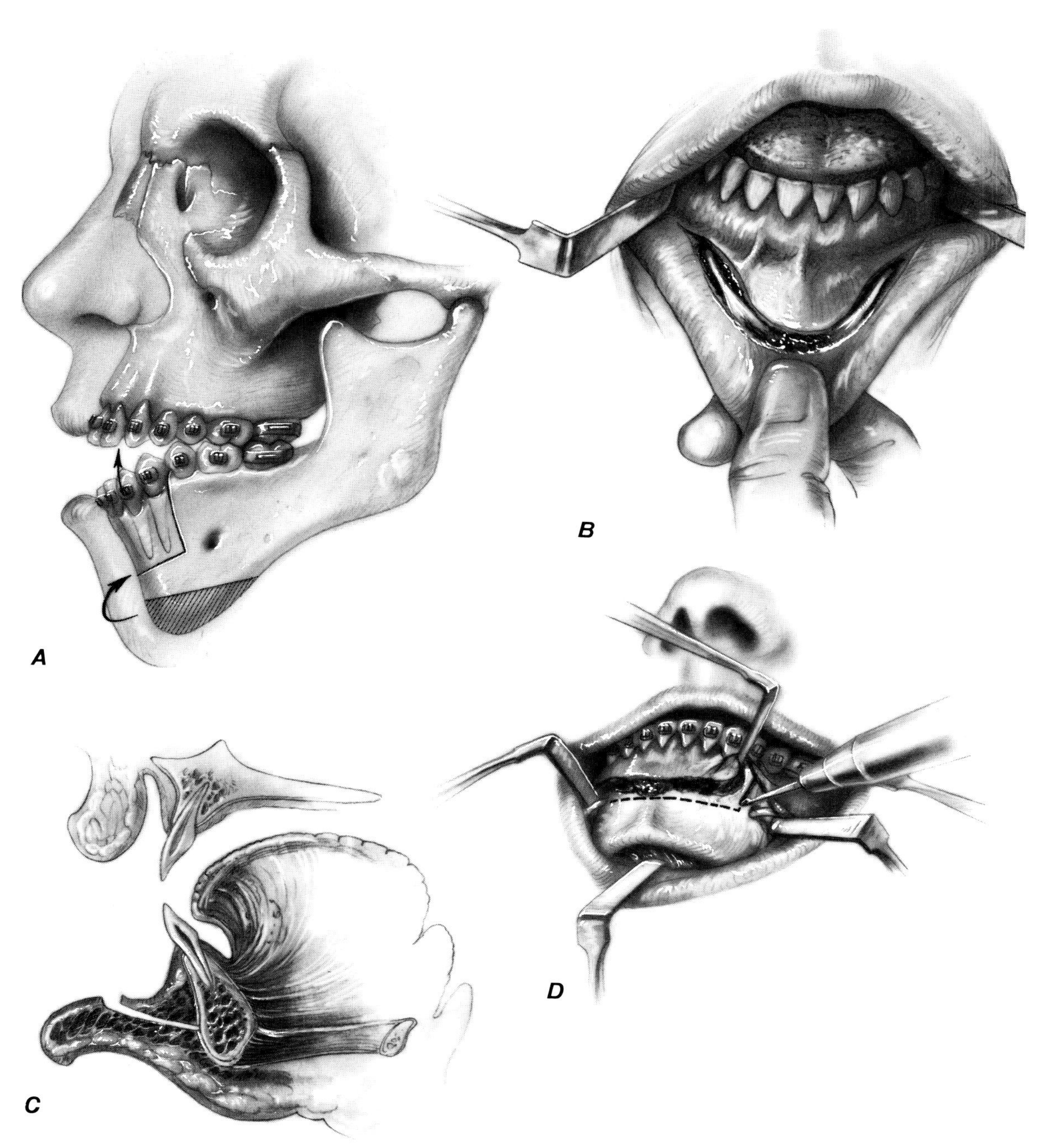

Figure 13–10. Correction of anterior open bite with excessive chin height by Köle modification of mandibular subapical osteotomy without extraction of teeth. *A,* Dental, skeletal, and facial features associated with open bite deformity with mandible in centric relation and lips relaxed. Arrows indicate planned directional movements of mandibular dentoalveolar segment to close anterior open bite and inferior portion of chin to fill bony gap created by closure of open bite. *B,* Soft-tissue incision for exposure of mandible. *C,* Incision through orbicularis oris muscle and mentalis muscles. *D,* With margin of mucobuccal flap raised with retractor, planned vertical and horizontal osteotomies are etched into bone with #701 fissure bur; inferior aspect of intended interdental osteotomy site is sectioned.

Illustration continued on the following page

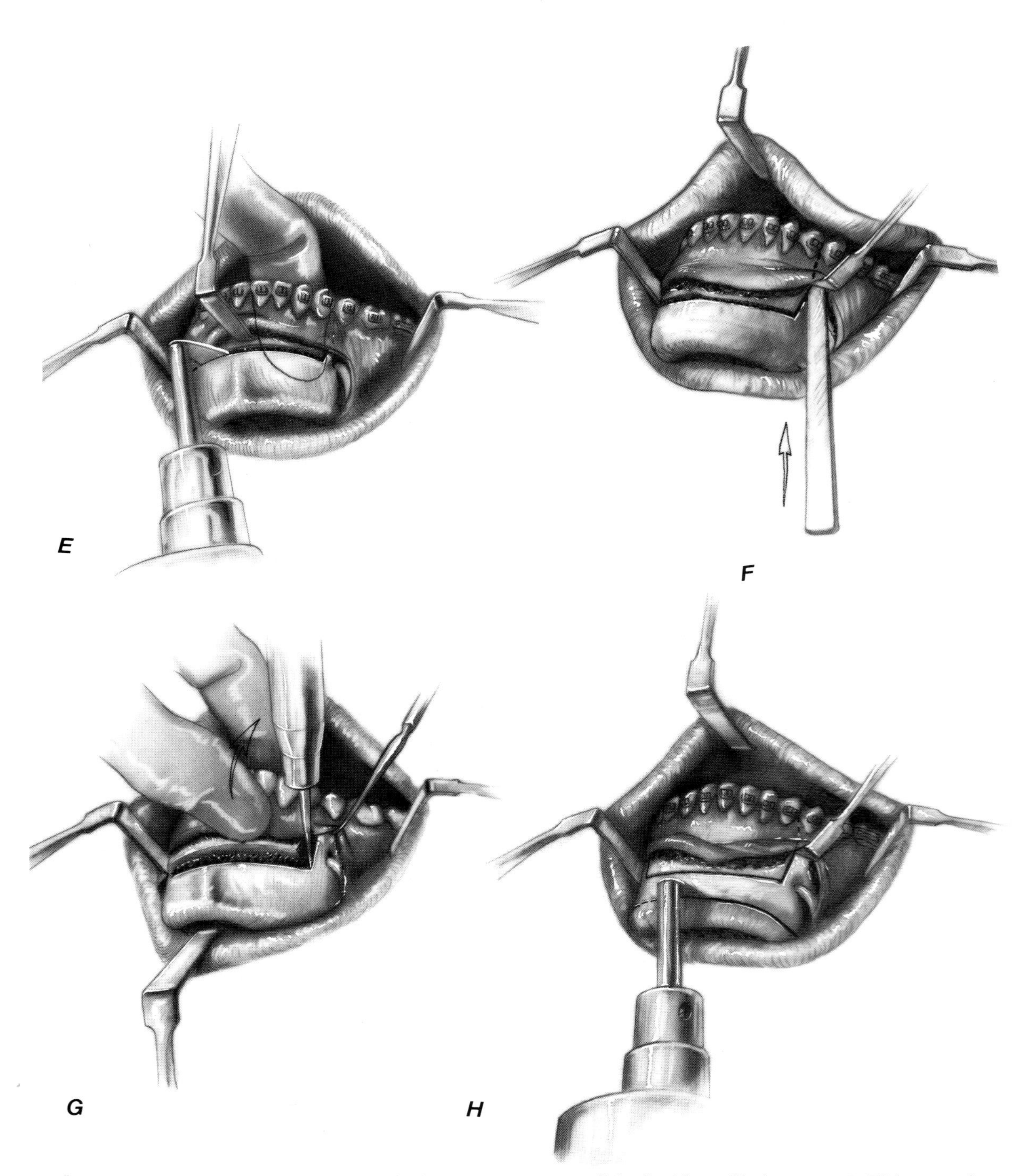

Figure 13–10 *Continued.* *E,* Subapical osteotomy accomplished with oscillating saw. *F,* Thin spatula osteotome is malleted into superior aspect of the interdental osteotomy site to facilitate fracturing of the interseptal and crestal alveolar bones. *G,* Mobilized segment tipped lingually to allow necessary bone sculpturing of inferior aspect of the mobilized segment at intersection of the horizontal and vertical bony cuts. *H,* Excision of inferior aspect of chin with oscillating saw blade.

Legend continued on the opposite page

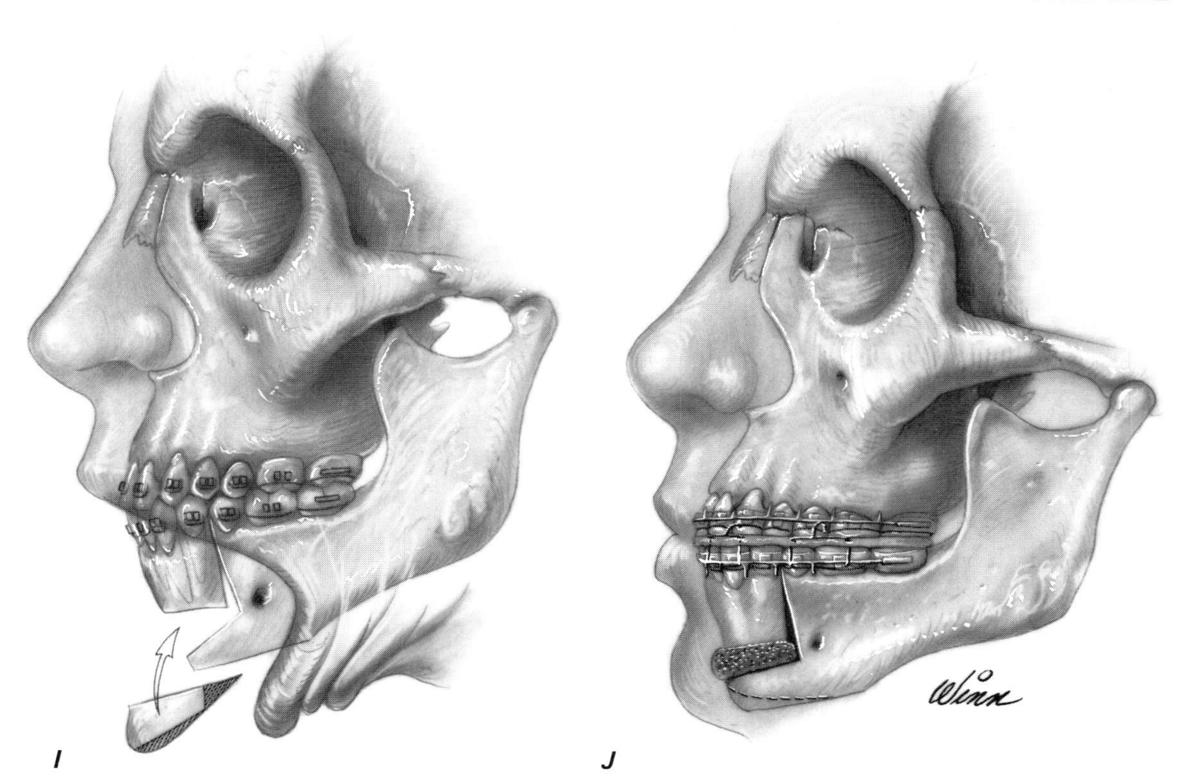

Figure 13–10 *Continued.* *I,* Excised bone is sculptured to proper dimensions to facilitate its placement into bony gap created by closure of open bite. *J,* Anterior mandibular segment fixed with wire ligatures that extend between the interocclusal splint and the mandibular arch wire.

tioned segment may be fixed with an arch wire or an acrylated arch bar without intermaxillary fixation.

Cephalometric prediction studies in concert with model surgery are essential for proper case analysis and will indicate the feasibility of closing the open bite in the premolar or molar extraction sites. A careful study of the positional changes of the horizontal and vertical reference lines drawn on the models before cuts are made will indicate the size of the bony defect created by raising the mandibular dentoalveolar segment, as well as its three-dimensional changes. These measurements are coordinated with similar measurements from cephalometric prediction studies. A paper template of the mandibular dentoalveolar segment to be repositioned is made and the planned movements for closing the open bite and extraction spaces are simulated. The bony gap produced by the positional change of the mandibular dentoalveolar segment should approximate the model study measurements.

The Köle procedure is feasible and indicated only when the distance between the apices of the mandibular anterior teeth and the inferior border of the symphysis is great. To operate when there is insufficient bone may invite pathologic fracture of the residual mandibular body. In patients considered for this surgical procedure, the chin height will usually exceed 50 mm; indeed, measurements in excess of 60 mm are not uncommon. The clinical parameters used to determine the amount of chin augmentation and chin height reduction are discussed in Chapter 14, Chin Surgery. The principal disadvantage of this procedure relates to the unpredictable soft-tissue profile and chin-height changes when virtually all the soft tissues are detached from the mental symphysis region as bone is excised from the chin. A well-placed pressure dressing maintained in place for approximately 7 days maximizes the soft-tissue change. In selected cases, cephalometric prediction studies may indicate that a more predictable and cosmetic result can be achieved when genioplasty is accomplished as a secondary procedure.

SURGICAL TECHNIQUE OF KÖLE MODIFICATIONS OF MANDIBULAR SUBAPICAL OSTEOTOMY (Figs. 13–9 and 13–10)

The surgery is accomplished under general nasoendotracheal anesthesia. Local anesthesia with vasoconstrictor is infiltrated into the planned soft-tissue incision lines for hemostasis. The surgical technique is very similar to the previous procedure for anterior mandibular subapical osteotomy described in Chapter 10. A horseshoe-shaped circumvestibular incision is made in the buccal and labial vestibule in the unattached mucosa terminating at least 1 cm posterior to the planned vertical osteotomy or ostectomy site. Anteriorly, the incision is made through the lower lip mucosa above the labial frenum midway between the depth of the labial vestibule and vermilion border of the lower lip. In the anterior region, the incision is carried sharply through the orbicularis oris muscle. The dissection is directed obliquely posteriorly and inferiorly through the mentalis muscle until contact is made with the mental symphysis 5 to 10 mm below the apices of the mandibular incisor teeth.

The anteroinferior tissue flap is retracted inferiorly to "deglove" the mental symphysis region completely. The mentalis muscle and submucosa are sharply incised posteriorly to an area opposite and above the apices of the canine teeth. The branches of the mental nerve which exist from the mental foramen are identified by subperiosteal tunneling beneath the anterior margins of the incised tissue. After the foramen has been located, the mental nerves are identified and carefully isolated by blunt dissection with mosquito hemostats through the margins of the vestibular incision. After the main branches of the nerve are identified and retracted inferiorly, an incision is made through the submucosal tissue above the nerve down to the underlying bone. The incisions may be extended posteriorly as far as necessary to accomplish the planned vertical osteotomies or ostectomies. After the mental symphysis from the mental foramen of one side to the contralateral mental foramen has been "degloved," the lateral part of the body of the mandible posterior to the foramen is similarly exposed. The mental symphysis, the inferior portion of the chin, and the lateral aspect of the mandible can be then clearly visualized.

From this point on, the mental nerves must be carefully retracted and protected as the vertical and subapical bone incisions are accomplished. Because the mental foramina are generally located inferior to the second premolar teeth in patients with the skeletal type of open bite, the horizontal and vertical osteotomies can be made with minimal danger to the contiguous teeth or nerves. The mandibular dentoalveolar segment is raised the amount necessary to level the mandibular arch and close the open bite as determined before surgery from cephalometric prediction studies and model surgery.

The desired horizontal osteotomy and vertical ostectomy sites are next etched into the mandible with a No. 701 fissure bur. The vertical bone etchings are made parallel to the long axis of the teeth to be extracted and carried to a point 3 to 5 mm inferior to their apices. The inferior ends of the two vertical marks are connected across the midline at least 3 to 5 mm below the nearest root apices. After the indicated extractions are accomplished, measured vertical segments of bone are excised with an oscillating saw blade or a fissure bur in a straight handpiece approximately 3 to 5 mm below the premolar and canine teeth. The index finger is positioned on the lingual mucosa to protect the tissue and feel the bur or saw blade as it transects the lingual cortex. A periosteal elevator may also be placed to preserve the lingual mucoperiosteum of the lingual cortical plate as the planned osteotomy is accomplished with a fissure bur.

The vertical bone incisions are connected by a horizontal bone incision accomplished for the most part with an oscillating saw blade, with the surgeon's index finger positioned on the lingual mucosa to feel the saw blade as it transects the lingual cortical plate. A fine, tapered osteotome is placed in the vertical and horizontal bone incisions to determine when the bone has been completely sectioned. When this is discernible, the dentoalveolar segment is mobilized by light digital pressure.

The lingual horizontal and vertical bony interfaces and the corner formed by the intersection of the horizontal and vertical bone cuts are the problematic sites which most frequently restrict moving the segment into the planned relationship. To facilitate the planned movements, the mobilized fragment is carefully tipped lingually to expose its inferior aspect. With a periosteal elevator positioned on the superior and lingual aspect of the mental symphysis segment, additional bone sculpturing is accomplished with a fissure bur to facilitate the desired anteroposterior and vertical movements. Similar manipulations are accomplished in the vertical ostectomy sites. The surgeon must be constantly vigilant to preserve the lingual mucosal pedicle to the mobilized segment.

Despite the fact that it may not be used after surgery, an interocclusal wafer splint is a necessary adjunct for keying the segment into the desired position and sculpturing the margins of the osteotomized segments. The mobilized dento-osseous segment is keyed into the desired occlusal relationship by ligating the interocclusal splint to the lower arch wire or arch bar. A horseshoe-shaped segment of bone is next excised from the inferior mental symphysis with an oscillating saw. The amount of height reduction is based on the preoperative cephalometric prediction studies. After appropriate scuplturing, the excised segment is mortised into the osseous gap created by raising the mandibular dentoalveolar segment. Depending on the results of the preoperative prediction studies, the chin may also be augmented in its anteroposterior dimension. The residual bone fragments may be used in conjunction with Proplast for additional augmentation of the anterior and/or lateral aspects of the chin.

A sequential closure of the dissected tissue planes is made using interrupted 3–0 plain catgut sutures for the mucosal incision. After the skin has been sprayed with tincture of benzoin, strips of elastic bandage (Elastoplast) are placed over the labiomental fold and below the chin to fix the raised soft tissues in position. This pressure dressing is secured with adhesive tape and maintained in place for 5 to 7 days.

MANDIBULAR BODY V, Y, OR SAGITTAL SPLIT OSTEOTOMY

Mandibular prognathism with concomitant anterior open bite is the principal indication for V, Y, or rectangular ostectomies, which are accomplished in a single stage through intraoral degloving incisions (Figs. 13–11, 13–12, and 13–13). The surgical techniques for body ostectomy are described and illustrated in detail in Chapter 11. The presence of a functional posterior occlusion in association with edentulous spaces also justifies use of the V body ostectomy if prognathism is associated with anterior open bite. Clinical and

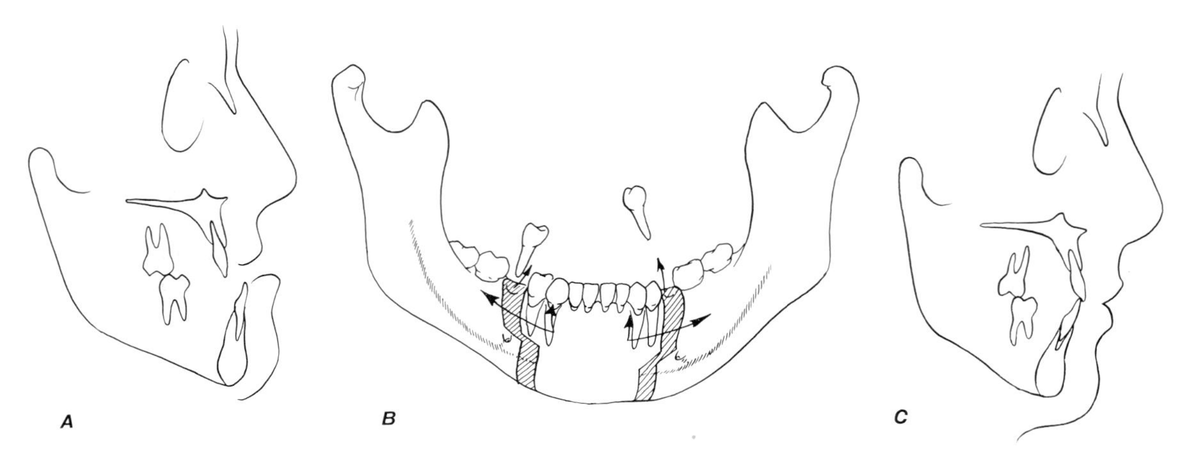

Figure 13–11. Mandibular body "step" ostectomy. *A,* Mandibular prognathism associated with anterior open bite; planned ostectomy in 2nd premolar region. *B,* Mandibular body "step" ostectomy to circumvent inferior alveolar nerve. Arrow indicates directional movement of anterior portion of mandible. *C,* Postoperative view.

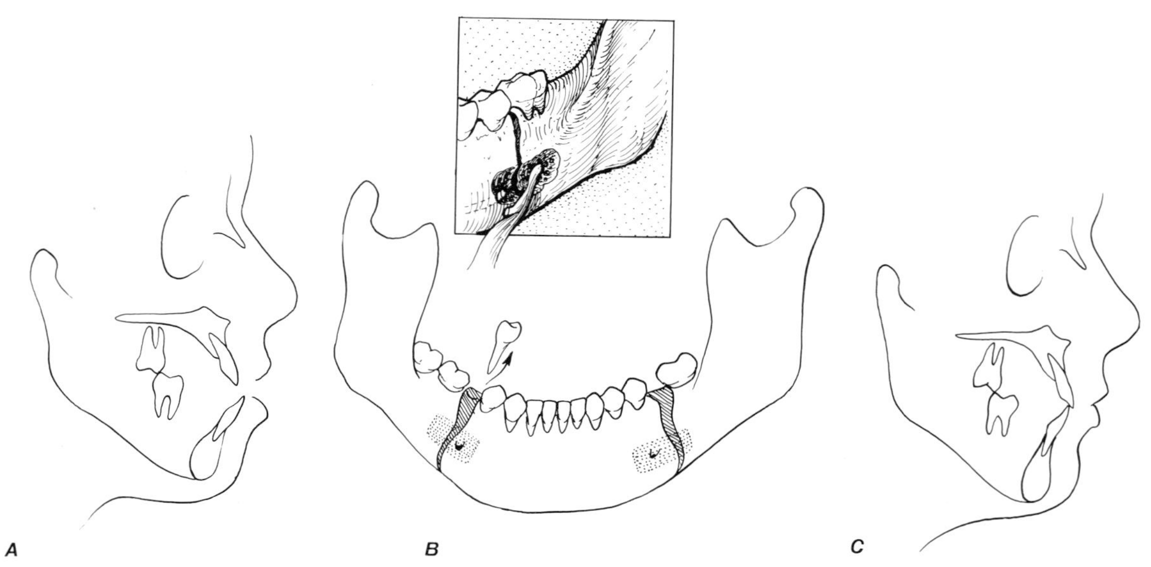

Figure 13–12. Mandibular body "V" ostectomy. *A,* Mandibular prognathism associated with anterior open bite. *B,* Mandibular body "V" ostectomy in 2nd premolar region; preservation of inferior alveolar nerve. *C,* Postoperative view.

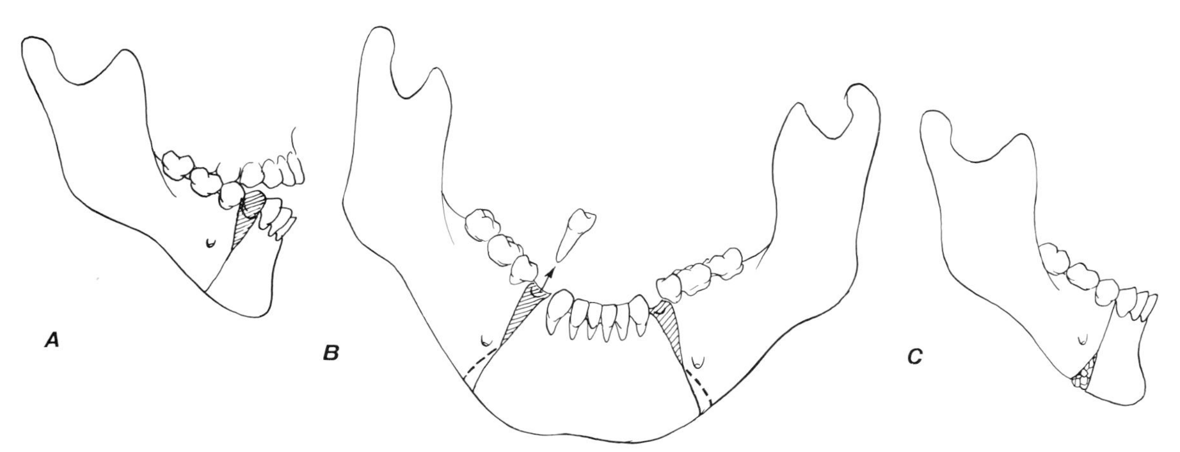

Figure 13–13. Mandibular body "Y" ostectomy. *A*, Mandibular prognathism associated with anterior open bite and reverse curvature of mandibular arch. *B*, Mandibular body "Y" ostectomy. *C*, Postoperative view.

cephalometric studies of candidates for the V body ostectomy will typically reveal a reverse curve in the mandible associated with open bite and a high mandibular plane angle. Some forward tipping of the mandibular anterior teeth by orthodontic forces may be necessary to improve the position of the lower anterior teeth with respect to their supporting basal bone. No attempt, however, is made to completely level a severe reverse curve in the mandibular arch by orthodontic treatment — such movement is accomplished by the body ostectomy or subapical osteotomy. When severe mandibular prognathism is associated with skeletal anterior open bite, surgical adjustment of the maxillary and the mandibular ramus may indeed be necessary to achieve occlusal balance and stability.

Despite the fact that mandibular ostectomy reduces the volume of the oral cavity and the mandibular arch length, postoperative studies have demonstrated stability with this procedure.[27] This stability has been attributed to the fact that the line of the ostectomies is anterior to the muscles of mastication. The influence of the masseter, temporalis, and internal pterygoid muscles is thereby obviated. If superior or anterior movement of the mobilized segment is great, however, or if there is evidence of restricted movement at the time of surgery because of attached muscles, geniohyoid and digastric myotomy are accomplished simultaneously with the body ostectomy through the degloving exposure.

The mandibular body Y ostectomy adds facility in treating patients with severe anterior open bite in whom the dysplasia manifests as a reverse curve in the mandibular arch. Model surgery and cephalometric prediction studies using templates to determine the resultant interface of repositioned bone segments are essential to determine the feasibility of the procedure and the need for bone grafting osseous defects at the inferior border of the mandible. The indications for the two procedures depend on a careful analysis of the individual case.

Model surgery may indicate that leveling a severe reverse curve of the mandibular occlusal plane by body osteotomy or ostectomy will produce contact of the anterior teeth but disocclusion of the premolars. In such cases, it is inadvisable to level the mandibular arch by presurgical orthodontics — this can be achieved more readily and predictably by postsurgical orthodontic extrusion of the premolars.

When anterior open bite is associated with interdental spacing between proclined maxillary or mandibular anterior teeth, the spaces are closed orthodontically before surgery to facilitate closure of the open bite and achievement of a satisfactory overbite and overjet.

SAGITTAL SPLITTING OF THE BODY OF THE MANDIBLE FOR CORRECTION OF ANTERIOR OPEN BITE (Fig. 13–14)

When feasibility studies indicate that surgery in the mandibular body would create a large osseous gap at the inferior border of the mandible, the body of the mandible may be split sagittally to correct the open bite.[13, 32] This technique preserves the integrity of the inferior aspect of the mandibular body and alveolar crest and obviates the need for bone grafting and the precise type of model surgery that is needed with conventional body osteotomies. Because the incisions are anterior to the muscles of mastication, stability is the rule. Additionally, the excellent interface of bone promotes early consolidation of the proximal and distal segments.

The surgery is easily accomplished intraorally in a single stage by any surgeon experienced with the sagittal split ramus osteotomy technique. The margins of the horizontal buccal vestibular incision are raised and retracted superiorly opposite the planned buccal osteotomy site; a lingual envelope flap is raised concomitantly to facilitate the necessary lingual bone incisions (Fig. 13–14).

Lingual and buccal vertical bone incisions are made to the area just inferior to the apices of the teeth. When the ostectomy is to be made in a residual molar extraction site or an edentulous area, the buccal bone incision is made somewhat *distal* to the lingual bone cut (Fig. 13–14*A* and *B*). Placing the buccal and lingual osteotomies at different levels allows overlapping of the proximal and distal segments. However, when body osteotomy between two closely spaced teeth without extraction of either of the contiguous teeth is planned, the superior portion of the vertical bone cuts is made at the same anteroposterior level and extended to a point some 3 to 4 mm below the level of the root apices; at this point, the two lines of osteotomy diverge (Fig. 13–14*C* and *D*). On the lingual side the bone incision is extended inferiorly to the inferior border of the mandible; the buccal bone cut, however, is directed obliquely to a point above the preangular notch where it is angled inferiorly to the inferior border of the mandible.

The sagittal bone incision is started by drilling into the vertical aspect of the crestal alveolar bone. Splitting of the mandible is accomplished by malletting a thin, tapered osteotome into the osteotomy sites. The osteotome is maintained in close proximity to the lingual aspect of the buccal cortex, so that the splitting is accomplished without damaging the inferior alveolar neurovascular bundle. The use of an interocclusal splint in combination with intermaxillary fixation usually obviates the need for direct wiring of the proximal and distal segments.

Posterior Maxillary Osteotomy

The skeletal type of anterior open bite is typically associated with a high and constricted palatal vault, excessive curvature of the maxillary occlusal plane, lip incompe-

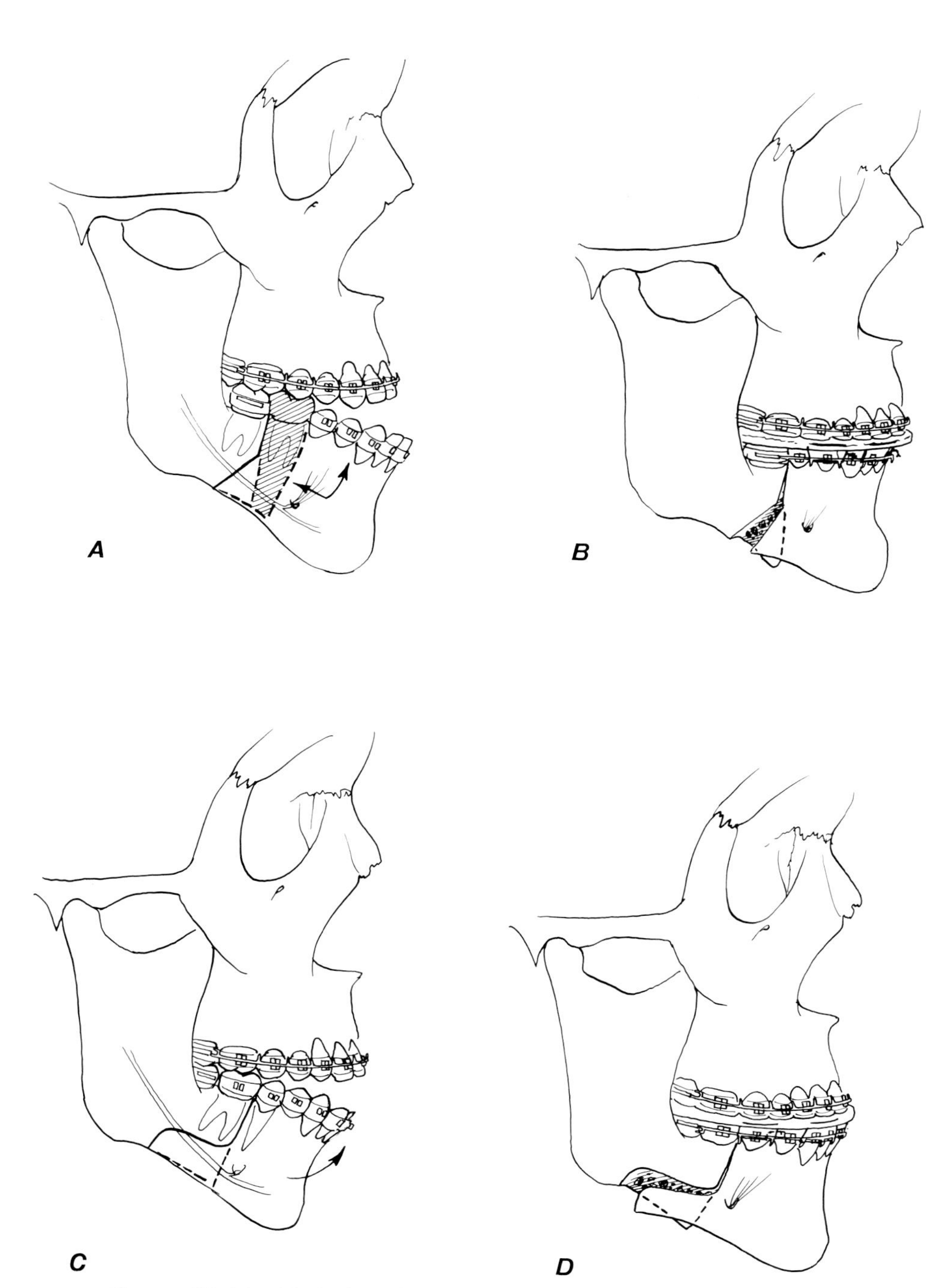

Figure 13–14. Technique for mandibular body sagittal split osteotomy. *A,* Mandibular body sagittal split osteotomy combined with ostectomy in 1st molar region. Solid line indicates buccal osteotomy; broken lines indicate lingual osteotomies. *B,* Postoperative view. *C* and *D,* Mandibular body sagittal split osteotomy without extraction of tooth. Solid line indicates buccal osteotomy; broken line indicates lingual osteotomy. *D,* Postoperative view.

tence, a high mandibular plane angle, and a long distance between the palatal root apices and the nasal floor. Although any one of three techniques of posterior maxillary osteotomy may be used to close the anterior open bite, the downfracture single-stage method of Kufner provides certain advantages when the dominant objective is to superiorly reposition the posterior maxilla.[26] This technique provides direct access to the superior aspect of the posterior maxilla to decrease the height of the posterior maxilla, close the open bite, and simultaneously advance, retract, narrow, or expand the posterior maxillary dentoalveolar segment. The three basic surgical techniques for repositioning the posterior portion of the maxilla and the criteria for the use of each method are described in Chapter 8, Maxillary Excess.

Surgical repositioning of the posterior portion of the maxilla alone to close an anterior open bite is indicated only when there is good anteroposterior, horizontal, and vertical balance between the maxillary anterior teeth, the upper lip, and the nose. Cephalometric and model surgery studies must indicate that a satisfactory overbite-overjet relationship can be achieved by posterior maxillary surgery combined with orthodontics and/or restorative procedures. When and if these studies indicate that closure of the open bite by posterior maxillary osteotomy is feasible, stable occlusal results can be achieved if the surgery is properly planned and executed.

Posterior maxillary osteotomy techniques are described and illustrated in this chapter as though they were being used to treat isolated clinical manifestations of posterior maxillary excess with anterior open bite. Such "pure" deformities, however, are relatively uncommon in clinical practice. The dysplasia will most frequently be manifest in the vertical, transverse, and anteroposterior planes of space.

LE FORT I OSTEOTOMY FOR CORRECTION OF ANTERIOR OPEN BITE (Figs. 13–15 and 13–16)

Contemporary surgical planning is concerned with designing an operation to meet the individual's functional and esthetic needs. Initially, this is a difficult concept for the clinician to accept because he has "grown up with" and practiced the old philosophy of adapting a "stock" surgical technique to an individual's problem. As a result, compromise was very common. When, however, the surgeon begins to plan treatment to achieve occlusal and facial harmony in all three planes of space, he or she will most frequently program surgery to reposition the anterior and posterior portions of the maxilla. Technically, the downfracture Le Fort I osteotomy technique, which is particularly useful when interdental osteotomies are indicated to level the maxillary occlusal plane and widen the maxillary arch, is less problematic, more versatile, and easier to execute than isolated anterior or posterior maxillary osteotomies.[4, 9] Presently, between 65 and 70 per cent of all dentofacial deformities treated at our institution are corrected by this operation, combined with adjunctive procedures. Approximately 90 per cent of patients with skeletal type open bite deformities are treated similarly.

The magnitude and direction of surgical movement of the maxilla to close an anterior open bite by total maxillary osteotomy is determined from a coordinated study of the patient utilizing lateral cephalometric tracings and model analysis. The biologic and surgical principles, diagnostic parameters, feasibility studies, and basic surgical technique are fully discussed and illustrated in Chapter 8, Maxillary Excess. It is suggested that the reader review Chapter 8 before undertaking the use of the downfracture Le Fort I osteotomy for correction of a skeletal type anterior open bite dentofacial deformity.

Special Considerations

A radiograph that delineates both soft and hard tissues is made with the mandible in centric relation and the lips in repose. The maxilla is moved superiorly the amount necessary to achieve 2 to 3 mm of maxillary incisor exposure with the upper lip at rest.[5] This may differ somewhat from the procedure used to treat vertical maxillary excess without open bite. The magnitude of superior movement of the posterior portion of the maxilla will usually be greater than the amount of superior movement of the anterior portion of the maxilla. This is necessary to level the maxillary occlusal plane and correct the anterior open bite. Consequently, there will be proportionally more autorotational movement of the mandible in the individual with skeletal type open bite than in the individual with vertical maxillary excess without open bite.

Closure of the Open Bite

A treatment plan for closing the open bite and leveling the maxillary occlusal plane must be programmed before orthodontic treatment is initiated. The selection of sites for the interdental osteotomy or ostectomy and the transverse palatal bone incision is based upon the location of the anterior open bite. Usually these procedures are accomplished in the first premolar–canine or canine–lateral incisor interdental spaces. The key to success with these procedures is to plan the appropriate interdental bone cuts before orthodontic treatment commences. When this is done, adequate space in the planned interdental osteotomy site can be maintained by orthodontic mechanics. It is not necessary for the orthodontist to level the arch, since this can be accomplished surgically. When extraction of premolars is indicated to facilitate arch alignment, the extraction spaces are not completely closed orthodontically; this allows more space for the surgical cuts. When the maxillary occlusal plane is to be leveled surgically, the planned interdental osteotomies are easily executed with the maxilla in the downfractured position.

The same basic surgical procedure is used routinely to correct anteroposterior, vertical, and horizontal manifestations of the open bite deformity. The downfractured maxilla, pedicled to the relatively inelastic palatal mucosa, can be widened between 6 and 10 mm. A horseshoe-shaped palatal bone incision facilitates lateral movement of the maxilla. When lateral expansion of the maxilla is more than 8 to 10 mm, the amount of movement may exceed the physiologic limits of the technique. In such cases, it is wise to program rapid maxillary expansion in coordination with lateral maxillary osteotomies to widen the maxilla the desired amount prior to the definitive surgical procedure. This treatment approach may also obviate the need for extractions by increasing the arch length to facilitate alignment of crowded and rotated anterior teeth. When premolars are extracted in an individual with minimal anterior open bite, the maxillary occlusal plane may be leveled by orthodontic closure of premolar extraction spaces. This, however, is not the general rule — correction of excessive curvature in the maxillary occlusal plane is accomplished by surgery.

No special effort is made to simplify surgery and correct the anterior open bite by one-piece Le Fort I osteotomy. Achieving such treatment by excessive extrusion of teeth increases the possibility of relapse and prolongs the treatment time unnecessarily. In addition, it may not be possible to maintain the desired axial inclination of the maxillary anterior teeth at the time of the definitive surgical procedure without segmentalizing the maxilla.

Text continued on page 1111

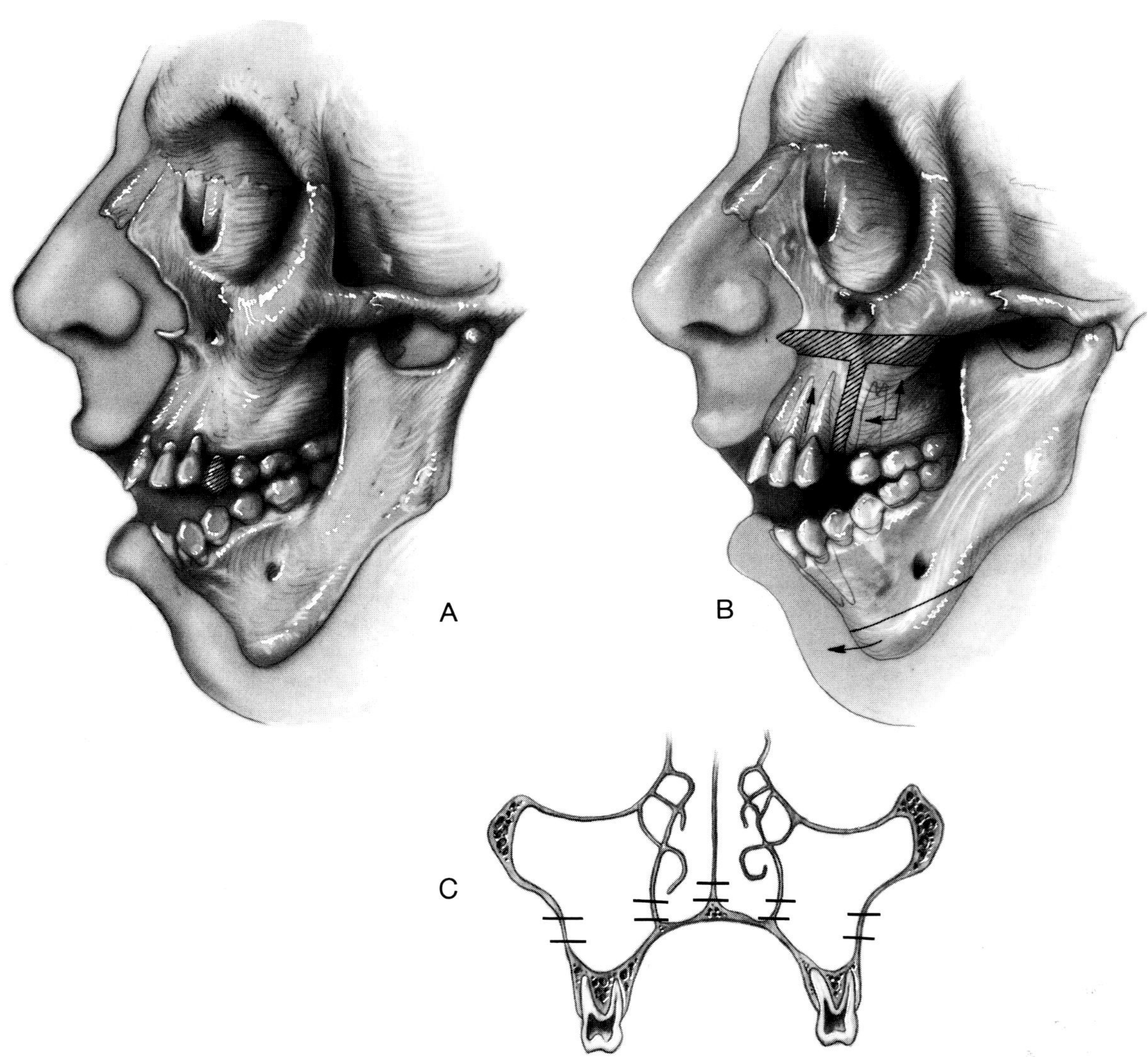

Figure 13–15. Surgical technique for correction of open bite deformity by segmentalized Le Fort I ostectomy through residual premolar extraction spaces. *A,* Typical features of open bite deformity with mandible in centric relation and lips relaxed. *B,* Premolar teeth have been extracted; extraction spaces are closed only the amount necessary to align anterior teeth. Cross-hatched areas indicate planned horizontal and vertical ostectomy sites. Arrows indicate directional movements of anterior and posterior maxillary segments and chin. *C,* Cross-sectional view of molar region showing planned lines of sectioning through lateral maxillary and nasal walls and nasal septum.

Legend continued on the opposite page

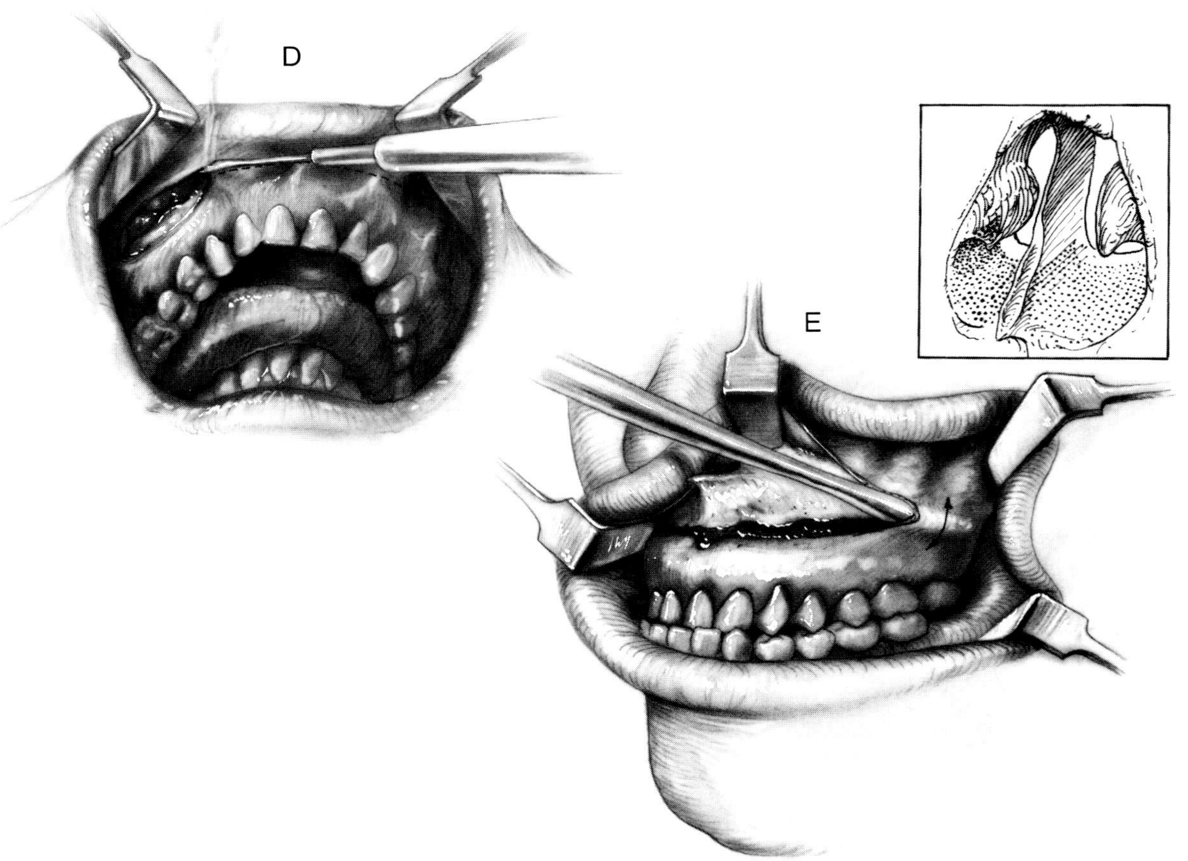

Figure 13–15 *Continued.* *D,* An electrosurgical cutting blade is used to make a horizontal incision in the maxillary vestibule above the mucogingival junction that extends from the 2nd molar region of one side to a similar area on the contralateral side. *E,* The margins of the superior flap are raised to expose the lateral walls of the maxilla, the zygomatic crests, the anterior nasal floor, the piriform aperture, and the pterygomaxillary junction. To assure maximum circulation to the maxillary bone and teeth, the inferior mucoperiosteal tissues are elevated just enough to visualize and palpate the bone encasing the apices of the teeth or to facilitate interdental osteotomies, the piriform aperture, and the pterygomaxillary junction. A right-angle retractor is placed anteriorly to facilitate visualization of the anterolateral portion of the maxilla. A curved Freer elevator is used to detach the mucoperiosteum from the nasal floor, the base of the nasal septum, and the lateral nasal walls superiorly to the base of the inferior turbinate. (Stippled areas of insert indicate areas of detached mucoperiosteum.) Since the anteroinferior margin of the piriform rim is usually elevated above the nasal floor, care must be taken to remain in a subperiosteal plane by dissecting inferiorly and posteriorly from the inferior piriform rim. The dissection is carried to the posterior aspect of the hard palate, onto the base of the nasal septum approximately 5 mm above the nasal floor, and then to the base of the inferior turbinate on the lateral nasal wall. The posterolateral portion of the maxilla is visualized by tunneling subperiosteally to the pterygomaxillary suture and then carefully positioning the tip of a curved right-angle retractor at the suture.

Illustration continued on the following page

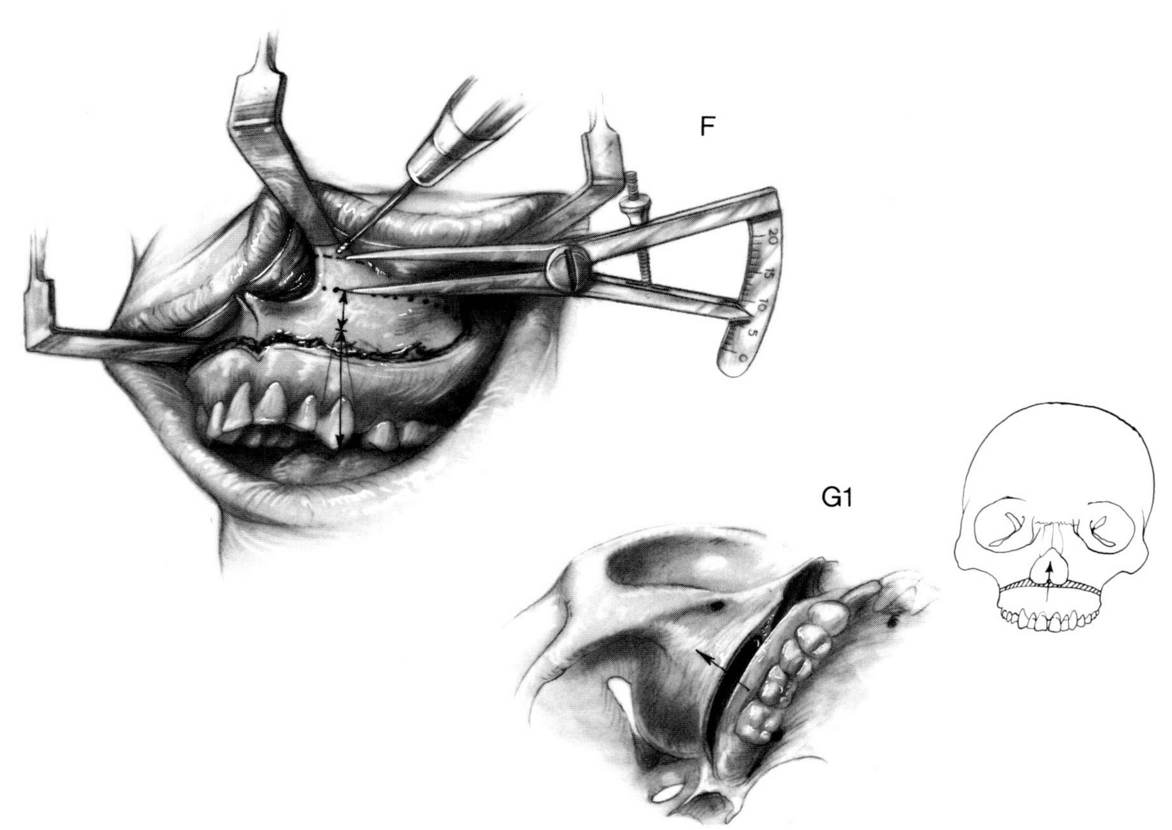

Figure 13–15 *Continued.* *F,* Anterior and posterior vertical reference lines are etched into the lateral maxilla. The inferior bone cut is positioned at a safe level above the apex of the maxillary canine tooth (small arrow), which can usually be visualized with minimal retraction of the inferior mucosal wound margins. A fissure bur is used to connect a series of holes drilled through lateral maxilla at the desired level for the superior osteotomy. The vertical distance between the inferior and the superior osteotomies is measured with a millimeter caliper. The planned superior osteotomy is then etched into the lateral maxilla at the desired level with a fissure bur. *G,* Effect of varying the position of lateral maxillary osteotomies on the stability of the superiorly repositioned maxilla. *1,* When osteotomies are made in the inferior aspect of lateral maxilla, where bony wall is vertically oriented, the margins of the proximal and distal segments are juxtaposed.

Legend continued on the opposite page

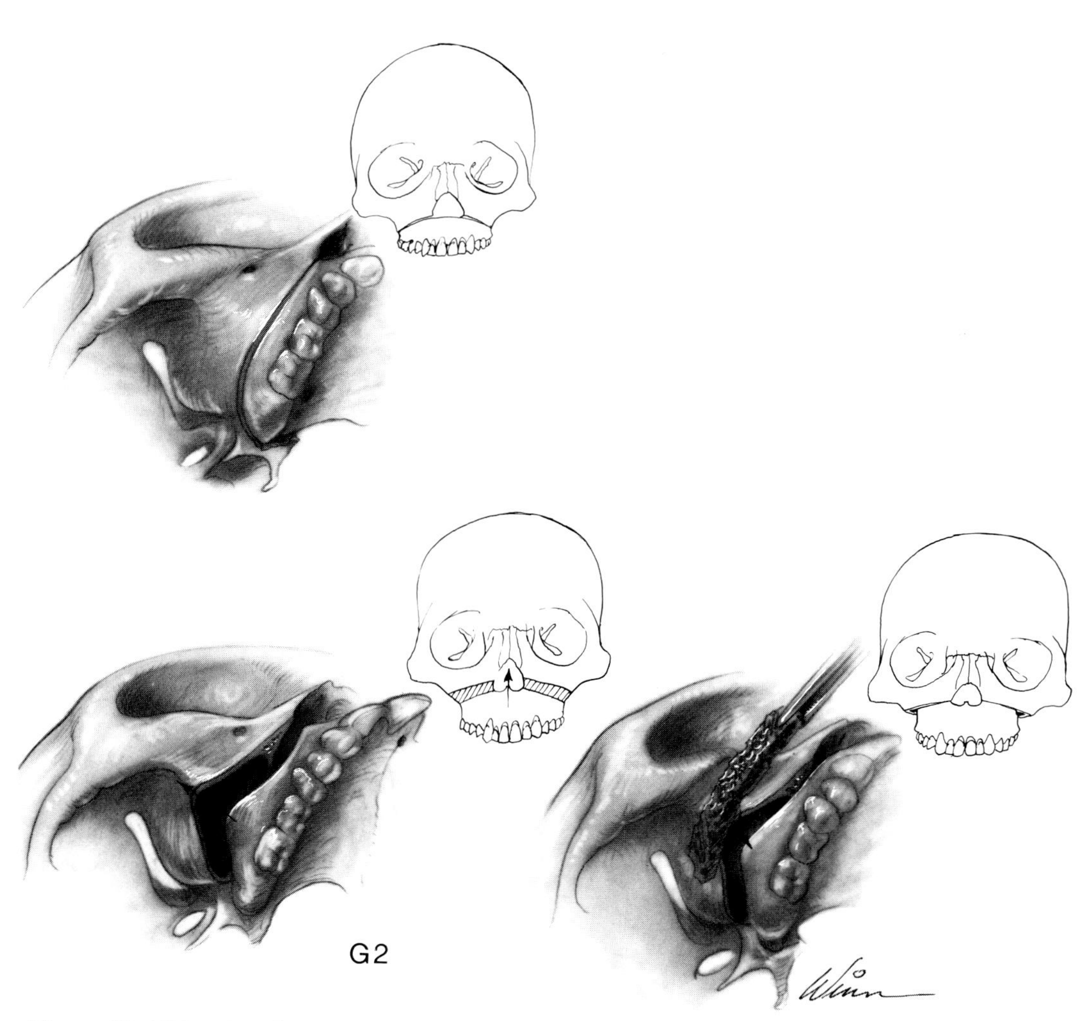

Figure 13–15 *Continued.* *G, 2,* When osteotomies are made in the superior aspect of the lateral maxilla, where bony walls are angular, the margins of the proximal and distal segments are not juxtaposed, allowing telescoping of the posterior maxilla into the maxillary antra and possible osseous instability and difficulty in stabilizing the repositioned maxilla by interosseous fixation. Improved stability of the repositioned maxilla can be achieved by interpositional autogenous cancellous bone grafts and suspension wires.

Illustration continued on the following page

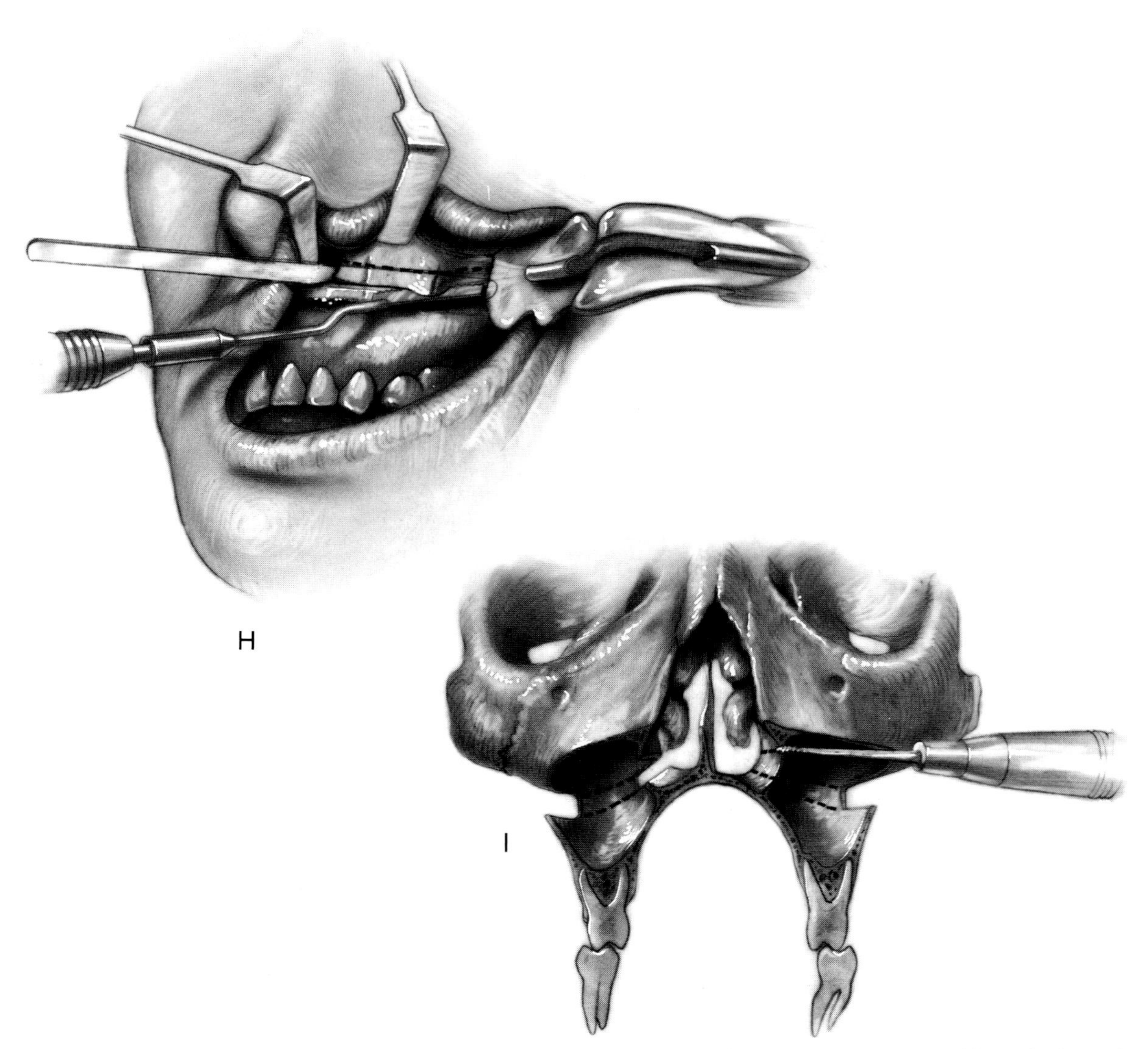

Figure 13–15 *Continued.* *H,* Anterior and posterior vertical reference lines are etched into the lateral maxilla. With a malleable retractor in place to protect the nasal mucoperiosteum, a horizontal section of bone is excised from the lateral maxilla from the piriform rim posteriorly to the pterygomaxillary fissure. Anteriorly, the horizontal bone incisions are carried through the lateral and medial aspects of the maxilla. *I,* The lateral nasal wall is sectioned above the nasal floor by directing a drill through the ostectomy site in the lateral maxilla.

Legend continued on the opposite page

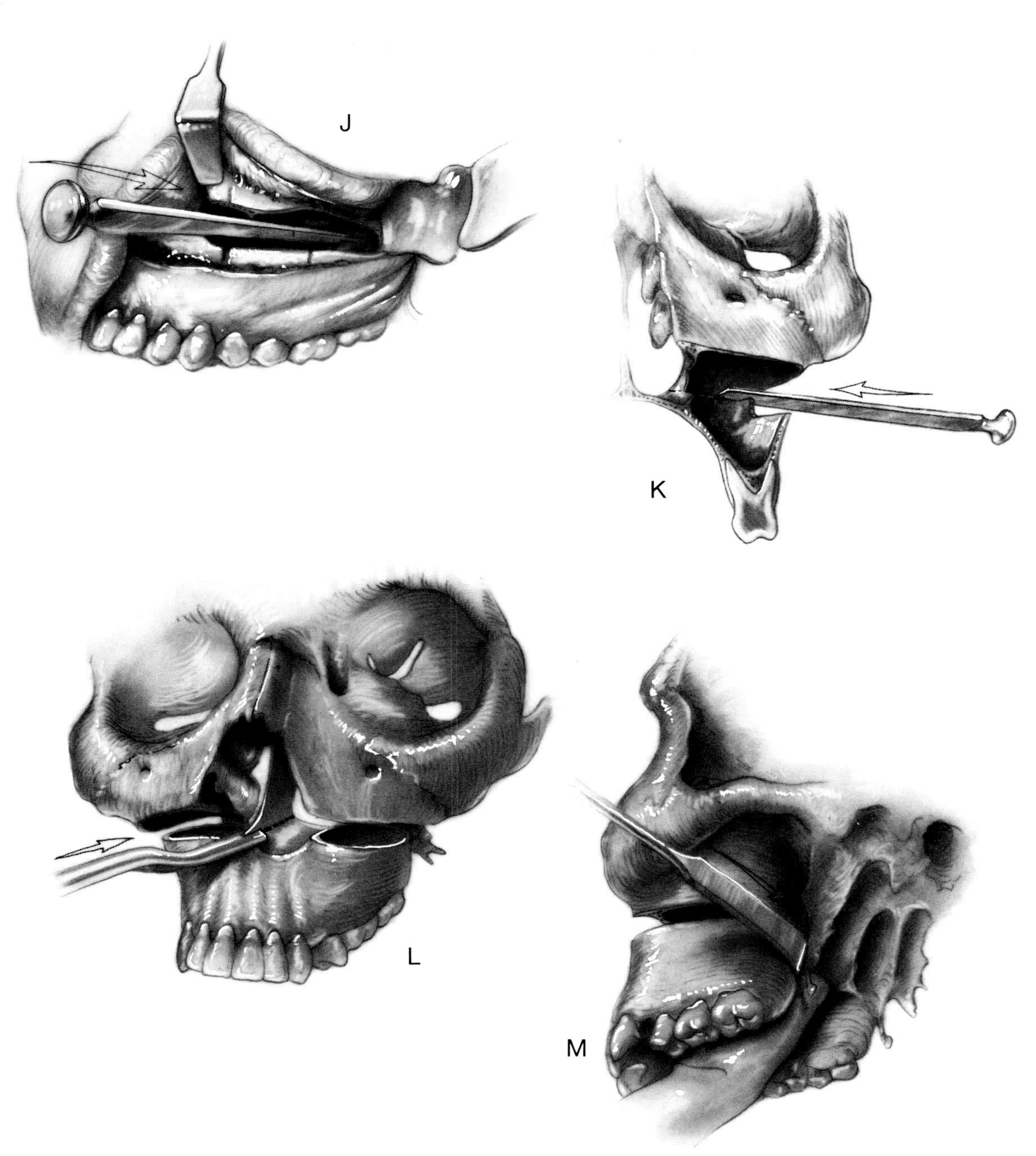

Figure 13–15 *Continued.* *J,* The posterior portion of the medial antral wall is sectioned with a thin spatula osteotome. *K,* Separation of posterior wall of maxillary antrum with an osteotome. *L,* Separation of nasal septum from superior part of maxilla with osteotome placed parallel to hard palate. *M,* Separation of maxilla from pterygoid plate with osteotome malleted medially and anteriorly. Surgeon's finger is positioned below palatal mucosa to feel osteotome as it transects bone.

Illustration continued on the following page

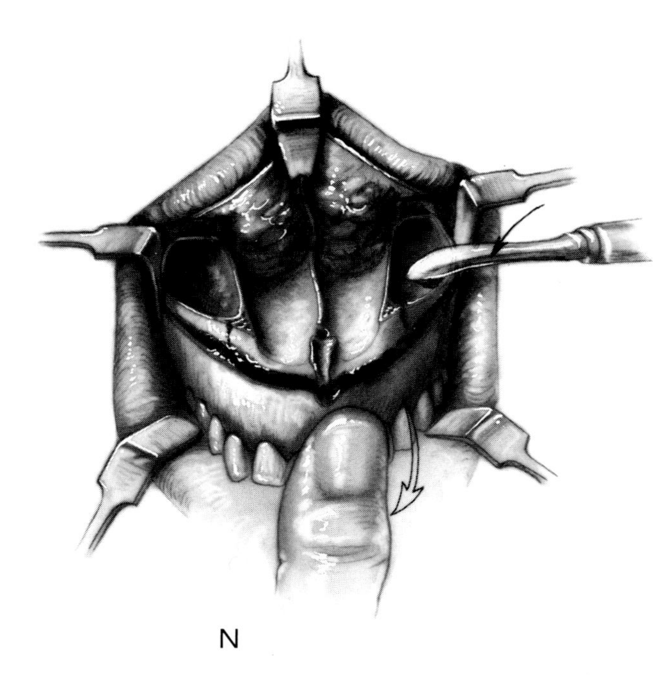

Figure 13–15 *Continued.* *N,* The mobilized maxilla is hinged inferiorly toward the mouth on an axis that passes through the condylar heads. As the maxilla is rotated downward and back, mucoperiosteum that has not already been detached is separated from the nasal surface of the maxilla and the horizontal plate of the palatine bone to facilitate "downfracturing."

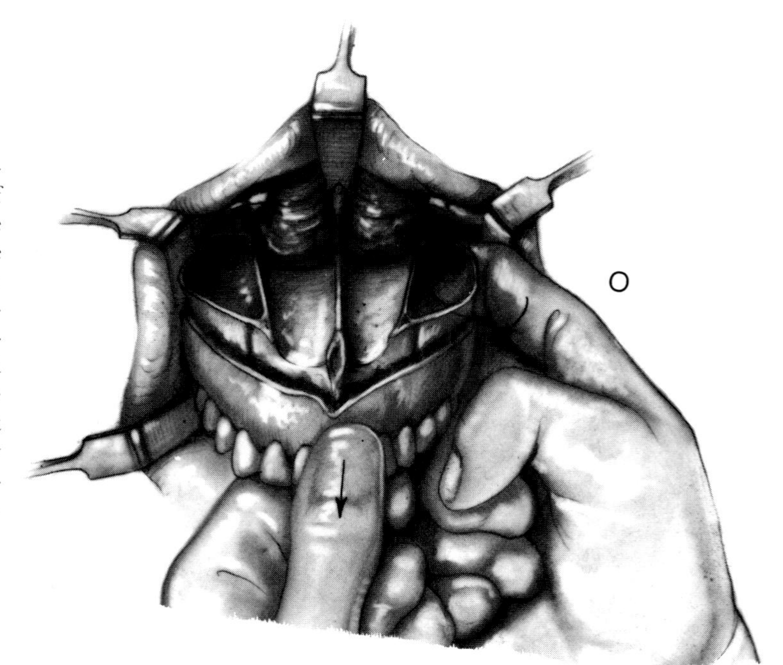

Figure 13–15 *Continued.*

O, The maxilla is mobilized by forward pressure of the index finger against the tuberosities to separate the posterior aspect of the maxilla from its remaining bony attachments. When this manipulation is ineffective, forward pressure of the concave side of a periosteal elevator against the tuberosity will usually achieve mobility and movement of the maxilla to the contralateral side.

Legend continued on the opposite page

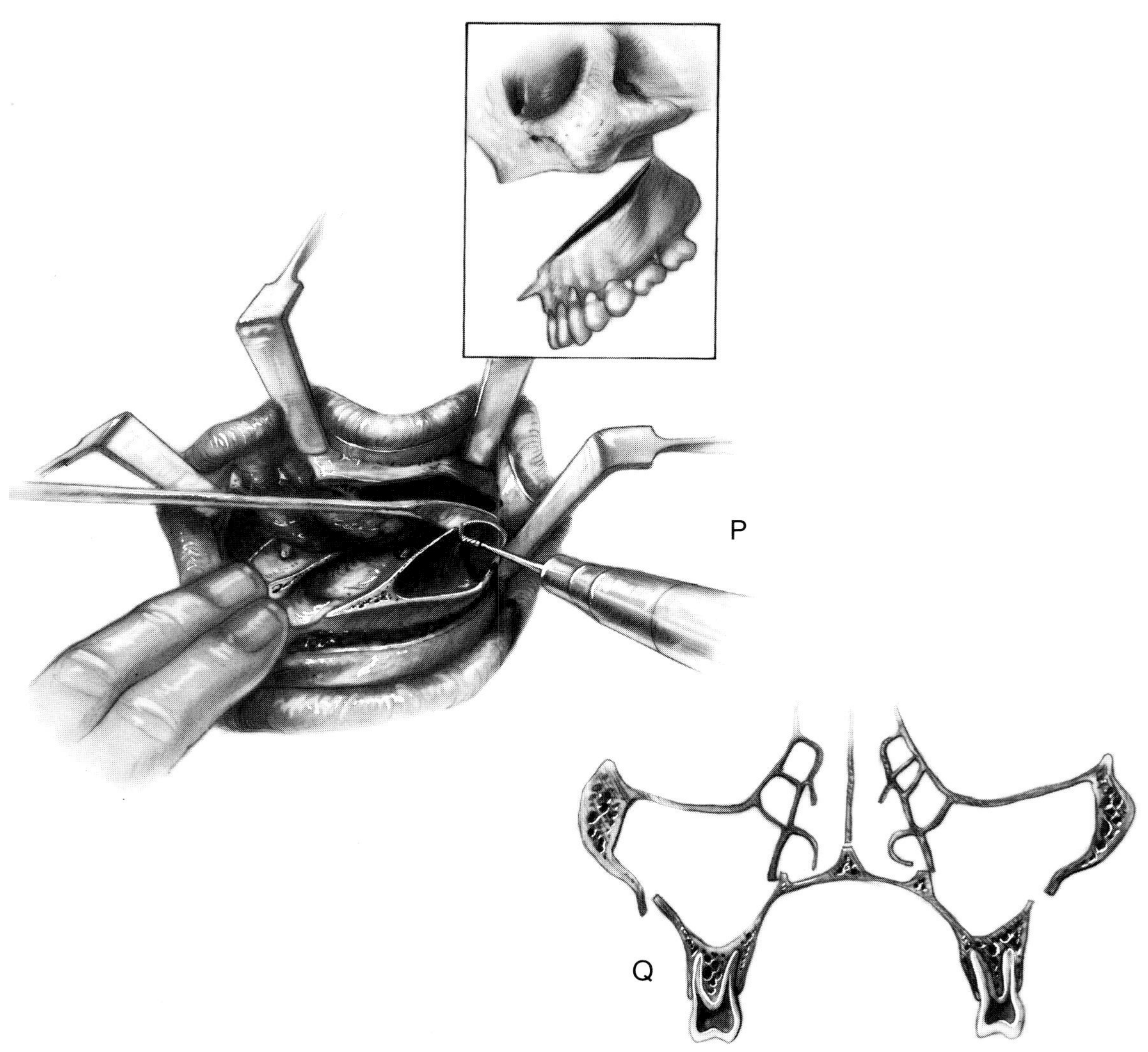

Figure 13–15 *Continued.* *P,* With the maxilla downfractured, the vertical dimension of the posterior aspect of the maxilla is reduced to facilitate the superior movement of the maxilla. Retractors are positioned appropriately to protect the contiguous soft tissues. *Q,* Cross-sectional view of molar region showing dentoalveolar portion of maxilla impacted into maxillary antra after ostectomies through lateral walls of maxilla, lateral nasal walls, and nasal septum.

Illustration continued on the following page

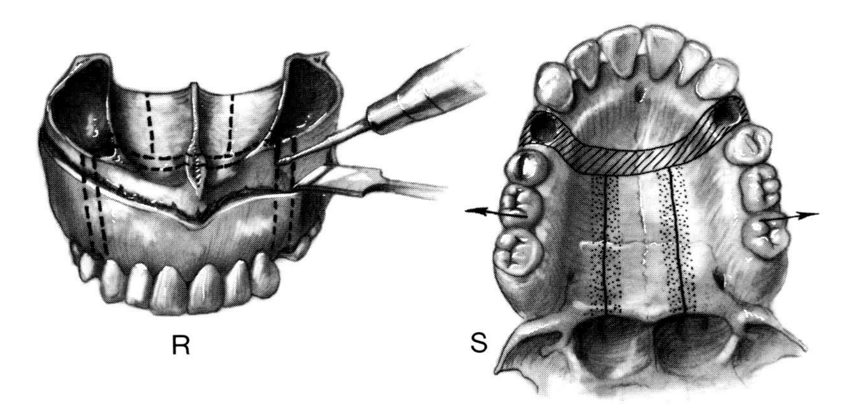

Figure 13–15 *Continued. R,* Vertical segments of bone are excised from the lateral maxilla in the 1st premolar residual extraction spaces and connected by a transverse palatal ostectomy distal to the incisive canal. The surgeon's finger is placed on the palatal mucosa to protect the vascular pedicle and to feel the bur as it transects bone. The maxilla is sectioned transversely to facilitate leveling of the maxillary occlusal plane and sagittally to increase the intercanine and intermolar width. *S,* The palatal portion of the maxilla is separated from the dentoalveolar portion of the maxilla by horseshoe-shaped circumpalatal bone cuts. The posterior maxillary dentoalveolar segments are moved superiorly to achieve the planned vertical movement. Superior movement of the maxilla may be facilitated by inferior turbinectomy when inferior turbinates restrict superior repositioning (see Chapter 8 for turbinectomy technique). Palatal mucoperiosteum is freed from the edges of the palatal segment and the posterior maxillary dentoalveolar segments. Stippled areas indicate where the mucoperiosteum may be undermined to facilitate lateral maxillary movement. Broken lines indicate palatal osteotomies; cross-hatched lines indicate palatal ostectomy.

Figure 13–15 *Continued. T,* The height of the bony nasal septum (vomer) is reduced an amount proportional to the planned superior movement of the maxilla. A midsagittal groove may be made in the superior aspect of the anterior maxilla to accommodate the nasal septum and to prevent its lateral displacement. Anteriorly, the maxillary nasal crest or cartilaginous nasal septum, or both, are reduced an amount that is proportional to the planned superior movement of the maxilla. Submucous resection of the cartilaginous nasal septum is accomplished to facilitate superior movement of the repositioned maxilla and to prevent buckling of the nasal cartilaginous septum. The height of the cartilaginous nasal septum is reduced an amount proportional to the planned superior movement. The mucoperiochondrium enveloping the inferior aspect of the cartilaginous nasal septum is easily incised after the mucoperichondrium is carefully detached bilaterally from the inferior lateral aspect of the cartilaginous nasal septum. The height of the cartilage is reduced an amount proportional to the planned superior movement of the maxilla. The maxilla may now be moved into the relationship without buckling the septum. The mucosal margins are closed with interrupted catgut sutures.

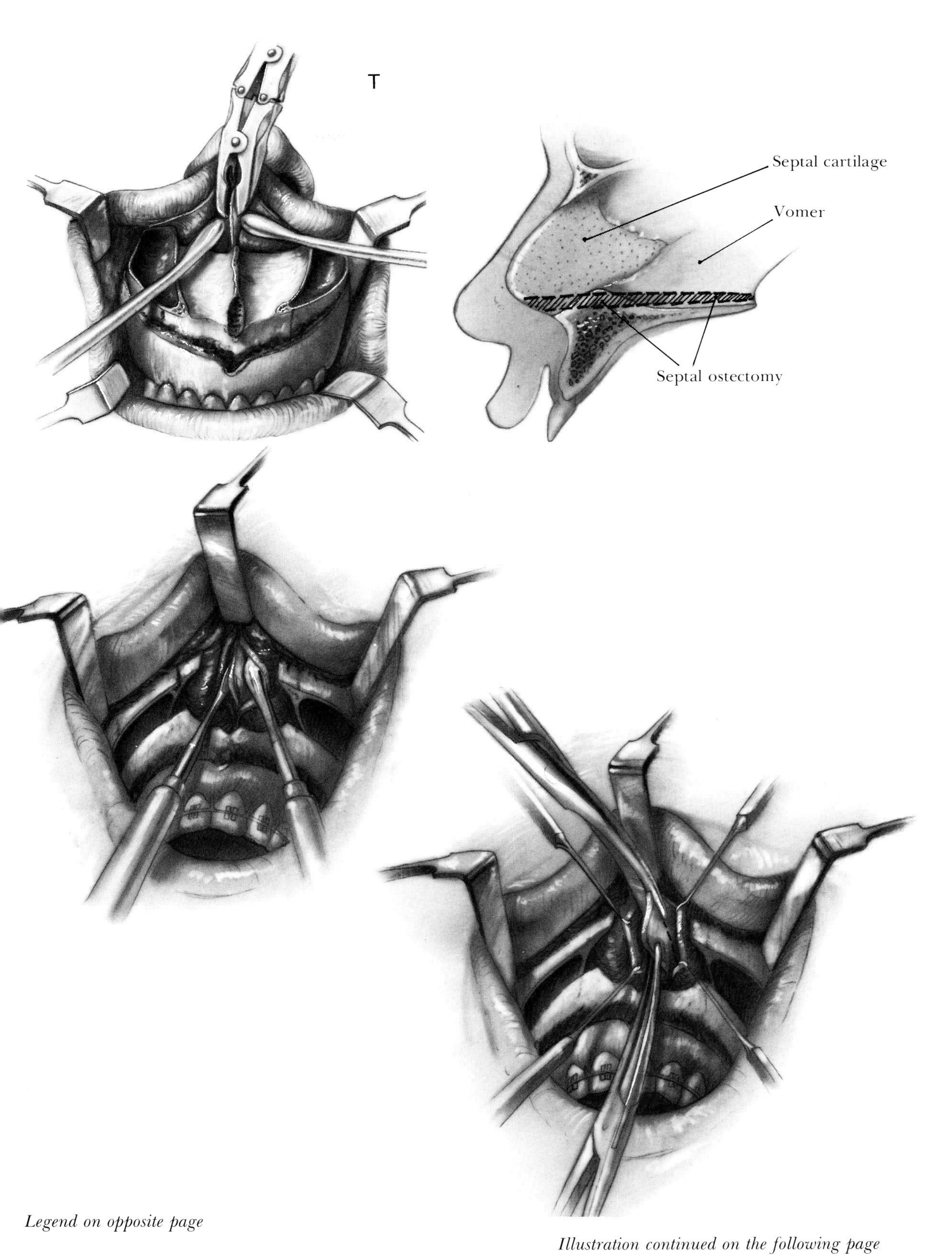

Legend on opposite page

Illustration continued on the following page

Figure 13–15 *Continued.* *U–AA,* Interosseous fixation of repositioned maxilla. *U,* A periosteal elevator is positioned subperiosteally along the anterior and inferior aspects of the lateral nasal wall to protect the nasal mucoperiosteum as a hole is drilled through the thickest portion of the nasal buttress with a #701 fissure bur. The interosseous wire hole is drilled through a similar area in the distal segment. *V,* Twenty-six gauge stainless steel wire is passed through the transosseous wire hole. The leading edge of wire is grasped with a clamp as the proximal portion of the wire is "fed" through the interosseous hole. *W,* The ends of the interosseous wires passed through the proximal and distal segments are twisted loosely to allow passive movement of the mobilized portion of the maxilla into the desired position. *X,* With the maxilla and mandible in intermaxillary fixation, the mandible is rotated closed until the margins of the osteotomized segments are juxtaposed. Then, the ends of the wires are twisted tightly and rosetted; segments of autogenous bone are onlayed along the lines of osteotomy if there is telescoping of the distal segment into the maxillary antrum or excessive instability. *Y,* The mandible is held in the most retruded position possible and rotated closed until the margins of the lateral maxillary osteotomies are juxtaposed. The margins of the posterior segments and superior aspect of the maxilla are carefully reduced until the mobilized segment can be placed into the planned position with light digital pressure.

U

V

W

X

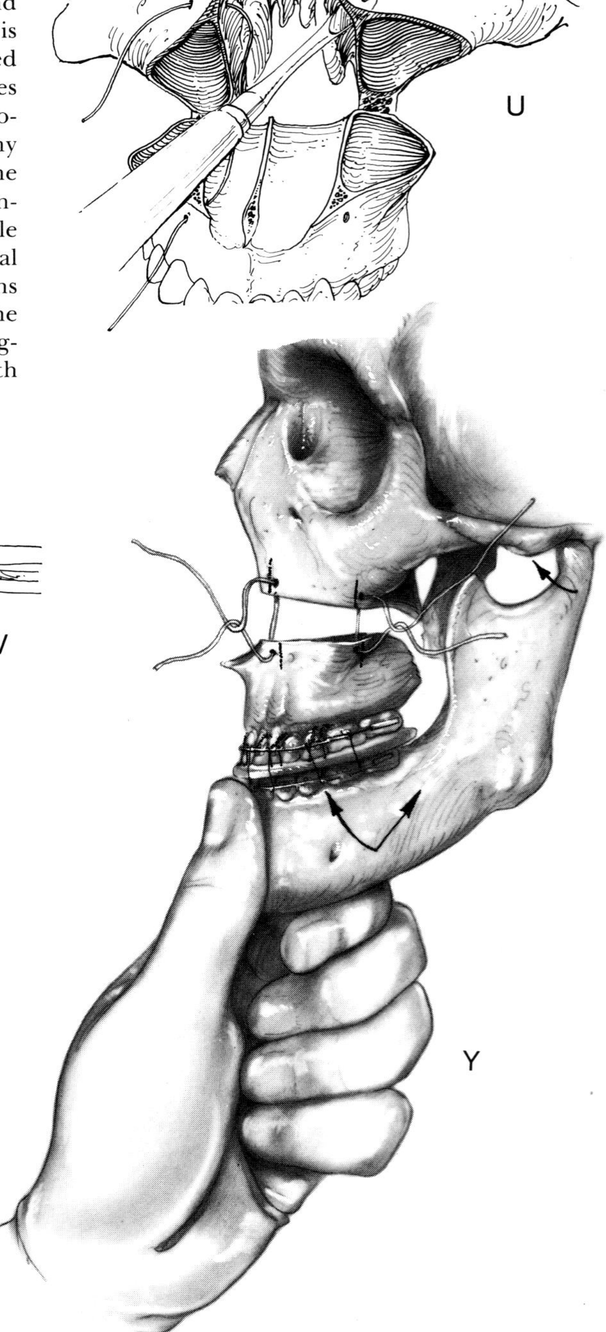

Illustration continued on the following page

Figure 13–15 *Continued.* *Z,* The repositioned maxilla is fixed to the piriform rims and zygomatic buttresses with transosseous wires. Suspension wire from the infraorbital rim to the maxillary arch wire provides additional support to the maxilla. The anterior maxilla has been repositioned directly superiorly, as evidenced by the vertical relationship of the anterior reference lines. The reference line in the posterior maxillary dentoalveolar segment is anterior to the previously made line in the lateral maxilla, indicating that the segment has been transposed anteriorly and superiorly. *AA,* Schematic illustration of intermaxillary fixation after three-piece Le Fort I osteotomy: "box" wire ligatures placed between vertical lugs soldered to rectangular arch wires for intermaxillary fixation: interocclusal wafer splint with occlusal impressions used to index maxilla in planned interocclusal relationship; suspension wires from nasal buttresses and zygomatic maxillary buttress to connect with another rosetted wire loop that has been passed around the arch wire. The repositioned maxilla is fixed into interocclusal splint with wire ligatures that pass through the splint and around the arch wire vertical lugs. Rectangular arch wire is ligated to the brackets and tied back from the vertical lug to the 2nd molar.

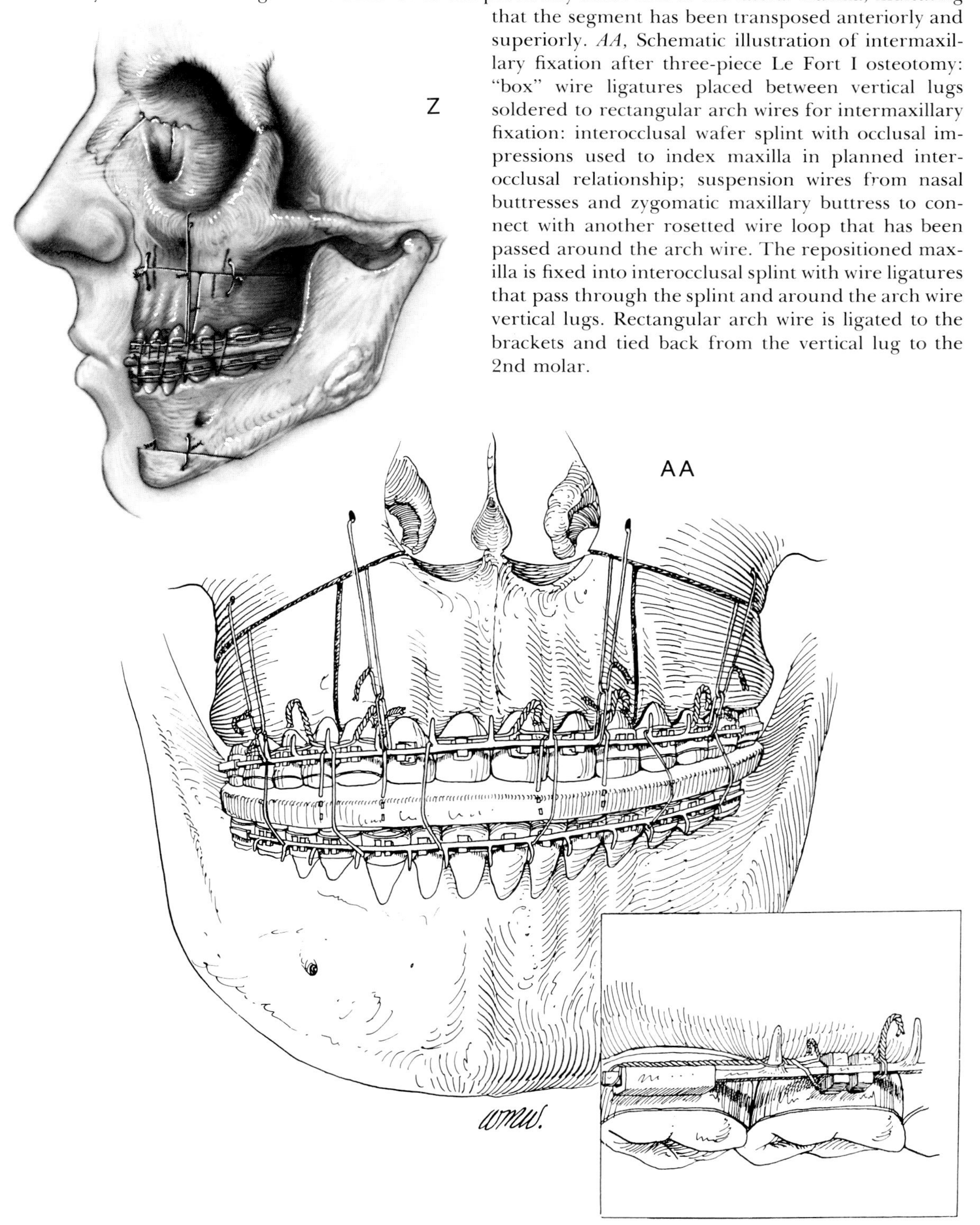

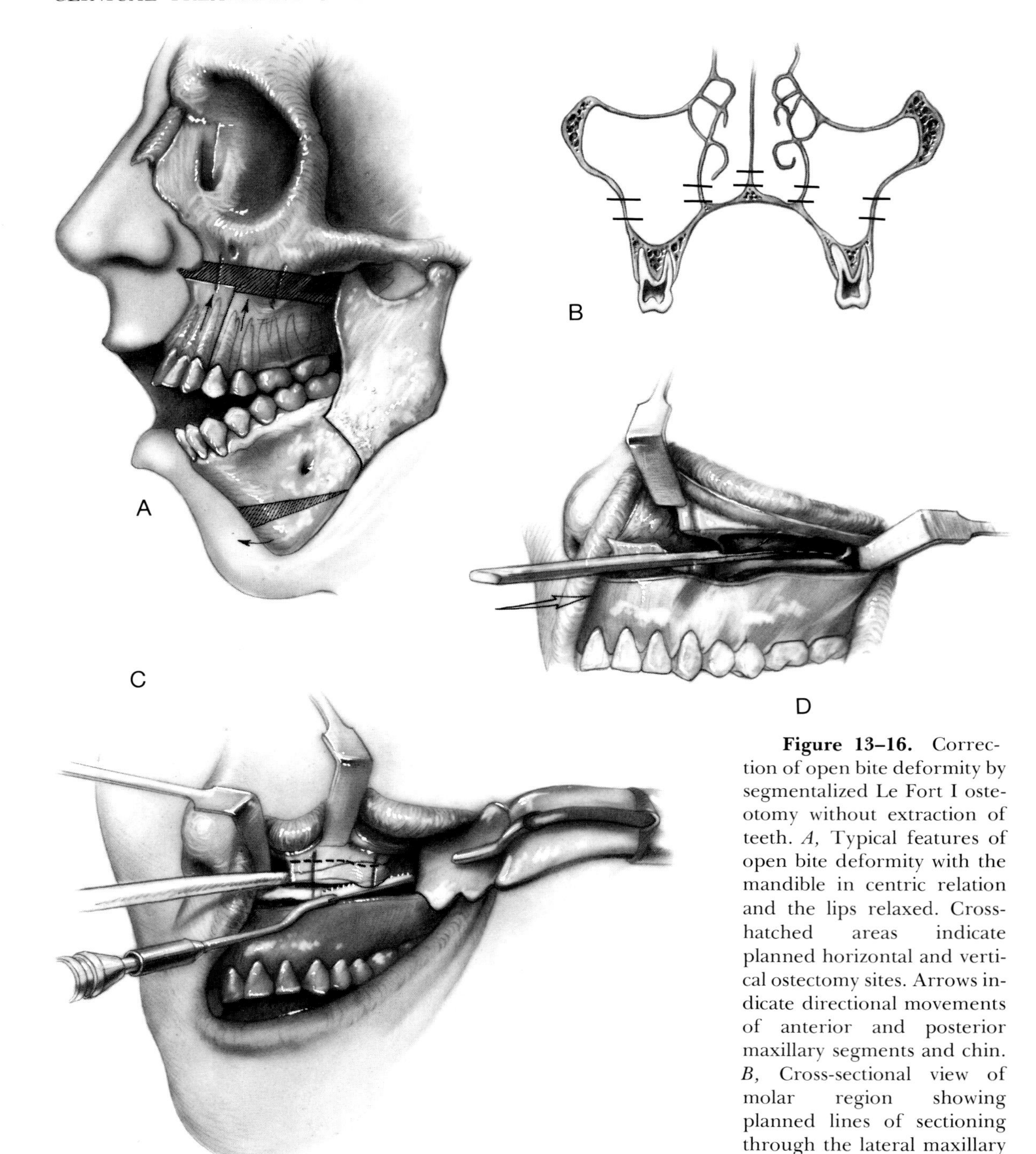

Figure 13–16. Correction of open bite deformity by segmentalized Le Fort I osteotomy without extraction of teeth. *A,* Typical features of open bite deformity with the mandible in centric relation and the lips relaxed. Cross-hatched areas indicate planned horizontal and vertical ostectomy sites. Arrows indicate directional movements of anterior and posterior maxillary segments and chin. *B,* Cross-sectional view of molar region showing planned lines of sectioning through the lateral maxillary and nasal walls and the nasal septum. *C,* Horizontal incision through the mucoperiosteum in the maxillary vestibule above the mucogingival reflection from the 2nd molar region of one side to a similar area on the contralateral side. Anterior and posterior vertical reference lines are etched into the lateral maxilla. With a malleable retractor in place to protect the nasal mucoperiosteum, a horizontal section of bone is excised from the lateral maxilla from the piriform rim posteriorly to the pterygomaxillary fissure. Anteriorly, the horizontal bone incisions are carried through the lateral and medial aspects of the maxilla. *D,* The medial antral wall is sectioned with a finely tapered straight osteotome.

Legend continued on the opposite page

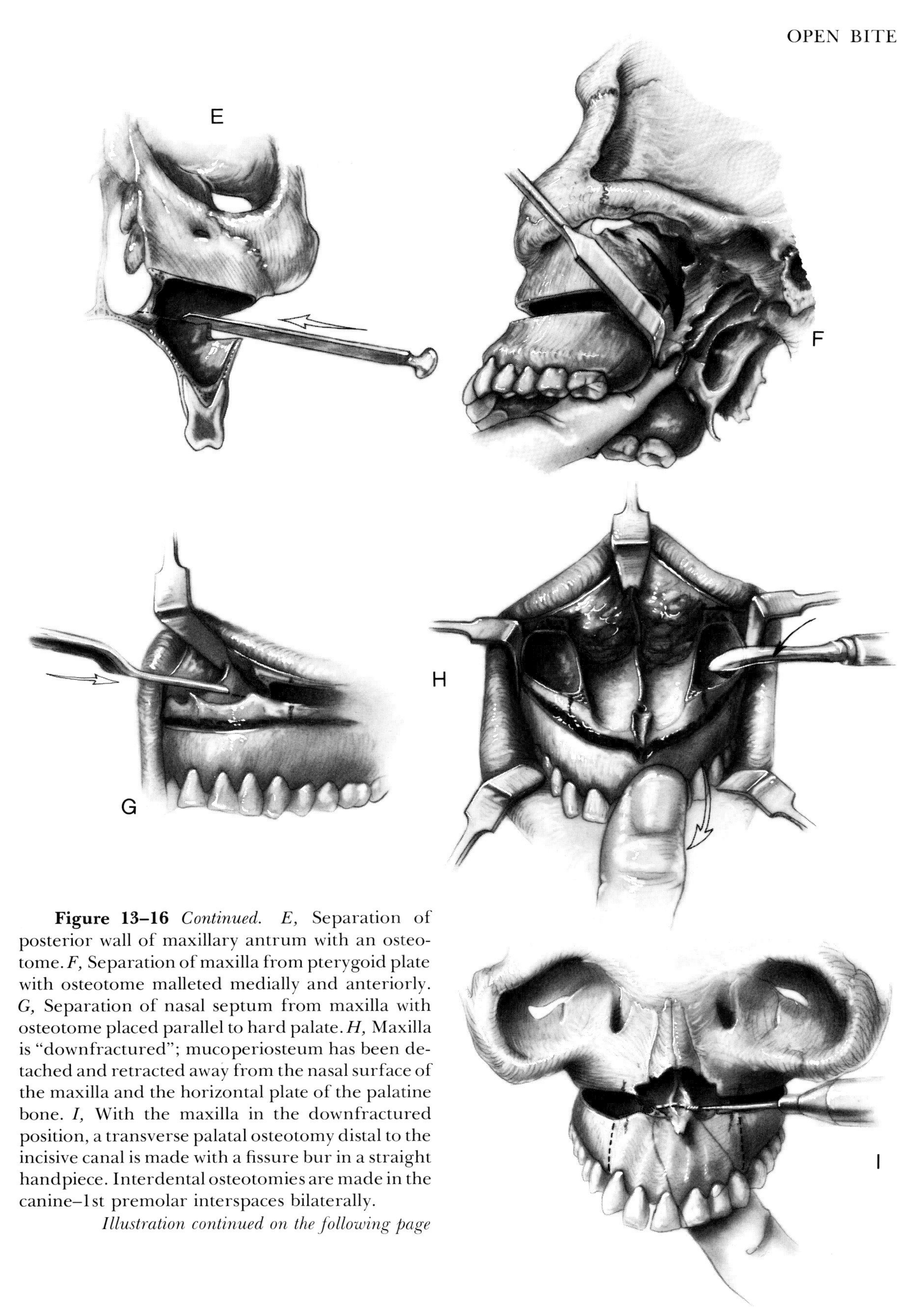

Figure 13–16 *Continued. E,* Separation of posterior wall of maxillary antrum with an osteotome. *F,* Separation of maxilla from pterygoid plate with osteotome malleted medially and anteriorly. *G,* Separation of nasal septum from maxilla with osteotome placed parallel to hard palate. *H,* Maxilla is "downfractured"; mucoperiosteum has been detached and retracted away from the nasal surface of the maxilla and the horizontal plate of the palatine bone. *I,* With the maxilla in the downfractured position, a transverse palatal osteotomy distal to the incisive canal is made with a fissure bur in a straight handpiece. Interdental osteotomies are made in the canine–1st premolar interspaces bilaterally.

Illustration continued on the following page

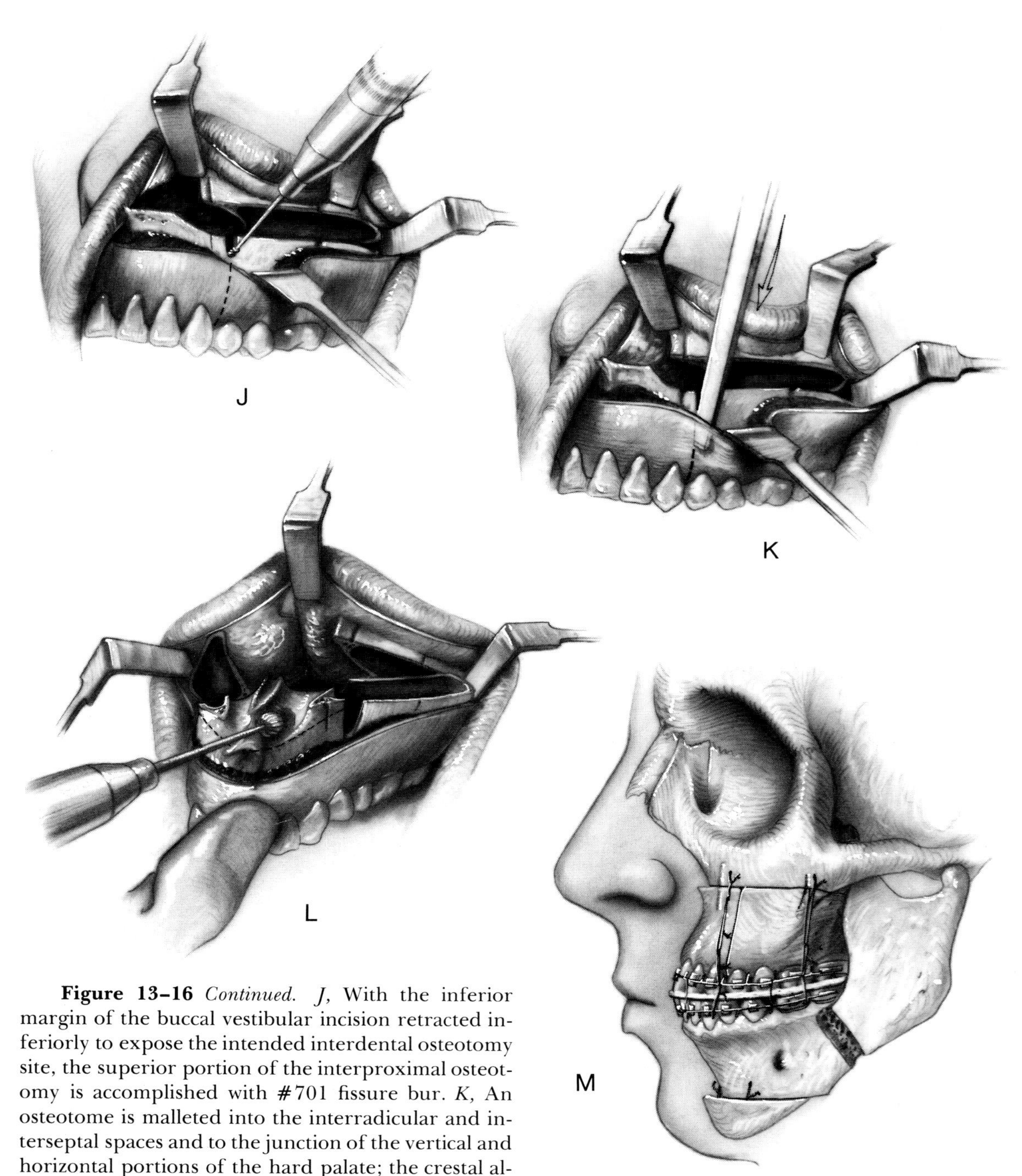

Figure 13–16 *Continued. J,* With the inferior margin of the buccal vestibular incision retracted inferiorly to expose the intended interdental osteotomy site, the superior portion of the interproximal osteotomy is accomplished with #701 fissure bur. *K,* An osteotome is malleted into the interradicular and interseptal spaces and to the junction of the vertical and horizontal portions of the hard palate; the crestal alveolar bone is *fractured* with osteotome rather than sectioned with burs. *L,* With the maxilla in the downfractured position, the vertical dimension of the nasal crest, superior aspect of the maxilla, and piriform rim is reduced to facilitate the planned superior movement of the maxilla. *M,* The repositioned maxilla is fixed to the piriform rim and zygomatic buttresses. Circumzygomatic suspension wires to the maxillary arch wire and interosseous wires in the nasal buttress and zygomaticomaxillary buttress regions provide support for the maxilla. The anterior and posterior maxilla have been repositioned directly superiorly, as evidenced by the vertical relationship of the anterior and posterior reference lines. The mandible has been surgically advanced to a Class I canine relationship after bilateral sagittal split ramus osteotomies. The mental symphysis segments have been repositioned and stabilized with interosseous wires.

Excellent stability has been achieved with the use of the Le Fort I osteotomy to correct vertical maxillary dysplasias associated with anterior open bite — it remains our surgical procedure of choice to manage the vertical, transverse, and anteroposterior manifestations of the open bite deformity.

Figures 13–15 and 13–16 illustrate the principal technical steps of the Le Fort I osteotomy to correct the open bite deformity with and without extraction of teeth, respectively. As illustrated in Figure 13–16, sagittal split ramus osteotomies and genioplasty are frequently combined with maxillary surgery. The patients in both these figures demonstrate the typical dental, skeletal, and facial features of the open bite deformity (Figs. 13–15*A* and 13–16*A*). Of note in both of these patients are the prominent nasal dorsum, the large distance between the apices of the maxillary teeth and the nasal floor, the excessive curvature of the maxillary occlusal plane, the high mandibular plane angle, the retropositioned mandible, the open bite, the contour deficient–chin, and the Class II malocclusion. The patient in Figure 13–15 also demonstrated an obtuse nasolabial angle and lip incompetency (Fig. 13–15*A*). The premolar teeth were extracted to facilitate correction of the crowded and malaligned teeth by orthodontic means (Fig. 13–15*B*). The patient in Figure 13–16 demonstrated an oblique nasolabial angle and a large interlabial gap in addition to those aspects of the deformity just mentioned (Fig. 13–16*A*). In both cases, the amount of bone to be excised was determined from cephalometric prediction studies and mock sectioning of study casts before surgery.

Everything being equal, large ostectomies in the angular superior aspect of the lateral maxilla to accomplish superior movement of the maxilla create larger spaces between the margins of the proximal and distal segments in the zygomaticomaxillary buttress than do small ostectomies—skeletal instability and difficulty in stabilizing the repositioned maxilla may result. Careful preoperative evaluation and knowledge of the involved anatomy will help the surgeon to predict when grafting of the osteotomy sites and bony gaps is necessary. Whenever the surgeon foresees a *possible* need for a bone graft at surgery, a preoperative patient consent should be sought. The hip is prepped and draped at the time of surgery contingent upon the actual need for bone (Fig. 13–15 G_1 and G_2).

Adjunctive Inferior Turbinectomy

Judicious inferior turbinectomy is a safe, predictable procedure for facilitating superior movement of the maxilla by Le Fort I osteotomy, At our institution, the technique has been accomplished without complication in 32 patients. Postoperative nasal breathing has remained unchanged or has even improved. This technique is discussed in detail and illustrated in Chapter 8, Maxillary Excess, pages 292 through 293.

Closure of Open Bite by Surgery in the Ascending Ramus

Success in treating anterior open bite with ramus surgery is variable and unpredictable. Numerous technical modifications, such as bone grafting and the sagittal split osteotomy technique, have consistently failed to prevent skeletal and dental relapse (see case reports 13-9 and 13-10). The initial relapse occurs during the period of intermaxillary fixation. Because this takes place without vertical separation of the teeth, such a change can easily go unnoticed unless the patient is monitored with cephalometric radiographs during the fixation period. After release from intermaxillary fixation, there may be a gradual positional change of the mandible which can eventually produce complete or partial relapse to the presurgical open bite condition.

The etiology of such relapse is difficult to explain. In the days before maxillary surgery was used routinely to close anterior open bite deformities, ramus surgery was used with very unpredictable results — although the occlusion of some patients remained quite stable, the majority of cases showed relapse. In view of our clinical experience and the parallel experience of many other investigators, it is not possible to account for relapse entirely on the basis of surgical technique or healing of the osseous segments. Biomechanical factors and lack of adaptation to the lengthening of the associated masticatory musculature are more reasonable explanations. Because of this theory and because maxillary osteotomies provide a predictable and stable means of closing an anterior open bite, ramus surgery is seldom selected as the primary or sole method of surgical correction. Ramus osteotomies do, however, serve an important function in correcting open bite deformities associated with severe mandibular deficiency or mandibular prognathism. In such cases, maxillary surgery shortens the lower anterior facial height; levels the maxillary occlusal plane; produces esthetic balance between the upper lip, teeth, and nose; and allows autorotation of the mandible. Additionally, and perhaps most importantly, ramus surgery allows the mandible to be repositioned anteriorly or posteriorly without causing it to rotate clockwise and without lengthening the associated masticatory musculature.

It is incumbent upon the clinician to predict patterns of skeletal instability and to plan treatment accordingly.[43] Ideally, skeletal relapse should be consistent with treatment objectives. When planning treatment for an open bite deformity that is associated with absolute mandibular deficiency, one must consider that maxillary surgery may potentiate skeletal stability because the superiorly repositioned maxilla tends to relapse superiorly. Repositioning the maxilla superiorly obviates counterclockwise surgical movement of the mandible to close the open bite and may offset the tendency of the surgically repositioned mandible to relapse posteriorly. The forward and upward movements of the maxilla and mandible are consistent with the usual treatment objectives for the individual with a skeletal type open bite and associated mandibular deficiency.

In order to achieve maximal stability with occlusal and esthetic harmony, the surgeon must be psychologically willing and technically able to perform combined maxillary and mandibular surgical procedures. When this kind of treatment is planned, certain technical considerations facilitate combined ramus and maxillary osteotomies. The bone incisions for sagittal split ramus osteotomies are initially accomplished without actually splitting the rami. Then, after the indicated maxillary surgery is accomplished and the maxilla has been repositioned, suspension wires are placed to maintain the maxilla in the desired anteroposterior and vertical position. At this time, the mandibular rami can be split with osteotomes with minimal trauma to the repositioned maxilla. After the mandible has been keyed into the desired relationship with the maxilla, intermaxillary fixation is accomplished.

With this type of maxillomandibular surgery, we do not routinely disocclude the posterior teeth with an interocclusal splint. Suprahyoid myotomy and a soft cervical collar are occasionally used as described in Chapter 10, Mandibular Deficiency, to offset the distracting forces associated with surgical advancement of the mandibular ramus or whenever there is an obvious indication at the time of surgery that the suprahyoid muscles are restricting the anterior movement of the mandible. If and when mandibular ramus surgery is used as the sole means of closing an anterior open bite, posterior overcorrection with an interocclusal splint, suprahyoid myotomy, and the use of a soft cervical collar after surgery should all be given serious consideration as means of offsetting the propensity for relapse.

ADJUNCTIVE SURGICAL PROCEDURES

Reduction of the Tongue

M. L. Allison, W. R. Wallace, and C. W. Miller

INDICATIONS FOR REDUCTION OF THE TONGUE

Reduction of the tongue rarely is a necessary part of orthognathic surgical procedures. Partial glossectomy is indicated as a primary procedure for patients with true macroglossia. Occasionally, lingual frenectomy or partial glossectomy is helpful in managing patients who have poor tongue posture or difficulty in controlling the tongue. The need for tongue surgery as an adjunct to jaw surgery depends on the physiologic adaptation of the tongue that can be anticipated as treatment (surgery or orthodontic) is completed. The more adaptable the patient's soft tissues and oral function, the less the need for tongue surgery.

Traditionally, oral surgeons and orthodontists, especially in Europe, have believed that large tongues, tongues with abnormal function, or both cause open bites (skeletal and dental) and cause reoccurrence of orthognathic abnormalities after they have been corrected. Function of the tongue may be altered by a change in form of the jaws and dental arches. More recent experience indicates that the size of the tongue often is not related to the problem.

Most of the literature on surgical tongue reduction has come from Europe. Becker,[2] in 1962, published as indications for tongue reduction the following (1) "Support of Conservative Treatment for Patients with "Prognathism and Tongue-Open Bite in Children . . . with not yet concluded Jaw Growth," and (2) "Prevention of Relapse in the Surgical Treatment of Prognathism in the Surgical Correction of Tongue-Open Bite"[2] These studies contained no method of determining whether a relapse would have occurred. Becker also gave as contraindications for tongue surgery "patients with neurotic tendencies and/or psychosis." Becker further stated:

> We agree with Wunderer that not every large tongue must cause a prognathism; as long as it is not possible for us to comprehend exactly tongue size, position, force and function, we also cannot say under what prerequisites the macroglossia affects a prognathism. On the basis of our investigation and observation, however, we are sure that the tongue represents an essential factor of the normal growth of the jaw and that a large tongue can cause a true prognathism.

In 1964, Egyedi and Obwegeser reviewed the history of surgical reduction of the tongue and listed criteria for surgical reduction.[14] Again, their criteria were opinions based only on clinical observations and experience. They classified the tongue as an etiologic factor:

> By these indications the tongue was looked on as the etiologic factor of the existing dysgnathism from the following three possibilities:
>
> 1. True macroglossia: in this besides a severe dysgnathism, there is usually a speech impediment also.
> 2. Relative macroglossia: the tongue lies like an amorphous mass in the floor of the mouth and shows tooth impressions. Often it seems relatively too large for the mandible itself and above all for the usually small maxilla.
> 3. Functional macroglossia: the tongue seems to us unremarkable in its size; however, in swallowing, it seems to have too little space for the oral cavity.

In the classification presented by Egyedi and Obwegeser, the first two types represent actual macroglossia, an anatomically large tongue, although tongue function and position may also be factors in the second, or "relative macroglossia" group. It is clear that "functional macroglossia" is a physiologic rather than an anatomic problem, being a matter of tongue function and position rather than size. The criteria for the diagnosis of "functional macroglossia" are not completely clear. It is apparent from the description of Egyedi and Obwegeser that the tongue is positioned forward during swallowing in these patients and that this tongue position is expected to persist following surgery and to contribute to relapse.

Recent research has added considerably to knowledge about the key elements in the concept of "functional macroglossia": the role of the tongue in etiology and relapse, and the extent of physiologic adaptation after treatment. For any patient with an anatomically normal tongue, considerable physiologic adaptation is required after orthognathic surgery. The surgical procedures, especially when open bite or mandibular excess is corrected, involve considerable reduction in the volume of the oral cavity. If physiologic adaptation did not occur, nearly every patient would have "functional macroglossia" postsurgically. In fact, nearly all patients adapt after surgery and "functional macroglossia" is difficult to substantiate clinically. The typical pattern of adaptation following mandibular surgery is shown in Figure 13–17. The position of the base of the tongue can be evaluated radiographically by following the position of the hyoid bone at rest. When oral cavity size is reduced by vertical ramus osteotomy, the mandible moves backward but the tongue moves downward.[19] After one year, tongue pressures usually increase to about the preoperative level.[44]

Some difficulty in physiologic tongue adaptation may occur in perhaps 10 per cent of patients on whom orthognathic surgery is performed. The condition is characterized by instability of incisor position, problems with speech and swallowing, or both. These complications appear in the first year after treatment. The difficulty may occur because the tongue was so large that adapatation is impossible, because a tight lingual attachment forces a forward tongue position, because of some physiologic maladaptive response. Continued vertical growth must be ruled out before any of these causes is considered seriously.

Open bite caused primarily by a large tongue (true macroglossia) is quite rare. When it does occur, the cause is resting pressure of the tongue against and between the teeth, not tongue pressure during swallowing. The precise effect will vary depending on whether the tongue rests between the teeth along the entire jaw or only in one area. Paradoxically, a "total open bite" produced by the tongue being between all the teeth may appear relatively mild clinically when the teeth do come into occlu-

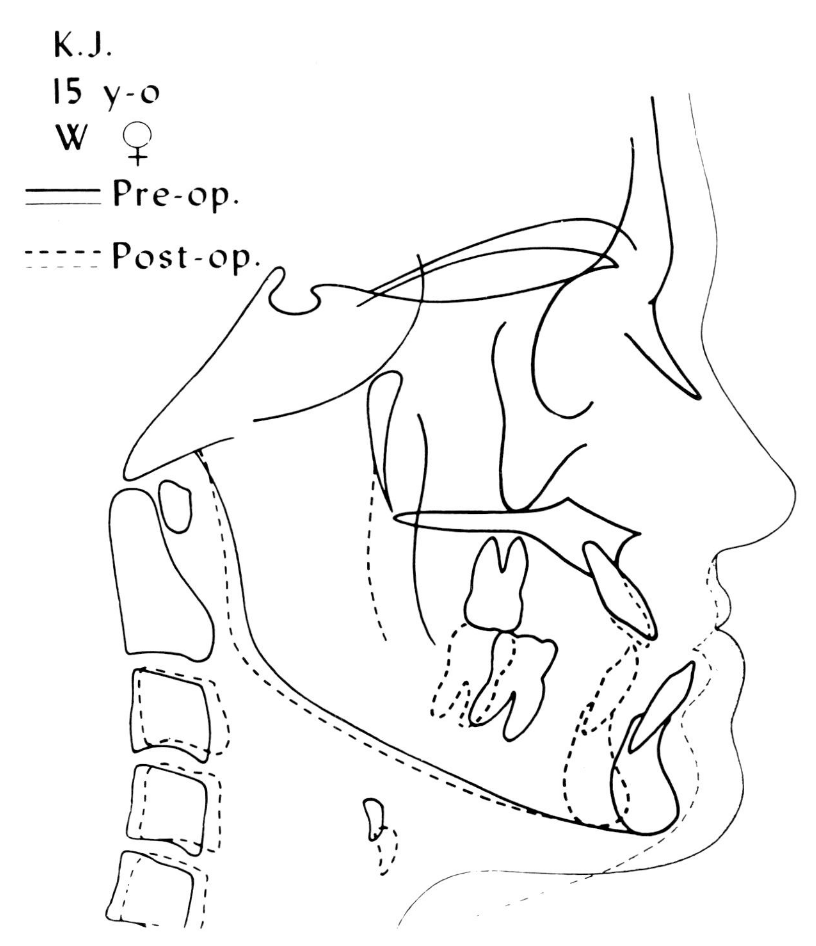

Figure 13–17. When the mandible is surgically moved back, physiologic adaptation is necessary to prevent the airway from being blocked as the tongue also goes posteriorly. The mechanism of this adaptation can be seen from the movement of the hyoid bone, which reflects the position of the base of the tongue. Note that as the mandible goes back, the hyoid bone moves downward, and the distance from the hyoid to the cervical vertebrae remains constant, demonstrating airway maintenance.

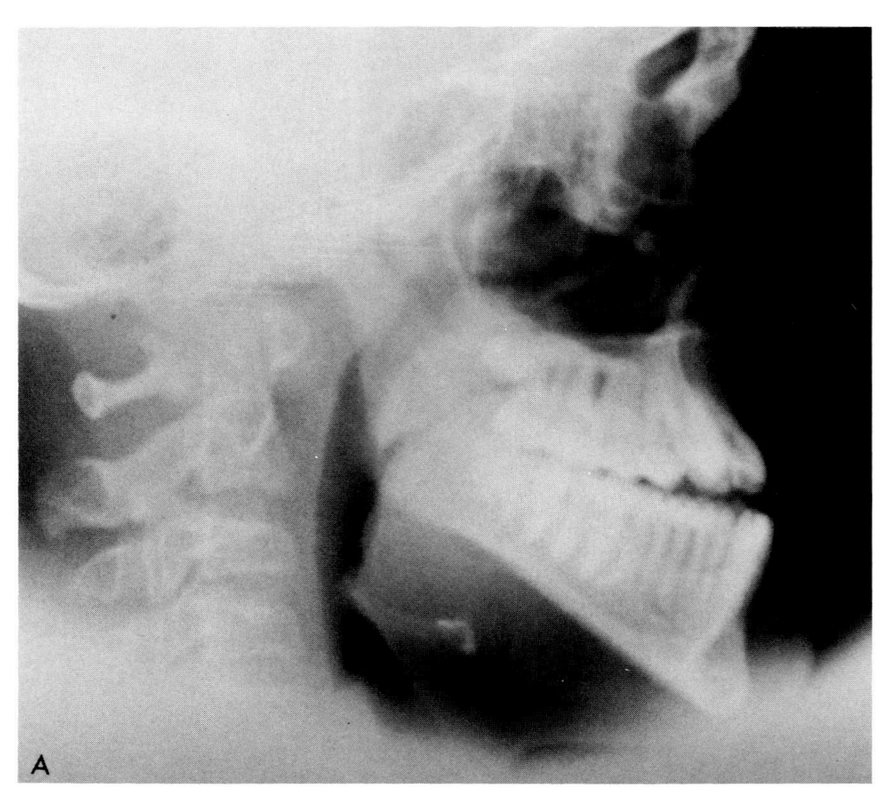

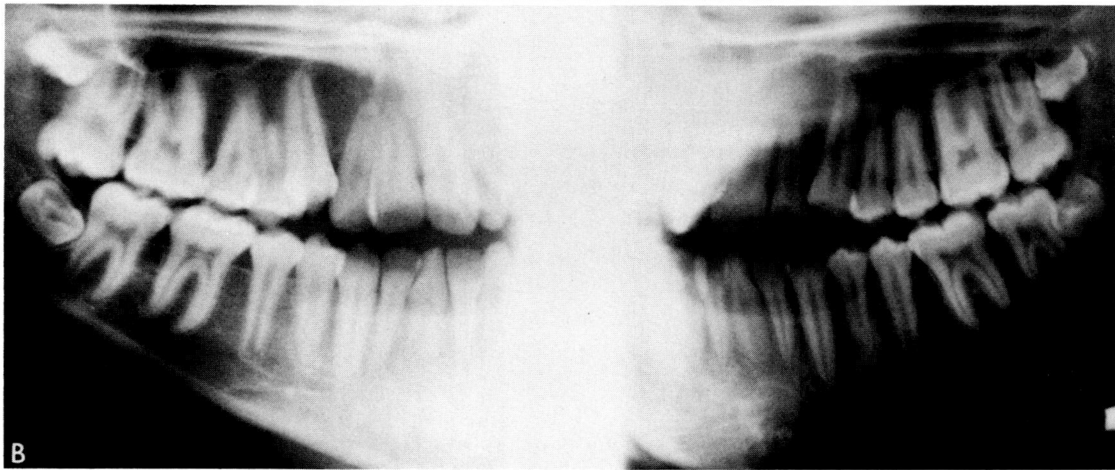

Figure 13–18. When the tongue is placed between the teeth at rest, eruption of teeth, particularly mandibular posterior teeth, is impeded. *A,* The resulting failure of vertical development can be seen in the lateral radiograph, by comparing the position of the root apex to the lower border of the mandible. *B,* Panoramic film of same patient showing lack of lower molar vertical development.

sion (Fig. 13–18). The condition can be recognized by failure of vertical development of the alveolar processes, especially in the mandibular arch (Fig. 13–18). Because of physiologic adaptation in the posture of the mandible, there may or may not be an increased freeway space. The patient can be expected to have mandibular protrusion when the teeth are in occlusion because the mandible rotates upward and forward upon closure. Frequently the maxilla is underdeveloped and there is true mandibular excess in addition to the horizontal excess in the lower third of the face that is produced by rotation. Surgical reduction of the tongue is indicated for such patients — relapse will occur if it is not done at the time of jaw surgery. Orthodontic extrusion of posterior teeth often is needed after surgery. Speech therapy is indicated, especially if speech problems existed before the operation.

If true macroglossia exists, partial glossectomy at the time of jaw surgery is indicated. "Functional macroglossia" is not an indication for tongue surgery, since the vast majority of patients do adapt very nicely following correction of dentofacial deformity and since there is no reliable way to predict which patients will not adapt well. In the few patients who prove unable to adapt postsurgically, either deep lingual frenectomy (to free the tongue so that repositioning can occur) or partial glossectomy may be needed as secondary surgical procedures to aid in adaptation. Patients must be followed closely for the first year following completion of treatment. If tongue position does seem to be causing relapse, any decision to perform tongue surgery should be weighed carefully by both the surgeon and the orthodontist.

THE V EXCISION FOR PARTIAL GLOSSECTOMY (Fig. 13–19)

After adequate preparation of the mouth and face, traction sutures are placed anteriorly as far as possible in the tongue just lateral to the anticipated margins of the incisions. The tongue is injected from its tip to the area of the circumvallate papilla with about 5 cc of solution containing a concentration of 1:100,000 epinephrine. A V excision of tongue mass is made from the front of the tongue lateral to the midline and extending posteriorly in nearly a straight line converging to the midline at about 4 mm from the circumvallate papillae (Fig. 13–19). The incision begins laterally in the tip of the tongue at a predetermined point depending upon the bulk of the tongue muscle to be removed and is directed from the dorsum of the tongue downward and slightly toward the midline through the ventral surface of the tongue. One half of the mass of the tongue muscle to be excised should be on each side of the midline of the tongue. The incision at the most posterior point on the dorsum of the tongue is posterior to the most posterior point of incision on the ventral surface of the tongue. At the posterior end of the incision, a scalpel with a No. 10 blade is directed downward and medially so that the incision on the ventral surface of the tongue ends anteriorly to the posterior limit of the incision on the dorsal surface and emerges at the reflection of the tongue mucous membrane and its juncture with the mucous membrane of the floor of the mouth just behind the orifices of the submandibular ducts. Excision of the lingual frenum may be necessary at this time. After bleeders are clamped or tied, traction sutures are used to stabilize both sides of the tongue. A similar incision is used through the other side of the tongue, and the mass of tongue muscle is removed.

The tongue is closed in layers using 3–0 chromic sutures on a round half-circle atraumatic needle for the first layer. A round needle is adequate to penetrate tongue

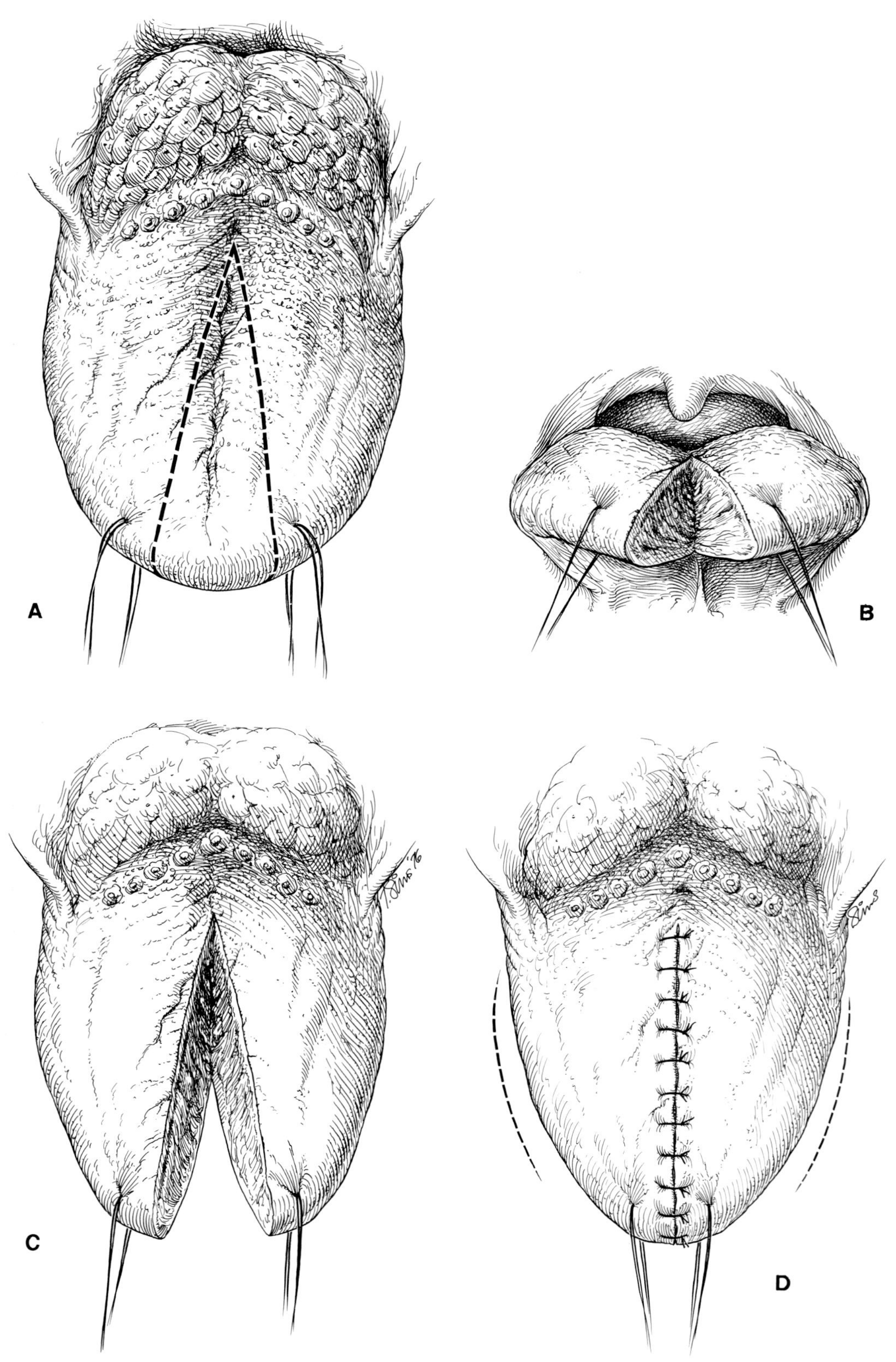

Figure 13–19. *See legend on the opposite page.*

muscle easily and produces less bleeding than a cutting needle. The first layer closed is the most central muscle mass of the tongue. Wound closure proceeds from the most posterior part of the wound forward to the tip. The traction sutures in the tips of the tongue help align the two sides correctly during closure so that the tips of the tongue come together equally.

The second layer of muscle is closed using 4–0 chromic sutures half-way between the center sutures and the dorsum of the tongue. Next, the incision margins of the dorsum of the tongue are closed with interrupted 4–0 sutures after the surgeon has ascertained that the two sides of the tongue come together equally. The tip of the tongue must be closed with the smooth mucous membrane of the ventral surface exactly matched in a manner not unlike closing the vermilion border of the lip evenly after surgery. The ventral surfaces of the tongue are usually sutured, in one layer, although sometimes a second layer of sutures is needed in the muscle half-way between the central suture layer and the ventral surface margins of the incision.

Taste is not altered by this V excision partial glossectomy. Taste buds are at the lateral margins of the tongue, circumvallate papillae, palate, tonsillar pillars, and pharynx. The lateral margins of the most anterior portion of the tongue are best suited for tasting "sweet" substances. However, even if most of these anterolateral buds are excised, other taste buds adapt to enable patients to taste "sweet" things. Tactile sensations of the tongue may be altered temporarily, but taste should remain normal for each patient.

KEYHOLE PROCEDURE FOR PARTIAL GLOSSECTOMY (Fig. 13–20)

A keyhole-shaped mass of muscle is excised when the tongue obviously is too large in the molar area and the anterior fourth is more nearly normal in size. The amount of muscle to be removed is determined individually for each patient. The "keyhole" must be large enough to allow the reduced tongue to fit naturally between the mandibular and maxillary arches.

The tongue is infiltrated with 10 cc of 1:100,000 epinephrine solution. Traction sutures are placed bilaterally in the tongue at the juncture of the anterior and middle thirds. The anterior portion of the incision begins at the tip of the tongue moving posteriorly until it reaches the area where the expanded part of the "keyhole" begins. The anterior part of the incision should go vertically completely through the tongue from the dorsal surface to the ventral surface. The posterior incision begins at the most posterior position of the "keyhole" in the midline of the tongue in front of the circumvallate papillae. This incision curves laterally and forward and then towards the midline until it joins the posterior end of the first incision just completed. Bleeding should be controlled at this point. The traction sutures are used to stabilize the

---

Figure 13–19. "V" excision for partial glossectomy. *A,* Traction sutures are placed anteriorly as far as possible in the tongue, just lateral to the anticipated margins of the incisions. Planned "V" excision is indicated by the broken line. *B* and *C,* An incision is made laterally in the tip of the tongue and directed from the dorsum of the tongue downward and slightly towards the midline through the ventral surface of the tongue. The incision at the most posterior point on the dorsum of the tongue is posterior to the most posterior point of incision on the ventral surface of the tongue. *C,* The incision on the ventral surface of the tongue emerges at the reflection of the tongue mucous membrane and its junction with the mucous membrane of the floor of the mouth just *behind* the orifices of the submandibular ducts. *D,* Closure of incision margins with interrupted sutures.

See illustration on the opposite page.

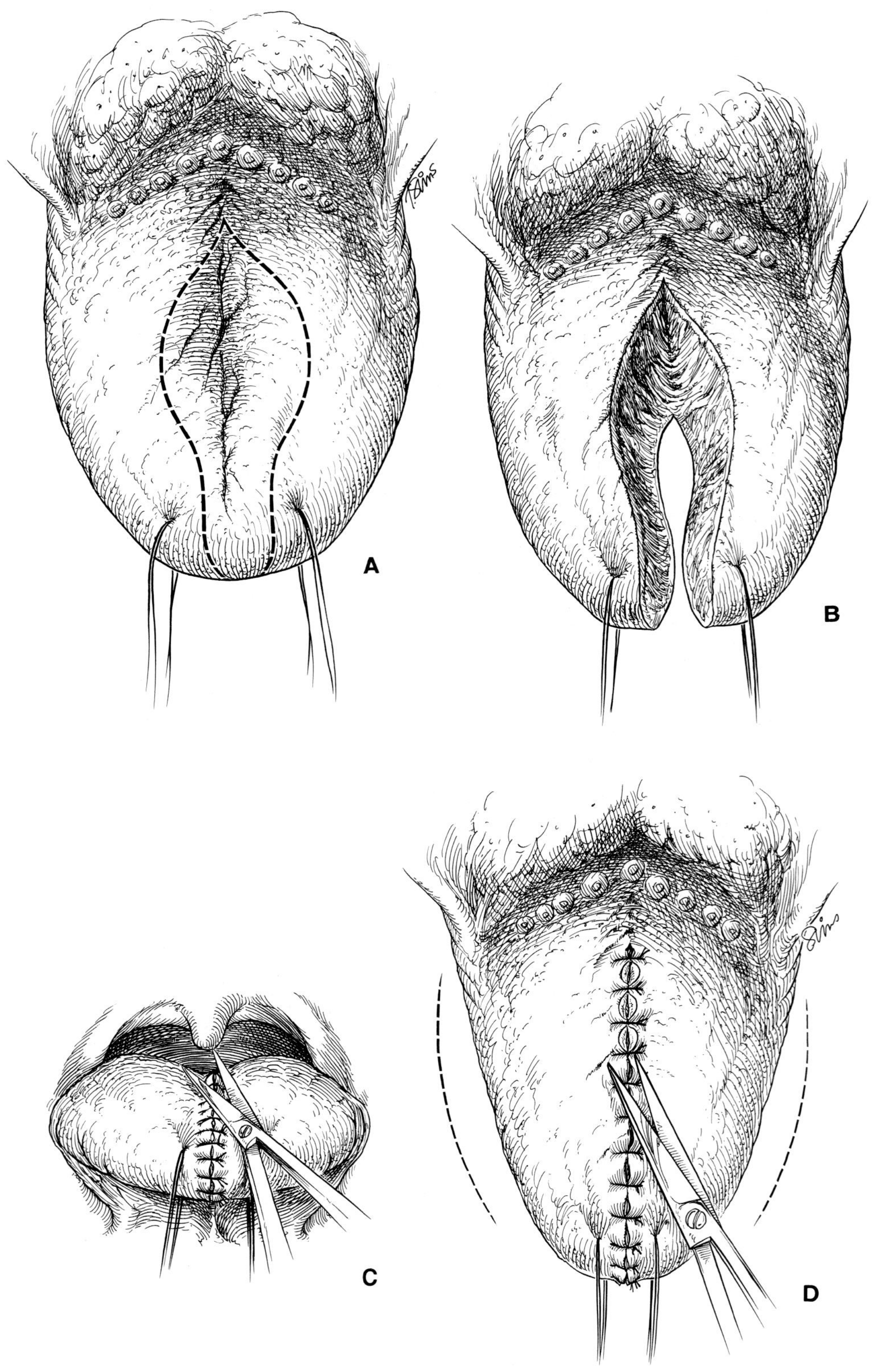

Figure 13–20. *See legend on the opposite page.*

Illustration continued on the opposite page.

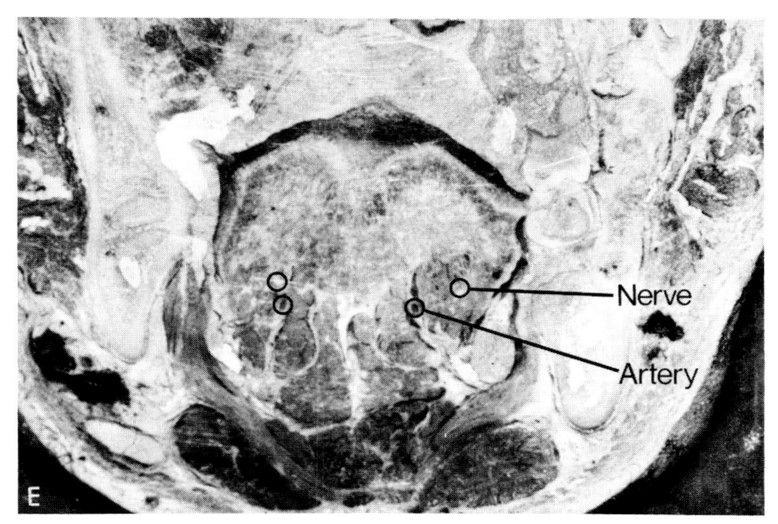

Figure 13–20. "Keyhole" procedure for partial glossectomy when tongue is too large in the molar region. *A,* Traction sutures are placed just lateral to the anticipated margins of the incisions. The planned "keyhole" excision is indicated by the broken line. *B,* The posterior "keyhole" portion of the incision is tapered like a funnel, wider at the dorsum of the tongue than at the ventral surface. The funnel tapers downward toward the midline and avoids cutting the principal branches of the lingual nerve, hypoglossal nerve, and lingual artery and veins. *C* and *D,* Closure of incision margins with interrupted sutures. After closure of the keyhole area with vertical mattress sutures, the everted tissue that is raised above the rest of the tongue surface is trimmed with a tissue scissor. *E,* Cross section of human skull in the 6-year molar area showing location of major vessels and nerves in the tongue. Tapering the incision toward the tongue midline from dorsal to ventral surface helps avoid cutting major vessels and nerves. See Figures 13–19*B* and *C*.

See illustration on the opposite page.

tongue while a mirror-image incision is made through its opposite side. This expanded posterior "keyhole" portion of the incision should taper like a funnel, wider at the dorsum of the tongue and less wide at the ventral surface. The funnel tapers downward toward the midline and avoids cutting the principal branches of the lingual nerve and hypoglossal nerve and the lingual artery and veins. After the tongue mass is excised from the "keyhole," all bleeding must be controlled before closure.

Using 3–0 chromic suture on a round half-circle atraumatic needle, the surgeon closes the wound starting posteriorly in the central muscle mass and suturing the central muscle tissue all the way to the tip of the tongue. A second layer of muscle is closed half-way between the first layer of sutures and the dorsal surface of the tongue. Simple interrupted sutures close the dorsal surface of the tongue starting at the tip. Vertical mattress sutures may be needed to close the surface where the largest amount of muscle has been removed — the "keyhole" area. Invariably, eversion of the surface occurs after the vertical mattress sutures close the "keyhole." The everted tissue raised above the rest of the tongue surface may be trimmed simply by cutting it away with a tissue scissor (Fig. 13–20). Mild surface bleeding may occur at this point and is controlled using single interrupted chromic sutures across the incision over the bleeding points. The ventral surface of the tongue can be closed in one layer. No mattress sutures are needed in the ventral surface.

Taste is not altered by the "keyhole" excision partial glossectomy. However, touch sensation is almost always lost, usually temporarily, in an area about 10 mm in diameter at the very tip of the tongue. This potential problem should be discussed with the patient *before* surgery. Patients soon adapt to this "numbness" at the tip of their tongues.

The jaws may be immobilized following partial glossectomy. The mouth then has a fixed volume and acts as a splint, limiting swelling. If jaw surgery is done along with tongue surgery, intermaxillary fixation may be required. Some surgeons believe that limiting tongue movement aids in the early phases of wound healing. Postoperative bleeding, excessive edema, and infection following partial glossectomy all are rare. Because of the potential for extensive edema, everything possible must be done to maintain hemostasis and minimize edema. Glucocorticosteroids and antibiotics are used routinely to reduce swelling and infection (see Chapter 7).

Egyedi reported side effects after 23 cases of surgical reduction.[14]

> In 23 operations severe post-operative swelling only occurred once. The airway, however, was not impaired and a tracheostomy was not necessary. Nevertheless, several times necrosis of the wound surfaces occurred which necessitated débridement and resuturing. The cause of this complication might have been an impaired blood supply to the anterior part. . . . We have also noted on several occasions a slight impairment in the function of the tongue after the healing had taken place. Reduced mobility has been frequently observed (16 cases) and the patients were not able to keep clean their buccal sulci in the upper molar areas. A slightly reduced sensitivity in the reconstituted tip of the tongue has been observed in three cases, and eight patients reported difficulty in pronouncing the letters *R* and *S*. Reduced mobility is probably the most unpleasant disturbance, although an increase in the caries rate in the affected regions has not yet been observed.

Allison believes that all these complications can be prevented except perhaps in patients with the most extreme macroglossia by the surgical technique of excising a V-shaped mass of muscle, wide at the dorsum and narrower at the ventral surface of the tongue, avoiding main trunks of motor and sensory nerves and vessels, and preserving the lateral muscle mass at the tip of the tongue (see Fig. 13–19).

In a series of 52 partial glossectomy procedures at Ohio State University, few side effects occurred. Most of the patients had little or no pain following the tongue reduction. They did suffer mild discomfort from edema of the tongue and discomfort from inability to open the mouth because the jaws were immobilized. (This was done for all patients. If only partial glossectomy was done, the jaws were immobilized for 10 to 14 days.) Sutures loosened in two patients, and about 15 mm of the wound dehiscence appeared at the tip of the tongue. In both cases, this condition was discovered at the end of the jaw immobilization when the mouth was opened the first time after surgery. The tongue edges on the open part of the incision already were healing. One patient, a 25-year-old woman, had been treated for mandibular prognathism, apertognathia, and macroglossia. Her jaw was immobilized for 6 weeks and on the day of mobilization, the tongue was found separated along the anterior portion of the incision for 15 millimeters. The tongue was prepared and resutured under local anesthesia. Following this, the patient used Class III training elastics for 4 weeks. During this period, the sutures of the anterior portion of the tongue again were loosened and the incision dehisced, requiring an additional secondary closure, which was successful.

Following partial glossectomy, patients may have difficulty in talking for 6 or 7 days because of stiffness and edema in the tongue. Incisions to remove a large, wide piece of the tongue tip seem to produce greater restriction of tongue mobility than do the midline incisions. Since reduction of tongue bulk rather than shortening the tongue usually is indicated, extensive reduction of the tongue tip should be avoided. Occasionally, the partial glossectomy is not symmetric, or sutures in the muscle masses of the tongue are not placed at equal depth on the right and left sides when the wound is closed. When this happens, the tongue may be unequal in size on the two sides immediately after the operation and may deviate right or left rather strongly when the patient protrudes it. In these cases, the tongue eventually becomes symmetric. With proper exercise of the tongue, the patient learns to protrude his tongue equally in all directions and without conscious effort.

Whether the jaws are immobilized after surgery or not, postoperative tongue exercises are recommended beginning about the fourteenth postoperative day or the same day the mandible is mobilized. (In certain individuals, speech articulation therapy may also be indicated.) After the tongue muscle is reduced in size by surgery, tongue function must be relearned. Soon after surgery, the tongue is firm, relatively immobile, and thick. During the first 12 postoperative weeks, it will become soft, pliable, mobile, thin, and, in most instances, normally tapered in shape.

Deep Lingual Frenectomy (Fig. 13–21)

A deep lingual frenectomy followed by a regimen of tongue exercises may be indicated when a "functional macroglossia" does not adapt following orthodontic treatment or jaw surgery. The anatomic shape of the lingual frenum can restrict tongue movement, forcing the tongue to function in the anterior part of the mouth.

Under local or general anesthesia, traction sutures are placed through the tongue near the tip. Once the tongue is elevated with the traction sutures, a linear excision of the mucosal portion of the thickened frenum is made with a knife or tissue scissors. Care must be taken to make the incision about 1 cm above the submandibular duct openings (Fig. 13–21).

Once the mucosa has been penetrated, dissection proceeds posteriorly into the genioglossus muscle. The line of incision should be confined to the midline, where the genioglossus muscle can be transected until the desired degree of mobility is attained. Bleeding in the depth of the mucosal opening is easily controlled with pressure or cautery. Multiple Z-plasties are cut in the mucosa to allow the wound to be lengthened at the time of closure. After transposition of the opposing flap margins, the wound is lengthened in a sagittal line and closed with interrupted sutures.

An exercise program must begin as soon as possible following surgery, preferably on the first postoperative day. Although any regimen that maintains tongue mobility is acceptable, the following is suggested. Have the patient hold a sugarless mint against the roof of the mouth with the tongue tip until the mint dissolves. This should be repeated as often as possible during waking hours (at least ten times each day). Exercises should be continued for at least 2 months after surgery.

Postoperative problems are minimal. No loss of tongue sensation occurs, and speech is not disturbed.

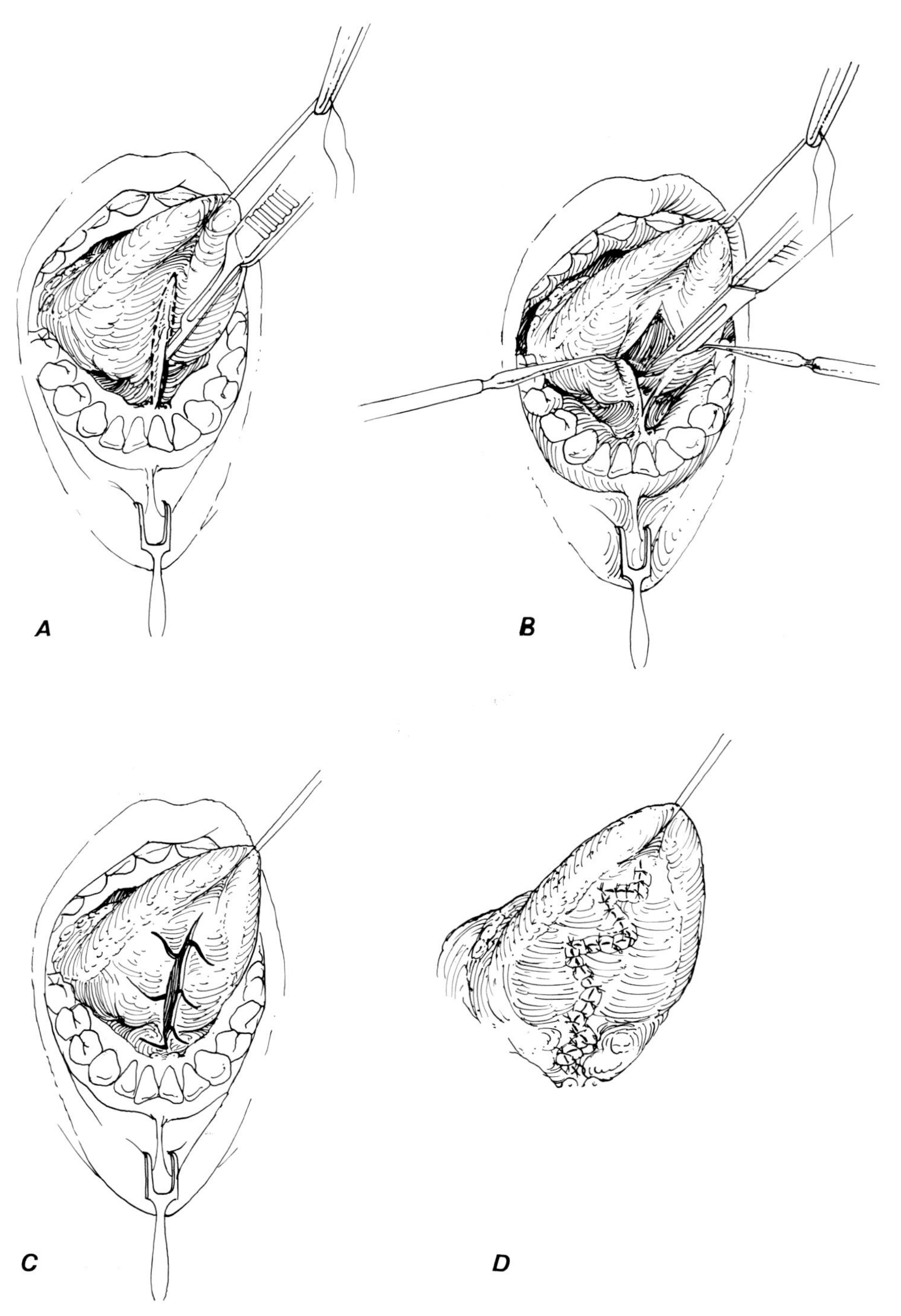

Figure 13–21. Deep lingual frenectomy by Z-plasty to correct ankyloglossia. *A,* With traction suture placed through tip of tongue, a linear excision of the mucosal portion of the thickened frenum is made. *B,* With the mucosal wound margins retracted, the fibrosed portion of the genioglossus muscle is transected until the desired degree of mobility is attained. *C,* Multiple Z-plasties are cut in the mucosa; care is taken to avoid the ducts and orifices of the submaxillary gland. *D,* After transposition of opposing flap margins, the wound is lengthened in a sagittal line and closed with interrupted sutures.

COMBINED SURGICAL AND ORTHODONTIC TREATMENT

Orthodontic Tooth Movement

The same general rules apply for combined treatment of open bite deformity as for other types of dentofacial deformity. The essential orthodontic preparation should be done before surgery, but it is permissible and indeed desirable to leave detailed orthodontic finishing until surgery has been completed.

Open bite does differ somewhat with reference to the second of the major rules for combined treatment that are discussed in Chapter 8: No orthodontic tooth movement that might contribute to relapse should be attempted after surgery. For patients who have had surgical correction of open bite, this rule contraindicates any type of tooth movement that would extrude the posterior teeth. Use of posterior cross-elastics to correct crossbite and use of Class II and Class III elastics should be avoided postoperatively, since they have the effect of opening the bite. Any tooth movement requiring their use should be completed before surgery. Orthodontic treatment for open bite differs from orthodontic intervention in other types of dentofacial deformity principally in that minor crossbites that would be corrected *after* surgery in most other patients should be corrected *before* surgery by rapid palatal expansion or *during* surgery by surgical expansion of the maxilla. The postsurgical result should not require the use of cross-elastics.

When extraction of maxillary teeth is contraindicated and it is necessary to increase the arch length to facilitate presurgical alignment of crowded and rotated teeth, rapid maxillary expansion is combined with lateral maxillary osteotomies (see Chapter 9, Maxillary Deficiency). Later, after the maxillary teeth are properly aligned and the arches coordinated (predicated on surgical change), the definitive vertical, transverse, and anteroposterior changes in the position of the maxilla are accomplished by total maxillary osteotomy (see Figs. 13–15 through 13–16).

More frequently, however, extraction of maxillary premolars is programmed to facilitate alignment of the maxillary teeth prior to surgery. The desired transverse, anteroposterior, and vertical positional changes of the maxilla are achieved by a segmentalized Le Fort I osteotomy (see Fig. 13–15). After the anterior teeth have been aligned and the rotations corrected, the maxillary occlusal plane is leveled by a transverse palatal ostectomy extending into the residual extraction spaces. The maxilla is expanded or narrowed simultaneously after sagittal, parasagittal, or horseshoe palatal osteotomies. Many other types of orthodontic tooth movement have an extrusive component, however, and the potential effect of extrusion should be evaluated carefully when the treatment plan is developed. (See Chapter 9 for treatment of transverse dimensions.)

The potential extrusive effects of the following types of tooth movement may be important:

1. *Maxillary expansion, including rapid maxillary expansion but also including use of cross-elastics and even lateral expansion arch wires.* As the maxillary molars move laterally, the different pattern of contacts of cusps with inclined planes inevitably means that some bite opening will occur. We routinely combine lateral maxillary osteotomy with rapid palatal expansion of the maxilla. In so doing, minimal or no opening of the bite is produced.

2. *Procedures to reposition incisors buccally or lingually, or to correct midline discrepancies, that would require interarch elastics.* It is difficult to complete many detailed positioning movements orthodontically without some use of interarch elastics, but Class II or Class III

elastic traction inevitably has a vertical component. If it is necessary to use such elastics postoperatively, it is important that anterior vertical elastics be used at the same time. Use of interarch elastics should be avoided if at all possible.

3. *Leveling the curve of Spee with arch wires or other mechanics.* This is likely to lead to some extrusion of molars as well as premolars, even though the mechanics may be directed at intrusion of incisors.

4. *Uprighting lower molars, which also tends to extrude them.*

When any of these tooth movements with an extrusive component are performed prior to surgery, the effect will be to make the open bite worse at that stage. Temporary worsening of the open bite prior to surgery is not a problem, since it will be corrected at the time of surgery. Sometimes it is difficult to grasp that presurgical orthodontic tooth movement, done as part of an overall surgical plan, is correct treatment when the immediate effect is to make the major problem worse. This, of course, is true in the correction of all types of dentofacial deformity, not just open bite.

The treatment plan for an open bite patient often calls for surgical intrusion of maxillary anterior and posterior segments. In this case, it is important that significant leveling of the maxillary arch *not* be done as part of preparatory orthodontic treatment. It may be necessary, as part of orthodontic preparation for surgery, to create a step in the occlusal plane at the point where the osteotomy later will pass through the alveolar process. All arch wires will have to incorporate a step to maintain the vertical difference. Otherwise, extrusion of incisor teeth will occur. If extrusion of maxillary incisor teeth does occur during the preparatory orthodontic phase of treatment, this does not defeat efforts at coordinated correction of the deformity because total maxillary osteotomy is usually indicated to intrude the anterior and posterior parts of the maxilla. Surgery can easily compensate for any extrusion of the maxillary incisors that might occur as a consequence of orthodontic mechanics.

Intrusion of maxillary posterior segments also tends to bring the root apices of posterior teeth closer to those of the anterior teeth. Because of this, separation of roots at the osteotomy site may be a necessary part of presurgical orthodontic preparation. An interdental osteotomy requires adequate space between the roots. If a premolar is to be extracted, root positioning is rarely a consideration; but if the cuts are to be made between adjacent teeth, it is usually necessary to "unparallel" the roots before surgery orthodontically. This is yet another example in which orthodontic tooth movement done as part of preparation for surgery is the opposite of the direction of tooth movement usually required for orthodontic treatment alone.

Surgical Stabilization

Patients with open bite are particularly likely to require combined anterior and posterior maxillary segmental surgery. In these cases, as in all other dentofacial deformity problems, the orthodontic appliance should be placed before operation, and orthodontic arch wires can be used for stabilization. It may be wise not to attempt to use a single continuous arch wire for stabilization. Instead, rectangular wire segments can be placed prior to operation, with the arch-wire segments separated as the teeth will be at the time of surgery. This allows free movement of the segments at surgery. When the segments are in place, they can be stabilized by tying the arch segments together across the osteotomy site or reinforced with arch bars across the osteotomy site if required. The mobilized segments are usually indexed into the desired relationship by an interocclusal splint. The segments are fixed to the splint with wires that ligate the brackets to the splint (see Chapter 9 for details).

With the foregoing exceptions, combined orthodontic and surgical treatment for open bite follows the guidelines discussed in connection with specific surgical procedures for the maxilla and mandible in Chapters 8 through 12.

SURGICAL TREATMENT DURING GROWTH

The timing of surgery is based upon the magnitude of the functional and esthetic deformity and its psychologic effects on the individual patient. Because many patients with skeletal type anterior open bite deformities continue to grow until age 21, it is often impractical to delay treatment until growth has terminated.

Technically, maxillary surgery is feasible when the permanent maxillary second molars are completely erupted. The vital question that remains to be answered, however, relates to whether or not growth of the maxilla is impaired by maxillary surgery during adolescence. Our preliminary results with total maxillary osteotomies to reduce facial height in adolescents have not shown a discernible adverse effect on facial growth. In such individuals the bite has remained closed even though the maxilla has continued to grow postoperatively. Patients who have been operated on as early as ages 12 and 13 have shown continued, apparently synchronous facial growth without recurrence of the open bite. Clearly, however, these results are preliminary, for the progress of only a relatively small number of individuals has been followed, and for less than 5 years. Latent vertical facial growth may yet become problematic and cause undesirable vertical and anteroposterior changes.

Familiarity with the growth and development pattern of the individual with a skeletal anterior open bite deformity, as well as with its clinical manifestations, is essential to effective correction. In the majority of such patients, the vector of maxillary and mandibular growth has a clockwise rotational component downward and backward.[4, 22] Clinically, this manifests as anterior open bite with increased anterior vertical facial height, a retropositioned mandible, and Class II or Class I malocclusion. By clinical examination and monitoring of facial growth by sequential cephalometric radiographs, it is possible to demonstrate the dominant vector of growth in early adolescence. Vertical facial growth frequently continues until after age 20. Shortening the facial height by maxillary surgery in such individuals has had only positive effects — closure of the open bite and forward and upper movement of the retropositioned mandible. If maxillary growth is "frozen" by surgery, this might actually be an asset to the individual who has this type of vertical jaw dysplasia.

Significant forward mandibular growth in the individual with Class I or II anterior open bite is unlikely. On the other hand, latent horizontal mandibular growth may compromise and complicate treatment of the individual with Class III open bite. Freihofer has shown that postoperative anteroposterior growth of the mandible played an important role in a large number of clinically unacceptable late results after ramus osteotomies in adolescence. The osteotomies had no discernible influence on the growth of the mandible.[15] Longitudinal growth studies of individuals with the long face syndrome are needed to provide guidance in planning the timing and sequence of treatment for individuals with this type of dentofacial deformity.

The psychologic effect of excessive vertical facial growth during adolescence can be very significant to the individual who experiences it. The surgeon must weigh the advantages of early correction against the possibility of latent mandibular growth after surgical correction by total maxillary osteotomy. When early surgical treatment is indicated because the occlusal and esthetic deformity is clinically significant and there are psychologic implications, both surgeon and patient must be aware of potential hazards and the possible need for secondary surgery.[15]

A retrospective study of surgical and orthodontic methods of treating open bite deformities reveals that multiple factors are indeed responsible for the poor results achieved in treating such individuals. Latent vertical facial growth, biomechanical factors associated with operating in the ramus (the "wrong jaw"), and limitations of orthodontic mechanics have each been responsible for many of the compromised results and failures in treating open bite deformities. The recent introduction of new techniques of maxillary and mandibular surgery for treatment of patients with dentofacial deformities has opened up many new possibilities for treating individuals who have received orthodontic treatment without surgery. When the surgeon or orthodontist evaluates an individual who has received previous orthodontic treatment, with or without a preconceived surgical plan, treatment is planned in a systematic manner after a comparative evaluation of pretreatment and post-treatment clinical records.

New therapy is programmed to achieve optimal function, facial esthetics, and stability. The best possible tooth-to-tooth, tooth-to-bone, and bone-to-bone relationships are accomplished by surgery and orthodontics. In some cases treatment may have already been completed and the orthodontic appliances removed. A retrospective analysis of the pretreatment and post-treatment records will reveal whether or not the orthodontic treatment has displaced teeth relative to their supporting bone to the extent that stability, function, or esthetics is compromised. Indeed, treatment in some cases will have resulted in probable occlusal instability of unknown proportions. If this is suspected, the wisest therapy may involve removing the appliances to permit occlusal relapse. After the teeth have assumed a more stable relationship within the next 6 to 12 months, new records are taken and therapy is planned to achieve optimum stability, function, and esthetics. At this time it may be necessary to reverse the results of treatment that was previously aimed at treating a skeletal problem by worsening the dental compensations that were already present before treatment was ever started. Such "reverse orthodontics" will necessitate rebanding the teeth or continuing orthodontic treatment if appliances are still in place. The goal will be to relate the teeth of each arch properly to their supporting bone, disregarding the occlusion, which will be corrected grossly by surgery and detailed by postsurgical orthodontic treatment.

In still other cases a retrospective analysis of pretreatment and post-treatment records may indicate that orthodontic therapy has been sound and designed to produce occlusal stability, but optimal facial appearance has not been achieved. In such cases the teeth are usually well related to their respective jaws and surgical treatment can be planned with minimal or no additional orthodontic treatment. On the basis of new treatment priorities, the maxilla, the mandible, or both are surgically repositioned to achieve optimum stability, function, and facial esthetics.

The case reports that conclude this chapter illustrate some of the many complications that may occur when skeletal open bite deformities are treated by orthodontics or by surgery in concert with orthodontics. Cases have been selected especially to demonstrate the great propensity for relapse following correction of such deformities by ramus osteotomies. Additionally, and perhaps more importantly, the results support the concept of using maxillary surgery to treat skeletal open bite and vertical maxillary excess deformities.

COMPLICATIONS

Surgical Complications

Several surgical procedures can be useful in management of open bite. Complications of all but one indicated surgical procedure are discussed in detail in the chapter in which a particular surgical technique is illustrated. For example, complications following total maxillary osteotomy, along with a more detailed description of the technique, are found in the chapter on maxillary excess (Chapter 8).

Complications of the Köle Procedure

The Köle procedure for elevating the mandibular incisor segments is the only surgical technique for which details of surgery are not presented in another chapter. Two major complications may arise following the Köle mandibular subapical osteotomy. These are:

1. *Loss of tissue related to inadequate postsurgical blood supply.* The anterior segment is pedicled to the lingual tissue, which provides an adequate blood supply. Experimental studies support the clinical experiences which indicate that this blood supply to the bone and teeth is adequate qualitatively.[8] There have been instances of inadvertent tearing of the lingual mucosa when the dento-osseous segment was being manipulated into position. If all soft tissue is detached, a free graft is created. In these instances, loss of tooth and bone may follow. Careful surgical planning and technique can prevent this unfortunate occurrence.

2. *Prolonged paresthesia of the lower lip.* Since the cuts used in the Köle procedure normally are superior to the mental foramen, damage to the nerve should occur only if there are anatomic variations and if adequate care was not taken to identify the position of the foramen and course of the neurovascular bundle. If the planned bone cuts will violate the integrity of the inferior alveolar nerve, the neurovascular bundle should be moved aside at the initial stages of surgery to allow the indicated bone cuts and preserve the sensory supply.

Both these complications with the Köle procedure are rare. Wound dehiscence may occur if wound closure is not meticulous. Proper pressure dressings placed immediately after surgery will help to avoid this problem. When dehiscence does occur, the wound must be irrigated daily until it heals secondarily. Scar revision and secondary vestibuloplasty with skin or mucosal grafting at a later date may be necessary in some instances.

Instability after Correction of Open Bite

Relapse into open bite following orthodontic correction has been a major problem in postadolescent patients with skeletal vertical dysplasias. Latent vertical growth of the face is now known to be a major factor in this type of relapse. Even in a relatively mild case of open bite, it may not be possible to obtain a stable and satisfactory result orthodontically until the patient is in the late teens because of the pattern of late vertical growth. Tongue activity (i.e., "deviate swallowing") is frequently cited as the cause of relapse, but this is of less importance than the pattern of vertical growth. Orthodontic treatment for open bite in such patients may have to continue much longer than with other problems, or, more practically, a final phase of orthodontic treatment may be required in the late teens. If anterior teeth are extruded orthodontically in young adults (after the late growth has occurred), the result is usually stable. In severe problems, however, the entire maxilla should be repositioned superiorly by Le Fort I osteotomy. This is usually an uncomplicated procedure because the teeth have already been aligned by the previous orthodontic treatment.

Relapse has also been observed in patients whose open bite was treated surgically. Patients who have had mandibular advancement with counterclockwise rotation of the anterior segment show a tendency toward relapse. This is discussed in some detail in Chapter 10 (Mandibular Deficiency). Such relapse is definitely related to the mandibular musculature and to incompletely understood biomechanical factors influencing the elevator muscles and the suprahyoid muscle group. These muscles tend to displace the proximal portion of the mandible during fixation and lead to an altered resting position after fixation is released. Relapse tendencies are the major reason that mandibular advancement to close an open bite usually is contraindicated unless it is done concomitantly with superior repositioning of the maxilla.

High-angle mandibular deficiency with vertical maxillary excess and open bite is the dentofacial deformity that manifests the greatest propensity for relapse following mandibular advancement. Marked skeletal relapse has been demonstrated when this deformity is corrected solely by mandibular advancement. In contrast, excellent skeletal stability has been demonstrated when lower anterior facial height is reduced by maxillary surgery. The complex and variable dentoskeletal and facial characteristics of many individuals with high-angle mandibular deficiency and vertical maxillary excess with open bite necessitate simultaneous superior repositioning of the maxilla and mandibular advancement. Their basic dentofacial deformity can be corrected to achieve occlusal and facial harmony by this type of bimaxillary surgery. Superior repositioning of the maxilla allows for autorotational advancement of the mandible that decreases the degree of absolute advancement and counterclockwise rotation of the distal segment. Mechanical efficiency of the mandibular elevators is improved subsequent to this type of bimaxillary surgery. In general, stability following simultaneous superior repositioning of the maxilla and advancement of the mandible with sagittal split ramus osteotomies has been good, with minimal to moderate tendency to relapse. Mandibular stability is primarily a function of the magnitude of advancement and the degree of superior movement of the maxilla. Careful assessment of the changes in the biochemical system must be included in the design of any operation to correct high-angle mandibular deficiency with open bite. Biomechanical influences are important considerations for the clinician as he plans surgical procedures to correct skeletal open bite deformities. Biomechanical alterations are easily predicted by simulating the planned changes with repositioning of acetate overlays. (See Chs. 6 and 8.)

As a general rule, anterior alveolar osteotomy to extrude maxillary or mandibular incisor segments produces remarkably stable correction of open bite.[6] If the open bite problem is caused by infraeruption of maxillary incisors, extrusion of the anterior segment is almost always stable. Similarly, if the problem is lack of eruption of mandibular incisors, the Köle procedure or mandibular subapical osteotomy to elevate the anterior segment gives very stable results. These procedures do not alter the posterior vertical dimension, and therefore the mandibular musculature has minimal effect on the result. In patients with anterior open bite, the tongue fills the anterior opening prior to surgery. After surgery, the tongue almost always adapts to the changed anatomic situation created by closing the open bite. In effect, the "tongue thrust" disappears. Tongue function and position adapt to the position of the teeth in the great majority of patients. In patients who do show relapse tendencies, the physiologic response will include an altered rest position of the mandible and further eruption of posterior teeth in addition to forward positioning of the tongue. An alteration in overall vertical dimension seems always to accompany relapse into open bite.

Clinicians have been concerned that when posterior maxillary intrusion is carried out alone or as part of total maxillary osteotomy, re-elongation of the maxillary teeth would occur because the operation would create excessive freeway space. In the initial reports of Schuchardt's posterior maxillary osteotomy, relapse tendencies were observed. Recent experience suggests that a key factor in superior movement of the maxilla is free mobility achieved by completely sectioning bony areas that would impede movement of the maxilla, so that the segment can be intruded freely without displacing the condyles from their articular fossae. When this is done, there seems to be little or no postoperative tendency toward re-elongation. When a total maxillary osteotomy is carried out the postsurgical tendency is toward slight continued intrusion of the maxilla, not extrusion. This can be exacerbated by pressure on the mandible in the fixation phase, such as would be produced by vertical-pull extraoral force or by a cervical collar. Accordingly, these retention techniques are contraindicated unless it is desired to intrude the maxilla further during the fixation phase or when ramus osteotomies are combined with maxillary surgery. A new rest position of the mandible typically is established after surgery, so that freeway space is not excessive.

When there is immediate reoccurrence of open bite at the time of release from intermaxillary fixation after posterior or total maxillary osteotomies (without mandibular surgery), it must be assumed that the maxillary surgery was not executed properly. Most frequently, at the time of surgery, the vertical dimension of the posterior maxilla was not adequately reduced. In an attempt to close the mandible into the planned intermaxillary relationship, the surgeon forces the mandible closed until the margins of the osteotomized maxilla are juxtaposed. As a consequence the mandibular condyles are distracted from the mandibular fossae. Later, when intermaxillary fixation is discontinued and the mandibular condyles are reseated into their normal spatial relationship in the articular fossae, there is immediate "relapse" and the open bite becomes manifest. Reoperation to *properly reduce the vertical dimension of the maxilla* is the only predictable means of managing this postoperative complication. A comprehensive review of complications and stability after maxillary surgery is discussed in Chapter 8.

Since physiologic adaptation seems to be the key to stability after correction of open bite, it is informative to look at what currently is known about the incidence of relapse. If patients treated by mandibular advancement are excluded, it appears that 85 to 90 per cent of patients with open bite can be treated surgically without concern for postoperative instability. This means that relapse will be a factor in 10 to 15 per cent. Relapse in these patients will be manifested as some combination of (1) instability of jaw or dentoalveolar segments, (2) alterations in the resting position of the mandible, with increase in posterior vertical dimension, and (3) repositioning of incisor teeth. The first problem can be prevented by choosing the appropriate surgical procedure and achieving technical success with it. If the second and third problems arise, surgical freeing of the tongue by a deep lingual frenectomy or reduction of the size of the tongue should be considered. Routine tongue surgery is not indicated.

Nasal Obstruction

Altered airflow patterns may be produced by distortion of the internal anatomy of the nose (i.e., the nasal septum). Such changes may cause the surface of the turbinate mucosa, where the air-flow is most rapid, to dry out. This serves as a stimulus for hypertrophy, and the turbinates become enlarged. Anosmia or diminution of the sense of smell occurs because the inspired air cannot reach the olfactory area.

Recurrent sinusitis and anosmia are two important complications of nasal obstruction that can occur after superiorly repositioning the maxilla without proper reduction of the nasal septum. When conservative means of treatment have failed, relief of symptoms can be achieved by septoplasty or submucous resection of the septum combined with turbinectomy.

When a patient who has had maxillary surgery complains of a persistently blocked nose, colds that "never go away," headaches above, behind, and between the eyes, aching in the cheeks and the bridge of the nose, and postnasal drip, the patient probably has maxillary sinusitis. If the nasal airway has been properly managed during and after surgery, postoperative nasal obstruction and maxillary sinus infection are rare (see Chapter 8). Indeed, many patients breathe better through their nasal passages after surgery than before. Airflow studies by Turvey and Hall corroborate these clinical observations.[10]

Postoperative Soft-Tissue Changes

The surgeon must exercise restraint about reoperating on a patient who appears to have a compromised esthetic result in the early postoperative period. Soft-tissue swelling, shortening and inversion of the lips, and lip incompetence are usually transient and may obscure the result that will ultimately be achieved after the interocclusal splint is removed, swelling diminishes, and the enveloping soft tissues assume their final drape. Stretching exercises of the lips and perioral musculature in the early postoperative period (after healing of the soft tissues and margins) may decrease the time necessary for this to take place. The final result may not be realized for 6 to 12 months after surgery because of a number of subtle changes in the soft tissues and settling of the repositioned maxilla.

CASE STUDIES

CASE 13–1 (Fig. 13–22)

M. H., a 38-year-old woman, sought correction of an open bite and treatment to decrease the prominence of her maxillary incisor teeth. The following problem list was evolved after appropriate clinical and laboratory examinations.

PROBLEM LIST

Esthetics

FRONTAL. Excessive exposure of the maxillary anterior teeth and gingiva in function and repose; bulging of upper eyelids caused by excessive periorbital fat and redundant skin.

PROFILE. Excessive lower-third facial height; retropositioned mandible; contour-deficient–chin; lip incompetence (10 mm); prominent nasal dorsum.

Cephalometric Analysis

1. Vertical maxillary excess — excessive lower anterior facial height.
2. High mandibular plane angle (SN–Mp 45°); 9° ANB difference.
3. Proclination of mandibular incisors with minimal labial alveolar bone support.
4. Proclination of maxillary anterior teeth.

Occlusion

DENTAL ARCH FORM. *Maxillary arch form:* tapered and constricted maxillary arch with high palatal vault and moderate curvature of occlusal plane.

DENTAL ALIGNMENT. Mandibular left lateral incisor missing as a result of a previous extraction; crowded and rotated maxillary and mandibular anterior teeth; blocked-out mandibular canine teeth.

DENTAL OCCLUSION. Class II malocclusion with 12-mm overjet and anterior open bite; excessive curvature of maxillary and mandibular occlusal planes.

TREATMENT PLAN

1. Reposition maxilla 6 mm superiorly in four segments to
   a. Shorten lower anterior face height.
   b. Reduce lip incompetence by shortening the skeletal framework.
   c. Decrease vertical exposure of teeth relative to length of upper lip.
   d. Allow autorotation of mandible, close open bite, and achieve maxillomandibular harmony.
   e. Correct maxillary constriction by surgical expansion of the maxilla in four segments.
2. Augment the contour-deficient–chin and deep labiomental fold with an alloplastic implant (Proplast).

Text continued on page 1140

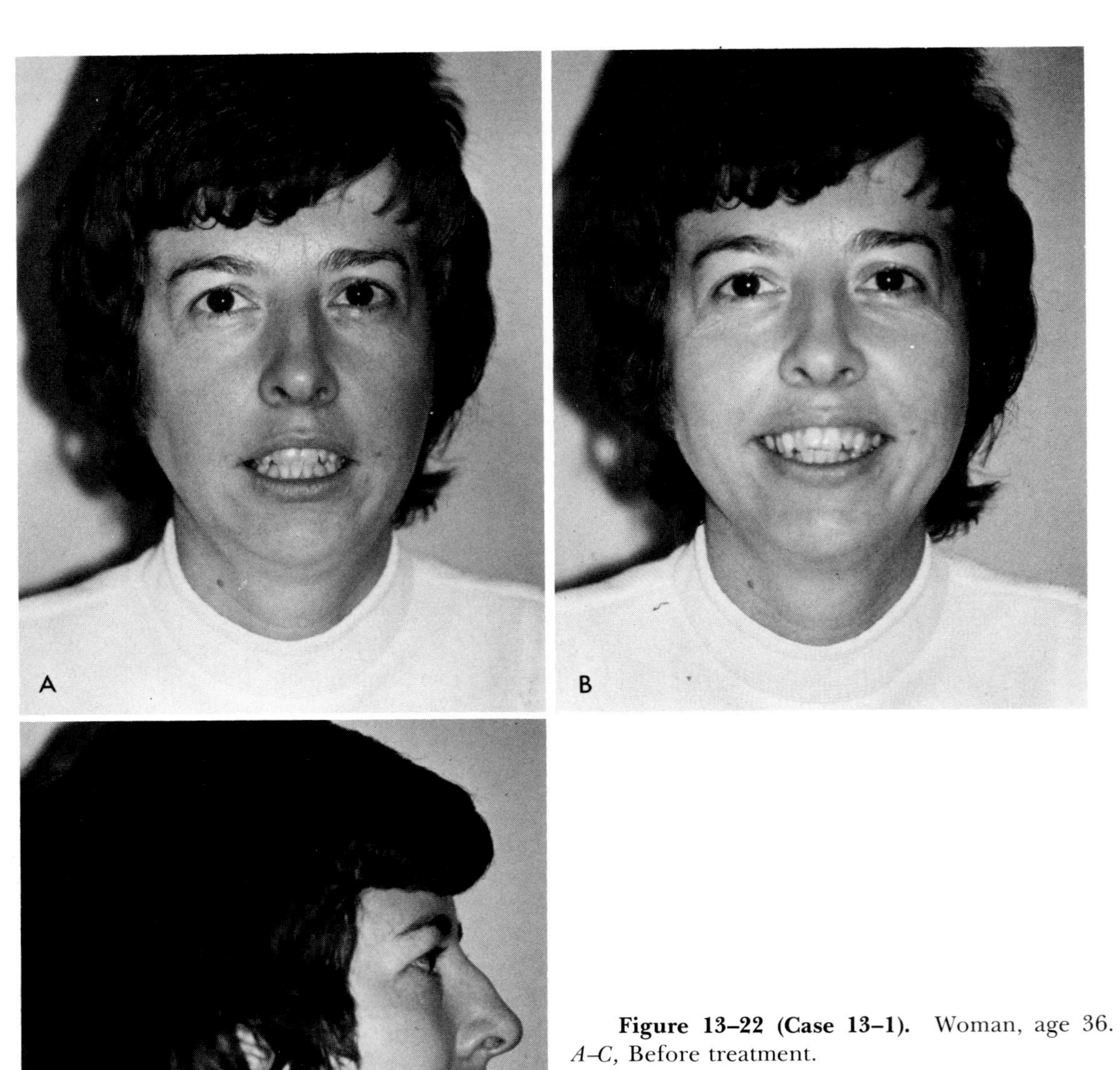

Figure 13–22 (Case 13–1). Woman, age 36. *A–C,* Before treatment.

Legend continued on the opposite page

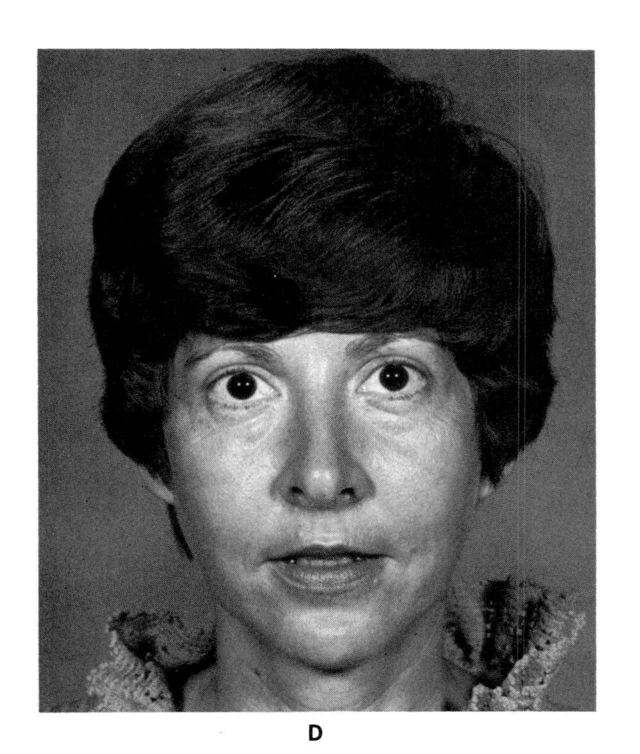

D

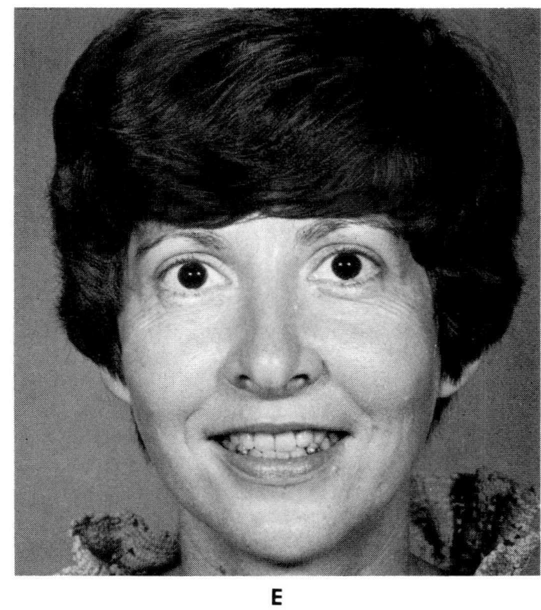

E

F

Figure 13–22 *Continued.* *D–F,* After maxillary surgery.

Illustration continued on the following page

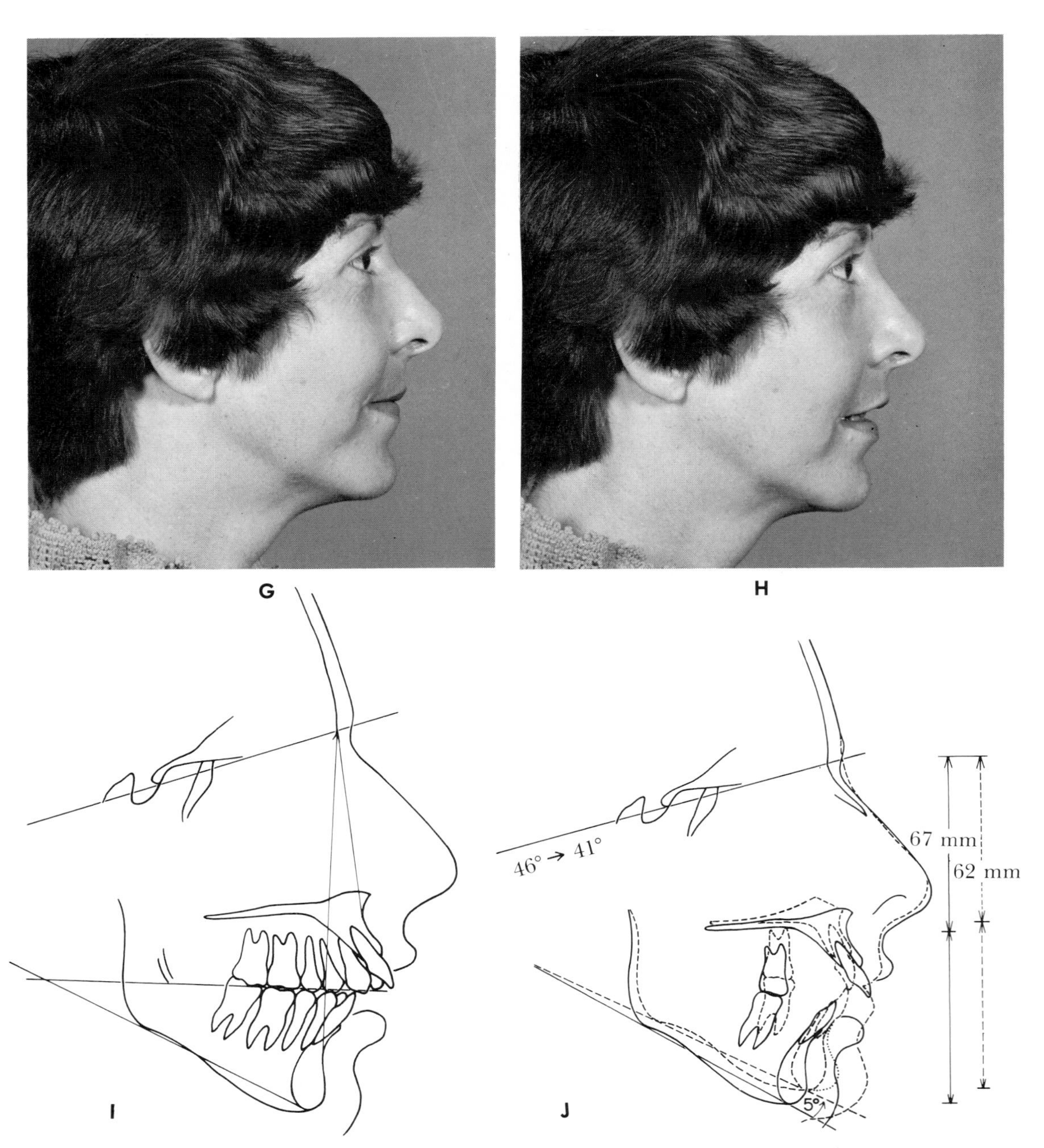

Figure 13–22 *Continued.* *G* and *H,* At end of treatment after rhinoplasty and genioplasty. *I,* Cephalometric tracing before treatment (age 36 years, 6 months). *J,* Composite cephalometric tracings before (*solid line,* age 36 years, 6 months) and after (*broken line,* age 38 years, 2 months) treatment, showing 5-mm reduction in anterior facial height.

Legend continued on the opposite page

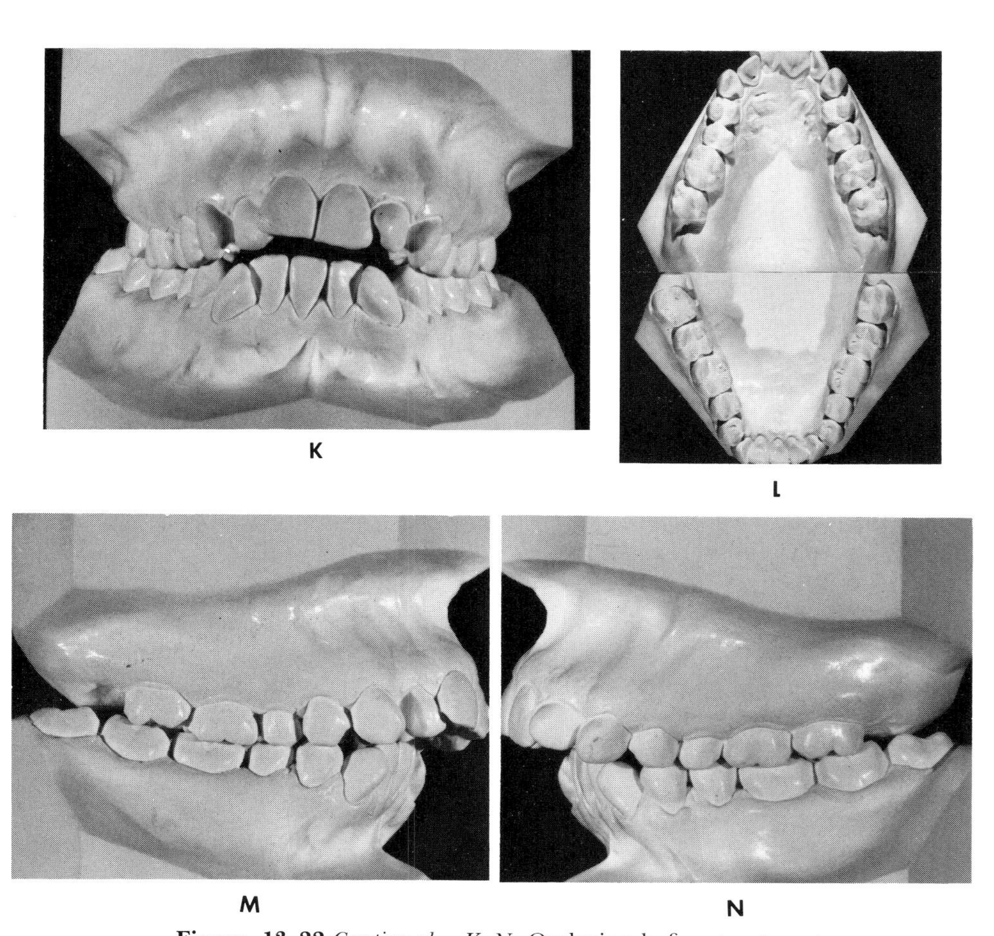

Figure 13–22 *Continued.* *K–N,* Occlusion before treatment.

Illustration continued on the following page

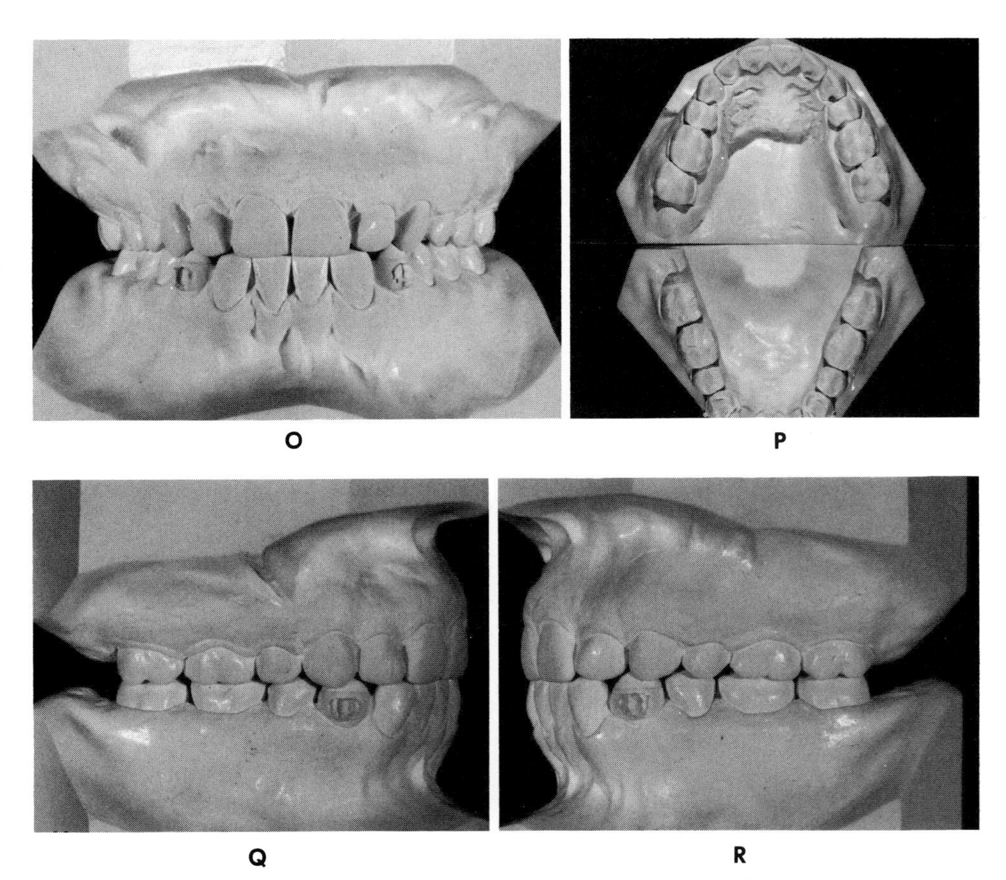

Figure 13–22 *Continued.* *O–R*, Post-treatment occlusion.

Illustration continued on the opposite page

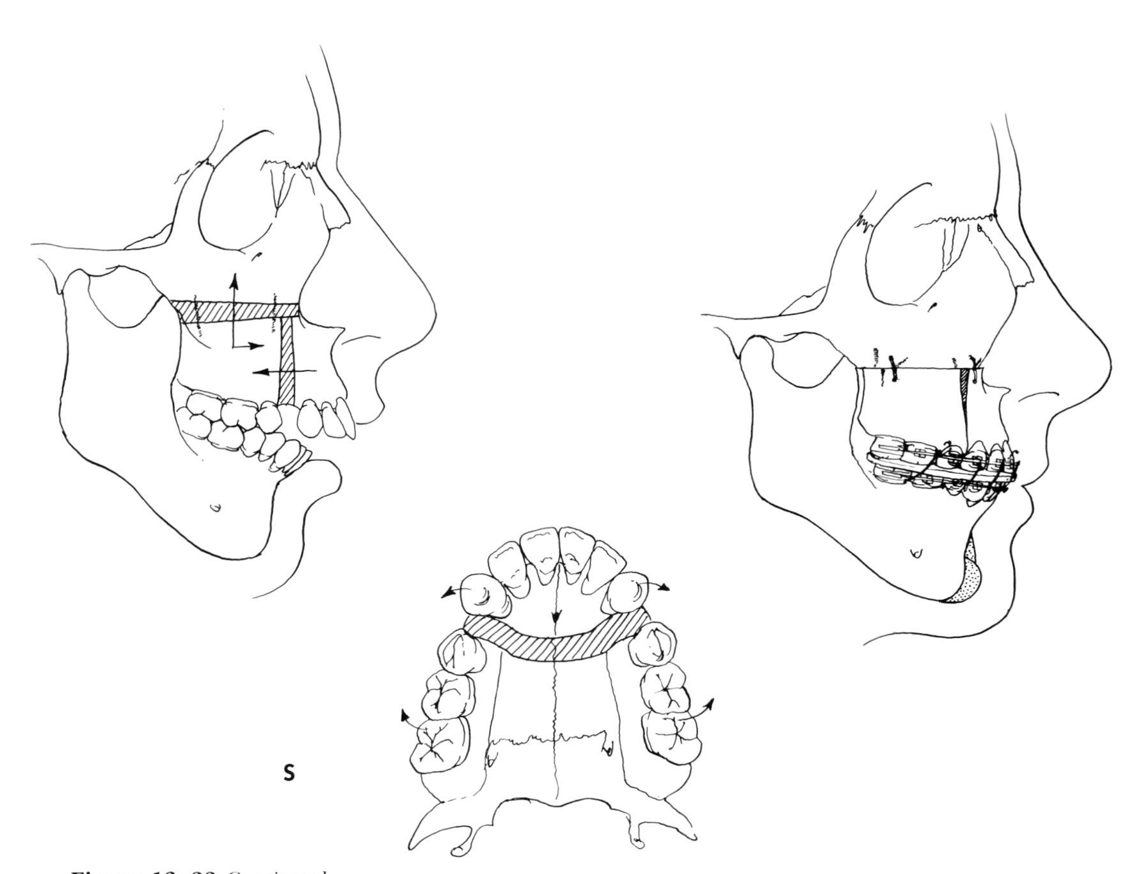

Figure 13–22 *Continued.*

S, Plan of surgery: four-piece Le Fort I osteotomy to reposition maxilla superiorly to close open bite, reduce lower anterior facial height and incisor tooth exposure, and level maxillary occlusal plane; anterior maxilla retracted; posterior maxilla advanced; intermolar and intercanine width increased; augmentation of chin with Proplast; 1st premolar teeth extracted to facilitate orthodontic alignment of crowded and rotated anterior teeth.

3. Reduce the prominent nasal dorsum by rhinoplasty.
4. Correct bulging upper and lower eyelids by blepharoplasties.
5. Treat patient orthodontically to
   a. Improve angulation of mandibular incisors after extracting the mandibular right lateral incisor.
   b. Relieve arch crowding and correct malalignment of teeth after extracting maxillary first premolars, one lower incisor, and mandibular third molars.
   c. Coordinate the dental arches.

FOLLOW-UP

Subjective

The patient's postoperative course was uncomplicated and associated with virtually no pain or swelling.

Objective

Since the mandibular left lateral incisor had been previously extracted, the mandibular right lateral incisor was also extracted to eliminate a 6-mm discrepancy in the mandibular arch. The canines were "slenderized" and reshaped to accommodate the positions of the missing lateral incisors.

Extraction of the maxillary first premolars provided space to align the six anterior teeth before surgery. During the 6-month period of presurgical orthodontic treatment, no attempt was made to level the maxillary occlusal plane or to close the extraction spaces completely. The anterior maxilla was surgically raised 6 mm and split into two segments to increase the intercanine width; the posterior portions of the maxilla were simultaneously repositioned superiorly 7 mm and advanced 2 mm to achieve a Class I canine and molar relationship, close the open bite, and achieve anteroposterior, horizontal, and vertical maxillomandibular harmony. Final cephalometric records showed a reduction in ANB, SN–MP, and lower-facial height. Final space closure and alignment were achieved by orthodontic means within 12 months after surgical intervention. Occlusal balance and facial harmony were achieved by the combined efforts of three disciplines over a period of 20 months.

Overall esthetic balance was gained by dimensional changes in the nose and chin associated with maxillary, nasal, and chin surgery. In addition, esthetic balance between the relaxed upper lip and incisors, a virtually unchanged nasolabial angle, and improved nose-lip-chin harmony were achieved by superior repositioning of the maxilla. With the lips sealed, there was mild contraction of the perioral musculature because of the 4-mm residual lip incompetence.

COMMENT

The extent of augmentation and the permanence of the improvements in the labiomental fold area with an alloplastic material are as yet poorly documented. Quantitative long-term follow-up studies are needed to document the effectiveness of the procedure and to determine whether or not resorption of bone encasing the incisal roots occurs as a result of pressure to the overlying implant and soft tissue. To date, the esthetic results have been good and there has been minimal discernible resorption below the implants in other patients whose cases have been followed for 2 years after surgery.

During the original case analysis, extraction of lower premolars in addition to one central incisor was considered to facilitate greater retraction of the lower anterior teeth. Such a treatment plan would have been potentially more problematic and would have necessitated mandibular advancement; the patient preferred the plan of treatment which included maxillary surgery, genioplasty, and rhinoplasty.

Surgeons: Larry Snider, Denver, Colorado; William H. Bell, Dallas, Texas.
Rhinoplasty and blepharoplasties: Jack Gunter, Dallas, Texas. *Orthodontist:* R. G. Alexander, Arlington, Texas.

CASE 13–2 (Fig. 13–23)

This young woman, L. P., was initially seen at age 13 years 8 months with chief complaints of protruding maxillary teeth and an inability to incise and chew properly. Full-face examination indicated facial features to be symmetric with the exception of the nasal tip, which veered to the right. The patient had incompetent lip closure and approximately 7 mm of central incisor crown exposed at rest; at a broad smile approximately 5 mm of gingival tissue was noted. The lower third of the face was excessively long and was retrognathic in appearance. Facial examination in profile indicated that the patient had a severely retruded mandible, increased lower-facial height, poor chin-neck contour, and incompetent lip closure with a deeply rolled lower lip.

Intraorally, poor oral hygiene and generalized dental caries with severe involvement of the mandibular first molars were noted. The patient's dentition was in a Class II relationship, with 7 mm of overjet and a 5-mm anterior open bite. Retained maxillary deciduous canines were still present and the permanent successors were blocked out of the arch. Both the maxillary and mandibular arches had 4 to 5 mm of crowding.

Cephalometric analysis supported the clinical impression of severe mandibular retrognathism, open bite, excessive lower anterior facial height, and maxillary and mandibular dental protrusion.

INITIAL PROBLEM LIST

1. Poor oral hygiene and dental caries with possible pulpal involvement of the mandibular first molars.
2. Severe mandibular retrognathism and retrogenia.
3. Anterior open bite.
4. Maxillary and mandibular protrusion.
5. Transverse maxillary deficiency.
6. Vertical maxillary excess.
7. Deviation of nasal tip and septum.
8. Maxillary and mandibular crowding.
9. Retained primary maxillary canines.

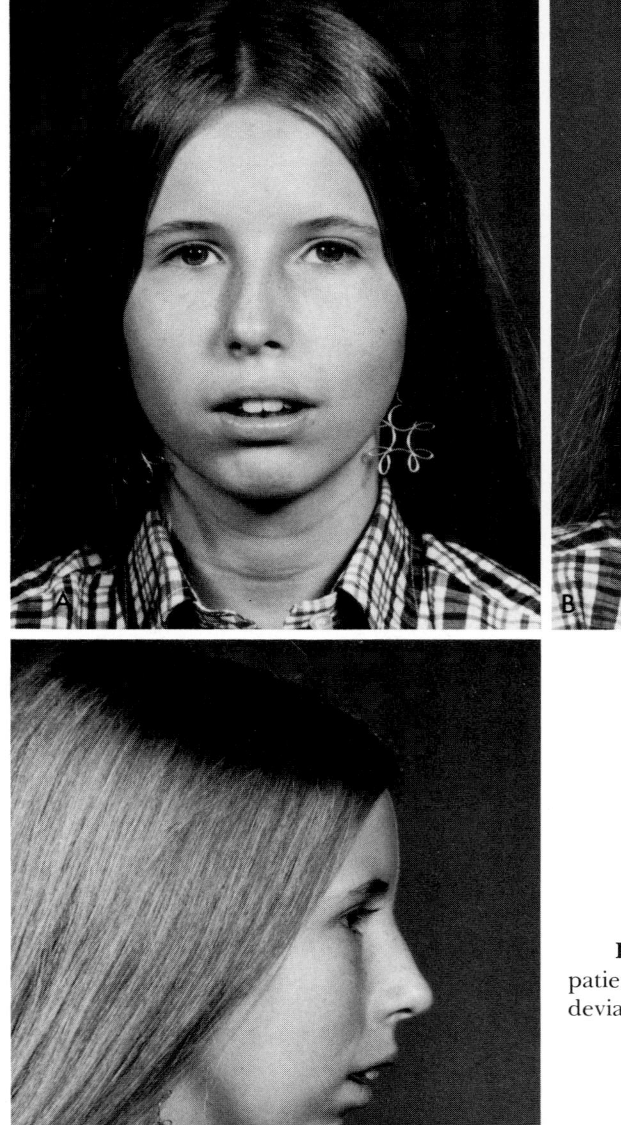

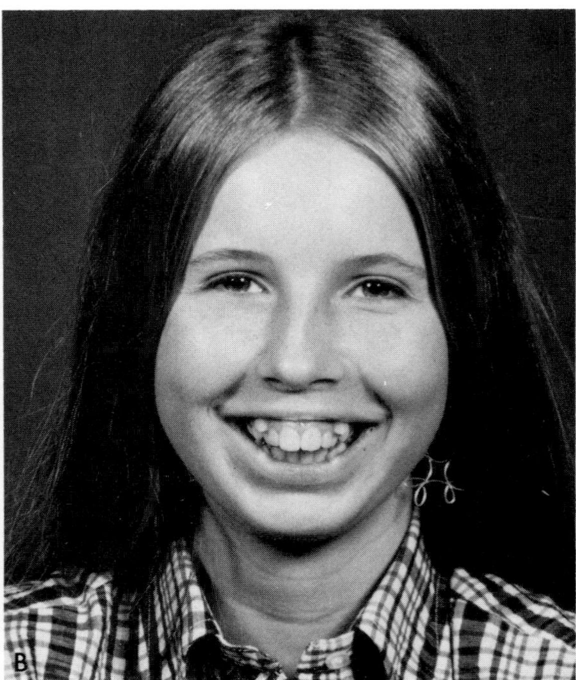

Figure 13–23 (Case 13–2). *A–C,* At age 13, the patient illustrates lower-face deficiency and nasal tip deviation.

Legend continued on the opposite page

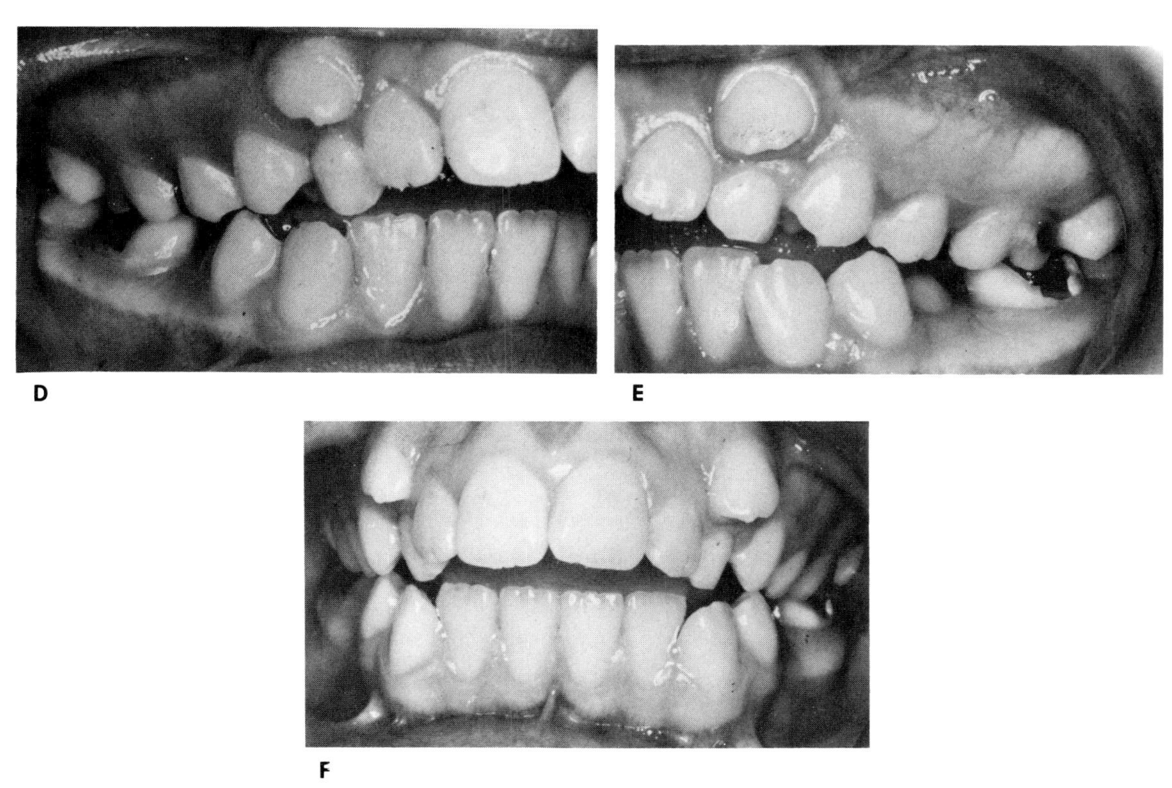

Figure 13–23 *Continued. D–F,* Occlusal views. The Class II molar and cuspid relationship, retained deciduous canine teeth in the maxilla, crowding in both the maxillary and the mandibular arches, anterior open bite, and 7 mm of overjet are apparent.

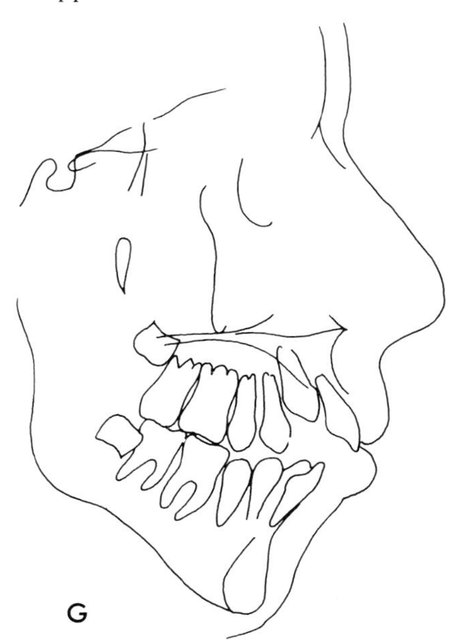

G, Cephalometric tracing confirms mandibular retrognathism, open bite, increased lower anterior facial height, and maxillary and mandibular dental protrusion.

Illustration continued on the following page

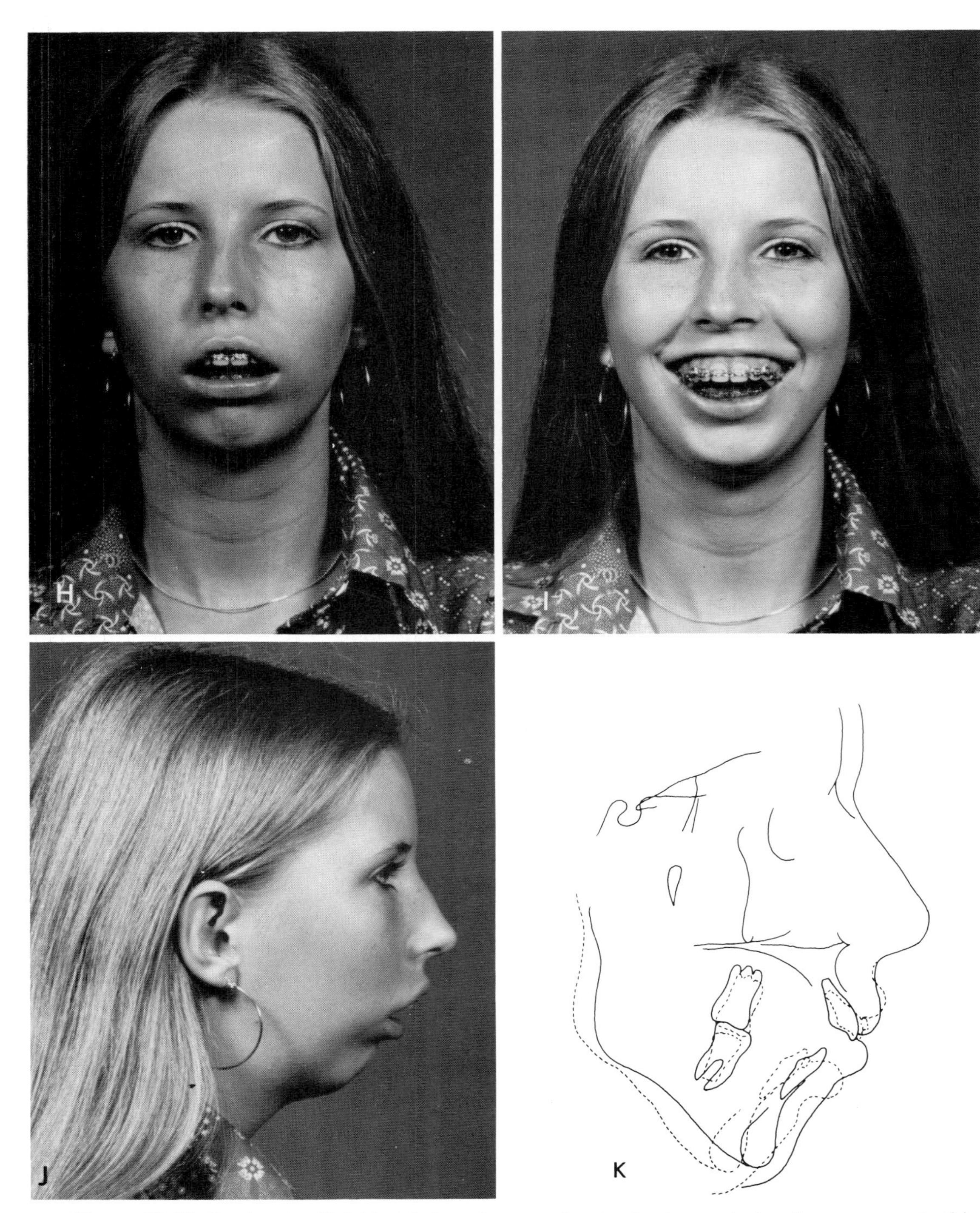

Figure 13–23 *Continued.* *H–J,* Facial views 2 years after beginning orthodontic treatment. At this time, the patient displays vertical maxillary excess, as is evidenced by her lip incompetence, inadequate lip coverage over the maxillary anterior teeth, long face, inferiorly and posteriorly rotated mandible, and constricted alar bases. Notice the excessive exposure of tooth and gingiva at broad smile and the severe retrogenia. *K,* Cephalometric tracings taken 3 years apart illustrate the changes that have taken place as a result of continued vertical maxillary growth and orthodontic preparation.

Legend continued on the opposite page

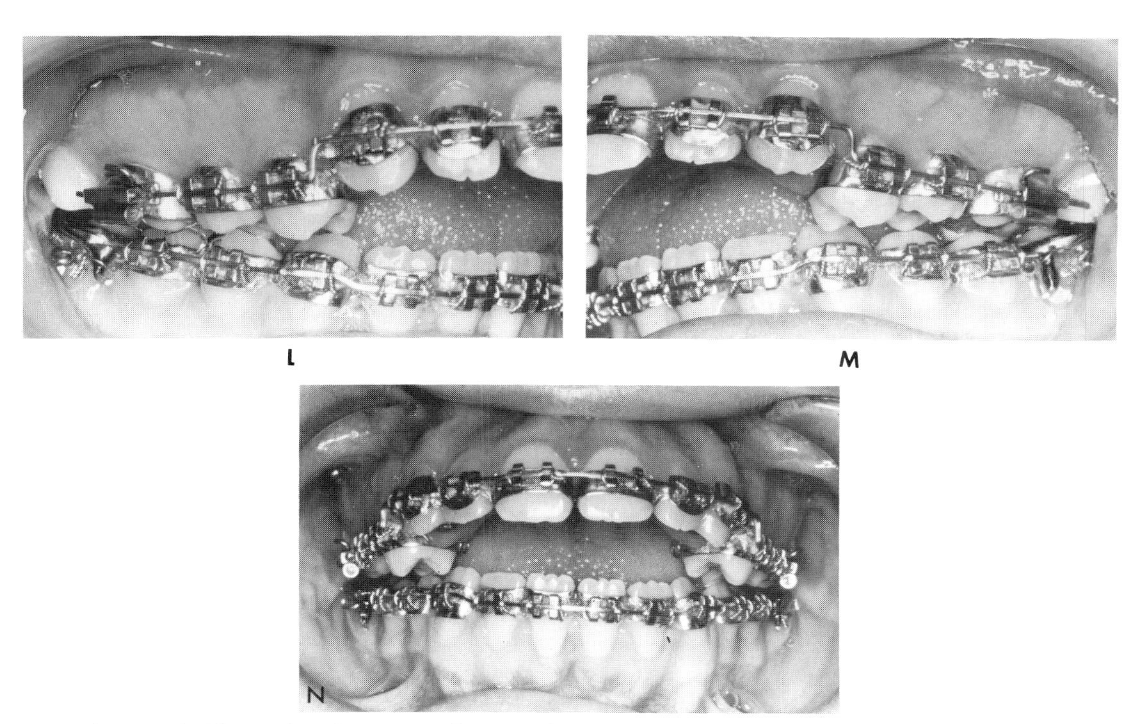

Figure 13–23 *Continued.* *L–N,* The step between the maxillary canines and premolars was maintained with each successive wire change. Note that no attempt has been made to level the maxillary arch since it is planned to move the arch in three different segments.

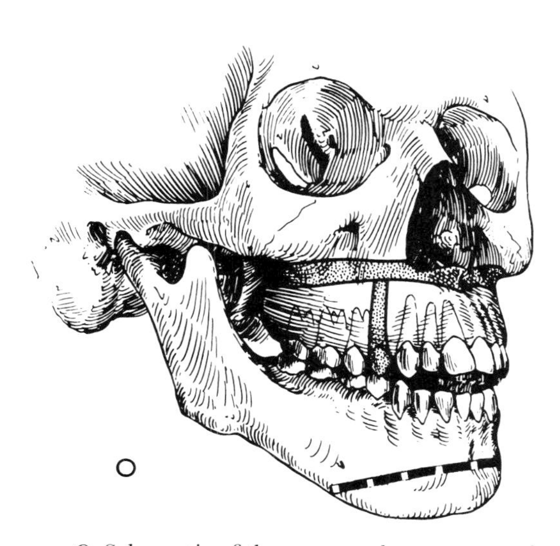

O, Schematic of the proposed surgery: total maxillary segmental osteotomy in three pieces, removal of 1st premolar teeth, and pedicled advancement genioplasty.

Illustration continued on the following page

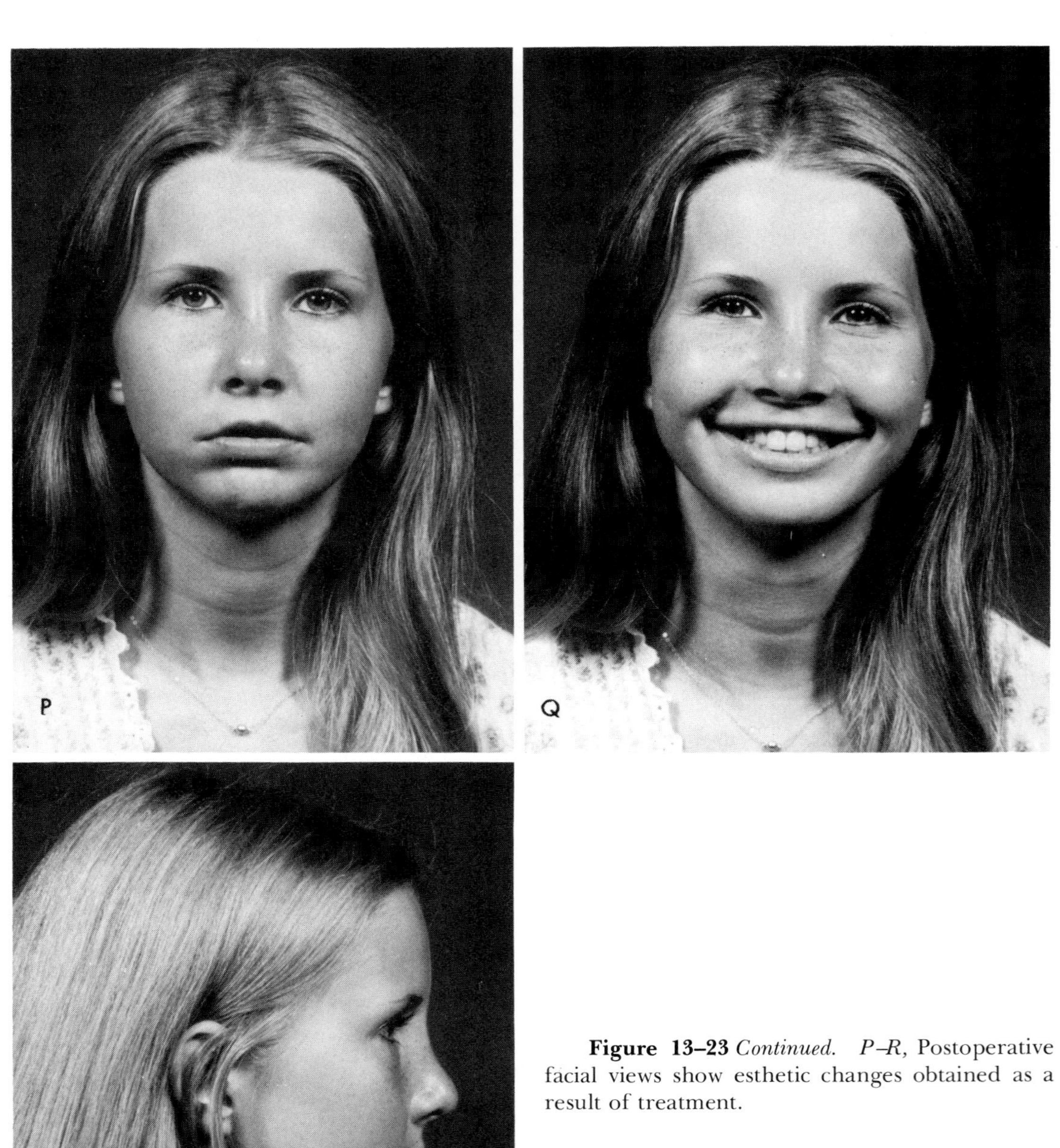

Figure 13–23 *Continued.* *P–R,* Postoperative facial views show esthetic changes obtained as a result of treatment.

Legend continued on the opposite page

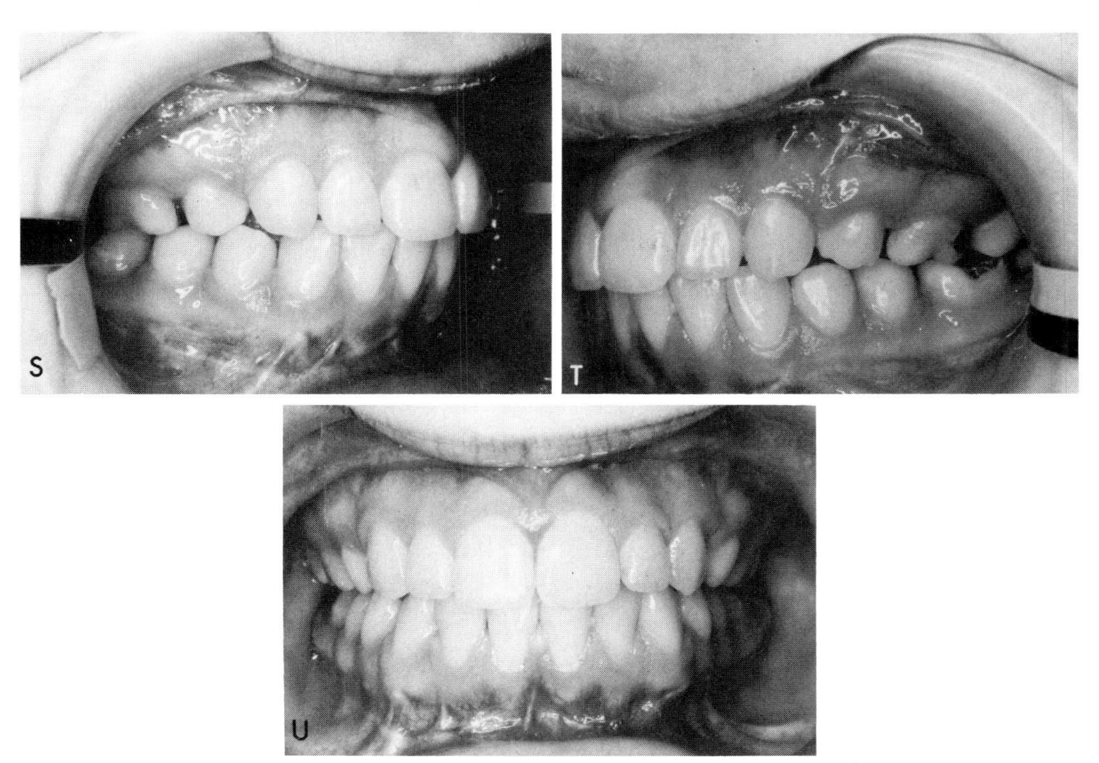

Figure 13–23 *Continued.* *S–U*, Occlusal views show that the Class I cuspid relationship and the closed bite have remained stable for 28 months.

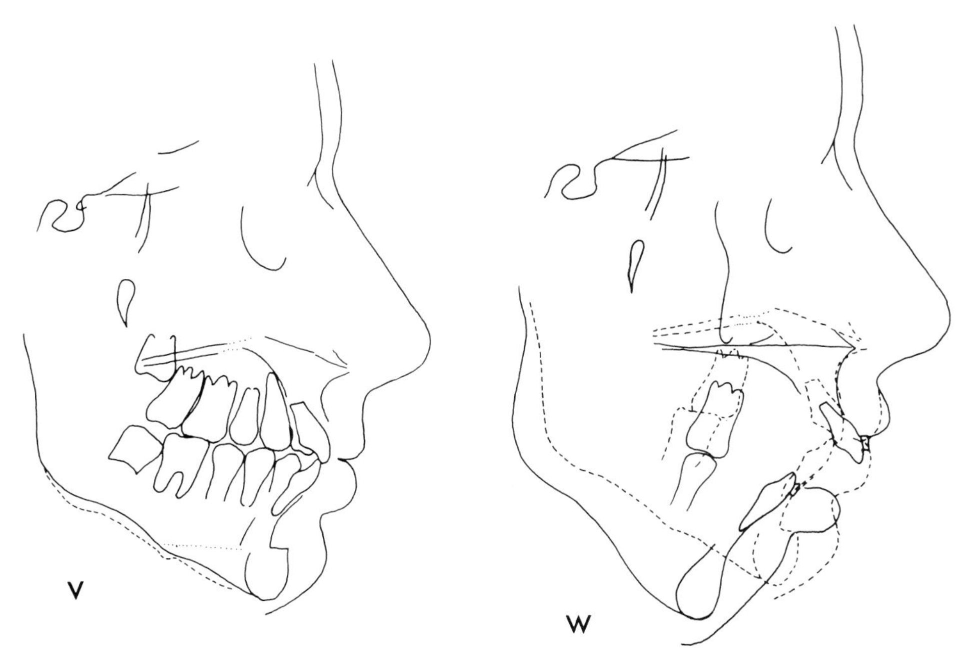

V and *W*, Postoperative cephalometric tracing *(V)* and superimposed immediate presurgical and postsurgical tracings *(W)* demonstrate the changes effected by total maxillary segmental osteotomy in three pieces and a genioplasty.

INITIAL TREATMENT PLAN

After consideration of the patient's concerns and the initial problem list, a treatment plan was formalized. It was decided that the patient's esthetic and malocclusal problems could best be managed by a combination of orthodontic and surgical treatment. The initial phases of treatment involved

1. Elimination of dental caries; oral hygiene instruction; and extraction of both mandibular first permanent molar teeth and maxillary deciduous canine teeth.
2. Full banding of both arches.
3. Closure of the mandibular extraction sites and correction of the crowding and rotations.
4. Rapid maxillary expansion and alignment of the maxillary arch.
5. Mandibular advancement and genioplasty.
6. Rhinoplasty.

The goal of the initial orthodontic treatment was to position the teeth in the maxilla and mandible to allow for maximum mandibular advancement. The maxilla was treated without extraction of permanent teeth and the mandibular extraction space was closed by retracting the anterior teeth. Rapid maxillary expansion was performed to allow the dental arches to be compatible in the transverse dimension when the mandible was advanced into a Class I canine relationship. It was realized that following initial orthodontic treatment, the patient's teeth would not occlude as well as they had previously and that facial esthetics would become worse. The patient was warned to expect these changes.

FINAL PROBLEM LIST

Approximately two years later, progress records were taken and reviewed. At that time, the mandibular extraction spaces were closed and the maxillary width was compatible with the mandibular width when the canines were articulated in a Class I relationship. Pertinent findings at this time included

1. Vertical maxillary excess.
   a. Lip incompetence.
   b. Inadequate lip coverage over the maxillary anterior teeth.
   c. Long face.
   d. Inferiorly and posteriorly rotated mandible.
   e. Constricted alar bases.
2. Horizontal maxillary excess evidenced by the protruded upper lip.
3. Retrogenia.
4. Anterior open bite.

Superimposed cephalometric radiographs indicated that the mandible had rotated open further during the initial orthodontic treatment. This occurred partially because of the orthodontic mechanics used and partially because of the continued vertical maxillary development.

FINAL TREATMENT PLAN

At this point, the treatment plan was revised to include

1. Total maxillary segmental osteotomy in three segments with superior repositioning.

2. Removal of maxillary first premolar teeth bilaterally and surgical retraction of the anterior segment.
3. Augmentation genioplasty.
4. Completion of orthodontic alignment.
5. Rhinoplasty.

The surgical plan was revised for several reasons. In our experience, mandibular advancement with counterclockwise rotation, when used to close an open bite, is an unstable procedure. In addition, mandibular advancement would do nothing to correct the maxillary vertical or horizontal excess. The proposed maxillary surgical plan would allow for correction of both the vertical and horizontal maxillary excess. The mandible would rotate closed, shortening the face and closing the bite. The genioplasty would provide good lower-face projection and enhance facial balance. Cephalometric predictions indicated that this treatment plan would result in closure of the open bite, correction of maxillary protrusion, improvement of the tooth-to-lip relationship, and shortening of the anterior facial height.

At this point, the maxillary arch wire was changed to maintain the step that existed between the canine and premolar teeth bilaterally. The step was maintained in each successive arch wire change, as wire size progressed to .021 by .025. An ideal .021 by .025 mandibular arch wire with fixation lugs was also placed approximately one month prior to surgery.

After this short period of preparation, the surgery was performed. The maxillary first premolar teeth were removed and the entire maxilla was mobilized. An ostectomy was performed through the extraction sockets and across the palate and nasal floor to facilitate posterior repositioning of the maxillary anterior segment. The anterior segment was superiorly repositioned 5 mm, while each of the posterior segments was independently moved 9 mm superiorly. A 10-mm advancement pedicled genioplasty was performed simultaneously.

Presurgical nasal examination revealed the presence of septal deviation and exostoses. Quantitative nasal airflow studies confirmed high airway resistance. At the time of maxillary surgery, a portion of the nasal septum was resected and the nasal crest of the maxilla was reduced to allow passive superior repositioning of the maxillary segments. In addition, the posterior segments were cut in the maxillary sinus and not the nasal floor. This permitted elevation of the segments with minimal change in the position of the nasal floor. The maxillary segments were positioned by means of an occlusal splint that had been fabricated on mock surgery models. These segments were stabilized by the placement of a .021 by .025 arch wire, which had also been prefabricated to fit the mock surgery models. The stabilized segments were then directly wired into place with interosseous wires. Intermaxillary fixation was applied for 6 weeks, and active orthodontic treatment was re-instituted shortly afterwards. Six months later, a rhinoplasty was performed.

Eighteen months after surgery, facial and occlusal photographs demonstrated the improved esthetic and functional results that were obtained from the combined orthodontic-surgical treatment of this patient. Preoperative and postoperative clinical and quantitative evaluation of nasal airway resistance revealed an increased capacity for nasal respiration as a result of the elimination of the septal deviation and exostoses.

Overall management of this patient illustrates several important aspects of treatment. This patient's continued vertical maxillary growth during her initial stages of orthodontic treatment made her deformity worse and was an instigating factor in the alteration of her overall treatment plan. A well-balanced dentofacial team must be flexible enough to change treatment plans in midcourse should problems be recognized that were not initially diagnosed or expected. Superior repositioning of the maxilla has proved to be a stable procedure for correction of this type of deformity. The procedure may be performed without adversely affecting nasal airflow; on the contrary, improvement may occur if the nasal septum and floor of the nose are judiciously managed.

Surgeon: Timothy A. Turvey, Chapel Hill, North Carolina. *Orthodontist:* David J. Hall, Chapel Hill, North Carolina.

CASE 13–3 (Fig. 13–24)

C. C., a 15-year-old female student, was initially seen in March 1974. All study parameters showed the typical facial esthetics commonly associated with a skeletal type of anterior open bite. The following problem list was evolved after appropriate clinical and laboratory examination.

PROBLEM LIST

Esthetics

FRONTAL. Excessive exposure of teeth and gingiva in repose and when smiling; lip incompetence as indicated by the 10-mm interlabial gap at rest.

PROFILE. Obtuse nasolabial angle; retropositioned mandible and contour-deficient chin; excessive anterior facial height.

Cephalometric Analysis

1. Excessive angulation of maxillary and mandibular incisors.
2. High mandibular plane angle.
3. Anterior open bite.
4. Excessive lower anterior facial height.
5. Supraeruption of mandibular incisors.
6. ANB difference 12°.

Occlusal Analysis

DENTAL ARCH FORM. Tapered and constricted maxillary arch with a high palatal vault.

DENTAL ALIGNMENT. Crowded and malaligned maxillary and mandibular anterior teeth.

DENTAL OCCLUSION. Full Class II canine and molar relationship with a 7-mm overjet and 5-mm anterior open bite.

Text continued on page 1157.

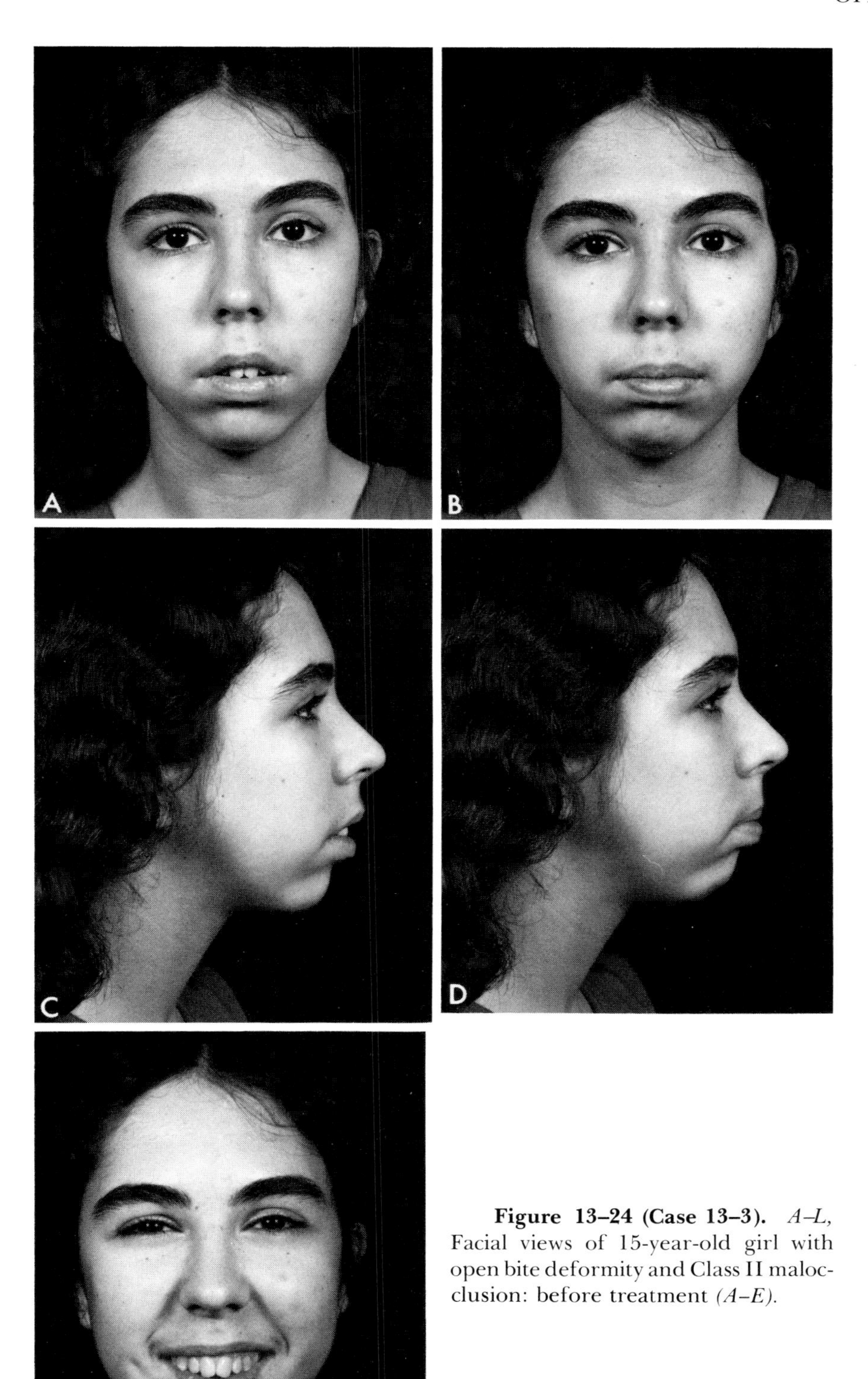

Figure 13–24 (Case 13–3). *A–L,* Facial views of 15-year-old girl with open bite deformity and Class II malocclusion: before treatment *(A–E).*

Illustration continued on the following page

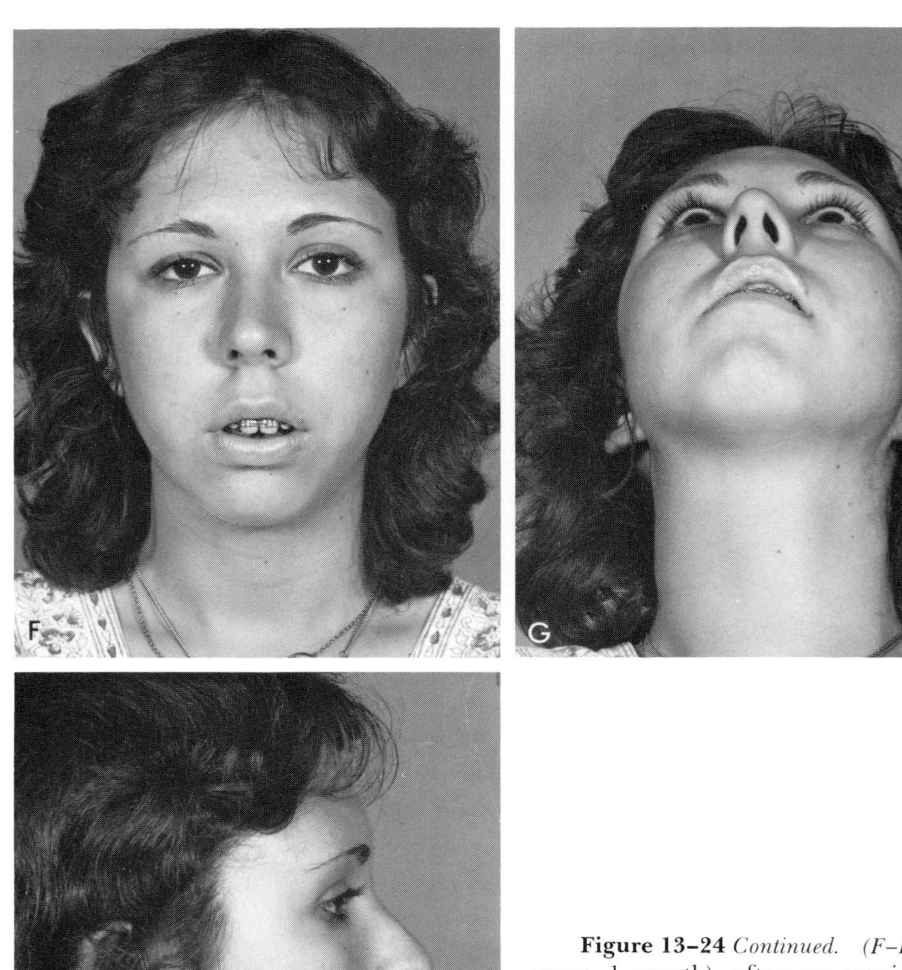

Figure 13–24 *Continued.* *(F–H)* (age 16 years, 1 month), after pre-surgical orthodontics.

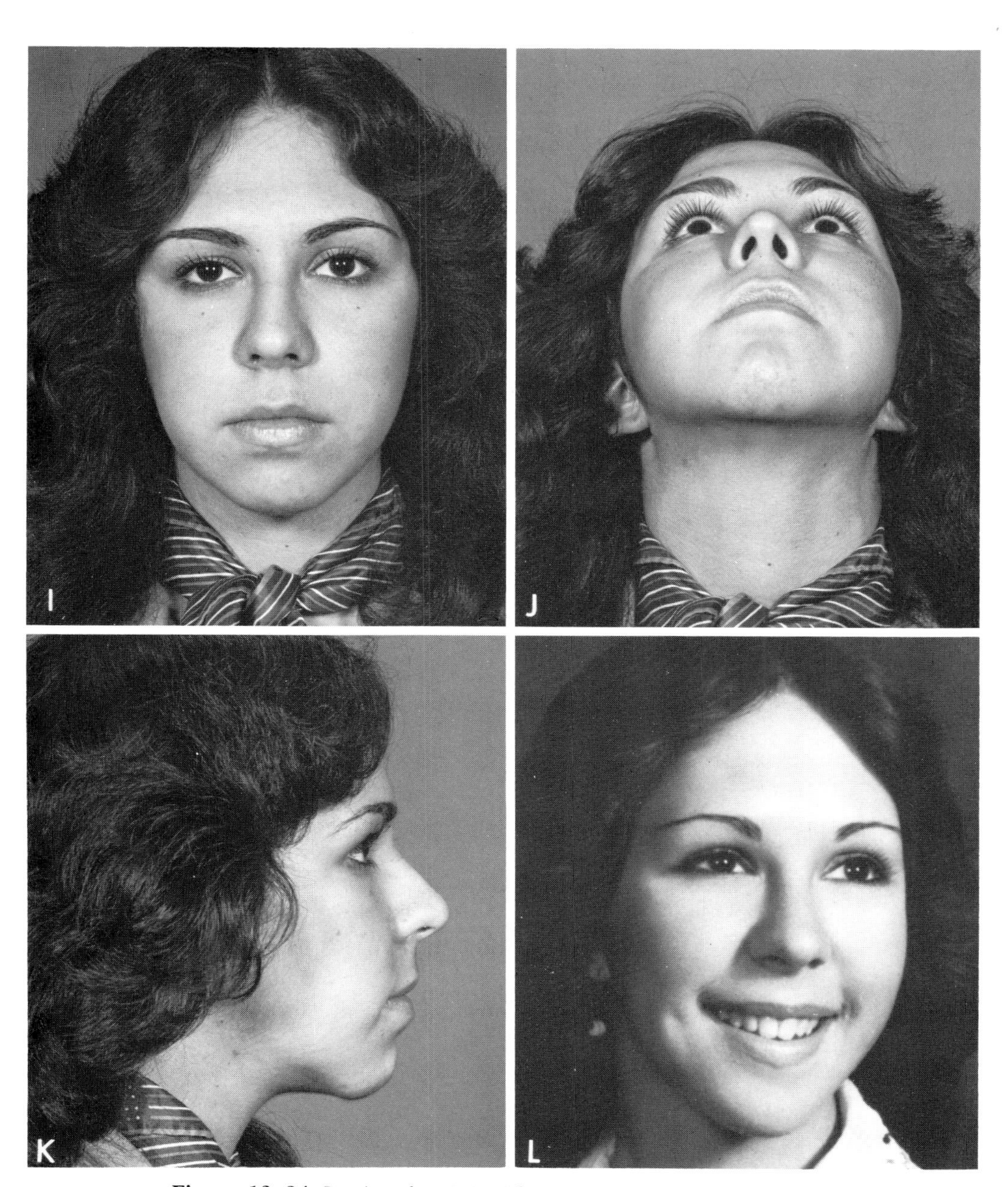

Figure 13–24 *Continued.* *(I–L)* After treatment (age 17 years).

Illustration continued on the following page

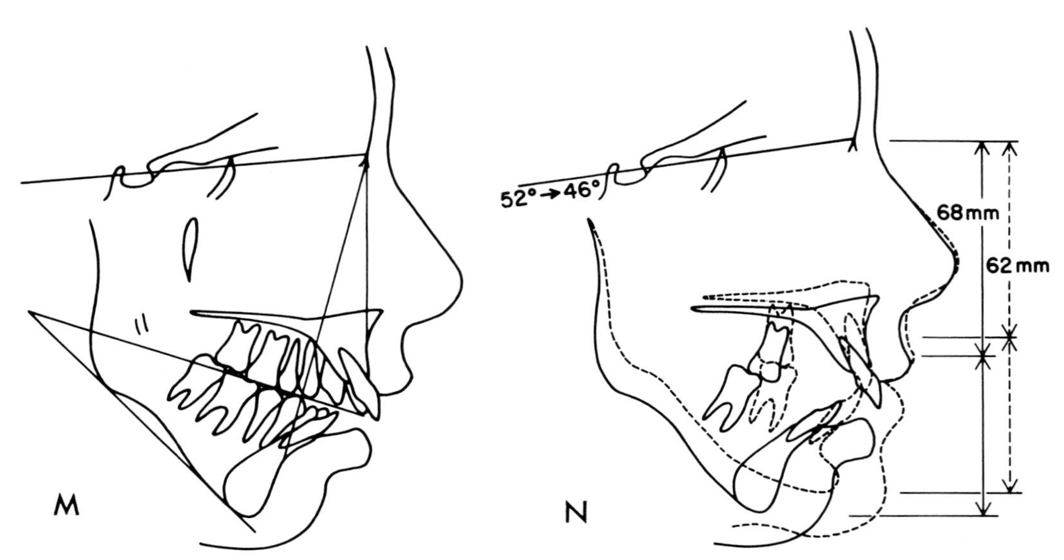

Figure 13–24 *Continued.* *M,* Cephalometric tracing before treatment (age 14 years, 10 months). *N,* Composite cephalometric tracings before (*solid line,* age 14 years, 10 months) and after (*broken line,* age 17 years) treatment show that maxilla was surgically repositioned superiorly and anteriorly; the mandible was surgically advanced into planned maxillomandibular relationship.

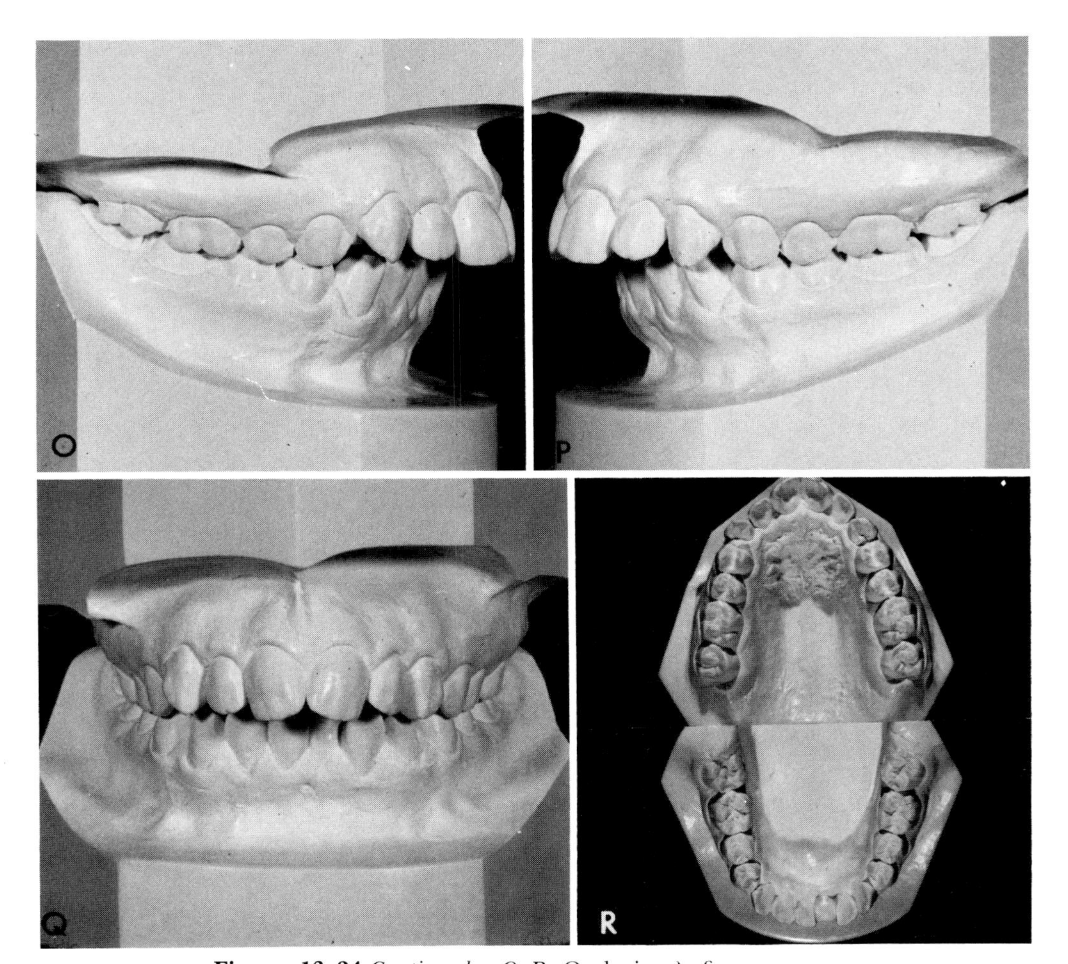

Figure 13–24 *Continued.* *O–R,* Occlusion before treatment.

Illustration continued on the following page

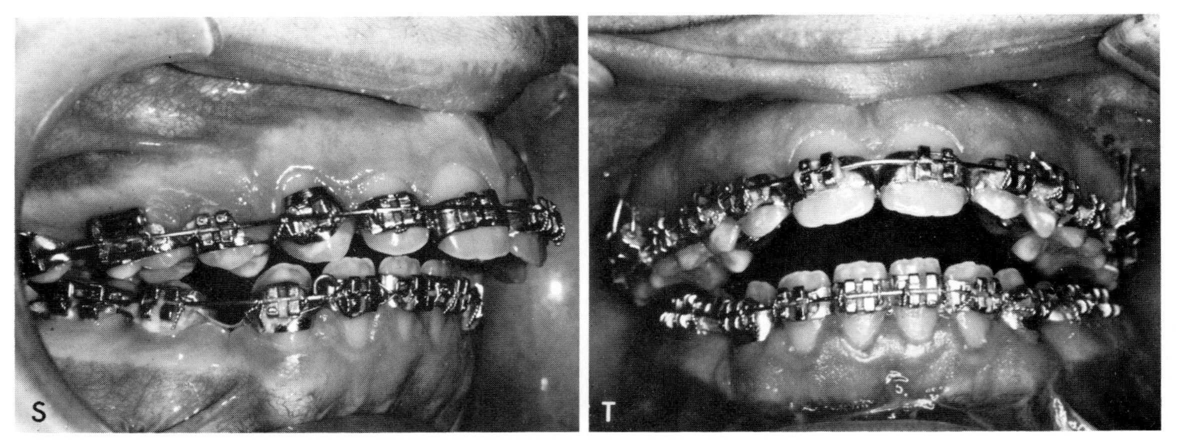

Figure 13–24 *Continued.* *S* and *T*, Occlusion after presurgical orthodontic treatment.

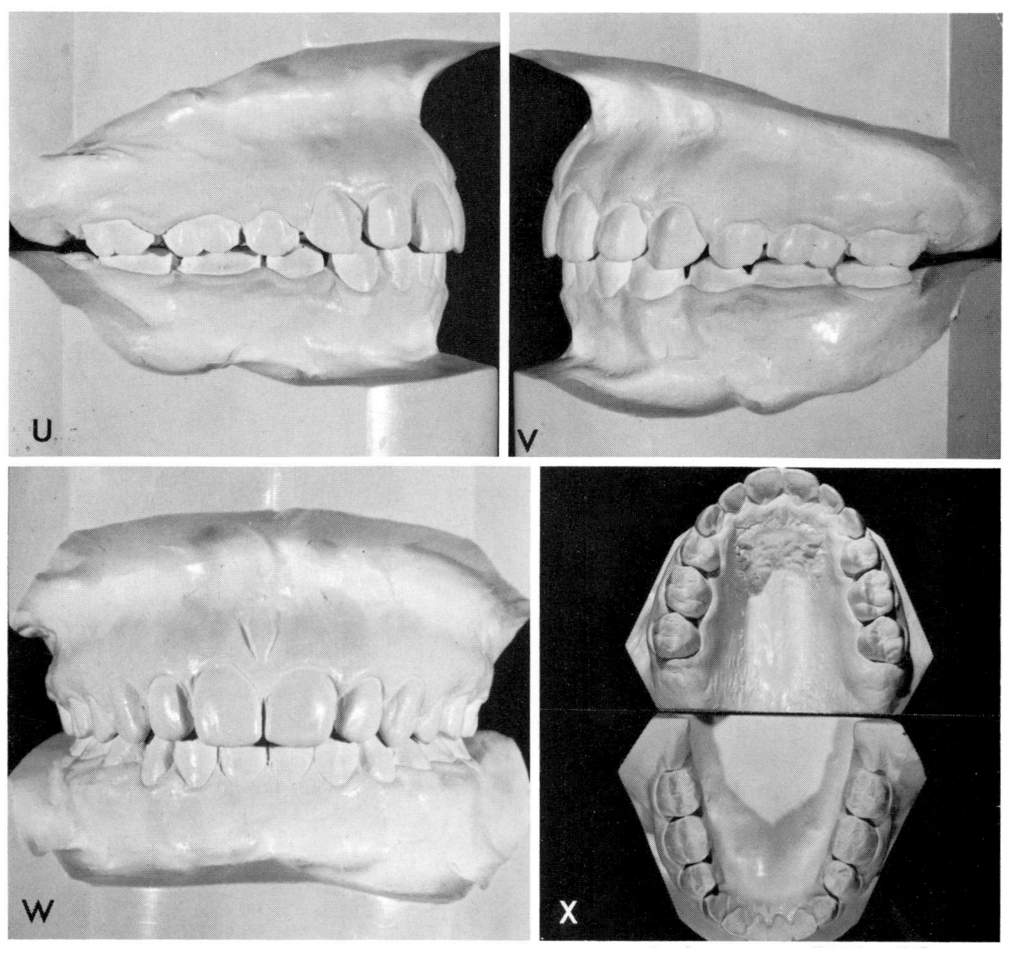

U–X, Occlusion immediately after orthodontic appliances were removed. A positioner was then worn 3 months to improve interdigitation of the maxillary and mandibular teeth.

Legend continued on the opposite page

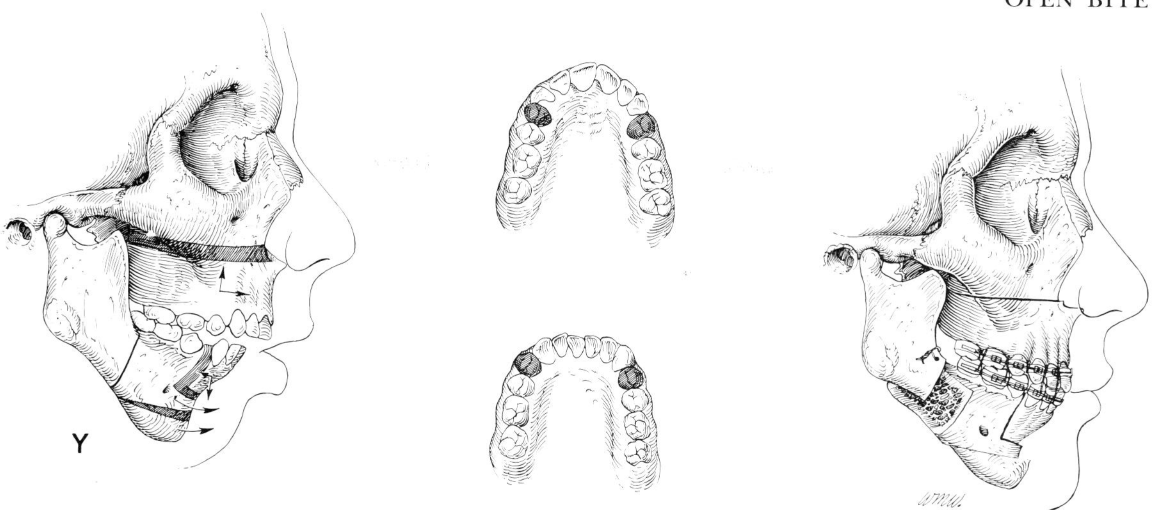

Figure 13–24 *Continued.* *Y*, Plan of surgery: Le Fort I osteotomy to reposition maxilla superiorly and anteriorly; mandibular subapical ostectomy to close residual extraction spaces and level mandibular occlusal plane; bilateral sagittal split ramus osteotomies to advance mandible into satisfactory maxillomandibular relationship; horizontal osteotomy of chin to increase chin prominence and decrease vertical height of mental symphysis. The 1st premolar teeth were extracted to facilitate orthodontic alignment of crowded and rotated anterior teeth.

TREATMENT PLAN

1. Reposition maxilla 6 mm superiorly and 4 mm anteriorly
   a. Reduce obtuseness of nasolabial angle and increase prominence of paranasal areas.
   b. Reduce exposure of teeth and gingiva.
   c. Shorten lower anterior facial height.
   d. Correct lip incompetence.
   e. Allow autorotation of the mandible and closure of open bite.
2. Advance the retropositioned mandible surgically to achieve maxillomandibular harmony.
3. Perform mandibular subapical ostectomy to lower supererupted mandibular anterior teeth.
4. Augment contour-deficient chin by genioplasty.
5. Treat patient orthodontically to
   a. Reduce angulation of maxillary and mandibular incisors after extracting maxillary and mandibular first premolars.
   b. Relieve arch irregularities.
   c. Coordinate the dental arches.

FOLLOW-UP

The postoperative course was uncomplicated, and the patient experienced relatively little pain. There were transient right and left hypoesthesias of the lower lip and chin following genioplasty and mandibular subapical osteotomy; normal feeling returned within 3 weeks of surgical intervention.

During the 12-month period of presurgical orthodontic treatment no attempt was made to level the maxillary and mandibular occlusal planes completely, close the mandibular extraction spaces, or correct the open bite. The surgical procedures were performed in two stages. (1) By Le Fort I osteotomy, the maxilla was raised 5 mm and advanced 4 mm; simultaneously, the mandibular anterior teeth were lowered 4 mm and retracted 3 mm by subapical osteotomy. After bilateral sagittal vertical ramus osteotomies, the mandible was advanced 13 mm into a Class I occlusal relationship with the maxilla. (2) Two months later, the chin was augmented and shortened by genioplasty. Final space closure and alignment of the arches was completed in another 8 months by orthodontic treatment. Post-treatment dental symmetry, normal overbite and overjet, and esthetic balance between the nose, lips, teeth, and chin were attained after approximately 24 months of treatment.

Cephalometric analysis after surgical intervention revealed minimal positional change of the surgically repositioned maxilla or mandible over an 18-month period of follow-up. Two different appliances were used after mandibular advancement to hyperextend the neck muscles and stabilize the repositioned mandible. A modified Pitkin collar was worn night and day, except when eating, for the first 5 months after surgery. Thereafter, a soft cervical collar was worn at night only for another 4 months. At the time of mandibular advancement, the digastric, geniohyoid, and mylohyoid muscle insertions were detached in an attempt to minimize the tendency for skeletal relapse.

CASE 13–4 (Fig. 13–25)

C. J., an eleven-year-old, moderately retarded girl, was seen in consultation with an orthodontist for treatment of her severe anterior open bite. The following problem list and treatment plan were developed in conjunction with the patient's orthodontist and general dentist.

PROBLEM LIST

Esthetics

FRONTAL. Excessive exposure of maxillary teeth when smiling and in repose; 11-mm interlabial space with lips relaxed; interalar width and intercanthal distances similar; slight paranasal deficiency.

PROFILE. Short and taut-appearing upper lip with slightly obtuse nasolabial angle; retropositioned mandible.

Cephalometric Analysis

1. SNA 86°; SNB 74°; ANB 12°.
2. High mandibular plane angle: SN–Go–Gn 41°.
3. Long lower anterior facial height.
4. Retropositioned mandible.
5. Vertical maxillary excess.
6. Skeletal-type anterior open bite.
7. Proclination of maxillary anterior teeth.

Text continued on page 1162

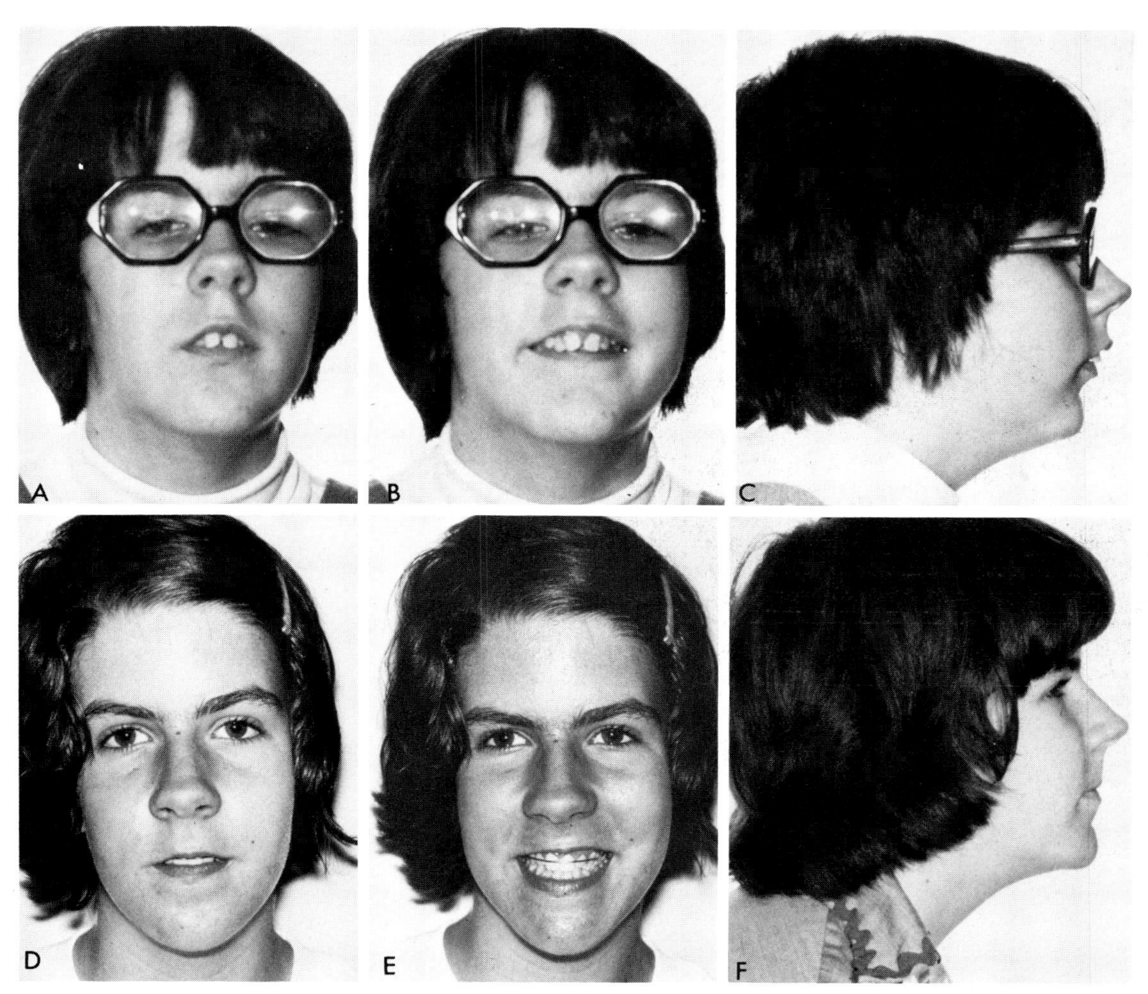

Figure 13–25 (Case 13–4). *A–F,* Facial appearance of 9-year-old girl with severe open bite associated with vertical maxillary excess and mandibular deficiency. *A–C,* Before treatment. *D–F,* After treatment.

Illustration continued on the following page

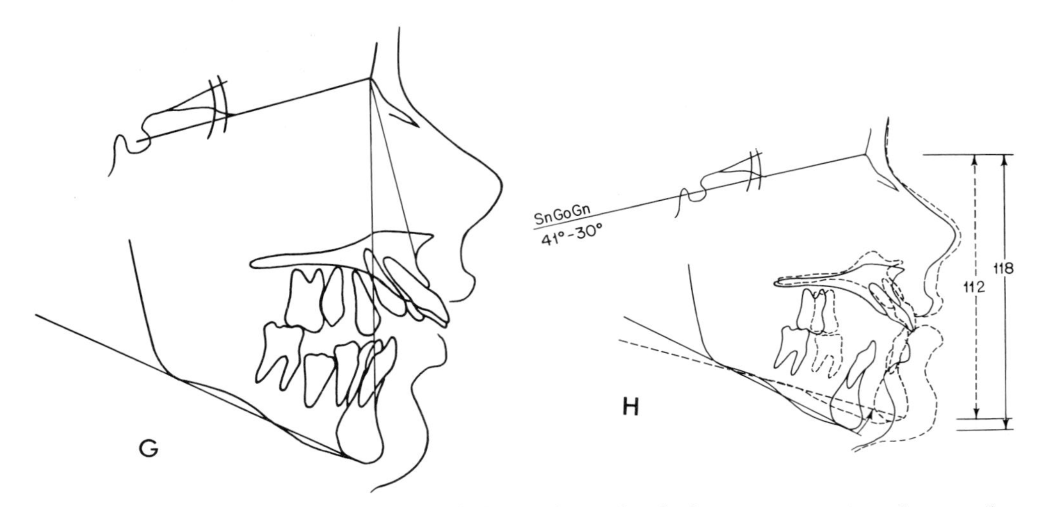

Figure 13–25 *Continued.* *G,* Cephalometric tracing before treatment (age 9 years, 5 months). *H,* Composite cephalometric tracings before (*solid line,* age 9 years, 5 months) and after (*broken line,* age 11 years, 5 months) treatment. Tracings show superior and anterior movements of the maxilla. The mandible was advanced by surgery to achieve maxillomandibular harmony.

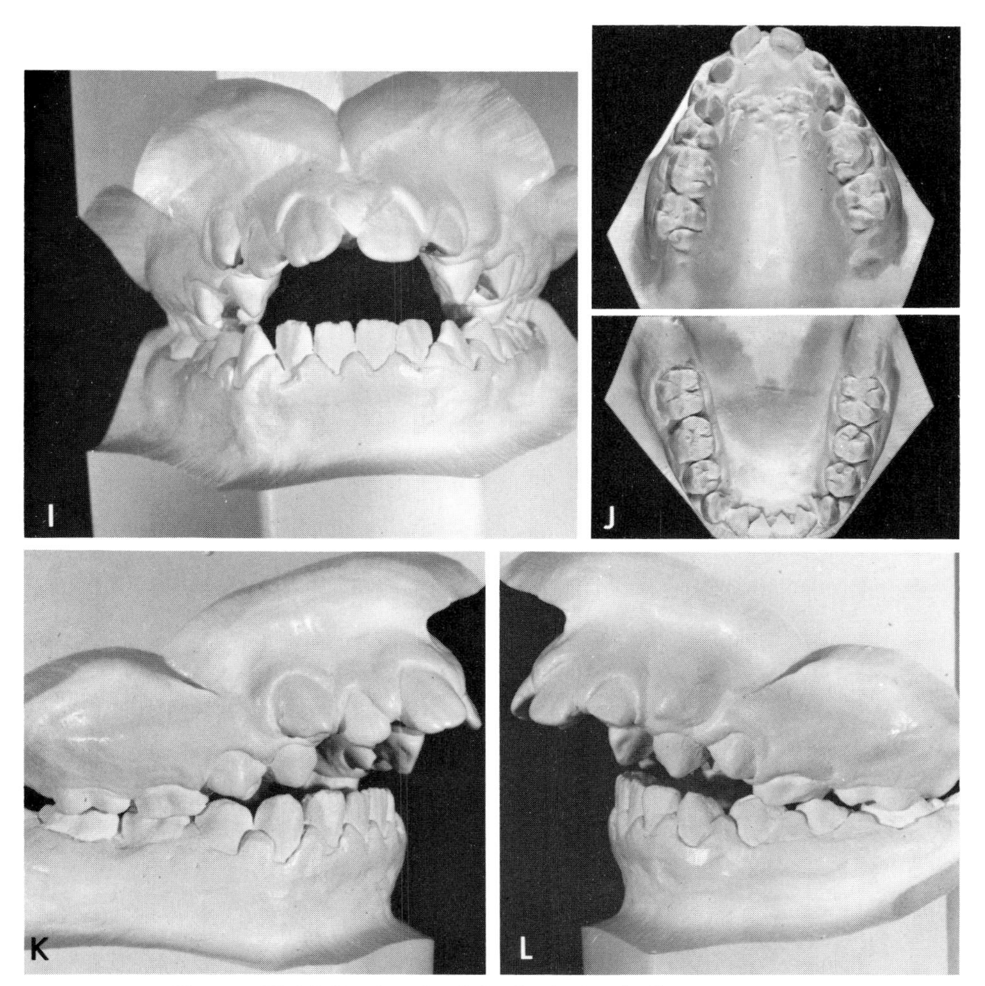

Figure 13–25 *Continued.* *I–L,* Occlusion before treatment.

Illustration continued on the following page

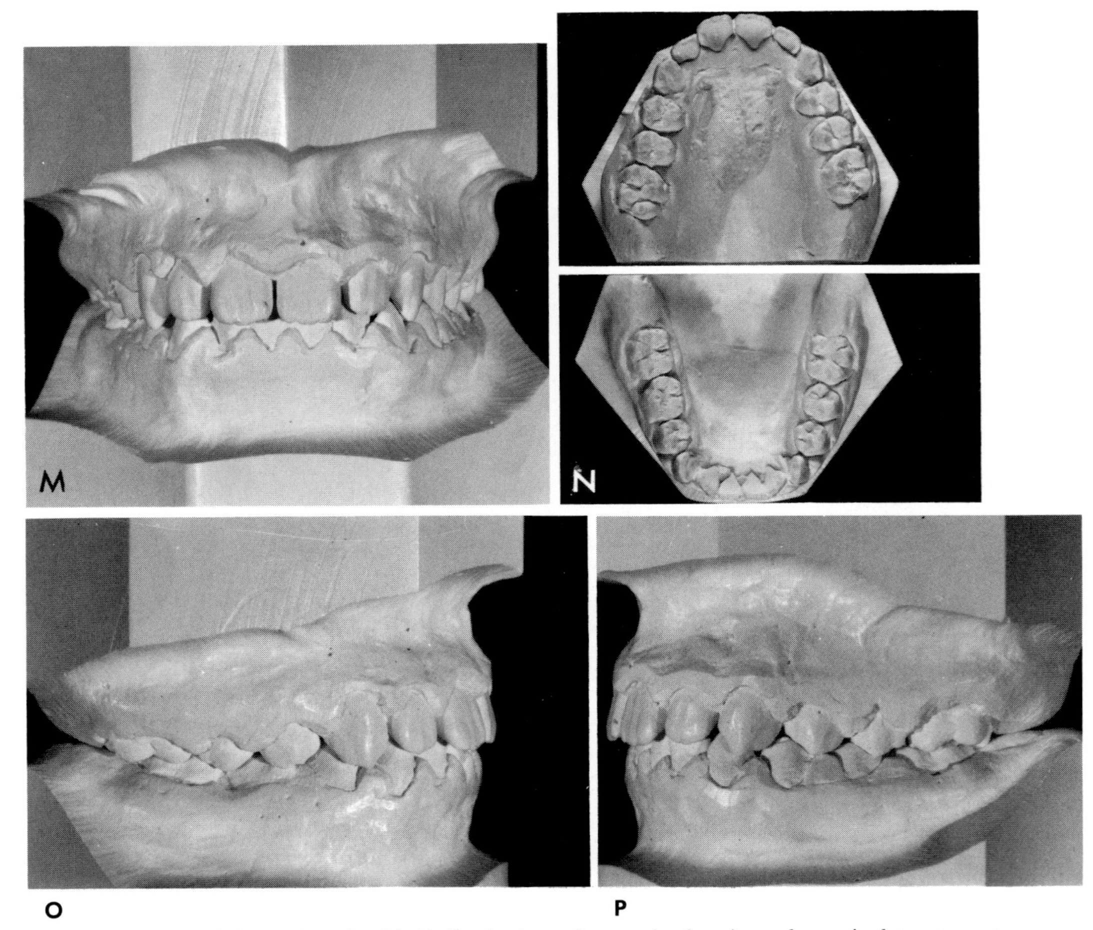

Figure 13–25 *Continued.* *M–P,* Occlusion after orthodontic and surgical treatments.

Occlusion

DENTAL ARCH FORM. *Maxilla:* constricted with high palatal vault. *Mandible:* square.

DENTAL ALIGNMENT. Retained maxillary primary molars and canines with poor eruption sequence; maxillary canines blocked out bilaterally; rotations and crowding of anterior teeth.

DENTAL OCCLUSION. Class II malocclusion with 12-mm overjet; excessive curvature of maxillary occlusal plane; bilateral anterior open bite starting in the second premolar region.

TREATMENT PLAN

Orthodontic Treatment

PRESURGICAL

1. Extract remaining maxillary deciduous teeth.

2. Place edgewise appliances on maxillary six anterior teeth. (Absence of patient cooperation because of her mental status precluded the placement of orthodontic bands on the posterior teeth.) Correct rotations and align anterior teeth. At the time of surgery, orthodontic bands were to be placed on the posterior teeth for intermaxillary fixation.

POSTSURGICAL

1. Complete alignment and finalization of occlusion.

Surgical Treatment

1. Reposition maxilla 3 mm superiorly and 3 mm anteriorly by Le Fort I osteotomy in three segments to
   a. Level maxillary occlusal plane by moving the buccal segments slightly higher than the anterior segments.
   b. Reduce lip incompetence and improve relationship between upper lip and maxillary incisors.
   c. Close the open bite.
2. Perform sagittal osteotomy of the mandibular ramus to advance the mandible 9 mm to
   a. Correct mandibular deficiency and achieve a satisfactory overjet.
   b. Achieve a Class I molar and canine relationship.
3. Utilize suprahyoid myotomies to reduce the possibility of relapse due to stretching of the suprahyoid musculature.

FOLLOW-UP

Subjective

Despite the limited amount of patient cooperation possible, the treatment progressed in an uncomplicated manner. The patient tolerated the surgical and orthodontic procedures without difficulty.

Objective

When this patient was first seen in November 1974 at the age of 9 she was in special educational classes. Her mental capacity and limited ability to cooperate were important considerations in planning therapy. The patient's future facial appearance and jaw function were paramount considerations to the child's family. It was hoped that orthodontic and surgical treatment would effect a significant change in her facial esthetics and achieve a serviceable occlusion.

Banding of the maxillary anterior teeth was a tedious task, as the patient was exceedingly apprehensive and difficult to manage. For this reason, orthodontic appliances were not placed on the mandibular teeth or the maxillary posterior teeth. Model surgery and cephalometric prediction studies indicated the feasibility of achieving a satisfactory occlusion with maxillary and mandibular surgery. The presurgical orthodontic treatment was carried out rather slowly so as to not frighten the child.

Superior and anterior movement of the maxilla in three segments decreased the amount of tooth exposure, gave additional prominence to the upper lip and paranasal areas, leveled the maxillary occlusal plane, and helped to close the open bite. A

Class I dental and skeletal relationship, lip competence, and nose-lip-tooth-chin balance were achieved by bilateral sagittal split ramus osteotomies to advance the mandible 9 mm.

At surgery, edgewise appliances were placed on the maxillary buccal segments. An arch wire was also placed to allow orthodontic consolidation and finalization of the occlusion after the intermaxillary fixation was discontinued. An arch bar was ligated to the lower teeth for intermaxillary fixation. When the intermaxillary fixation was removed after five and one-half weeks the patient wore a soft cervical collar for five months to reduce the possibility of relapse secondary to lengthening the suprahyoid muscles. The patient is presently wearing a maxillary removable Hawley retainer. Clinical and cephalometric studies 18 months postoperatively revealed essentially no change from the immediate postoperative position.

COMMENT

Marginal patient cooperation necessitated a flexible plan of therapy for this young patient. Flexibility, practicality, compromise, and innovation are the prerequisites for successful treatment of this type of individual. The poor prognosis for future mandibular growth gave support to early surgical intervention to advance the mandible and harmonize the occlusion (see Chapter 21). During treatment, the patient went through her pubertal growth spurt. Postoperative cephalometric studies showed evidence of continued maxillary and mandibular growth after surgical intervention. Such findings support the theory that maxillary surgery does not significantly affect growth and development of the jaws.

Surgeon: Douglas Sinn, Dallas, Texas.

CASE 13–5 (Fig. 13–26)

A gradually progressive open bite developed in C. C., a 23-year-old woman who was initially seen some eight years after orthodontic treatment for her Class I deep bite malocclusion. The cause of the open bite was obscure and may have been unrelated to previous orthodontic treatment. After evaluation of the patient's clinical records, a problem list was developed.

PROBLEM LIST

Esthetics

FRONTAL. Large interlabial gap (11 mm); excessive tooth exposure; inadequacy of upper-lip coverage; gingival exposure on smiling.

PROFILE. Normal nasolabial angle and a retropositioned mandible with deficiency of the soft-tissue chin prominence were the dominant features revealed by clinical analysis of the patient's profile with her lips in a relaxed posture.

Cephalometric Analysis

1. Steep mandibular plane (49°).
2. Anterior open bite.
3. Excessive anterior vertical facial height.

Text continued on page 1168.

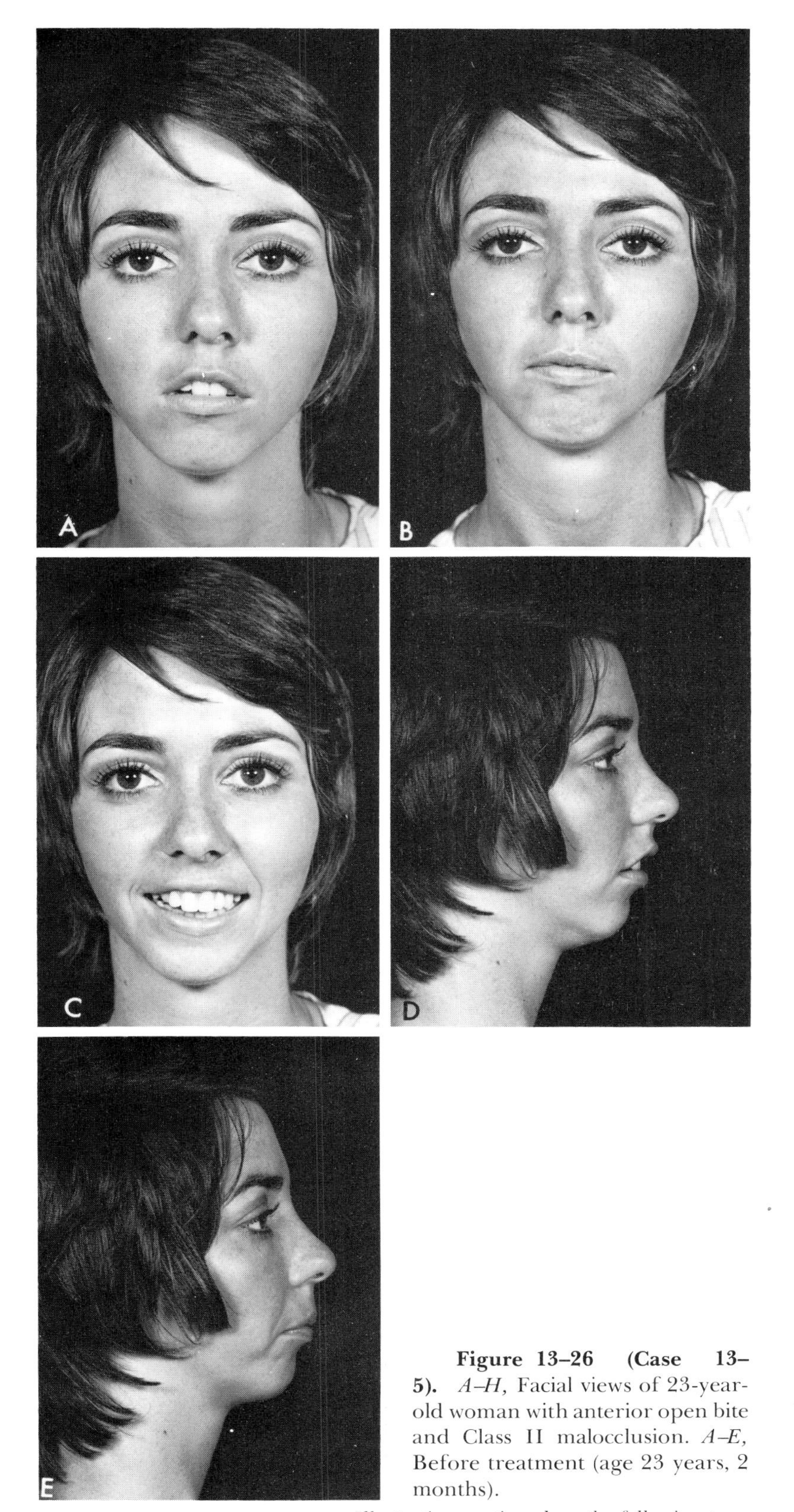

Figure 13–26 (Case 13–5). *A–H,* Facial views of 23-year-old woman with anterior open bite and Class II malocclusion. *A–E,* Before treatment (age 23 years, 2 months).

Illustration continued on the following page

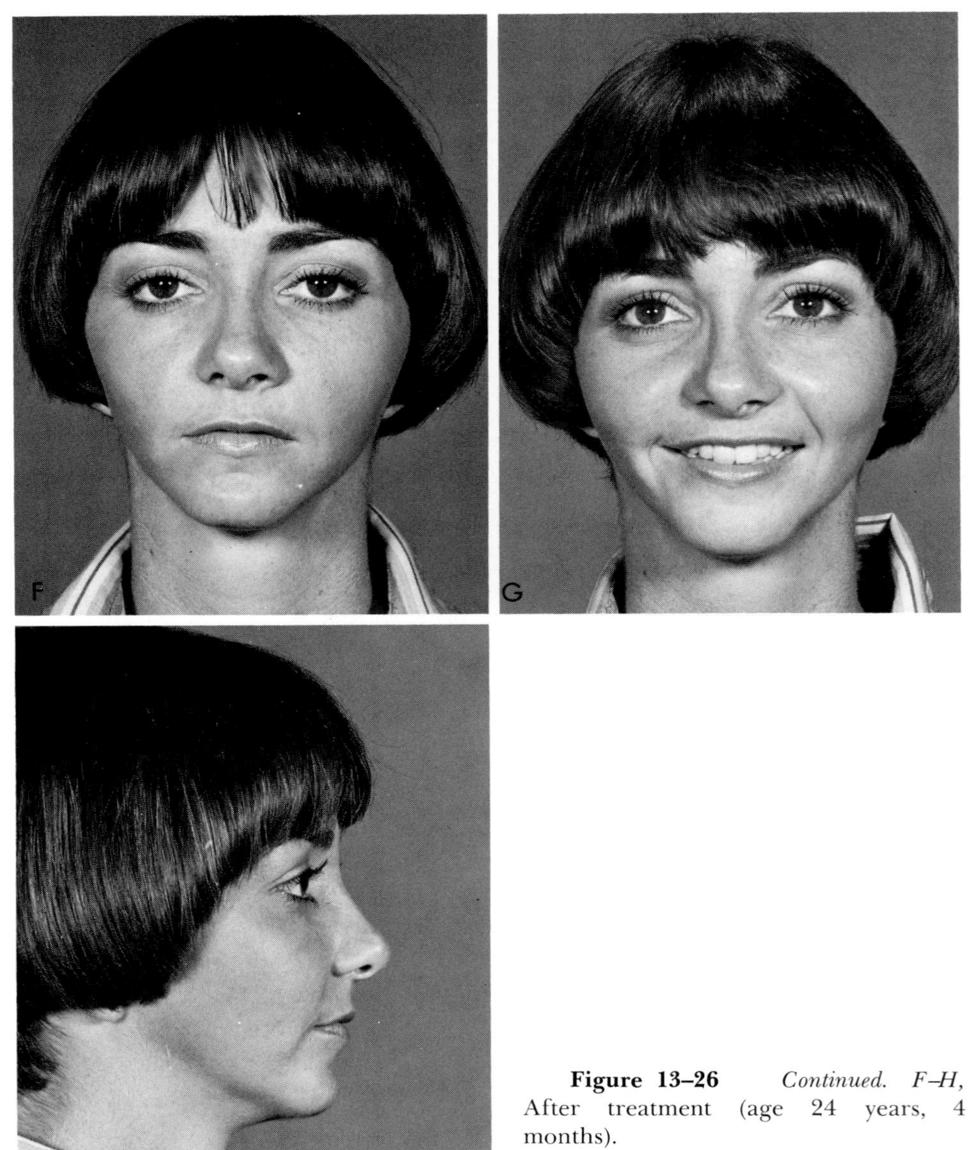

Figure 13–26 *Continued. F–H,* After treatment (age 24 years, 4 months).

Legend continued on the opposite page

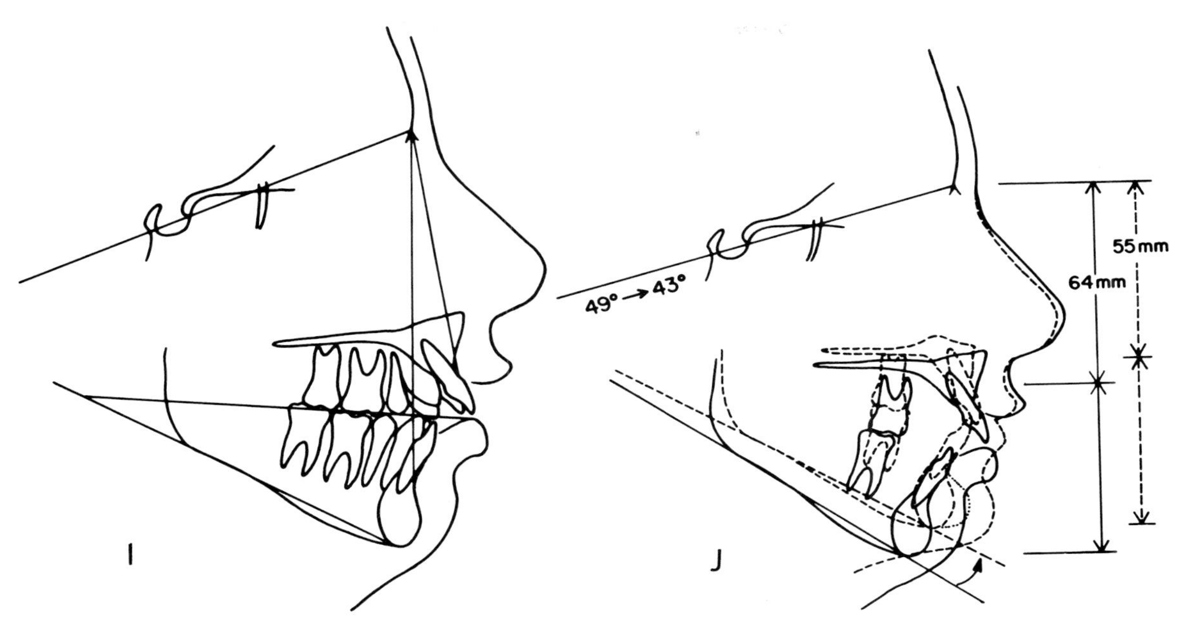

Figure 13–26 *Continued.* *I,* Cephalometric tracing before treatment (age 23 years, 2 months). *J,* Composite cephalometric tracings before (*solid line,* age 23 years, 2 months) and after (*broken line,* age 24 years, 4 months) maxillary surgery show 9-mm reduction in anterior facial height, augmentation of chin by genioplasty and reduction of nasal prominence by rhinoplasty.

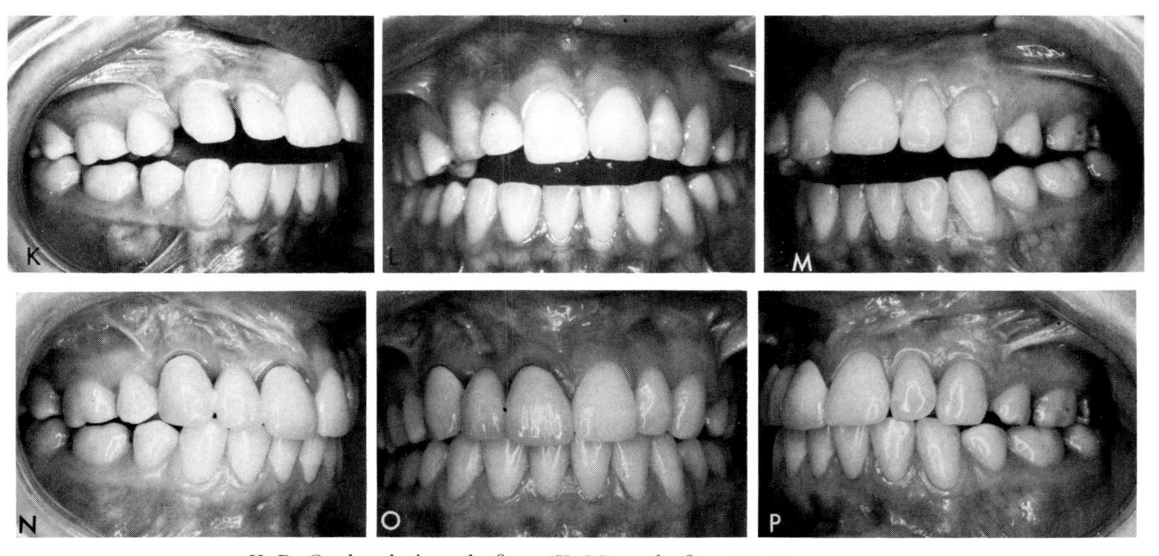

K–P, Occlusal views before *(K–M)* and after *(N–P)* treatment.

Illustration continued on the following page

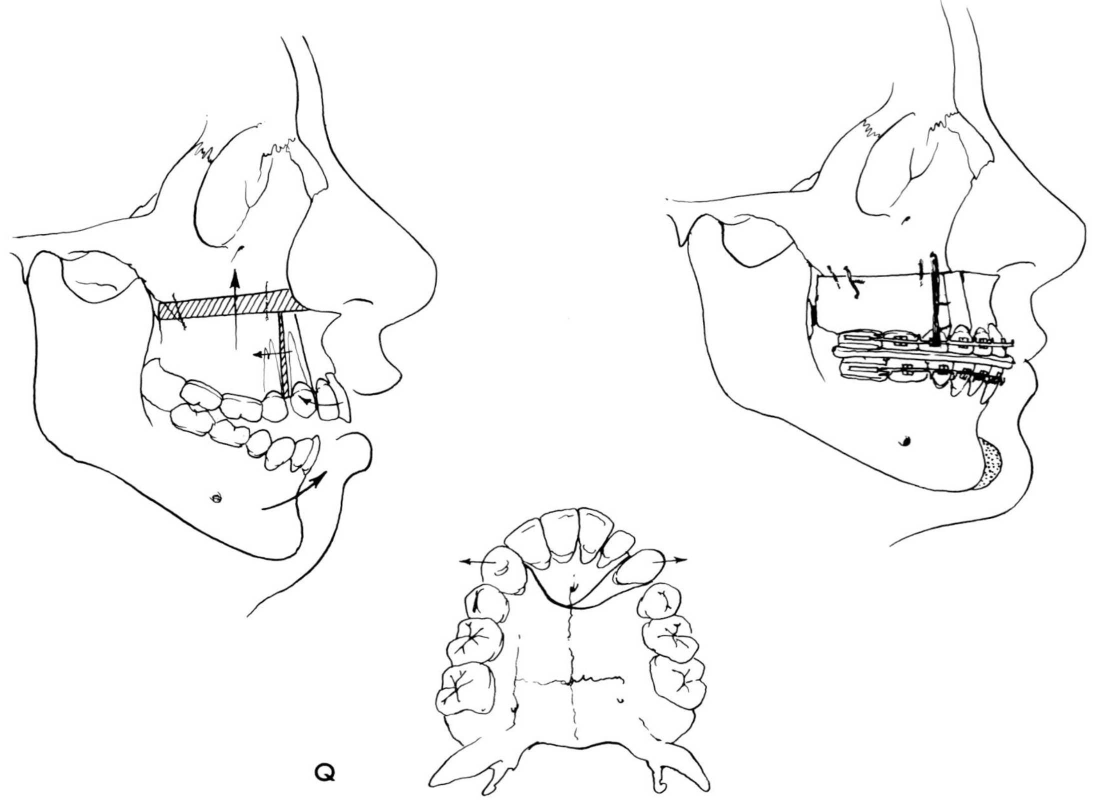

Figure 13–26 *Continued.* *Q,* Schematic plan of surgery: multiple maxillary osteotomies to raise maxilla, level maxillary occlusal plane, close anterior open bite, increase intercanine width and close interdental spacing; augmentation genioplasty with Proplast.

4. Inferior margin of upper lip in relaxed posture approached cervical margin of incisor teeth.
5. ANB difference 10°.

Occlusal Analysis

DENTAL ARCH FORM. Maxilla and mandible symmetric; slight constriction of maxillary arch.

DENTAL ALIGNMENT. Interdental spacing in right anterior maxillary quadrant.

DENTAL OCCLUSION. Class II malocclusion with 5-mm overjet; bilateral open bite between maxillary and mandibular teeth starting in the molar region.

TREATMENT PLAN

A cephalometric prediction analysis and model surgery indicated the feasibility of the following treatment plan.

Surgical Treatment

1. Reposition the maxilla 8 mm superiorly by Le Fort I osteotomy to
   a. Reduce exposure of teeth and gingiva.
   b. Shorten facial height.
   c. Correct lip incompetence.
   d. Close open bite.
   e. Allow autorotation of the retropositioned mandible.

2. Reposition maxillary right canine (single-tooth segment) and the maxillary central and left lateral incisors (three-tooth segment) to achieve a Class I canine relationship and correct interdental spacing.
3. Augment contour-deficient chin with 5-mm thick alloplastic implant (Proplast).

Orthodontic Treatment

1. Postsurgical alignment of mandibular anterior teeth.

Prosthodontic Treatment

1. Crown and bridge restorative procedures on anterior teeth to improve dental esthetics and replace extracted right lateral incisor.

FOLLOW-UP

Subjective

The patient's postoperative course was complicated by splaying of the alar bases and buckling of the nasal septum. Two months after maxillary surgery, good nasal appearance was achieved by rhinoplasty.

A Class I dental and skeletal relationship, lip competence, and an esthetic nose-lip-tooth-chin balance were achieved by shortening the lower facial height. There has been no discernible change in the skeletal, soft-tissue, or dental structures over a postoperative follow-up period in excess of 5 years.

COMMENT

Surgical reduction of lower-facial height by excision of osseous tissue in the maxilla tends to balance the soft tissue in the lower face and may minimize bone resorption below the alloplastic chin implant because of reduced tension of the perioral and mentalis musculature.

The surgery was carried out in two stages to achieve the planned positional and dimensional changes without jeopardizing the viability of the teeth and bone in the small dentoalveolar segments. Today, however, all the surgery would be carried out in a single stage by the Le Fort I downfracture technique.

Surgeon: William H. Bell, Dallas, Texas. *Orthodontist:* Martin Shirling, Dallas, Texas.

CASE 13–6 (Fig. 13–27)

L. K., a 16-year-old boy, was seen on consultation in 1976 for correction of his severe malocclusion, prominent lower jaw, and excessive facial height. Clinical, cephalometric, and panographic studies substantiated the following list of problems and the treatment plan.

PROBLEM LIST

Esthetics

FRONTAL. Prominent chin and lower lip; "short-appearing" upper lip; prominent nasal dorsum with deviation to the right; narrow constricted anterior nares; long lower third of the face with bilateral flattening of the canine fossae.

PROFILE. Long nose with prominent dorsum and drooping tip; "short" upper lip; anteroposterior deficiency.

Cephalometric Analysis

1. Skeletal type Class III open bite deformity.
2. Anteroposterior deficiency (ANB −4°, SNA 65°, SNB 69°).
3. Anterior open bite.
4. Steep mandibular plane angle (SN-GoGn 55°) and excessive facial height.
5. Retroclined maxillary and mandibular incisors ($\underline{1}$ to SN 85°, $\overline{1}$ to GoGn 76°).
6. Bilateral anterior open bite beginning in the first molar regions.

Occlusion

DENTAL ARCH FORM. Constricted maxillary arch with high palatal vault; tapered mandibular arch with moderate curve of Spee.

DENTAL ALIGNMENT. *Maxilla:* Moderate crowding with premature loss of the right canine; 5-mm midline shift of maxilla to the right; retroinclination of the maxillary incisors. *Mandible:* Crowding and retroinclination of the anterior teeth.

DENTAL OCCLUSION. Class III molar relationship with 5-mm reverse overjet and 5-mm anterior open bite beginning in the first molar areas with complete crossbite.

TREATMENT PLAN

Orthodontic Treatment

PRESURGICAL
1. Level and align the maxillary and mandibular arches.
2. Expand maxillary premolars and molars bilaterally.

POSTSURGICAL
1. Obtain final interdigitation and tooth position.

 Text continued on page 1176.

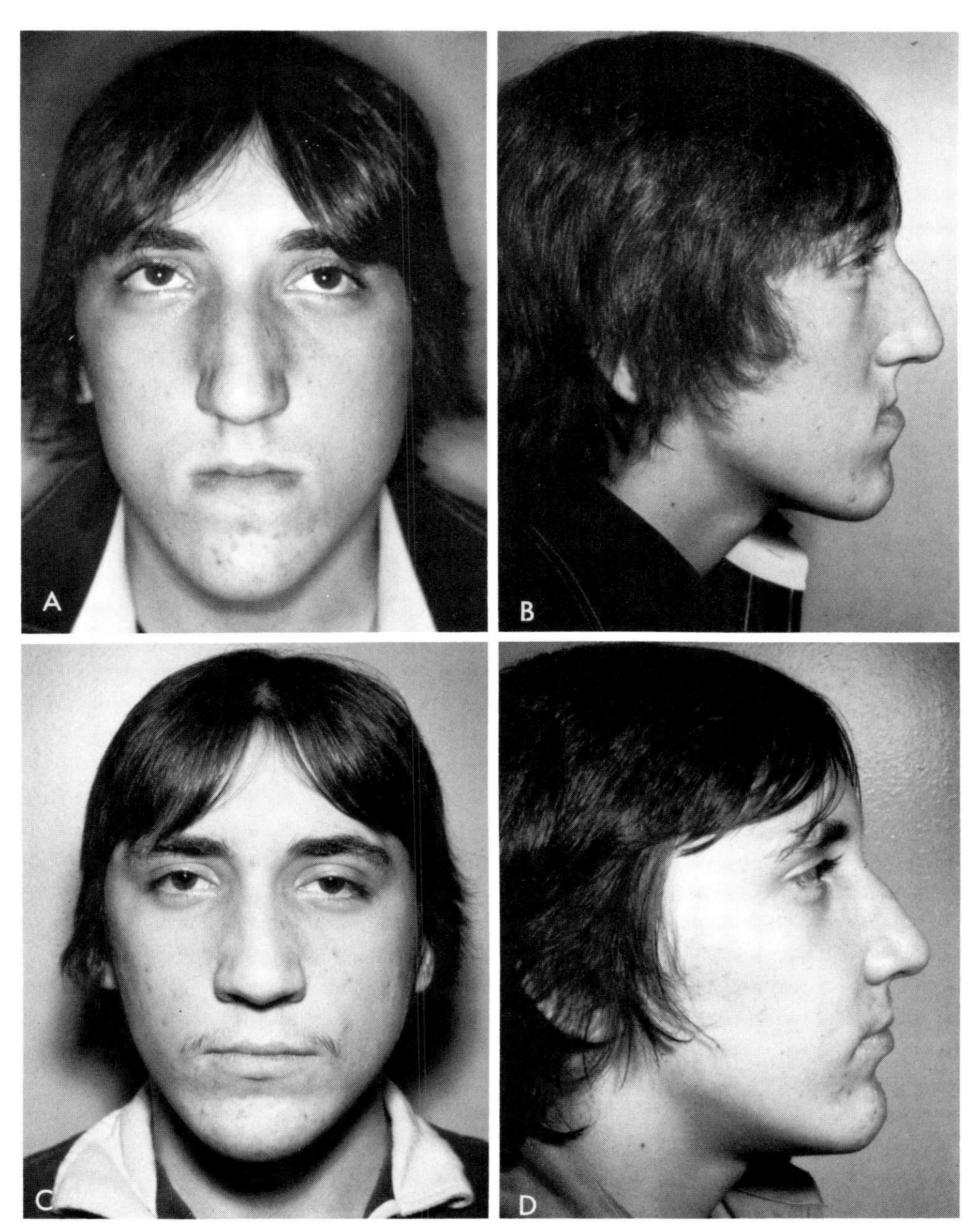

Figure 13–27 (Case 13–6). *A–D,* Facial views of 16-year-old boy before (*A* and *B*) and after (*C* and *D*) treatment.

Illustration continued on the following page

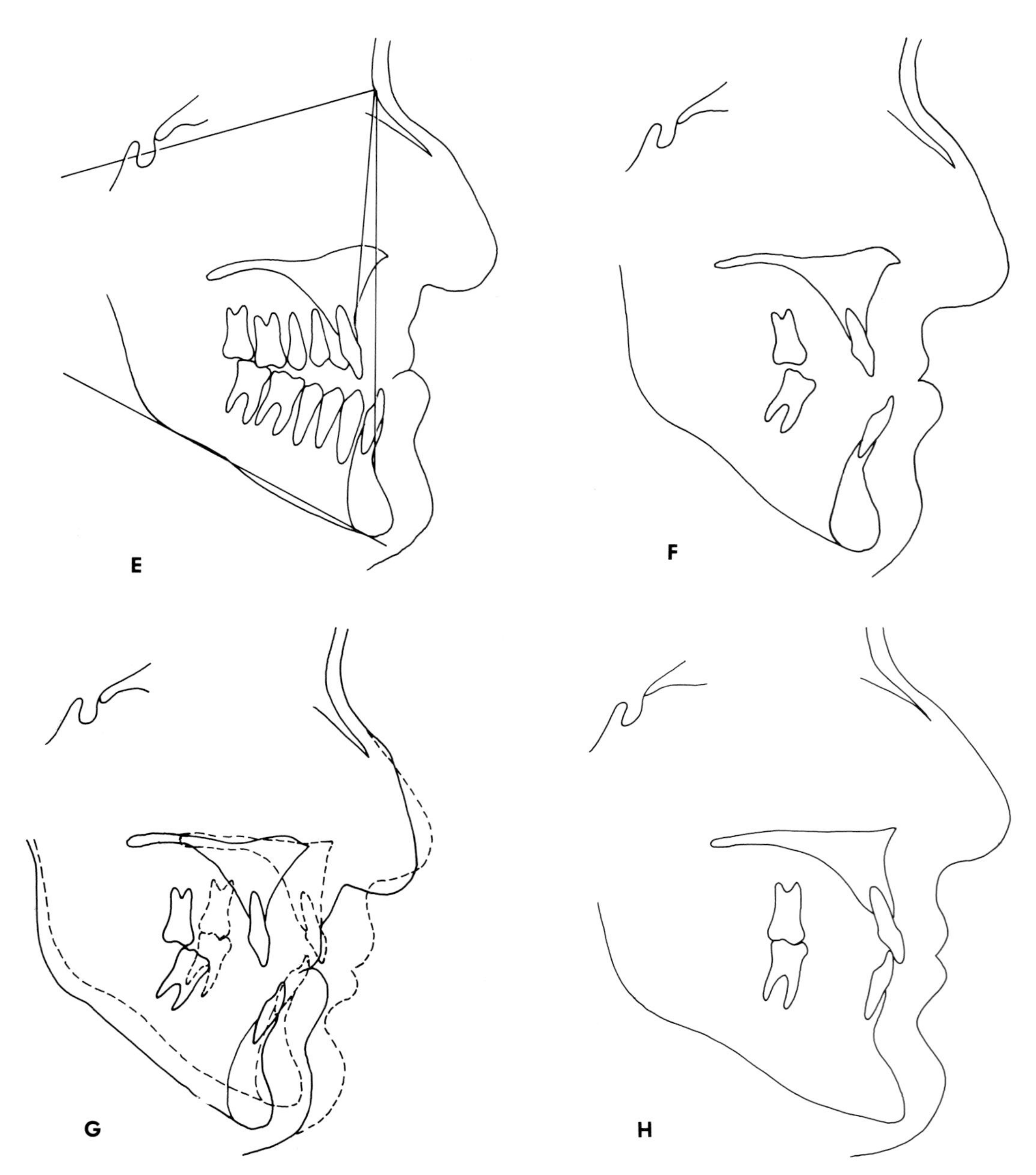

Figure 13–27 *Continued.*

E, Cephalometric tracing before treatment (age 16 years, 1 month). *F,* Cephalometric tracing before surgery after 6 months of orthodontic treatment (age 16 years, 7 months). *G,* Composite cephalometric tracings before (*solid line,* age 16 years, 1 month) and after (*broken line,* age 16 years, 11 months) surgery show 7-mm reduction in anterior facial height, closure of open bite, advancement of maxilla 17 mm, and improvement in nasal and labial profiles. *H,* Cephalometric tracing 10 months after removal of orthodontic appliances (age 17 years, 9 months).

Legend continued on the opposite page

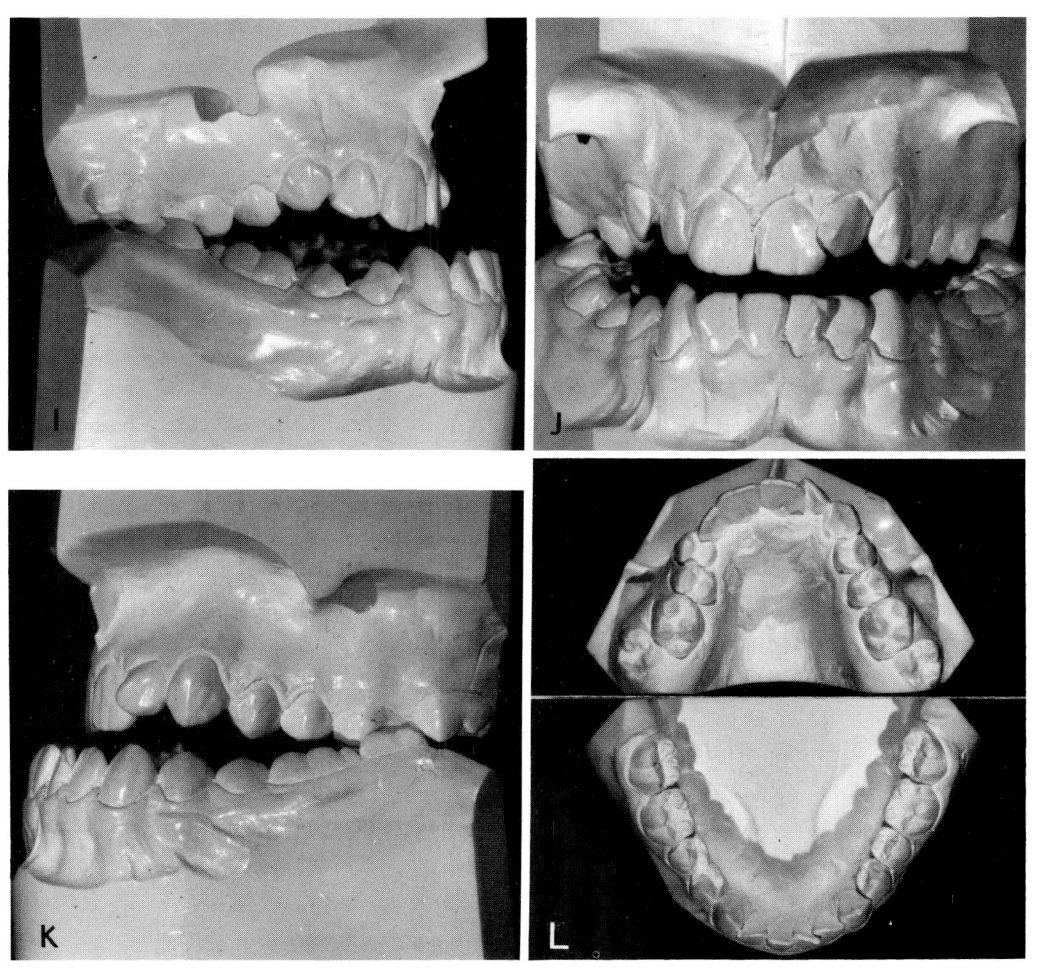

Figure 13-27 *Continued.* *I-L,* Occlusion before treatment.

Illustration continued on the following page

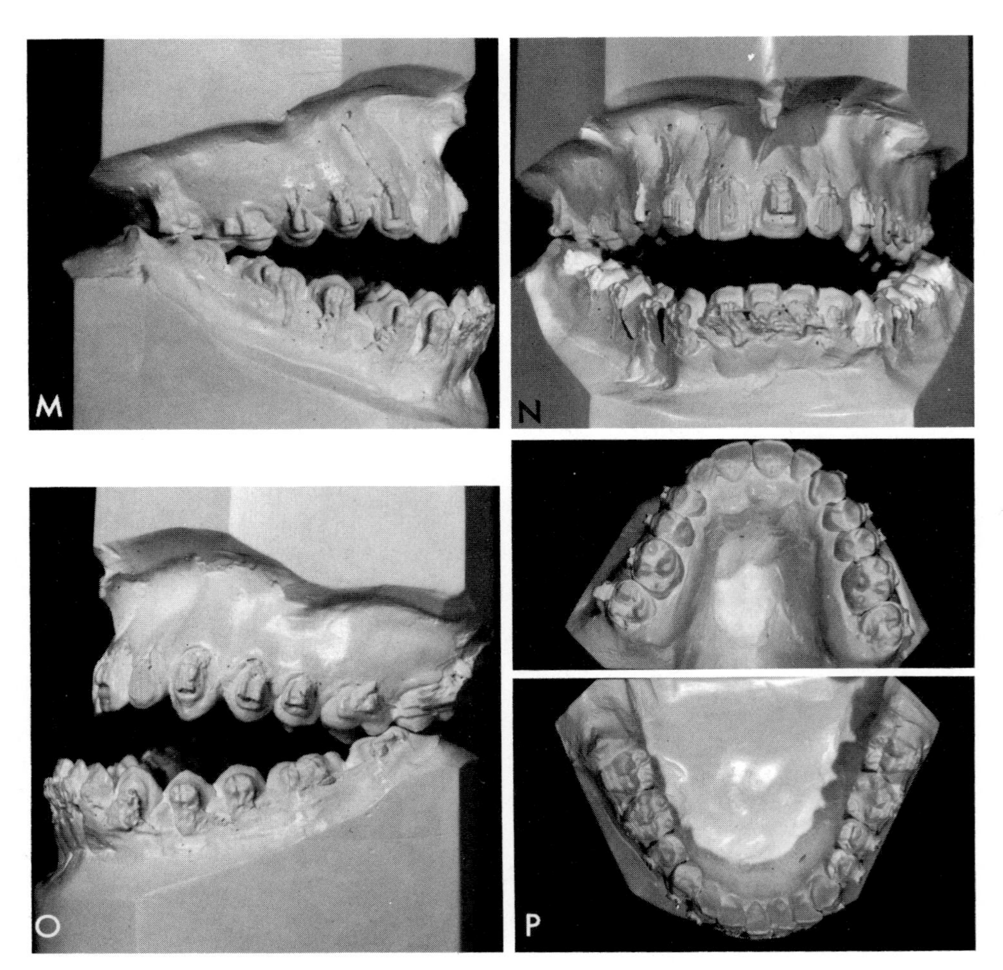

Figure 13–27 *Continued.*
M–P, Occlusion before surgery, after 6 months of orthodontic treatment.

Legend continued on the opposite page

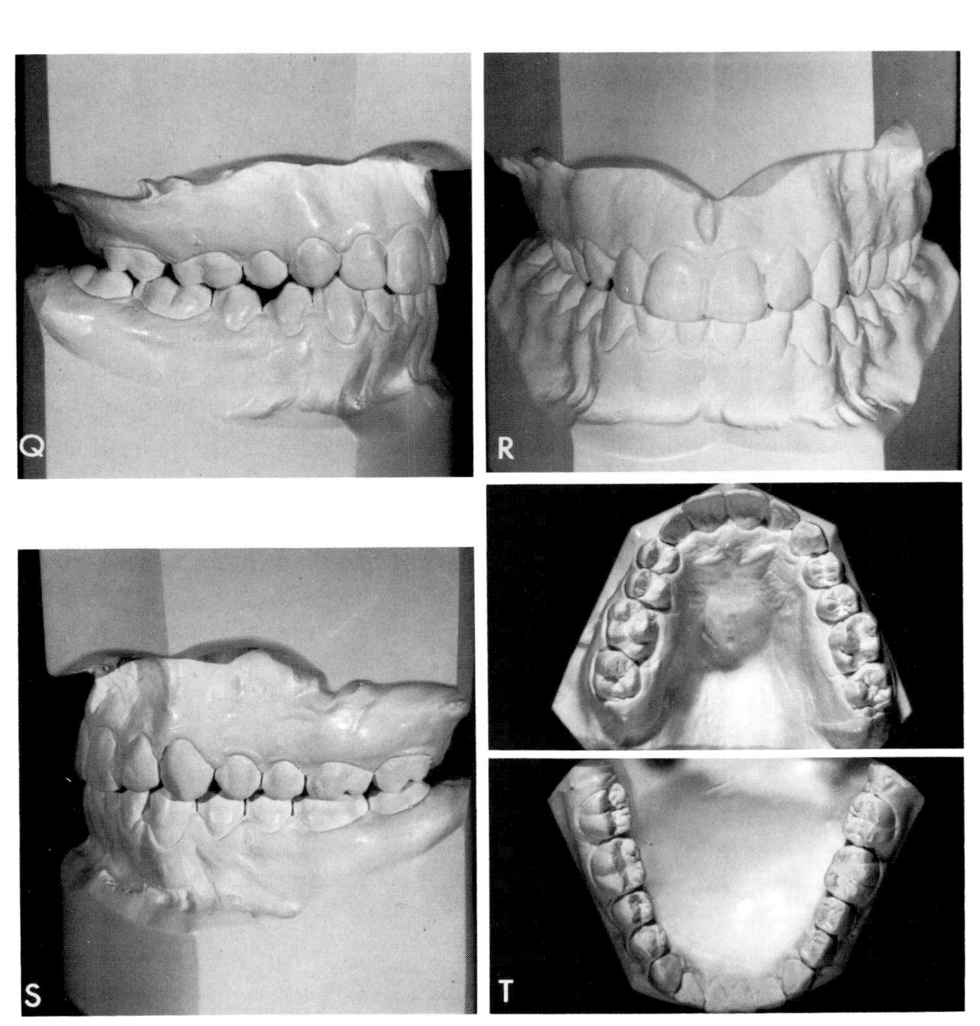

Figure 13–27 *Continued.*

Q–T, Final occlusion (10 months after completion of postsurgical orthodontic treatment).

Surgical Treatment

1. Reposition the maxilla superiorly and anteriorly by Le Fort I osteotomy to
   a. Correct the anteroposterior maxillary deficiency and anterior open bite.
   b. Decrease the nasolabial angle.
   c. Decrease lower anterior facial height.
   d. Improve balance between nasal dorsum and tip of the nose.

FOLLOW-UP

Subjective

The postoperative course was uncomplicated and associated with virtually no discomfort. There was transient bilateral infraorbital nerve hypoesthesia associated with the placement of infraorbital rim suspension wires. Normal sensation returned within four weeks, however. Maxillomandibular fixation was discontinued after seven and one-half weeks, at which time the maxilla was stable.

Objective

During the six months of presurgical orthodontic treatment, no attempt was made to close the open bite. After Le Fort I osteotomy and downfracture, the maxilla was advanced 14 mm on the left and 17 mm on the right, and raised 4 mm posteriorly. As a consequence, the mandible autorotated anteriorly and superiorly to correct the anteroposterior maxillary deficiency, close the open bite, and decrease the facial height 7 mm. Overall esthetic balance was gained by dimensional changes in the nose, maxilla, and chin associated with the maxillary surgery and autorotational movement of the mandible. Trapezoidal blocks of autogenous bone from the iliac crest were placed along the defects of the lateral maxilla and the pterygoid plate–maxillary tuberosity areas bilaterally.

Postoperative cephalometric studies revealed an SNA 77°, SNB 73°, SN–GoGn 48°, and a 7-mm decrease in facial height. There was minimal postoperative movement of the repositioned maxilla. Despite excellent skeletal stability demonstrated by sequential cephalometric tracings there was some compromise in the transeverse dimension of the maxilla arch. Retrospective occlusal studies indicated that this was probably a consequence of orthodontic expansion of the maxillary premolars and molars before surgery. In retrospect, this problem might have been obviated by employing rapid maxillary expansion and total maxillary osteotomies. Such treatment would have facilitated correction of the horizontal maxillary deficiency and alignment of the maxillary teeth without extractions. Another treatment option was extraction of maxillary premolars to allow orthodontic alignment of the maxillary teeth and subsequent maxillary surgery (four-piece Le Fort I osteotomy) to level the maxillary occlusal plane, widen the maxillary arch, and achieve the desired anteroposterior and vertical position of the maxilla.

COMMENT

The limit of anterior movement of the maxilla is not known and probably depends on a number of factors for each individual patient. In planning for the surgery, it was decided that a mandibular procedure be performed if the extreme anterior movement of 17 mm could not be accomplished. However, the total movement was performed in a single operation without major difficulty. The anterior nasal spine was removed to allow a more natural draping of the lip, to facilitate soft-tissue closure without tension, and to prevent distortion of the nasal tip.

The choice of operating in the maxilla in this particular patient was based upon the individual's esthetic needs and desires and the fact that superior repositioning of the maxilla to close the anterior open bite was calculated to produce a more stable result than mandibular surgery for the same purpose. If cephalometric prediction studies had indicated that the maxilla or mandible would be too prominent after maxillary surgery, mandibular surgery would have been programmed to retract the mandible concomitantly.

Surgeons: David S. Topazian and Paul L. Wineland, Milford, Connecticut. *Orthodontist:* Albert D'Onofrio, New Haven, Connecticut

Case Studies Illustrating Complications Encountered in Treatment of Open Bite

CASE 13–7 (Fig. 13–28)

R. B., a 23-year-old man, sought treatment to correct his open bite.

PROBLEM LIST

Esthetics

FRONTAL. Symmetric facial contours; width of nasal base corresponded with intercanthal distance; 7-mm interlabial gap.

PROFILE. Retropositioned chin; adequate nasolabial angle.

Cephalometric Analysis

1. Steep mandibular plane angle (48°).
2. ANB difference 4°, $\underline{1}$ to NA 6 mm.; $\overline{1}$ to NB 5 mm.

Occlusal Analysis

DENTAL ARCH FORM. Maxilla and mandible symmetric.

DENTAL ALIGNMENT. Slight crowding in anterior part of maxillary and mandibular arches.

DENTAL OCCLUSION. Class I occlusion with bilateral anterior open bite commencing in the canine region.

TREATMENT PLAN

Orthodontic Treatment

1. Extract maxillary and mandibular first premolars to facilitate closure of open bite by tipping the maxillary and mandibular incisors lingually about their apices.
2. Align anterior teeth.

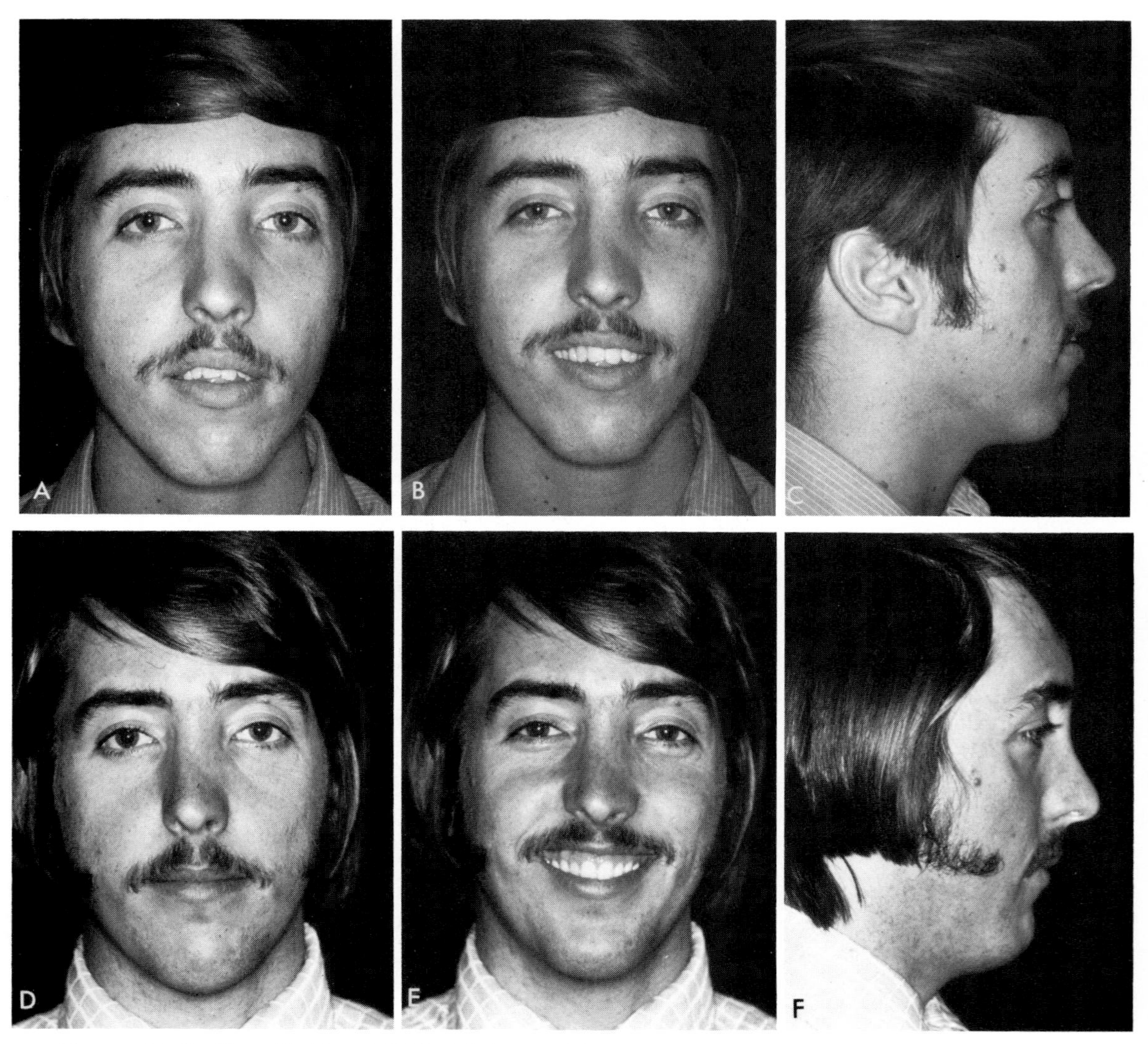

Figure 13–28 (Case 13–7). *A–F,* Facial views of 23-year-old man with skeletal type of anterior open bite and Class I malocclusion. Before *(A–C)* and 30 months after *(D–F)* treatment. Lip incompetence is still evident, maxillary incisors are too long in relation to the upper lip, and excessive gingiva is displayed when the patient smiles.

Legend continued on the opposite page

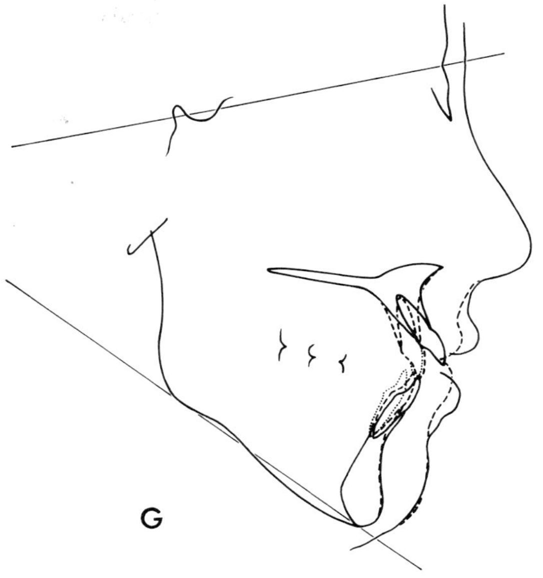

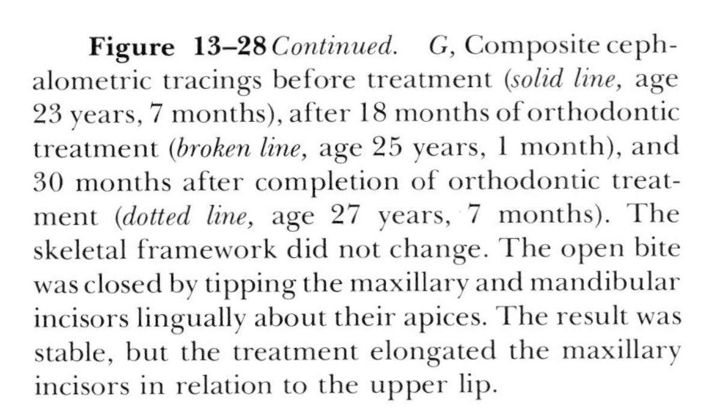

Figure 13–28 *Continued.* *G,* Composite cephalometric tracings before treatment (*solid line,* age 23 years, 7 months), after 18 months of orthodontic treatment (*broken line,* age 25 years, 1 month), and 30 months after completion of orthodontic treatment (*dotted line,* age 27 years, 7 months). The skeletal framework did not change. The open bite was closed by tipping the maxillary and mandibular incisors lingually about their apices. The result was stable, but the treatment elongated the maxillary incisors in relation to the upper lip.

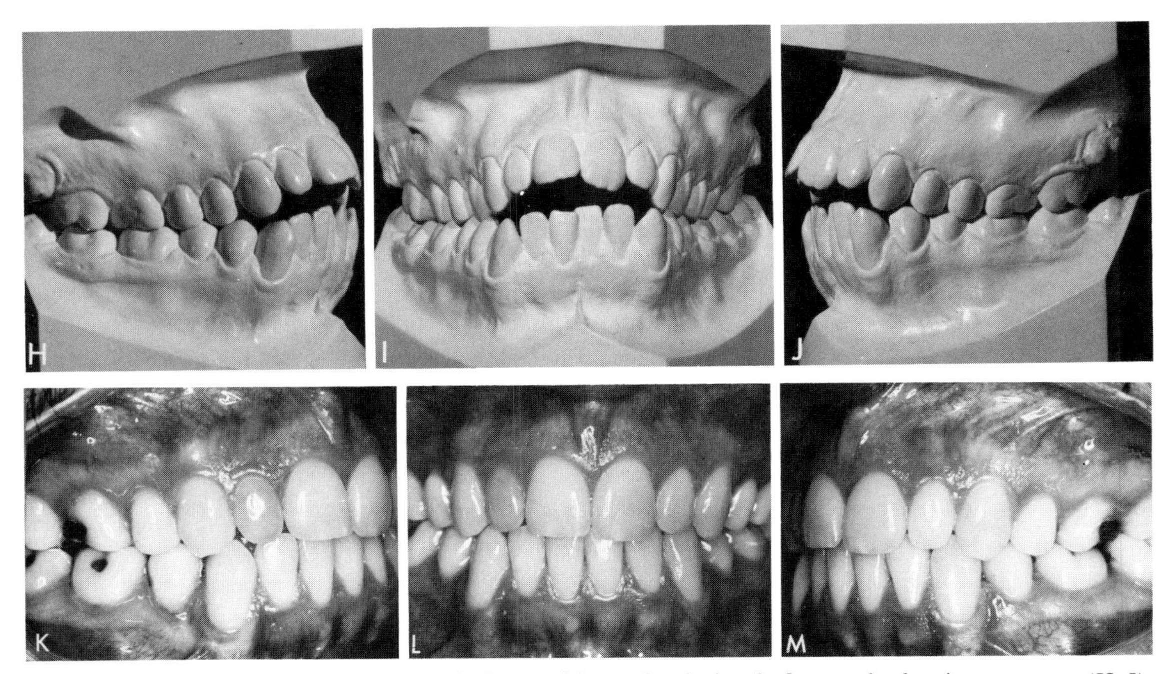

H–M, Occlusal views. Class I crowded open bite malocclusion before orthodontic treatment *(H–J)*. Occlusion 30 months after completion of orthodontic treatment, which required 18 months *(K–M)*. All four 1st premolars were extracted.

ACTIVE TREATMENT

After extraction of all four first premolars, the arches were aligned and coordinated and the open bite closed within a period of 18 months. The occlusion remained stable over a 30-month period of post-treatment follow-up. Despite the stable occlusal result, facial esthetics were compromised because treatment elongated the maxillary incisors relative to the upper lip. As a consequence, there was excessive lip strain when the patient sealed his lips and inordinate exposure of gingiva when he smiled. In addition, he continued to manifest a contour-deficient chin.

COMMENT

In nongrowing individuals such as this patient, a functional and stable result may be achieved by orthodontics alone, but usually only at the expense of compromising facial appearance. The orthodontist should project the various available treatment options to the patient when discussing the esthetic and occlusal goals of treatment.

Orthodontist: Thomas Creekmore, Houston, Texas.

CASE 13–8 (Fig. 13–29)

T. L., an 11-year-old boy, was initially seen for treatment of his malocclusion in June 1955. All study parameters showed the typical facial appearance commonly associated with a Class II long-face condition without open bite. The following problem list was evolved after appropriate clinical and laboratory examinations.

PROBLEM LIST

Esthetics

FRONTAL. Excessive exposure of teeth and gingiva in repose and when smiling; lip strain with lips sealed.

PROFILE. Obtuse nasolabial angle; retropositioned mandible and contour-deficient chin; excessive anterior facial height.

Cephalometric Analysis (Two-Year Pretreatment Growth Study)

1. High mandibular plane angle (39°) increased 3° to 42°.
2. Anterior dental height increased 6 mm.
3. Incisors erupted in compensation, maintaining a nonopen-bite occlusion.

Occlusal Analysis

DENTAL ARCH FORM. Tapered and constricted maxillary arch with high palatal vault.

Text continued on page 1186.

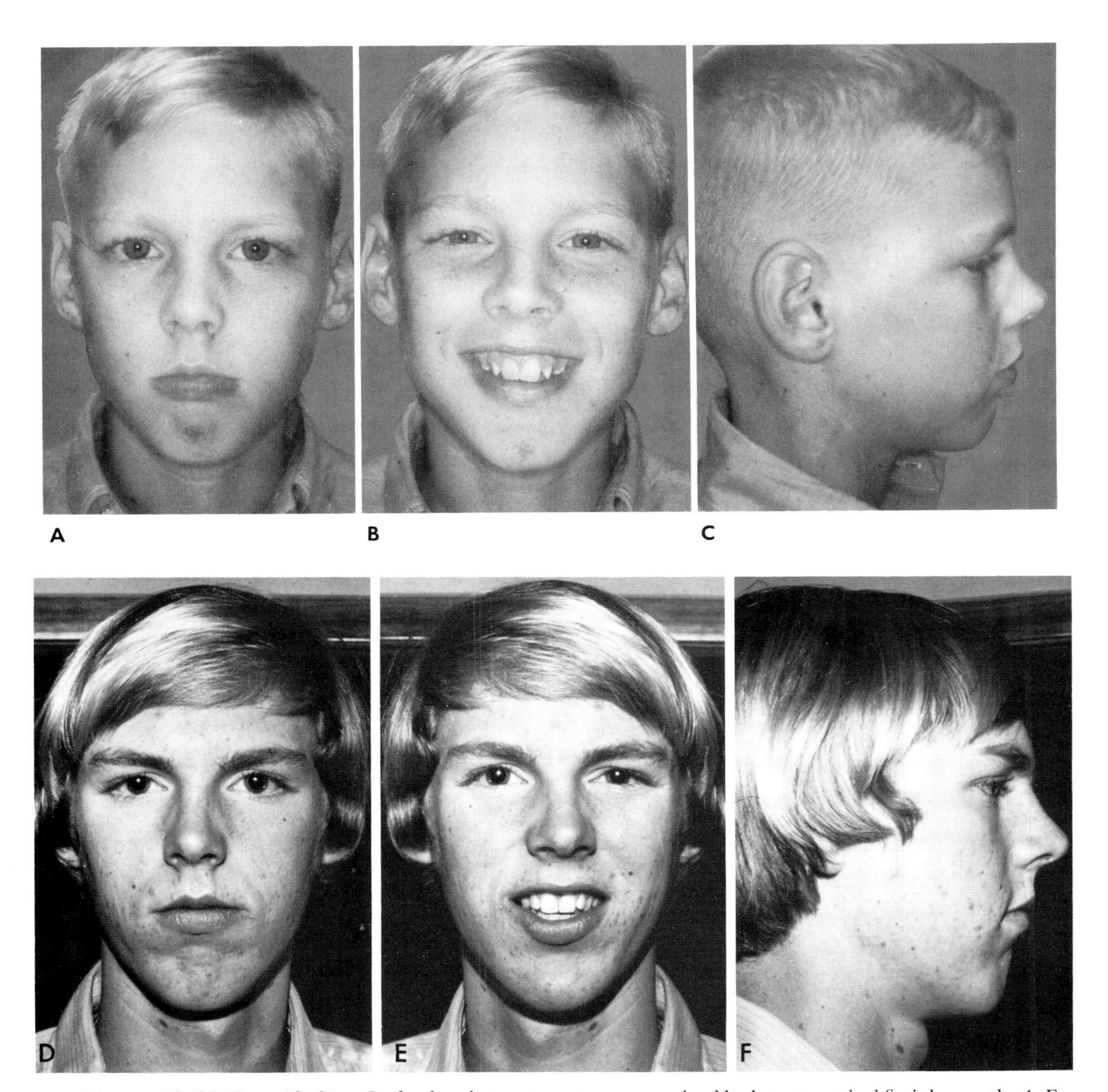

Figure 13–29 (Case 13–8). Orthodontic treatment compromised by latent vertical facial growth. *A–F,* Facial views. *A–C,* Appearance of 11-year-old boy with Class II long face non–open bite condition before orthodontic treatment shows lip incompetence and excessive exposure of teeth and gingiva when smiling. *D–F,* Facial appearance 4 years, 6 months after orthodontic treatment (age 17 years, 6 months). Lip incompetence has increased. Upper lip line to incisor relation has remained the same. Mandible is more retropositioned. The patient's face appears to be very long.

Illustration continued on the following page

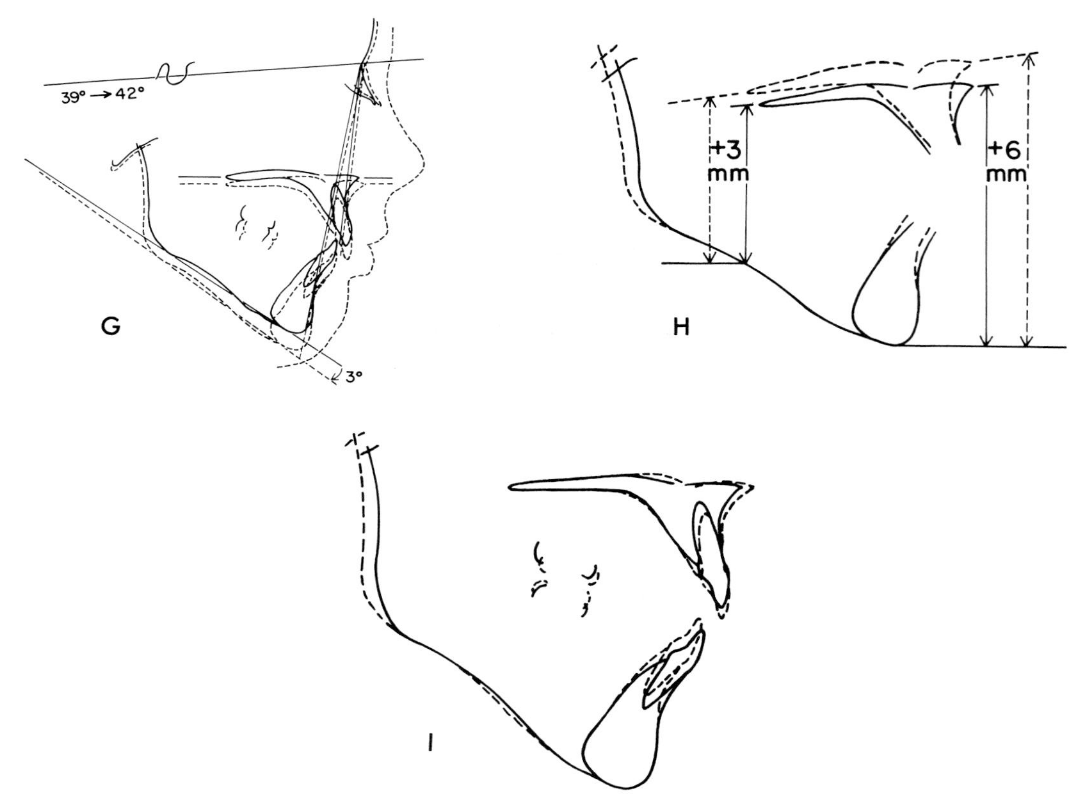

Figure 13–29 *Continued.* *G–I,* Two-year pretreatment growth study. Mandibular plane angle increased 3° *(G)*. Anterior dental height increased 6 mm *(H)*. Incisors erupted in compensation, maintaining a non–open bite occlusion *(I)*.

Legend continued on the opposite page

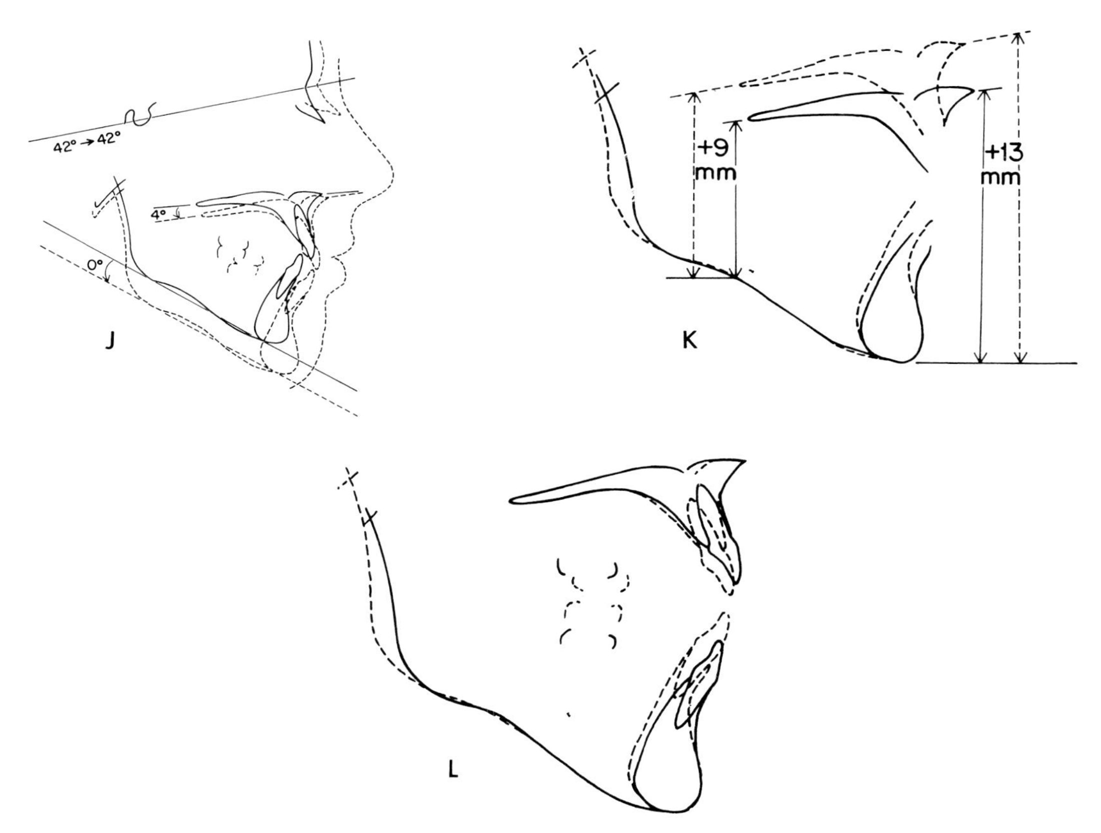

Figure 13–29 *Continued.* *J–L,* Composite cephalometric tracings before 22 months of orthodontic treatment and 26 months after treatment. Mandibular plane angle remained unchanged at 42° *(J).* Anterior dental height increased 13 mm *(K).* Bite started opening slowly after treatment *(L).*

Illustration continued on the following page

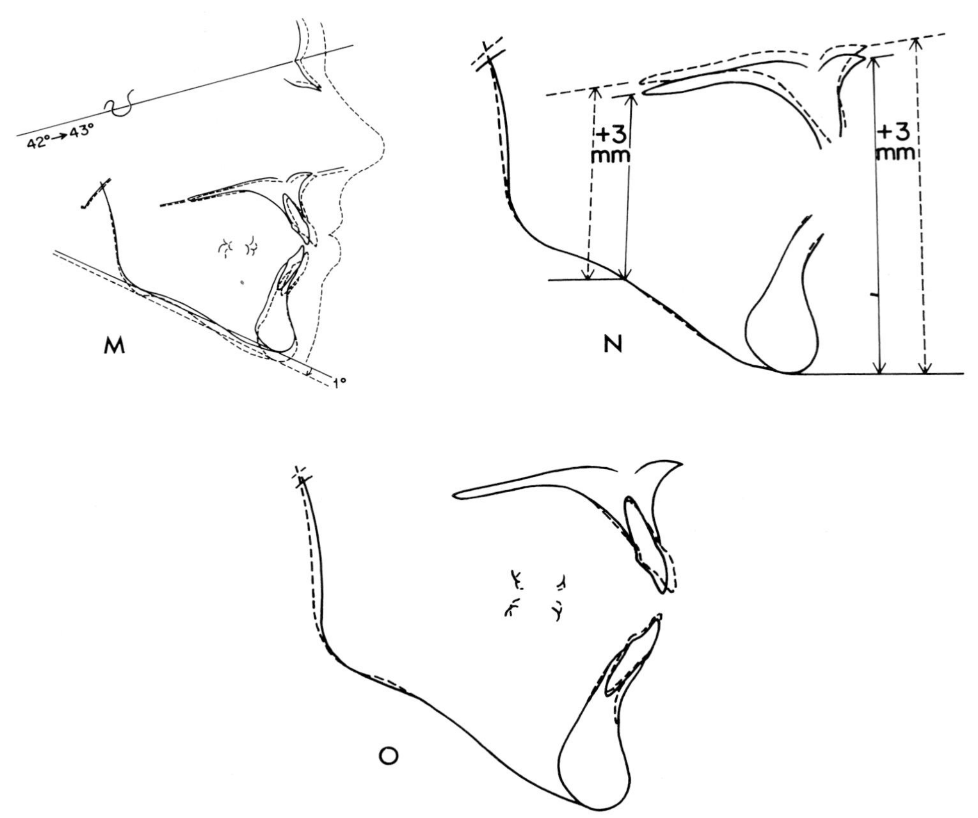

Figure 13–29 *Continued.* *M–O,* Continued post-treatment growth similar to that seen in pretreatment growth study. Anterior facial height continued to increase more than did posterior facial height.

Legend continued on the opposite page

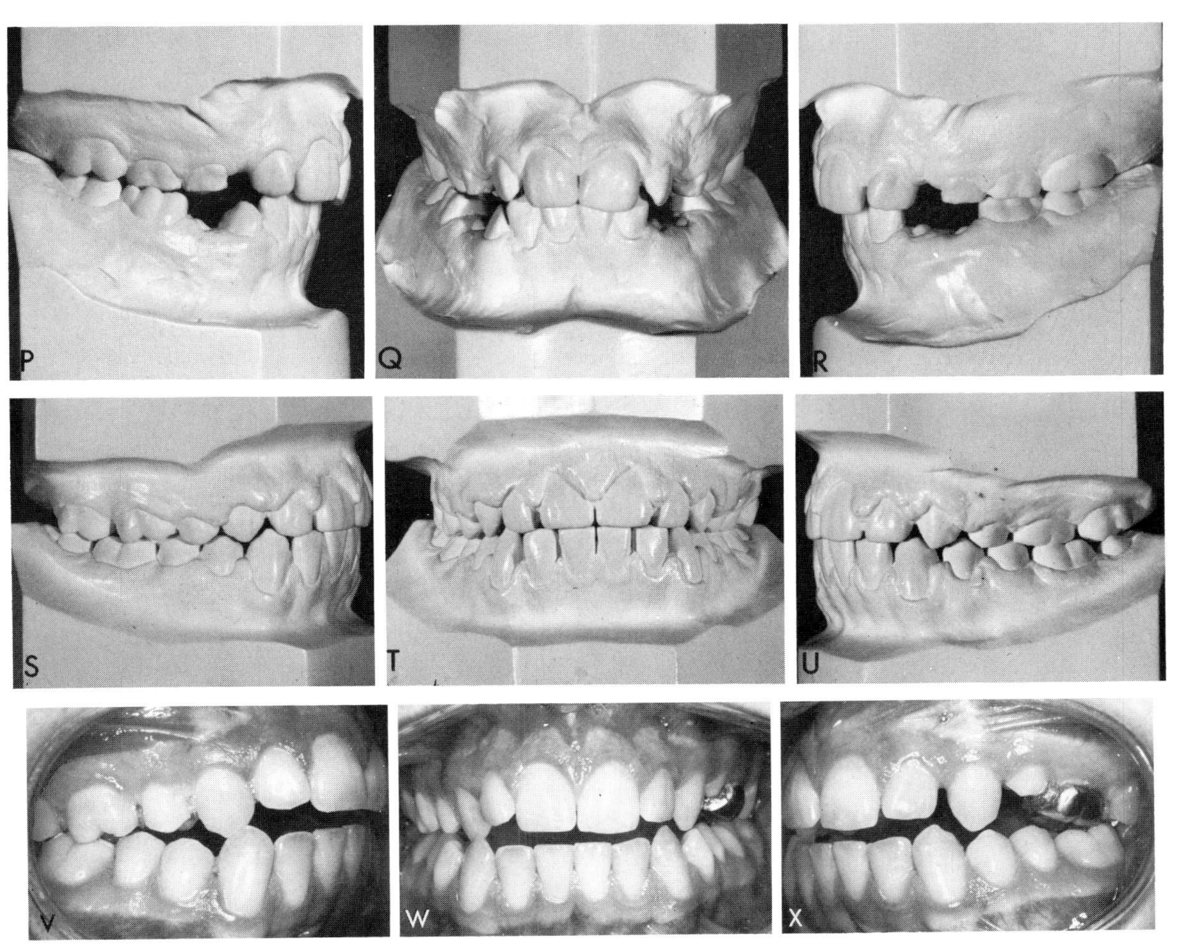

Figure 13–29 *Continued.* *P–X,* Occlusal views. Occlusion at age 11 years *(P–R).* Occlusion after 22 months of orthodontic treatment *(S–U).* Maxillary 1st premolars were extracted. High pull face-bow was worn to inhibit posterior maxillary development. Occlusion 4 years, 6 months after treatment *(V–X).* The position of the ankylosed maxillary left 1st premolar that was in occlusion at completion of treatment indicates the amount of eruption of the teeth, yet the teeth anterior to the 1st molars are still not in occlusion.

DENTAL ALIGNMENT. Crowded and malaligned maxillary and mandibular anterior teeth.

DENTAL OCCLUSION. End-to-end canine and molar relationship.

TREATMENT PLAN

Orthodontic Treatment

1. Band all maxillary and mandibular teeth with edgewise orthodontic appliance.
2. Extract maxillary first premolars to facilitate alignment of maxillary arch.
3. Use high-pull facebow to inhibit posterior maxillary development.
4. Relieve arch irregularities.
5. Coordinate the dental arches.

ACTIVE TREATMENT AND FOLLOW-UP

After extraction of the maxillary first premolars, the arches were aligned and coordinated within 22 months. Cephalometric monitoring revealed essentially no change in the 42° mandibular plane angle. Because of continued vertical facial growth, the anterior facial height increased 13 mm. As a consequence, the bite started opening slowly after treatment. Post-treatment growth similar to that observed in the pretreatment growth study continued, with the result that anterior facial height continued to increase more than posterior facial height. Compensatory eruption of the anterior teeth was insufficient to compensate for the excessive anterior vertical facial growth. As a result, the bite opened despite orthodontic treatment. Sequential clinical, cephalometric, and occlusal studies showed the effects of this latent vertical facial growth (see Fig. 13–29).

Orthodontist: Thomas D. Creekmore, Houston, Texas.

CASE 13–9 (Fig. 13–30)

This case illustrates orthodontic treatment of open bite complicated by latent vertical facial growth.

J. A., a 17-year-old boy, was seen in consultation with an orthodontist for treatment of his severe anterior open bite. He had received orthodontic treatment at age 11. A retrospective study of his clinical, cephalometric, and occlusal records revealed the following problems at the time when orthodontic treatment was initiated in 1972.

PROBLEM LIST

Esthetics

FRONTAL. Excessive exposure of teeth in repose and when smiling.

PROFILE. Prominent upper lip; retropositioned mandible and contour-deficient chin; long face; severe lip strain with lips sealed.

Text continued on page 1190.

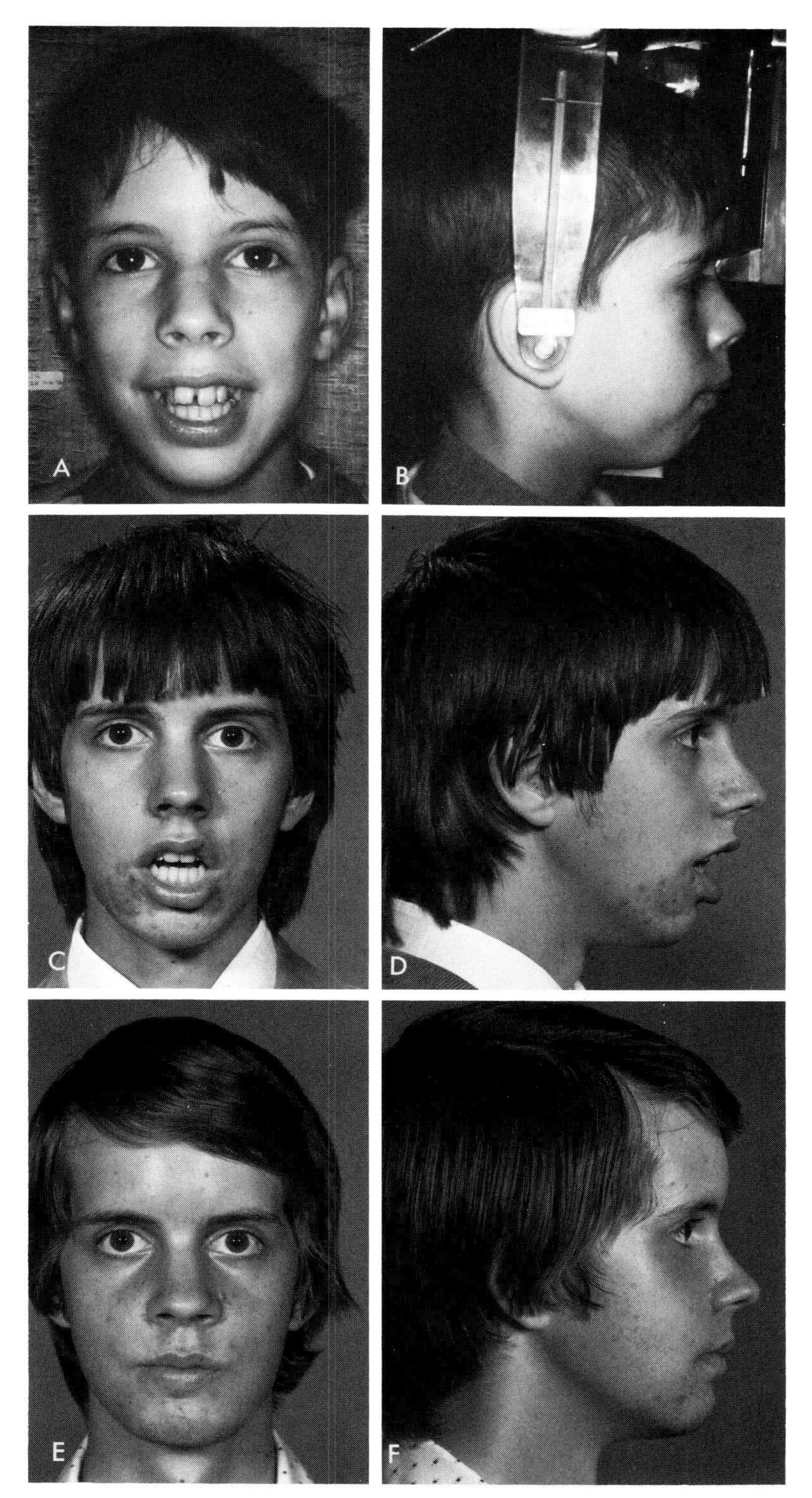

Figure 13–30 (Case 13–9). *A–F,* Facial views. *A* and *B,* Before orthodontic treatment, age 11 years. *C* and *D,* At age 17, 4 years after orthodontic treatment was completed. *E* and *F,* Facial appearance after Le Fort I osteotomy and horizontal sliding genioplasty (age 18 years, 5 months).

Illustration continued on the following page

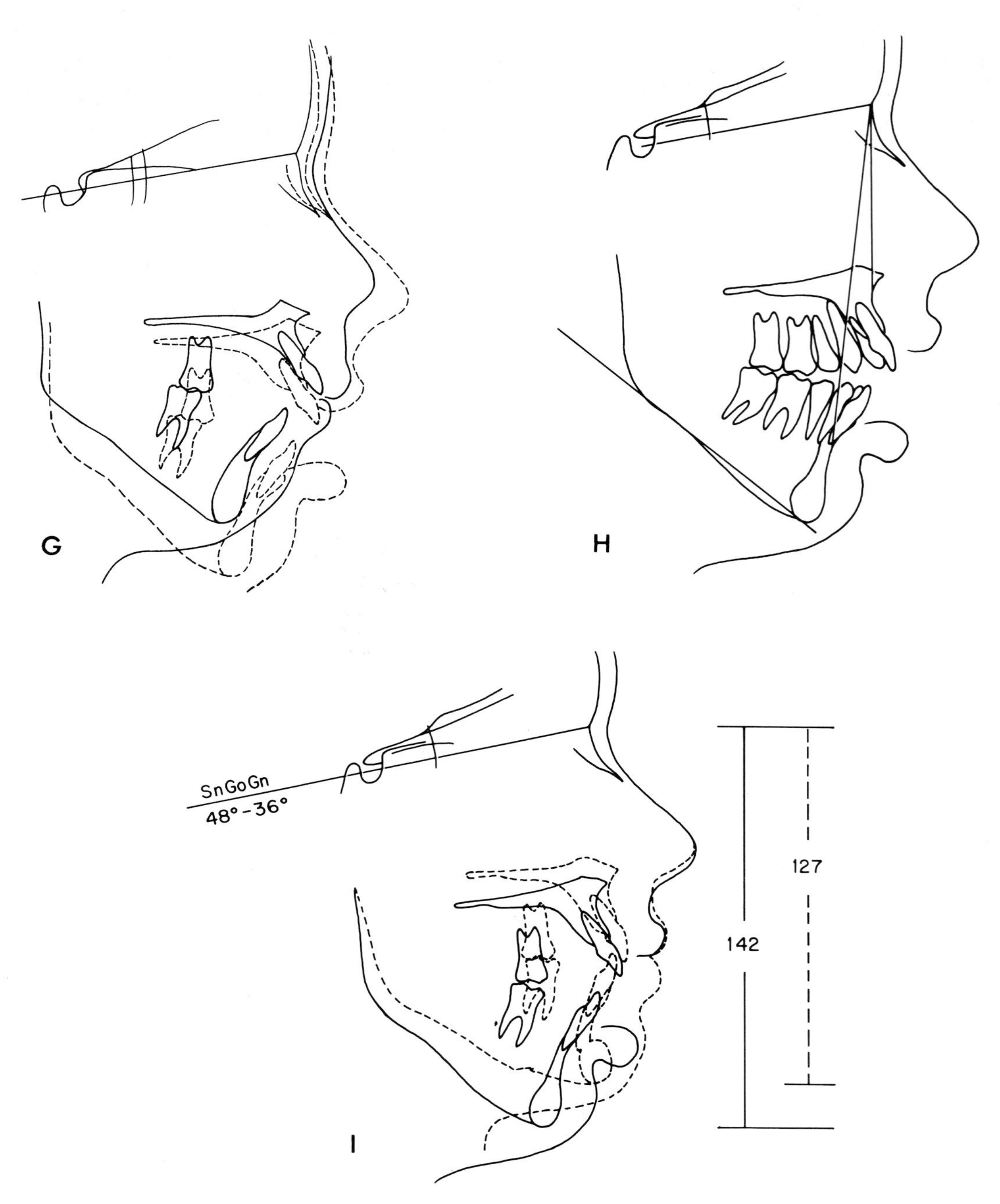

Figure 13–30 *Continued.*

G, Composite cephalometric tracings after orthodontic treatment and recurrence of open bite (*solid line,* age 13 years) and 4 years later (*broken line,* age 17 years, 3 months) demonstrating latent vertical facial growth that caused recurrence of the anterior open bite. *H,* Cephalometric tracing before surgery (age 18 years, 3 months). *I,* Composite cephalometric tracings before surgery (*solid line,* age 18 years, 3 months) and after Le Fort I osteotomy and genioplasty (*broken line,* age 18 years, 5 months).

Legend continued on the opposite page

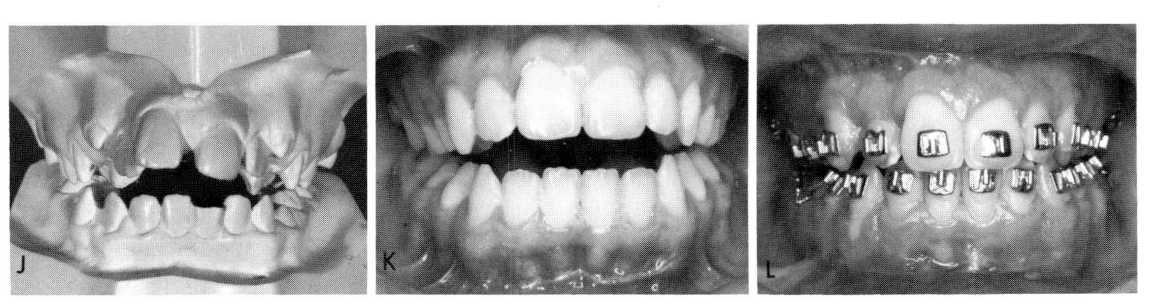

Figure 13–30 *Continued.* *J–L,* Occlusal views. Before orthodontic treatment *(J)*. Anterior open bite 4 years after completion of orthodontic treatment *(K)*. (This case study is incomplete because all the patient's records were not available for study.) Occlusion after surgery *(L)*. Open bite has remained closed and postoperative result stable over a 2-year postoperative follow-up period. Long-term postoperative view is not available.

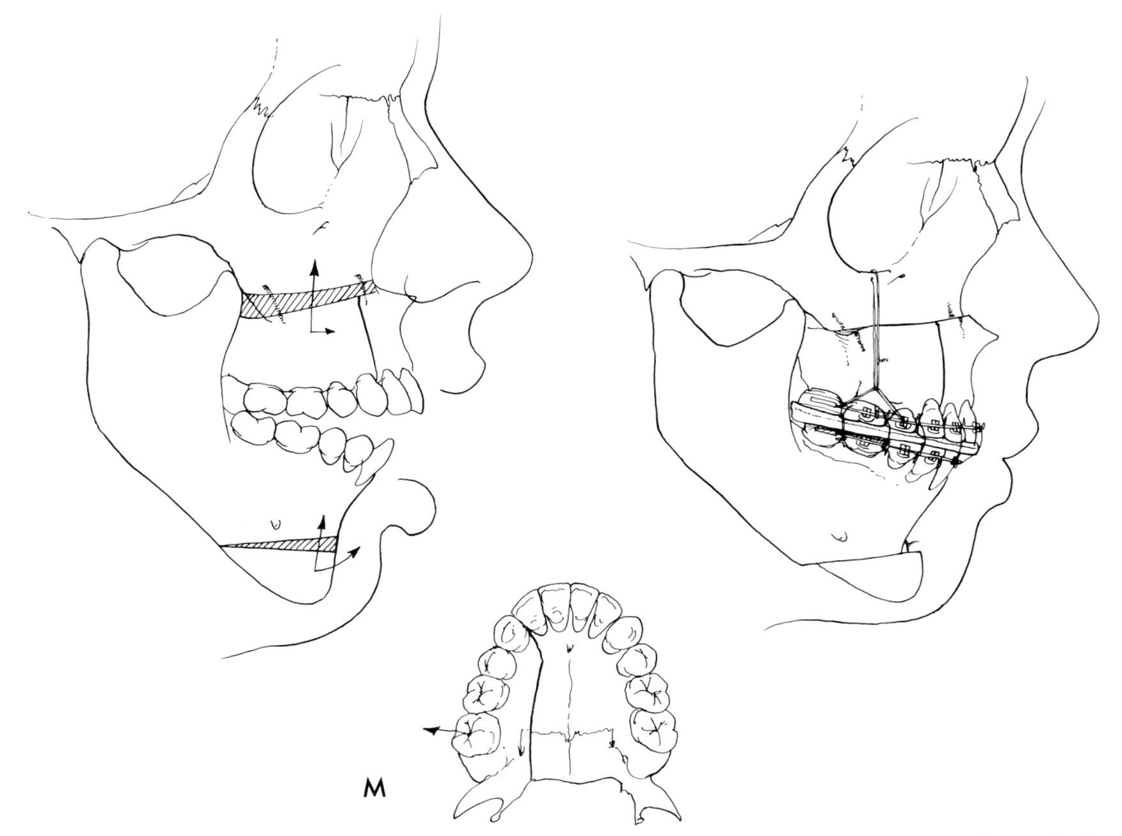

M, Plan of surgery: Le Fort I osteotomy (two-piece) to reposition maxilla superiorly and anteriorly to shorten lower anterior facial height, close open bite, and widen maxilla; horizontal sliding osteotomy of inferior border of mandible to increase chin prominence and decrease vertical height of mental symphysis.

Cephalometric Analysis

1. High mandibular plane angle; SN–GoGn 47°.
2. Excessive lower anterior facial height.
3. SNA 78°; SNB 72°; ANB 6°.
4. $\underline{1}$ to NA 33°, 12 mm; $\overline{1}$ to NB 26°, 10 mm; Po to NB 0 mm.
5. Anterior open bite deformity.
6. Retropositioned mandible.
7. Excessive curvature of maxillary occlusal plane.

Occlusal Analysis

DENTAL ARCH FORM. *Maxilla*: Tapered and constricted with high palatal vault. *Mandible*: U-shaped.

DENTAL ALIGNMENT. Crowded and malaligned maxillary and mandibular anterior teeth.

DENTAL OCCLUSION. Class II canine and molar relationship with 10-mm overjet; 5-mm anterior open bite extending from molar region of one side to contralateral molar region; congenitally missing mandibular second premolars; excessive curvature of maxillary occlusal plane; partially erupted maxillary canines.

TREATMENT PLAN

Orthodontic Treatment

1. Extract maxillary deciduous canines, permanent first premolars, and mandibular second deciduous molars to facilitate alignment of maxillary and mandibular arches and closure of open bite.
2. Place edgewise appliances on maxillary and mandibular teeth.
3. Apply Class II elastic traction.

TREATMENT AND FOLLOW-UP

After the necessary extractions were accomplished, the arches were aligned and coordinated and the anterior open bite was closed with box elastics and Class II elastic traction within 24 months. Despite the use of a positioner and continuous myotherapy after active orthodontic treatment was completed, the anterior open bite gradually reoccurred. Within two years, a 6-mm anterior open bite and a 7-mm overjet appeared. The patient manifested most of the typical facial and skeletal features associated with an open bite deformity. His teeth, however, remained remarkably well aligned and the dental arches remained nearly coordinated. A 20-mm interlabial gap, severely retropositioned chin, excessively long face, and an anterior open bite prompted him to seek surgical treatment. Cephalometric and model studies indicated the feasibility of correcting his occlusal and esthetic problems by Le Fort I osteotomy to advance the maxilla and superiorly reposition it in two segments, close the anterior open bite, increase the intercanine and intermolar width, and reduce the height of the lower face and the interlabial gap. (The posterior maxilla was raised 10 mm; the anterior maxilla was raised 3 mm). The patient's contour-deficient chin would be augmented 6 mm by horizontal sliding osteotomy.

Closure of the anterior open bite and improved nose-lip-chin balance were achieved by the surgical treatment. Postsurgical orthodontic treatment, which was started at release from intermaxillary fixation three weeks after surgery, was completed within six months.

COMMENT

A retrospective analysis of the patient's growth after orthodontic treatment by sequential cephalometric tracings indicated that latent vertical facial growth had outstripped compensatory tooth eruption. As a consequence, the anterior open bite reoccurred. In males with this type of dentofacial deformity, vertical facial growth may continue until after age 21. As a result, there is the possibility of operating before growth has terminated. Psychologic factors and the magnitude of this individual's problem far outweigh this consideration and militate against any delay in surgical treatment.

Surgeon: William H. Bell, Dallas, Texas.

CASE 13–10 (Fig. 13–31)

This case illustrates relapse after bilateral sagittal osteotomies of vertical rami to advance mandible and close anterior open bite.

J. M., a 23-year-old woman, was first seen in August 1970. She complained of pain in the area of her temporomandibular joints. She reported a six-month history of bilateral temporomandibular joint pain that was more severe on the right side. Examination revealed tenderness in the right masseter muscle and arthralgia in the right temporomandibular joint. The pain was treated by a conservative regimen of rest, diazepam, and a disocclusion splint. Serologic tests for rheumatoid factor were within normal limits. During the following two weeks there was complete resolution of the pain and joint tenderness.

PROBLEM LIST

Esthetics

FRONTAL. Symmetric ovoid face.

PROFILE. Moderate facial convexity with contour-deficient chin; 7-mm lip incompetence; 5-mm tooth exposure with lips in relaxed posture.

Cephalometric Analysis

1. Vertical maxillary excess with anterior open bite.
2. Moderately high mandibular plane angle, SN–GoGn 50°.
3. Relative mandibular retrusion; ANB 9°; SNA 80° SNB 71°.

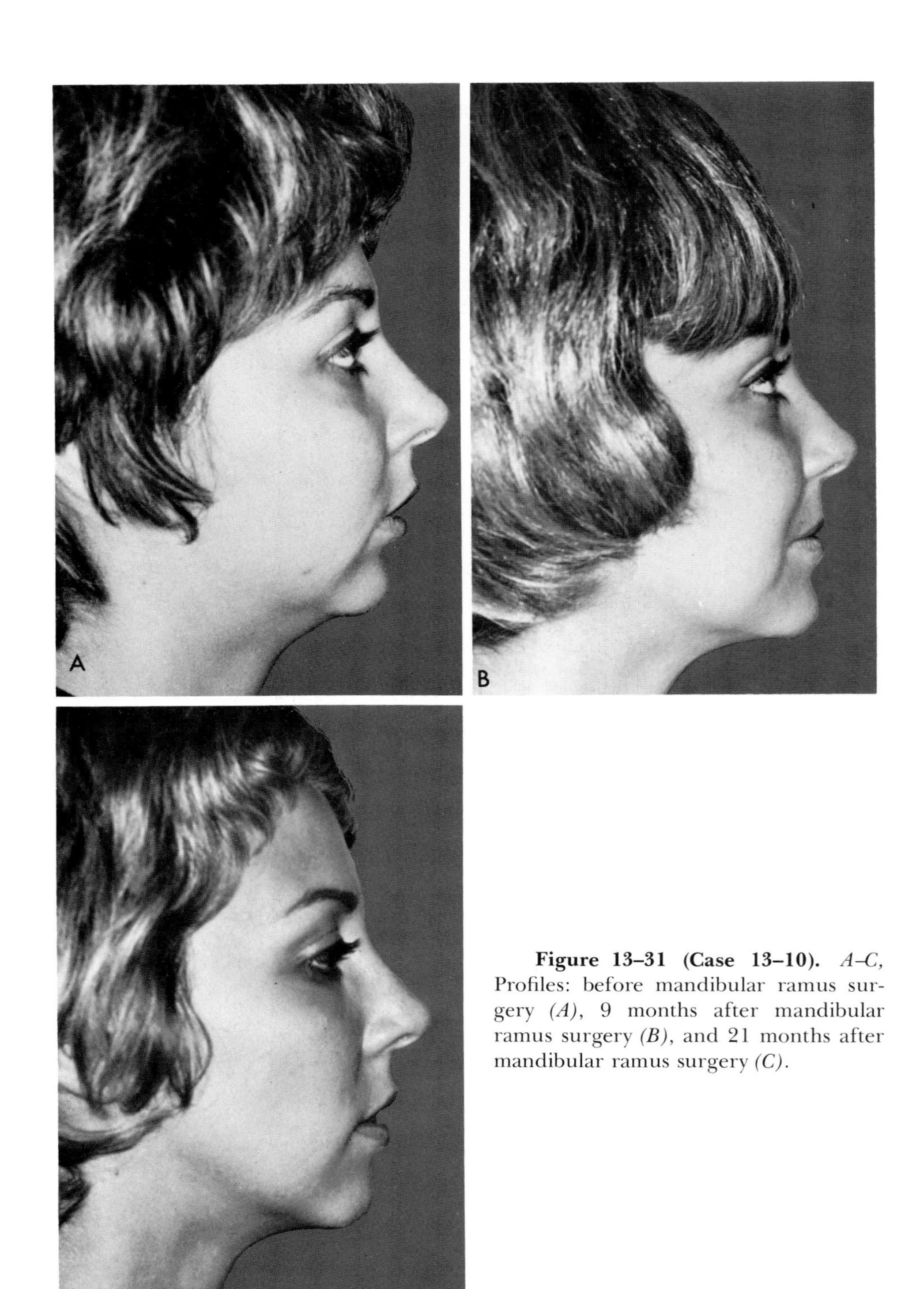

Figure 13–31 (Case 13–10). *A–C,* Profiles: before mandibular ramus surgery *(A)*, 9 months after mandibular ramus surgery *(B)*, and 21 months after mandibular ramus surgery *(C)*.

Legend continued on the opposite page

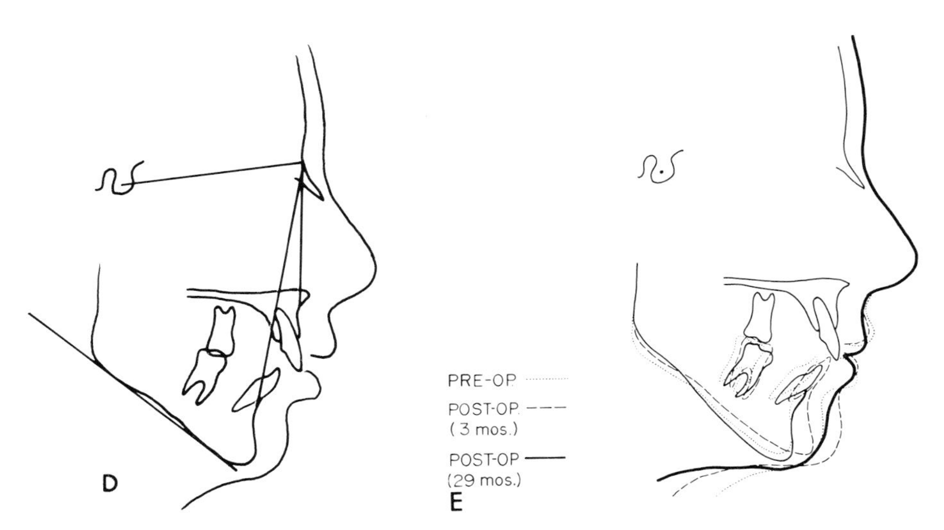

Figure 13–31 *Continued.* *D,* Preoperative cephalometric tracing, age 23 years. *E,* Composite cephalometric tracings before mandibular ramus surgery (*dotted line,* age 23 years), 3 months after ramus surgery (*broken line,* age 23 years, 3 months), and 29 months after ramus surgery (*solid line,* age 25 years, 5 months).

Illustration continued on the following page

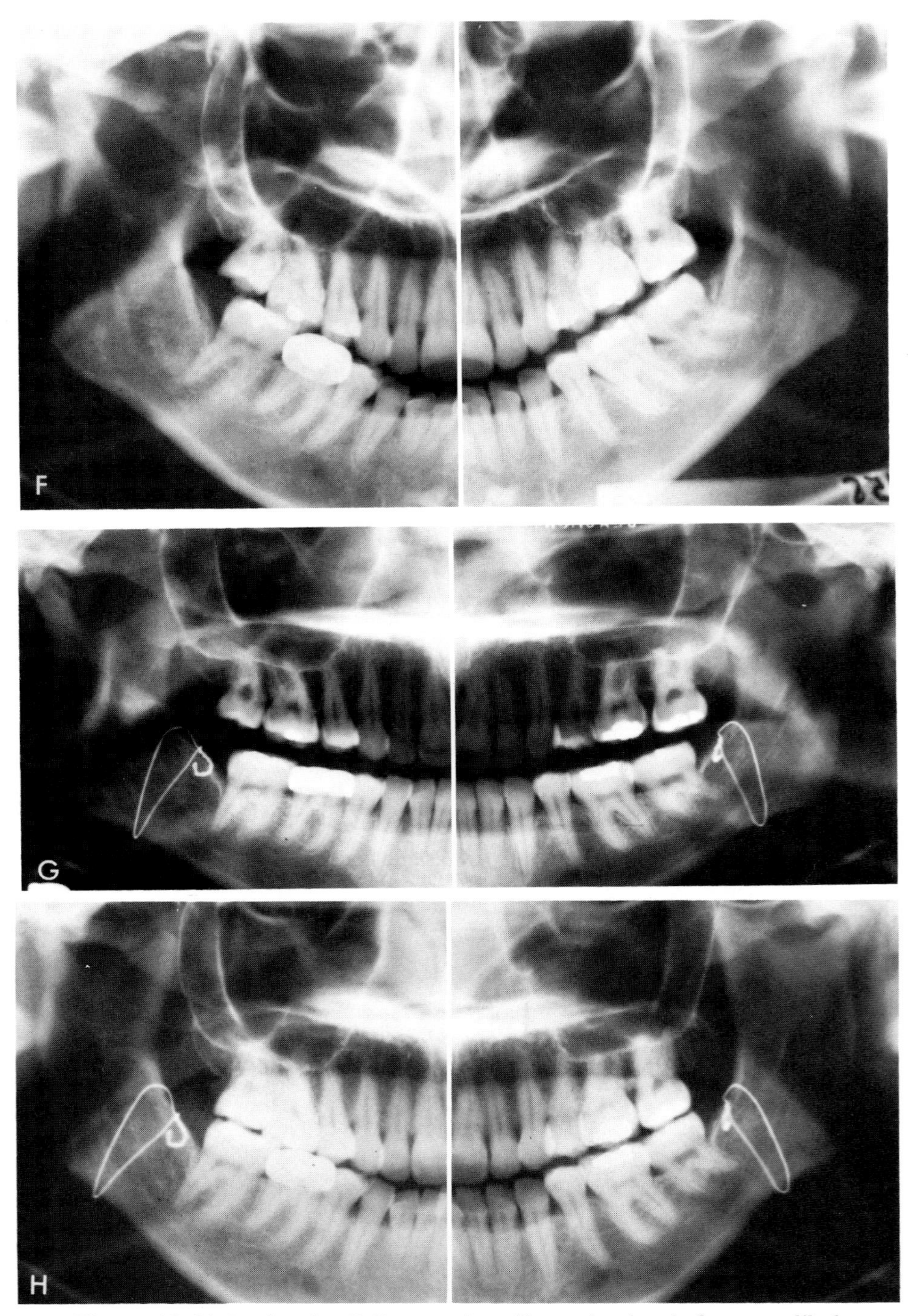

Figure 13–31 *Continued.* *F,* Panoramic radiograph taken before mandibular surgery. *G,* Panoramic radiograph taken 3 months after ramus surgery. *H,* Panoramic radiograph 21 months after ramus surgery, showing marked diminution in size of condyles.

Legend continued on the opposite page

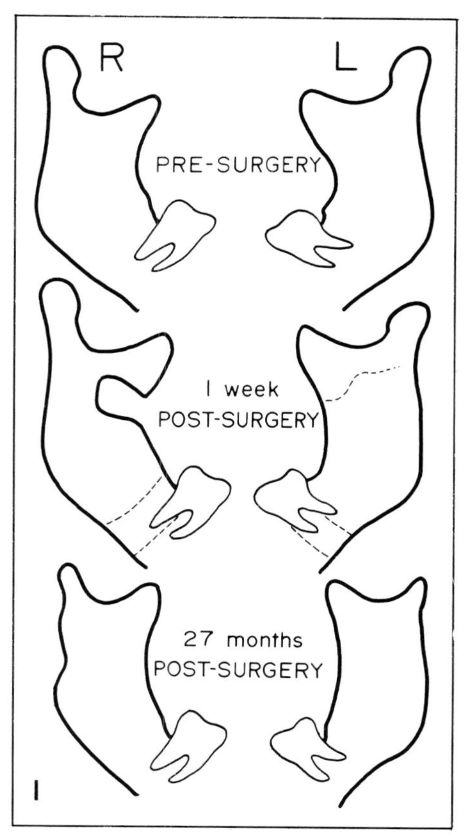

Figure 13–31 *Continued. I,* Composite tracings of representative panoramic radiographs.

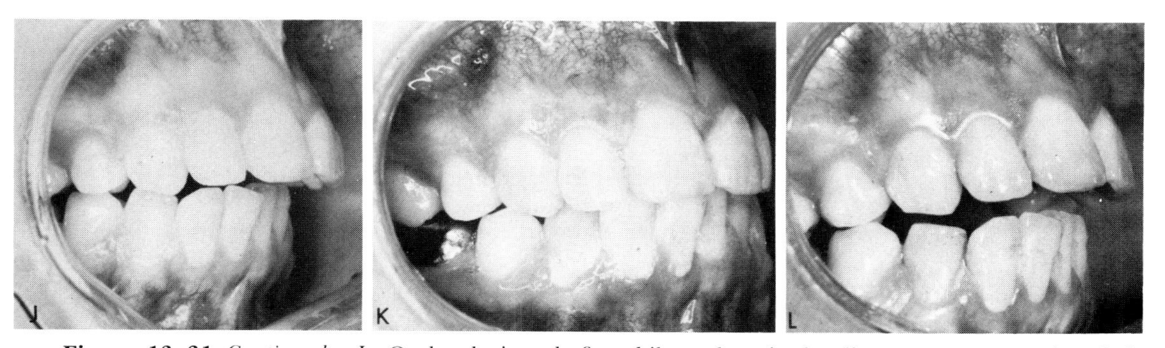

Figure 13–31 *Continued.* *L,* Occlusal view: before bilateral sagittal split ramus osteotomies. *J,* 9 months after ramus surgery (*K*), and 21 months after ramus surgery (*L*).

Illustration continued on the following page

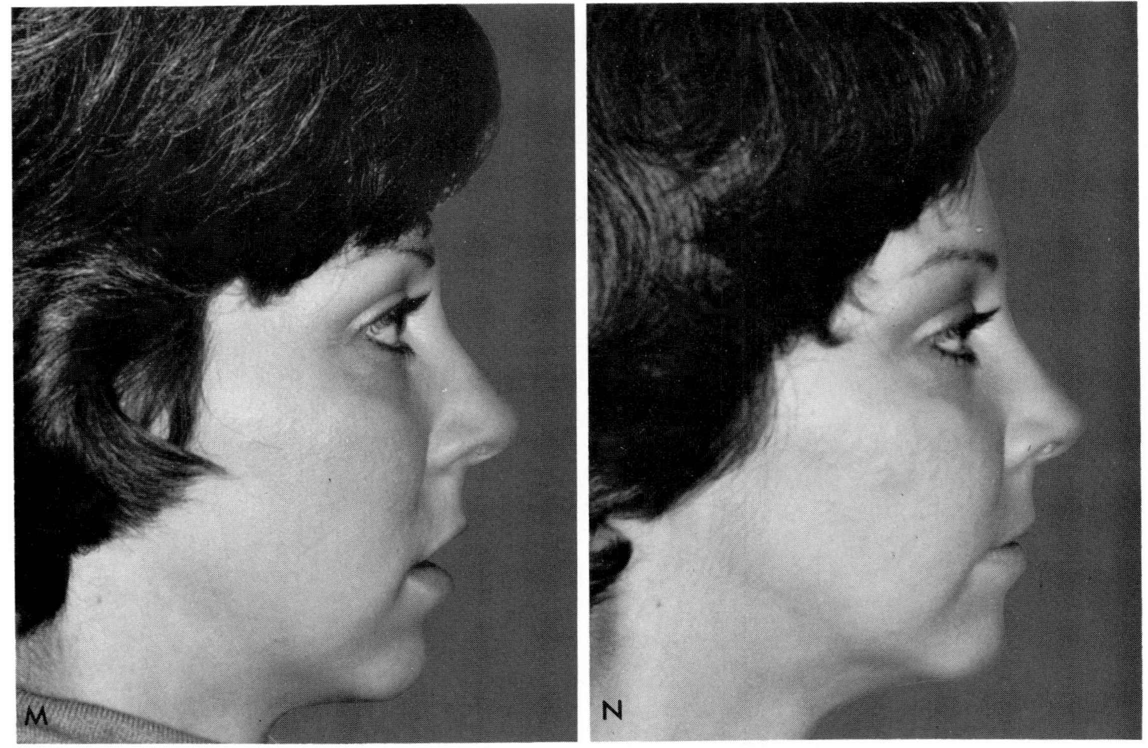

Figure 13–31 *Continued.* *M,* Profile 6 years, 6 months after original mandibular ramus surgery. *N,* Profile 3 months after correction of anterior open bite by Le Fort I osteotomy.

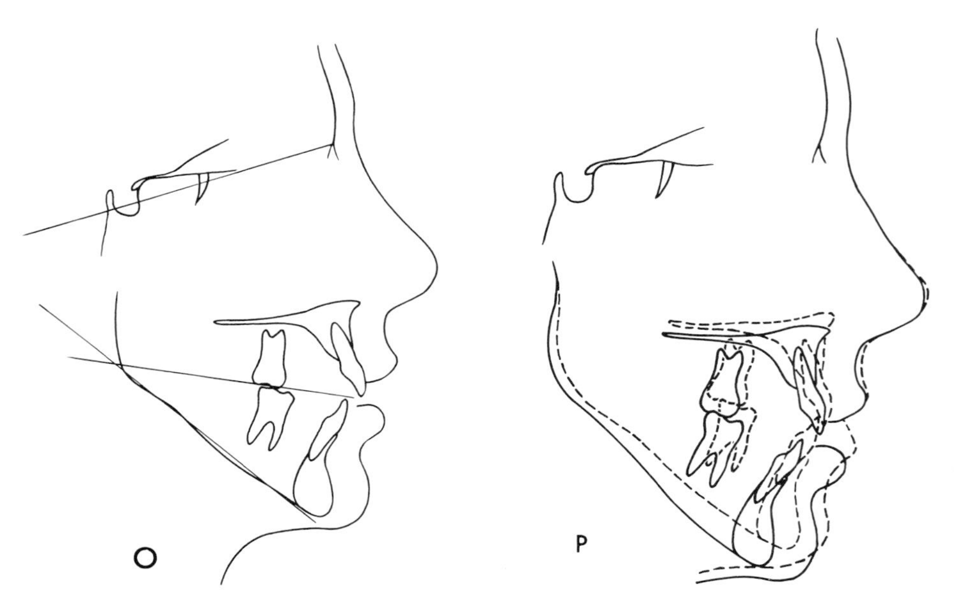

Figure 13–31 *Continued.* *O,* Cephalometric tracing 6 years, 6 months after mandibular ramus surgery. *P,* Composite cephalometric tracings before (*solid line,* age 29 years, 6 months) and after (*broken line,* age 30 years, 9 months) Le Fort I osteotomy to close anterior open bite and allow autorotational movement of mandible.

Illustration continued on the following page

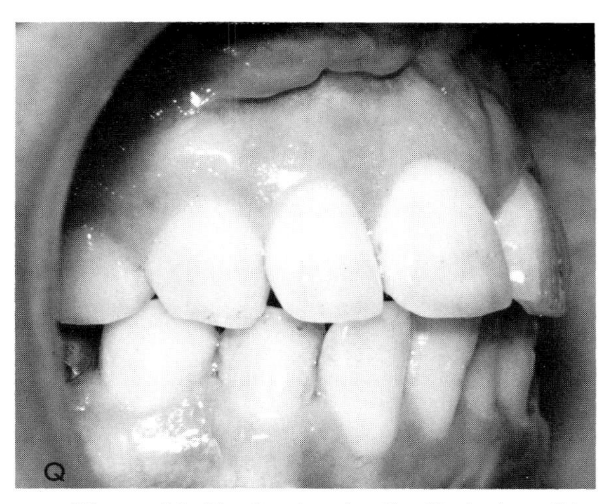

Figure 13–31 *Continued.* *Q,* Occlusion 24 months after Le Fort I osteotomy to close anterior open bite.

Occlusal Analysis

DENTAL ARCH FORM. Maxillary arch tapered and constricted; mandibular arch tapered.

DENTAL ALIGNMENT. Crowding of mandibular anterior teeth.

DENTAL OCCLUSION. End-to-end canine and molar relationship with anterior open bite.

TREATMENT PLAN

Surgical Treatment

1. Bilateral sagittal osteotomies of vertical rami to advance the mandible 6 mm into Class I canine and molar relationship and rotate the mandible to close the open bite.

TREATMENT AND FOLLOW-UP

On September 30, 1970, a sagittal split ramus osteotomy was performed bilaterally. The mandible was repositioned anteriorly 6 mm and rotated slightly. The pterygomasseteric sling was detached from its bony insertions to minimize relapse and facilitate the bone incisions. After the proximal and distal bone fragments were approximated with circumramus wires, care was taken to insure proper positioning of the mandibular condyles in the glenoid fossae as the wires were tightened.

On the seventh postoperative day, a panoramic radiograph showed the condyles to be well seated in the glenoid fossae. Intermaxillary fixation was maintained for five weeks after surgery, by which time there was clinical union of the ramus segments. Three months following surgery, the occlusion appeared stable with no clinical evidence of relapse. Nine months following surgery, after adjustment of occlusal prematurities, the occlusion appeared to be stable and the patient was free of temporomandibular joint pain. Radiographic examination indicated early signs of bilateral atrophy of the mandibular condyles.

The patient did not keep her recall appointments and was not seen again until 21 months following surgery. At this time, she was observed to have a total relapse with additional anterior open bite deformity. Because of the suspicious radiographic appearance of the mandibular condyles, a diagnosis of rheumatoid arthritis was reconsidered. Results of a complete series of rheumatoid arthritis studies, however, were all within normal limits. The patient was virtually free of temporomandibular joint pain during the next three years of close follow-up. A careful retrospective review of study models, radiographs, and clinical findings revealed that relapse occurred during the first 27 months following surgery. The radiographic changes are summarized by tracings of representative radiographs in Figure 13–31.

Increased tension of the geniohyoid and anterior digastric muscles has been suggested as a cause of skeletal relapse following mandibular advancement. In addition to release of the pterygomasseteric sling, various procedures have been suggested to prevent relapse. These include the use of posterior bite-opening interocclusal splints, neck braces, longer periods of intermaxillary fixation, overcorrection of the occlusion, stripping of the internal pterygoid muscle from the mobilized distal bone fragment, and suprahyoid myotomies. In this case, pterygomasseteric sling detachment only was used.

Six and one-half years after the original mandibular surgery, the patient was reevaluated. Clinical, cephalometric, and occlusal findings were similar to the records that had been taken after relapse. Clinical analysis, model surgery, and cephalometric prediction studies indicated the feasibility of correcting the dentofacial deformity by maxillary surgery.

SECONDARY SURGICAL PLAN

1. Le Fort I osteotomy (one-piece) to
   a. Raise maxilla 4 mm.
   b. Close open bite.
   c. Reduce lip incompetence.
   d. Reduce amount of maxillary incisor tooth exposure.
   e. Allow autorotational movement of mandible.
2. Possible secondary genioplasty if chin remains contour-deficient after maxillary surgery.

TREATMENT AND COMMENTS

Occlusal balance and improved facial appearance were achieved by Le Fort I osteotomy. As with all surgical procedures designed to advance the mandible, relapse can occur following sagittal split ramus osteotomies. Although a definite etiology could not be established, a biomechanical phenomenon based on increased muscle tension was the most likely causative mechanism. Maxillary surgery frequently provides the clinician a feasible and practical means of treating individuals who have been unsuccessfully treated by mandibular surgery and/or orthodontics. We have successfully treated the occlusal and esthetic problems of numerous patients who have had such treatment with subsequent relapse. Occlusal and skeletal stability have been routinely achieved in such patients.

Surgeon: Rod Phillips, Beaumont, Texas.

CASE 13–11 (Fig. 13–32)

R. T., an 18-year-old boy, desired treatment to improve the contour of his face and to correct his open bite, which had been present since the eruption of his permanent teeth. He reported having had asthma and hay fever for more than five years. His speech was abnormal because of his difficulty with sibilant sounds. Analysis of his clinical records revealed the following problem list.

PROBLEM LIST

Esthetics

FRONTAL. Adequate exposure of the maxillary anterior teeth and gingiva in function and repose; prominent upper and lower lips.

PROFILE. Excessive facial convexity with lack of chin prominence; 7-mm interlabial gap; prominent, everted lower lip.

Text continued on page 1203.

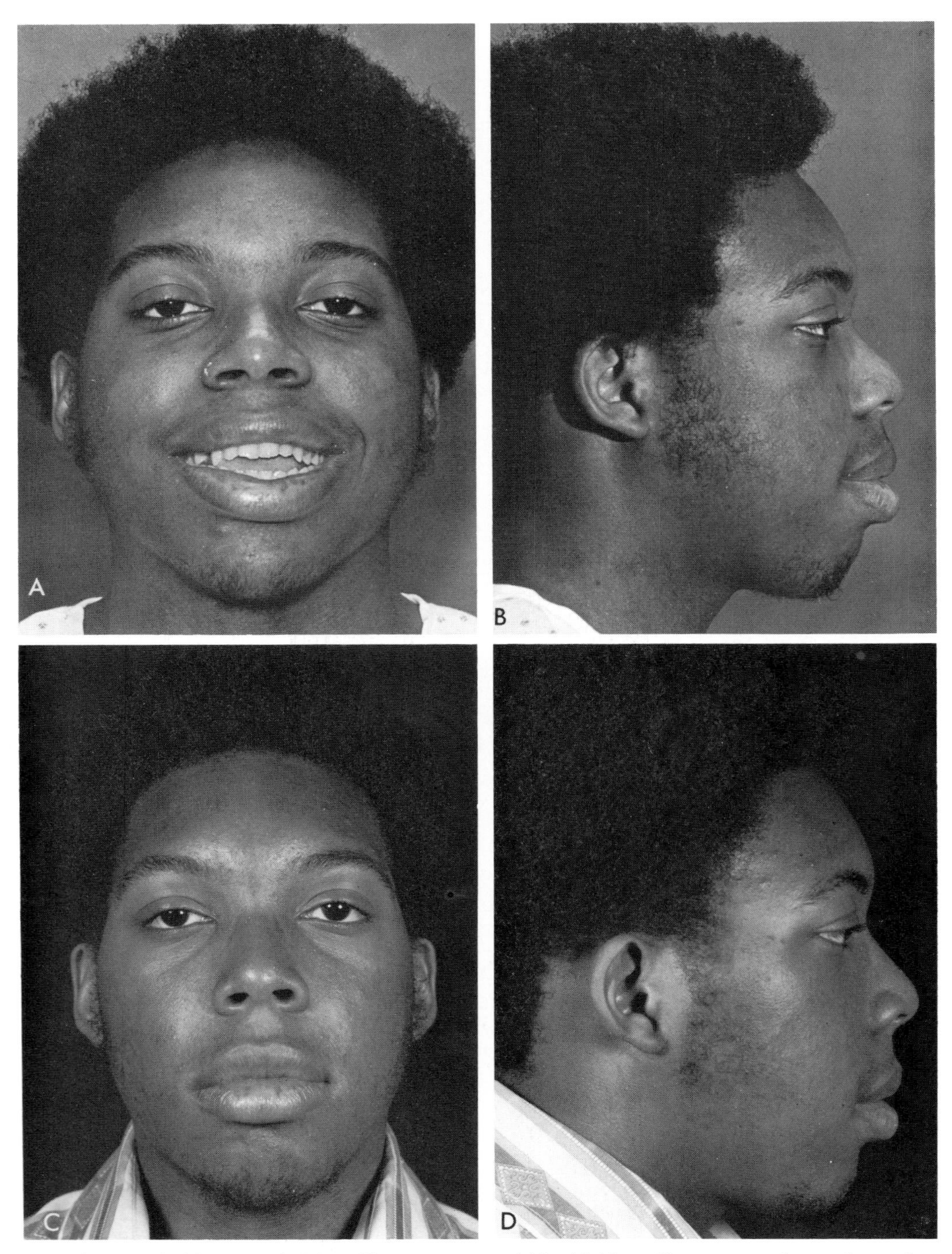

Figure 13–32 (Case 13–11). Young man aged 18 with bimaxillary protrusion and associated anterior open bite. *A–D,* Facial views before (*A* and *B*) and after (*C* and *D*) treatment.

Legend continued on the opposite page

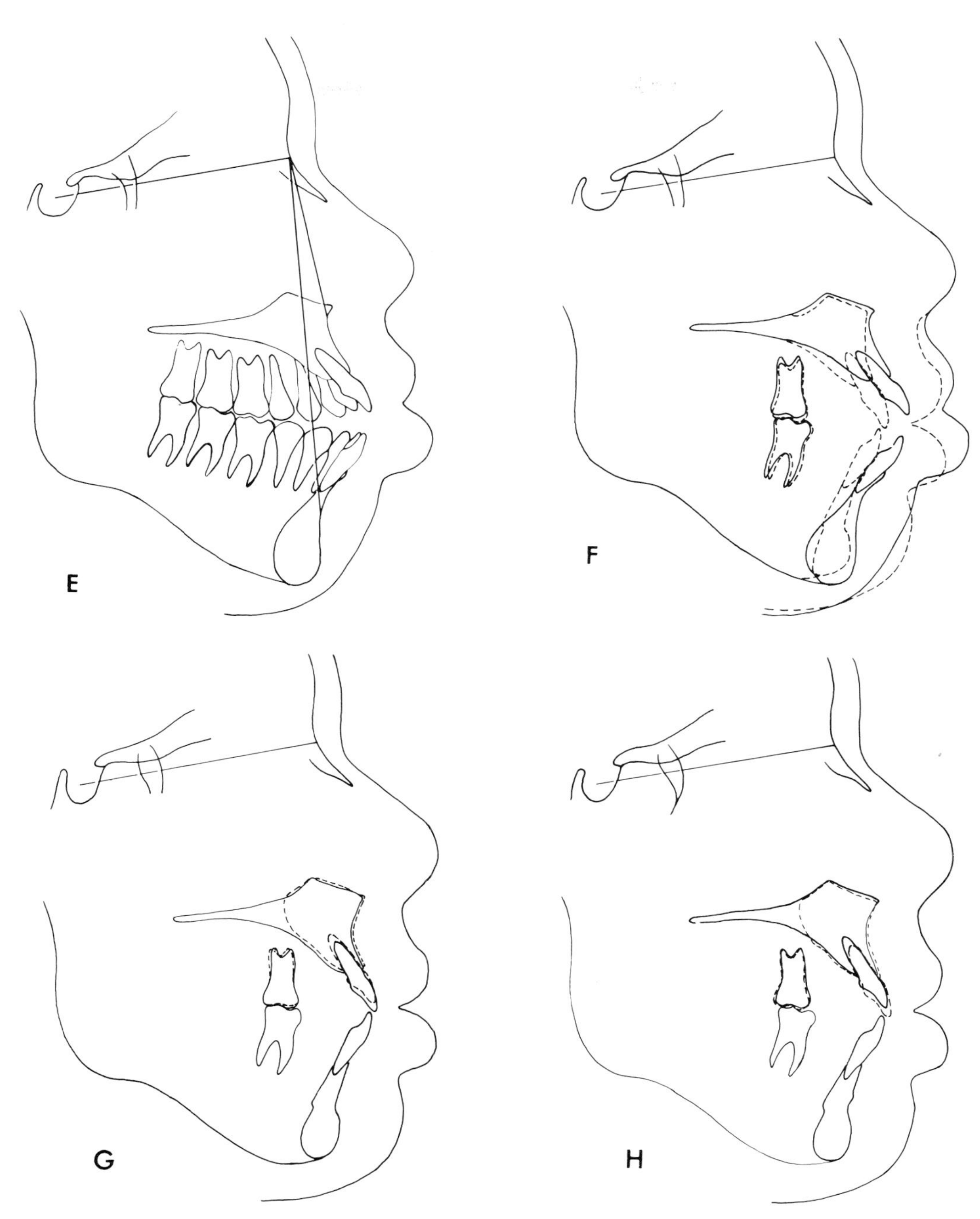

Figure 13–32 *Continued.* *E,* Cephalometric tracing before treatment (age 18 years, 2 months). *F,* Composite cephalometric tracings before (*solid line,* age 18 years, 2 months) and after (*broken line,* age 18 years, 4 months) correction by anterior maxillary and mandibular subapical osteotomies. *G,* Cephalometric tracing 5 months after surgery demonstrating relapse. *H,* Composite cephalometric tracings 5 months after jaw surgery (*solid line,* age 18 years, 7 months) and 1 month after partial glossectomy (*broken line,* age 18 years, 8 months), showing spontaneous correction within 1 month. Four years after partial glossectomy correction was stable.

Illustration continued on the following page

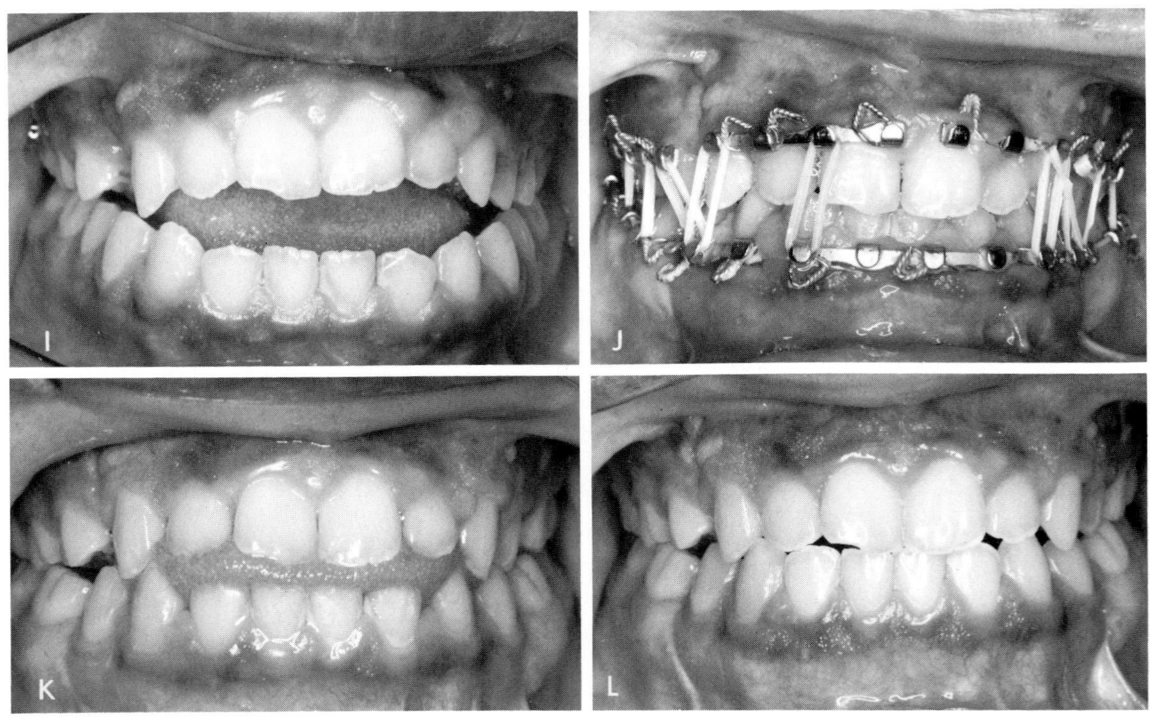

Figure 13–32 *Continued.* *I,* Occlusion before treatment. *J,* Occlusion 2 months after surgical closure of anterior open bite. *K,* Recurrent open bite 3 months after release from intermaxillary fixation. *L,* Occlusion 1 month after partial glossectomy showing spontaneous correction of open bite, which has remained closed over a 4-year postoperative period of follow-up.

Cephalometric Analysis

1. Procumbent maxillary and mandibular incisors.
2. Seven-millimeter interlabial gap.
3. SNA 86°; SNB 87°; ANB difference 8°; $\underline{1}$ to NA 6°; $\overline{1}$ to NB 15°.
4. Steep mandibular plane angle, 46°.
5. Anterior open bite, 7 mm.
6. Excessive curvature of maxillary occlusal plane.
7. Reverse curvature of mandibular occlusal plane.

Occlusal Analysis

DENTAL ARCH FORM. Tapered maxillary arch with high palatal vault.

DENTAL ALIGNMENT. Satisfactory alignment of maxillary and mandibular teeth.

DENTAL OCCLUSION. Class I molar and canine relationship with 7-mm anterior open bite extending from the second premolar region forward to the incisors; macroglossia; tongue thrust when swallowing; frequent posturing of tongue between anterior teeth when in repose and swallowing.

TREATMENT PLAN

Surgical Treatment

1. Anterior maxillary and mandibular ostectomies in second premolar areas to
   a. Reduce facial convexity.
   b. Close anterior open bite.
2. Augmentation genioplasty with 8-mm thick alloplastic implant (Proplast).
3. Secondary cheiloplasty to reduce prominence of lower lip for better harmony with upper lip.
4. Partial glossectomy to reduce size of tongue should the open bite recur after maxillary and mandibular ostectomies.

TREATMENT

Anterior maxillary and mandibular ostectomies were performed simultaneously with the patient under general nasoendotracheal anesthesia. Maxillomandibular fixation was maintained for seven weeks, after which light night-time elastics were worn for another four weeks. Despite the fact that the upper and lower retention appliances were worn for an additional three months, there was a gradual and progressive opening of the bite in the anterior region. Posturing of patient's large tongue between the anterior teeth was implicated as the cause of his recurrent open bite. Within the next two months (five months after removal of intermaxillary fixation), a "keyhole" partial glossectomy was performed to reduce the size of the tongue and eliminate the patient's habit of posturing his tongue between his anterior teeth. A 6-cm by 5-cm wedge resection was accomplished under general anesthesia. The use of Solu-Medrol appeared to reduce the amount of postoperative tongue swelling.

Within a period of four to five weeks after an uneventful postoperative recovery, the open bite gradually closed spontaneously. One year after jaw surgery, an 8-mm thick Proplast implant was placed to augment the patient's contour-deficient chin. The surgery was accomplished simultaneously with a reduction cheiloplasty.

FOLLOW-UP

A Class I canine relationship with a satisfactory overbite and overjet were accomplished by the maxillary and mandibular ostectomies. During a four-year period of postoperative follow-up, the bite has remained closed with no discernible change in the position of the mobilized segments or the occlusion.

The result of the reduction cheiloplasty was probably compromised by the fact that it was performed simultaneously with the augmentation genioplasty. Ideally, it should be performed independent of, and after, chin surgery. The patient's tongue, which previously did not "fit" into his mouth, appeared to be of average size and functioned normally after treatment. More importantly, he ceased to posture his tongue between his anterior teeth when speaking or in repose. His speech was improved as evidenced by his lack of difficulty with sibilants.

Surgeon: William H. Bell, Dallas, Texas.

CASE 13–12 (Fig. 13–33)

R. F., a 39-year-old woman, desired treatment to improve the contour of her face and to correct her open bite. Because of alveolar bone loss, the general condition of the periodontium, and the age of the patient, a satisfactory occlusal and esthetic result could not be obtained by orthodontic treatment alone. Consequently, the following problem list and plan of treatment were developed.

PROBLEM LIST

Esthetics

1. Prominent lips.
2. Stretching of the perioral and mentalis muscles with the lips sealed.
3. Contour-deficient chin.

Cephalometric Analysis

1. Maxillary and mandibular teeth tipped forward off their skeletal bases. $\underline{1}$ to NA 37°, 9 mm; $\overline{1}$ to NB 36°, 8 mm.
2. Interincisal angle 115°.

Occlusal Analysis

DENTAL ARCH FORM. Maxilla and mandible tapered and symmetric.

DENTAL ALIGNMENT. Crowding in anterior part of maxilla and mandible.

DENTAL OCCLUSION. Unilateral Class II bimaxillary dental protrusion with 3 mm anterior open bite, extending from canine to canine.

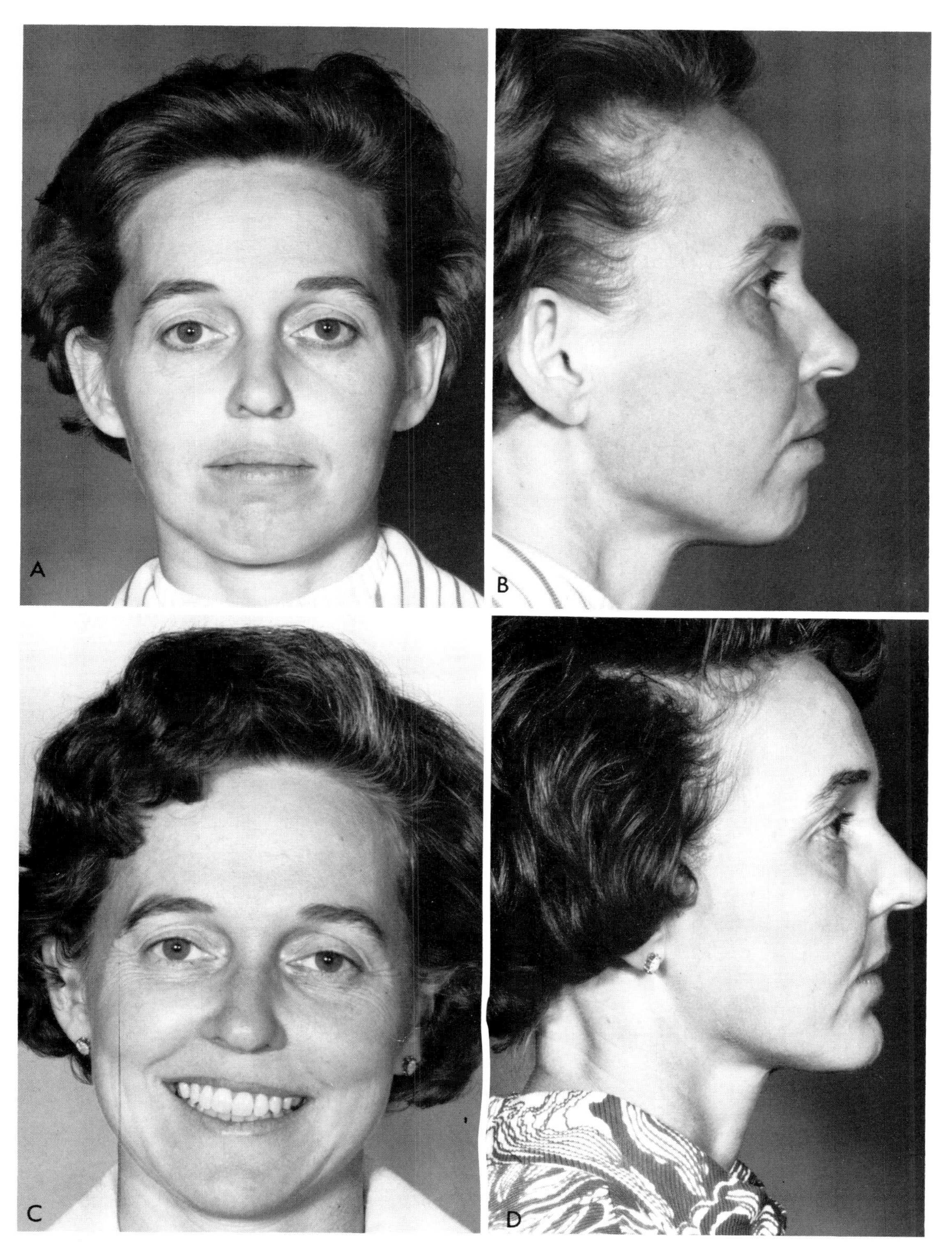

Figure 13–33 (Case 13–12). Woman, aged 39, with bimaxillary dental protrusion and open bite. Before (*A* and *B*) and after (*C* and *D*) treatment.

Illustration continued on the following page

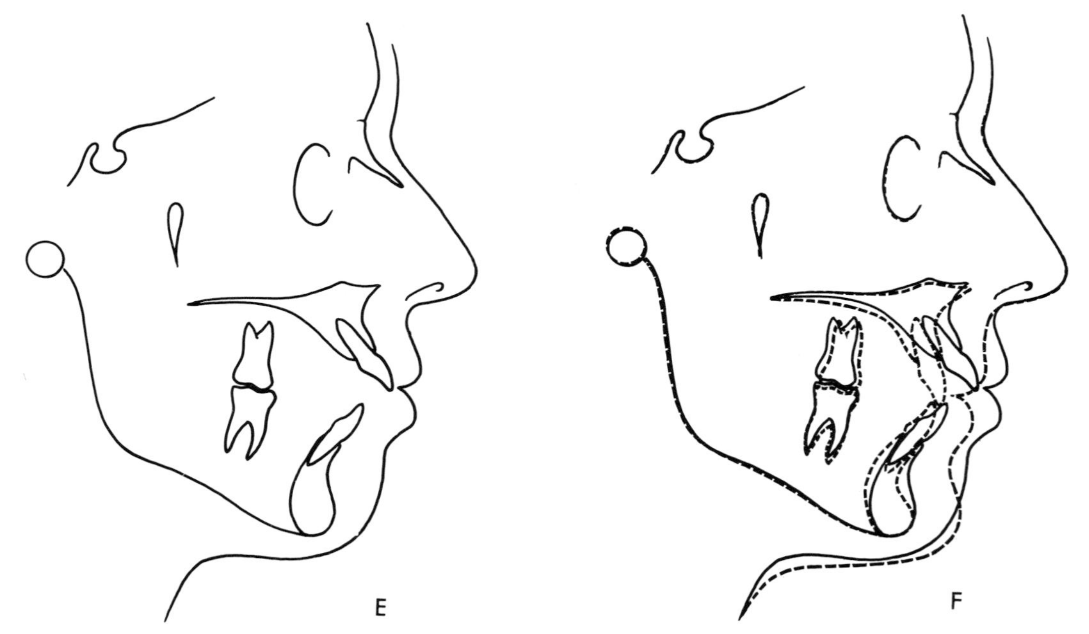

Figure 13–33 *Continued.* *E,* Cephalometric tracing before treatment (age 39 years). *F,* Composite cephalometric tracings before (*solid line,* age 39 years) and after *(broken line)* treatment, showing closure of anterior open bite by orthodontic treatment and anterior subapical ostectomies.

Legend continued on the opposite page

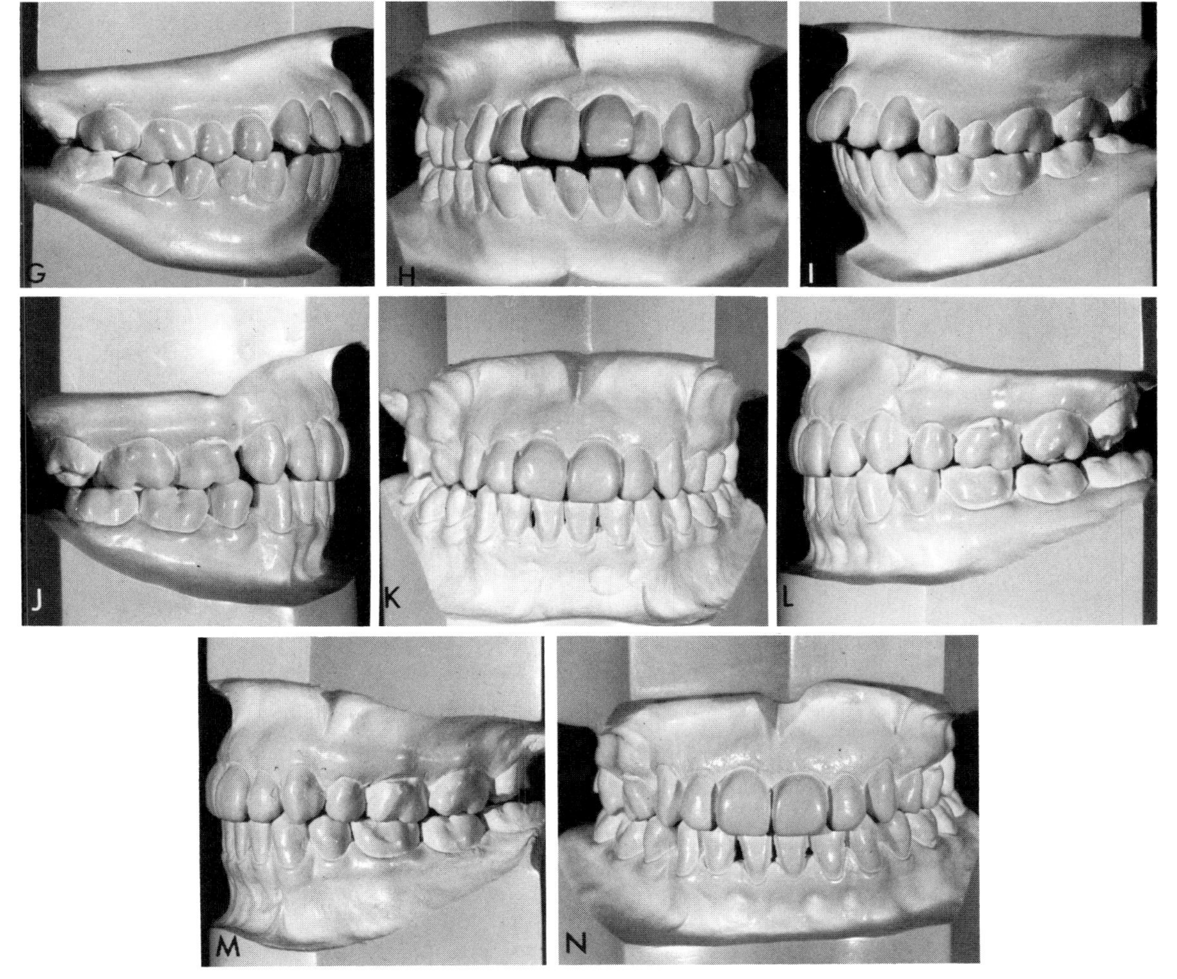

Figure 13–33 *Continued.* *G–N*, Occlusal views: before. *(G–I)*, immediately after *(J–L)*, and 10 years after *(M* and *N)* treatment.

TREATMENT PLAN

Orthodontic Treatment

PRESURGICAL

1. Band all teeth except the first premolars (to be extracted), with full edgewise orthodontic appliance.
2. Extract maxillary and mandibular first premolars to facilitate alignment of anterior teeth and position incisors in good relationship to skeletal base.
3. Align the maxillary and mandibular teeth and correct rotated canines.

POSTSURGICAL

1. Obtain final space closure and alignment of the dental arches.

Surgical Treatment

1. Perform anterior maxillary and mandibular ostectomies to close residual open bite and extraction spaces.

ACTIVE TREATMENT

After the first premolars were extracted, the teeth were aligned and the canines were retracted by coil springs approximately half the distance of the extraction spaces. The spacing created in the incisor region was used to correct rotations of the incisors. After the anterior rotations were corrected, the incisors and canines were consolidated and stabilizing arch wires were placed. The presurgical orthodontic preparation was accomplished within 12 months. Trial sectioning of articulated progress study casts indicated the feasibility of closing the residual open bite and extraction spaces by anterior subapical ostectomies after extraction of the maxillary right second premolar.

When intermaxillary fixation was discontinued six weeks after surgery, the anterior maxillary and mandibular segments were stable. Postsurgical orthodontic treatment accomplished final space closure and alignment of the arches.

Postoperative records showed satisfactory balance between the nose, lips, and chin, a pleasing smile line, and occlusal balance. The stability of the segmental surgery was demonstrated by a ten-year follow-up study of the occlusion and by cephalometric radiographs, which revealed dental and skeletal stability.

The occlusal stability achieved in this case is typical of cases treated by properly planned and executed maxillary and mandibular segmental osteotomies. The time of treatment, however, was quite lengthy (30 months). Today, treatment time would be significantly reduced by Le Fort I osteotomy to simultaneously reposition the anterior and posterior segments into the desired relationship and concomitantly close the residual extraction spaces. Complete closure of extraction spaces in adults by orthodontic treatment may require a lengthy treatment time.

Surgeon: William H. Bell, Dallas, Texas. *Orthodontist:* Cliffort Condit, Houston, Texas.

REFERENCES

1. Alexander RG: The effects on tooth position and maxillofacial vertical growth during treatment of scoliosis with the Milwaukee brace. Am J Orthod *52*:161–189, 1966.
2. Becker R: Results in the treatment of prognathism and open bite with simultaneous tongue reduction. Deut Zahnarzt Zeitschr, *17*:892–903, 1960.
3. Bell WH: Correction of the short-face syndrome — vertical maxillary deficiency: a preliminary report. J Oral Surg *35*:110–120, 1977.
4. Bell WH: Le Fort I osteotomy for correction of maxillary deformities. J Oral Surg *33*(6):412–426, 1975.
5. Bell WH, Creekmore TD: Surgical correction of the long face syndrome. Am J Orthod *71*:40–67, 1977.
6. Bell WH, Dann JJ: Correction of dento-facial deformities by surgery in the anterior part of the jaws. Am J Orthod *64*(2):162–187, 1973.
7. Bell WH, Epker BN: Surgical-orthodontic expansion of the maxilla. Am J Orthod *70*:517–528, 1976.
8. Bell WH, Fonseca RJ, Kennedy JW III, Levy BM: Bone healing and revascularization after total maxillary osteotomy. J Oral Surg *33*:253–260, 1975.
9. Bell WH, McBride KL: Correction of the long face syndrome by Lefort I osteotomy. Oral Surg, *44*:493–520, 1977.
10. Burstone CJ: Lip posture and its significance in treatment planning. Am J Orthod *53*:262, 1967.
11. Conn-Stock G: Die chirurgische Immediate-Gulierung der Kiefer, speizule die chirorgische Behändlung der Prognathie. Vjscher Zahnhk *37*:320–39, 1921.
12. Cupar I: Die chirurgische Behändlung der Form-und-stellungs Veränderungen des Oberkiefers. Ost Z Stomatol *51*:565, 1954; Bus Sc Cons Acad RPF Yougosl *2*:60, 1955.
13. Delaire J: Sagittal splitting of the body of the mandible (Mehnert's technique) for correction of open bite and deep over bite. J Maxillofac Surg *5*:93–158, 1977.
14. Egyedi P, Obwegeser H: Zur operativen Zungenverk-Leinerung. Dtsch Zahn Mund Kieferheilk *41*:16, 1964.
15. Freihofer HPM Jr: Results of osteotomies of the facial skeleton in adolescence. J Maxillofac Surg *5*:267–297, 1977. Stuttgart: Georg Thieme Verlag.
16. Harvold EP, Vargervik K, Chierici G: Primate experiments on oral sensation and dental malocclusion. Am J Orthod *63*:494–508, 1973.
17. Haryett RD, Hansen FC, Davidson PO:

Chronic thumb sucking: a second report on treatment and its psychological effects. Am J Orthod *57*:164–178, 1970.
18. Haryett RD, Hansen FC, Davidson PO: Chronic thumb sucking: the psychological effects and relative effectiveness of various methods of treatment. Am J Orthod *53*:569–585, 1967.
19. Hofer O: Operation der Prognathie und Mikrogenie. Dtsch Zahn Mund Kieferheilk *9*:121, 1942.
20. Hogeman KE, Wilmar K: Die Vorverlangerung des Oberkiefers zur Korrektion von Gebissanomalien. Fortschr Kiefer Gesichts *12*:275, 1967.
21. Hullihen SP: Case of elongation of the underjaw and distortion of the face and neck, caused by burn, successfully treated. Am J Dent Sci *9*:157, 1849.
22. Isaacson JR, Isaacson RJ, Speidel MD, Worms FS: Extreme variations in vertical growth and associated variations in skeletal and dental relations. Angle Orthod *41*:219–229, 1971.
23. Kelley JE, Harvey CR: An assessment of the occlusion of teeth of youths 12–17 years. National Center for Health Statistics, US Public Health Service (DHEW Pub No HRA 77–1644), 1977.
24. Kelley JE, Sanchez M, Van Kirk GE: An assessment of the occlusion of teeth of children 6–11 years. National Center for Health Statistics, US Public Health Service (DHEW Pub No HRA 74–1612), 1973.
25. Kole H: *In* Reischenback, Kole, Brueckel (Eds). Chirurgische Kieferorthopädie. Leipzig: Barth, 1965.
26. Kufner J: Four year experience with major maxillary osteotomy for retrusion. J Oral Surg *29*:549, 1971.
27. Lash SM: Comprehensive Evaluation of Long Term Results of Two Types of Surgical Correction for Mandibular Prognathism. Thesis, University of Michigan, July 1972.
28. Lear CSC, Moorrees CFA: Bucco-lingual muscle force and dental arch form. Am J Orthod *56*:379–393, 1969.
29. Limberg AA: Treatment of open bite by means of plastic oblique osteotomy of the ascending rami of the mandible. Dent Cosmos *67*:1191, 1925.
30. McNamara JA: Neuromuscular and skeletal adaptation to altered function in the orofacial region. Am J Orthod *64*:578–606, 1973.
31. Mason RM, Proffit WR: The tongue thrust controversy: background and recommendations. J Speech Hear Dis *39*:115–132, 1974.
32. Mehnert H: Progenieoperation durch sagittalstuformige Osteotomie in horizontalen ast bei bezahntem Unterkiefer. Dtsch Zahn Mund Kieferheilk *4*:88, 1967.
33. Moyers RE: Handbook of Orthodontics, ed 3. Chicago: Yearbook Medical Publishers, 1973.
34. Obwegeser HL: Surgical correction of small or retrodisplaced maxilla: the "dish-face" deformity. Plast Reconstr Surg *43*:351, 1969.
35. Proffit WR: Equilibrium theory revisited. Angle Orthod (In press.)
36. Proffit WR: Muscle pressures and tooth position: findings from studies of North American whites and Australian aborigines. Angle Orthod. *45*:1–11, 1975.
37. Proffit WR, Mason RM: Myofunctional therapy for tongue thrusting: background and recommendations. J Am Dent Assoc *90*:403–411, 1975.
38. Proffit WR, Norton LA: The tongue and oral morphology: influences of tongue activity during speech and swallowing. J Speech Hear Res ASHA Reports, No. 5, 106–115, 1970.
39. Schendel SA, Eisenfeld JH, Bell WH, Epker BN: Superior repositioning of the maxilla: stability and soft tissue osseous relations. Am J Orthod *70*:663–674, 1976.
40. Schuchardt K: Formen des offenen Bisses und ihre operativen behandlungsmöglechkeiten. *In*: Schuchardt K: Fortschrift Kiefer und Gesichtschirurgie. Stuttgart: Thieme I, 1955.
41. Schudy FF: The rotation of the mandible resulting from growth: its implications in orthodontic treatment. Angle Orthod *35*:36–50, 1965.
42. Wassmund M: Frakturen und Luxationen des Gesichtsschädels. Berlin, 1927.
43. West RA, McNiell RN: Maxillary alveolar hyperplasia, diagnosis and treatment planning. J Maxillofac Surg *3,4*:239–249, 1975.
44. Wickwire NA, White RP, Proffit WR: The effect of mandibular osteotomy on tongue position. J Oral Surg *30*:184–190, 1972.
45. Worms FW, Meskin CH Isaacson RJ: Open bite. Am J Orthod *59*:589–595, 1971.
46. Wunderer S: Erfahrungen mit der operativen Behandlung hochgrädiger Prognathien. Dtsch Zahn Mund Kieferheilk *39*:451, 1963.

SELECTED READINGS

Bell WH: Correction of skeletal type of anterior open bite. J Oral Surg *29*:706–714, 1971.

Brammer J, Finn R, Bell WH, Sinn D, Reisch J, Dana K: Stability following bimaxillary surgery to correct vertical maxillary excess and mandibular deficiency. J Oral Surg. In press.

Finn RA, Throckmorton GS, Bell WH, Legan HL: Biomechanis of mandibular deficiency. J Oral Surg. In press.

Throckmorton GS, Finn RA, Bell WH: Biomechanics of differences in lower facial height. Am J Ortho. In press.

Chapter 14

CHIN SURGERY

Kevin L. McBride and William H. Bell

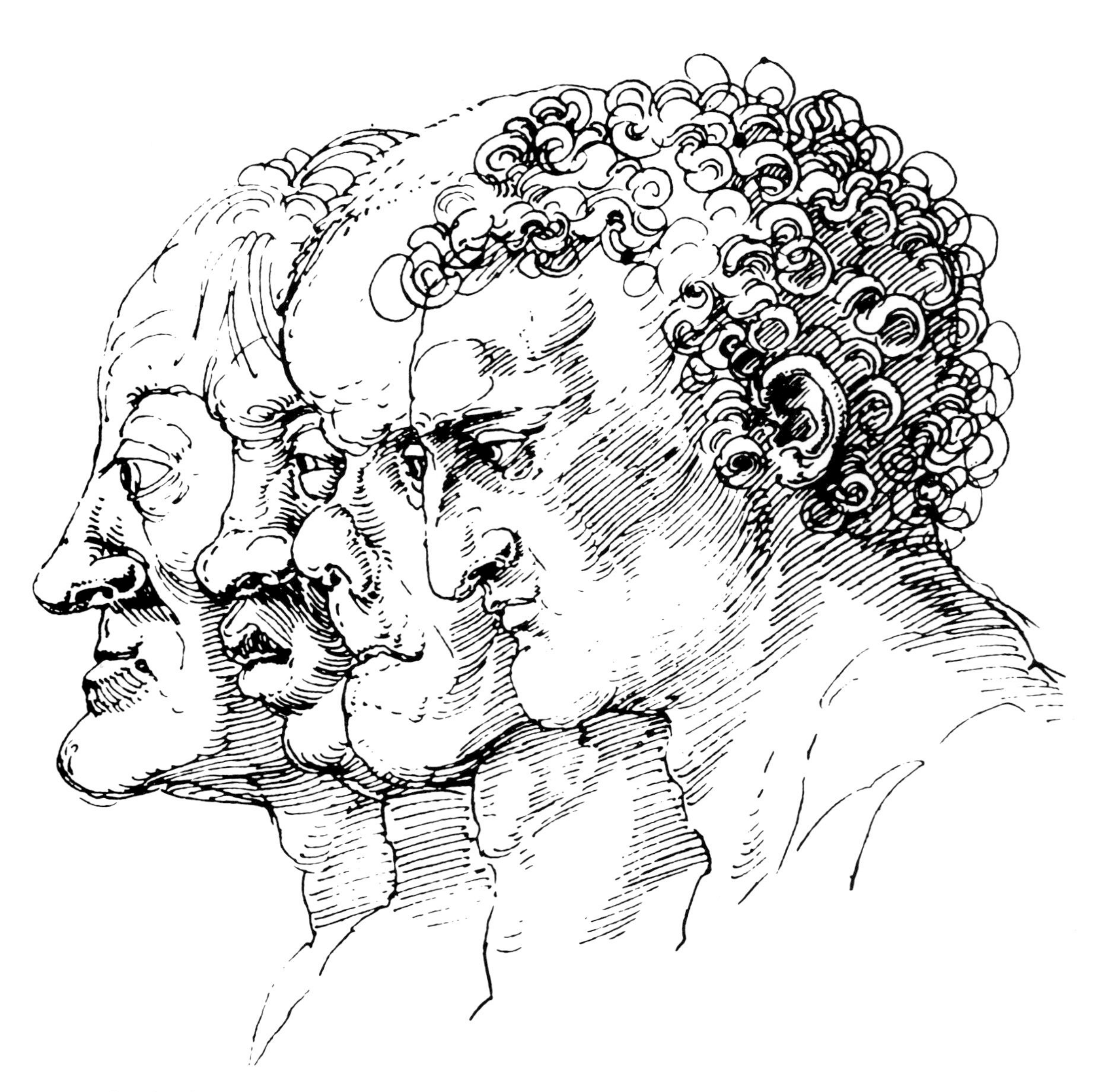

Four Heads, Albrecht Dürer, circa 1503

The chin, which is one of the most obvious facial structures, has long been the object of curiosity, the basis for judging "human character," and a challenge to the surgeon interested in facial esthetics. The important role that the chin plays in facial appearance has been recognized since antiquity — ivory, bovine bone, and alloplastics are but a few of the materials that have been used clinically with variable success to augment the contour of the chin.[1] Only within the last quarter century have surgical techniques been perfected to alter the chin contour in a reliable manner.[7, 11, 19, 29] During the period when modern techniques of chin surgery were being developed, modalities for soft-tissue analysis evolved concurrently.[2, 12, 15] Today, by prudent application of artistic sense, knowledge of the principles of facial esthetics, and proper execution of contemporary techniques of genioplasty, the maxillofacial surgeon can achieve almost any variation of three-dimensional changes in chin contour and proportions.

The characteristics that are considered esthetically pleasing vary according to culture, ethnic type, and even historical period. There is evidence, however, that the general characteristics associated with a beautiful face have changed very little throughout the history of Western European culture. This is also true of many other cultures — what was considered a beautiful face 2000 years ago is still looked on as esthetically pleasing today.

Western society associates certain facial characteristics with an individual's personality. A person with a "weak" or deficient chin may subconsciously be expected to have a timid, nonathletic, unaggressive, or indecisive personality, whereas an individual with a "strong" or prognathic chin may be expected to be bold, athletic, aggressive, and decisive. The fact that our culture uses the words "weak" and "strong" to describe the chin implies subconscious association with "character," or personality trait. The hallmarks of a "normal" or "balanced" face are a slightly protruding chin associated with a nose of normal proportions.

In general, a "weak" or retruded chin is associated with femininity; a strong or prominent chin with masculinity. Because undesirable characteristics are associated with a weak chin, society seems to prefer facial forms with at least *some* chin prominence — more in men than in women. Even though the general public appreciates the fact that some people have more esthetically pleasing chins than others, many people do not yet realize that chin contour can be altered by surgery.

Historically, attention given to chin contour has emphasized the lateral aspect, because the retrusive chin was the most obvious and common deformity. As a consequence, results of genioplasties were evaluated on the basis of profile only. Unfortunately, the esthetic change when viewed from the way the patient actually sees himself (frontally) was sometimes compromised. Patients with the most conspicuous microgenia received the most impressive profile change, but frontal appearance was compromised unless particular attention was directed to augmenting the lateral contour during advancement.

SYSTEMATIC DESCRIPTION OF THE DEFORMITY

In evaluating facial form from an esthetic viewpoint, the absolute measurements of facial structures are not as important as the relative size and proportion of each structure when compared with the others. Harmony of facial structures (facial balance) is the primary determinant of good facial esthetics.

A face is balanced when the upper, middle, and lower thirds are approximately equal in size and the structures within each segment are proportional in size and prominence.[3] The lips and chin should be in harmony with one another as well as with the structures in the middle third of the face. The prominence of the lips and chin in relation to one another and in relation to the midfacial structures has much to do with the esthetic appeal of the lower face.

Anatomically, the chin is the area below the labiomental fold. This is also true clinically when the patient is viewed from the lateral aspect. However, when viewing the face from the frontal aspect, it becomes difficult to separate the chin from the lower lip area; consequently the eye assesses the whole complex from the labial angle to soft-tissue gnathion. The examiner must therefore consider the entire lower lip–chin complex, which consists of the lower lip, labiomental fold, and chin, rather than simply the "chin." It is difficult to isolate parts of this complex because the examiner evaluates the position, size, and shape of each component in relation to the other. In addition, a surgical procedure that alters the "chin" frequently alters the lower lip and labiomental fold.

Each component of the lower lip–chin complex is affected by numerous soft-tissue and hard-tissue characteristics. The lower lip is influenced by maxillary and mandibular incisor position, the amount of overbite and overjet, tone of the mentalis and orbicularis oris muscles, and bony chin projection. Undoubtedly, other factors are also involved. A deep bite with excessive overjet frequently results in a lower lip that is pushed down and rolled out by the maxillary incisors. When the patient opens his mouth, the lower lip rolls back into a better position.

Hyperfunction of the mentalis muscle must be properly diagnosed, because it may lead to an inaccurate assessment of chin esthetics. This condition may be so habitual that it may be very difficult to obtain a cephalometric radiograph with the lips relaxed. Mentalis muscle hyperfunction can be recognized on the lateral cephalometric radiograph by a prominent mentalis bulge, elevation of the margin of the lower lip above the incisial edges of the mandibular anterior teeth, and a flattened labiomental fold. Conversely, poor orbicularis oris muscle tone may contribute to a rolled-out procumbent lower lip that exposes the mandibular anterior teeth. This kind of lip morphology is frequently seen in black patients with bimaxillary protrusion and in both white and black adults with Class II malocclusion.

Soft-tissue chin contour is influenced by bony chin projection and length, mentalis muscle thickness, and soft-tissue chin thickness.[4, 5] The shape of the labiomental fold is influenced by all the factors that control lower-lip contour and soft-tissue chin contour because the fold is formed by confluence of these structures. The general contour, depth, and height of the fold determine the esthetic appeal. The fold should have a sigmoid shape with a smooth transition between the lip and chin. A deep angular fold is unesthetic from both the frontal and lateral views, particularly if the patient has a short face. The most desirable depth of the fold varies with the height of lower lip–chin complex and the degree of facial protrusion. A long complex balances better with a deep fold, whereas a short complex balances better with a shallow fold.

An individual with a protrusive midface generally looks better with a relatively deep fold because it balances with the prominent curves of the cheeks, lips, and nasolabial areas; a shallow fold, conversely, generally harmonizes with flat midfacial structures.

The vertical position of the deepest point of the fold has considerable effect on the appearance of the chin. For good balance, it should be located near the midpoint between the superior border of the lip and inferior border of the chin. This point corresponds to the juncture between the lower and middle thirds of the lower third of the face (Fig. 14–1).

Treatment planning for chin surgery involves a three-dimensional analysis of chin esthetics that integrates problems noted in the anteroposterior, vertical, and tranverse planes. In the interest of simplicity, soft-tissue analysis, treatment planning, and surgical technique are considered separately for each plane of orientation. The reader should appreciate the fact that most individuals with dentofacial deformities do not have pure deformities in a single plane but have components of varying severity in all three planes. The final surgical plan is based upon a synthesis of data obtained from analyses of the three individual planes.

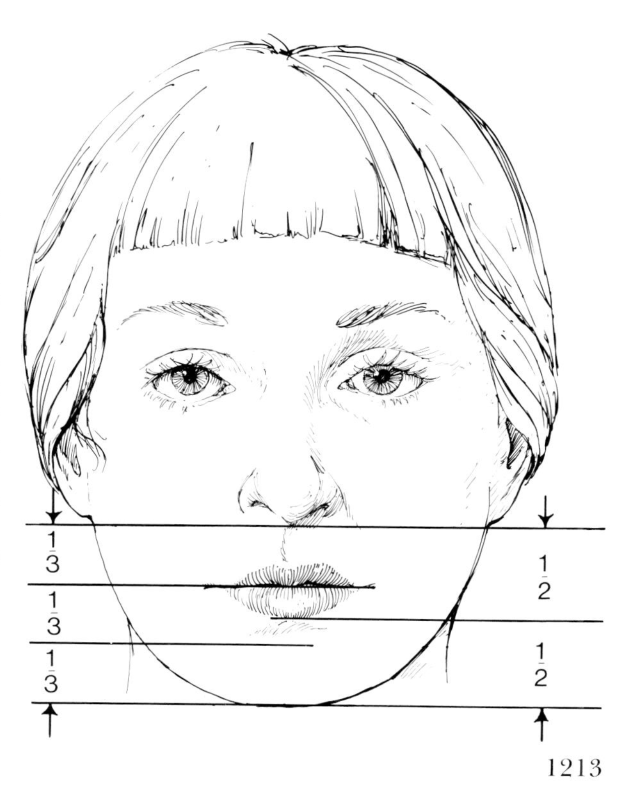

Figure 14–1. Vertical balance of lower third facial structures. A balanced lower-third face may be divided into equal thirds by lines passing through the subnasale, the stomion, the deepest point of the labiomental fold, and the most inferior point on the soft-tissue chin. Equal halves are established by lines through the subnasale, the mucocutaneous junction of the lower lip, and the most inferior point of the soft-tissue chin. The lower third of the face, from the subnasale to the most inferior point on the soft-tissue chin, is divided into equal thirds by lines passing through the stomion and the deepest point of the labiomental fold; equal halves are established by a line through the mucocutaneous junction of the lower lip.

ANTEROPOSTERIOR (PROFILE) DEFORMITIES

For the purpose of clinical analysis, it is assumed that facial structures other than the chin are esthetically pleasing or will be surgically moved to produce a pleasing effect. Techniques for predicting frontal and profile soft-tissue changes following movement of other facial structures are described in the chapters dealing with the specific deformities involved.

The concept of relating lower facial structures to a vertical line to establish a straight facial profile is well-founded. Studies have shown that both the general public and those trained in facial esthetics prefer such a profile.[20, 21] They consider that the structures of the lower face, including the chin, lips, and subnasal region, should lie very close to a straight line that represents a vertical plane. The majority of previous attempts to use linear and angular cephalometric esthetic guides[14-19] have been predicated on the use of fixed intracranial reference lines and points.[13, 16, 23-25, 27] The inconstancy of craniofacial anatomy and the almost infinite variety of human geometry prevent such cephalometric systems from working consistently.[22] Interpretation of facial profile esthetics should be based on the relationship of facial structures to external landmarks rather than on variable intracranial landmarks.[17] Since the way human beings normally posture their heads is remarkably constant, natural head position is used as a point of orientation.

All cephalometric radiographs are taken in natural head position to orient the head to natural horizontal and vertical planes. A natural vertical is any vertical line constructed perpendicular to the normal horizontal visual axis of the patient.[17] With the cephalometric radiographs taken in natural head position, the natural vertical is parallel to the lateral edges of the film. By constructing a natural vertical line through subnasale, the relative prominence of the nose, lips, and chin may be assessed. Ideally, the chin should lie on this line and the lips slightly anterior to it. The proposed position and contour of the chin may be drawn tangential to the natural vertical reference line.

There is obviously considerable variation in individual profiles, and all patients cannot be made to fit a specific stereotype. A vertical reference line on a cephalometric radiograph provides a convenient, reproducible mechanism for determining the relationship of the chin to the remainder of the facial profile. Analysis of facial esthetics, however, is more complex than simply using a single profile reference line. A multitude of complex inter-relationships among other facial structures must be considered when altering the position of any part of the face. Consequently, the final decision as to where to position the chin must be made by evaluating the patient in a clinical setting. The nasolabial angle, thickness of the upper and lower lips, cheek prominence, total length of the face, and even general body build will affect the final decision as to what chin contour and prominence complement an individual's face. For example the face of a female with fine facial features, a small nose, thin lips, and flat midfacial structures will be better balanced with a relatively retrusive chin. The 6-foot male, on the other hand, prefers a relatively prominent chin.

ANTEROPOSTERIOR DEFICIENCY

Clinical and cephalometric analyses with the patient in natural head position are used to determine the amount of soft-tissue advancement needed to establish a balanced facial profile. A natural vertical reference line through subnasale is constructed on the

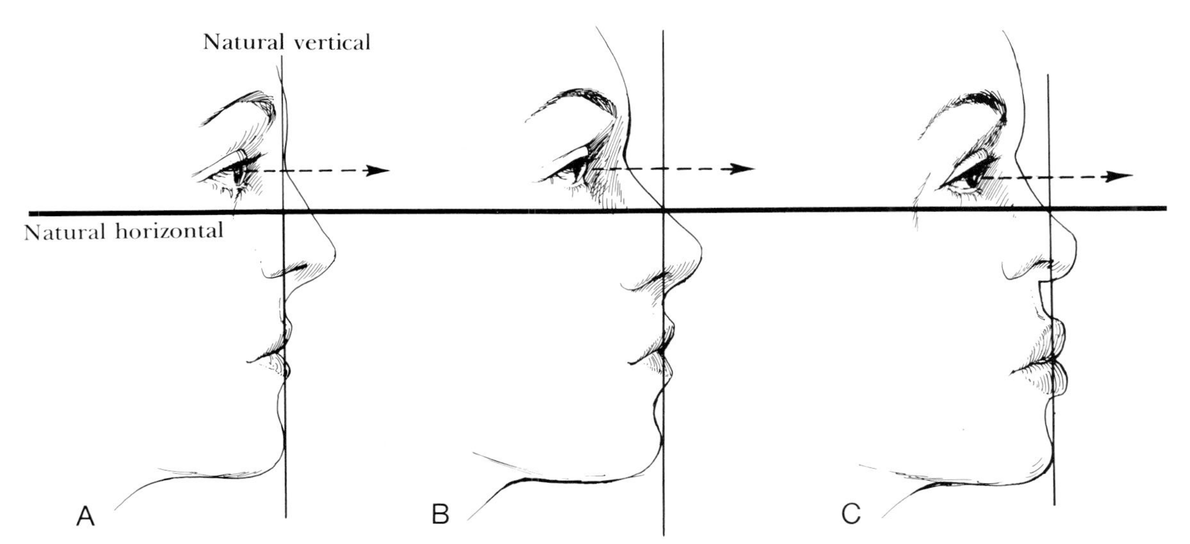

Figure 14–2. Natural vertical reference line for evaluation of profile esthetics. *A,* A natural vertical reference line is constructed to pass through subnasale. In the balanced, relatively straight face, this line passes near or through soft-tissue nasion and soft-tissue pogonion. The upper and lower lips are slightly anterior to this line. *B,* In more protrusive caucasoid profiles, the natural vertical through subnasale is tangent to soft-tissue pogonion but passes anterior to soft-tissue nasion. *C,* For Negroid profiles the vertical line is moved anteriorly to a point midway between the subnasale and the anterior prominence of the upper lip. Soft-tissue pogonion should be close to this line. The lower lip should be slightly behind the upper lip.

cephalometric tracing. Subnasale, the most posterior superior point on the curve formed by the nose and upper lip, is arbitrarily selected as the point of reference in Caucasians because it is a relatively stable landmark that moves relatively little when maxillary surgical procedures such as the Le Fort I osteotomy are performed. The facial profile is usually balanced when subnasale and chin fall on the same line and the lips are slightly anterior to it (Fig. 14–2). If the nose and lips are particularly prominent, the vertical reference line is moved anterior to subnasale to establish appropriate balance with the chin. This is usually necessary for Negroes, who frequently manifest variable degrees of bimaxillary protrusion and lip prominence (Fig. 14–2*C*). In such patients, the vertical reference line should lie about halfway between subnasale and the anterior prominence of the upper lip. When the chin is constructed on this line, the lips will appear less prominent, and better facial balance will be achieved. When the vertical line lies anterior to the more prominent lip, it may be desirable to move the line posteriorly to a point tangential with the more prominent lip, which then becomes the reference point for the anteroposterior position of the chin. The line is moved a few millimeters posteriorly for women, in whom a "softer" profile is preferred.

By tracing the present or proposed profile for the middle third of the face and utilizing the landmarks and criteria suggested for establishing balanced facial esthetics, the proposed profile of the lower lip and chin is drawn. The horizontal difference between the preoperative soft-tissue chin position and the planned position as sketched on the profile tracing represents the amount of soft-tissue augmentation required. These measurements serve as the basis for selecting the appropriate surgical procedure to effect the desired change. The final "result" is approved or disapproved by the surgeon, who relies on his or her artistic sense of what a balanced facial profile should look like. Using this artistic sense, the surgeon may choose to simulate additional facial contour changes.

A proportioning device consisting of a clear plastic grid with horizontal and vertical reference lines can be an aid in evaluating frontal and profile facial esthetics (Fig. 14–3). Such clinical studies are made with the patient's head in a natural head position (Fig. 14–3).

ADVANCEMENT GENIOPLASTY

A variety of surgical techniques are available to augment a contour-deficient chin. These techniques include several variations of horizontal sliding osteotomy,[6, 8, 18, 22, 26] free autogenous onlay bone grafts,[7] implantation of an alloplastic material,[16] and combinations of these methods. The horizontal sliding osteotomy of the mandibular symphysis with advancement of the mobilized segment is the technique of choice for correction of anteroposterior deficiency because the results are predictable and stable. In studying the results attained with horizontal sliding osteotomy, Bell and Dann found a consistent relationship between bone and soft-tissue change of 1:0.6.[2] Soft-tissue advancement was approximately 60 per cent of bone advancement. These figures, however, related to

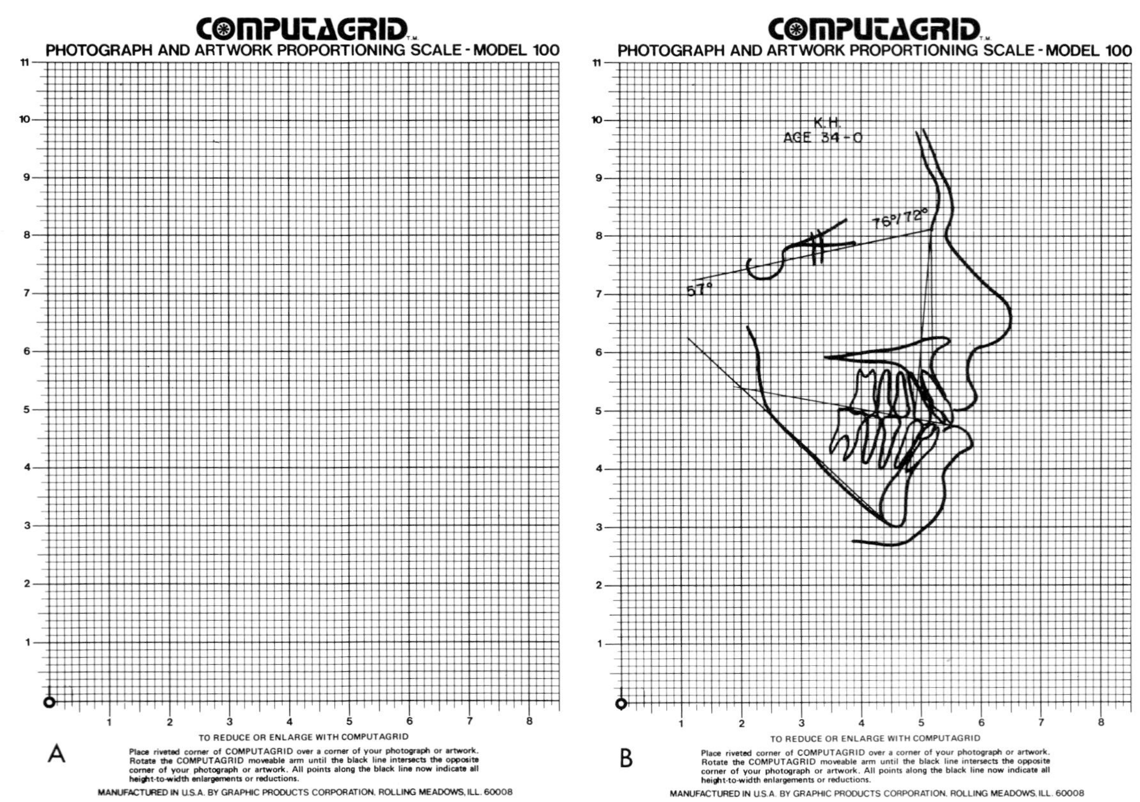

Figure 14–3. Use of the Computagrid. *A,* The Computagrid is a photographic and artwork proportioning device consisting of a grid of horizontal and vertical lines scribed on an 11 inch × 9 inch clear plastic sheet. It provides a series of coordinates to aid in evaluating frontal and profile facial esthetics. It is manufactured by Graphic Products Corporation, Rolling Meadows, Illinois, 60008, and is sold in many art and photographic supply houses. *B,* Analysis of profile esthetics is facilitated by orienting a clear acetate grid over the cephalometric tracing so that grid lines parallel the natural horizontal and vertical reference lines. By following a line that passes through subnasale, the relative prominence of the lips and chin may be measured.

genioplasties performed with more soft-tissue detachment than we presently use. Our more recent results indicate that minimal soft-tissue detachment allows closer correlation between bone and soft-tissue movement. We now expect the soft tissue to advance 75 per cent of the bone advancement. This observation has recently been confirmed by McDonnel and associates.[15] By monitoring the horizontal advancement of the soft-tissue chin brought about by advancement genioplasty and subsequent change, they concluded that for the purposes of prediction, the ratio between the initial surgical horizontal advancement of the symphysis and the ultimate horizontal advancement of the soft-tissue chin was 4:3.[15]

SLIDING HORIZONTAL OSTEOTOMY

After the proposed chin contour is sketched on the cephalometric tracing, a template of the chin segment to be advanced is traced on an additional piece of acetate tracing paper. The soft tissue anterior and inferior to the mobilized segment and a natural horizontal line passing about 4 mm below the mental foramen are added to this template.

The position of the horizontal osteotomy is controlled by the level of the mental

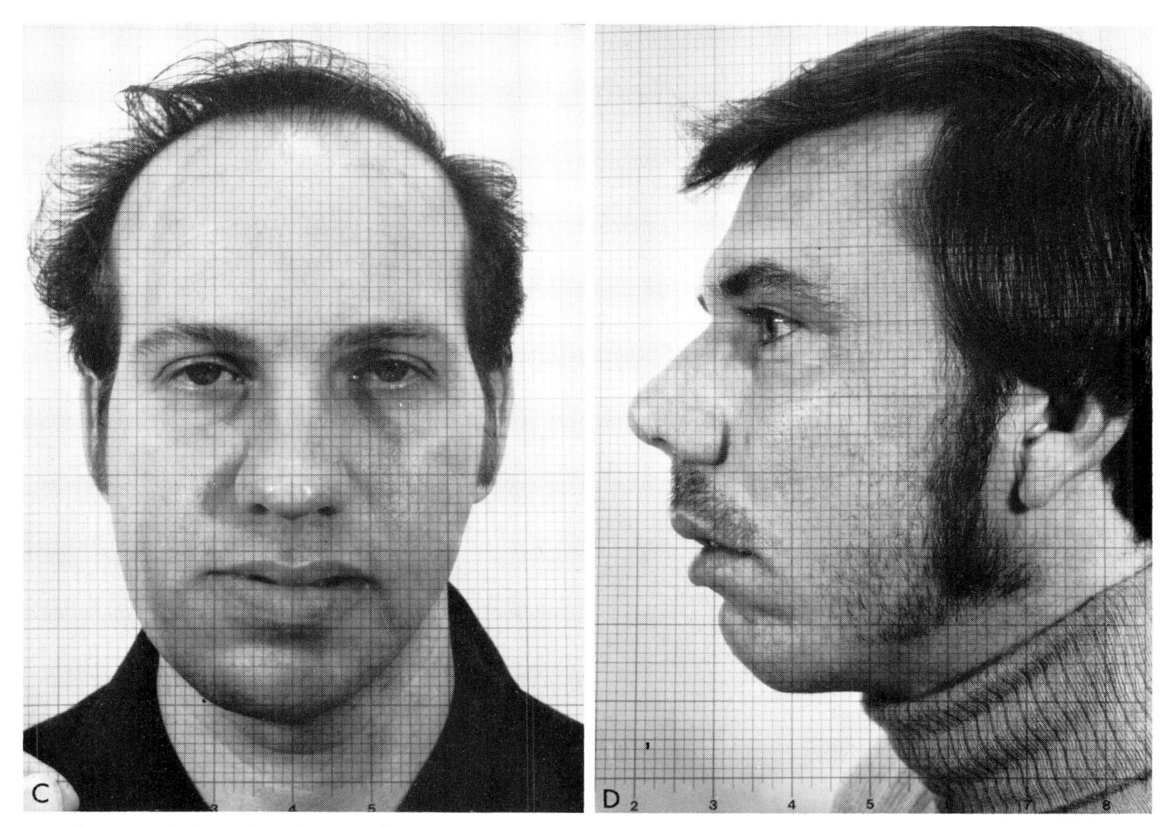

Figure 14–3 *Continued.* *C,* Clear plastic grid held in front of patient: Horizontal line on grid is oriented to natural horizontal passing through orbital rims, balance and symmetry of facial structures is evaluated in relation to vertical lines, and vertical relationships are evaluated in relation to horizontal lines. *D,* Clear plastic grid held up to lateral aspect of patient whose head is held in a natural head position: A horizontal line is oriented to the natural horizontal through the infraorbital rims, and the anteroposterior balance of the nose, lips, and chin is evaluated in relation to vertical lines.

foramen and inferior alveolar canal. The fact that the inferior alveolar canal curves superiorly as it approaches the mental foramen makes it mandatory to position the horizontal osteotomy 3 to 4 mm below the inferior edge of the mental foramen to prevent injury to the neurovascular bundle. The inferior alveolar canal can usually be identified on the cephalometric radiograph so that the distance the canal extends below the foramen can be measured. This measurement is recorded for use at surgery and determines the posterior height of the osteotomy. The anterior height of the osteotomy is dictated by the direction in which the segment must move to produce the desired chin contour and prominence. If only horizontal augmentation is desired, the osteotomy should be made parallel to the natural horizontal. Horizontal and vertical augmentation may be accomplished by directing the anterior part of the osteotomy below the natural horizontal. Shortening is produced by directing the anterior bone incision above the natural horizontal.

The exact angle of the osteotomy is determined by advancing the chin template to coincide with the outline of the proposed chin. The template must be advanced beyond the proposed outline to compensate for the fact that the soft tissue advances only 75 per cent of the bone advancement. A line is constructed between the point where the natural horizontal line intersects the labial cortical bone on the repositioned template and a point 3 to 4 mm below the mental foramen. This line represents the position of the osteotomy needed to achieve the proposed result.

Chin augmentation by horizontal sliding osteotomy is limited by the thickness of the symphysis, angulation of the osteotomy, and anterior soft-tissue attachments. Because the amount of advancement that can be achieved with sliding horizontal osteotomy is limited by the thickness of the mental symphsis at the level of the proposed cut, this dimension is measured on the preoperative cephalogram. If movement greater than the thickness of the symphysis is carried out, there will be no bone contact in the midline, and the possibility of instability of the repositioned segment, delayed healing, and relapse will be greater.

The height of the advanced segment will range between 10 and 15 mm at the anterior aspect of the symphysis. If the segment is too short, a pointed unesthetic soft-tissue chin may result; if the vertical dimension of the segment is too long, a large knobby chin and elevation of the labiomental fold result. The specific thickness should balance with the overall height of the chin from lip margin to soft-tissue gnathion. A point about 2 mm above pogonion is usually selected for the anterior extent of the osteotomy when the angulation permits.

When it is not feasible to direct the osteotomy at the necessary angle and still maintain the desired thickness of the segment, a wedge ostectomy may be used to shorten the chin and alter the direction of forward movement (Fig. 14–4). An interpositional bone graft likewise permits lengthening the chin while maintaining ideal segment thickness.

Degloving Exposure for Horizontal Osteotomy of the Inferior Border of Mandible (Fig. 14–5)

The operation is performed in the operating room with the patient under general nasoendotracheal anesthesia. When hypotensive anesthesia is not used, local anesthetic with vasoconstrictor is infiltrated into the labiobuccal vestibule to aid in hemostasis. The

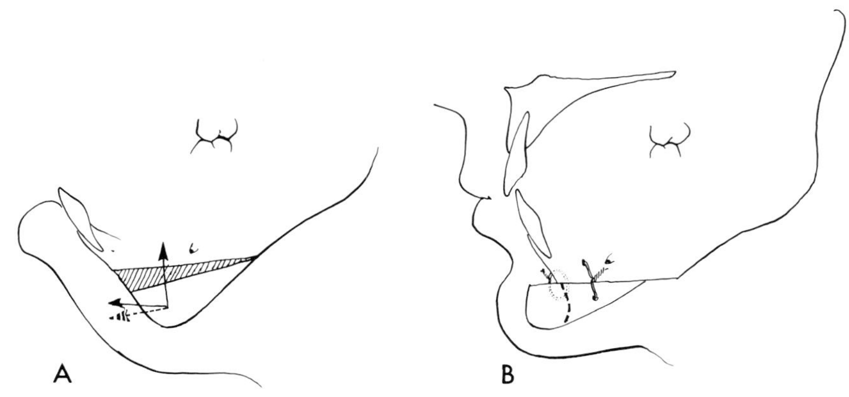

Figure 14–4. Altering directional movement of chin by wedge ostectomy to maintain same effective chin height. *A,* Chin lengthened by downward and forward movements after horizontal sliding osteotomy without wedge ostectomy (broken arrow). Directional movement of chin altered by combining small wedge ostectomy (cross-hatched area) and horizontal sliding osteotomy (solid arrow). *B,* Repositioned inferior segment has been moved straight forward and fixed to body of mandible with interosseous wires.

incision for genioplasty is designed to maintain circulation to the mobilized portion of the inferior border of the mandible by means of an intact soft-tissue pedicle of genial and digastric muscles and periosteum. Anteriorly, the incision is made through the lower-lip mucosa above the labial frenum midway between the depth of the labial vestibule and the vermilion border of the lower lip (Fig. 14–5*A* and *B*). The incision is carried into the most lateral part of the buccal vestibule and as far posteriorly as necessary to gain sufficient exposure of the bone and mental nerves. The incision is usually terminated in the second premolar or first molar region, opposite the most posterior portion of the planned horizontal osteotomy. In the premolar region, the initial incision is made through the mucosa only, to prevent damage to branches of the mental nerves. When genioplasty is accomplished independently or simultaneously with intraoral ramus osteotomies, the vestibular incision may be carried posteriorly to connect with the soft-tissue incision used to expose the ramus.

The anterior portion of the circumvestibular incision is carried sharply through the mucosa only; the mucosa is then raised from the underlying orbicularis oris muscle of the lower lip. From this point the dissection is directed obliquely posteriorly and inferiorly through the mentalis muscle and periosteum until contact is made with the mental symphysis 5 to 10 mm below the apices of the mandibular incisor teeth. The mentalis muscle and the submucosa are incised sharply posteriorly to an area opposite and above the apices of the canine teeth. Branches of the mental nerve, which exit from the foramen, are identified by subperiosteal tunneling beneath the anterior margins of the incised tissues (Fig. 14–5*C*). The mental foramen is localized with the aid of carefully oriented periapical and panoramic radiographs. When the foramen has been located, the mental nerves are identified and carefully isolated by blunt dissection with a mosquito hemostat through the margins of the previously made vestibular incision. After the main branches of the nerve are identified and retracted inferiorly an incision is made through the submucosal tissue above the nerve down to the underlying bone. The incision may be extended posteriorly as far as necessary to accomplish the planned osteotomy. Next, the osteotomy site is "exposed" from the mental foramen of one

Text continued on page 1225.

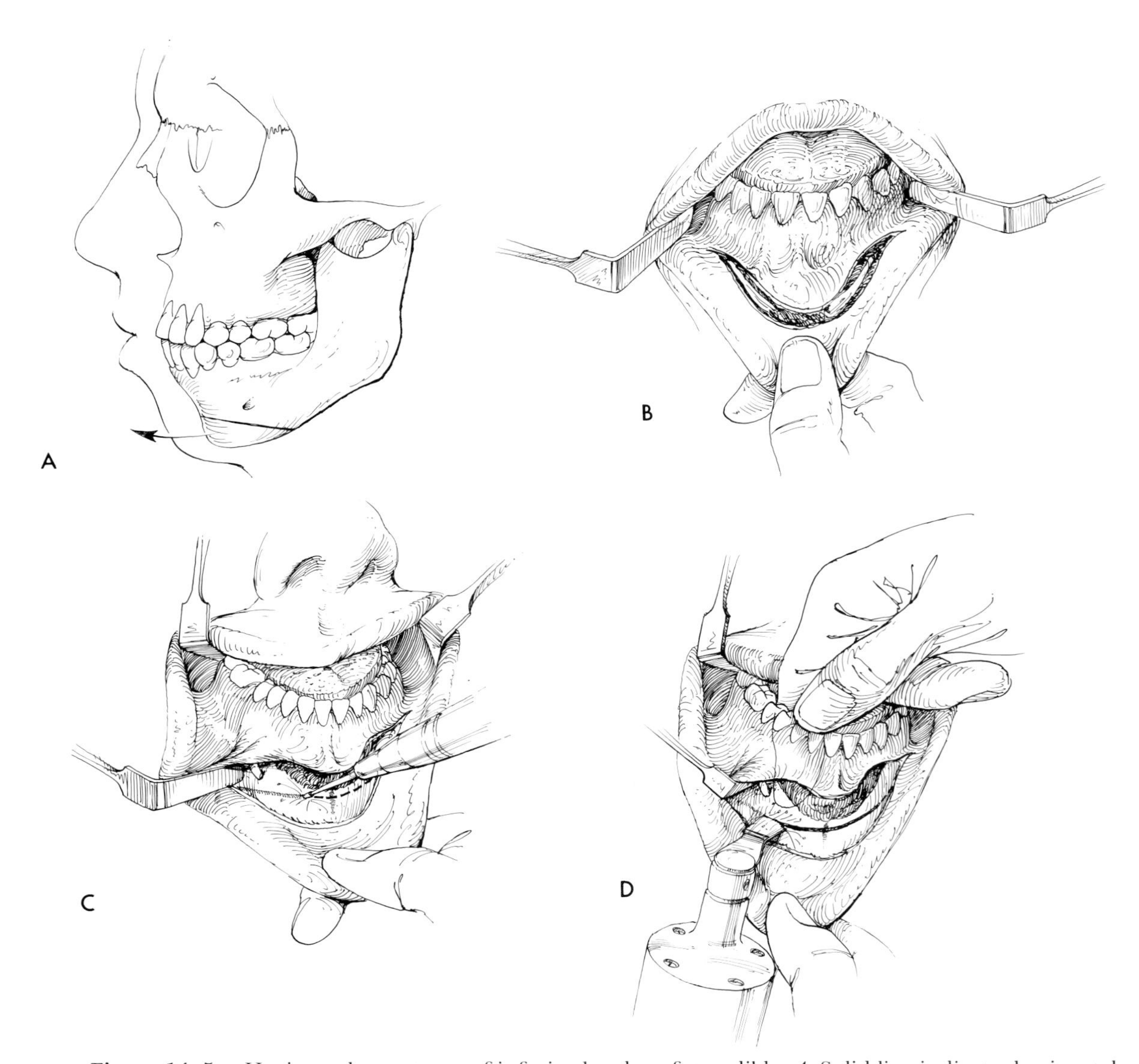

Figure 14–5. Horizontal osteotomy of inferior border of mandible. *A*, Solid line indicates horizontal osteotomy; arrow indicates directional movement of inferior segment. *B*, Soft-tissue incision for exposure of mandible; superficial branches of mental nerves exposed. *C*, Chin prominence degloved from mental foramen of one side to contralateral mental foramen; planned osteotomy etched into mandible with #701 fissure bur. *D*, Midline vertical reference line etched into midsagittal plane of the chin across the area of planned horizontal osteotomy; horizontal osteotomy in the anterior region accomplished with oscillating saw. *E*, Mental nerve and contiguous soft-tissue flap retracted and protected while planned osteotomy extended laterally and posteriorly with small oscillating saw blade. *F*, Reciprocating saw blade used to extend osteotomy posteriorly, 3 to 4 mm inferior to the mental foramen. *G*, Fine tapered osteotome placed in horizontal line of osteotomy to determine if the lingual cortex has been completely sectioned. When osteotomy is complete in all areas the inferior segment is easily downfractured by torquing the instrument between the proximal and distal margins of the sectioned bone. *H*, Inferior segment pedicled to geniohyoid and digastric muscles and periosteum is advanced a measured distance with bone-holding clamp. *I*, Holes drilled into proximal and distal segments to maintain advanced position of chin. In *H* and *I*, instrumentation is illustrated without trying to show the attachment of the integument to the anterior and inferior borders of the mandible. As shown in *Q*, the largest possible soft-tissue pedicle to the inferior segment is maintained while still providing accessibility for the planned osteotomy.

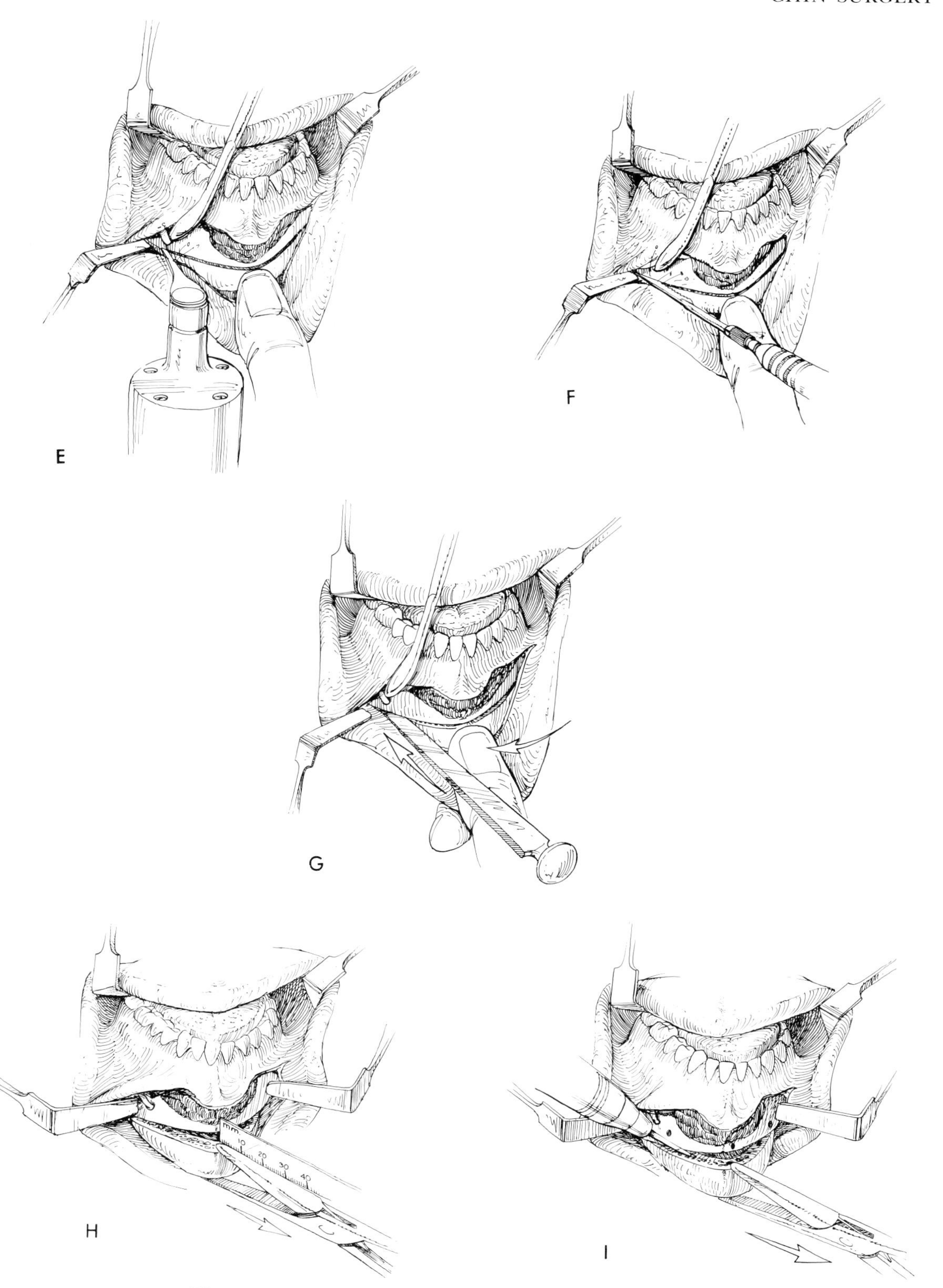

Figure 14–5 *Continued.* See legend on the opposite page.

Illustration continued on the following page

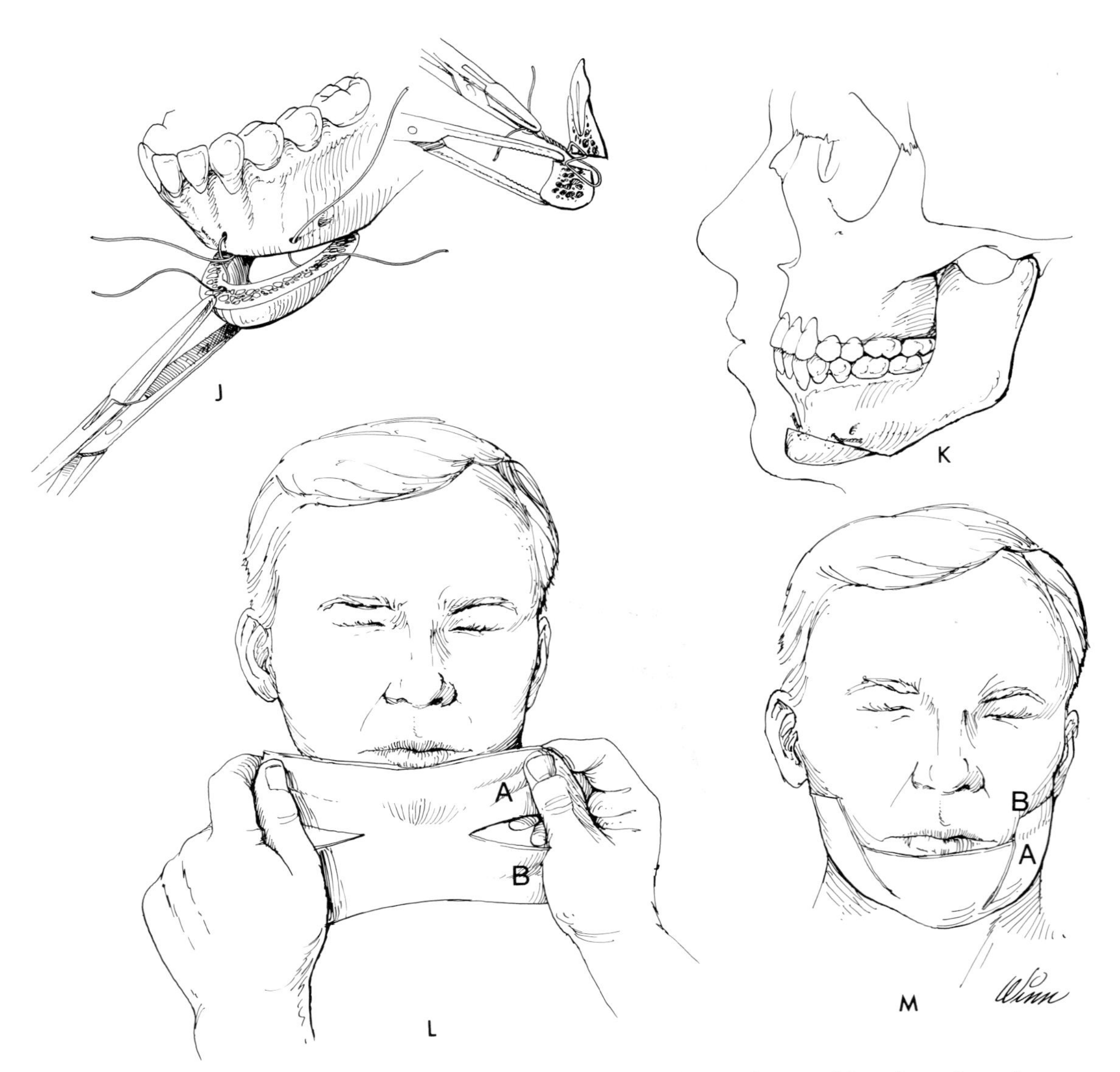

Figure 14–5 *Continued.* *J* and *K*, Interosseous fixation with one figure of 8 and two lateral mattress wire ligatures to maintain chin in preplanned position. *L* and *M*, Pressure dressing of Elastoplast secured to face with adhesive tape.

Legend continued on the opposite page.

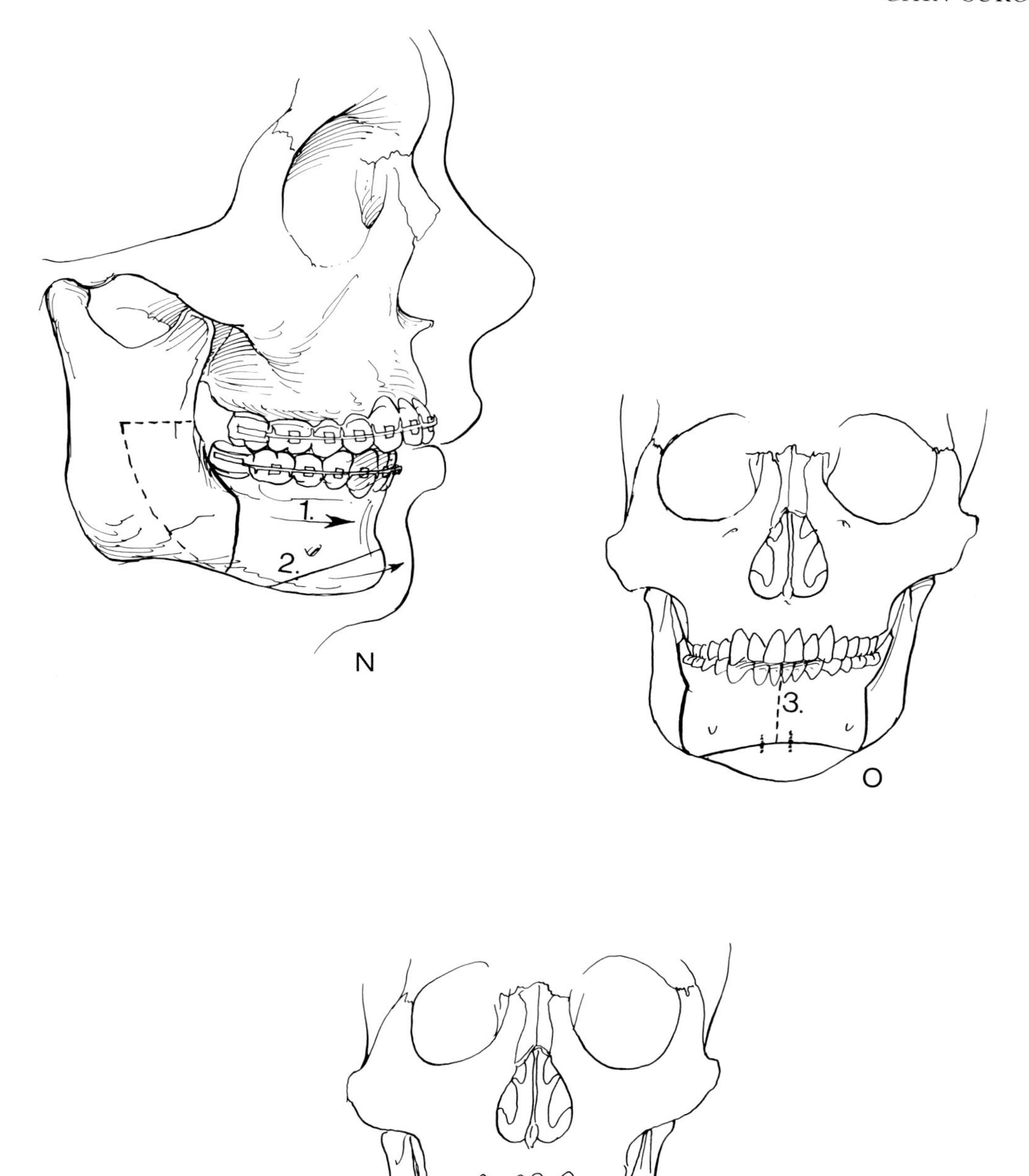

Figure 14–5 *Continued. N–T,* Simultaneous advancement and narrowing of mandible and augmentation of chin. *N* and *O,* Preoperative deformity: mandibular deficiency (absolute), contour-deficient chin, and transverse maxillary deficiency. Plan of surgery: sagittal split ramus osteotomies to advance mandible (1), genioplasty to augment contour-deficient chin (2), and interincisal osteotomy to facilitate narrowing of mandible (3). Arrows indicate planned positional movements of mandible and chin. *P,* After mandibular advancement, transverse maxillary deficiency is manifest as lingual crossbite.

Illustration continued on the following page.

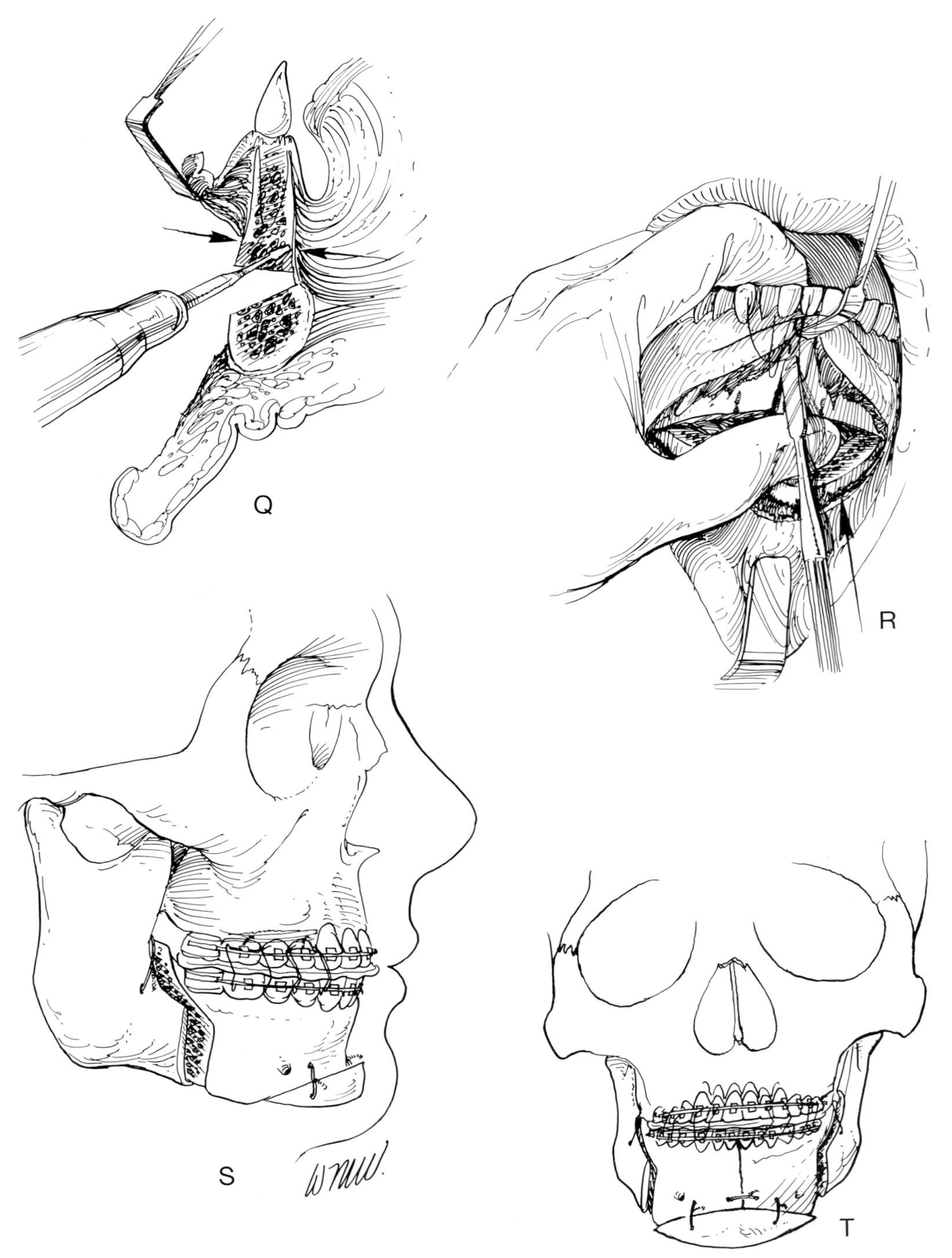

Figure 14–5 *Continued.* *Q,* Genioplasty is accomplished after degloving exposure of mental symphysis. With mental symphysis segment positioned inferiorly and superior margin of soft tissue flap retracted, the labial cortical plate and alveolar bone immediately below the level of incisor apices is sectioned with a #701 fissure bur (vertically oriented cross-hatched lines indicate where bone is sectioned; arrows indicate level of interdental osteotomy). *R,* The symphysis is halved by malleting a spatula osteotome into the partially sectioned interdental osteotomy site. *S* and *T,* Repositioned mandible immobilized with intermaxillary wire ligatures. Mandible and chin fixed in planned relationship after mandibular advancement, advancement genioplasty, and narrowing of mandible.

side to the contralateral mental foramen; the lateral part of the body of the mandible posterior to the foramen is exposed similarly. Now, the mental symphysis and lateral aspect of the mandible can be clearly visualized (Fig. 14–5*C*).

The mental nerves must be bluntly dissected clear of investing tissues and carefully retracted and protected as the planned osteotomies or ostectomies are accomplished. With meticulous care, the bone incisions can be made with impunity to the mental nerves. Occasionally, when the planned bone incisions cannot be designed to bypass the nerves, the nerves are decorticated to uncover the neurovascular bundle and preserve the integrity of the nerve. The inferior alveolar nerve, severed from its incisive branch, is reflected superiorly with the contiguous soft-tissue flap to facilitate the planned osteotomy. (See Chapter 11, Mandibular Excess, for further details.)

Surgical Technique of Horizontal Sliding Osteotomy for Anteroposterior Augmentation

A midline vertical reference line is etched into the midsagittal plane of the chin across the area of the planned horizontal osteotomy for orientation after the inferior mental symphysis is mobilized. The planned horizontal osteotomy (or ostectomy) is then etched into the mandible with a No. 701 fissure bur (Fig. 14–5*C*). The vertical distance from the anterior horizontal bone incision to the inferior border of the mandible, angulation and configuration of the bone cut,[3] amount of bone to be excised, and posterior extension of the bone incision are determined preoperatively from cephalometric prediction studies (see section on preoperative planning). The height and angulation of the horizontal ostectomy is varied to produce the desired anteroposterior, vertical, and transverse changes in the individual's chin.

The anterior portion of the horizontal osteotomy is accomplished with an oscillating saw blade (Fig. 14–5*D*). Ideally, this osteotomy is made just above the point of greatest chin prominence. The surgeon's finger may be positioned on the lingual mucosa to feel the saw blade as it initially transects the lingual cortical plate. With the mental nerves and the contiguous soft-tissue flap carefully retracted and protected, the planned osteotomy is extended laterally and posteriorly. Osteotomies of the lateral cortex, which may be extended from 0.5 to 2.0 cm posterior to the mental nerves, are made with a small oscillating saw blade or a sharp reciprocating blade, approximately 3 to 4 mm inferior to the mental foramina (Fig. 14–5*E* and *F*). A fine instrument is placed in the horizontal line of osteotomy to determine when the lingual cortex has been completely sectioned (Fig. 14–5*G*). The posteromedial aspect is the most difficult area to osteotomize completely and is potentially problematic. If it is incompletely cut, an undesirable fracture of the inferior border of the mandible distal to the planned osteotomy site may occur. Such fractures are comparable to the "splitting of a log" and may extend posteriorly the entire length of the mandible. *Complete* sectioning of the segment to be repositioned is the key to preventing this complication. When the osteotomy is accomplished in this manner, the segment is easily downfractured and mobilized by teasing a periosteal elevator or thin tapered osteotome between the proximal and distal segments. If there is resistance to fracturing, the osteotomy sites are carefully examined to determine where the inferior border of the mandible has been incompletely sectioned. The mobilized segment, pedicled to the geniohyoid and digastric muscles and periosteum, is grasped with a bone-holding clamp and moved into the preplanned position (Fig. 14–5*H*). The inferior segment is repositioned with the least possible subperiosteal detachment of the suprahyoid muscles and periosteum. Occasionally it is impossible to advance the segment the desired distance without detaching some of the soft tissue enveloping the anterior portion of the inferior segment. Usually, however, gradual and continual anterior pressure on the inferior segment with a bone-holding forceps allows the segment to be repositioned the planned amount. Vertical relief incisions through the reflected periosteum facilitate advancement of the pedicled inferior segment and closure of the wound. The amount of forward movement is determined by measuring the bony step created between the proximal and distal segments (Fig. 14–5*I*). With a periosteal elevator positioned on the lingual aspect of the mobilized segment to protect the soft tissue at the floor of the mouth, additional bone sculpturing may be accomplished to facilitate the desired anteroposterior and vertical movements (Fig. 14–5*Q*).

The repositioned segment is fixed to the body of the mandible with three or four direct transosseous wires (Fig. 14–5*J* and *K*). Proper placement of the wires assures stability of the mobilized segment (Fig. 14–5*J*). With the distal segment positioned inferiorly, a No. 703 fissure bur is used to drill obliquely through the labial cortex into the cancellous margin of the sectioned proximal segment; similar holes are drilled obliquely through the margins of the sectioned distal segment through the lingual cortex (Fig. 14–5*I*). Drill holes are positioned in the lateral aspect of the distal and proximal segments so that the interosseous mattress sutures will tend to hold the advanced segment forward (Fig. 14–5*J*). To accomplish this, holes are drilled in the posterior portion of the inferior segment and the anterior portion of the proximal segments. By strategically altering the position of the vertical drill holes in the proximal and distal margins of the osteotomized bone one or two figure-of-8 wire sutures are placed in the anterior region, and two lateral mattress wire ligatures maintain the advanced segment in the planned position.

A double-layered closure of the mucosa and muscles is made with interrupted 3-0 catgut sutures. After the skin overlying the chin, the inferior border of the mandible, and the lateral aspect of the face has been painted with tincture of benzoin, a pressure dressing in secured to the skin. This dressing is kept in place for 5 to 7 days (Fig. 14–5*L* and *M*). Elastoplast strips, secured by strips of adhesive tape, serve to anchor the soft tissues to the underlying bone and to decrease dead space. Secondary infection associated with dissolution of a hematoma is thereby minimized.

Surgical Technique of Double Horizontal Sliding Osteotomy (Fig. 14–6)

A double horizontal osteotomy technique may be considered when the amount of advancement desired exceeds the thickness of the symphysis.[3] In such cases the vertical chin height must be sufficient to create two separate bone segments, each of which is at least 7 to 8 mm thick. Each segment may be advanced the full thickness of the symphysis so that almost twice as much bone advancement may be achieved compared with what is possible with a single slide. Both segments remain pedicled to lingual periosteum and muscle. Because the anterior bellies of the digastric muscles are stretched farther than they are with a single slide, considerable care must be exercised when wiring the segments to ensure adequate stabilization. Additional particulate marrow grafts may be placed along the lines of osteotomy on the newly created labial "steps" and between the

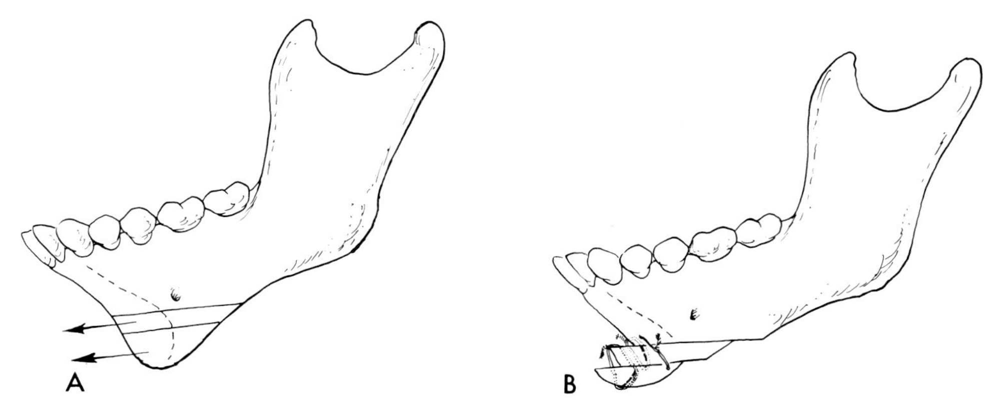

Figure 14–6. Augmentation genioplasty by double-step osteotomy. *A,* Two horizontal osteotomies of inferior border of mandible. Solid lines indicate horizontal osteotomies; arrows indicate directional movement of segments. *B,* Segments maintained in preplanned advanced position with multiple interosseous wires.

segments to promote better healing and consolidation of the repositioned segments and augmentation of the labiomental region.

Surgical Technique of Hinge Sliding Osteotomy
(Fig. 14–7)

When the mental symphysis is relatively thin, it may be impossible to advance the chin the desired amount or direction. As the lingual cortex of the mobilized distal segment is repositioned anteriorly, it will pass labial to the labial cortex of the proximal segment. Consequently, stabilization of the segment may be difficult, if not impossible.

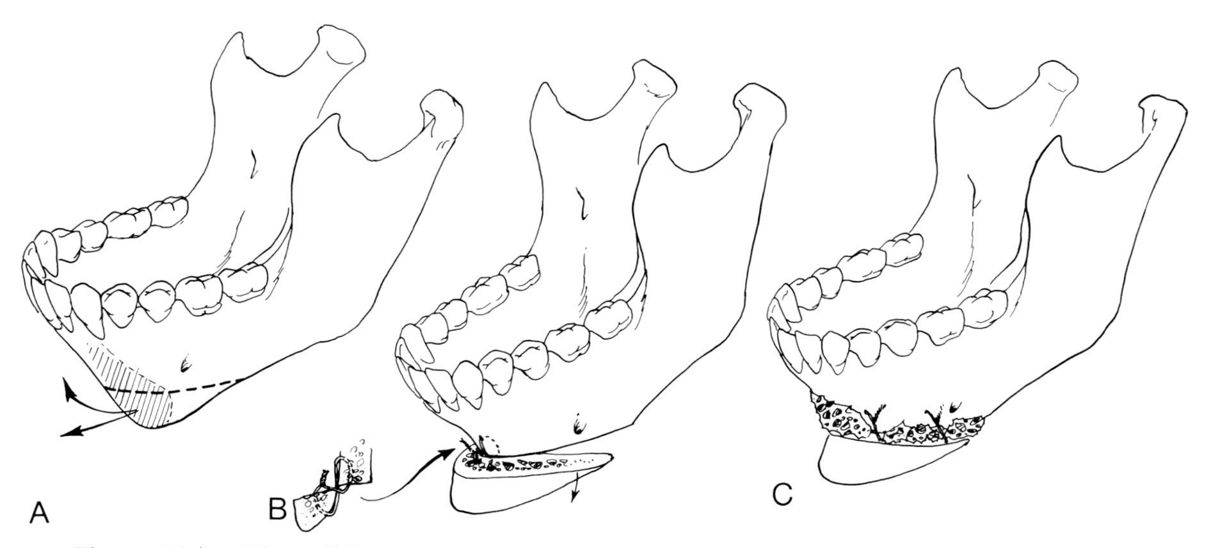

Figure 14–7. Hinge sliding osteotomy. *A,* Solid line indicates horizontal osteotomy. Arrow indicates directional movement that increases amount of chin advancement. *B,* Anterior end of chin is rotated superiorly around labial cortex of the body of the mandible; particulate marrow bone graft interposed between the proximal and distal segments to maintain the advanced position of chin.

The hinge sliding osteotomy, another modification of the horizontal sliding osteotomy may be used to increase the amount of "effective" chin.[8] Rotation of the chin can significantly increase the amount of bone contour. The chin is hinged upward and forward with a midline wire that is passed between the mandibular lingual and labial cortices. A higher horizontal cut for the same degree of rotation will create even more prominence.

In very high mandibular plane angle cases with relatively little chin height, the anterior end of the osteotomy must be directed inferiorly to avoid injury to the roots of the incisor teeth. Because of the downward and forward inclination of the line of osteotomy, the mobilized segment is moved downward and forward only to increase the chin height. To overcome this tendency to lengthen the chin and simultaneously to increase the amount of advancement, the anterior end of the segment may be rotated superiorly around the labial cortex of the superior segment by hinge sliding osteotomy. This rotation advances and superiorly repositions the inferior border of the segment while lowering the posterior end.

A particulate marrow bone graft is interposed between the proximal and distal segments to achieve and maintain the advanced position of the chin. Trial repositioning of cephalometric templates is essential to determine whether the procedure is feasible and desirable and will indicate the exact amount of forward movement that can be achieved.

Autogeneous Bone Grafts or Alloplastic Implants as Adjuncts to Horizontal Advancement Osteotomy

When preoperative studies indicate that the hinge-sliding, oblique-sliding, or double-step osteotomy is not feasible, will not produce the necessary advancement, or is precluded by insufficient bone in the vertical and horizontal dimensions of the chin, an autogenous bone graft or Proplast alloplastic implant may be used in addition to the horizontal advancement osteotomy. Autogenous cancellous bone from the ilium may be used to fill the void between the lingual surface of the inferior segment and anterior

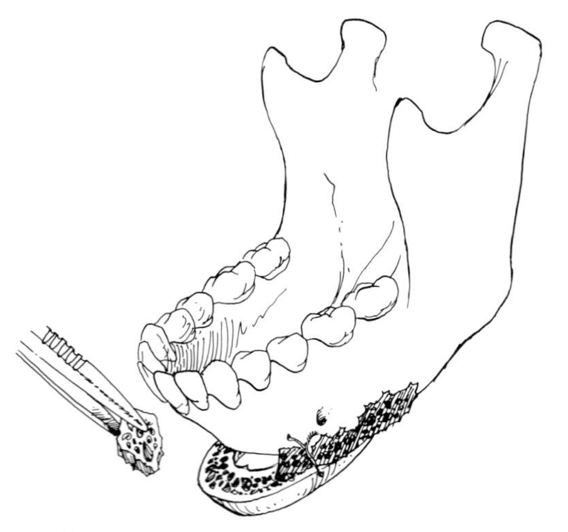

Figure 14–8. Autogenous cancellous bone graft placed at junction of the advanced inferior segment and anterior aspect of the proximal segment to allow additional advancement of the chin, consolidation of the repositioned segment, and augmentation of the labiomental region.

surface of the symphysis (Fig. 14–8). Placing additional bone chips at the juncture of the advanced inferior segment and the anterior aspect of the proximal segment creates subtle contour changes in the labiomental region. Onlay corticocancellous bone grafts (Fig. 14–8) or Proplast (Fig. 14–9) may be placed over the lateral aspects of the body of the mandible and the anterior and lateral aspects of the repositioned inferior segment.

Horizontal sliding advancement osteotomy is precluded in a few individuals with severe mandibular deficiency and excessively small chins in whom the deformity is manifest in all three planes of space. In such individuals, large free whole bone grafts from the ilium supplemented by particulate marrow grafts are used to augment the contour of the chin. Contour restoration of the chin in this manner may be associated with partial progressive resorption of the graft necessitating subsequent serial grafting with onlay corticocancellous bone. When this kind of large graft is placed in the site of an earlier operation, an extraoral submental approach to the operative site may be preferable to the intraoral degloving exposure.

Proplast may be added to the front of an advanced segment to produce more augmentation than can be attained with a horizontal slide alone. The amount of Proplast to be added to the front of the advanced segment equals the difference between the maximal bone advancement and the desired soft-tissue augmentation plus a small amount to compensate for the difference between hard-tissue and soft-tissue advancement. The Proplast to soft tissue advancement ratio is about 1:0.8. The contour of the chin is altered by carving the Proplast to the desired shape. To broaden the chin, the implant is sculptured to produce more lateral prominence. A tapered chin is produced by the addition of a narrow implant that is thick in the middle and tapers laterally to a feather edge.

The possibility of postoperative hematoma formation and infection associated with excessive dead space may be decreased by operating in two stages. The horizontal sliding osteotomy is initially accomplished under general anesthesia. Six to eight weeks later, the esthetic result is reassessed and the chin is additionally augmented with Proplast under general or local anesthesia.

AUGMENTATION OF THE LABIOMENTAL FOLD

Corticocancellous autogenous bone or Proplast may be inserted above a sliding osteotomy to prevent formation of a deep angular labiomental fold (see Case Reports 14–4 and 14–5 respectively). The more extensive the advancement, the greater the tendency to produce such a defect because of the larger step created above the advanced segment. By sculpturing autogenous bone or Proplast to fit this step from cuspid to cuspid, the resulting soft-tissue fold may be contoured to the desired form. We prefer the use of autogenous bone whenever feasible if the area to be augmented involves the alveolar bone encasing the mandibular anterior teeth. Proplast, besides having a greater propensity for infection (periodontal) may also cause bone and root resorption if placed over the roots of the mandibular anterior teeth.

Surgical Technique of Augmentation Genioplasty Employing Proplast

Proplast is a highly porous alloplastic material intended for augmentation of facial bony contour in patients with congenital, developmental, or acquired deficiencies.[29, 30] It

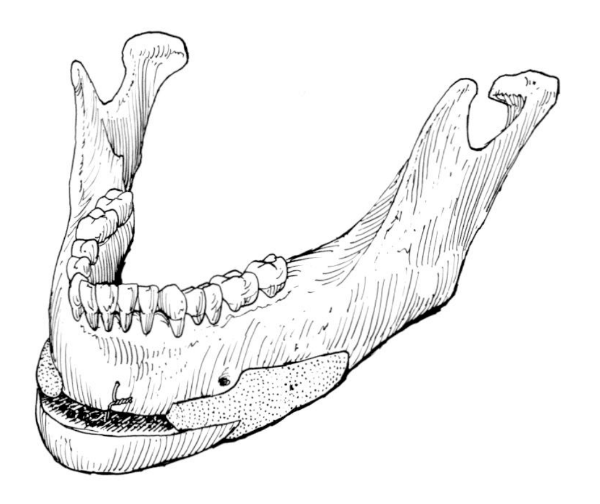

Figure 14–9. Horizontal sliding advancement genioplasty with lateral augmentation by Proplast. Carved Proplast implants positioned over midbody of the mandible provide lateral augmentation and eliminate the notch at the inferior border of the mandible created by the advancement genioplasty.

is prepared from Teflon fluorocarbon polymer and vitreous carbon fibers. The pores, which compose 70 to 90 per cent of the total material volume, permit tissue ingrowth, which aids in stabilization. The material may be easily carved to the desired shape with a sharp scalpel blade at the time of surgery. Compression of Proplast should be avoided as much as possible throughout its preparation and surgical implantation, because excessive manipulation and compression will collapse the pores. The material is sterilized by wrapping it in a lint-free material and inserting it into a standard gravity autoclave for 30 minutes at 250° F (15 PSI).

Proplast may be used for anteroposterior chin augmentation when horizontal sliding osteotomy of the mandibular symphysis is not feasible (Fig. 14–10). Anterior mandibular subapical osteotomy may preclude simultaneous horizontal osteotomy of the mandibular symphysis because of insufficient bone to maintain adequate strength of the mental symphysis. The amount of augmentation is determined by prediction studies. Proplast is inserted via a subperiosteal degloving exposure of the mandibular symphysis (Fig. 14–10). Maximal soft-tissue attachment is maintained at the inferior border of the

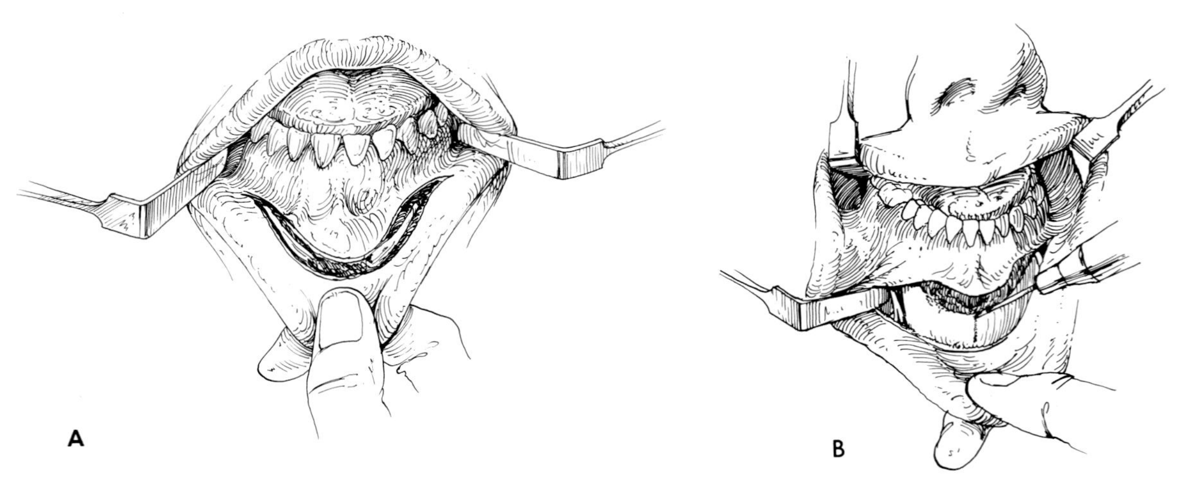

Figure 14–10. *A–D,* Increasing chin prominence by Proplast implant. (Proplast is considered as an adjunct to horizontal osteotomy of the inferior border of the mandible. It is also used when horizontal osteotomy of the inferior border of the mandible is not feasible.) *A,* Soft-tissue incision for exposure of mandible; superficial branches of mental nerves exposed. *B,* Chin prominence degloved between the mental foramina; bilateral subperiosteal tunnels extended to the 2nd molar region below the mental foramen; midline vertical reference line etched into midsagittal plane of the chin.

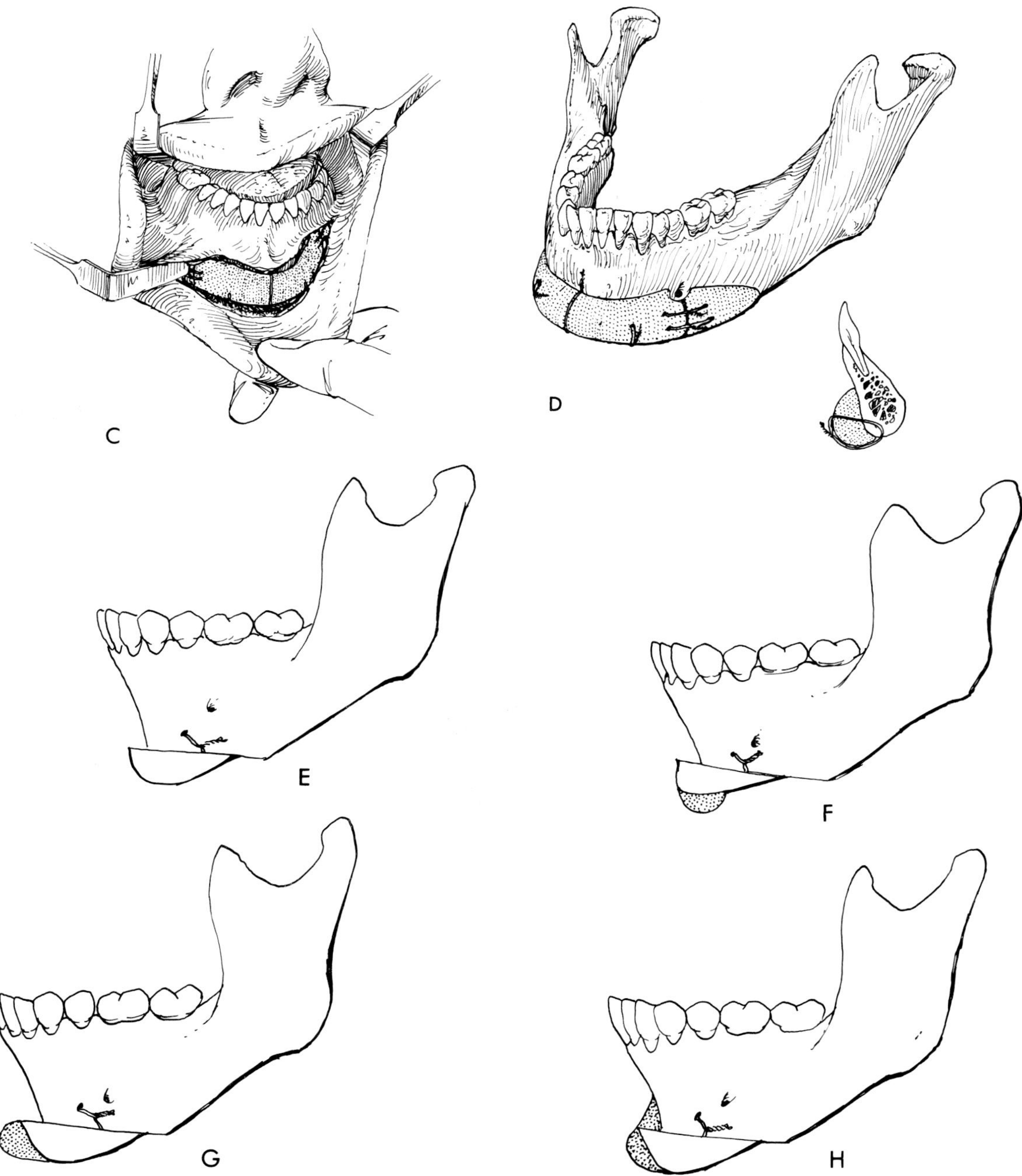

Figure 14–10 *Continued.* *C,* Carved Proplast implant inserted into subperiosteal pocket and secured with transosseous sutures or wires; lateral augmentation is achieved by extending the implant into the subperiosteal tunnels posterior to the mental foramina. *D,* Position of segmental Proplast blocks used to increase chin prominence and provide lateral augmentation; the blocks used for lateral augmentation are sutured to the anterior block to prevent migration; anterior block secured to mandible with transosseous wires or sutures. *E–H,* Augmentation of chin prominence by horizontal sliding osteotomy plus Proplast. *E,* Horizontal sliding osteotomy to increase horizontal chin prominence. *F,* Horizontal sliding osteotomy with Proplast under mobilized segment to increase horizontal and vertical dimensions. *G,* Horizontal sliding osteotomy with Proplast added to anterior surface of advanced segment to achieve additional horizontal augmentation. *H,* Horizontal sliding osteotomy with Proplast added above and on front of the advanced segment to decrease the depth of the labiomental fold and to achieve additional horizontal augmentation. Proplast is not placed over bone that encases the mandibular anterior teeth.

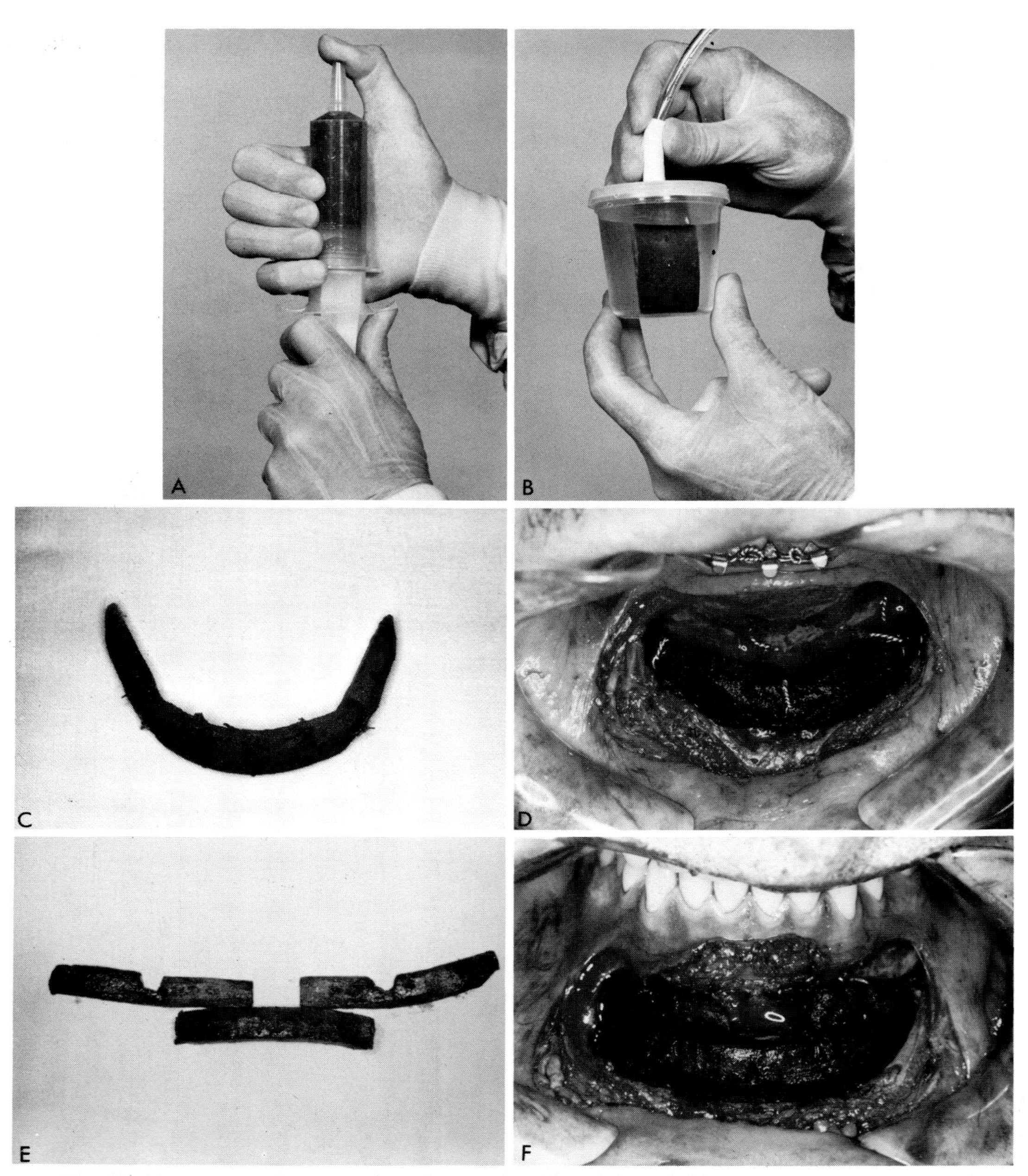

Figure 14–11. *A,* Prior to carving, the Proplast block is inserted into a 50- or 60-ml syringe filled with antibiotic solution. The syringe outlet is occluded and traction is exerted on the plunger, creating a vacuum that causes the air within the Proplast to expand and come to the surface. The syringe is tapped with an instrument to force the antibiotic solution into the Proplast. The cycle is repeated until the Proplast block sinks, indicating that it is saturated with solution. *B,* An alternate method employs a disposable plastic specimen container with a small hole cut in the lid. Antibiotic solution and Proplast are placed in the container; the end of the suction tubing is alternately placed over the hole in the lid and released. Bubbles that form are forced to the surface by tapping the container. The cycle is repeated until the Proplast sinks. *C,* Three-piece Proplast block carved to desired contour for lateral and anterior augmentation. Proplast sutured together to prevent displacement of lateral implant segments. *D,* Carved Proplast implant wired to the anterior aspect of the repositioned mental symphysis to provide additional augmentation. *E,* Three-piece carved Proplast implant prepared for insertion; middle piece is inserted in front of horizontal sliding osteotomy to increase anteroposterior augmentation. Upper pieces are inserted above osteotomy to fill in labiomental fold and provide lateral augmentation. *F,* Three-piece implant shown in *E* secured to advanced bony segment. Proplast implant should not be placed over alveolar bone that encases and supports mandibular anterior teeth. Implants are placed over the hard-tissue chin to minimize bone resorption below the implant and the possibility of infection secondary to periodontal disease.

mandible. After exposure of the mandibular symphysis, a block of Proplast of appropriate thickness is selected and placed in a 50-cc or 60-cc syringe filled with an antibiotic solution containing 1 gram of cephalosporin in 50 ml sterile saline (Fig. 14–11a). After air is evacuated from the syringe, a finger is held over the end opening and the plunger is pulled out to create a vacuum within the syringe. This causes the air within the Proplast to expand and form bubbles on the surface. The syringe is tapped with an instrument to free the bubbles, which then rise to the surface. The plunger is released and antibiotic solution is drawn into the Proplast to replace the evacuated air. The plunger is repeatedly pulled and released until the Proplast sinks to the bottom of the syringe, indicating that it is saturated with solution.

The Proplast block is then removed and sculptured to the desired shape. It is tried in position with the soft tissue drape repositioned. Additional carving and trial positioning are performed until the desired soft-tissue contour is achieved. Additional pieces of Proplast may be carved to provide lateral augmentation. These pieces are inserted into subperiosteal tunnels developed below the mental nerves. Adequate stabilization of the Proplast used for lateral augmentation is usually obtained from the periosteal envelope, but in certain cases it may be desirable to suture the lateral segments to the anterior segments to ensure exact positioning. After the anterior segment is fixed to the mandible with two or three fine transosseous wires, a layered closure of the soft-tissue wound is accomplished. Finally, a pressure dressing is applied to the chin.

REDUCTION OF CHIN PROMINENCE (ANTEROPOSTERIOR EXCESS)

The natural vertical reference line is used to plan surgery to reduce chin prominence in the same manner described for anteroposterior deficiency. By following the present or proposed profile for the middle third of the face and utilizing the landmarks and criteria suggested for establishing good facial esthetics, the proposed profile of the lower lip and chin is traced. The horizontal difference between the preoperative soft-tissue chin position and the planned soft-tissue position as sketched on the profile tracing represents the needed soft-tissue change. Horizontal sliding osteotomy is the technique of choice for reducing chin prominence.

Surgical Technique of Horizontal Sliding Osteotomy for Anteroposterior Reduction (Fig. 14–12)[20]

A reduction of chin prominence and soft-tissue redraping is accomplished by horizontal osteotomy of the inferior border of the mandible when the attachment of the soft tissue to the inferior and anteroinferior portions of the repositioned segment is maintained.

Currently, prediction of the desired surgical bony movement is difficult owing to the great variability of soft-tissue to hard-tissue change (40 to 75 per cent) even when a maximal soft-tissue pedicle is maintained.

By varying the angulation of the ostectomy, the chin height can be concomitantly shortened or lengthened somewhat. The magnitude of movement and the angulation of the horizontal osteotomy are determined by trial repositioning of a template of the bony and soft-tissue chin. At surgery the amount of posterior movement of the most prominent portion of the chin is not necessarily reflected by the step produced by retraction of

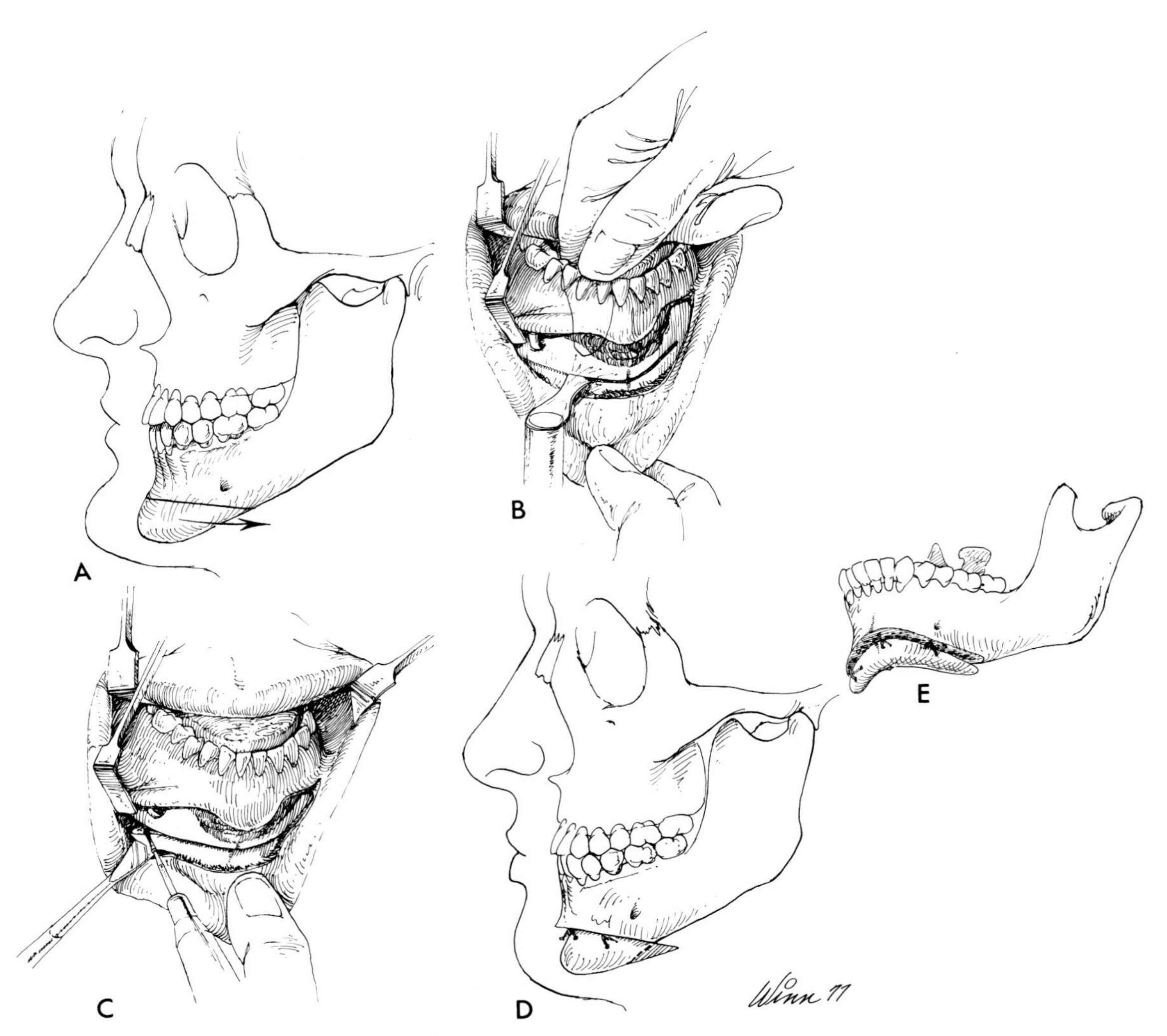

Figure 14–12. Reduction of chin prominence by horizontal sliding osteotomy. *A,* Horizontal sliding osteotomy for decreasing chin prominence. Arrow indicates directional movement of inferior segment. *B,* Chin prominence degloved from mental foramen of one side to contralateral mental foramen; midline vertical reference line etched into midsagittal plane of the chin across the planned horizontal osteotomy. Maximal soft-tissue attachment is maintained to the inferior and anteroinferior portions of the repositioned segment to optimize the result. *C,* Posterior position of the inferior segment shortened to maintain normal contour of the skin at the inferior border of the mandible. *D* and *E,* Inferior segment retracted and fixed into planned position with interosseous wires. Near 1:1 changes of movement of soft tissue to movement of underlying osseous segment are achieved when we preserve the largest possible soft-tissue pedicle to the inferior and anteroinferior aspects of the repositioned segment.

the mobilized segment. This step, however, should be virtually the same as the one produced on the cephalometric prediction study.

After the anterior portion of the chin is exposed as previously described, the midline of the chin and the planned horizontal osteotomy are inscribed into the chin (Fig. 14–12*A* and *B*). Vertical reference lines may also be inscribed into the lateral aspect of the mandible to indicate when the planned amount of posterior movement of the inferior segment has been achieved. The distance between vertical reference lines on the proximal and distal segments before and after the inferior segment is moved posteriorly serves as a guide to the amount of posterior movement. When the amount of retraction is in excess of 3 or 4 mm, the posterior portions of the mobilized segments are usually shortened to maintain the desired contour of the skin at the inferior border of the mandible (Fig. 14–12*C*). Small posterior movements have minimal effect on the contour of the inferior border of the mandible. Gradual remodeling of the repositioned segment restores the contour of the inferior border of the mandible to normal.

The repositioned inferior segment is fixed to the body of the mandible with interosseous wires, which resist further posterior displacement of the mobilized segment by either extraoral pressures or the muscles that attach to the lingual and inferior aspect of the segment (Fig. 14–12*D*). The labiomental fold may be maximized by removing bone from the superior edge of the step after retraction of the symphysis. By sticking with a "game plan" based upon the results of preoperative cephalometric prediction studies, bony changes are programmed to achieve rapid, predictable, and stable changes in the soft-tissue drape.

Posterior repositioning of the mobilized segment may be limited by the thickness of the symphysis at the level of the proposed cut. If the mobilized segment is moved posteriorly a large distance, a point may be reached where the segment becomes positioned distal to the lingual cortex of the mandibular body. When this occurs, stabilization of the segment could become difficult. Furthermore, the procedure could have an adverse effect on the soft-tissue contour at the inferior border of the mandible. To alleviate these problems, the mobilized segment may be widened by midsymphysis sectioning. After expansion, stabilization and bone contact are improved. So far, we have not used this procedure, and in clinical practice it is probably indicated only rarely.

Excessive removal of bone or retraction of the inferior border of the mandible will tend to obliterate the labiomental fold that is so essential for good esthetic balance in the lower third of the face. A disparate thickness of the soft-tissue and bony chin can also produce unpredictable results.

Surgical Technique of Recontouring the Chin by Removal of Bone

When there is minimal prominence of the chin associated with a distinct labiomental fold in an individual who cannot be hospitalized for horizontal osteotomy of the inferior border of the mandible under general anesthesia, reduction of chin prominence by removal of bone may be feasible. Preoperative cephalometric prediction studies will indicate the desired soft tissue result so that the surgeon can continually work toward this goal. Such studies *do not* provide a *quantitative* estimate of the amount of bone to be removed. Because of the unpredictable change in the soft tissue associated with removing excess bone in this manner, the amount of chin reduction is based principally on clinical judgment at the time of surgery as to what constitutes balance between the chin, lips, and nose. Subtle anterior recontouring of the mental symphysis area can be achieved satisfactorily when the surgery is accomplished in a systematic manner and when the distinct limitations of the technique are appreciated. When a great reduction in the prominence of the chin is desired, this method does not produce predictable results; in addition, the excessive detachment of the submental integument may produce a "witch's chin" appearance. Posterior transpositioning of the inferior border of the mandible, pedicled to its enveloping tissues, minimizes the chance that this will occur.

The surgery is ideally accomplished with the patient in a sitting position under local anesthesia. When the surgery is done without an endotracheal tube in place, the facial morphology can be constantly evaluated, and the chin is sculptured until the desired result is achieved.

VERTICAL DEFORMITIES

By analyzing the spatial relationships among the structures of the lower third of the face, the segment responsible for the deformity can be determined. Care must be taken to ensure that the clinical analysis is undertaken with the lips relaxed and the teeth in occlusion. The apparent deformity is not only the abnormal length of the chin but the equally important unesthetic contour of the lip and labiomental fold associated with an abnormally long or short chin.

The lower third of the face can be divided into two or three equal segments.[3] When it is divided into three segments, the distances between subnasale and the labial angle, the labial angle and the depth of the labiomental fold, and the labiomental fold and soft-tissue gnathion are equal (see Figure 14–1). When the lower third of the face is divided into two equal segments, the distance from subnasale to the vermilion border of the lower lip is equal to the distance from the vermilion border of the lower lip to soft-tissue gnathion. The total height of the lower third should equal the height of the middle and upper thirds. Therefore, the components of the lower third must not only be in balance with one another, but the entire lower third must blend with the upper and middle thirds. It is relatively difficult to alter the height of the middle third more than a few millimeters, whereas the lower third may be shortened or lengthened more than a centimeter. Consequently, surgical procedures are directed toward altering the lower third to achieve balance with the middle third.

Treatment Planning in Vertical Deficiency

Individuals with severe mandibular deficiency secondary to deficient mandibular growth or skeletal type deep bite may clinically manifest a lack of chin height, a relatively short distance between the edge of the lower lip and soft-tissue gnathion, a deep labiomental fold, a compressed lower lip and inferiorly directed labial angles. The lower lip–chin complex may be anatomically short at rest when compared with the other facial segments or it may only appear short when the teeth are in occlusion because the lower lip is compressed as a result of a deep bite. In the latter case, the appearance of having a short chin may be corrected by appropriate dentoalveolar surgery, by complete subapical osteotomy or a mandibular ramus procedure to achieve a satisfactory overjet–overbite relationship.

Treatment planning for correction of vertical deficiency utilizes the same techniques employed for anteroposterior deficiency. A tracing is made of the present or proposed middle-third facial profile. Using the criteria suggested for establishing vertical facial balance, the clinician sketches the proposed profile for the lower lip and chin onto the drawing to make the lower facial third equal to the middle and upper thirds. The vertical difference between the preoperative soft-tissue chin position and the planned soft-tissue position represents the needed augmentation and serves as the basis for selecting the appropriate surgical procedure. The vertical dimension of the chin can be increased predictably by pedicled horizontal osteotomy supplemented by insertion of an interpositional horseshoe-shaped wedge of cancellous bone from the ilium.[6] Bone chips may be placed anteriorly or laterally for additional augmentation. Proplast or bone may be placed below the inferior border of the chin, or the mobilized segment may be moved inferiorly and anteriorly to lengthen and augment the chin during horizontal osteotomy.

The desired increase in chin length is determined from cephalometric prediction tracings, which serve as a basis for drawing the proposed profile. A transparent template of the preoperative soft-tissue and bone contour is traced from the cephalograph. A horizontal line then is drawn on the bony chin about 4 mm below the mental foramen to represent the osteotomy. An identical line is drawn on the prediction drawing. The template is repositioned so that the preoperative soft-tissue chin profile coincides with the planned profile. The space between the horizontal line on the prediction drawing and the line on the template represents the size and shape of the bone graft needed to fill the anticipated gap. Measurements of the length and the anterior and posterior heights of the gap are recorded and used at surgery to help contour the graft. It is our clinical impression that the lower lip may be slightly lowered as a result of this procedure. Unfortunately, we do not presently have follow-up data on a sufficient number of cases to permit prediction of this change.

Surgical Technique of Horizontal Osteotomy with Interpositional Bone Graft (Fig. 14–13)

When it is necessary to increase the vertical dimension of the chin, a corticocancellous iliac crest bone graft may be used to supplement horizontal osteotomy of the

Figure 14–13. Horizontal sliding osteotomy combined with interpositional autogenous bone graft to increase chin height and alter labiomental fold. *A,* Preoperative short face syndrome deformity. Solid line indicates planned horizontal osteotomy. *B,* Postoperative.

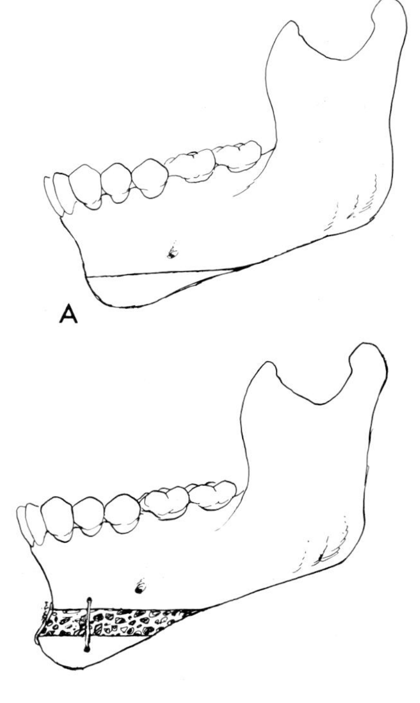

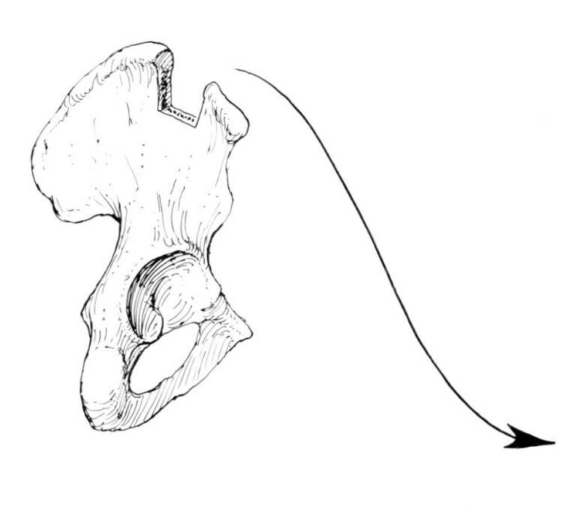

mental protuberance. Individuals who manifest a Class II deep bite or extreme mandibular deficiency are the most logical candidates for such surgery. The bone graft sculptured to the preplanned dimensions and the mobilized chin segment are fixed to the body of the mandible by direct interosseous wires. To maximize the vertical change of the soft tissues, the surgery is accomplished by maintaining as much soft tissue as possible to the inferior and inferoanterior portions of the mobilized segment.

An alternative method of increasing chin height involves placement of Proplast below the inferior border of the mandible through a degloving exposure. A piece of Proplast proportional in size to the proposed increase in chin height is carved to the desired contour and wired to the inferior border of the mandible. Although the technique is quite simple, the soft-tissue change may not be proportional to the thickness of the implant, and therefore the outcome of this method is not as predictable as that of the "sandwich technique."

Treatment Planning in Vertical Excess

The individual with an excessively long chin frequently has a flat labiomental fold, mentalis muscle hyperfunction, and excessive bone height between the apices of the mandibular incisors and the inferior border of the mandible. The soft tissue of the lower lip and chin may be deficient, normal, or excessive in height. The total height of these soft tissues appears to shorten as the bony symphysis is reduced in height; consequently, it is difficult to raise the margin of the lower lip by raising the inferior border of the mandible. Shortening of the excess soft tissue with vertical reduction genioplasty, however, permits establishment of facial balance.

The surgical plan is developed by tracing the present or proposed upper-third and middle-third facial profile and sketching the proposed lower-third facial profile as suggested for establishing vertical facial balance. A clear template of the preoperative bony and soft-tissue chin is prepared as described in the section on anteroposterior treatment planning. The template is repositioned to coincide with the proposed chin position. The vertical difference between the preoperative and postoperative soft-tissue chin profile represents the amount of bone that must be removed from the mental symphysis. The design and angulation of the proposed ostectomy are determined from these cephalometric studies.

The height of the chin may be reduced by removing bone from the inferior border of the symphysis, excising a wedge of bone from the midportion of the symphysis, or angling the bone cut superiorly as part of a sliding augmentation genioplasty. Excision of bone from the inferior border is relatively ineffective and unpredictable, owing to swelling of the soft tissue below the inferior border, which compensates for the bone reduction. A relatively minor vertical change, less than 5 mm, may be obtained by oblique angulation of the osteotomy during advancement genioplasty. Therefore, a wedge ostectomy of the mandibular symphysis is utilized routinely to reduce chin height.

Surgical Technique of Wedge Ostectomy (Fig. 14–14)

Many variations of the horizontal sliding osteotomy may be adapted to meet an individual's esthetic needs. A moderate decrease of the vertical dimension of the chin

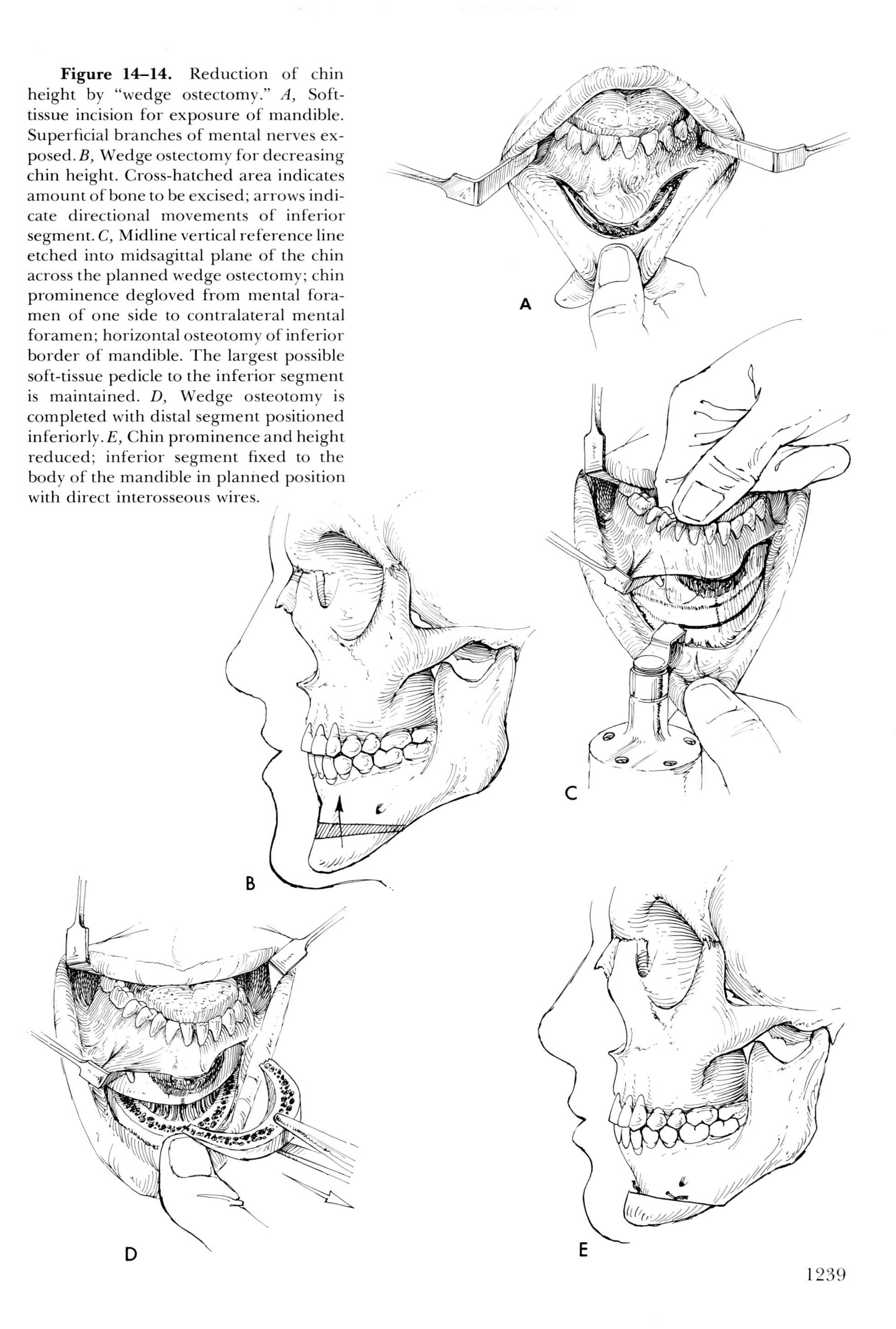

Figure 14–14. Reduction of chin height by "wedge ostectomy." *A,* Soft-tissue incision for exposure of mandible. Superficial branches of mental nerves exposed. *B,* Wedge ostectomy for decreasing chin height. Cross-hatched area indicates amount of bone to be excised; arrows indicate directional movements of inferior segment. *C,* Midline vertical reference line etched into midsagittal plane of the chin across the planned wedge ostectomy; chin prominence degloved from mental foramen of one side to contralateral mental foramen; horizontal osteotomy of inferior border of mandible. The largest possible soft-tissue pedicle to the inferior segment is maintained. *D,* Wedge osteotomy is completed with distal segment positioned inferiorly. *E,* Chin prominence and height reduced; inferior segment fixed to the body of the mandible in planned position with direct interosseous wires.

can be achieved by oblique sliding osteotomy. By angling the bone cut superiorly, the inferior segment can be transposed forward and upward to reduce the chin height approximately 5 mm. When larger height reductions (in excess of 5 mm) are indicated, however, a horizontal wedge of bone is removed above the horizontal sliding osteotomy. An additional advantage of reducing chin height in this manner relates to the improved lower lip–tooth relationship as a consequence of decreased tooth exposure. Cephalometric prediction studies are essential to determine the new position of the pogonion, the amount of bone to be excised, and the design and angulation of the horizontal sliding osteotomy.

When feasible, the genioplasty is simplified and made less problematic by excising a wedge of bone anterior to the mental foramina. The horizontal sliding osteotomy, however, will generally extend posterior to the foramina. After the planned lines of osteotomy and ostectomy are etched into the chin, the horizontal sliding osteotomy is completed. Then, with the pedicled inferior segment retracted inferiorly, the ostectomy is accomplished. After appropriate sculpturing of the bony margins to allow optimal interfacing of the proximal and distal segments, the mobilized segment is fixed into the planned position.

Several technical modifications simplify the surgical technique of reducing chin height and make it more predictable and less problematic. After the circumvestibular incision is accomplished, the chin is minimally "degloved" to maximize attachment of the integument to the anterior and inferior border of the mandible, while still providing accessibility for the planned bone incision. Preserving the soft-tissue attachment to the anterior aspect of the mobilized segment maximizes the soft-tissue change in the vertical facial dimension and provides predictable treatment planning (ratio between soft tissue and hard tissue change is approximately 0.8:1). More predictable changes in the soft tissue are achieved by keeping the soft tissue attached to the inferior border of the repositioned segment.

TRANSVERSE DEFORMITIES

Evaluation of transverse chin esthetics is best accomplished with the patient in the clinical setting where the complex curvatures of the nose, lips, chin, and cheeks may be studied in three dimensions during smiling and in repose. Well-oriented photographs may be used as reminders when the patient is not available, but photographs cannot be relied on for final surgical planning. Posteroanterior cephalometric radiographs are particularly useful in evaluating the bony architecture of patients with facial asymmetry.

Tranverse Deficiency and Excess

There are relatively few guidelines to aid the examiner in evaluating the width of the chin. The examiner must use artistic sense and must analyze the transverse dimension and contour for balance with other facial structures. In the frontal view, the periphery of the face may be described as round, oval, square, tapering, or any combination of these shapes. The outline form of each third of the face should be recorded along with the surgical changes that are needed to bring the lower third into harmony with the middle and upper thirds. Transverse reduction of the corners of a square chin to establish harmony with oval upper and middle facial thirds or broadening of a narrow tapered chin to establish balance with a square midface are examples of typical treatment plans. The amount of reduction or expansion may be estimated preoperatively but the final determination is made intraoperatively when the surgeon can observe the actual change.

Widening the Chin (Transverse Deficiency)
(Fig. 14–15*A*)

The chin may be widened by midline sectioning following horizontal osteotomy of the inferior border of the mandible. This is generally unnecessary when the horizontal osteotomy is extended posteriorly to the molar region. The lateral protuberance of the posterior ends provides important contour to the lateral aspect of the face.

Forward advancement of a pointed chin may not produce the desired amount of lateral or anteroposterior augmentation. In such cases, Proplast or onlay-bone grafts are carefully sculptured and used in concert with the sliding advancement genioplasty.

Narrowing the Chin (Transverse Excess)
(Fig. 14–15*B*)

The chin may be made more tapered by midline sectioning and excision of a triangular section of bone from the lingual aspect of the mobilized segment following horizontal osteotomy of the inferior border of the mandible. If the advanced segment is narrowed, the apposition of the proximal and distal segments is improved, the inferior segment can be advanced farther, and tension on the mental nerves is decreased. A very broad chin can be narrowed by excising a rectangular segment of bone from the midsymphyseal region. To maximize the effect on the soft tissue, the surgery is usually accomplished by maintaining as much soft-tissue attachment as possible to the lateral and inferior aspects of the repositioned segments. In clinical practice, however, it is undesirable to narrow the posterior ends of the segments, which provide a symmetric, subtle increase in contour to the lateral aspect of the face as the inferior segment is advanced. The lateral protuberance of the posterior ends may *appear* too prominent at the time of surgery and may indeed stretch the mental nerves. The surgeon, however, should resist the temptation to remove these lateral protuberances, for the increased prominence is usually desirable and is an important reason for extending the horizontal osteotomy posteriorly to an area below the molar teeth.

Asymmetry

Chin asymmetry is rarely an isolated entity; more frequently, the entire mandible is involved. Indeed, there may be compensatory changes in the midface (see Chapter 20, Hemifacial Microsomia, and Chapter 21, Maxillary Asymmetry). A facial midline is established by marking several points on the soft tissue. The middle of the forehead, the midpoint of the interpupillary distance, and the middle of the columella may be used if the midface is symmetric. Points on the lower third of the face that should intersect with this line include the middle of the philtral column, the middle of the upper and lower lips, the midpoint of the chin, and the maxillary and mandibular dental midlines. The structures on either side of the midsagittal plane should be equal in size, form, and proportion. By comparing the actual midline of the chin to the true facial midline, a measure of the necessary correction may be made. Similar measurements should be made from the true facial midline to each gonial angle. The use of a grid has proved to be a useful adjunct in localizing and quantifying the amount of the asymmetric manifestation (see Figure 14–3).

Surgical Treatment Planning

If the gonial angles are asymmetric, the appropriate procedure is planned to establish symmetry. Usually at least one ramus osteotomy is indicated (see Unilateral Mandibular Excess, Part B of Chapter 12). Maxillary osteotomies may also be required to correct occlusal and bony deformities associated with the mandibular asymmetry. Such osteotomies may significantly affect chin symmetry. The proposed mandibular move-

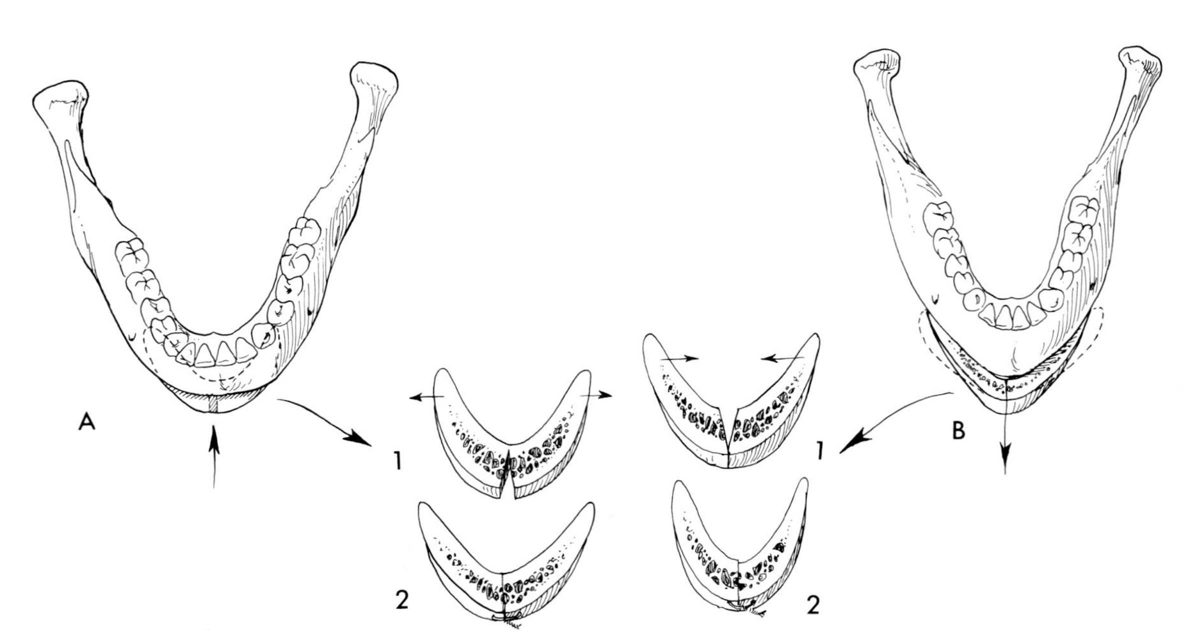

Figure 14–15. Altering horizontal dimension of chin by horizontal osteotomy of inferior border of mandible. *A,* Widening the chin by midline sectioning of the chin after reduction genioplasty. *B,* Narrowing the chin by excising triangular-shaped segment of bone from the mobilized segment after horizontal osteotomy of inferior border of the mandible. *C,* Excessively wide chin associated with flaring of inferior border and excessive vertical dimension of chin. Plan of surgery: Reduction of excessive chin height by horizontal ostectomy; reduction of chin width by midline ostectomy of mobilized inferior segment. Vertical reference marks are inscribed into bone; cross-hatched areas indicate planned ostectomy sites. *D,* Horizontal and vertical segments of bone excised from chin. *E,* Repositioned segments stabilized with transosseous wires; positional changes of vertical reference lines indicate amount of narrowing achieved.

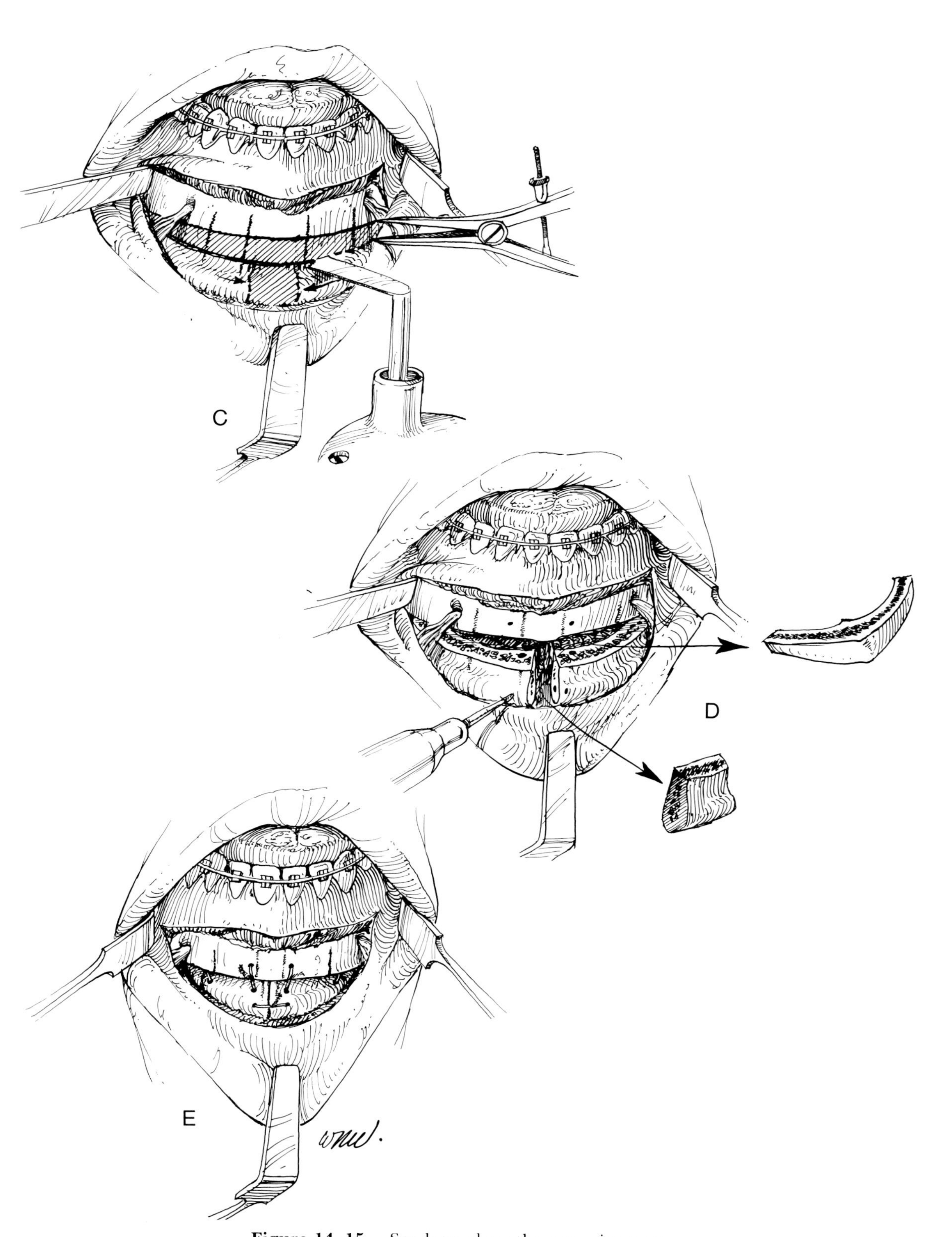

Figure 14–15. See legend on the opposite page.

ment will partially correct the chin midline discrepancy. Frequently the mandibular angles are symmetric when the mandibular dental midline coincides with the true facial midline. The relative difference between the chin, facial, and dental midlines must be carefully calculated by clinical examination of the patient with the head postured in natural head position.[17] A careful correlative study between these differences is the basis for selecting the appropriate surgical procedure and calculating the positional change of the chin.

By having the patient move his mandible so that the lower dental midline corresponds to the true facial midline, the surgeon may gain perspective on the anticipated soft-tissue changes associated with ramus surgery. With the mandible held in this position, the additional lateral repositioning of the chin required to establish chin symmetry may be planned. This also provides perspective regarding the need for augmentation of flattened or contour-deficient areas. Horizontal osteotomy of the mandibular symphysis with lateral repositioning is the procedure of choice for correcting most chin asymmetries. Maximal soft-tissue attachment is maintained to optimize soft tissue:bony change. The osteotomy may be extended posteriorly to the second molar region if correction of midbody asymmetry is needed. A vertical reference line is inscribed in the center of the chin to determine the exact amount of lateral movement of the inferior segment. A smooth contour on the contralateral side of the asymmetric chin is achieved by resecting a portion of the protruding bone. Small residual contour-deficient areas can be augmented by carefully shaped portions of the resected bone or by Proplast.

In many chin asymmetries the problem is manifest vertically as well as horizontally. When this is the case, a transverse wedge ostectomy is accomplished in conjunction with the horizontal osteotomy of the mandibular symphysis to permit shortening of the long side of the chin and leveling of the inferior border.

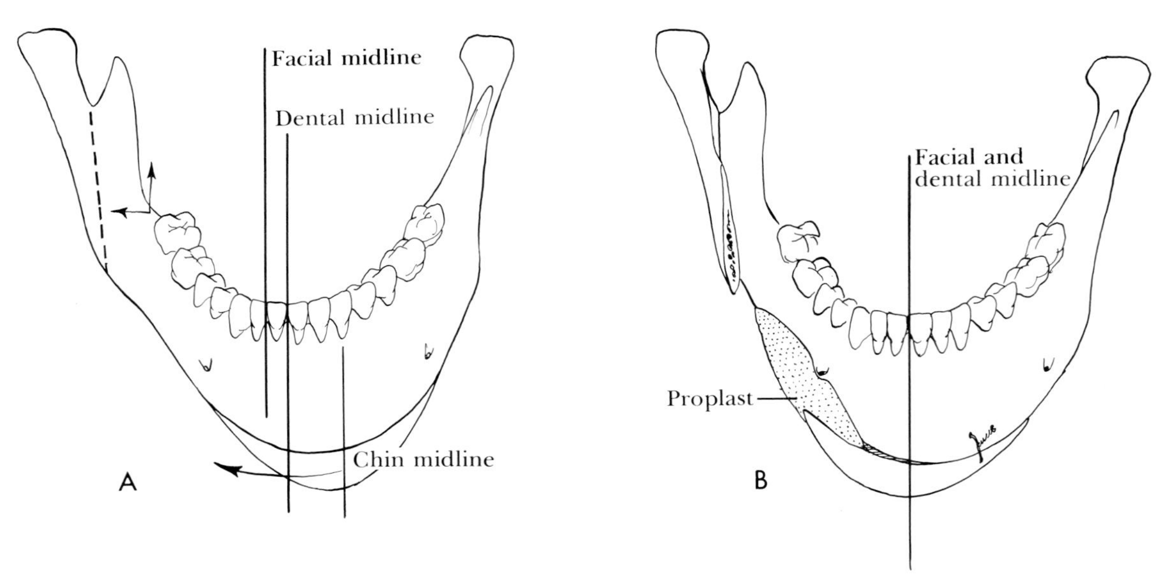

Figure 14–16. Correction of mandibular asymmetry by ramus osteotomy, transverse sliding osteotomy, and lateral augmentation with Proplast. *A,* Mandibular asymmetry with discrepancy between dental, chin, and facial midlines. *B,* Ramus osteotomy corrects the dental and facial midline discrepancy and partially corrects the chin asymmetry; transverse sliding osteotomy establishes facial and chin symmetry; midbody contour deficiency is augmented by Proplast implant.

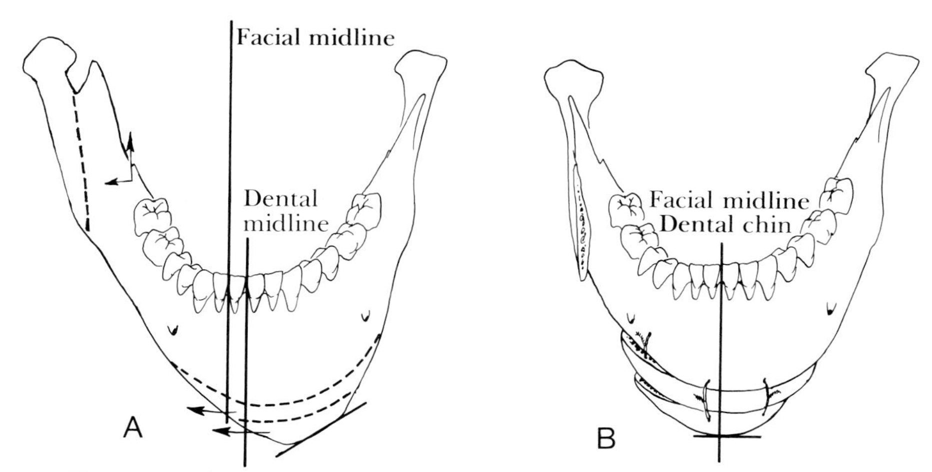

Figure 14–17. Double lateral sliding osteotomy. *A,* Double lateral sliding osteotomy for correction of asymmetry. Vertical ramus osteotomy helps to level the occlusal plane, coordinates the dental and facial midlines, and establishes ramus symmetry. Arrows indicate directional movement of ramus and chin segments. *B,* Mandible shifted by ramus osteotomy to establish dental and ramus symmetry; chin segments repositioned laterally and stabilized to establish chin symmetry.

Surgical Technique for Correcting Chin Asymmetry

The degloving exposure for horizontal sliding osteotomy to correct chin asymmetry is designed to maintain blood circulation to the mobilized portion of the inferior border of the mandible by maximizing the soft-tissue pedicle of genial and digastric muscles and periosteum. The circumvestibular incision is carried into the most lateral part of the buccal vestibule and as far posteriorly as necessary. In many instances the incision is extended to the anterior aspect of the vertical rami for simultaneous exposure of the angle region where the mandibular asymmetry is also manifest. Symmetry of the mandible is restored by a single, two-segment or three-segment transverse sliding genioplasty (Figs. 14–16, 14–17, and 14–18).[18]

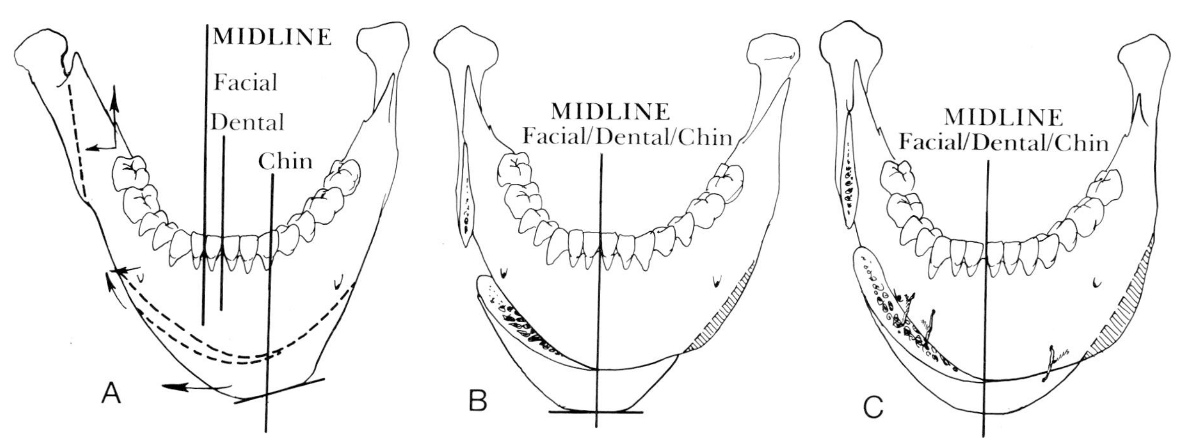

Figure 14–18. Oblique sliding wedge ostectomy. *A,* Oblique sliding wedge ostectomy to correct chin asymmetry; vertical ramus osteotomy for establishing dental and ramus symmetry and leveling occlusal plane. Arrows indicate directional movement of ramus and chin segments; area between dotted lines is proposed wedge ostectomy. *B,* Mandible shifted by ramus osteotomy to establish dental and ramus symmetry. Chin leveled by wedge ostectomy and midline corrected by lateral shift of segment; chin segment maintained under mandibular segment. Hatch marks indicate area of possible lateral ostectomy to achieve final contour. *C,* Mandible shifted by ramus osteotomy; chin leveled, maximal lateral augmentation achieved by stabilizing chin segment lateral to labial cortex of superior segment. Possible ostectomy indicated by hatch marks.

A midline vertical reference line is inscribed into the midsagittal plane of the chin across the area of the planned horizontal osteotomy for orientation after the inferior border of the mandible is mobilized. The surgery must be accomplished so that the segments to be repositioned are adequate in size to accomplish the desired clinical result. When aberrant vertical growth is associated with chin asymmetry, careful measurements are made from the panographic* and lateral cephalometric prediction tracings to determine the feasibility of single, double, or triple segment transverse sliding genioplasty and the amount and location of vertical reduction necessary. On the basis of these studies, the planned lines of osteotomy are inscribed into the mandible. Despite the emphasis given these quantitative measurements, the "clinical eye" is a vital determinant of the "final" result. In correcting many severe asymmetries of the lower third of the face, the optimal esthetic result can only be achieved by operating in two or three stages. The refinements and subtle changes necessary for excellent facial balance usually defy treatment by a single procedure.

COMPLICATIONS OF CHIN SURGERY

When chin surgery is well planned and executed and accomplished with competent assistance and adequate control of blood pressure during surgery, complications are relatively uncommon. The majority of problems are the result of inadequate planning.

Infection

Infection after either horizontal sliding osteotomy or augmentation genioplasty with Proplast is relatively uncommon. Antibiotics are routinely used at surgery and postoperatively until there is clinical evidence of healing of the mucosal wound margins. Just as there may be with any "degloving" exposure of the mandible, superficial dehiscence of the mucosal incisions with or without exposure of the underlying bone or implant may occur. When there is dehiscence of the wound margins or clinical evidence of infection postoperatively, the surgical wound is irrigated daily through the mucosal wound margins. An antibiotic mixture of polymixin, bacitracin, and neomycin may be used as an irrigating solution, although normal saline may be equally effective. The "flushing" action of the irrigant contributes to the effectiveness of this treatment, which is continued until there is spontaneous closure of the wound margins. Culture and sensitivity tests and antibiotic therapy based upon the results of these analyses are maintained for 1 to 2 weeks after there is no clinical infection and the wound margins are joined with granulation tissue and have re-epithelialized.

Infection of a pedicled mobilized bone segment is relatively rare — if suppuration should occur in the surgical wound, aggressive treatment with daily irrigations is started immediately and will usually control the infection with minimal loss of bone. In contrast, however, if and when a Proplast augmentation genioplasty becomes secondarily *infected,* the implant will more than likely be lost. Treatment with daily irrigations of the surgical wound and implant may be attempted for a short period; in most cases, however, the

*See technique described by R. V. Walker in Part B of Chapter 11, Mandibular Excess.

implant must be removed. Intraoral dehiscence and infection are minimized by atraumatic surgery, meticulous double-layer closure, good oral hygiene, and the use of pressure dressings.

Neurologic Problems

Paresthesia of the mental nerves occurs to some degree in almost all cases. Unless the patient is willing to accept the risk of paresthesia, and is warned about this possible complication before surgery, the surgery should not be done.

If no major branches of the mental nerves have been transected, paresthesias are only transient (usually a matter of weeks). Poor exposure, excessive retraction, and inadequate protection of the mental nerves at the time of horizontal osteotomy inferior and posterior to the mental foramina are the most common causes for such neurologic complications. The responsibility for assisting at such an operation should be delegated to an experienced surgeon who is continually vigilant and concerned about preserving the continuity of the mental nerves. Careful and meticulous surgical techniques will prevent unnecessary transection of the superficial branches of the mental nerves as the incision is carried through the lower lip mucosa.

Changes after Horizontal Sliding Osteotomy

McDonnel and associates[15] made a retrospective cephalometric analysis of osseous and soft-tissue changes associated with advancement of the chin by means of horizontal osteotomy of the mandibular symphysis in 15 adults. They consistently found an osseous remodeling pattern of resorption at pogonion and bony apposition at B-point and in the region of the inferior mandibular border where the horizontal osteotomy was completed. The major portion of the advanced segment, however, was maintained during the postoperative follow-up period. Studies to date indicate that the duration of postsurgical follow-up and extent of postsurgical horizontal resorption have little effect on the long-term prominence of the soft-tissue chin.[2, 15] The procedure has been proved stable for the patients studied over a follow-up period of 18.2 months[2] and 20 months.[15] Within a few months after surgery and for an additional 6 to 12 months, the edges of the advanced segment remodel and round off; the anterior projection of the segment, however, remains remarkably stable. The progress of one of the patients included in the original study by Bell and Dann has been followed for 9 years (Case 14–3). Treatment consisted of horizontal sliding osteotomy and wedge ostectomy to augment the chin contour and reduce facial height. Subsequent staged anterior and posterior maxillary osteotomies were used to close the open bite, reduce facial height, and improve the relationship of the upper lip line to the incisors. The pedicled sliding genioplasty in this case has been stable for 9 years as evidenced by sequential cephalometric tracings, which have shown minimal skeletal change.

Blood Loss

Horizontal osteotomy of the inferior border of the mandible, which should be routinely done in the operating room, must never be considered a benign procedure.

Significant blood loss with this operation may occur as a consequence of persistent oozing from detached muscles; transection of the submental, mylohyoid, or intramedullary vessels; or inadequate intraoperative control of the blood pressure. Local anesthesia with vasoconstrictor is infiltrated into the labiobuccal sulcus and floor of the mouth for hemostasis. Once the horizontal osteotomy is started, the bone is sectioned completely as soon as possible with oscillating and reciprocating saw blades. When hemorrhage is poorly controlled a full unit of blood may be lost in a relatively short time. When the systolic blood pressure is maintained below 100 mm of mercury by properly administered anesthesia, capillary oozing and bleeding are minimized. The anesthesiologist must be apprised of the surgeon's needs before anesthesia is started so that optimal operating conditions are present.

Soft-Tissue Changes

Excessive subperiosteal dissection of the inferior mental symphysis area to facilitate the removal of bone, suprahyoid myotomy, or surgical advancement of the mandible tends to produce unpredictable changes in the soft-tissue drape. Chin ptosis (witch's chin) manifest as a double-chin appearance may occur as a consequence. The possibility of this complication's arising after genioplasty is minimized by maintaining as large a soft-tissue attachment to the inferior and anterior aspects of the mental symphysis as is consistent with the objectives of surgery. If the soft tissue does not adapt to the surgical changes, submental lipectomy may be necessary to achieve an optimal drape of the integument.

Desirable shortening of the lip usually occurs when the vertical dimension of the chin is reduced by wedge ostectomy (pedicled). The soft-tissue drape shortens as the chin height is reduced to effect the desired esthetic change. This effect makes it difficult to raise the level of the lower lip by wedge reduction genioplasty. Undesirable shortening of the lower lip may also be produced by genioplasty. This is especially true with posterior and *inferior* repositioning of the chin by pedicled horizontal sliding osteotomy of the inferior border of the mandible. Such untoward changes can be obviated by careful preoperative simulation studies of the planned movements of the chin utilizing cephalometric prediction templates.

Bone Resorption below Alloplastic Implants

Bone resorption beneath alloplastic chin implants has been observed by numerous clinical investigators, whether the implant is placed above or below the periosteum. Indeed, it is a rare case in which no resorption is observed below the implant. Bone erosion below preformed Silastic implants has been a consistent postoperative finding. Superior displacement of the implant and penetration into the mandible has been observed frequently. When this type of migration occurs, the implant may penetrate the outer cortical bone and damage the roots of the incisor teeth; this kind of displacement may occur rather rapidly. In such cases the implant must be removed. If sufficient bone is still present in the mental symphysis, a horizontal sliding osteotomy, with or without an autogenous particulate marrow bone graft, may be used to augment the chin. In certain instances the bony resorption may be so severe as to preclude horizontal osteotomy of the mandibular symphysis. In these cases, free onlay bone grafts from the ilium may be the only recourse. For these reasons alloplastics should not be positioned over the roots of the incisor teeth.

It was initially hoped that Proplast would not migrate or displace into the bone. Because of its porous nature, Proplast is receptive to superficial ingrowth of tissue, which leads to an integration of the implant with the host. Postoperative migration of Proplast has not been observed when the material has been used to augment the chin. Variable amounts of bone resorption, however, have been observed beneath the majority of Proplast implants which have been placed entirely beneath the periosteum. To date, the amount of bone resorption has not necessitated removal of any of the implants, but these observations must be considered preliminary — in time, some of the Proplast implants may require removal as have preformed Silastic implants.

Patients who have had alloplastic genioplasties should be periodically monitored with cephalometric radiographs until the amount of bone erosion stabilizes. Proper case selection appears to be an important factor in preventing or minimizing the amount of resorption. If the soft tissues that overlie the implant are very tight (e.g., when lip incompetency is associated with an open-bite deformity), the pressure of the enveloping tissues may be the primary cause of the bone erosion. For this reason it is important to program treatment that will reduce lip incompetence and facial height. This can usually be best accomplished by maxillary surgery to reposition the maxilla superiorly and by pedicled wedge ostectomy of the chin. Progressive resorption may also be minimized by placement of the implant over the resistant cortical bone of the mental symphysis.

CASE REPORTS

CASE 14–1 (Fig. 14–19)

G. B., a 12-year-old girl, was evaluated for orthodontic treatment to correct her protruding teeth.

PROBLEM LIST

Facial Esthetics

Good facial contour and symmetry, with marked facial convexity related to a well-developed nose and moderately deficient chin.

Cephalometric Analysis

1. Moderate skeletal Class II malocclusion due to a combination of maxillary protrusion and mandibular deficiency.

Occlusal Analysis

1. Unilateral Class II malocclusion, with mandibular midline off to right.

TREATMENT PLAN

Orthodontic Treatment

Nonextraction orthodontic treatment utilizing unilateral headgear and unilateral Class II elastics; premolar extraction to be re-evaluated after 6 months.

ACTIVE TREATMENT

After 6 months, progress seemed good. After 15 months, good alignment and interdigitation of the teeth had been obtained, but examination of the cephalometric film and facial contours made it clear that this had occurred primarily through protrusion of the mandibular dentition. The lower incisor position was considered unstable and the facial esthetics were unsatisfactory, making further treatment mandatory.

At this stage, premolar extraction and further orthodontic treatment to retract the incisors was one possibility, but maxillary incisor retraction was undesirable, since if this were done, rhinoplasty would be needed because of the large nose. The alternative was augmentation genioplasty, which would provide a pleasing appearance and also would alter lip pressures against the lower incisors, possibly making them stable in their present position.

With the orthodontic appliance still in place but passive, a pedicled osteotomy on the lower border of the mandible was used to augment the chin. In addition, autologous freeze-dried bone (cadaver bank bone) was placed superior to the pedicled segment to improve contour of the labiomental fold. After waiting another 3 months to be sure the occlusion was stable, the orthodontist placed a maxillary removable retainer and a mandibular bonded canine-to-canine retainer. The esthetic result was quite pleasing.

COMMENT

There are no long-term data on the stability of lower incisors as related to augmentation genioplasty. At present, using genioplasty to improve incisor stability seems feasible on the basis of what is known about influences on tooth position. Esthetically, genioplasty produced a more pleasing result for this patient than the alternative, premolar extraction followed by rhinoplasty, would have.

Orthodontist: William R. Proffit, Chapel Hill, North Carolina. *Surgeon:* Ronald D. Baker, Chapel Hill, North Carolina.

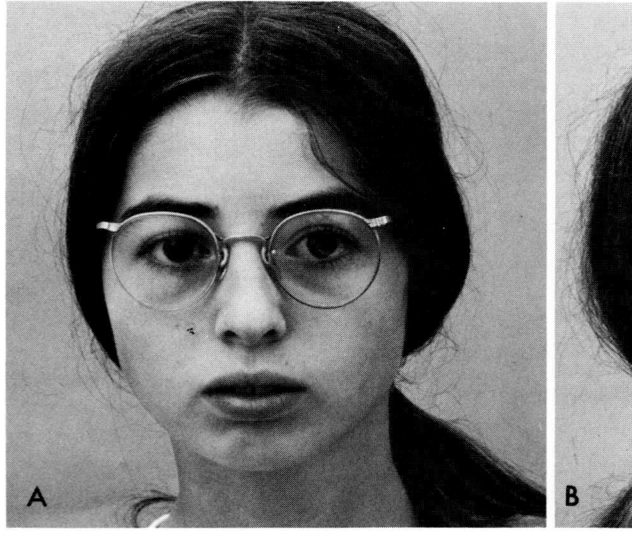

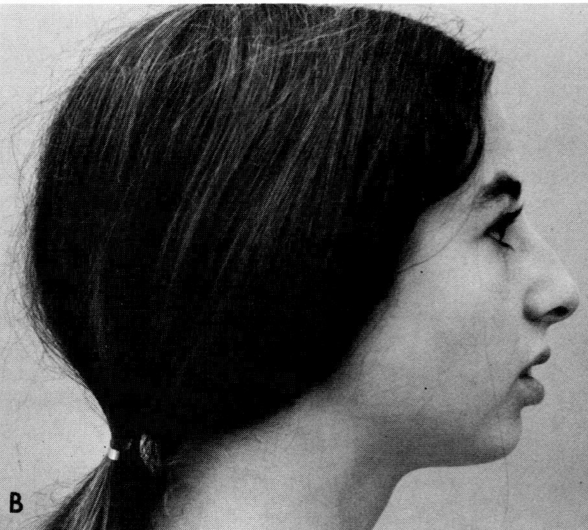

Figure 14–19 (Case 14–1). *A* and *B*, Pretreatment facial views.

Legend continued on the opposite page.

Figure 14–19 *Continued.* *C,* Pretreatment cephalometric tracing. *D–G,* Pretreatment intraoral views. *H–J,* Intraoral views after nonextraction orthodontic treatment.

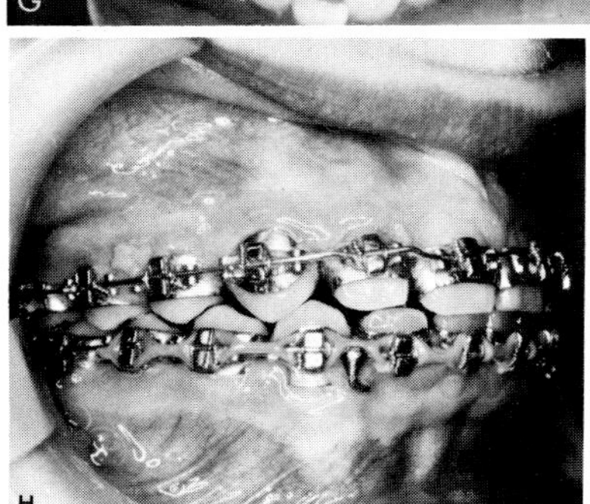
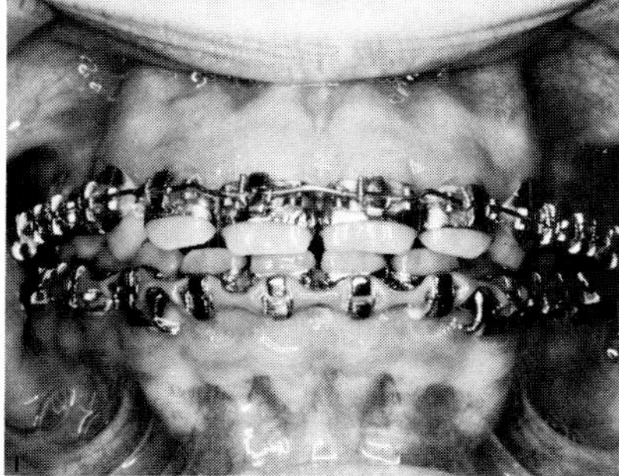
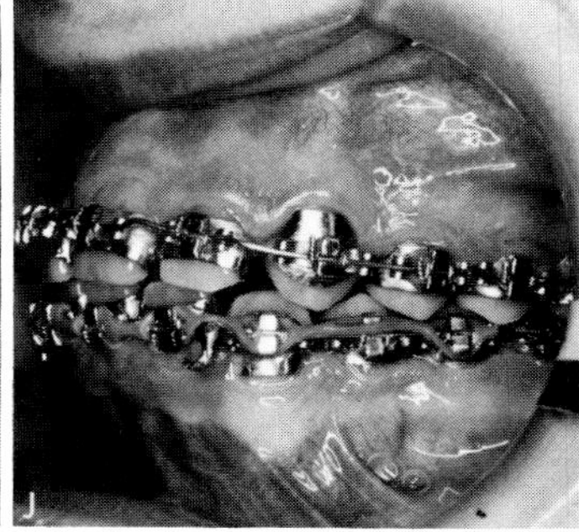

Illustration continued on the following page.

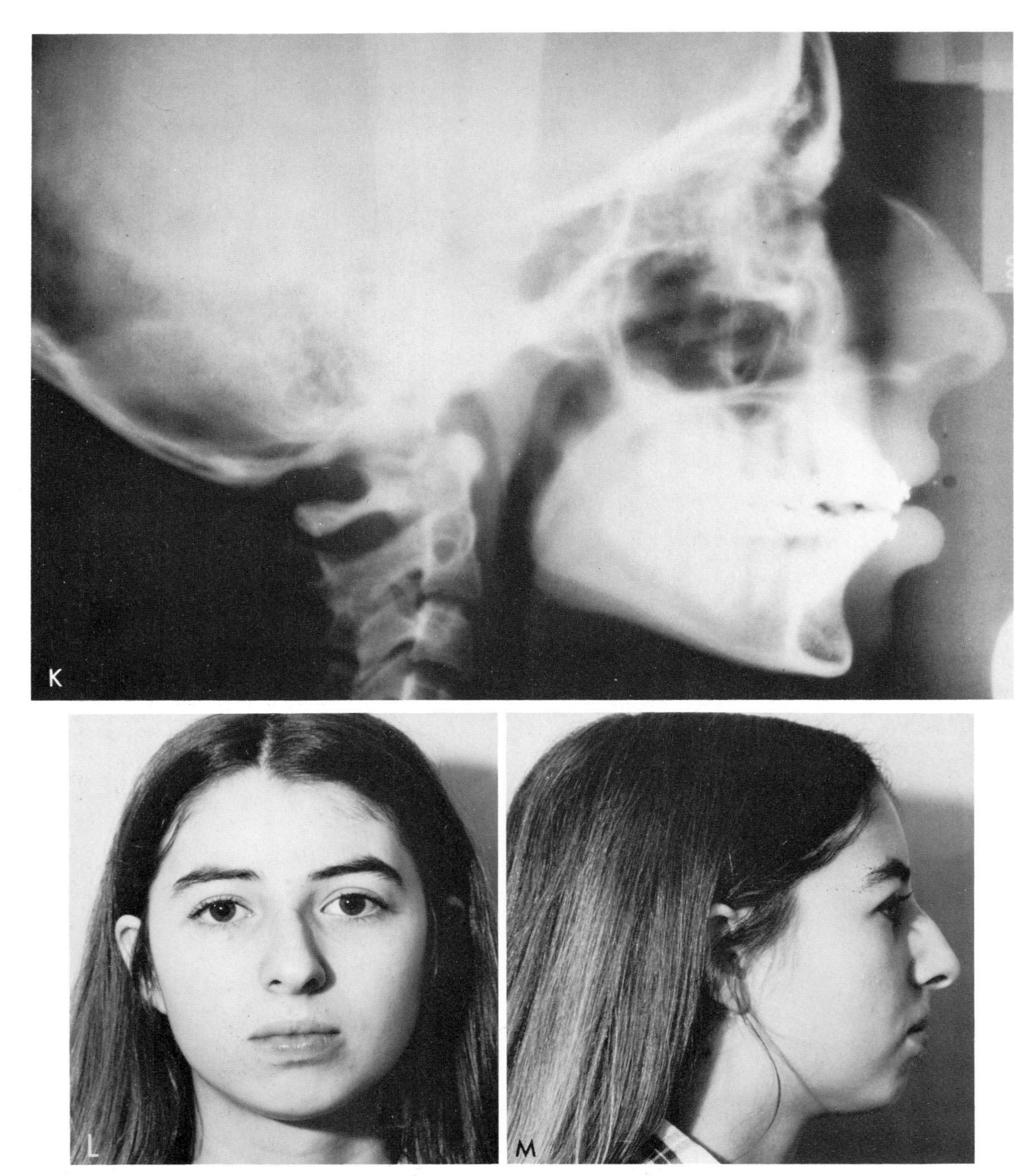

Figure 14–19 *Continued.* *K,* Cephalometric film after orthodontic alignment. *L* and *M,* Facial views after nonextraction orthodontic treatment.

Legend continued on the opposite page.

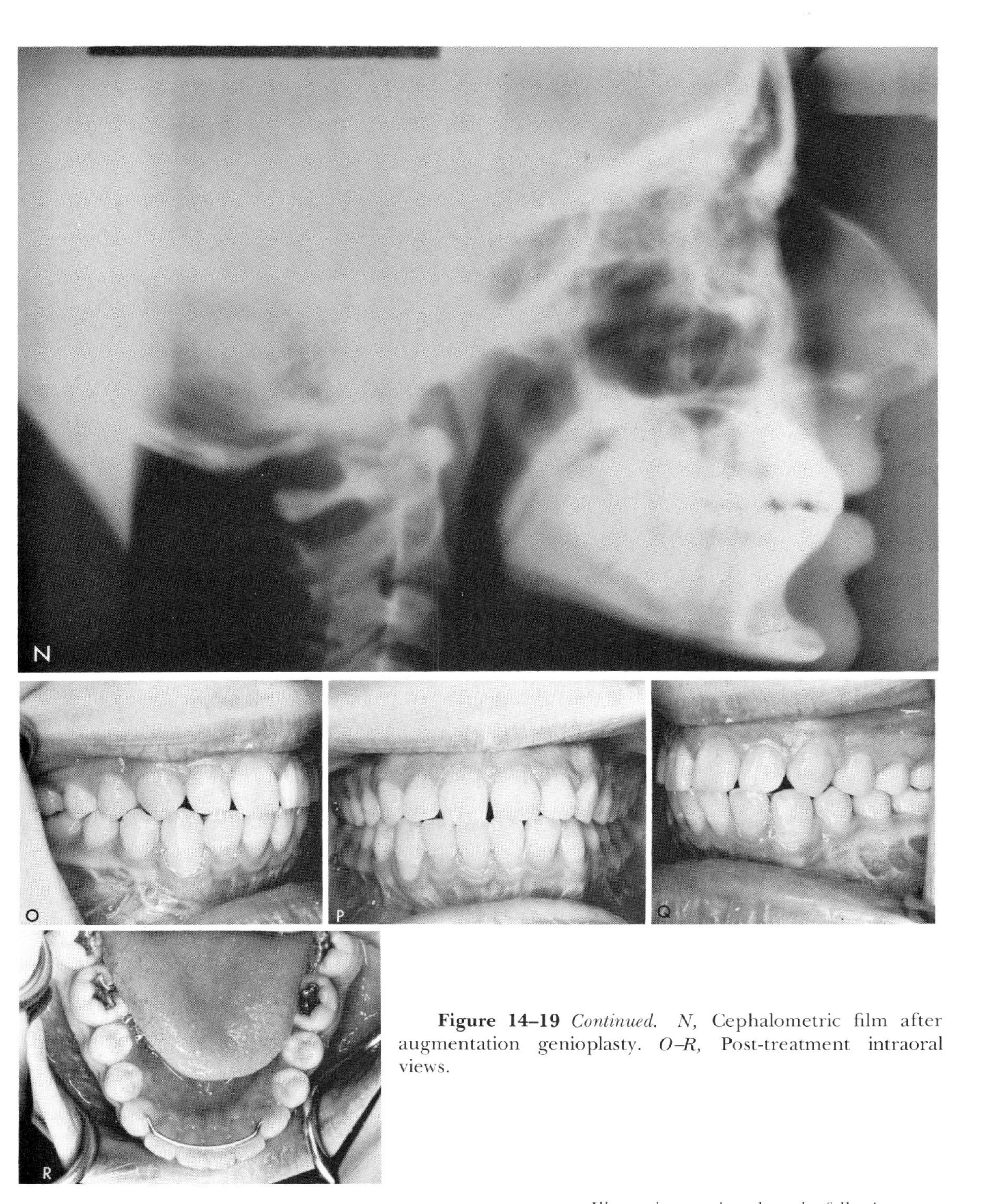

Figure 14–19 *Continued. N,* Cephalometric film after augmentation genioplasty. *O–R,* Post-treatment intraoral views.

Illustration continued on the following page.

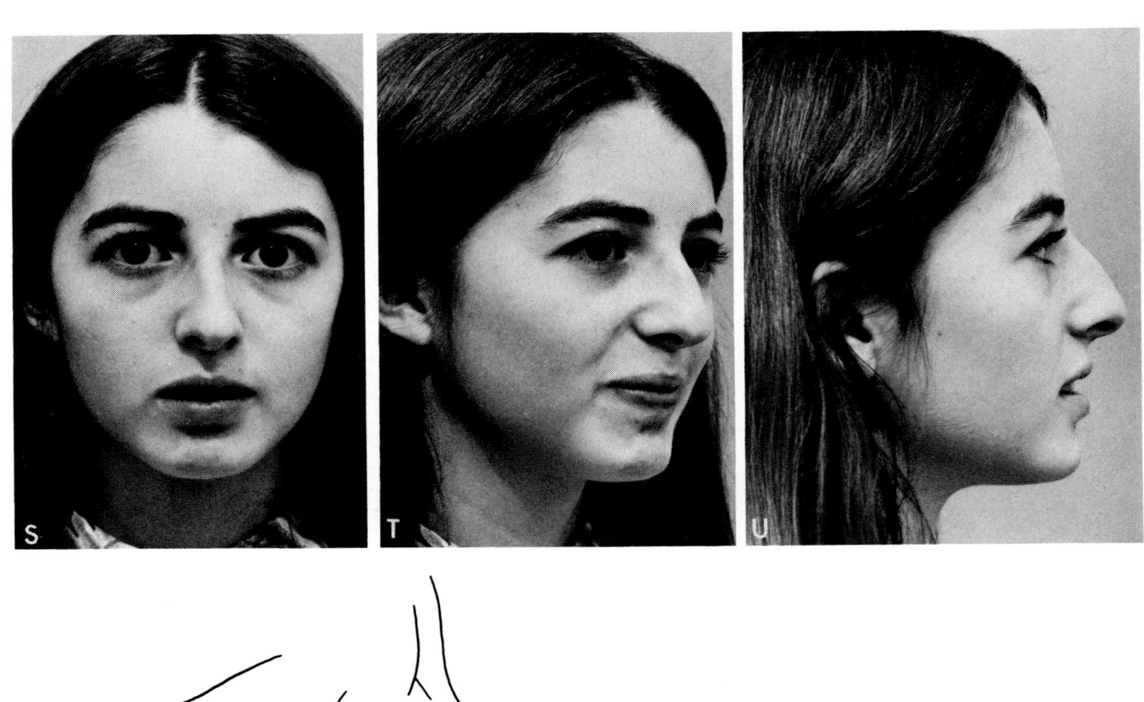

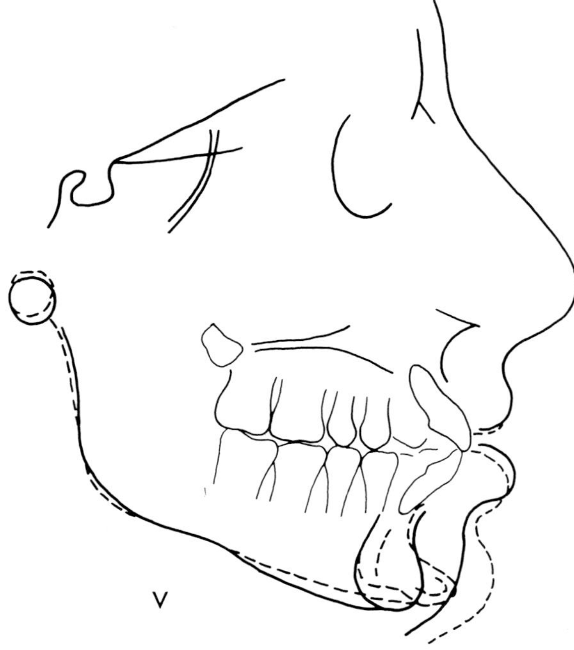

Figure 14–19 *Continued. S–U,* Facial views after genioplasty. *V,* Cephalometric superimposition before (*solid line*) and after (*broken line*) genioplasty.

CASE 14–2 (Fig. 14–20)

D. C., a 25-year-old man, desired correction of his anterior open bite and weak chin.

PROBLEM LIST

Esthetics

FRONTAL. Adequate smile line; overall facial symmetry; long face.

PROFILE. Marginal nasolabial angle; anteroposterior mandibular deficiency, anteroposterior chin deficiency, vertical chin excess.

Cephalometric Analyses

1. Moderately high mandibular plane angle: SnGoGn 41°.
2. Increased lower anterior facial height with 7 mm anterior open bite.
3. ANB 3°.

Occlusal Analysis

DENTAL ARCH FORM. *Maxillary arch:* Tapered and constricted; excessive curvature of occlusal plane. *Mandibular arch:* Ovoid with reverse curve of Spee.

DENTAL ALIGNMENT. Crowding of maxillary and mandibular anterior teeth.

DENTAL OCCLUSION. Class I molar and canine relationship with 7-mm anterior open bite; bilateral palatal crossbite.

TREATMENT PLAN

Surgical Treatment

1. Posterior maxillary osteotomies to:
   a. Close open bite.
   b. Correct bilateral crossbite.
   c. Level maxillary occlusal plane.
   d. Shorten facial height.
   e. Advance posterior maxillary dentoalveolar segments to close residual extraction space.
2. Genioplasty to:
   a. Increase chin prominence
   b. Decrease chin height.

Orthodontic Treatment

1. Extract mandibular second premolars.
2. Retract mandibular incisors to align the mandibular arch and achieve final interdigitation.
3. Extract maxillary first premolars.
4. Align maxillary arch.
5. Maintain anteroposterior and vertical position of the incisors.

FOLLOW-UP

The maxillary surgery technique shown in Fig. 14–20 was used to close the open bite and partially close the first premolar extraction spaces by superior and anterior movement of the posterior maxillary dentoalveolar segments. Genioplasty was done simultaneously.

Because of the satisfactory nose-lip-tooth balance, treatment was designed to close the open bite and shorten the facial height without altering the anteroposterior or vertical position of the maxillary anterior teeth. Initially, the patient declined orthodontic treatment. Ideally, premolar extractions and alignment of the anterior teeth would have preceded surgery. Despite the sequence of treatment, a serviceable occlusion was achieved. Cephalometric and occlusal studies 5 years after surgery (4 years and 6 months after band removal) showed virtually no positional change of the posterior segments and the repositioned inferior mental symphysis.

Surgeon: William H. Bell, Dallas, Texas. *Orthodontist:* Patrick Alessandra, Houston, Texas.

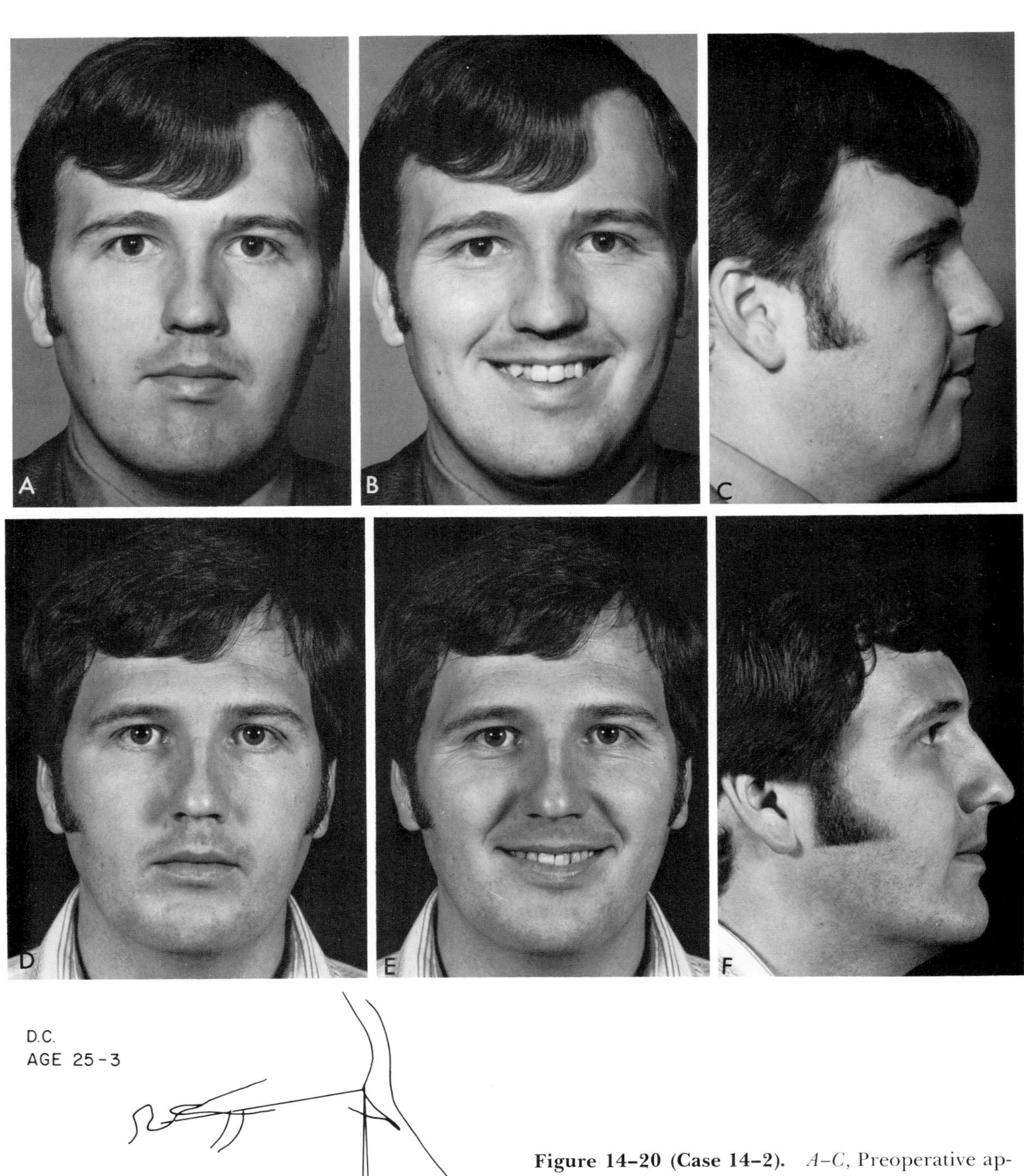

Figure 14–20 (Case 14–2). *A–C*, Preoperative appearance of 25-year-old man. *D–F*, Postoperative appearance after posterior maxillary osteotomy and genioplasty as illustrated in *J*. *G*, Cephalometric tracing (age 25 years, 3 months) before treatment.

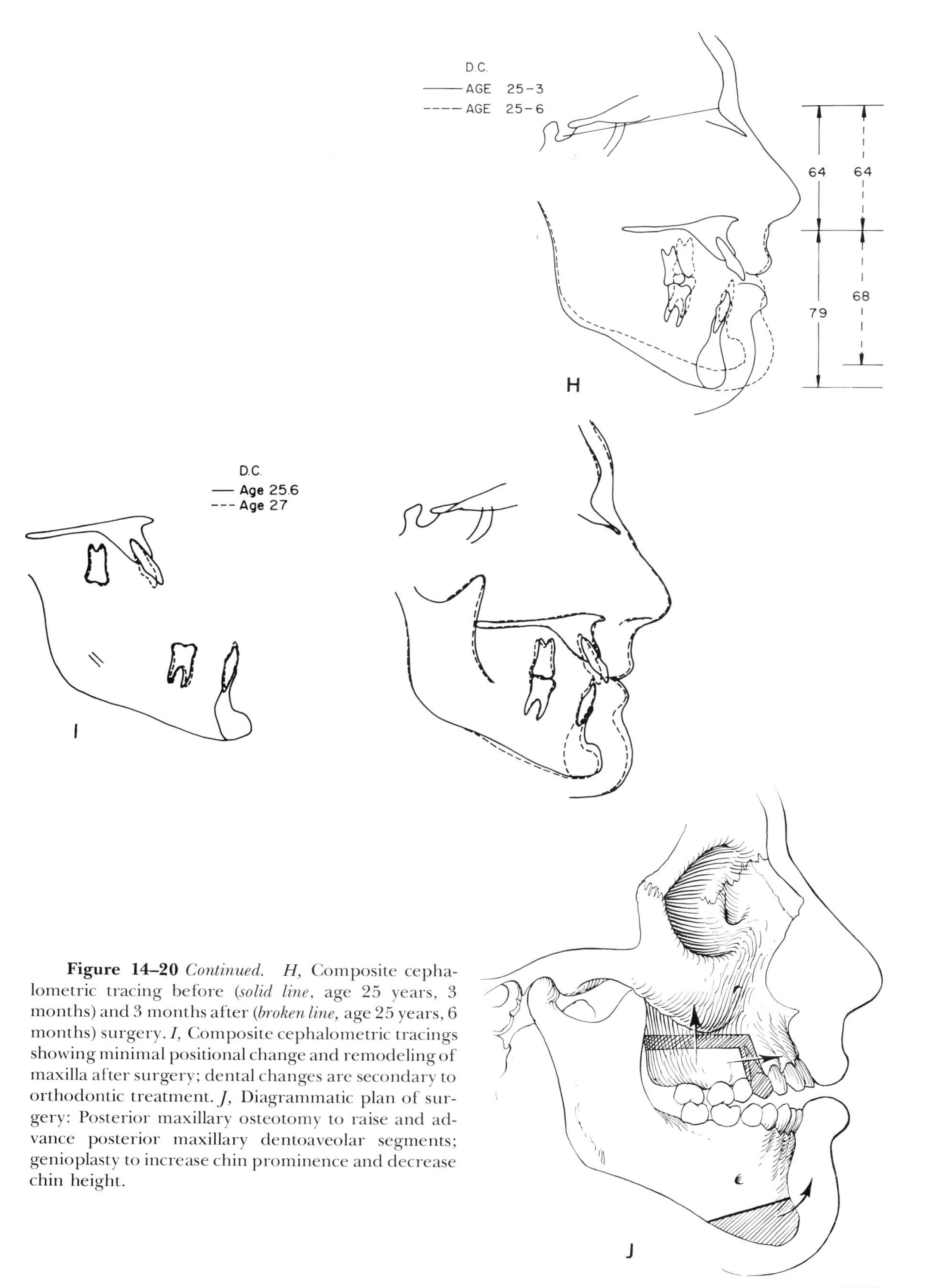

Figure 14–20 *Continued. H,* Composite cephalometric tracing before (*solid line,* age 25 years, 3 months) and 3 months after (*broken line,* age 25 years, 6 months) surgery. *I,* Composite cephalometric tracings showing minimal positional change and remodeling of maxilla after surgery; dental changes are secondary to orthodontic treatment. *J,* Diagrammatic plan of surgery: Posterior maxillary osteotomy to raise and advance posterior maxillary dentoaveolar segments; genioplasty to increase chin prominence and decrease chin height.

CASE 14–3 (Fig. 14–21)

This case illustrates correction of chin deformity manifest in the anteroposterior (deficiency) and vertical (excess) planes of space.

R. M., a 24-year-old man, desired treatment to improve the contour of his face and to correct his open bite.

PROBLEM LIST

Esthetics

1. Lip incompetence.
2. Excessive exposure of teeth and gingiva in repose and function.
3. Acute nasolabial angle.
4. Relative mandibular anteroposterior deficiency.
5. Anteroposterior chin deficiency, vertical chin excess.

Cephalometric Analysis

1. Severe skeletal Class II open bite.
2. GoGn to SN 62°; NB to Po 0 mm.

Occlusal Analysis

1. Symmetric Class II malocclusion with severe crowding of anterior teeth.

TREATMENT PLAN

Orthodontic Treatment

1. Full-banded edgewise orthodontic appliances with extractions in both arches to facilitate alignment of teeth.

Surgical Treatment

1. Anterior and posterior maxillary osteotomies to
   a. Close anterior open bite.
   b. Reduce lip incompetence.
2. Horizontal sliding osteotomy of inferior border of mandible to:
   a. Augment contour of chin.
3. Wedge ostectomy to:
   a. Reduce chin height.

ACTIVE TREATMENT

The anterior open bite and Class II malocclusion were treated within 14 months by surgery and orthodontics. The chin was reduced approximately 12 mm in height and advanced 9 mm by genioplasty. Gradual healing and progressive consolidation of the repositioned inferior segment were observed.

A 9-year postoperative follow-up revealed typical remodeling changes and excellent stability of the repositioned inferior segment. Minimal change in the occlusal relationship over this period suggested that augmentation genioplasty may have had a stabilizing effect on the lower incisiors. Facial balance has also been maintained.

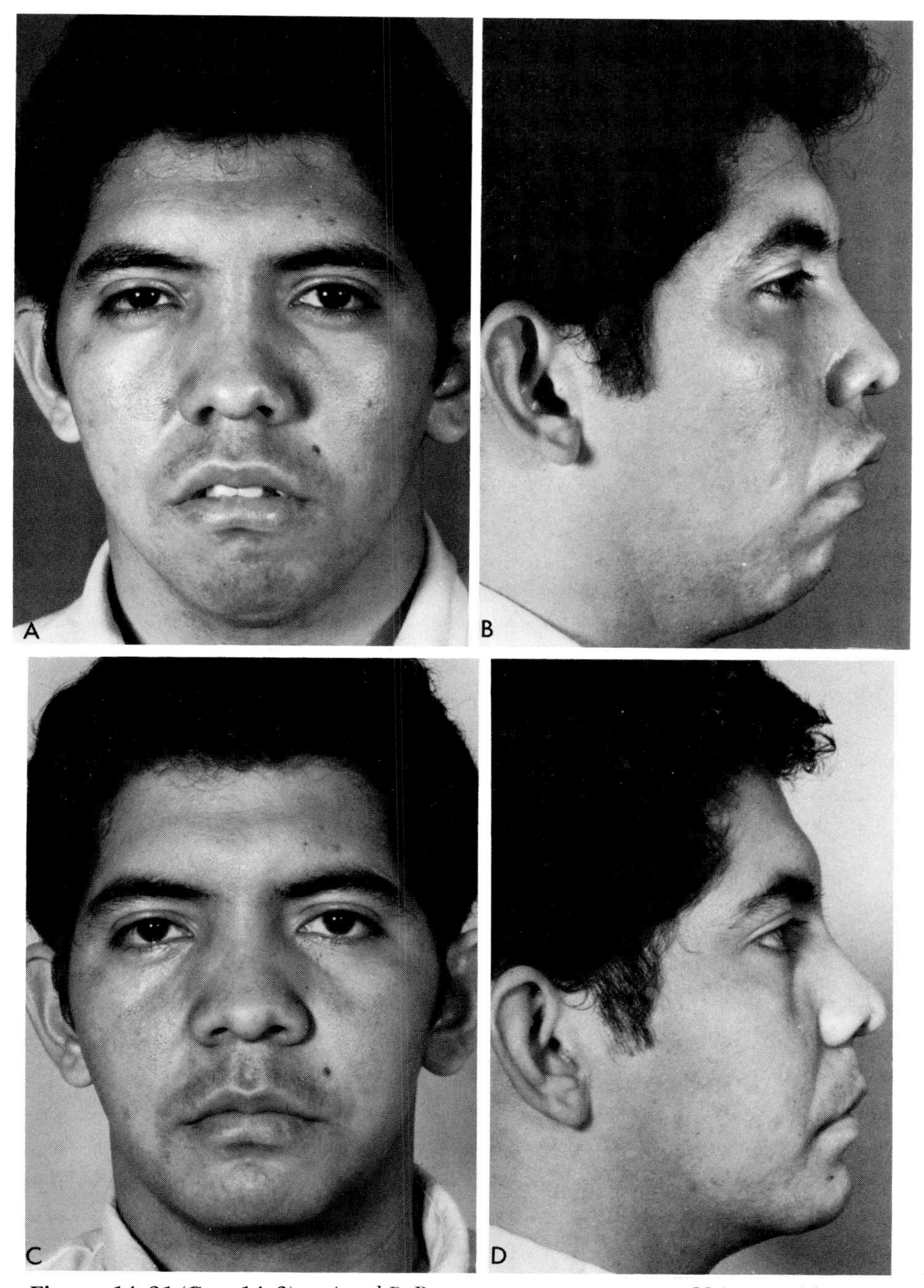

Figure 14–21 (Case 14–3). *A* and *B*, Pretreatment appearance of 24-year-old man. *C* and *D*, Facial appearance after treatment. *Illustration continued on the following page.*

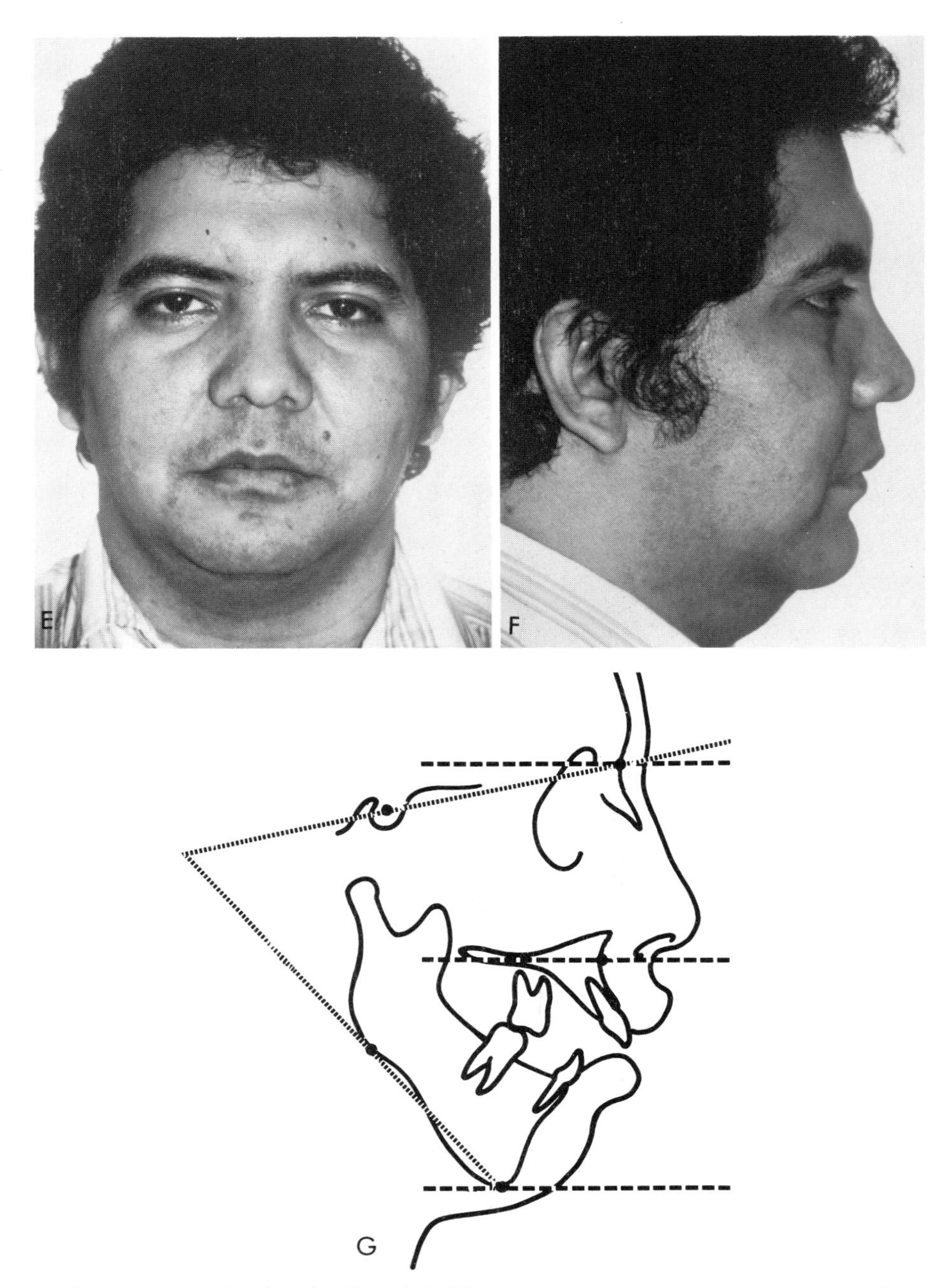

Figure 14–21 *Continued.* *E* and *F*, Nine-year post-treatment appearance. *G*, Cephalometric tracing before treatment.

Legend continued on the opposite page.

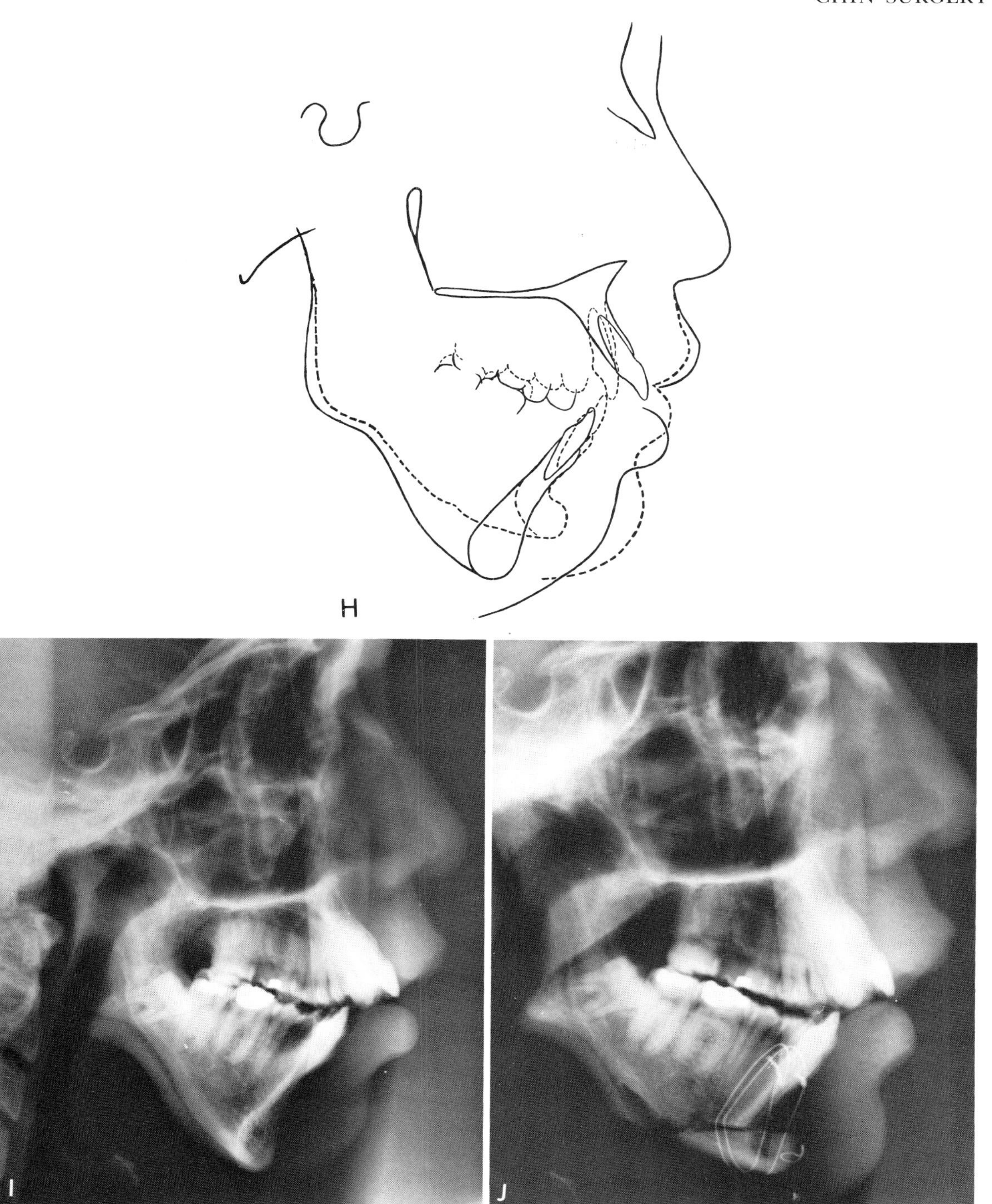

Figure 14–21 *Continued.* *H,* Composite cephalometric tracings before (solid line) and two years after *(broken line)* treatment, showing 14-mm reduction of anterior facial height, restoration of chin contour, closure of open bite, improved lip posture and lip seal, and leveled maxillary occlusal plane. *I–K,* Sequential radiographs showing remodeling and consolidation of repositioned chin and stability over postoperative period of follow-up. *I,* Preoperative radiograph. *J,* Radiograph after genioplasty; chin height reduced 12 mm and mental symphysis segment transposed anteriorly 9 mm.

Illustration continued on the following page.

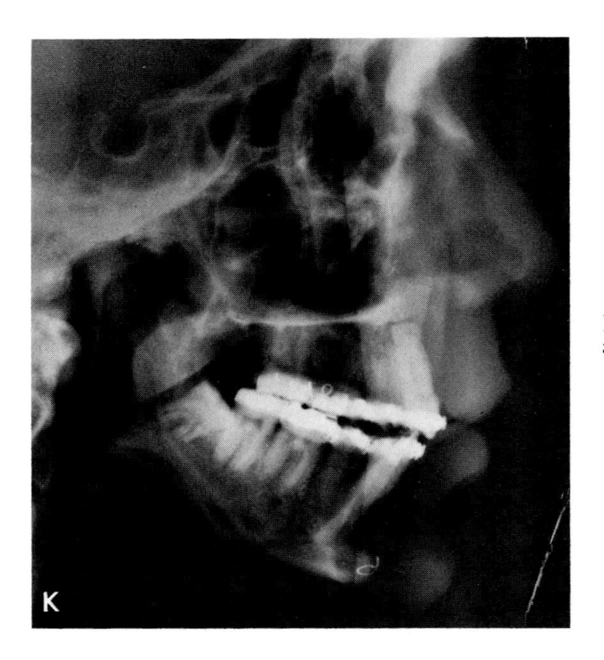

Figure 14–21 *Continued.* *K*, Consolidation of repositioned inferior mental symphsis segment 1 year after genioplasty.

COMMENT

Long-term occlusal and skeletal stability was maintained by the overall approach to treatment of this individual's dentofacial deformity. Closure of the anterior open bite, reduction of facial height and lip incompetence by maxillary surgery, and genioplasty to reduce facial and chin height additionally achieved overall balance between the skeletal structures and their enveloping musculature. Treatment planning concerned with the individual's entire dentofacial deformity ana not just the chin deformity achieved a state of functional homeostasis and as such maintained occlusal and skeletal stability.

Surgeon: William H. Bell, Dallas, Texas. *Orthodontist:* Thomas Creekmore, Houston, Texas.

CASE 14–4 (Fig. 14–22)

This case illustrates correction of anteroposterior chin deficiency by means of a horizontal sliding osteotomy combined with implantation of Proplast.

A. C., a 28-year-old man, requested surgery to improve the appearance of his chin.

PROBLEM LIST

Esthetics

Good midfacial contour; good balance between nose and upper and lower lips; chin anteroposteriorly contour-deficient.

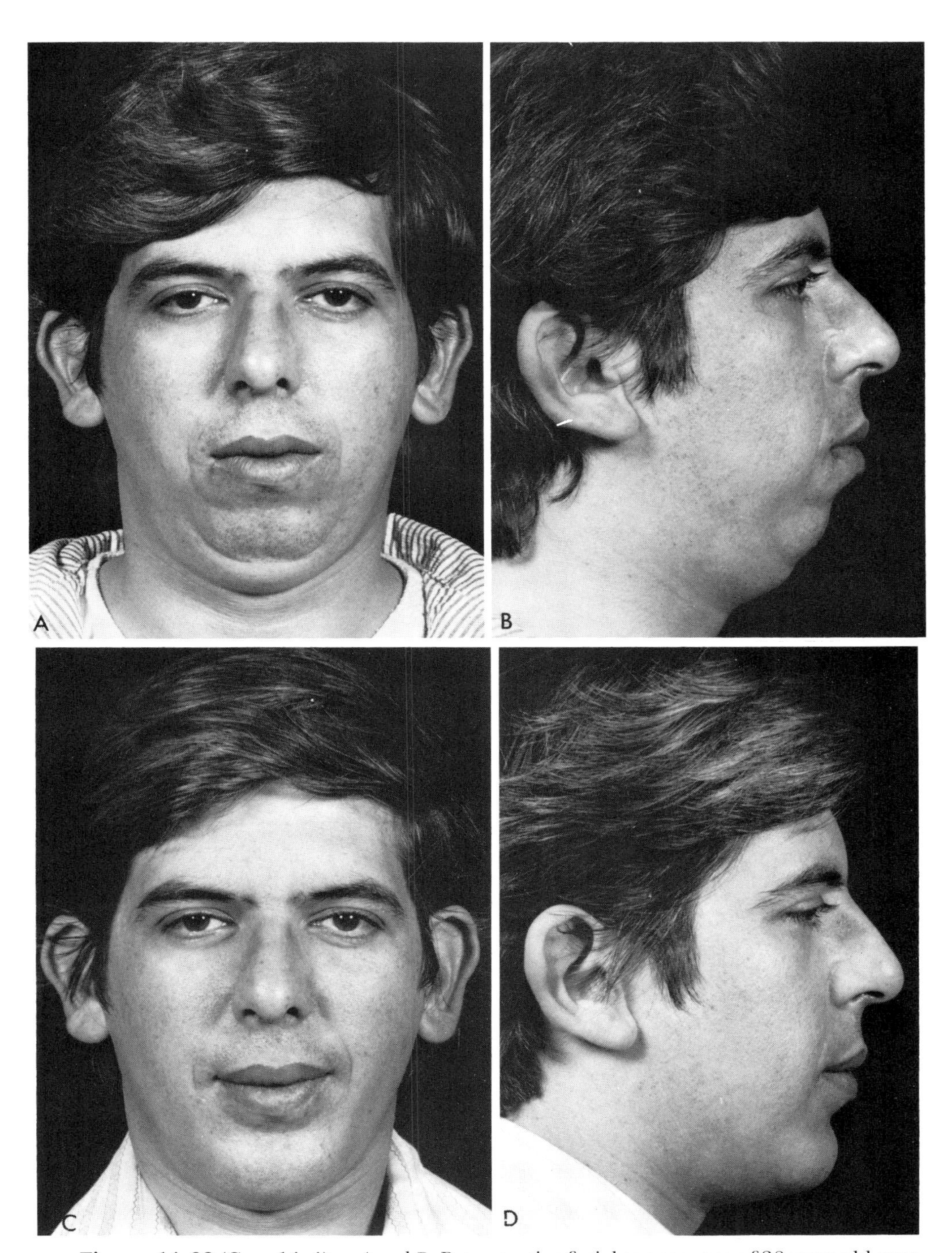

Figure 14–22 (Case 14–4). *A* and *B*, Preoperative facial appearance of 28-year-old man with deficient chin projection. *C* and *D*, Appearance 2 years after horizontal sliding augmentation genioplasty with Proplast onlayed to the anterior aspect of the advanced segment.

Cephalometric Analysis

1. Mandibular deficiency (SNA 85°; SNB 77°; ANB 8°; NB to Po 0 mm.
2. High mandibular plane angle (SNGoGn 42°).

Occlusal Analysis

Bilateral Class I cuspid and molar relationship.

TREATMENT PLAN

Surgical Treatment

1. Augmentation genioplasty with combined horizontal sliding osteotomy and insertion of proplast.

ACTIVE TREATMENT

The pedicled bony symphysis was advanced 15 mm by means of a horizontal sliding osteotomy 16 mm above the inferior border of the mandible. To achieve maximal augmentation, the segment was advanced to lie outside the labial cortex of the superior segment. A 5-mm-thick piece of Proplast was wired to the anterior aspect of the advanced segment. Thus, the combined hard-tissue advancement totaled 20 mm.

During the first few postoperative weeks, the anterior end of the bony segment rotated inferiorly as a result of inadequate stabilization and the position of the segment lateral to the labial cortex. This rotation resulted in a 5-mm increase in chin height. Fortunately, this did not detract from the final esthetic result. Two years postoperatively, a total soft-tissue advancement of 14 mm was maintained.

Surgeons: Larry Snider, Denver, Colorado; Kevin McBride, Dallas, Texas.

CASE 14–5 (Fig. 14–23)

This case illustrates correction of vertical excess and anteroposterior chin deficiency by wedge ostectomy of the mandibular symphysis and advancement genioplasty.

J. M., a 24-year-old man, requested treatment for his anterior open bite and excessive gingival exposure during smiling.

PROBLEM LIST

Esthetics

1. Lip incompetence at rest (10 mm).
2. Excessive mentalis muscle function.

3. Long lower-third facial height (middle third, 75 mm; lower third, 90 mm).
4. Excessive chin height, anteroposterior chin deficiency, and chin asymmetry.

Cephalometric Analysis

1. High mandibular plane angle (SnGoGn 44°).

Occlusal Analysis

1. Class I cuspid and molar on right; Class III cuspid and molar on left.
2. End-to-end occlusion around entire arch.
3. Anterior open bite (1 mm).

TREATMENT PLAN

Surgical Treatment

1. Le Fort I ostectomy in five pieces with superior repositioning and expansion to:
   a. Shorten the lower third of the face.
   b. Correct the end-to-end bite:
2. Horizontal wedge ostectomy of mandibular symphysis to:
   a. Shorten (5 mm).
   b. Advance chin (7 mm).
3. Lateral augmentation of chin with proplast to correct asymmetry.

ACTIVE TREATMENT

Good alignment of the teeth in bilateral Class I cuspid and molar occlusion and 7 mm reduction of lower facial height with elimination of lip incompetence was achieved by means of maxillary surgery. Advancement and vertical reduction of chin height established balance between middle-third and lower-third facial structures. Proplast (30 mm × 4 mm × 6 mm) was inserted above the advanced chin segment to decrease the depth of the labiomental fold. Proplast (20 mm × 4 mm × 3 mm) was adapted to the left inferoanterior aspect of the chin to correct the mild asymmetry.

COMMENT

A 6-mm vertical bony chin reduction resulted in a 3-mm soft-tissue reduction after 8 months. Thickening of the soft tissue below the bony chin resulted in a bone to soft tissue change of 1:0.5. The insertion of Proplast to correct the asymmetry at the left inferoanterior aspect of the mobilized segment necessitated greater soft-tissue detachment than usual. This was a possible explanation for the poor hard-tissue to soft-tissue change.

Surgeons: Paul Vedtoffee, Copenhagen, Denmark; Kevin McBride, Dallas, Texas.

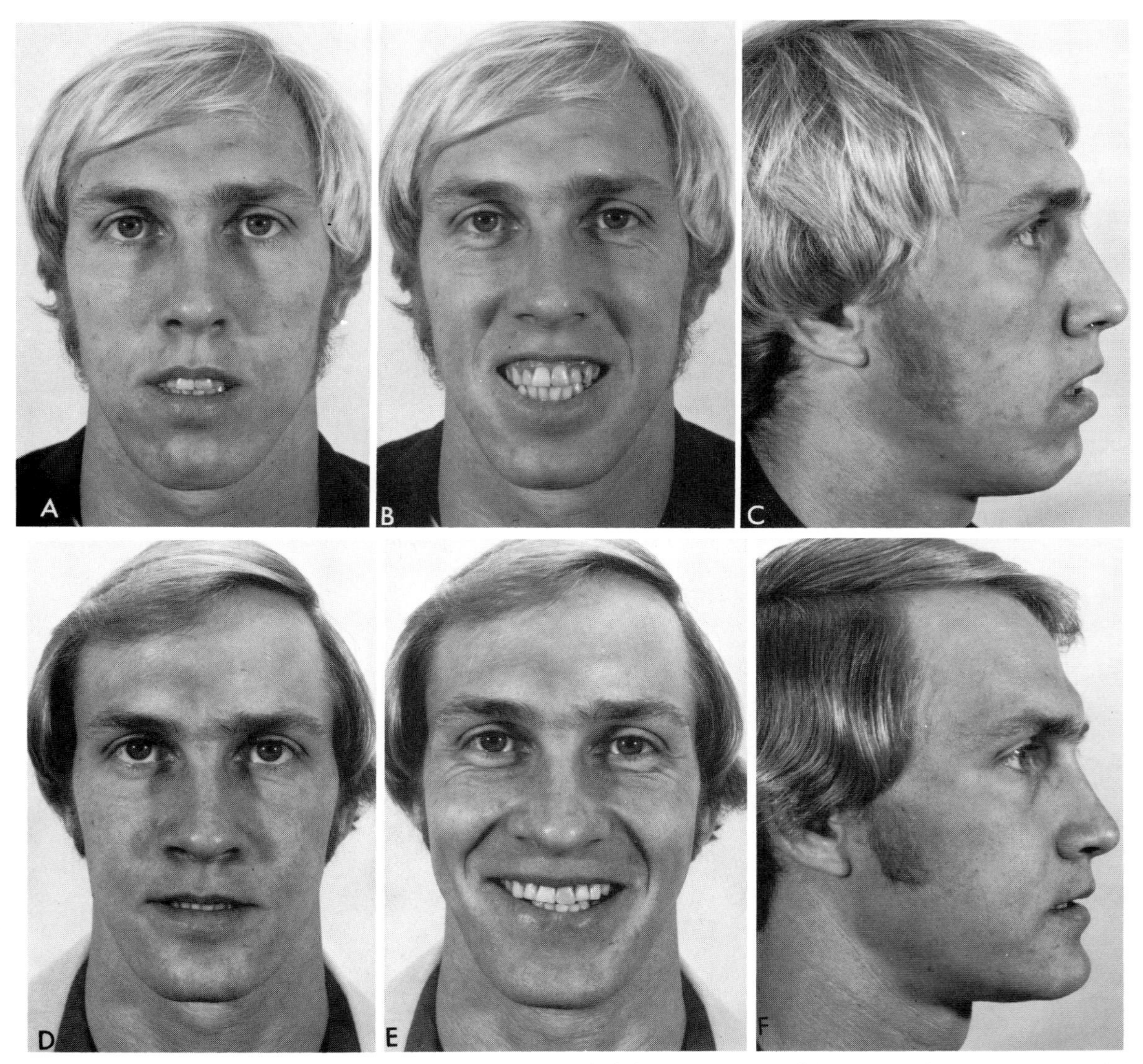

Figure 14–23 (Case 14–5). *A–C,* Preoperative facial appearance of 24-year-old man. *D–F,* Facial appearance 8 months after Le Fort I osteotomy to reposition the maxilla superiorly and genioplasty to reduce the vertical dimension of the chin and to increase the prominence of the chin. A small piece of Proplast was added to the left inferior border of the chin to correct the vertical asymmetry.

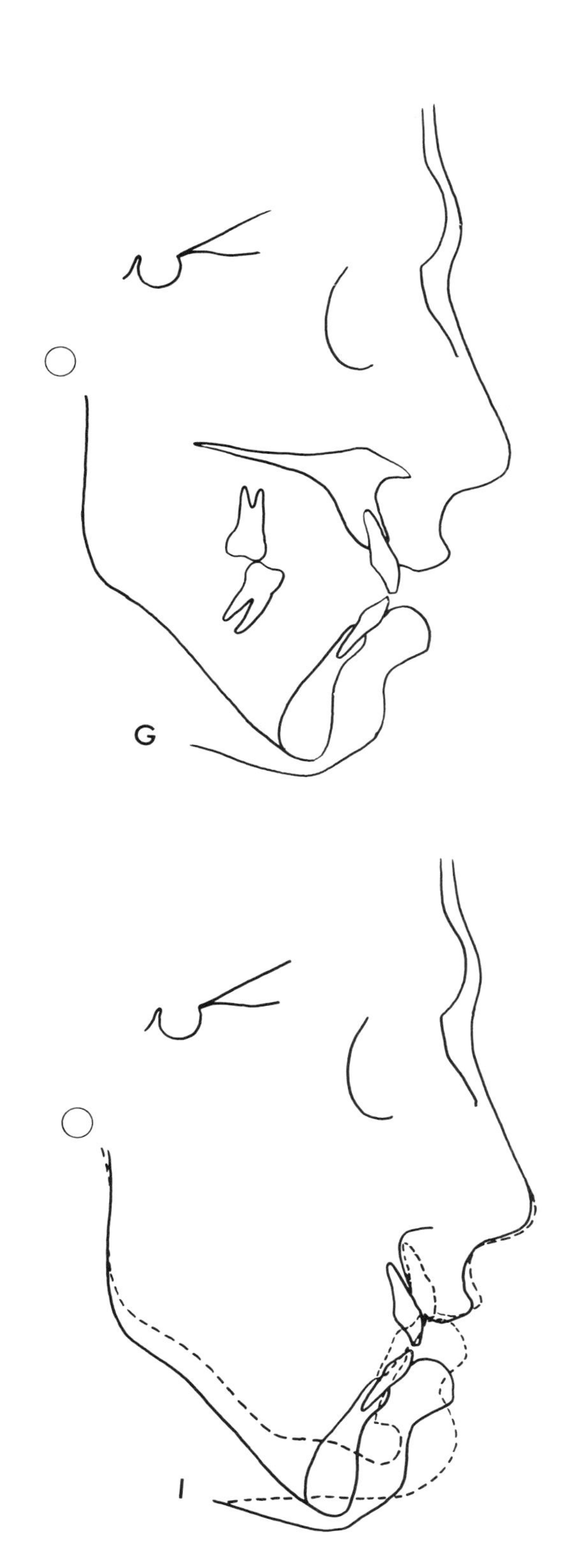

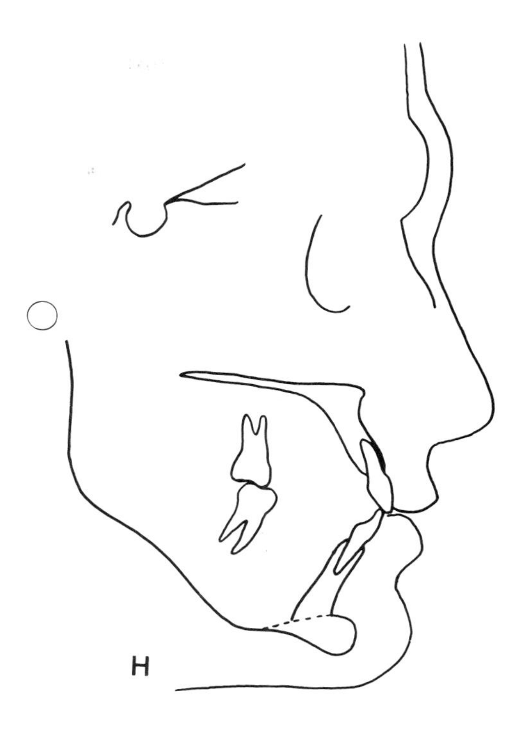

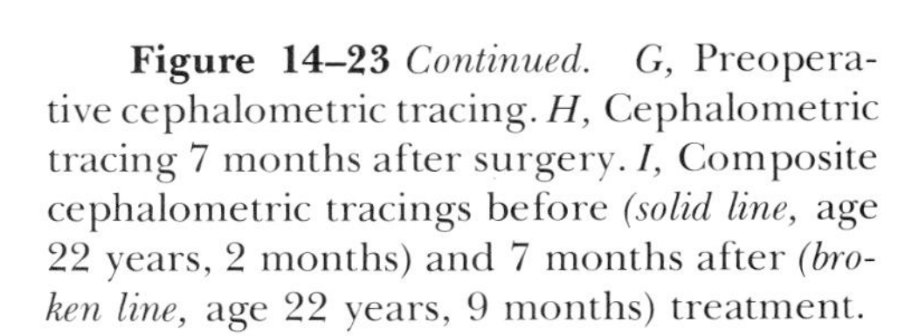

Figure 14–23 *Continued.* *G,* Preoperative cephalometric tracing. *H,* Cephalometric tracing 7 months after surgery. *I,* Composite cephalometric tracings before *(solid line,* age 22 years, 2 months) and 7 months after *(broken line,* age 22 years, 9 months) treatment.

CASE 14–6 (Fig. 14–24)

This case illustrates correction of chin prominence by reverse horizontal sliding osteotomy.

K. W., a 16-year-old girl, was evaluated for treatment to correct her malaligned teeth and prominent chin.

PROBLEM LIST

Esthetics

1. Good midfacial contour and symmetry.
2. Prominent chin in the anteroposterior plane of space.

Cephalometric Analysis

1. Class I malocclusion associated with prominent chin in anteroposterior plane of space.
2. SN to mandibular plane angle 25° $\underline{1}$ to NA 5 mm; $\overline{1}$ to NB 3 mm; NB to Po 8 mm.

Occlusal Analysis

1. Class I malocclusion with moderate crowding and malalignment of maxillary and mandibular teeth.

TREATMENT PLAN

Orthodontic Treatment

1. Nonextraction orthodontic treatment with edgewise orthodontic appliances.

Surgical Treatment

1. Horizontal sliding osteotomy of inferior border of mandible with posterior repositioning of segment to reduce chin prominence.

ACTIVE TREATMENT

Good alignment and interdigitation of the teeth was accomplished within 12 months by orthodontic treatment. A 6-mm reduction of chin prominence was achieved by a pedicled horizontal sliding osteotomy of the inferior border of the mandible. The amount of chin reduction was consistent with the preoperative plan (hard-tissue chin retracted 6 mm; soft-tissue chin retracted 3.5 mm). Over a postoperative follow-up period of approximately 24 months there has been no discernible change in the patient's profile.

Surgeon: William H. Bell, Dallas, Texas. *Orthodontist:* William Wyatt, Hurst, Texas.

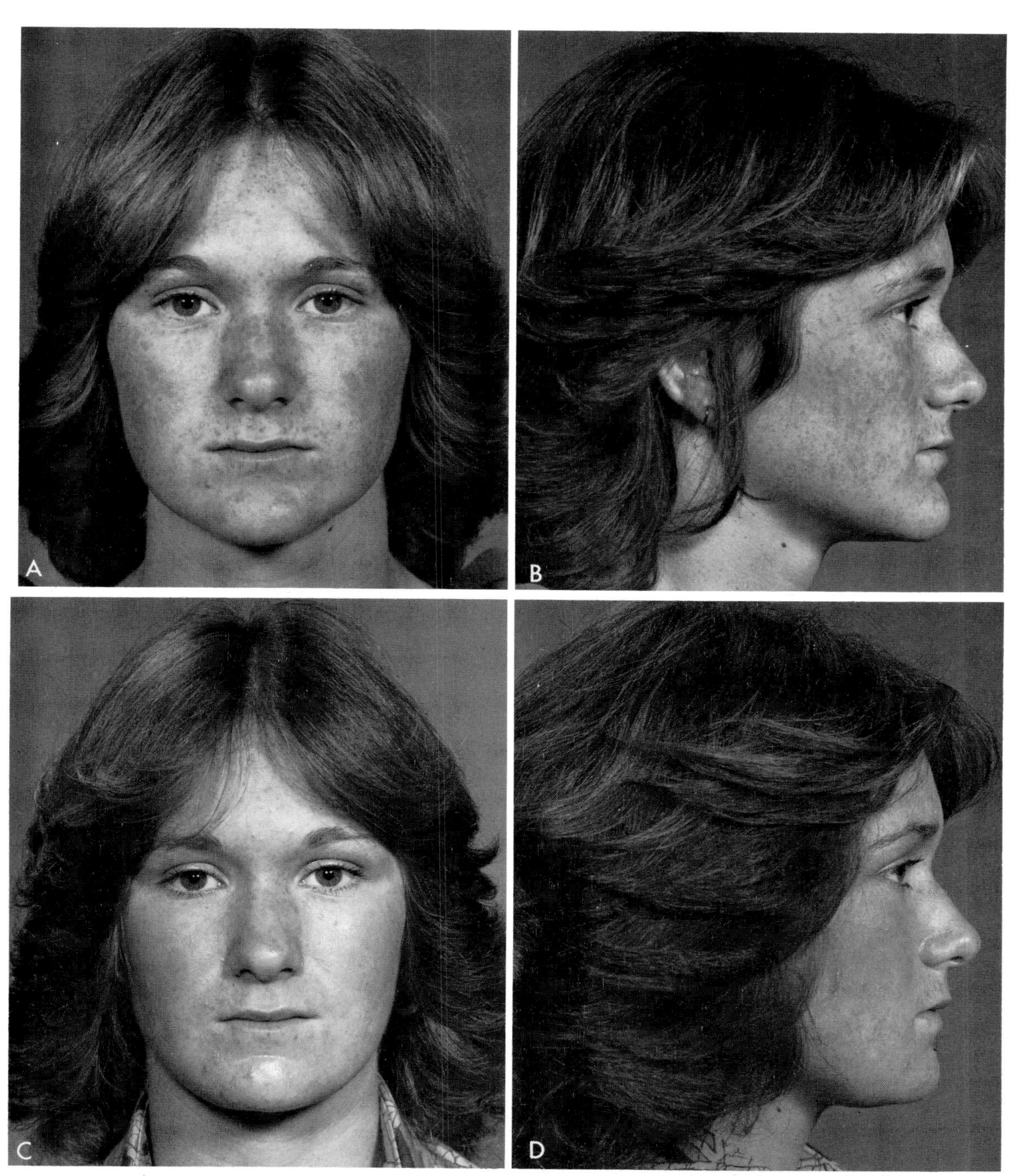

Figure 14–24 (Case 14–6). *A* and *B*, Preoperative appearance of 16-year-old girl. *C* and *D*, Postoperative appearance after reducing chin prominence by reduction genioplasty (horizontal sliding osteotomy).

Illustration continued on the following page.

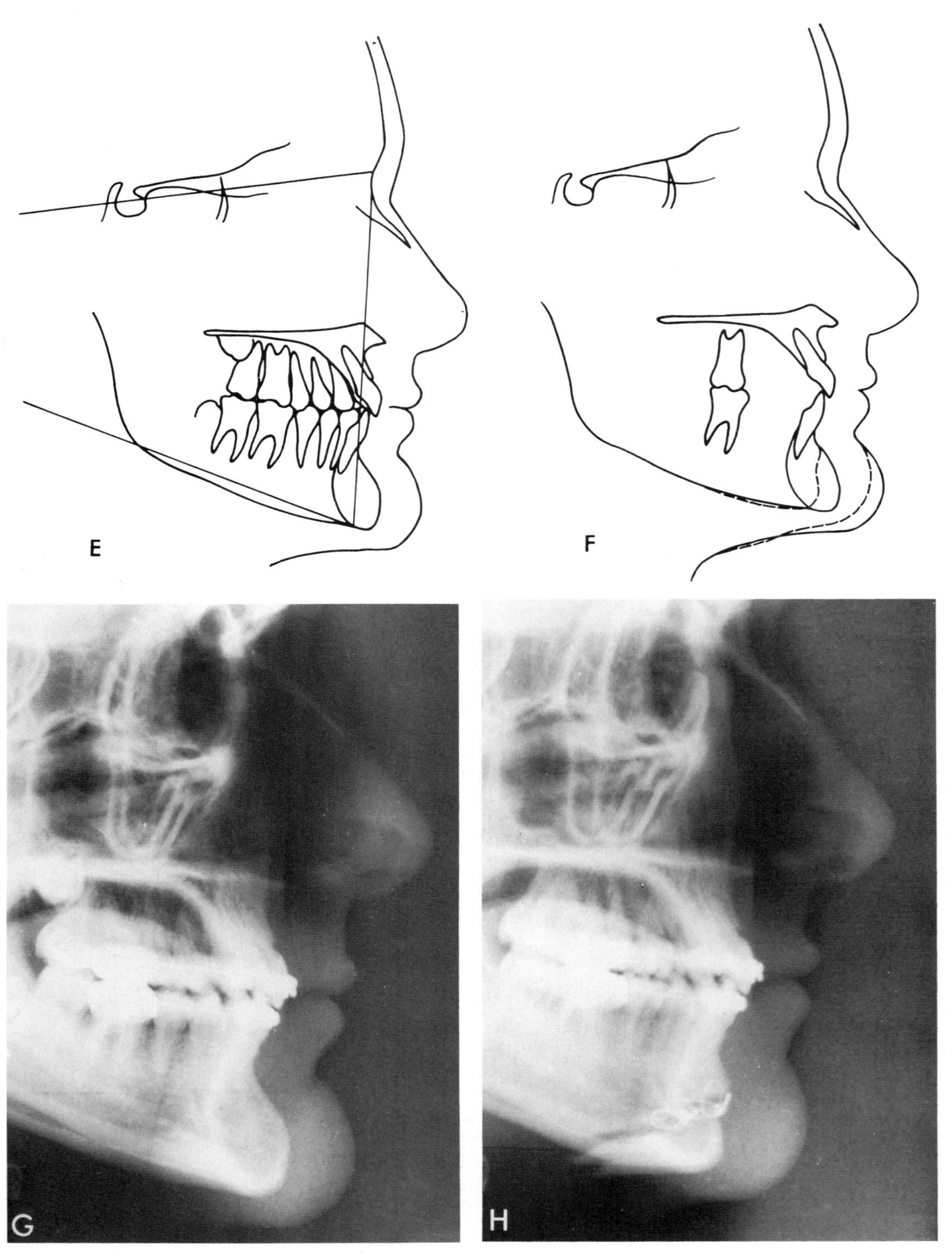

Figure 14–24 *Continued.* *E,* Cephalometric tracing before surgery (age 15 years, 10 months). *F,* Composite cephalometric tracings before *(solid line,* age 15 years) and after *(broken line,* age 16 years 1 month) surgery. *G,* Lateral head radiograph before surgery. *H,* Lateral head radiograph 2 months after surgery.

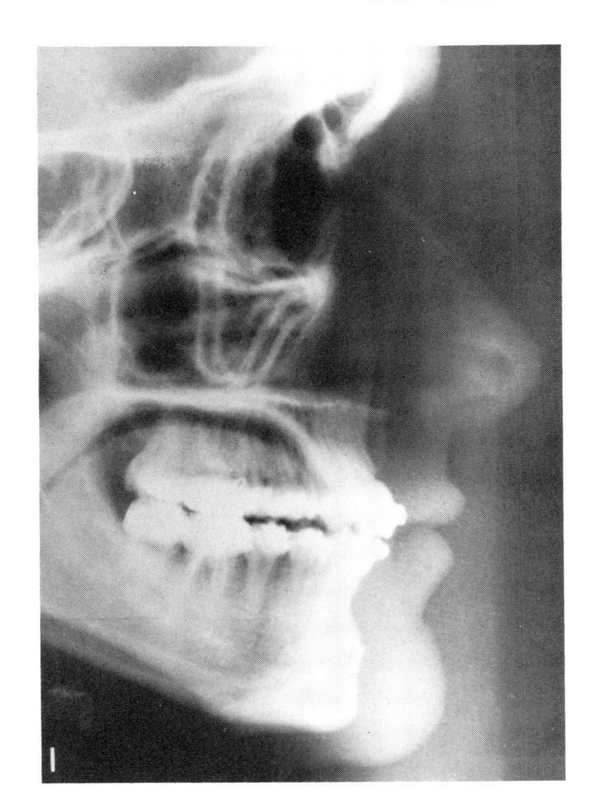

Figure 14–24 *Continued.* *I*, Lateral head radiograph 18 months after surgery.

CASE 14–7 (Fig. 14–25)

K. J., a 26-year-old woman, was evaluated for correction of her prominent chin.

PROBLEM LIST

Esthetics

1. Good overall facial symmetry.
2. Esthetic balance between the nose and upper lip. Everted lower lip and deep labiomental fold.

Cephalometric Analysis

1. Moderate skeletal deep bite pattern — low mandibular plane (NB to Po 6 mm).
2. Hard-tissue chin thickness 16 mm; soft-tissue chin thickness 12 mm.

Occlusal Analysis

1. Class II, division 1 malocclusion.

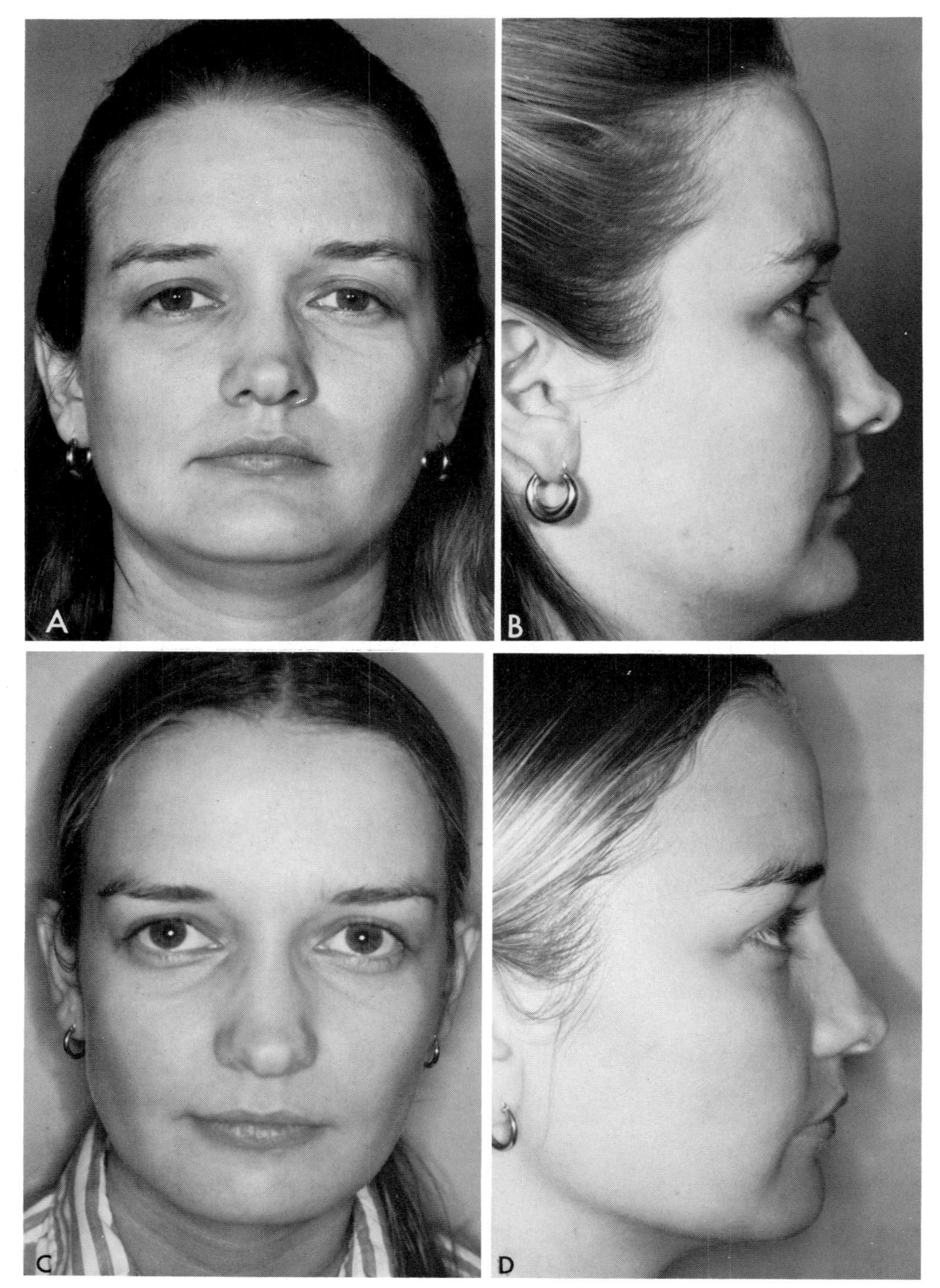

Figure 14–25 (Case 14–7). *A* and *B*, Preoperative appearance of 27-year-old woman. *C* and *D*, Postoperative appearance.

ACTIVE TREATMENT

An 8-mm reduction in the anteroposterior dimension of the chin was accomplished by mentoplasty done under local anesthesia with the patient in a sitting position. A number of subtle changes in the soft-tissue drape softened the soft-tissue

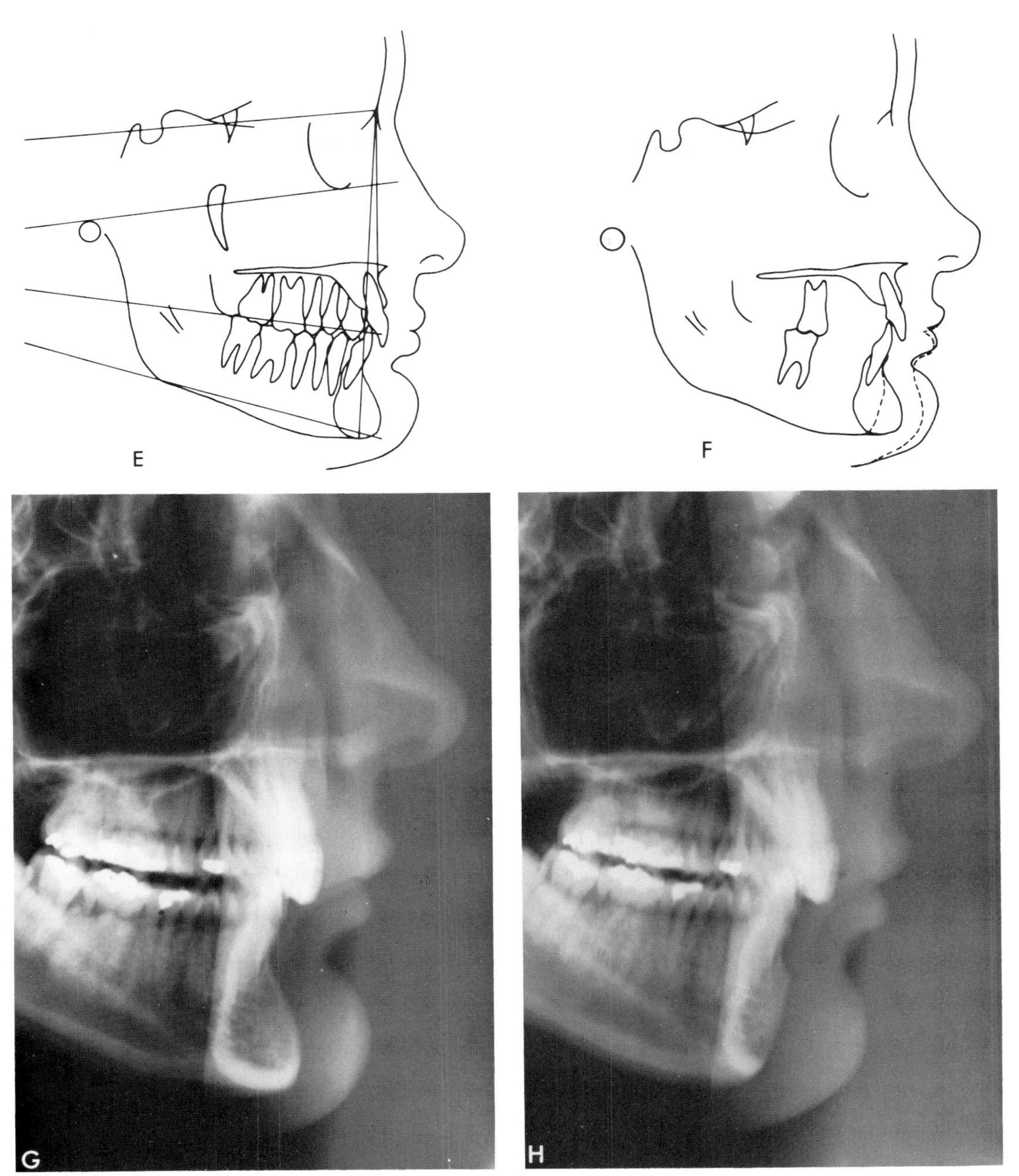

Figure 14–25 *Continued.* *E,* Cephalometric tracing before mentoplasty. *F,* Composite cephalometric tracings before *(solid line,* age 26 years, 2 months) and 18 months after *(broken line,* age 27 years, 8 months) surgery. *G,* Lateral cephalograms before surgery (age 26 years, 2 months). *H,* Lateral cephalogram 18 months after surgery (age 27 years, 8 months).

profile and provided good balance between the chin, lips, and nose. A 4-mm reduction of the soft-tissue chin prominence was associated with flattening of the labiomental fold produced by a 2-mm anterior movement of the skin overlying the labiomental fold.

Surgeon: William H. Bell, Dallas, Texas.

CASE 14–8 (Fig. 14–26)

This case illustrates correction of chin asymmetry by lateral sliding osteotomy of chin and ramus osteotomy.

K. K., a 31-year-old man, requested treatment for his prominent asymmetric mandible and his malocclusion.

PROBLEM LIST

Esthetics

1. Good midfacial contour.
2. Prominent lower lip and chin.
3. Mandible deviated to right.
4. Oral commissure lower on left.

Cephalometric Analysis

1. Mandibular excess (SNA 83°; SNB 90°; ANB −7°).
2. Maxillary dentoalveolar protrusion ($\overline{1}$ to NA 49° and 13 mm).

Occlusal Analysis

1. Class III cuspid and molar relationship bilaterally.
2. Right maxillary palatal crossbite.
3. Anterior crossbite (overjet −5 mm).
4. Mandibular dental midline 5 mm to right of facial and maxillary dental midlines.
5. Canted maxillary occlusal plane (lower on right than left).

TREATMENT PLAN

Orthodontic Treatment

1. Rapid maxillary expansion.
2. Nonextraction alignment and coordination of arches.

Surgical Treatment

1. Before orthodontic treatment:
   a. Lateral maxillary and pterygomaxillary osteotomies to facilitate rapid maxillary expansion.
2. After orthodontic arch coordination:
   a. Bilateral ramus osteotomies to posteriorly reposition mandible and correct ramus asymmetry.
   b. Horizontal sliding genioplasty to correct chin asymmetry and provide augmentation to improve chin to lip relationship.
   c. Right posterior maxillary ostectomy to level maxillary occlusal plane.

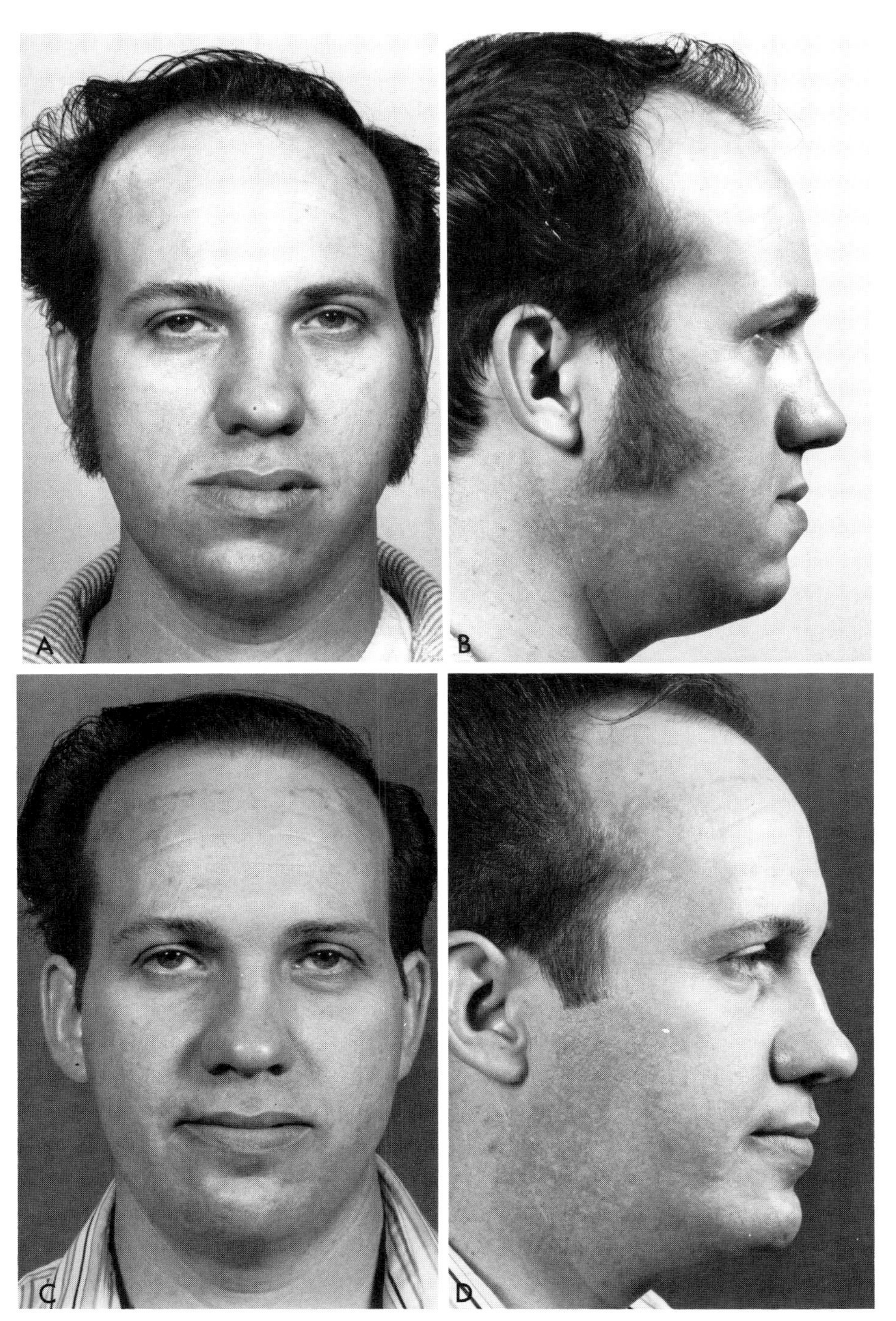

Figure 14–26 (Case 14–8). *A* and *B*, Preoperative facial appearance of 33-year-old man. *C* and *D*, Appearance 6 months after correction of facial asymmetry and mandibular prognathism by bilateral manibular ramus osteotomies and transverse sliding genioplasty. Correction of relative chin deficiency was achieved by advancing the laterally repositioned chin segment.

ACTIVE TREATMENT

Coordination of the maxillary and mandibular arches was facilitated with rapid maxillary expansion. Facial symmetry and balance were achieved by means of maxillary and mandibular osteotomies. Bilateral mandibular ramus osteotomies achieved partial correction of the chin asymmetry. Horizontal sliding osteotomy of the mandibular symphysis with lateral and anterior repositioning completed correction of the asymmetry and established anteroposterior balance between the chin and lower lip.

Surgeons: Stephen Hill, Dallas, Texas. Kevin McBride, Dallas, Texas. *Orthodontist:* Martin Sherling, Dallas, Texas; Harry Legan, Dallas, Texas; Francis Miller, Rockwall, Texas.

CASE 14–9 (Fig. 14–27)

I. P., a 33-year-old woman, was evaluated for treatment to correct her deficient chin.

PROBLEM LIST

Esthetics

1. Moderate facial convexity with contour-deficient chin.
2. Short lower anterior face.

Cephalometric Analysis

1. With mandible rotated closed, proportionately short lower face.
2. Mandibular deficiency (SNA 84°; SNB 74°; ANB 10°; NB to Po 0 mm.

Occlusal Analysis

1. Class II, division 2 malocclusion with minimal overjet.
2. Retroclined maxillary incisors and proclined mandibular incisors compensated for maxillomandibular dysplasia.

TREATMENT PLAN

Orthodontic Treatment

1. Nonextraction orthodontic treatment in upper arch.
2. Orthodontic treatment with extraction of premolars in lower arch.

Surgical Treatment

1. Surgical advancement of mandible.
2. Possible advancement genioplasty.

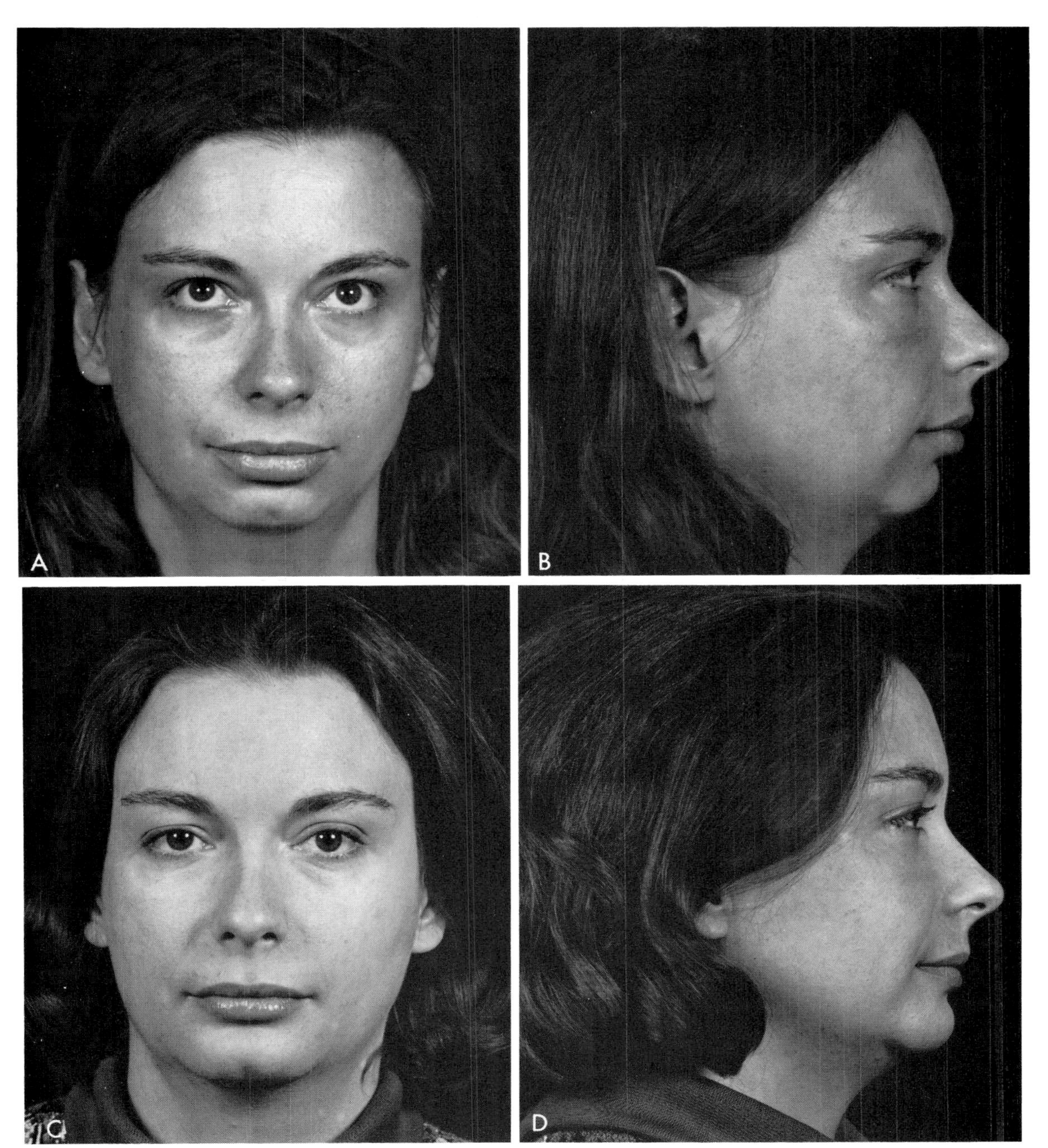

Figure 14–27 (Case 14–9). *A* and *B*, Pretreatment facial views. *C* and *D*, Post-treatment facial views.

Illustration continued on the following page.

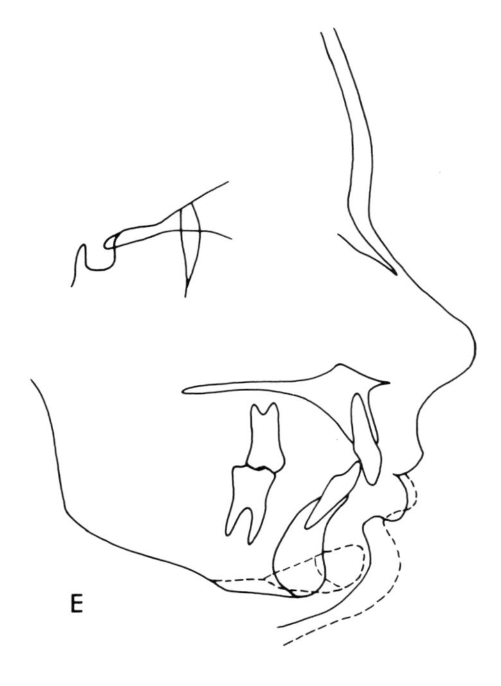

Figure 14–27 *Continued. E,* Composite cephalometric tracings before *(solid line,* age 35 years, 2 months) and after *(broken line,* age 36 years, 3 months) horizontal osteotomy advancement genioplasty.

ACTIVE TREATMENT

Because the patient declined orthodontic treatment and surgical advancement of the mandible, horizontal osteotomy of the inferior border of the mandible was considered a viable alternative to manage the patient's primary concern — her contour-deficient chin. A 1-cm pedicled horizontal sliding advancement genioplasty 12 mm above the inferior border of the mandible was accomplished under general anesthesia. This operation effectively masked the patient's basic problem, mandibular deficiency. Because of the patient's proportionately short lower face and tapered chin, the horizontal osteotomy was designed to extend posteriorly to the second molar region. The chin was moved straight forward without decreasing facial height. Additionally, the lateral portions of the advanced segment made the lower lateral portions of the face more prominent.

Surgeon: William H. Bell, Dallas, Texas.

REFERENCES

1. Aufricht G: Combined plastic surgery of the nose and chin. Am J Oral Surg *95*:231–236, 1958.
2. Bell WH, Dann JJ III: Correction of dentofacial deformities by surgery in the anterior part of the jaws. Am J Orthod *64*(2):162–187, 1973.
3. Broadbent BH: The face of the normal child. Angle Orthod 7:209–233, 1937.
4. Burstone J: Integumental contour and extension patterns. Am J Orthod *29*:(2):93–104, 1959.
5. Burstone CJ: Lip posture and its significance to treatment planning. Am J Orthod *53*:262–284, 1967.
6. Converse JM, Wood-Smith D: Horizontal osteotomy of the mandible. Plast Reconst Surg *34*:464, 1964.
7. Converse JM, Horowitz SL, Wood-Smith D: Deformities of the jaws. *In* Converse JM (Ed): Reconstructive Plastic Surgery. 2nd edition. Philadelphia, WB Saunders Co. 1977, p. 1386.
8. Fitzpatrick BN: Genioplasty with reference to resorption and the hinge sliding osteotomy. Int J Oral Surg *3*:247–251, 1974.
9. Hinds EC, Homsy AC, Kent JN: Use of a Biocompatible Interface for Combining Tissue and Prostheses in Oral Surgery. Presented to the meeting of Fourth Inter-

national Association of Oral Surgeons, Amsterdam. The Netherlands, May 1971.
10. Hinds EC, Kent JN: Genioplasty: the versatility of horizontal osteotomy. J Oral Surg *27*: 690–700, 1969.
11. Hofer O: Operation der Prognathie und Microgenie. Dtsch Zahn Kieferheilkd *9*:121, 1942.
12. Hohl TH, Epker BN: Macrogenia: a study of treatment results, with surgical recommendations. Oral Surg Med Pathol *41*(5):545–567, 1976.
13. Holdaway R: *In* Hambleton RS: The soft tissue covering of the skeletal face as related to orthodontic problems. Am J Orthod *50*:405–420, 1964.
14. Homsy CS, Kent JN, Hinds EC: Materials for oral implantation — biological and functional criteria. J Am Dent Assoc *86*:817, 1973.
15. McDonnell J, McNeill W, West R: Advancement genioplasty, a retrospective cephalometric analysis of osseous and soft tissue changes. J Oral Surg *35*:640–647, 1977.
16. Merrifield LL: The profile line as an aid in critically evaluating facial esthetics. Am J Orthod *52*(11):804–822, 1966.
16. Millard DR: Chin implants. Plast Reconstr Surg *13*:70, 1954.
17. Moorrees C, Kean M: Natural head position, a basic consideration in the interpretation of cephalometric radiographs. Am J Phys Anthropol *16*:213–214, 1958.
18. Neuner O: Correction of mandibular deformities. Oral Surg Med Path *36*(6):779–789, 1973.
19. Obwegeser H: *In* Trauner R, Obwegeser H: The surgical correction of mandibular prognathism and retrognathia with consideration of genioplasty. Part I. Oral Surg *10*:677, 1957.
20. Peck H, Peck S: A concept of facial esthetics. Angle Soc Orthod (4):284–318, 1969.
21. Poulton DR: Facial esthetics and Angle Orthod *27*:133–137, 1957.
22. Rabey GP: Current principles of morphoanalysis and their implications in oral surgical practice. Br J Oral Surg *15*:97–109, 1977–1978.
23. Ricketts RM: Planning treatment on the basis of the facial pattern and an estimate of its growth. Angle Orthod *27*(1):14–37, 1957.
24. Riedel RA: An analysis of dentofacial relationships. Am J Orthod *43*(2):103–119, 1957.
25. Steiner C: *In* Hambleton RS: The soft tissue covering of the skeletal face as related to orthodontic problems. Am J Orthod *50*:405–402, 1964.
26. Trauner R, Obwegeser H: The surgical correction of mandibular prognathism and retrognathia with consideration of genioplasty. Part II. Operating methods for microgenia and distocclusion (cont'd). Oral Surg Med Pathol *10*(9):899–909, 1957.
27. Tweed C: Frankfort–mandibular incisor angle (FMIA) in orthodontic treatment planning and prognosis. Angle Orthod *24*:121, 1954.

SELECTED READINGS

Bell W H: Correction of skeletal type of anterior open bite. J Oral Surg *29*:706–714, 1971.

Bell W H, Brammer J A, McBride K L, Finn R A: Reduction genioplasty—soft tissue changes after modified technique. J Oral Surg (in press).

Bell W H, Scheideman G B, Legan H L: Correction of mandibular prognathism by mandibular setback and augmentation genioplasty. Am J Orthod (in press).

SPECIAL CONSIDERATIONS

Section III

Chapter 15

MANAGEMENT OF NASAL DEFORMITIES

Jack P. Gunter and William H. Bell

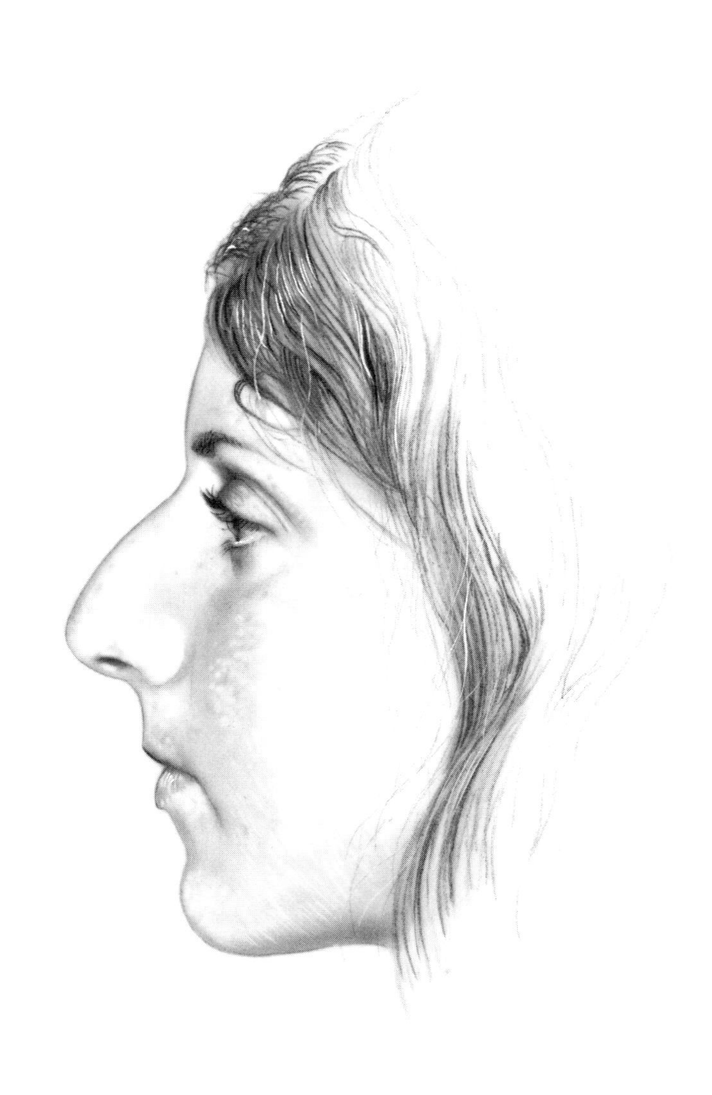

Surgeons who are interested in correcting dentofacial problems must consider the most exposed and prominent feature of the face — the nose. The nasal area plays an important part in individual recognition and a major role in facial esthetics. The relationship between the nose and other structures of the face must be harmonious if appearance is to be esthetically pleasing. Thus, a thorough evaluation of the nasal area must be included in the diagnostic and planning phases of the treatment of dentofacial deformity.

Rhinoplasty for the treatment of nasal deformity is the oldest form of reconstructive surgery — the first recorded information on this subject dates as far back as 2500 B.C. In India and Egypt, nasal reconstruction was performed using skin from the forehead, cheeks, and buttocks to replace missing tissue.[1] It was not until the late 1800s, however, that rhinoplasty to improve nasal appearance without external incisions was described. Only in the last quarter-century has rhinoplasty developed into a practical and predictable procedure.

SYSTEMATIC DESCRIPTION OF THE DEFORMITY

Nasal deformities range from mild cosmetic to severe congenital anomalies, e.g., congenital clefts. This chapter deals principally with deformities considered to be developmental in origin. Although some authors believe that trauma at the time of birth is the causal agent, it is apparent that heredity also plays a dominant role in the pathogenesis of nasal deformity.

Cosmetic nasal deformity is relative. That is, a nose may be viewed as being deformed by the patient or his peers but might be considered normal in appearance by another culture or ethnic group. Noses may vary considerably in shape (measurement) and size (proportion) from one individual to another and still be considered "normal" for that particular individual. A nose that is considered to be attractive in one person might be unsightly in another. The esthetic value of the nose is determined by its proportions and its relationships to the other facial structures (features).

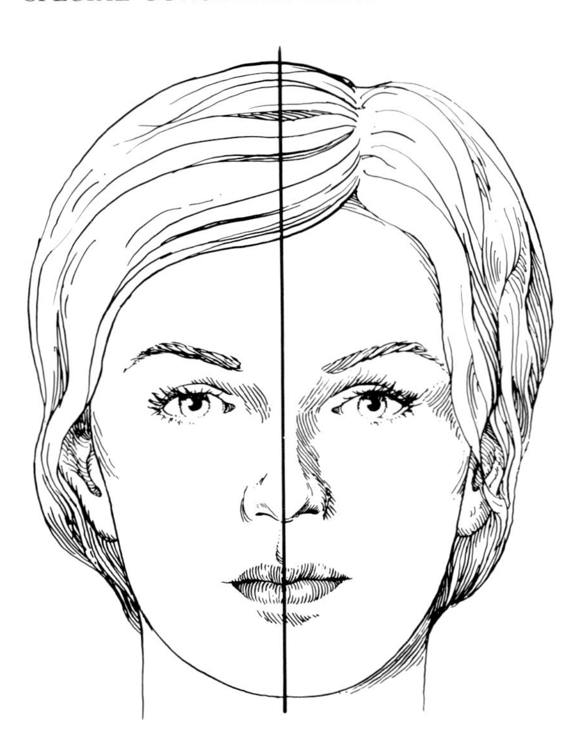

Figure 15–1. Evaluation of nasal position. The nose should be halved by a line running from the center of the glabellar region, through the midpoint of the cupid's bow, to the midpoint of the chin.

Realizing that a normal-looking nose may take many forms and sizes, one can use some general guidelines to assess nasal appearance. Guidelines discussed in this chapter are for Caucasians. Esthetic values differ among the races and even differ within the same race for the male and female, and this must be considered in any application of guidelines.

On frontal view, the nose should be positioned in the center of the face. If both sides of the face are symmetric, the nose is halved by a line running from the center of the glabellar region through the midpoint of the cupid's bow to the midpoint of the chin (Fig. 15–1). Deviation of the nose from this line usually indicates a deviated nasal septum, displaced nasal bones, or both. If the face is asymmetric, it is more attractive if the nose corresponds with the glabellar–mid cupid's bow line. The midpoint of cupid's bow should correspond to the space between the maxillary central incisors. If the two do differ, it is more esthetically pleasing for the nasal tip to be in line with the cupid's bow, even though the relationship of the nose to the teeth will appear abnormal when the patient smiles. These facts must be kept in mind when considering a change in the position and shape of the nose from a frontal view.

The nose should have a pyramidal shape (Fig. 15–2). The width of the base should correspond to the distance between two vertical lines drawn through the inner canthi (intercanthal distance), which should in turn equal the distance between the inner and lateral canthi on either side (Fig. 15–3). Visually, the nose should be divided into a body and a tip that appear as two separate anatomic entities (Fig. 15–4). This perspective gives the nose more character and better definition. The nose itself should present as a well-defined entity separate from the rest of the face. In persons with middle-third facial deficiency (maxillary hypoplasia), the nasomaxillary groove may be ill-defined, making it hard to tell where the lateral walls of the nose stop and the maxillae begin. This is undesirable, as it detracts from facial appearance.

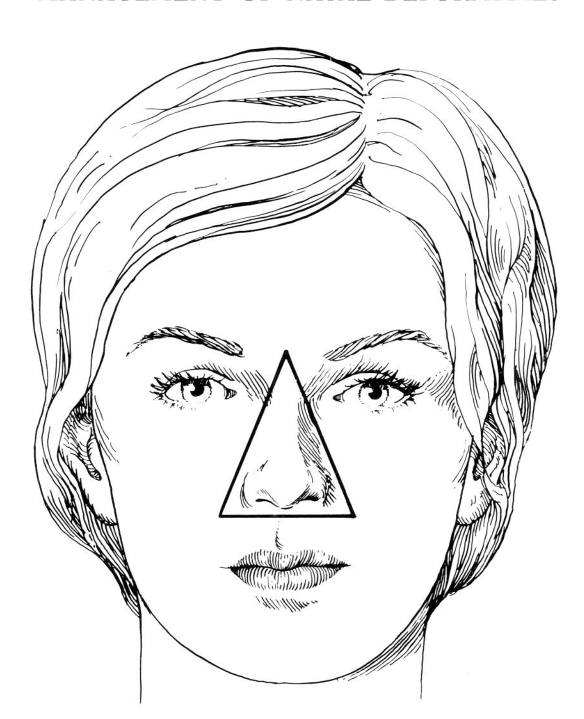

Figure 15–2. Evaluation of nasal shape. The nose should be pyramidal.

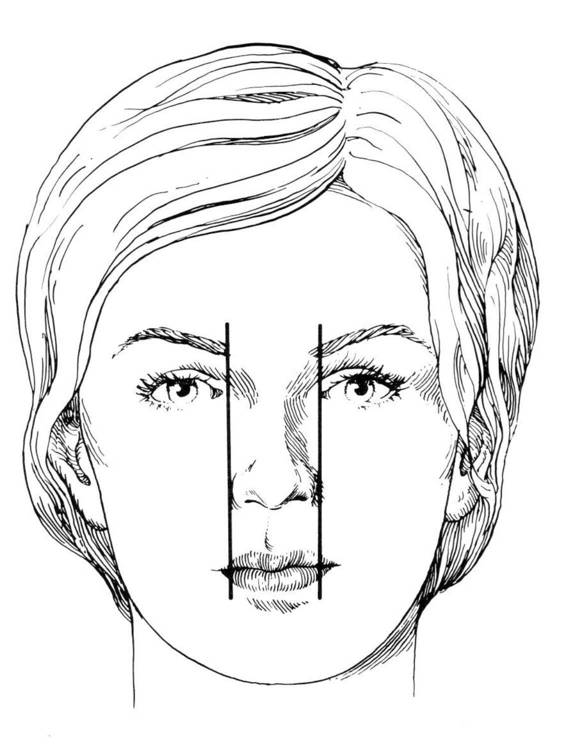

Figure 15–3. Evaluation of nasal width. The width of the nose should correspond to the distance between two vertical lines drawn through the inner canthi.

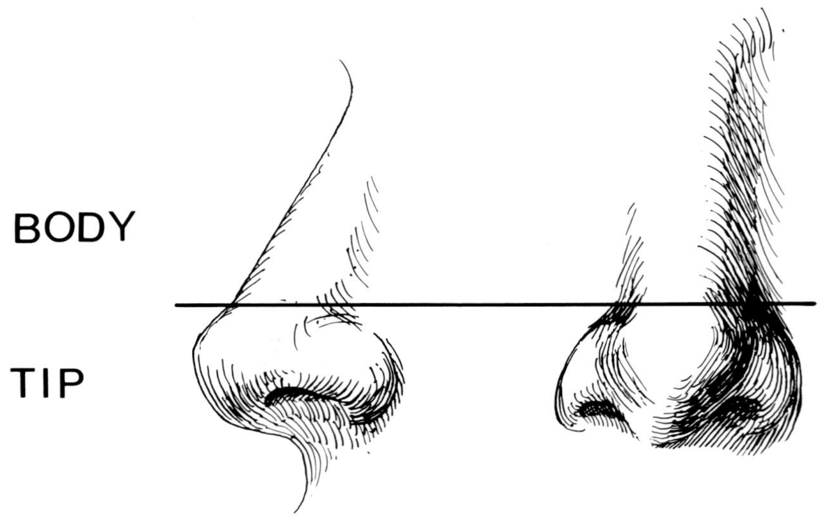

Figure 15–4. Visual delineation of nose into two separate entities—the nasal body and nasal tip.

On profile view, the important considerations are: (1) the amount by which the nasal body and nasal tip project, and (2) the nasofacial (i.e., the nasofrontal and nasolabial) angles (Fig. 15–5). The tip should be the most projecting part of the nose. At the juncture of the tip and the body there should be the slightest suggestion of an angle; the "supratip break." This subtle break occurs because the dorsum of the tip lies in a slightly more horizontal plane than the dorsum of the body, allowing the tip to appear separated from the body on the profile view. The juncture of the root of the nose with the forehead (the nasofrontal angle) is another well-defined landmark, denoting the upper limit of the nose. If the forehead projects more than the root of the nose, creating a groove in this area, the nasofrontal angle is well-delineated. This groove can be too deep, but it is impossible to give specific measurements, and the evaluator must depend on his own esthetic sense as he views the patient's problem.

Nasal projection is evaluated by the angle formed between the line extending along the most projecting part of the dorsum and the true vertical (line perpendicular to Frankfort horizontal), as shown in Figure 15–6. Ideally, this angle of nasal projection is between 30° and 37°. Inclination of the nasal base (or the amount of rotation of the nasal tip) is measured by the angle between the true vertical and a line through the long axis of the nostril (Fig. 15–7). The angle varies from about 90° in men to as much as 110° in women.

The inclination of the nose may fall within normal limits but appear abnormal because of excess fullness at the columella-lip juncture. This variation is caused by a prominent nasal spine or a retroinclination of the upper lip resulting from lack of support by palatally positioned maxillary incisor teeth. Such an increased nasolabial angle (or columella-labial angle) is seen occasionally following orthodontic treatment of Class II malocclusion and in individuals with vertical maxillary excess. The skin is more firmly attached along the length of the columella toward the nasal tip and looser in the nasal spine area. Because of this, the angle between the nasal tip and the lip increases and tends to be obliterated when the lip is pulled down.

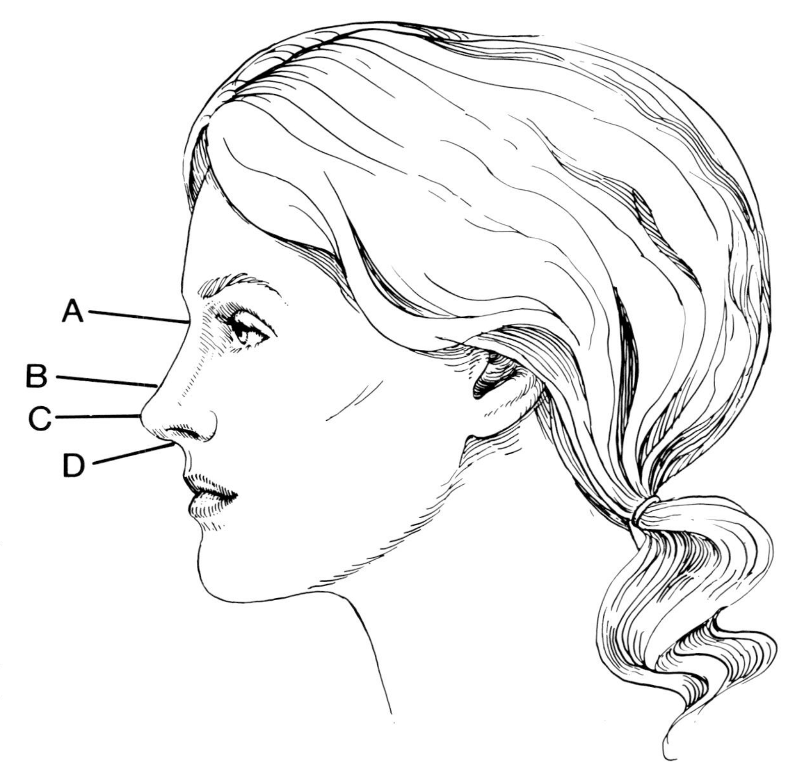

Figure 15–5. Important nasal landmarks for evaluation of nasal esthetics. *(A)* Nasofrontal angle junction of the root of the nose with the forehead should be well defined. *(B)* "Supratip break" — slight angle formed at juncture of nasal tip and body. *(C)* Nasal tip. *(D)* Nasolabial angle.

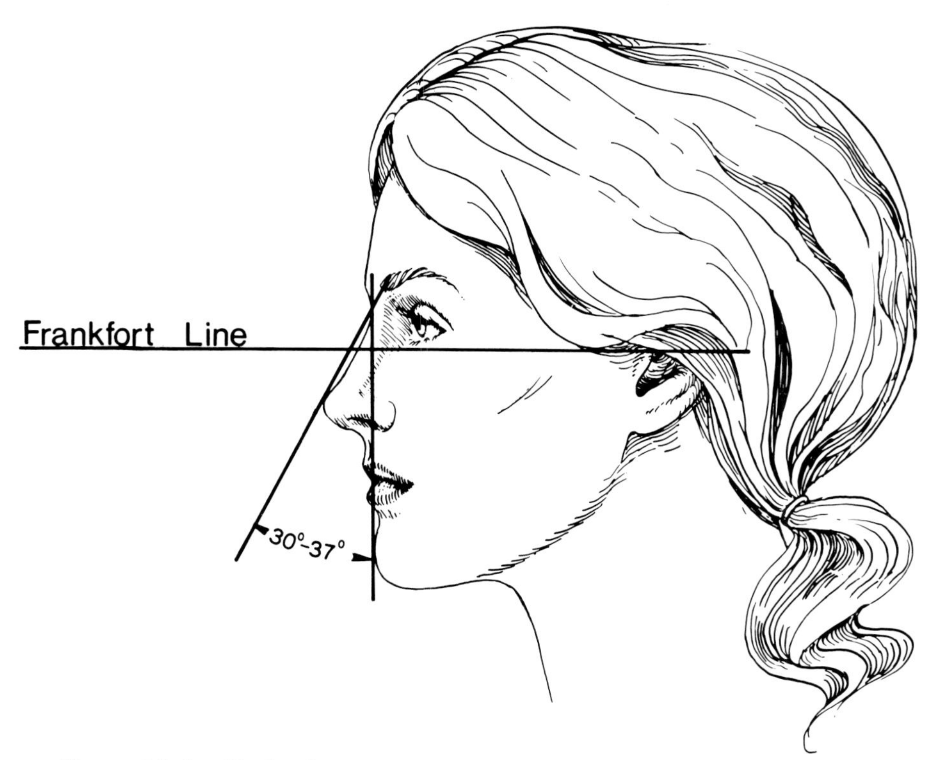

Figure 15–6. Evaluation of nasal projection. Ideal angle of nasal projection is usually between 30 and 37°

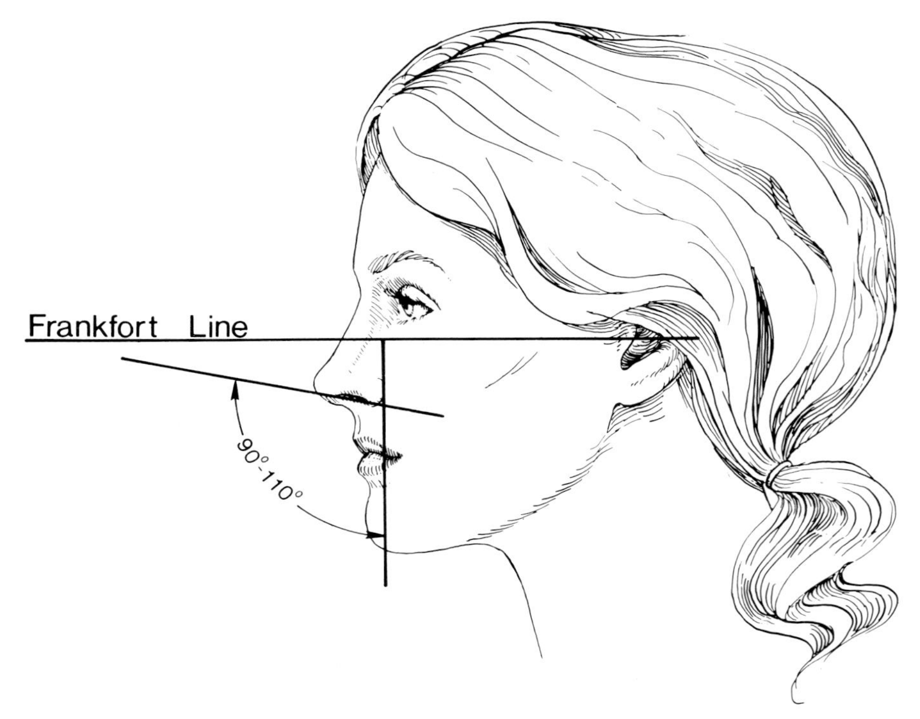

Figure 15–7. Evaluation of nasal base inclination. Should vary between 90° in males to as much as 110° in females.

The most common cosmetic nasal deformity is a nose that is large and out of proportion to the rest of the face (Fig. 15–8). The entire nose or only a part of it may be too large. Other common deformities that can be corrected with endonasal rhinoplasty are: a prominent dorsal hump, a drooping nasal tip, a long nose, too much projection of the tip, a bulbous-appearing tip, a wide dorsum, a wide nasal base, or a crooked nose. These conditions may appear alone or in combination.

SURGICAL TREATMENT APPROACHES

The goal of the surgeon performing rhinoplasty is to produce an attractive, natural-looking, normally functioning nose that is in balance and harmony with the rest of the face.

When a patient has a nasal deformity that can be improved by rhinoplasty, the operation should be performed after the nose has reached its full growth, usually around age 15 in girls and age 17 in boys. Performing a rhinoplasty on a developing nose may alter the growth pattern of that nose, and the long-term result will be unpredictable.

The ideal face for a rhinoplasty has a high, prominent maxilla with good proportions on frontal view in addition to a correctable nasal deformity. On profile, the glabellar region should be the most projecting part of the forehead, with the rest of

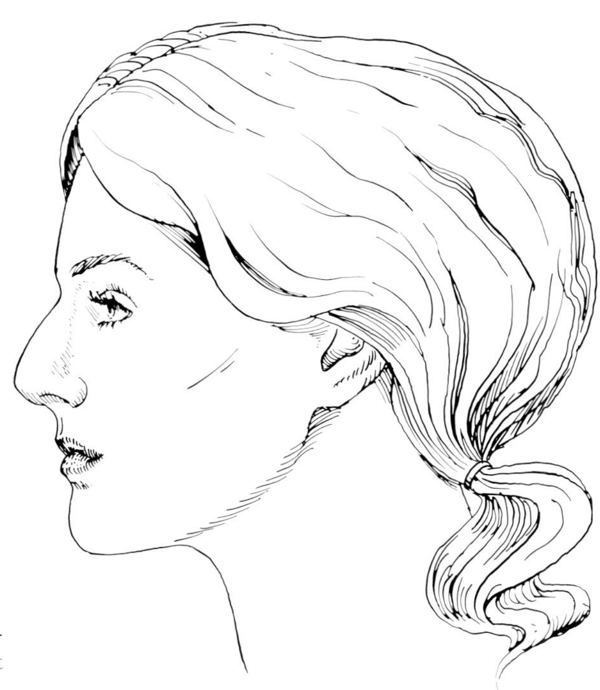

Figure 15–8. The most common cosmetic nasal deformity. Nose is too large and out of proportion with rest of face.

the forehead gradually sloping backward to the brow line. A definite nasofrontal angle is desirable, as this angle is difficult to create surgically. The upper lip should be slightly concave with the vermilion border and mucosal surface in slight projection. The lower lip should rest in a slightly more posterior plane than the upper, and there should be a groove between the lower lip and the chin to define them as separate entities. The most projecting part of the chin should lie on a vertical plane at the same level as or just posterior to the most projecting part of the lower lip.

The usual reasons for performing rhinoplasty are to (1) straighten a crooked nose, (2) reduce a dorsal hump, (3) narrow a wide nose, (4) remodel the nasal tip or change its position, or (5) correct a combination of the above. Conditions that most readily lend themselves to surgical correction are a large dorsal hump, a bulbous nasal tip, a wide nasal dorsum, a drooping nasal tip, and an abnormal relationship of the nose to the lips.

The basic steps in the rhinoplastic procedure are:

1. Separate the dorsal skin from the underlying bones and cartilages through endonasal incisions.
2. Remodel the nasal tip cartilages.
3. Remove bony and cartilaginous hump.
4. Straighten the nasal septum.
5. Perform medial and lateral osteotomies to infracture the nasal bones.
6. Redrape the skin over this newly constructed framework.

The way the results of these steps relate to each other at the end of the operation determines the final results. During the procedure each step may be modified, but because one step is usually dependent on the others, it is rare that a partial rhinoplasty is successful.

During the rhinoplasty, additional steps may be taken to improve the results.

Deepening the nasofrontal angle, narrowing the base of the nose, correcting columellar deformities, and changing the projection of the nasal spine are not routine steps in the rhinoplastic procedure but can be added when needed.

ADDITIONAL CONSIDERATIONS

Not all nasal deformities are amenable to surgical correction. Although there are exceptions, it is accepted that a narrow nose cannot be widened and a short nose cannot be lengthened by rhinoplasty as it is performed routinely. A very large nose can be reduced in size only a certain amount, and a small nose cannot be enlarged. Noses with very thick, oily skin can be reduced in size, but the skin usually will not redrape over the remodeled supporting structures to give the definition desired, especially in the nasal tip area.

A rhinoplasty is contraindicated if a patient is a poor candidate psychologically (see Chapter 4). This does not necessarily mean a patient who suffers a psychiatric disorder. Some patients' desires are not realistic, and they may expect too much from the operation. The patient must accept an improvement and understand that perfection is not possible. Great care must be taken when operating on patients whose noses are minimally deformed. Although at times the results may be very gratifying, there is very little margin for error. In such situations the surgeon must be certain that he has all factors in his favor, that he realizes his own capabilities, and that the patient has realistic expectations.

Many patients who present with dentofacial deformities have combined nasal, jaw, and occlusal deformities. These deformities must be evaluated in relationship to each other if optimal results in treatment are to be achieved. Such evaluation is best accomplished by a multidisciplinary team approach. Each specialist involved should evaluate the patient independently. The team should then meet to discuss the findings and formulate an all-inclusive treatment plan. When combined surgical and orthodontic treatment is indicated, the rhinoplasty should be the last step in the treatment plan. Since the desired position and shape of the nose are determined by its surrounding structures, it is best that these structures be in their permanent position before the rhinoplasty is performed. Changes in the position of the anterior maxilla may alter the shape of the nasal tip; thus, perfect rhinoplasty may be compromised if it is followed by anterior maxillary surgery. The surgeon performing rhinoplasty attempts to change the appearance of the nose so that the nose is in harmony with the rest of the face. If the position of the jaws or teeth changes after the rhinoplasty, the nose may appear out of balance.

Occasionally, orthognathic surgery and rhinoplasty may be performed at the same time, particularly if the orthognathic procedure does not result in compromise of the oral airway or repositioning of the anterior nasal spine or nasal septum. If the jaws have to be wired together following the surgical procedure or if the anterior maxilla is repositioned, rhinoplasty should be postponed. Mentoplasty, sliding genioplasty, reduction genioplasty, posterior maxillary osteotomy, and mandibular operations that do not require intermaxillary fixation all are compatible with concomitant rhinoplasty.

COMPLICATIONS OF RHINOPLASTIC SURGERY

Edema and Related Complications

Following rhinoplasty there is always some degree of swelling, ecchymosis, and nasal congestion. These sequelae usually subside within two weeks following the surgery, and those that remain are inconspicuous. It takes several months and sometimes up to a year for all the edema to subside completely. During this time, the small amount of edema present may hide small irregularities (imperfections) and asymmetries. For this reason, the final evaluation of a rhinoplasty should not take place until at least one year after the operation.

Occasionally the nose may remain edematous for several weeks following rhinoplasty for reasons that cannot be explained. Most authors feel this edema is due to a low-grade infection, such as periostitis along an osteotomy site or necrosis of bony splinters that were not removed. If the cause is known it is treated accordingly; if not, the patient is observed until the swelling eventually subsides. This waiting period can be very frustrating for both the surgeon and the patient.

Hemorrhage

Hemorrhage is occasionally a complication of rhinoplasty. When bleeding does occur, it is usually within the first 48 hours or else 10 to 14 days postoperatively, when the protective crusts start to separate from the incision sites. Bleeding can usually be controlled with light packing using a material soaked with a vasoconstrictive solution such as epinephrine. Rarely, it may be necessary to place a posterior nasal pack.

Skin Disorders

Minor skin complications may sometimes be seen following rhinoplasty, e.g., a tape reaction or skin pustules forming beneath the dressing. Formation of telangiectasis of the skin has been reported, as have forms of hypo- and hyperpigmentation of the nasal skin. Pigmentation changes are seen most often in patients whose skin is exposed to sun for prolonged periods within the first two months after surgery. A more serious complication is skin necrosis due to an improperly applied dressing. An area of skin necrosis may heal without much scarring if it is small. If more extensive scarring occurs, secondary surgery may be required.

Unsatisfactory Esthetic Appearance

The item of most concern following rhinoplasty is a result that is less than satisfactory esthetically. Such a result may be due to faulty planning, faulty technique, lack of patient cooperation during the postoperative period, or variations in the healing process over which the surgeon has no control, e.g., the excessive formation of scar tissue in the supratip area or thick oily skin that does not redrape and contract as expected. A surgeon is sometimes guilty of being concerned only with the nasal deformity and failing to evaluate thoroughly enough the other facial features that affect the final result. Before rhinoplasty is performed the entire facial structure must be evaluated. At times even the body structure is important: an upturned nose is not as desirable for a tall individual as it might be for a short one. A missed diagnosis is possible with the best planning and evaluation. For example, a patient may appear to have an excessive nasal dorsal hump. Further evaluation may reveal that the nasal dorsum is not actually in excess but that the nasal tip does not project far enough. Increasing the projection of the tip may improve the relationship so that hump removal is unnecessary.

ERRORS OF SURGICAL TECHNIQUE

The most common errors of surgical technique in rhinoplasty are related to faulty management of a deviated nasal septum and of the supratip area. The surgeon performing rhinoplasty must be able to correct internal as well as external deformities. A deviated nasal septum, if left uncorrected, may result in deviation of the external nose or widening of the nasal bone area. Function must be considered also, since improper treatment may result in nasal airway obstruction. The supratip area remains an enigma to rhinoplastic surgeons. Noses that appear to have a good contour at the end of the operation occasionally develop a rounding in the supratip area referred to as a "parrot's beak" deformity. Many factors may be responsible for this development, but it is much less of a problem to those who understand the dynamics of nasal tip surgery and the factors that influence nasal tip projection.

Other errors in technique, such as incomplete osteotomies or overzealous removal of supporting structures and mucosal lining, can occur, but these are rare.

Although proper preoperative study and planning are very important in rhinoplasty, the operation cannot be planned with numbers and measurements like many of the maxillary and mandibular procedures. Even if one could measure the exact amount by which the dorsal hump should be reduced, the nasal tip should be projected, or the nose should be narrowed, it is impossible to control the operation to meet exact figures. When the local anesthetic agent is injected, some distortion occurs, and anatomic landmarks that could be used for references change position. Because there are no immobile landmarks to use as reference points for measurement, the rhinoplasty operation is dependent on the surgeon's understanding of what he wants to accomplish and what is necessary to obtain the desired results. During the operation, the most important factors are the surgeon's clinical judgment and his understanding of how each step affects the subsequent steps.

Rhinoplasty in properly selected patients achieves good results. It often produces dramatic changes, not only in the patient's appearance but also in his outlook on life. The case studies that follow describe patients with combined deformities of nose and jaws that were treated by a coordinated plan including orthodontic treatment, orthognathic surgery, and rhinoplasty.

CASE 15–1 (Fig. 15–9)

C. M., a 26-year-old woman, desired treatment to improve her facial appearance.

PROBLEM LIST

Esthetics

The patient's nasal deformity included a moderately sized dorsal hump and an excessively projecting nasal tip that lacked definition. She also had a slightly receding chin.

PLAN OF TREATMENT

1. Rhinoplasty.
2. Genioplasty employing 6-mm intraoral solid Silastic implant.

FOLLOW-UP

A good postoperative result was obtained from the rhinoplasty. The chin augmentation increased the chin prominence, created better definition between the lip and chin, and improved the balance between the middle and lower thirds of the face.

Surgeon: Jack P. Gunter, Dallas, Texas.

CASE 15–2 (Fig. 15–10)

C. L., a 28-year-old woman, was initially seen for treatment of her malocclusion.

PROBLEM LIST

Esthetics

All study parameters showed the typical dentofacial features of mandibular prognathism. The patient's prominent "hooked" nose necessitated a treatment plan combining orthodontic treatment, mandibular surgery, and rhinoplasty.

PLAN OF TREATMENT

1. Orthodontic treatment to correct malalignment of teeth.
2. Bilateral mandibular body ostectomies to retract mandible.
3. Rhinoplasty.

ACTIVE TREATMENT

Treatment was planned so that bilateral mandibular midbody ostectomies (5 mm left side; 8 mm right side) to retract the mandible were done concomitantly with the rhinoplasty. Orthodontic arch wires were used to affix the mandibular bony segments

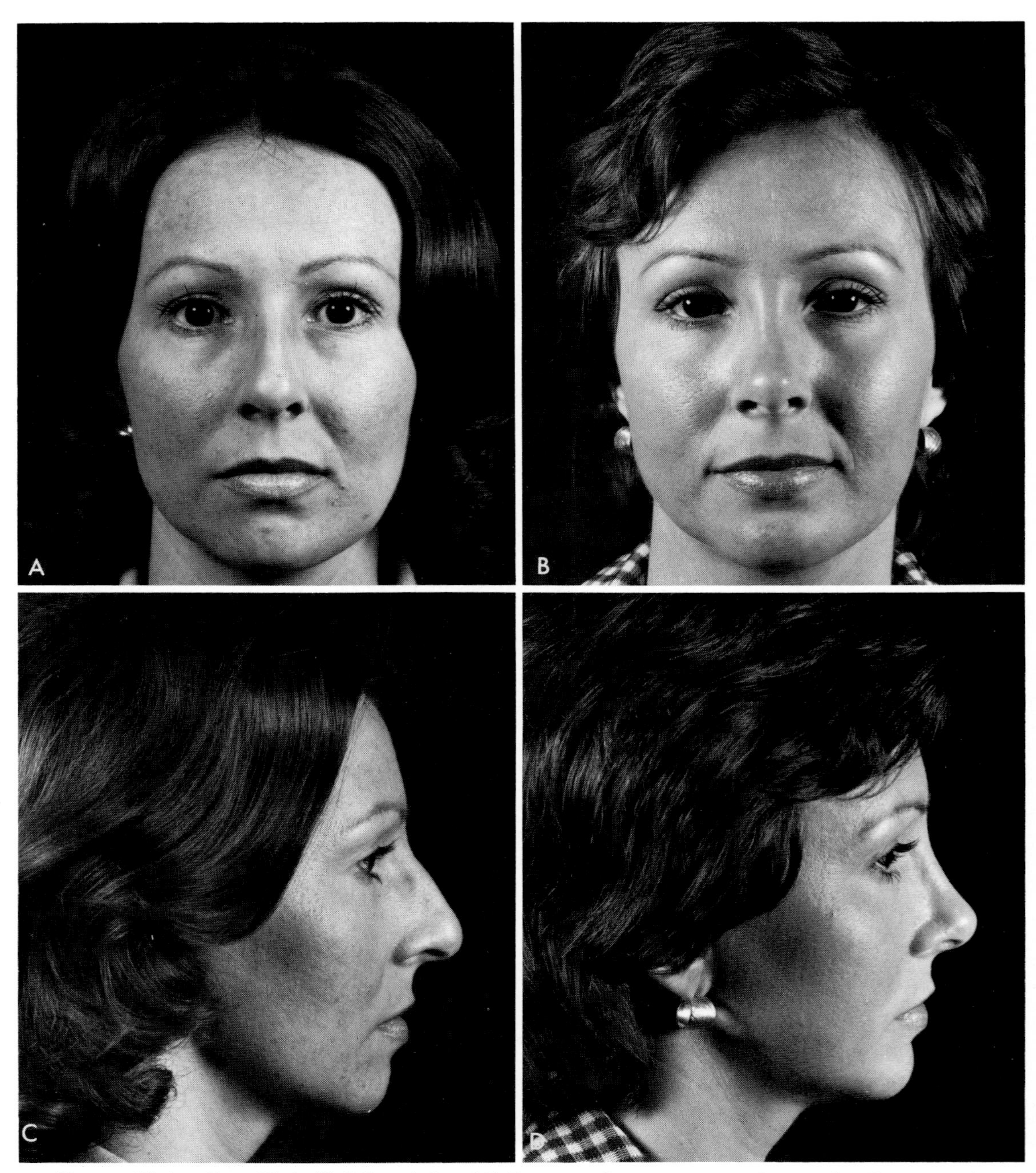

Figure 15–9. Case 15–1. (C. M.). *A, C* and *E,* Preoperative appearance. *B, D,* and *F,* Postoperative appearance.

Illustration continued on the opposite page

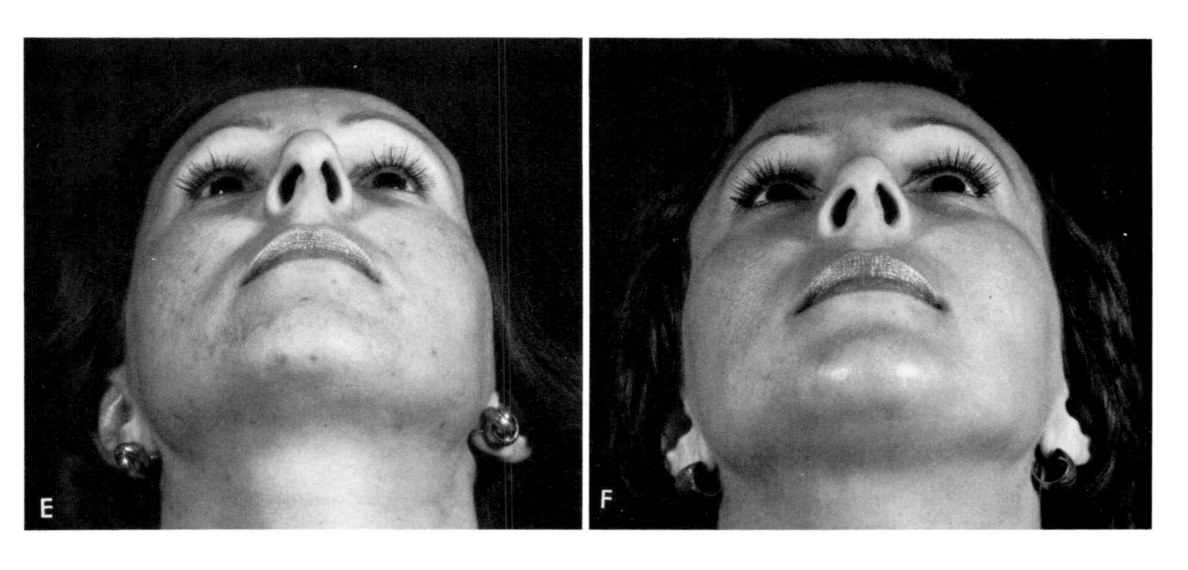

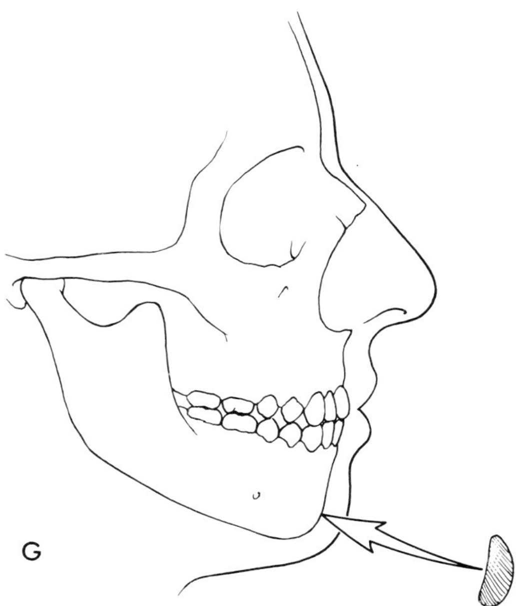

Figure 15–9 *Continued.* *G,* Diagrammatic plan for chin implant insertion.

in the desired position at the time of surgery and in the immediate postoperative period when the nasal airway was compromised. This treatment plan facilitated rhinoplasty by obviating the immediate need for intermaxillary fixation. Five days after surgery, when the nasal airway was patent, the mandible was immobilized in the desired position.

FOLLOW-UP

Twenty-four months of treatment produced a balanced soft-tissue profile, facial symmetry, and occlusal balance.

Rhinoplasty: Jack P. Gunter, Dallas, Texas. *Mandibular surgery:* William H. Bell, Dallas, Texas.

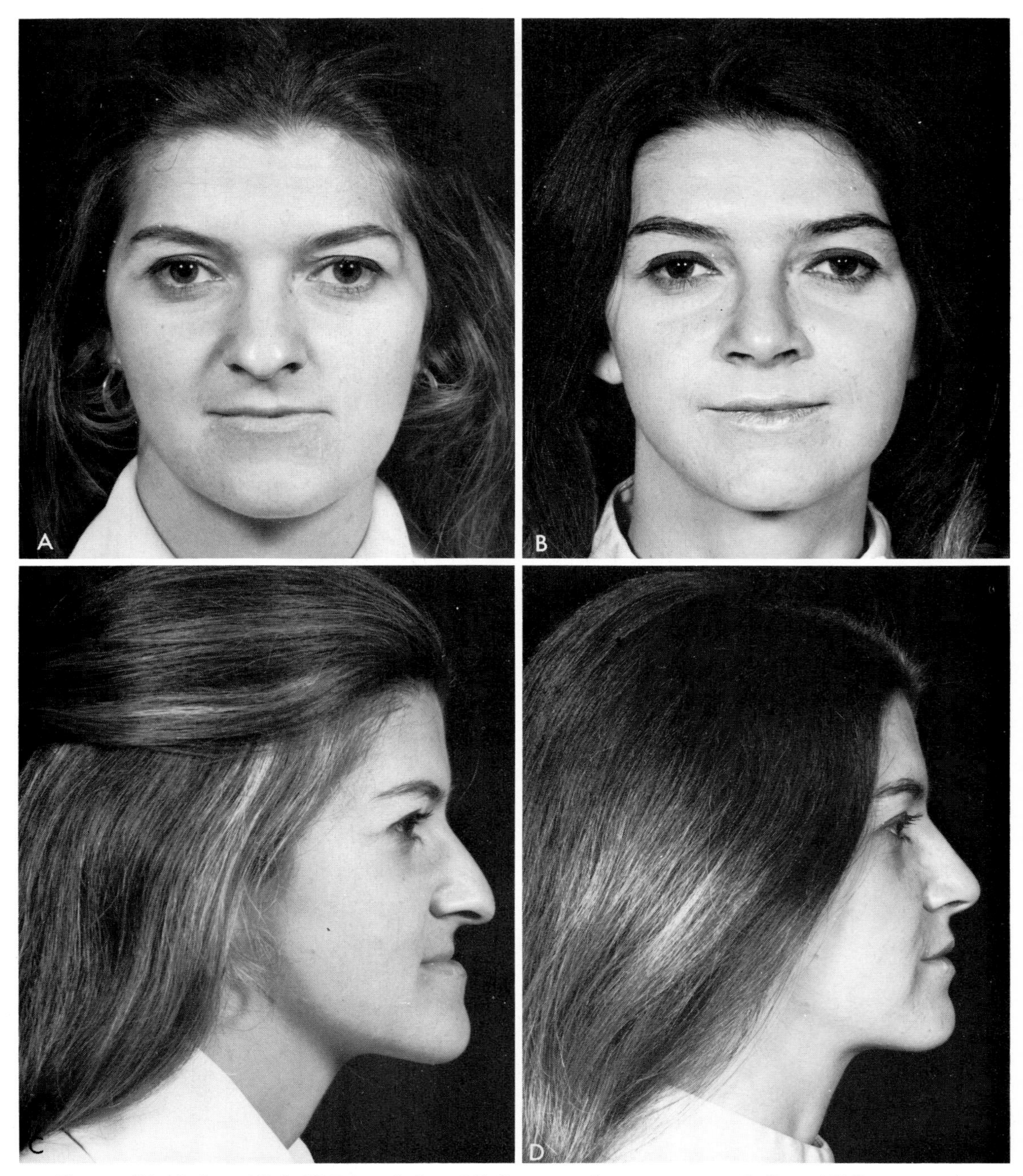

Figure 15–10. Case 15–2. (C. L.). *A, C,* and *E,* Preoperative appearance. *B, D,* and *F,* Postoperative appearance.

Illustration continued on the opposite page.

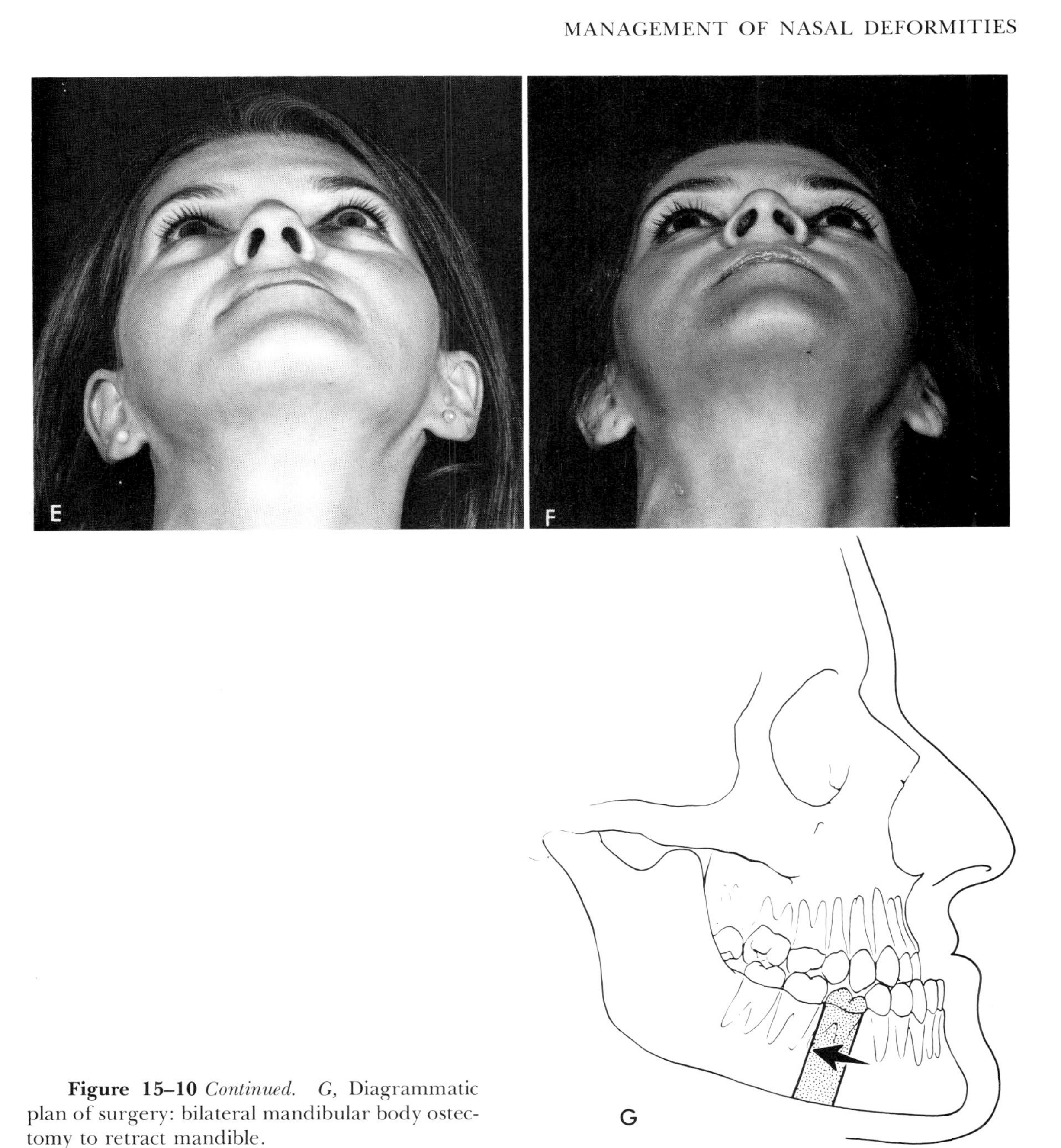

Figure 15–10 *Continued.* *G,* Diagrammatic plan of surgery: bilateral mandibular body ostectomy to retract mandible.

CASE 15–3 (Fig. 15–11)

G. G., a 21-year-old woman, sought treatment to decrease the "prominence" of her maxillary teeth and improve the contour of her face.

PROBLEM LIST

Esthetics

Clinical and cephalometric analysis disclosed total maxillary alveolar hyperplasia, increased height of the face, lip incompetence, Class II malocclusion, a contour-

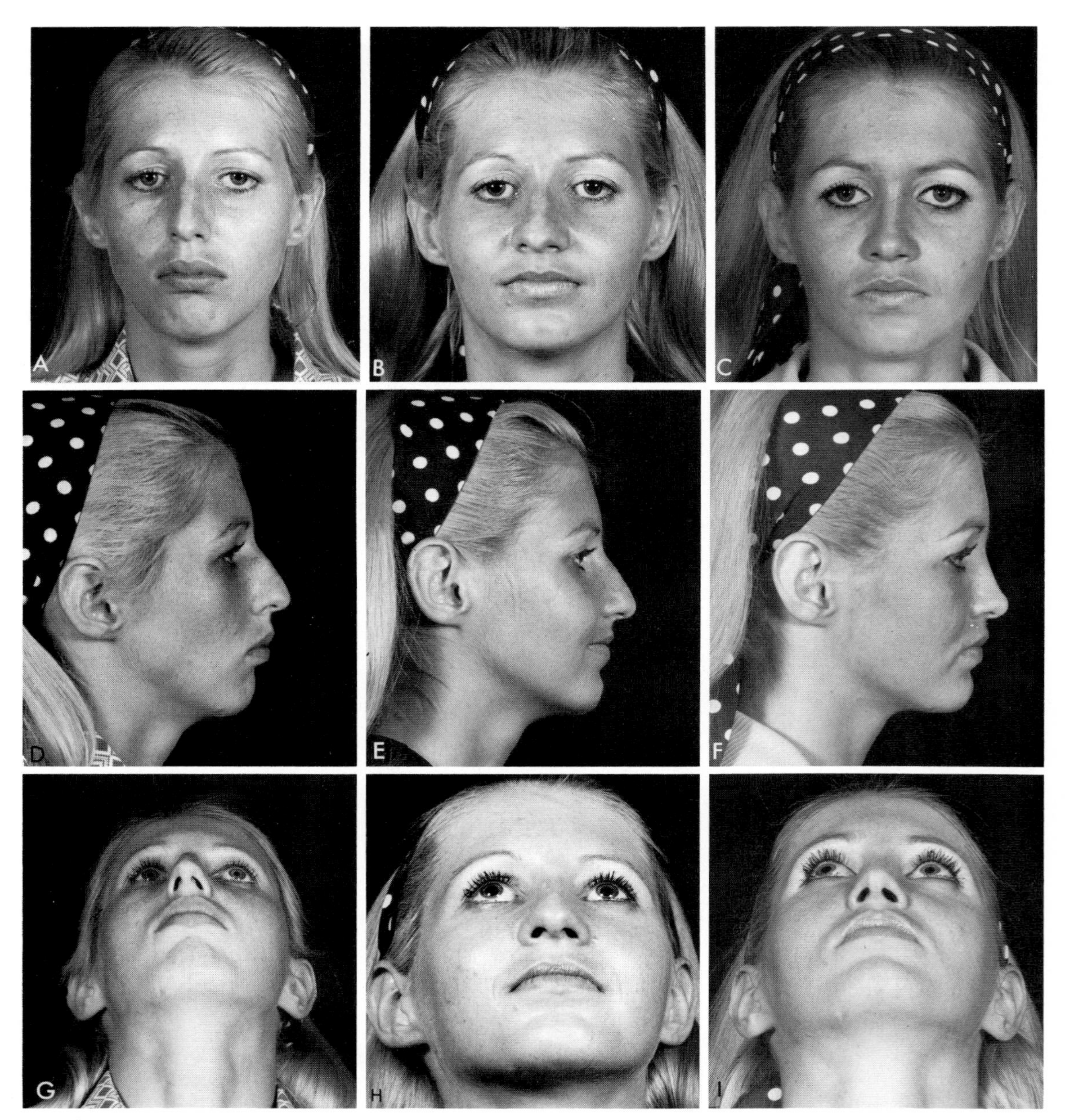

Figure 15–11. Case 15–3. (G. G.). *A, D,* and *G,* Preoperative appearance with lips sealed. *B, E,* and *H,* Postoperative appearance after maxillary surgery showing splaying of alar bases (technique for maxillary surgery shown in Fig. 15–11*J*). *C, F,* and *I,* Facial appearance 6 months after rhinoplasty and 2 years after maxillary surgery.

Illustration continued on the opposite page.

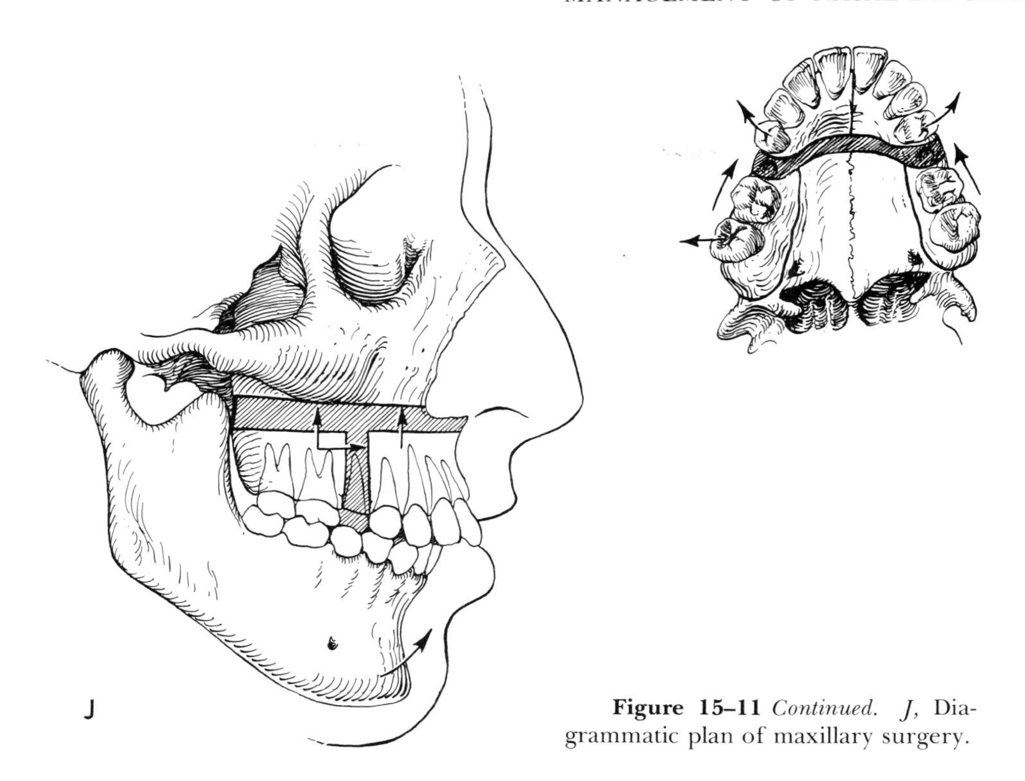

Figure 15–11 *Continued.* *J,* Diagrammatic plan of maxillary surgery.

deficient chin, and lack of prominence in the midfacial region. The patient's maxillary anterior teeth were positioned 7 mm anterior to the mandibular anterior teeth. The nose was deviated and had a prominent dorsal hump and a small nasolabial angle.

TREATMENT PLAN

1. Le Fort I osteotomy to:
   a. Reduce facial height.
   b. Facilitate autorotation of mandible and increase chin prominence.
   c. Widen maxilla.
   d. Improve interdigitation and alignment of teeth.
2. Rhinoplasty to reduce prominence of nose.

FOLLOW-UP

The anterior maxilla was superiorly repositioned 7 mm and the posterior maxilla 9 mm to facilitate forward and superior movement of the mandible. This shortened the face, improved the upper lip line–tooth relationship, corrected the malocclusion, and increased the chin prominence. Raising the maxilla increased the prominence of the cheeks and widened the nose.

Several months later, rhinoplasty was performed to correct the nasal deformity. Although the rhinoplasty reduced the dorsal hump and rotated the nasal tip, there was some external deviation and splaying of the nasal base.

Rhinoplasty: Jack P. Gunter, Dallas, Texas. *Maxillary surgery:* William H. Bell, Dallas, Texas.

CASE 15–4 (Fig. 15–12)

G. G., a 21-year-old woman, had the typical dentofacial characteristics of mandibular prognathism associated with anteroposterior maxillary deficiency.

PROBLEM LIST

Esthetics

A broad nose with a bulbous tip, a hypoplastic appearing midfacial region, and prominent chin were the dominant facial features (Fig. 15–12*A* and *D*). Cephalometric studies corroborated the clinical findings. The lower anterior teeth were positioned approximately 12 mm anterior to the maxillary dentition.

TREATMENT PLAN

1. Le Fort I osteotomy (Fig. 15–12*G*) to:
    a. Advance maxilla to increase prominence of midface.
    b. Achieve maxillomandibular harmony.
2. Bilateral mandibular body ostectomies (Fig. 15–12*G*) to retract mandible and improve arch form.
3. Orthodontic treatment to correct malalignment of teeth.
4. Rhinoplasty to reduce nasal width.

FOLLOW-UP

After preliminary orthodontic treatment, the maxilla was surgically advanced 6 mm by Le Fort I osteotomy and the mandible simultaneously retracted 7 mm by bilateral mandibular body ostectomies (Fig. 15–12*G*). Eight months following orthognathic surgery, the patient had a better lower facial relationship, but the nasal deformity had become more pronounced owing to splaying of the alar bases as a result of the maxillary advancement.

Overall facial balance was achieved by rhinoplasty performed five months later to narrow the nasal body and reshape the tip. Modified Weir procedures were performed as part of the rhinoplasty to narrow the nasal base.

Jaw surgery: William H. Bell, Dallas, Texas. *Rhinoplasty:* Jack P. Gunter, Dallas, Texas.

CASE 15–5 (Fig. 15–13)

C. L., a 34-year-old woman, desired surgery to correct her severe jaw and nasal deformity.

PROBLEM LIST

Esthetics

Clinical and cephalometric analysis revealed severe mandibular retrognathism, Class II malocclusion, proclination of the maxillary anterior teeth, excessive curvature

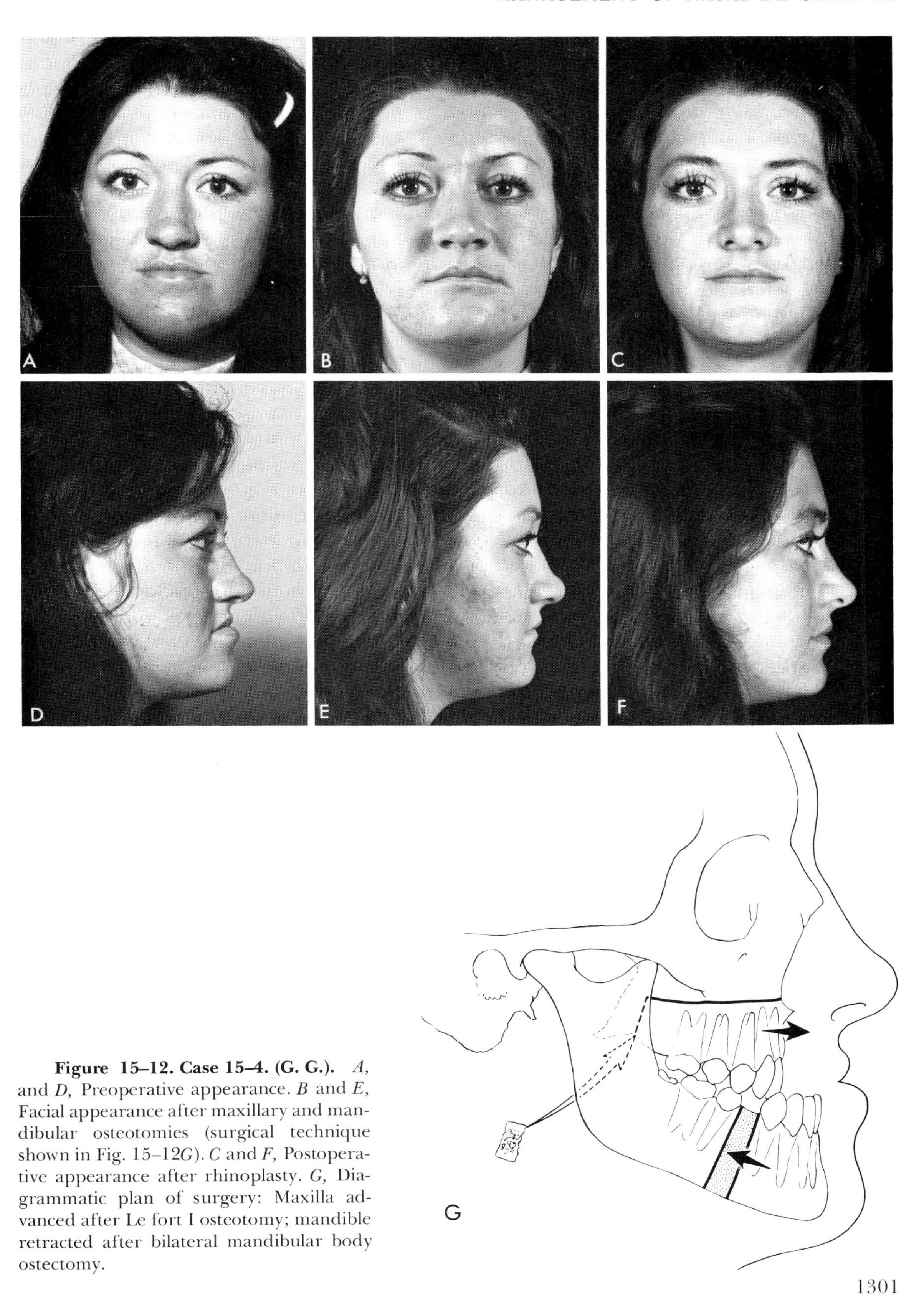

Figure 15–12. Case 15–4. (G. G.). *A,* and *D,* Preoperative appearance. *B* and *E,* Facial appearance after maxillary and mandibular osteotomies (surgical technique shown in Fig. 15–12*G*). *C* and *F,* Postoperative appearance after rhinoplasty. *G,* Diagrammatic plan of surgery: Maxilla advanced after Le fort I osteotomy; mandible retracted after bilateral mandibular body ostectomy.

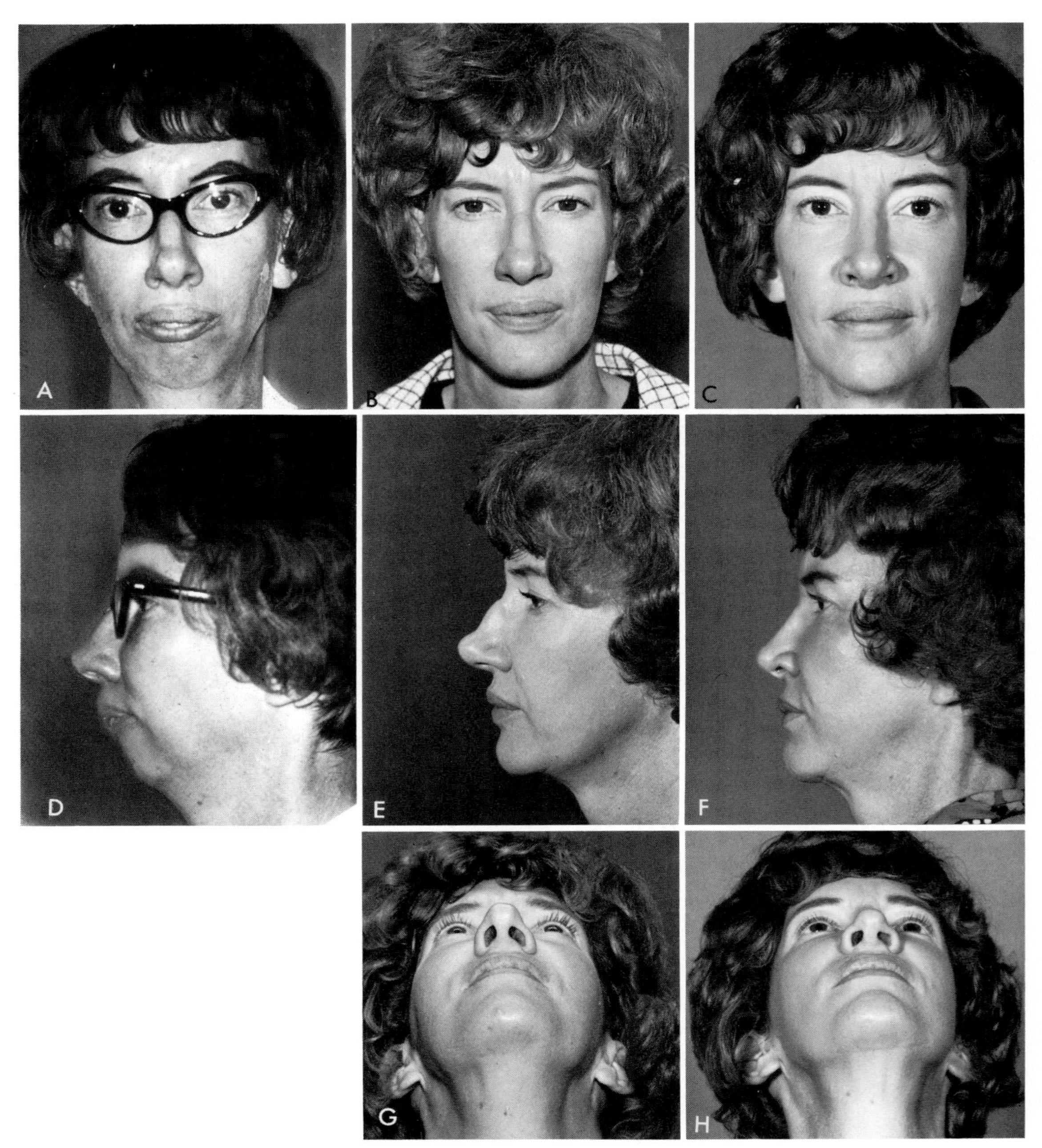

Figure 15–13. Case 15–5. (C. L.). *A* and *D,* Preoperative appearance. *B, E,* and *F,* Facial appearance following jaw surgery. *C, F,* and *H,* Facial appearance following rhinoplasty.

Illustration continued on the opposite page.

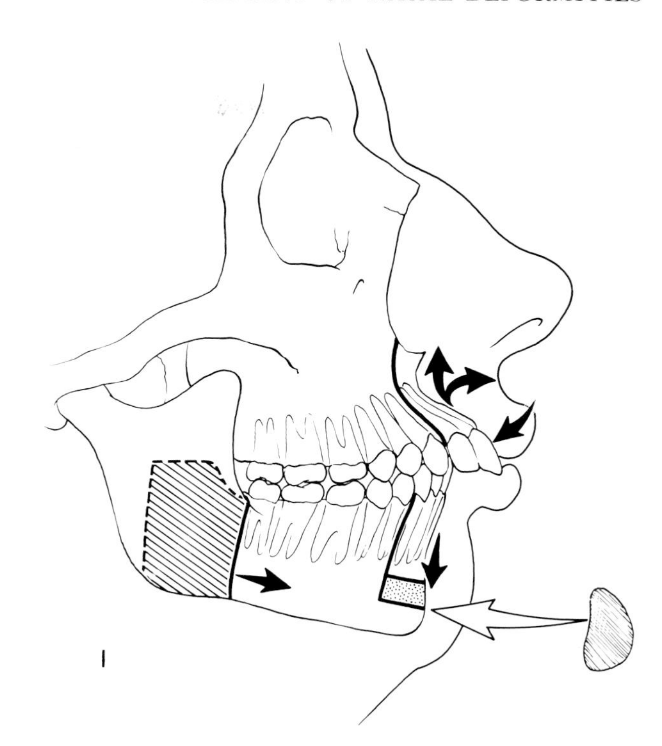

Figure 15–13 *Continued.* *I,* Diagrammatic plan of jaw surgery: Anterior maxillary and mandibular osteotomies; chin augmentation; and bilateral sagittal split ramus osteotomies.

of the mandibular occlusal plane, and lip incompetence. The nose had a large bulbous tip with excessive projection and a moderately sized dorsal hump.

TREATMENT PLAN

1. Anterior maxillary osteotomy to upright maxillary incisor teeth.
2. Bilateral sagittal split mandibular ramus osteotomy to advance mandible 13 mm.
3. Mandibular body osteotomies to level mandibular occlusal plane.
4. Ten-mm Silastic implant to augment contour-deficient chin.
5. Rhinoplasty.

FOLLOW-UP

After the orthognathic surgery was completed, the need for rhinoplasty was more apparent.

Three months later, the rhinoplasty was performed. In addition to routine hump removal tip remodeling, a portion of the columella was resected to decrease the nasal tip projection. Although this was successful, it resulted in a bowing of the alar rims, which could have been avoided by means of modified Weir procedures.

Rhinoplasty: Jack P. Gunter, Dallas, Texas. *Maxillomandibular surgery:* Noel G. Stoker, Fresno, California; Bruce N. Epker, Fort Worth, Texas.

REFERENCE

1. Denecke HJ, Meyer R: Plastic surgery of the head and neck in correction and reconstructive rhinoplasty. Correction and Reconstructive Rhinoplasty, vol 1, Chap 1. New York: Springer-Verlag, Inc, 1967.

Chapter 16

MANAGEMENT OF SOFT TISSUES

Timothy A. Turvey and Raymond J. Fonseca

Improved techniques for correction of dentofacial deformities allow the surgeon the option of moving the entire facial skeleton, or any part of it, to achieve good facial balance and to obtain improved functional relationships. An appreciation of each patient's soft-tissue anatomy is critical since moving the underlying skeleton will alter the overlying soft-tissue drape to varying degrees. This chapter discusses management of soft tissues when designing skin incisions for access to the facial bones and describes several soft-tissue procedures that, when performed in conjunction with osseous surgery, can enhance facial balance. The focus in the chapter is selective: only problems commonly faced when correcting dentofacial deformities are discussed. Major problems of soft-tissue reconstruction are not within the scope of this chapter, and texts devoted to complicated soft-tissue problems should be consulted for detail.

PLACEMENT OF SKIN INCISIONS FOR ACCESS TO THE FACIAL SKELETON

The oral cavity is used often for surgical access to facial bones, which can be easily achieved when mucosal incisions are designed properly. One of the most significant benefits of using the oral route is the elimination of facial scarring. When the oral approach is not feasible, or if it will not allow sufficient exposure for the surgical procedure, then skin incisions are indicated. If skin incisions are used, it is imperative that every effort be made to minimize the resulting facial scar. Skin incisions can be acceptable cosmetically if general principles of soft-tissue management are observed:[9]

1. *Utilization of strategic locations for the placement of incisions.* Such locations include natural skin folds; along lines of tension, which usually run perpendicular to the underlying functional muscle groups ("favorable lines"); hair-bearing portions of the eyebrow or scalp; areas adjacent to the face such as the neck; and the junctures of two anatomic areas such as the ear and the cheek or the lips and the nose.

2. *Meticulous handling of all soft tissues.* Incisions should be made with sharp scalpel blades and generally at right angles to the skin surface. If hair-bearing tissue is utilized, the incision should parallel the hair follicles to avoid injury to these structures and a resulting non-hair-bearing scar. The tissues should be handled with fine sharp instruments as atraumatically as possible. In addition, attention must be directed to using aseptic techniques, providing adequate hemostasis, and assuring adequate blood supply to the wound edges.

3. *Careful approximation of the tissues during wound closure.* For best results, all dead space should be obliterated and a tension-free approximation of wound edges with eversion should be accomplished.

The availability of a wide variety of monofilament and braided suture material in different sizes with choice of needles allows for precise selection of sutures to suit the operative area and the desires of the surgeon. For example, areas such as the submental region are under more tension than infraorbital regions and require larger suture material (4-0 to 5-0 rather than 6-0). The suturing technique itself will vary according to the region of the face. It should be stressed that the atraumatic handling of tissue is more important to the overall appearance of the scar than the instruments or suture materials used during the surgery.

Basic principles of wound care must be applied in managing the operative site during the postoperative period to insure proper healing. A petroleum-based ointment should be placed over the suture lines immediately following wound closure to provide protection. The wound can be protected further by dressing it with a nonadhesive (cellophane) pad. Pressure dressings of fluffed gauze sponges and elasticized bandages may be applied also to aid hemostasis, decrease edema, and splint the wounds. The application of wound dressings depends on the specific surgical site and judgment of the surgeon. In general, dressings may be eliminated on the first or second postoperative day. Suture lines should be cleansed several times daily with a dilute solution of hydrogen peroxide and water (1:4); following each cleansing, petroleum-based ointment should be reapplied. Since the facial region is well vascularized, healing progresses more rapidly if dermal closure is adequate and tension-free. In general, sutures may be removed on the fourth or fifth postoperative day and adhesive strips may be applied to splint the wound edges for the next week. The importance of adhering to a strict and thorough postoperative care regimen cannot be overemphasized.

Approaches to the Mandible

Mandibular Body and Ramus

Extraoral approaches for mandibular surgery are preferred when limited mandibular opening or microstomia makes it difficult to expose the ramus or body of the mandi-

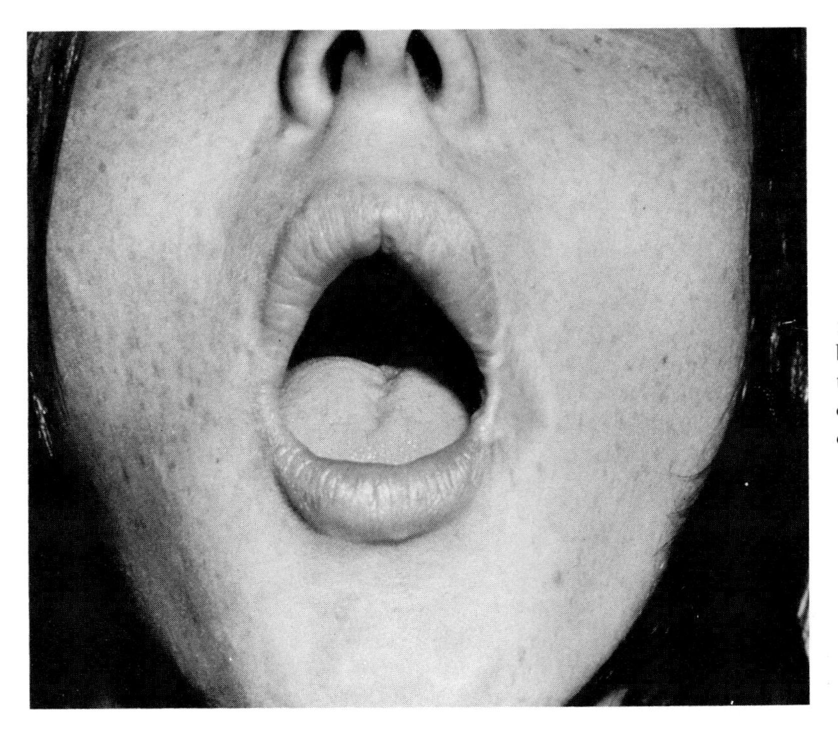

Figure 16–1. Microstomia secondary to an electrical burn scar at the commissure of the lip is an indication for an extraoral approach to the mandibular ramus.

ble by an oral approach (Fig. 16–1). Likewise, excessive mandibular prognathism (greater than 15 mm) may be treated more easily by an extraoral approach to the mandibular ramus to facilitate the posterior repositioning of the distal segment. To approach the mandibular ramus and body through the skin of the neck, the incision should be placed a finger's breadth below and parallel with the inferior border of the mandible. Preferably, the incision should be made in a natural skin crease and should be long enough to permit instrumentation (approximately 3 cm).

Technique (Fig. 16–2)

A line of incision should be enscribed on the neck with the blunt tip of a scalpel blade, and two or three cross-hatches perpendicular to this mark will provide a guide for accurate approximation of the skin edges at the time of closure. Following infiltration with a dilute solution of a vasoconstrictor (epinephrine, 1:100,000 or 1:200,000), an incision should be made through the skin to the superficial fascial layer. Sharp dissection will be enhanced by placing the area to be incised under tension. The skin should be undermined through the superior and inferior aspects of the incision with dissecting scissors or scalpel to define the cutaneous plane. Sharp dissection may be used to deepen the wound to the platysma muscle; blunt dissection through the platysma and superficial layer of the deep cervical fascia may avoid injury to the branches of the facial nerve that run just superficial to this fascial layer. In cadavers, the marginal mandibular branch of the facial nerve has been found by dissection to be cephalad to the inferior border of the mandible in the region of the angle and body in 81 of 100 specimens.[2] These data, obtained from normal specimens, may not necessarily apply to patients with dentofacial deformities since these patients also may have other anomalies. The facial artery and vein are almost always located anterior to the masticator sling in the superficial layer of the deep cervical (investing) fascia, and these vessels should be retracted out of the field or clamped and tied. The facial nerve anterior to the masticator sling is usually lateral to the facial vein but varies in its relationship to the facial artery. Once the masticator sling is incised and the subperiosteal dissection completed, adequate exposure to the mandibular vertical ramus, mandibular body, coronoid process, and neck of the condyle can be obtained. Properly designed retractors and adequate lighting are necessary for optimum exposure and visibility of these areas. Closure of the wound in layers will be enhanced by carefully defining each plane of dissection (masticator sling, fascia, platysma, subcutaneous tissues, and skin), and hematomas can be avoided by meticulous hemostasis during the dissection, closure of all dead space, and postsurgical application of a pressure dressing.

Mandibular Symphysis

Most deformities in the area of the mandibular symphysis can be approached transorally, but on rare occasions it is necessary to approach the mandibular symphy-

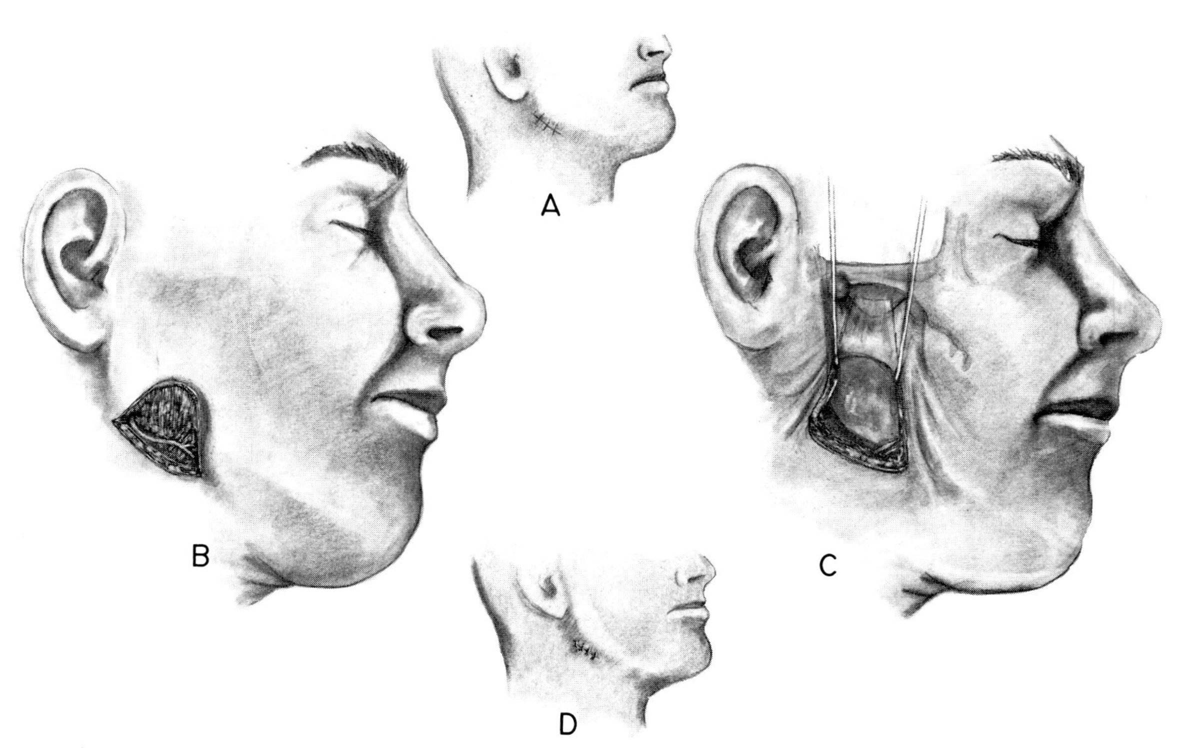

Figure 16–2. Extraoral approach to the mandibular body and ramus. *A,* A 3-cm incision scribed on the neck in a natural wrinkle line and crossed-hatched perpendicular to this mark to facilitate accurate approximation of the wound edges. *B,* Soft-tissue dissection demonstrating the relationship of the marginal mandibular branch of the facial nerve lateral to the facial artery and vein at the antegonial notch. *C,* Exposure of the mandibular angle, body, and ramus; the coronoid process; and the condylar neck. *D,* Closure of incision with interrupted permanent sutures.

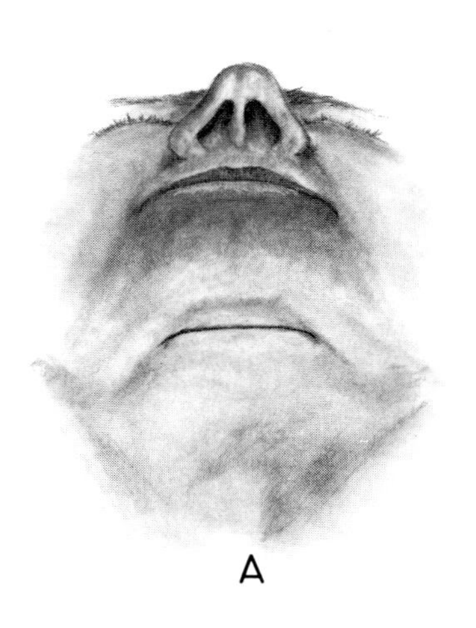

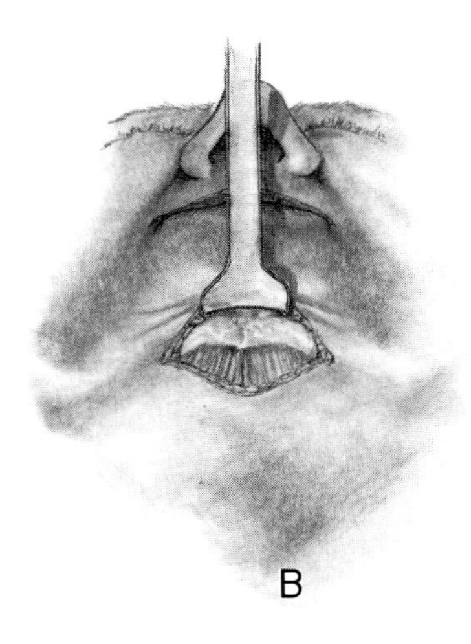

Figure 16–3. Extraoral approach to the mandibular symphysis. *A*, Incision placed in a natural submental skin crease. *B*, Exposure of the inferior border of mandible can be obtained without injuring any major anatomic structures.

sis extraorally. An incision along natural skin lines at the inferior border of the mandible, confined to the submental crease, will permit exposure to the area (Fig. 16–3). Locating this incision below the symphysis results in a well-concealed scar. Good results are obtainable when the planes of dissection are defined, the tissues are handled carefully, and meticulous wound closure is performed. This dissection can be performed without fear of damaging any major nerve or vascular structures.

Mandibular Condyle

Surgical procedures involving the temporomandibular joint require exposure of the articular surface of the mandibular condyle and the joint space. The preauricular approach, with an anterosuperior extension in the hair-bearing area of the scalp, allows good surgical access and will result in a satisfactory postoperative appearance.

Technique (Fig. 16–4)

Preauricular hair and the hair of the scalp superior and anterior to the outer helix of the ear must be shaved in the preparation immediately before surgery. An occlusive dressing placed in the external auditory canal prevents blood from accumulating along the canal and tympanic membrane. After the incision has been marked on the skin and cross-hatched with the reverse side of a scalpel blade, the entire region should be infiltrated with a dilute solution of vasoconstrictor (epinephrine 1:100,000 or 1:200,000).

The incision should extend from just anterior and superior to the earlobe to 5 to 6 mm above the tragus and then curved anteriorly and superiorly at 45° into the scalp. When the incision is placed approximately 5 to 6 millimeters anterior to the tragus, as advocated by Walker,[16] there is direct access to the joint and the superficial temporal vessels remain posteriorly. Once the skin is incised, it should be undermined anteriorly and sutured back to the cheek for self-retention.

The dissection is deepened to the fascia overlying the zygomatic arch and hemostasis is obtained. Care should be taken to avoid the branches of the facial nerve that normally course anterior to the plane of dissection at the level of the parotidomasseteric fascia. If the transverse facial artery impedes access to the joint, it should be ligated, transected, and retracted. The superficial temporal vessels should be identified and retracted posteriorly or ligated and transected. The auriculotemporal nerve also may be identified with the vessels and retracted out of the field.

Some surgeons believe that interruption of the auriculotemporal nerve will minimize postoperative joint pain, but we do not recommend that the nerve be transected. The potential complications of this neural interruption (e.g., gustatory sweating) may outweigh the benefits. Pain referred from distant visceral structures may focus in the temporomandibular joint even if the auriculotemporal nerve is interrupted.[7] Since this nerve supplies only part of the sensory innervation of the joint, interrupting its course may not provide total relief.

When the zygomatic arch is reached and the joint capsule is identified, an intra-articular injection of a vasoconstrictor (epinephrine 1:100,000) should precede a cruciate or T-shaped incision through the capsule, which will provide adequate exposure of the condyle. After completion of the condylar procedure, the joint capsule should be approximated with absorbable sutures and the wound closed in layers. The dressing should be removed from the external ear canal and the canal should be irrigated to remove any blood that may have collected during the procedure. A pressure dressing should be applied to the operative site to assist in the prevention of hematoma formation and to support the wound in the first few postoperative days.

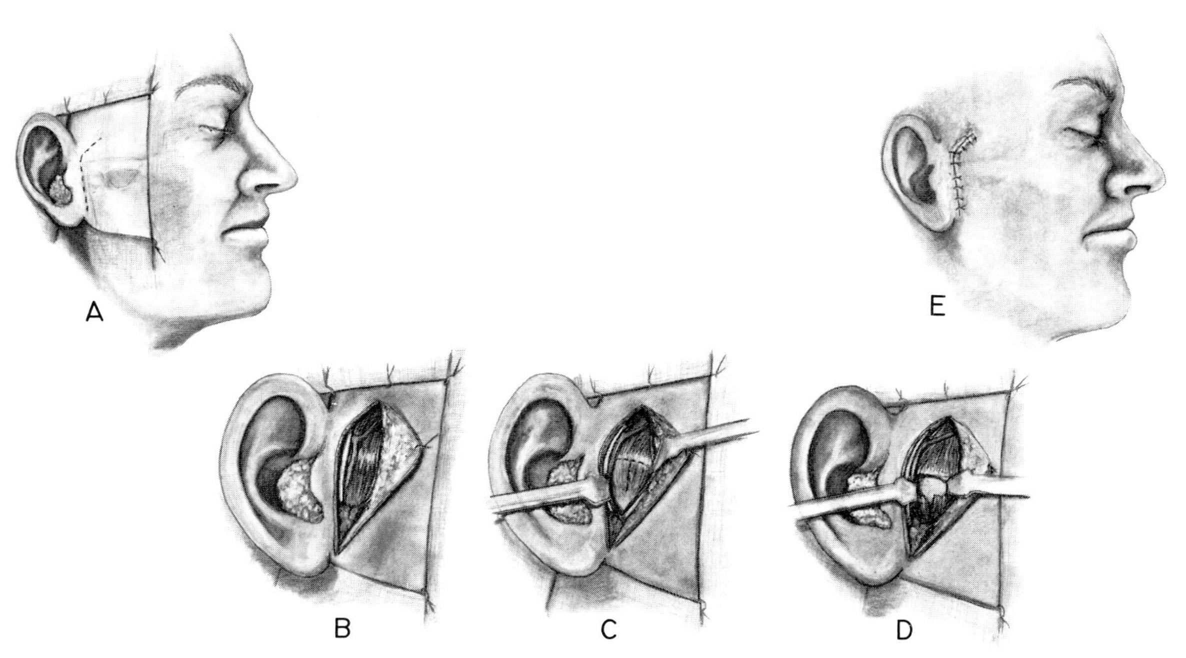

Figure 16–4. Preauricular approach to the temporomandibular joint and mandibular condyle. *A,* Outline of incision, 5 to 6 mm anterior to tragus, extending superiorly from the earlobe and carried anteriorly into the scalp. *B,* Note the posterior relationship of the superficial temporal vessels and the auriculotemporal nerve and the anterior relationship of the facial nerve. *C,* T-shaped incision enscribed on the joint capsule. *D,* Exposure of the condylar head. *E,* Closure with interrupted permanent sutures.

Approach to the Midface

Several surgical procedures require access to the upper midfacial region. Congenital deformities such as craniofacial synostosis (Crouzon's syndrome, Apert's syndrome), developmental deformities, and acquired deformities such as malunited midfacial fractures are managed through midfacial incisions. Adequate exposure can be obtained through incisions placed in the scalp or in skin folds. The area of the middle face lends itself well to concealing incisions, and there should be no hesitation to use skin incisions routinely when transoral exposure is not adequate (Fig. 16–5).

Inferior Lid Incision

The inferior orbital rim, the orbital floor, and the lateral wall of the maxilla can be approached by an incision made in the inferior eyelid. This standard incision also can be modified to provide access to adjacent structures. A stepped incision in the lid avoids a unified scar that shortens the lid height and a possible postoperative ectropion.

Technique (Fig. 16–6)

The inferior lid should be studied to identify natural skin folds. Placing the incision in a natural skin crease 5 to 8 mm inferior to the lid margin (more inferior laterally than medially) will conceal the scar well and provide for good venous and

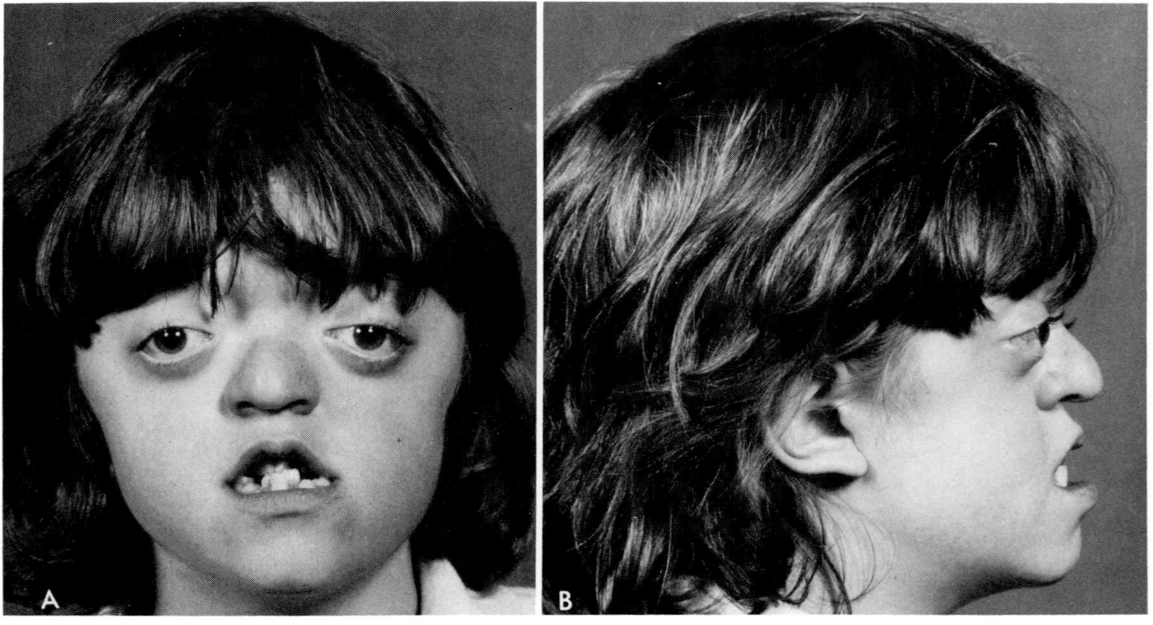

Figure 16–5. Example of a patient with Apert's syndrome requiring access to the upper midfacial region during surgical correction of the facial deformities. *A,* Full face view. *B,* Profile.

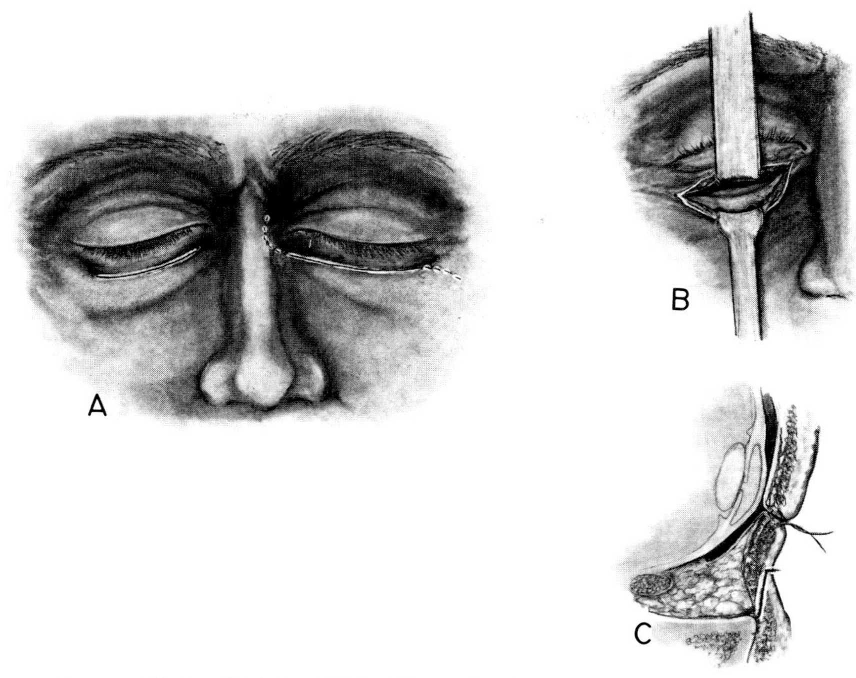

Figure 16–6. Inferior lid incision. *A*, The incision is placed 5 to 8 mm inferior to the lid margin in a natural crease extending lower laterally than medially; note on the right the lateral and medial extensions of this incision if greater access is required. *B*, Exposure of inferior orbital rim, orbital floor, and lateral maxilla. *C*, Lateral view illustrating the stepped dissection of the inferior lid through skin and orbicularis oculi muscle but superficial to septum orbitale.

lymphatic drainage. Once the incision is made through the skin, it should be undermined inferiorly and the dissection should be deepened through the orbicularis oculi muscle at a more caudal level than the skin incision. Care must be taken not to violate the septum orbitale (the extension of the orbital periosteum into the lid itself). When the level of the orbital rim is reached, an incision is made through the remaining orbicularis oculi muscle and the overlying periosteum just inferior to the rim. Subperiosteal dissection into the orbit and around the rim will expose the orbital rim, the floor of the orbit, the inferior orbital fissure, the lateral maxilla, and the infraorbital neurovascular bundle.

Extending the skin incision farther laterally and inferiorly in a natural wrinkle line provides access to the inferior lateral orbital rim and zygomatic buttress and arch (Fig. 16–7).

Carrying the incision medially and superiorly along the frontal process of the maxilla and the nasal bone exposes the medial orbital wall, the nasal bones, the frontonasal suture, the medial canthal tendon, and the lacrimal apparatus. The angular artery and vein usually are encountered during this medial approach and must be ligated. When using this modification, one should take care to place the incision far enough away from the medial canthus to avoid severing the medial canthal tendon and to avoid webbing postoperatively.

When the procedure has been completed the incision must be closed in two layers: the periosteum should be apposed with interrupted absorbable sutures,

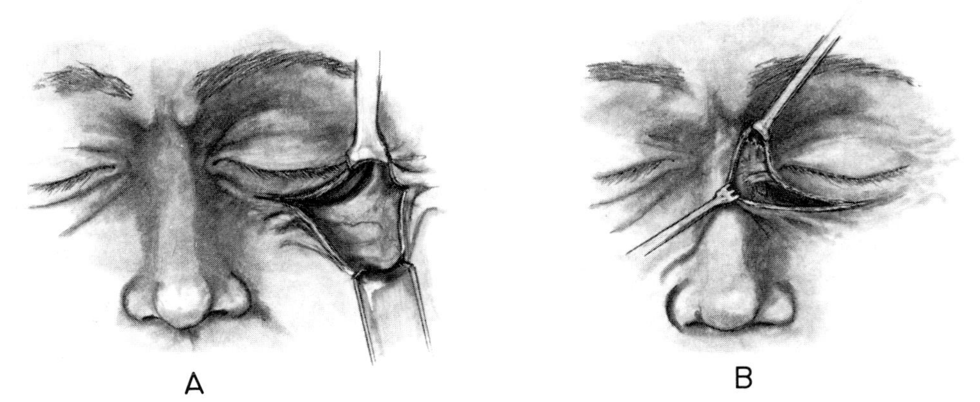

Figure 16–7. Lateral and medial extensions of the lid incision. *A,* Lateral extension exposing the lateral orbital wall and the zygomatic buttress and arch. Note the incision follows the natural skin lines. *B,* Medial extension exposing the medial orbital wall, nasal bones, frontonasal suture, medial canthal tendon, and nasolacrimal apparatus.

whereas the loose skin of the lid can be approximated with removable sutures in a horizontal mattress fashion for eversion of the skin edges (Fig. 16–8). The closure provides good esthetic results when principles of soft-tissue management are followed.

Brow Incision (Fig. 16–9)

Access to the superior lateral orbital rim, lateral orbital wall, and inferior orbital fissure can be gained by an incision in the inferior portion of the eyebrow along the orbital rim. Since the incision is placed in the unshaven hair-bearing portion of the brow, the residual scar remains well camouflaged if the incision follows the direction of the hair follicles (Fig. 16–10). Terminal branches of the superficial temporal vessels commonly are encountered during the dissection; these should be clamped and tied or retracted. Following closure of the periosteum, the remaining tissues can be apposed in one or two layers to assure a thin scar.

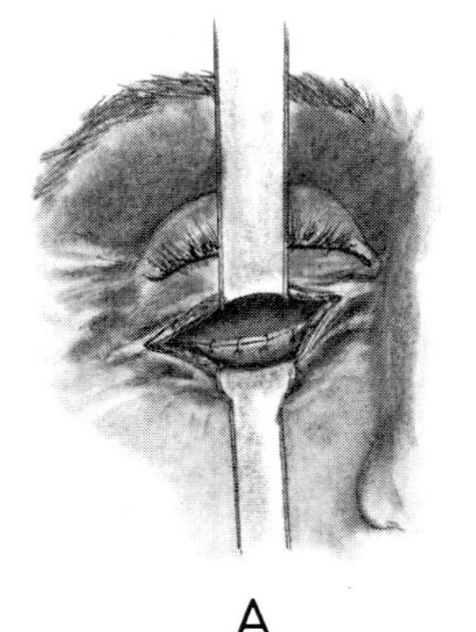

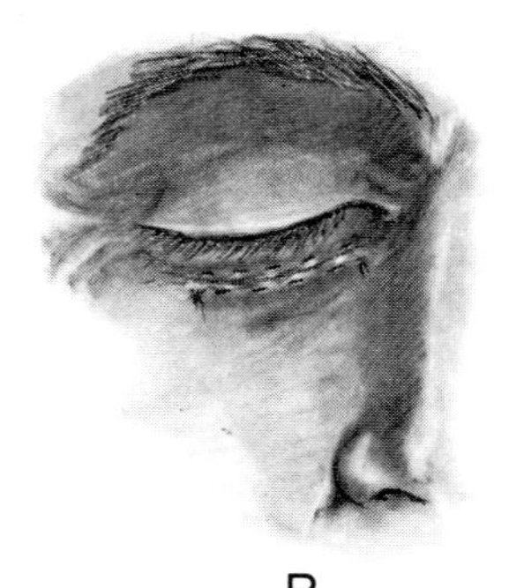

Figure 16–8. Layered closure of the inferior lid incision. *A,* Periosteum apposed with interrupted absorbable sutures. *B,* Skin closure with permanent horizontal mattress sutures to obtain eversion of skin edges.

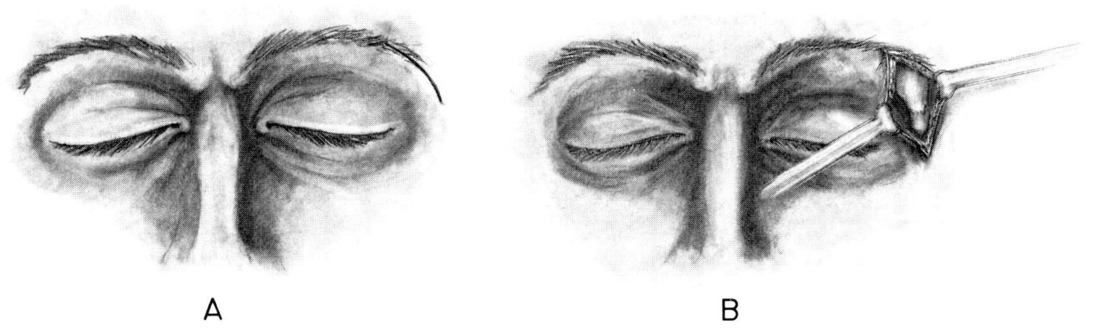

Figure 16–9. Brow incision. *A,* The incision is partially concealed in the hair-bearing portion of brow. *B,* Exposure of the superior lateral orbital rim and lateral orbital wall.

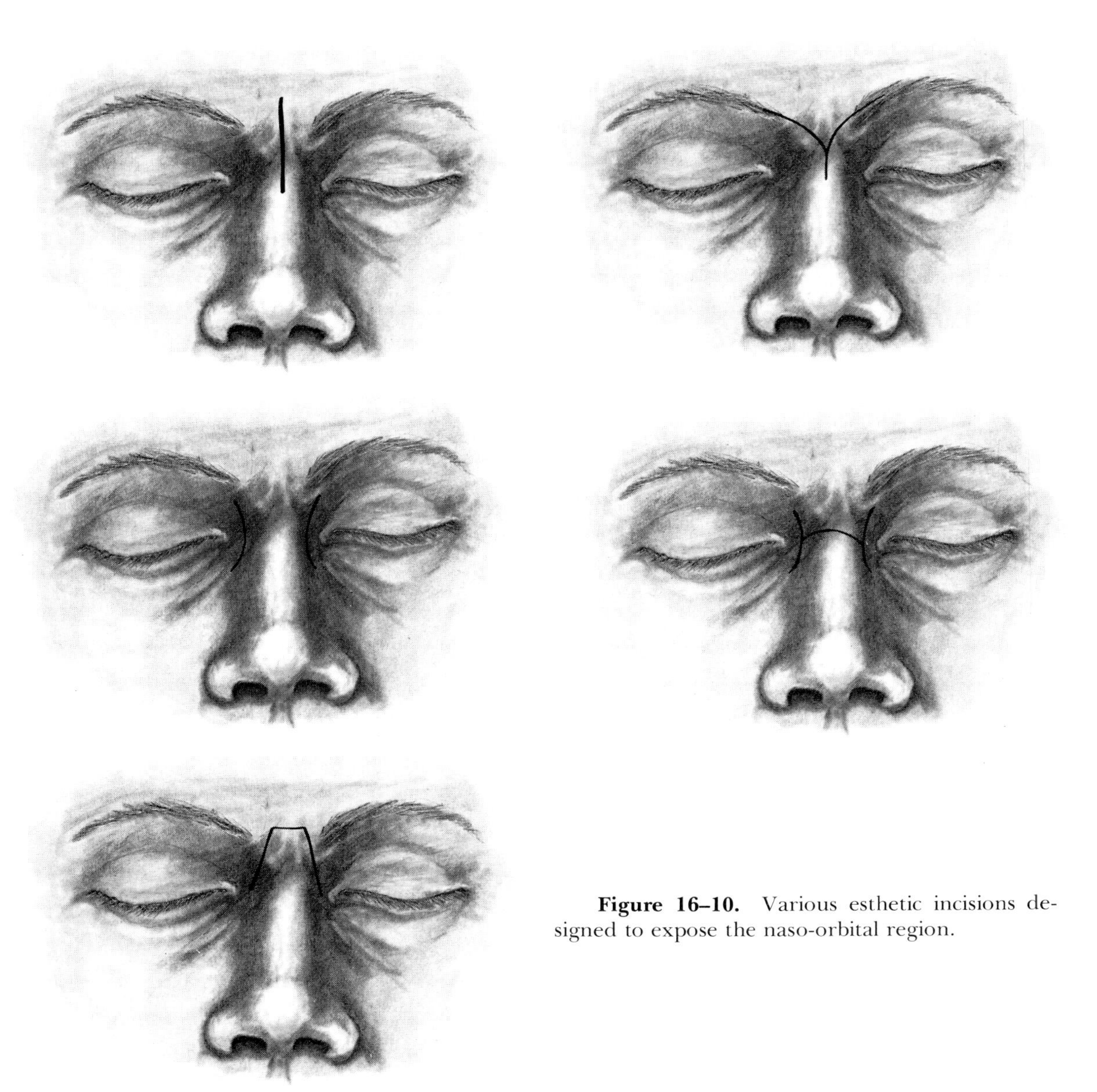

Figure 16–10. Various esthetic incisions designed to expose the naso-orbital region.

Naso-orbital Incisions

The frontonasal region can be exposed by a medial superior extension of the inferior lid incision, (see Fig. 16–7), by a separate incision on the nasal dorsum, or by a bitemporal flap. When access to this region alone is necessary, the first two approaches will afford adquate exposure, but when the superior orbital rims and forehead must be exposed, a bitemporal flap is suggested.

Various incisions on the nasal dorsum have been described, but because this area is very prominent and noticeable, care must be taken to minimize the effect of scarring. The tissues overlying the dorsum of the nose are thin and comparatively fixed. Dissection in this region can be executed in one layer. Bleeding may occur if the supratrochlear or dorsalis nasi vessels are violated during the procedure. The wound should be closed in one or two layers.

Figure 16–10 illustrates the various facial incisions for approaching the naso-orbital region. All have been found to provide adequate exposure for instrumentation of this area.

BITEMPORAL FLAP

The bitemporal flap provides access to the forehead, the superior orbital rims, the naso-orbital region, the lateral orbital rims, and the zygomatic areas. It leaves few visable traces of the incision. The tissues of the flap are pedicled to the skin of the face and remain well vascularized by the numerous collateral blood vessels supplying the face and orbit. Elevation of the scalp provides visualization of the forehead, frontonasal region, superior orbital rim, supraorbital neurovascular bundle, medial orbital wall, medial canthal tendon, lacrimal apparatus, lateral canthal tendon, and lateral orbital rim, and of the lateral orbital wall to the inferior orbital fissure and zygomatic buttress and arch. When the bitemporal flap is combined with an inferior lid incision, the entire orbit and midfacial osseous structure can be exposed.

Technique (Fig. 16–11)

The scalp should be shaved from the anterior hairline to 2 cm posterior to the ear. The injection of a copious amount of saline into the supraperiosteal layer of the scalp prior to the incision will aid the dissection and in hemostasis. The incision is begun just anterior to the superior attachment of the outer helix of the ear and is carried superiorly across the midline of the scalp to the same position on the opposite side. It may be extended further inferiorly and anteriorly if greater access to the medial portions of the zygomatic buttress and inferior orbital rim is needed. The incision is made superficial to the temporalis fascia and the periosteum. Bleeding should be controlled on both sides of the dissection with scalp clips as the flap is reflected. The supraperiosteal plane should be utilized to carry the dissection to the forehead anteriorly. The periosteum should then be incised and the remainder of the dissection should be completed subperiosteally to the orbits, nasal bones, and zygoma. The supraorbital neurovascular bundle can be identified exiting from its foramen and can be dissected, and protected.

A large W incision through the periosteum overlying the forehead will facilitate

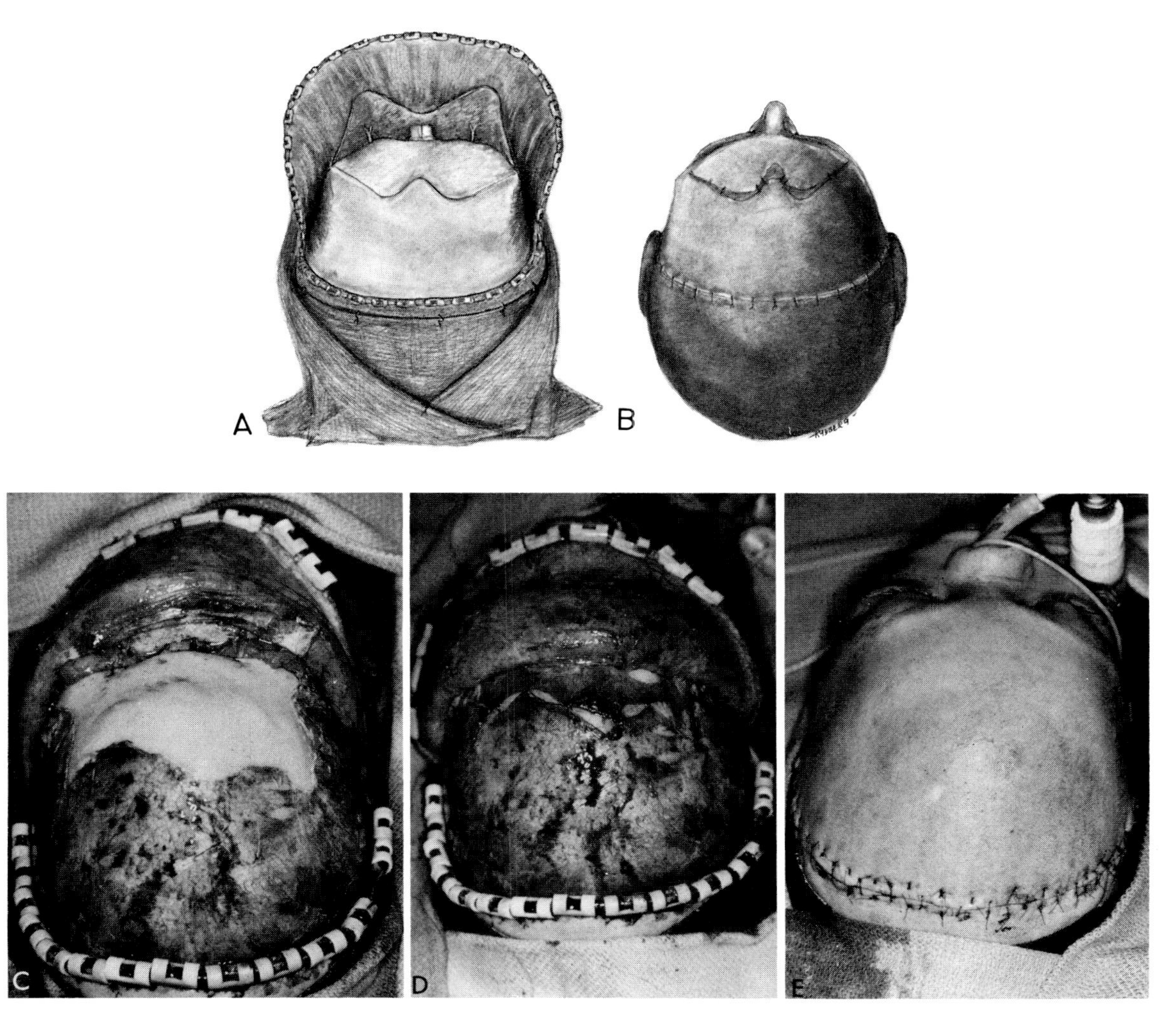

Figure 16–11. Bitemporal flap. *A,* Exposure of the forehead, superior orbital rims, naso-orbital region, lateral orbital rims, and zygomatic area is possible; note the superior orbital neurovascular bundle extending from the foramen into the flap. *B,* W-shaped periosteal incision closed at points following midfacial advancement leaves defects distant from the remainder of the scalp closure. *C–E,* Clinical photographs illustrating bitemporal flap and closure technique.

periosteal approximation when the middle face has been advanced or when grafts have been placed on the superior orbital rims. This incision maintains a distance between the scalp closure site and the periosteal defects and any bone graft or surgical defect. The remainder of the scalp can be stretched if necessary to achieve primary closure at a site distant from the area of surgery. When the operation of the upper midface is completed and closure has begun, the periosteum should be apposed with absorbable or permanent sutures.

Midfacial advancement or onlay bone grafts placed on the supraorbital rims or forehead will cause periosteal defects to persist. Point closure of the W incision in the periosteum will correct this deficiency somewhat in some instances but will leave defects over a portion of the calvaria in others. The remainder of the scalp can be closed in the subcutaneous and skin layers. A pressure dressing should be applied to prevent hematoma and to keep the scalp well adapted to the underlying skull. Drains may also be placed at the discretion of the surgeon if adequate hemostasis cannot be obtained.

MANAGEMENT OF MEDIAL CANTHAL TENDONS AND THE LACRIMAL APPARATUS

When osteotomies are performed on the medial orbital walls, the lacrimal sac must be identified, dissected, and protected. The anterior and posterior parts of the medial canthal tendon occasionally are detached from the anterior and posterior lacrimal crests (Fig. 16–12). The anterior slip of the tendon, which is the larger of the two, attaches to the frontal process of the maxilla along the anterior lacrimal crest. According to Robinson and Stranc,[14] the attachment is approximately 25 mm^2 in size and accounts for the sharpness of the medial portion of the palpebral fold. The posterior part of the tendon contains the small Horner's muscle, which inserts on the posterior lacrimal crest of the lacrimal bone. The lacrimal sac lies between the two tendon attachments and must be protected during surgery (see Fig. 16–12).

As the wound is closed, the anterior portion of the canthal tendon *must* be reattached in order to prevent or minimize telecanthus. The technique of canthopexy as advocated by Wolford and Epker[18] consists of a mattress suture through each tendon (Fig. 16–13). These sutures are then passed transnasally through small drill holes on the anterior lacrimal crests to the opposite tendon where they are secured in mattress style. Additional transnasal sutures are passed through the skin overlying the tendon, thus securing each tendon and the skin of the opposite medial canthal region. These sutures are tied over bolsters to provide more medial support for the tendons and to help readapt soft tissues around the medial portions of the orbit and nose. After being properly secured, each tendon is supported by three sutures, two of which will remain in place. The sutures tied over the bolsters may be removed in five days. Stainless steel wires, and more recently, Supramid and Prolene sutures, have been successfully used for this canthopexy technique.

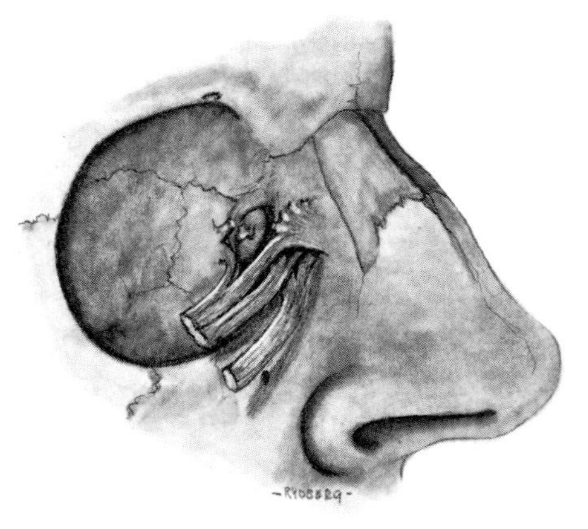

Figure 16–12. Medial canthal tendon and lacrimal apparatus. The relationship of the anterior and posterior slips of the medial canthal tendon to the lacrimal apparatus and medial orbital wall is illustrated. The lacrimal sac lies between the anterior and posterior slips of the medial canthal tendon. Note the larger anterior slip of the tendon, which is primarily responsible for the sharp medial palpebral fold.

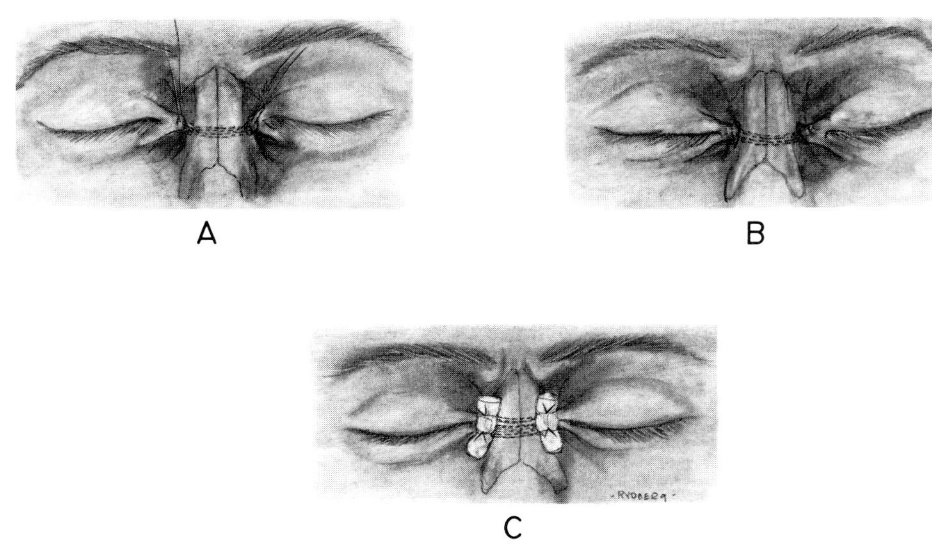

Figure 16–13. Medial canthopexy technique. *A,* Bilateral horizontal mattress sutures ligate the medial canthal tendons and are passed transnasally to the opposite tendons. *B,* Transnasal horizontal mattress sutures securing medial canthal tendons to each other. *C,* Additional transnasal canthopexy sutures exit the skin and are tied over cotton bolsters to provide extra medial support to the medial canthal tendons and overlying tissues.

ADJUNCTIVE SOFT-TISSUE PROCEDURES

When soft-tissue deformities and skeletal abnormalities exist concomitantly, they must be distinguished and considered separately. The timing and sequencing of osseous surgery and soft-tissue corrective procedures are important for achieving satisfactory and predictable results. The underlying skeletal framework usually is corrected first, and soft-tissue procedures are deferred until a later time; occasionally it is possible to do both simultaneously. The patient who has a cleft lip and palate with resultant maxillary deficiency and a compromised soft-tissue veneer is a classic example. Surgical-orthodontic or surgical-prosthetic reconstructive procedures should be performed initially to be followed by lip and nasal revisions. If the sequence were reversed, the osseous surgery could distort an excellent soft-tissue result. The remainder of this chapter describes various soft-tissue procedures that can be performed in conjunction with dento-osseous repositioning or as secondary procedures to improve esthetics and enhance facial balance.

Chin-Neck Contour

In the normally contoured chin and neck, an angle at the level of the hyoid bone represents an alteration in the direction of the skin drape from horizontal to vertical (Fig. 16–14). Patients who present with a straight or very obtuse throat form should be examined carefully to ascertain the cause. Four anatomic situations can contribute to the lack of chin-neck contour: (1) retrogenia, (2) hypertrophy of the submental fat

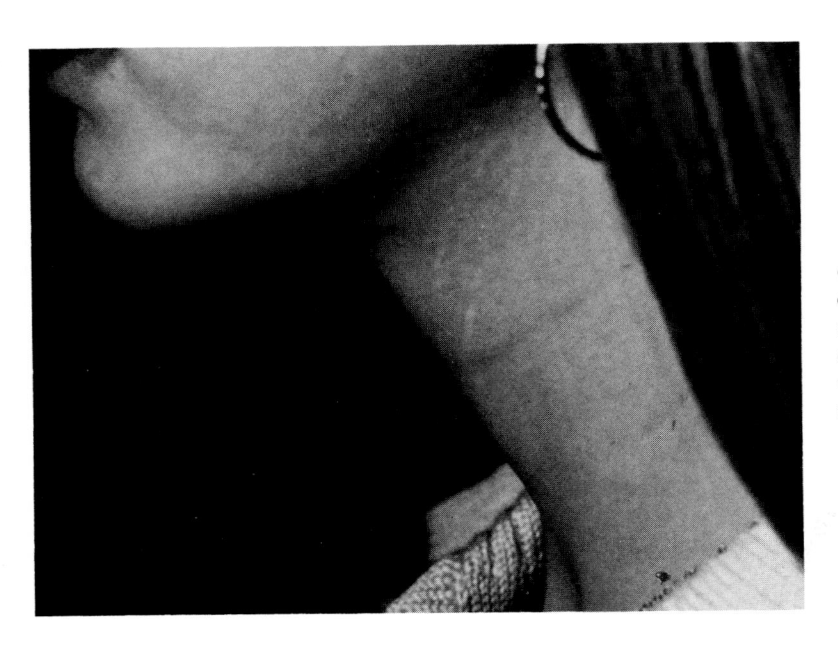

Figure 16–14. Normal chin-neck contour. This angled contour represents an alteration in the direction of skin drape from a horizontal to a vertical direction at the level of the hyoid bone.

pad, (3) inferior positioning of the hyoid bone, and (4) aging cutaneous tissues. If any of these conditions is present either individually or in combination, the patient's appearance will be compromised. The first two conditions can be corrected with the expectation that results will be stable. When the hyoid bone is involved, however, long-term successful correction of the inferior position is doubtful. This bone is freely suspended by multiple muscle groups, and its position is determined by resting muscle posture. According to Mareno and associates,[12] its normal position is at the level of the fourth cervical vertebra, placing it superior to the inferior border of the mandibular symphysis in most patients. The position of the hyoid bone is shifted temporarily by some maxillary and mandibular surgical procedures, but it tends to return to its original position after several months. Although stable correction of the source of the deformity (inferior position of the hyoid bone) is doubtful, submental lipectomy, augmentation genioplasty, or both may improve chin and neck contour in such patients if retrogenia and hypertrophy of submental fat are present.

The problem of chin-neck contour deformity caused by aging cutaneous tissues is beyond the scope of this chapter. Face lifting procedures may be beneficial in correcting this deformity if cervical and facial tissues are sagging. Best results in correcting this problem by rhytidectomy can be obtained when the hyoid bone is in a normal or superior position. Improvement will be limited if the hyoid bone is inferiorly positioned.[9]

The chin and neck area must be carefully evaluated when treating mandibular excess, especially in obese patients, for the patient who trades his mandibular prognathism for a "turkey gobbler" postoperative appearance may be less than satisfied (Fig. 16–15). If such a problem is anticipated, alternative dento-osseous maneuvers may prevent the occurrence of this deformity or plans may be made to correct it secondarily. If other procedures do not produce satisfactory functional and cosmetic results, the excess soft tissue can be managed by submental lipectomy with resuspension of the skin or, as reported by Neuner,[13] an ellipsoid excision of the redundant tissue of the neck followed by plication. If an abnormally large submental fat pad is present, it can be removed easily through a submental incision (Fig. 16–16). This approach should be used only in those patients with an isolated hypertrophied fat pad and should be avoided in patients with generalized obesity. Such patients should be reevaluated and treated only after they have lost weight. The procedure may be combined with an augmentation genioplasty or other soft-tissue procedures to improve the contour.

Technique (Fig. 16–17)

A 3-cm horizontal incision is made in the submental crease and carried through the skin into the subcutaneous tissues, maintaining hemostasis. Two planes of dissection should be established with the fat pad in between. The superficial level should include skin and a thin layer of fat. The deeper plane should be superficial to the platysma muscle and should include another thin layer of fat. Leaving the skin and muscle layers lined with fat will prevent the skin from healing directly to the muscle. If skin-muscle healing takes place, the improved contour will distort during function. The dissection may be deepened through the platysma muscle if there is an additional pad of fat under this structure. Care must be taken when entering the deeper plane to avoid injury to branches of the facial nerve.[17]

The fat pad is dissected and removed, and several subcutaneous sutures are placed in strategic locations to achieve the desired angular contour (Fig. 16–17). These sutures should be directed from the subcutaneous plane posteriorly and su-

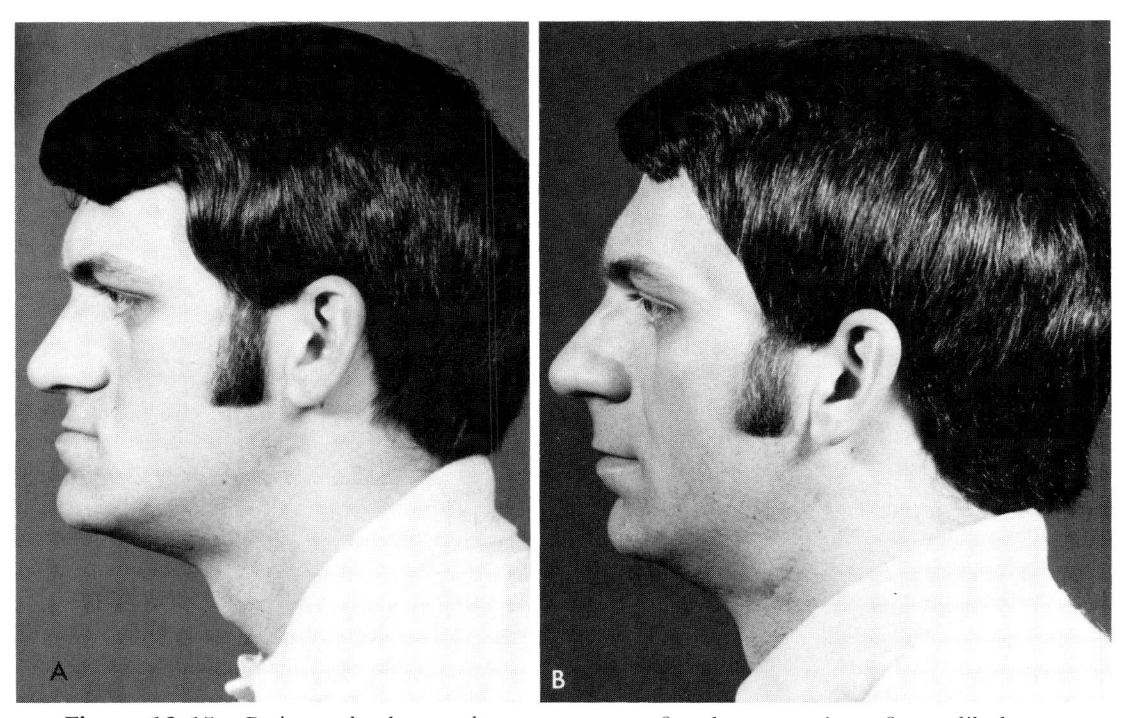

Figure 16–15. Patient who has undergone surgery for the correction of mandibular excess. Resultant "turkey gobbler" neck appearance detracts from the final esthetic result. *A,* Preoperative. *B,* Postoperative.

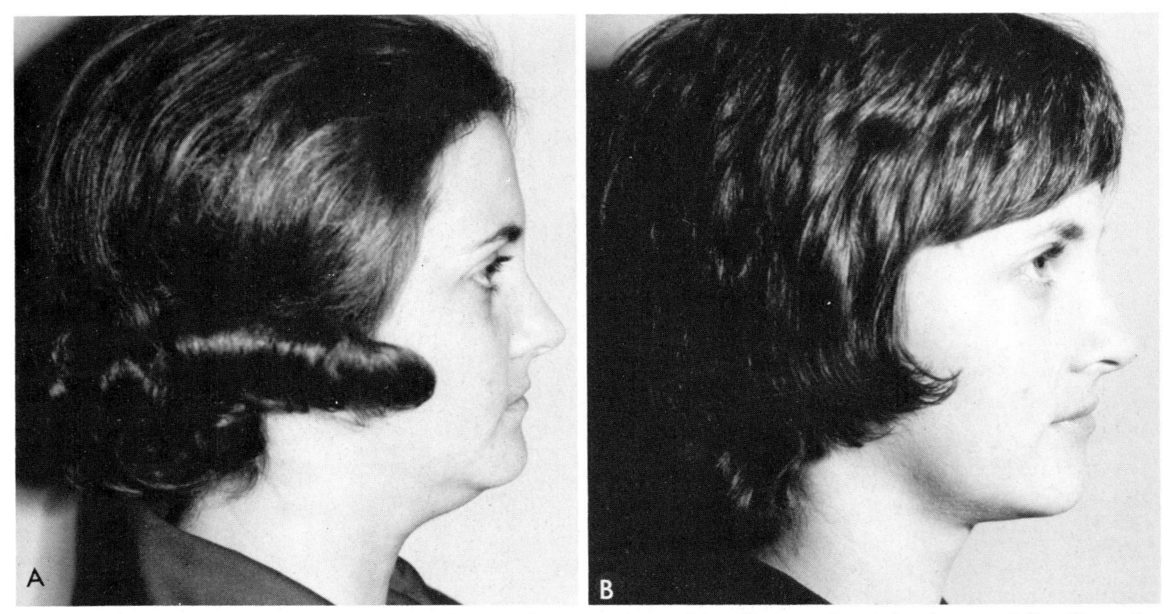

Figure 16–16. Patient with poor chin-neck contour resulting from enlarged submental fat. Note the preoperative and postoperative changes following maxillary surgery and submental lipectomy as described in Figure 16–17. *A*, Preoperative. *B*, Postoperative.

periorly and embedded in the deep tissues of the neck. Judicious placement of these key sutures will properly suspend the skin, stabilize neck contour, and prevent hematoma formation. The skin must not be dimpled by the sutures, since unnatural folds will detract from the result. The remainder of the incision should be closed in two layers, and a pressure dressing should be placed over the operative site.

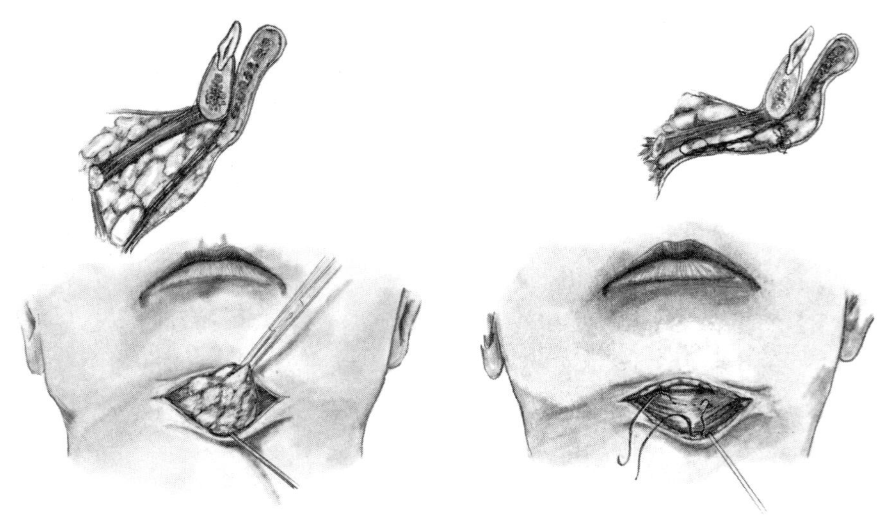

Figure 16–17. Submental lipectomy technique illustrating the removal of excess fat superficial and deep to the platysma muscle and resuspension of the cutaneous tissues posteriorly and superiorly.

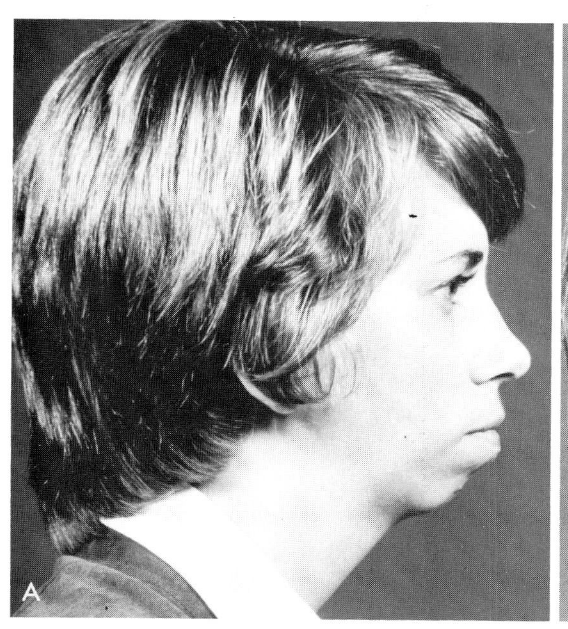

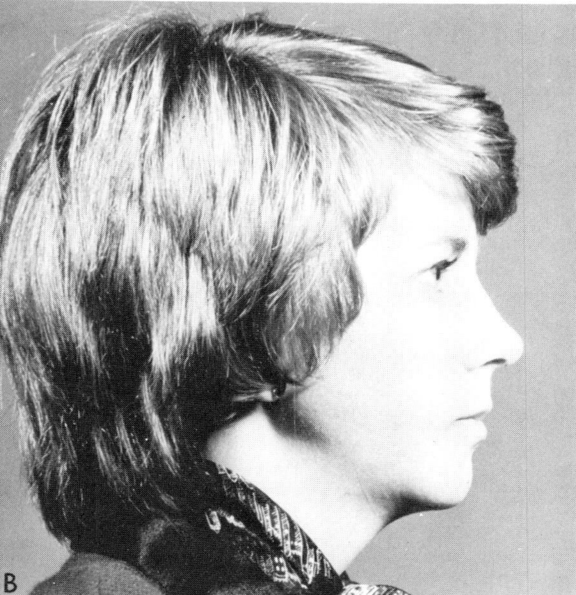

Figure 16–18. Abnormal chin-neck contour coexisting with retrogenia. Note preoperative and postoperative changes following anterior maxillary osteotomy, mandibular subapical osteotomy with retraction of both segments and augmentation genioplasty. *A*, Preoperative. *B*, Postoperative.

Augmentation genioplasty dramatically improves the straight chin-neck contour when it coexists with retrogenia (Fig. 16–18). Alloplastic materials or a pedicled osseous graft used to augment the chin will stretch the soft tissues of the neck and chin and result in a more pleasing and normal form. Surgical techniques for chin augmentation are described in Chapter 14.

Correction of Soft-tissue Ptosis of the Chin

Even distribution of fat and muscle around the face enhances facial contours and esthetics. Hypertrophied soft tissues underlying the mandibular symphysis, with or without an osseous deformity, will produce an unattractive facial appearance. A long and flabby chin may exaggerate the submental crease, whereas a hypertrophied fat pad may deaccentuate or obliterate it. The chin area must be examined while the patient's lips are relaxed, because lip strain will produce an unnatural soft-tissue drape. Lateral facial radiographs will help to distinguish between primary deformities of soft tissues of the chin and those due to underlying osseous deformities. A vertically enlarged, unsightly soft tissue mass should be dealt with directly, because restructuring the underlying skeleton will not correct this abnormality. Gonzales-Ulloa[5] describes a procedure that corrects vertical overhanging tissue of the chin (Fig. 16–19); this procedure can be combined with a submental lipectomy or augmentation genioplasty where indicated (Fig. 16–20). The procedure removes the excess tissue and closes the defect in a Y pattern, eliminating ptosis and projecting the soft-tissue pogonion forward slightly.

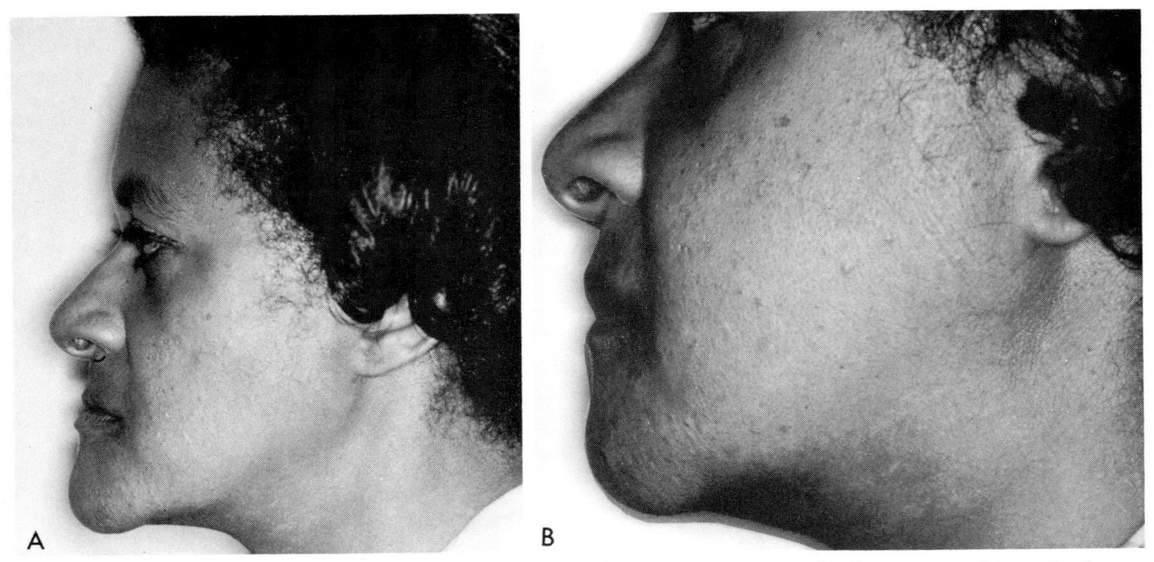

Figure 16–19. *A,* Soft-tissue ptosis of the chin coexisting with mandibular prognathism. *B,* Same patient after mandibular retropositioning procedure and correction of soft-tissue ptosis by technique illustrated in Figure 16–21.

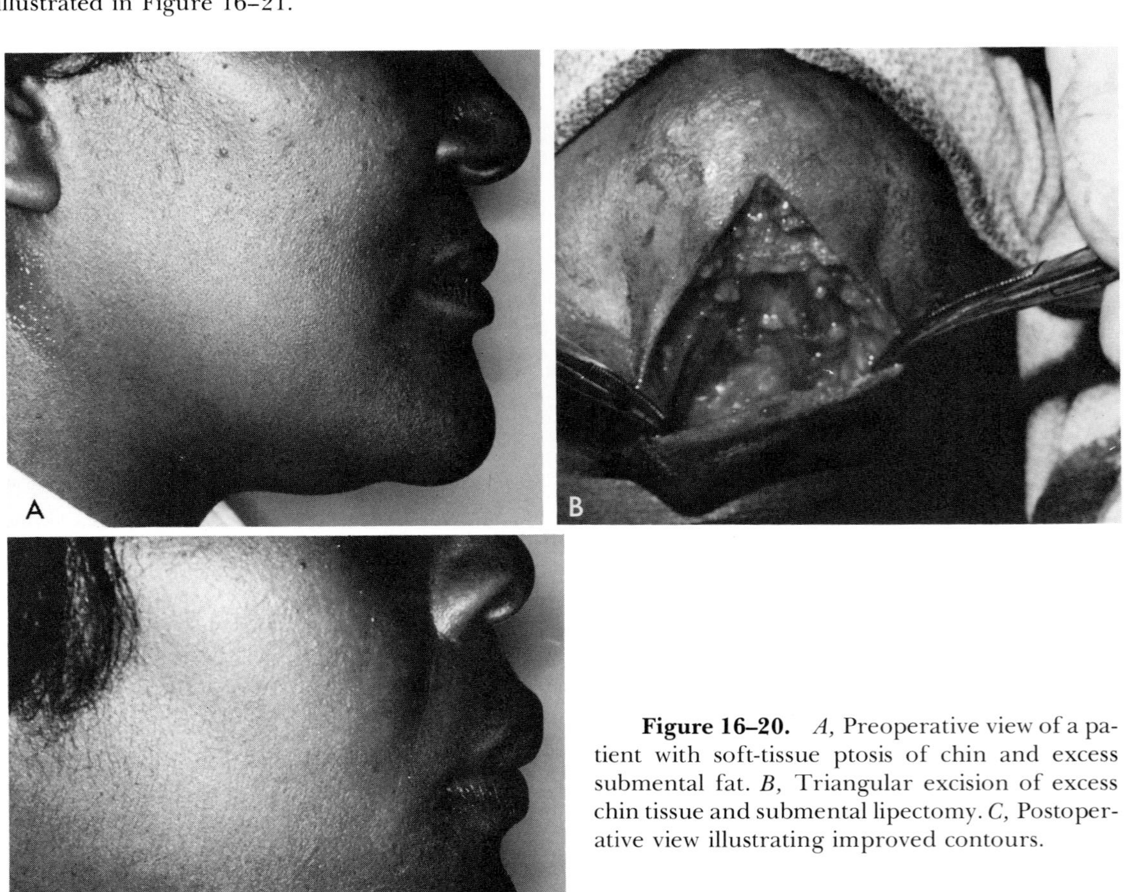

Figure 16–20. *A,* Preoperative view of a patient with soft-tissue ptosis of chin and excess submental fat. *B,* Triangular excision of excess chin tissue and submental lipectomy. *C,* Postoperative view illustrating improved contours.

Technique (Fig. 16–21)

The midline of the soft-tissue symphysis is identified, and a point midway on the curvature of the inferior border is marked. The submental crease is identified, and the two ends are marked where the crease runs across the subsymphyseal region. The triangle that is formed by connecting the three points indicates the amount of tissue to be removed. The amount of curvature of the two sides of the triangle whose apex is the point on the symphysis is inversely proportional to the amount of tissue to be excised; the greater the curvature of the two sides of the triangle, the less soft tissue will be removed.

The tissue is incised on a bevel, removing a greater amount of subcutaneous tissue than skin. The incisions are carried through the subcutaneous layer to a point just superficial to the periosteum, and the triangular mass of tissue is dissected and discarded. Undermining should be done at the periosteal level. In closure, the first suture is the most critical; it engages the midpoints of the sides of the triangle whose apex is on the symphysis. Once the suture has engaged the full thickness of skin on each side of the wound, it is tacked to the mandibular periosteum in the midline. The beveled excision allows the subcuticular tissues to be suspended from the mandibular periosteum. Closure of the remainder of the wound can be completed in two layers, and the skin sutures can be removed on the fifth postoperative day. The application of a pressure dressing is advised to aid in proper skin suspension and to help prevent hematoma formation.

When hypertrophy of the submental fat pad coexists with chin ptosis, it may be eliminated by an extension of this approach. Care must be taken to resuspend the soft tissues of the neck posteriorly and superiorly as previously mentioned.

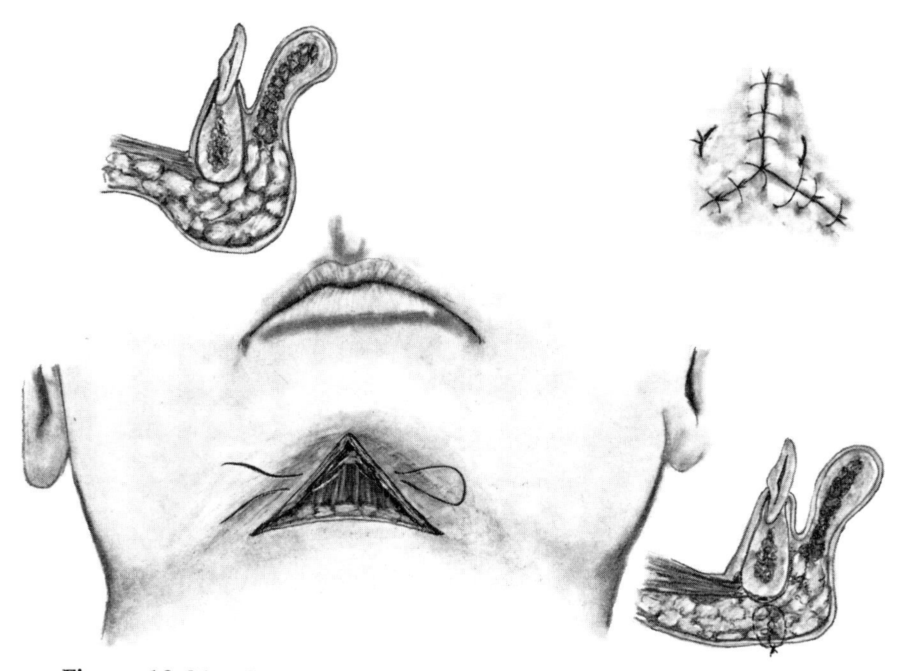

Figure 16–21. Correction of soft-tissue ptosis of the chin. A triangular excision of excessive tissue closed in a Y pattern and suspended to the mandibular periosteum in the midline.

Management of the Labiomental Fold

Many patients with a Class II malocclusion have deep labiomental folds. The posture of the lower lip in relation to the maxillary anterior teeth must be evaluated before any therapy to improve this condition is initiated. The lower lip may be pressed forward by the maxillary incisors, in which case the lower lip will retract and assume better balance as the maxillary teeth are repositioned. High muscle attachments must be suspected if the labiomental fold is abnormally deep and the dentition is not the cause. A shallow mandibular labiomucosal vestibule confirms the existence of the condition (Fig. 16–22).

Steep labiomental folds have been treated successfully by using a prosthetic device to augment the fold, but the disadvantages of such an appliance are obvious: it is inconvenient, unhygienic, and uncomfortable. Hamula[10] has reported a procedure for lengthening the vestibule by performing multiple myotomies and using a stent for an extended period to maintain the vestibular depth gained at surgery. Proplast implants also have been used to correct this problem, and more details can be found in Chapter 14. A modification of Hamula's technique[15] involves careful dissection and suturing

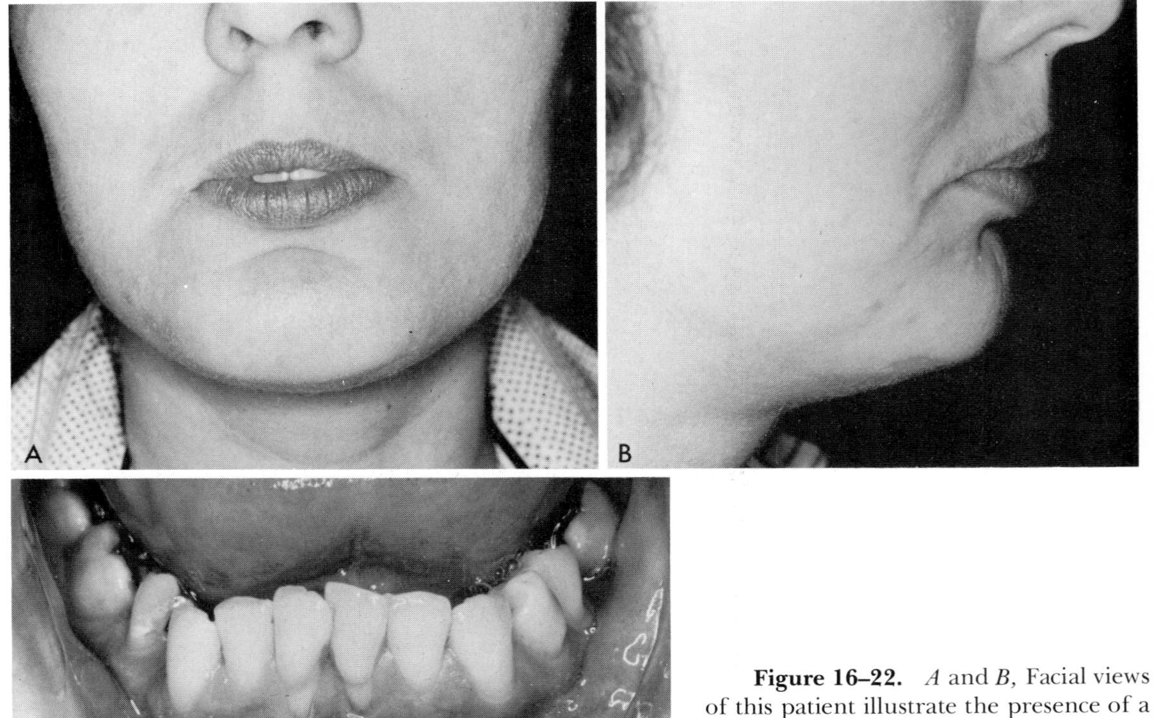

Figure 16–22. *A* and *B*, Facial views of this patient illustrate the presence of a deep labiomental fold due to high muscle attachments, confirmed by oral examination (*C*).

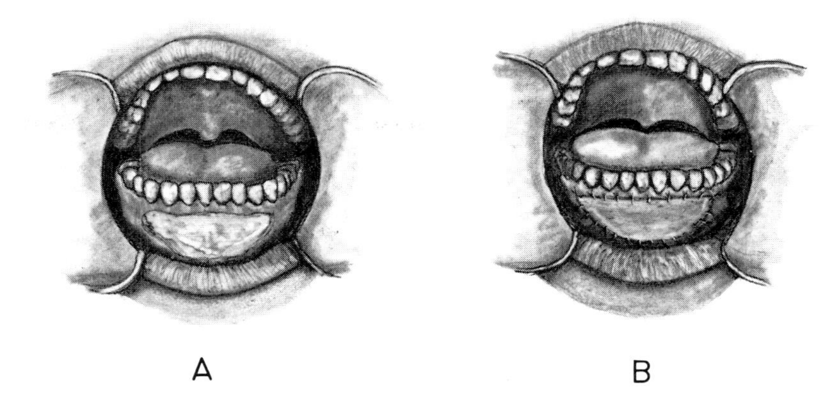

Figure 16–23. This procedure may correct the deep labiomental fold when caused by high muscle attachments: supraperiosteal dissection displacing the high muscle attachments inferiorly and placement of a mucosal or palatal graft.

of a palatal or mucosal graft to the denuded area at the symphysis; this technique eliminates the need for a prosthesis and insures that the depth of the fold will be maintained.

Technique (Fig. 16–23)

The vestibule is infiltrated with a dilute vasoconstrictor solution (epinephrine, 1:100,000) supraperiosteally. The mandibular mucosa is incised from canine to canine at the mucogingival junction, down through muscle to a supraperiosteal plane. Once this plane is established, the dissection is carried inferiorly toward the pogonion. All muscle attachments must be removed over the denuded periosteum, because any intact muscle encourages reattachment at a higher than desirable level after wound closure. No attempt is made to dissect to the inferior border, since this may produce undesirable esthetic changes (chin ptosis, abnormal projection of pogonion). Once the dissection is completed, the labial flap is inferiorly repositioned and sutured in place at the depth of the dissection. A palatal or buccal mucosal graft is sutured to place without stenting. The graft must be sutured to the periosteum at the depth of the incision in the labial vestibule to prevent muscle reattachment at a higher level after healing.

MANAGEMENT OF THE LIPS

Inadequacy of lip tissue or the inability of a patient to achieve lip contact at rest (lip incompetence) is a problem that plagues both surgeon and orthodontist. The inability to achieve lip contact at rest most often occurs because of skeletal and dental abnormalities and not because of inadequate lip tissue or length. Lip incompetence is a widespread deformity, and when it coexists with a dentofacial deformity, the patient's appearance may be unacceptable. Lip incompetence secondary to skeletal or dental problems should be managed by correcting the primary problems and not the soft tissues. Lengthening of the superior lip in patients with a congenitally short lip has been reported, but results of the procedures are difficult to assess. Bloomquist[1] reported minimal alterations with his experiments on primates, in which he detached and repositioned all the midfacial muscles of expression inferiorly in an attempt to lengthen the upper lip.

Lack of muscle tone that causes the lower lip to assume an everted posture will contribute to lip incompetence. This deformity may be altered surgically by reduction cheiloplasty as subsequently described. It is beyond the scope of this chapter to discuss problems related to patients with clefts of the lip and other major lip defects. Interested readers should consult a textbook on this subject.[6]

Enlargement of the Lip

Hyperplasia or hypertrophy of fat, salivary glands, or muscles can cause abnormally enlarged lips. In addition, macrocheilia or distention of the lymphatic space of the lip, replacement of normal tissue by granulomatous and edematous fibrous tissues (as seen in Melkersson-Rosenthal syndrome), or redundant tissue (as seen in Ascher's syndrome) can all contribute to lip enlargement. Lack of muscle tone will contribute to ptosis of the inferior lip, producing an apparent increased thickness of the lip. Although increased lip thickness has been reported to be a characteristic of certain racial groups, Fonseca[4] did not find a significant difference in lip thickness between Negro and Caucasian subjects, but he reported greater vermilion exposure to be a characteristic of the Negro lip. This finding should not be misinterpreted to represent lip thickness.

Each case of suspected lip enlargement, excessive vermilion exposure, or abnormal eversion must be evaluated individually with consideration of the patient's concerns and ethnic background. When contemplating correction simultaneously with dento-osseous surgery, it is important to predict lip posture alterations that will occur as a result of the osseous movement effected by surgery. If there is any question of lip inadequacy following dento-osseous repositioning, reduction cheiloplasty should be deferred for three to six months, and a secondary procedure should be considered after the soft tissues have adapted to their new position and the surgeon is able to evaluate the postoperative situation.

The results of reduction cheiloplasty are unpredictable. Lehnert[11] studied ten patients who underwent reduction cheiloplasty concomitantly with osseous surgery either primarily or as a secondary procedure. He reported little consistency of results. In osseous surgery, lip position can be predicted from certain quantitative measurements with a fair degree of accuracy, but the posture of the lips following reduction is variable, inconsistent, and difficult to predict. When reduction of lip bulk, vermilion exposure, or lip eversion is indicated, a horizontal wedge resection should be employed (Fig. 16–24). The amount of bulk to be removed is arbitrary and must depend on the surgeon's judgment.

Technique (Fig. 16–25)

The wet line of the lip (point demarcating lip mucosa that is continuously bathed with saliva from that which is exposed) to be reduced is marked from commissure to commissure. This line constitutes one edge of an ellipse, and another matching line scribed on the mucosal surface of the lip will complete the ellipse, indicating the amount of tissue to be removed. After injection of a dilute solution of vasoconstrictor (epineph-

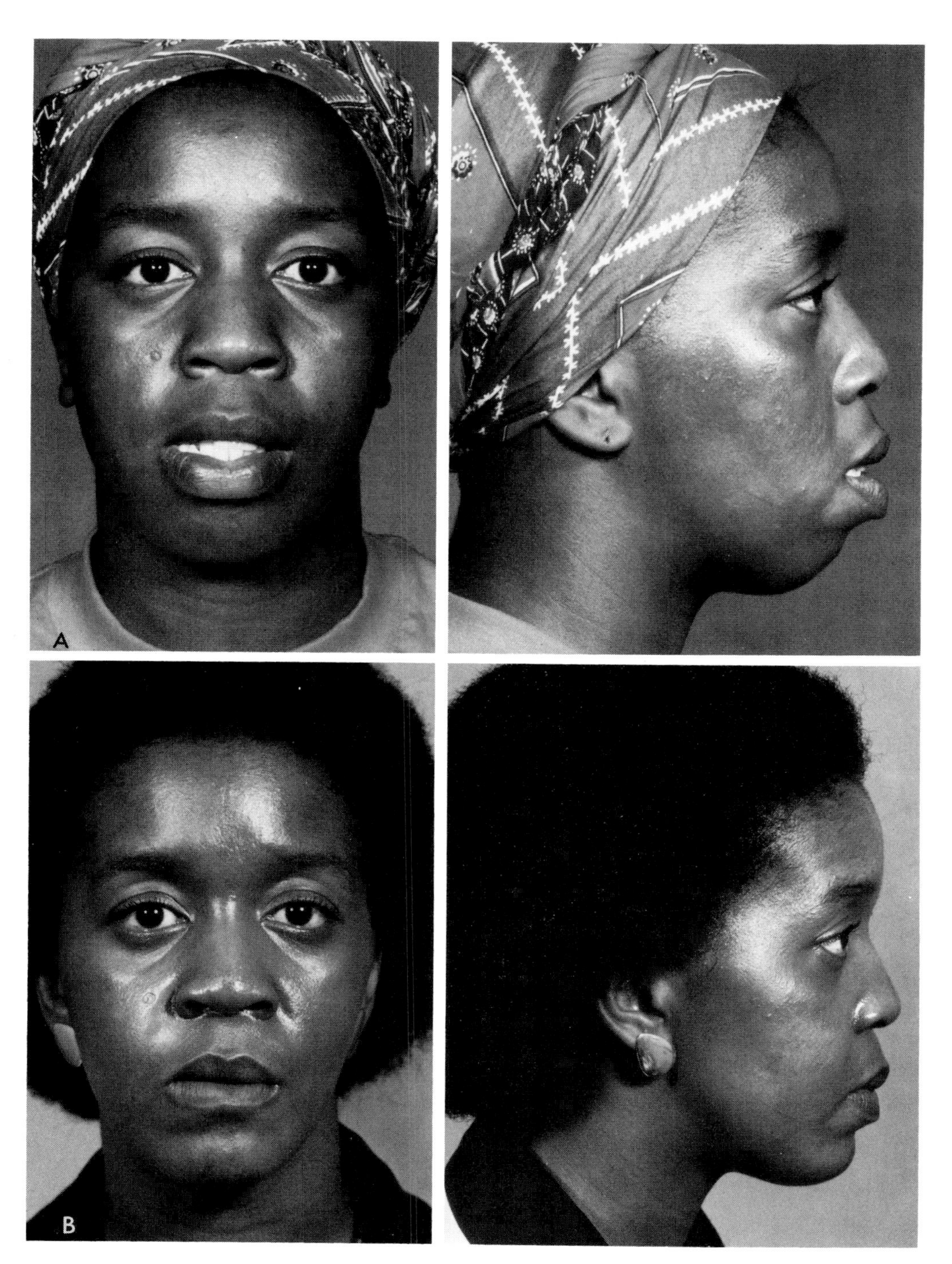

Figure 16–24. Example of a patient with lower lip enlargement. *A*, Preoperative. *B*, Postoperative changes following horizontal wedge excision of excessive lip tissue.
Surgeon: William H. Bell, Dallas, Texas.

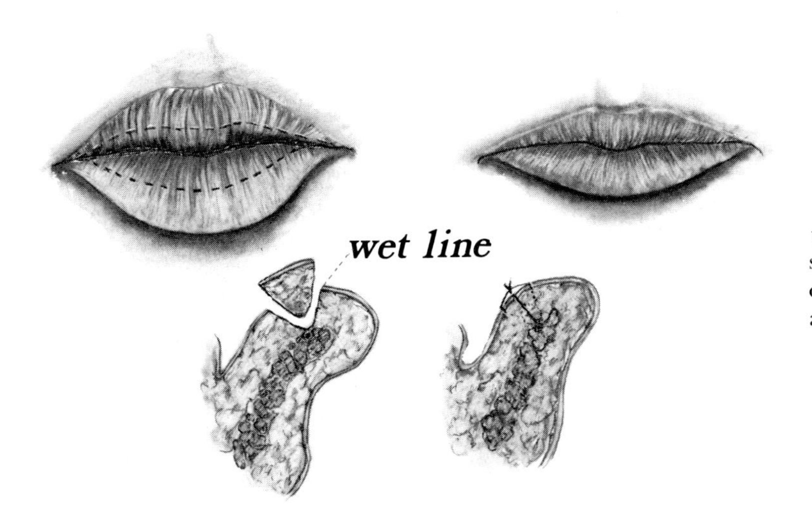

Figure 16–25. Horizontal wedge excision of lip bulk and closure without undermining will reduce lip bulk, vermilion exposure, and lip eversion.

rine, 1:100,000 or 1:200,000), a wedge of mucosa and submucosa is excised. The labial artery is almost always violated, but bleeding can be controlled by applying pressure on both sides of the lip lateral to the area of hemorrhage until the vessels can be ligated. When hemostasis has been obtained, the soft tissues are closed in two layers without undermining, to help achieve the desired postural inversion of the lip. Immediately following surgery, lip incompetence will persist, even after small tissue reductions, but once the swelling has decreased and function has resumed, the posture of the lip will improve in a matter of weeks. Stretching and various lip exercises may help to restore normal lip posture, function, and esthetics in some difficult cases.

REFERENCES

1. Bloomquist DS: Investigation of the surgical lengthening of the superior lip on primates. Presented at the 57th Annual Meeting of the American Society of Oral Surgeons. Washington DC, 1975.
2. Dingman RO, Grabb WC: Surgical anatomy of the mandibular ramus of the facial nerve based on the dissection of 100 facial halves. Plast Reconstr Surg *29*:266, 1962.
3. Farino R. Currey E: Labial malocclusion. Br J Plast Surg *23*:254, 1970.
4. Fonseca RJ, Klein WD: A cephalometric evaluation of American Negro women. Am J Orthod *73*:152, 1978.
5. Gonzales-Ulloa M: Ptosis of the chin. Plast Reconstr Surg *50*:54, 1972.
6. Grabb WC, Rosenthal SW, et al.: *Cleft Lip and Palate.* Boston: Little, Brown and Co, 1971.
7. Gregg JM: Personal communication, March 1977.
8. Gunter JP: Camouflaging scars in the head and neck area. In press. Am J Otolaryngol.
9. Gunter JP: Personal communication, May 1976.
10. Hamula W: Surgical alteration of muscle attachments to enhance esthetics and denture stability. Amer J Orthod *57*:327, 1970.
11. Lehnert MW: Reduction cheiloplasty—its role in the correction of dentofacial deformities. Presented at the 58th Annual Meeting of the American Society of Oral Surgeons. New York, 1976.
12. Mareno H, Galeano J, Gandolfo EA: Plastic correction of double chin. Plast Reconstr Surg *31*:45, 1963.
13. Neuner O: Surgical correction of mandibular prognathism. Oral Surg Med Path *42*:415, 1976.
14. Robinson RJ, Stranc MF: The anatomy of the medial canthal ligament. Br J Plast Surg *23*:1, 1970.
15. Turvey TA, Epker BN: Soft tissue procedures adjunctive to orthognathic surgery for improvement of facial balance. J Oral Surg *32*:572, 1974.
16. Walker RV: TMJ degenerative joint disease—a common contemporary matter. Chalmers J Lyons Memorial Lecture presented at the 58th Annual Meeting of the American Society of Oral Surgeons. New York, 1976.
17. Weisman PA: Simplified technique in submental lipectomy. Plast Reconstr Surg *48*:443, 1971.
18. Wolford L, Epker BN: Personal communication, April 1977.

Chapter 17

RESIDUAL ALVEOLAR AND PALATAL CLEFTS

Daniel E. Waite and Ralph B. Kersten

Clefts of the prepalate and palate were described in the literature of antiquity. There is a report of successful closure of the lip by a Chinese surgeon as early as A.D. 390. Records exist of surgical repairs done in the 16th century. Le Monnier,[24] a dentist, performed one of the early successful repairs of a cleft of the palate in 1776. Early successful repairs of clefts performed in the United States have been credited to Dr. J. C. Warren of Boston in 1820 (reported in 1828)[34] and Dr. J. P. Mettauer of Virginia in 1827 (reported in 1837).[11]

In the history of medicine, progress in the treatment of cleft lip and palate is expressed primarily in the form of a series of improving surgical techniques, usually identified by the name of the surgeon who originated or refined the technique. These names have become synonymous with cleft palate treatment: Von Graefe (1817),[31] Roux (1819),[25] Mirault (1844),[18] Dieffenbach (1845),[6] von Langenbeck (1861),[32] Hagedorn (1892),[10] Veau (1922),[30] Dorrance (1925),[7] Wardill (1928),[33] Le Mesurier (1949),[14] and Millard (1958).[17]

Although progress in treatment for clefts had primarily been in the form of surgical techniques until the 1940s, another major advance occurred when techniques of anesthesia were refined. The problems resulting from the lack of proper anesthesia perhaps are best suggested by Rogers' description of the positioning used in the 15th century by Braunschweig, an Alsatian army surgeon, whose patient was placed on the table and fastened to it by three hand towels while undergoing a lip repair.[24] Rogers also describes the positioning of an infant for a lip repair by Warwich in the 17th century; the child was placed in the lap of a "discreet person." Another person stood behind to hold the child's head, and the hands were tied down. The child was kept awake for 12 hours before the surgery so that he would be "disposed to sleep from exhaustion."

DESCRIPTION OF THE DEFORMITY

Generally, cleft lip and palate are discussed together, although embryologically these are separate entities. Although various classifications have been developed to categorize cleft lip and palate deformities, perhaps the most practical and easiest to understand is a classification based on anatomic antecedents and defined according to location — right, left, or bilateral — and extent. Cleft of the prepalate, according to extent, can include the lip and the alveolar process to the incisive foramen (Fig. 17–1). Cleft of the palate includes, according to extent, the soft palate and the hard palate to the incisive foramen (Fig. 17–2). Approximately 25 per cent of all clefts involve part or all of the prepalate. Another 25 per cent of clefts involve part or all of the palate. The remaining 50 per cent of clefts are combined prepalatal and palatal clefts; thus cleft of the prepalate is a consideration in about 75 per cent of all cleft disorders (Fig. 17–3).

SURGICAL TREATMENT

Importance of the Team Approach

The problems encountered in rehabilitation of patients with cleft lip and palate are unique among problems presented by major congenital defects. Because of the anatomic features of the defect, treatment and care must include consideration of appearance, speech, hearing, mastication, and deglutition, and, as a result of the interrelation of these multiple factors, the emotional and social development of the child. Despite the complex problems presented, the outlook for total rehabilitation in all areas — physical, emotional, and vocational — is extremely good, provided that care is undertaken in the proper sequence. Although this is a matter of major importance no consensus exists about the sequence of treatment.

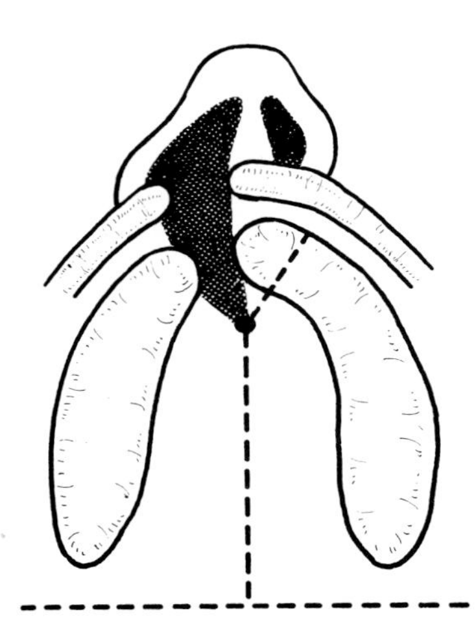

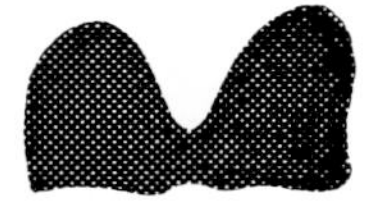

Figure 17–1. Schematic drawing of cleft of the prepalate, extending from the incisive foramen through the alveolar process, the lip, and the floor of the nose.

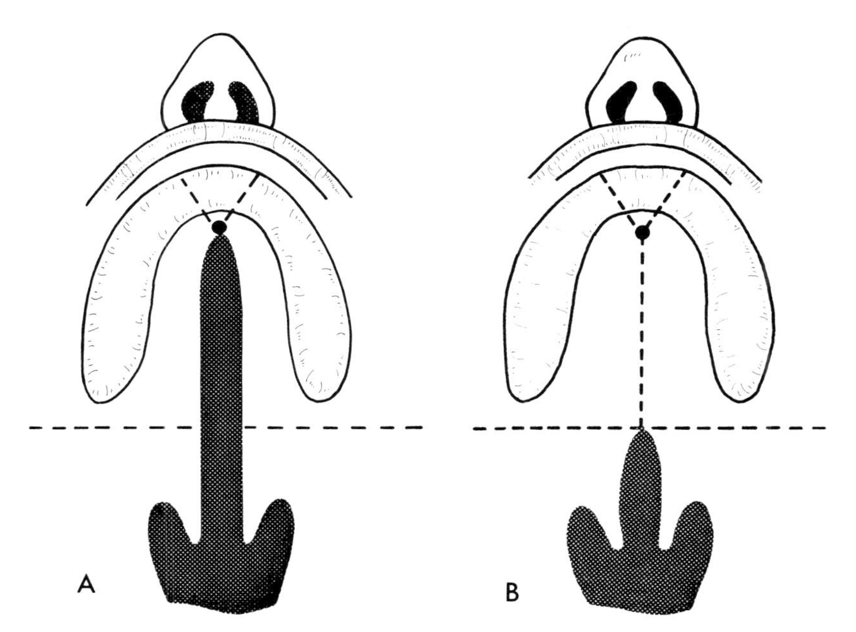

Figure 17–2. *A*, Complete cleft of the soft and hard palate with the incisive foramen as the anterior limit. *B*, Cleft of the soft palate only is shown extending to the posterior border of the hard palate.

It is understandable that there is controversy concerning the treatment of cleft disorders, since so many professional disciplines must become involved: pediatrics, reconstructive surgery, restorative dentistry, orthodontics, prosthodontics, oral surgery, otolaryngology, plastic surgery, audiology, speech pathology, and at times social service and psychiatry. Unfortunately, no one person can be proficient enough in all these special disciplines to provide total treatment planning and treatment for the patient. This is where the cleft palate team, with representatives of all involved specialties, plays a vital role.

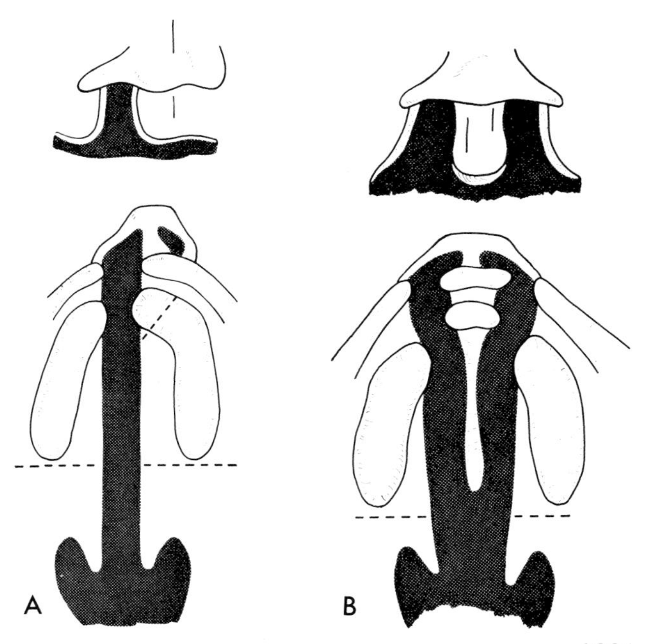

Figure 17–3. *A*, Unilateral cleft of the lip and palate, extending from the soft palate to the incisive foramen and the floor of the nose. *B*, Bilateral cleft lip and palate.

Historically, patients with cleft lip and palate have generally been treated by the surgeon alone. Occasionally the dentist and speech therapist became involved. It was by chance that Dr. James Mabie, a maxillofacial surgeon, and Dr. Albert MacDougal, an orthodontist, jointly established an office in Bangor, Maine, to form what turned out to be the first functioning cleft palate team. Dr. Herbert Cooper, a dentist practicing in Lancaster, Pennsylvania, established the first recognized cleft palate clinic in the United States. This was one of the first steps toward adoption of the current concept of team treatment of patients with cleft lip and palate, which possibly is the most significant advance in this field in the last few decades.

Despite all the advances that have been made in surgical correction of cleft lip and palate, the development of the interdisciplinary team, increased understanding of growth and development, and improved techniques in orthodontics, prosthodontics, and restorative dentistry, too many patients with cleft lip and palate are still seen with residual defects and associated oronasal fistulae that seriously compromise facial and dental appearance and/or prevent proper function. Thus, the lack of continuity of the maxillary alveolar arch and possible related fistulae continue to pose problems requiring the expertise of the oral surgeon in addition to that of other disciplines.

Related Problems

Anterior palatal and alveolar ridge defects usually do not present early severe complications; however, as the patient grows, numerous problems can arise to complicate further surgery, orthodontic treatment, and even speech production. More specifically, one or several of the following problems may be present:

1. If the cleft extends into the floor of the nose, the alar cartilage on that side is flared, and the columella of the nose is pulled toward the noncleft side. The lack of support for the alar base at the site of the cleft causes facial asymmetry (Fig. 17–4).

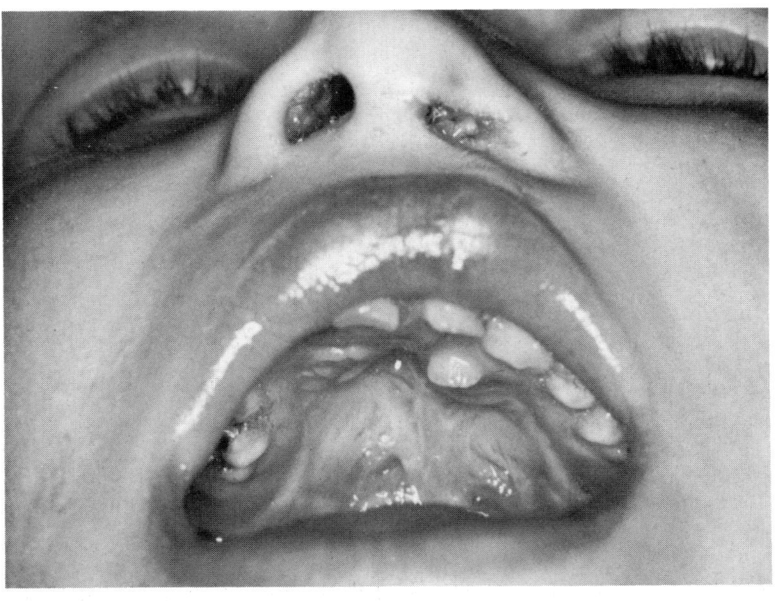

Figure 17–4. When the patient has an oronasal or labionasal fistula, unsightly crusting of the nostrils is frequently present. Note also alar flare.

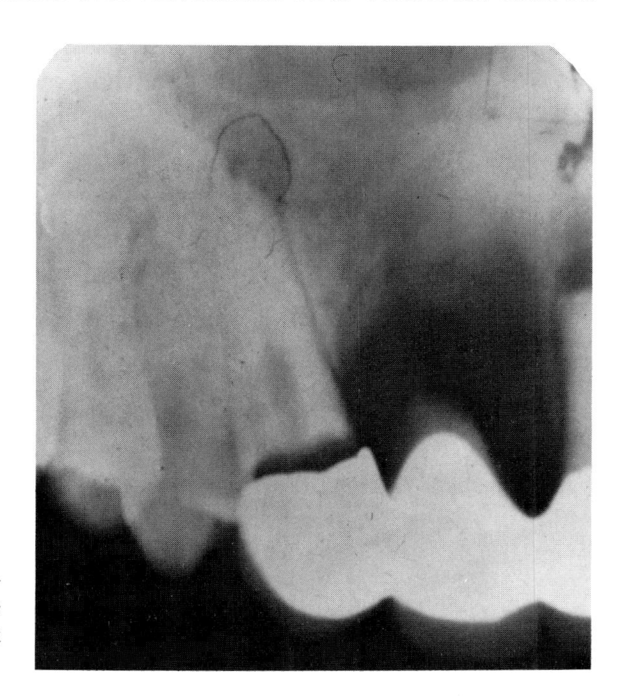

Figure 17–5. Radiograph shows a typical example of loosening of an abutment of a fixed bridge caused by mobility of the maxillary segments not stabilized by bone grafting the alveolar defect.

2. If the cleft involves the alveolus, the alveolar ridge is displaced palatally on the cleft side, and the teeth in the area of the cleft frequently erupt out of alignment. In some cases, the teeth — most often the lateral incisor adjacent to the cleft — are congenitally absent. Conversely, supernumerary teeth are frequently found in the cleft area. Timing of the removal of a supernumerary tooth should be determined by its effect on the total treatment plan, with special emphasis on its relationship to bone grafting in the area. If it is part of the deciduous dentition, the tooth usually can be allowed to exfoliate normally. If it is part of the permanent dentition, it can be allowed to remain until just before bone grafting in order to preserve as much alveolar bone as possible and to avoid bone resorption that occurs following tooth extraction.

3. Permanent teeth adjacent to the cleft are usually deficient in bone along the root surfaces near the cleft; that is, the distal aspect of the central incisor root and the mesial aspect of the canine root have minimal or no bony support. The lateral incisor, if still present, frequently has inadequate bony support. Early bone loss around these teeth due to periodontal disease further contributes to loss of the teeth adjacent to the cleft.

4. Because the teeth are frequently maloccluded and malaligned, rampant caries occurs because adequate oral hygiene is difficult to achieve.

5. In patients with bilateral cleft lip and palate, the premaxilla is mobile, frequently protrudes, and often is displaced inferiorly. At other times, it may be inclined lingually. Both posterior maxillary segments frequently collapse medially, causing a bilateral crossbite. Both anterior and posterior crossbites may be present.

6. Whether clefts are unilateral or bilateral, the maxillary segments are sufficiently mobile to make long-term use of fixed prosthodontic appliances impractical. Too frequently, one or both abutments of the fixed bridge break loose because of this mobility (Fig. 17–5). Removable appliances also prove less than ideal, since they further contribute to irritation of the residual cleft and also interfere with good oral hygiene for the remaining teeth.

7. The contour of the upper arch also may influence speech production. A narrow arch may restrict tongue activity, and an irregular arch may present a hazard to precise articulation of sibilant sounds such as /s/, /z/, /sh/, /ch/, /j/ as in "jaw," and /j/ as in "azure."

8. Residual fistulae also pose problems. In normal persons, the oral and nasal cavities are separated by the bony maxilla and flexible soft palate. Although both the oral and the nasal cavities are functionally related to respiration and speech, each has a different basic role to play. The primary functions of the oral cavity are deglutition and mastication, whereas the primary roles of the nasal cavity are air conditioning and olfaction. When these cavities are not separated, as in the case of a cleft or an oronasal fistula, neither cavity functions normally or adequately, and their function in producing speech is adversely affected.

9. During speech, the nasal cavity of normal persons is separated from the oral cavity and throat. The soft palate acts as a valve in the posterior pharynx to separate these two cavities. If an oronasal fistula exists, however, it can affect the development of oral pressure during the production of most consonants, causing unacceptable nasal emission, hypernasality during speech production, or both.

10. Communication between the oral cavity and the nasal cavity through a fistula is not hygienically acceptable. Oral secretions and nasal secretions must be separated. When there is communication between the two cavities as a result of an oronasal or labionasal fistula, unsightly crusting in the nostrils is frequently observed (Fig. 17–4).

Bone Grafting in Cleft Palate Patients

According to Maisels,[15] the first bone grafting procedure in an alveolar defect resulting from clefting was done by R. Drachter in 1914. In 1952, Axhausen performed the procedure, and in the years immediately following, others reporting their procedures for bone grafting included Schmidt in 1955,[26] Nordin and Johanson in 1955,[20] Nordin in 1957,[19] and Schuchardt in 1961.[16] These procedures for the most part involved grafting during infancy, whereas Brauer in 1962,[4] Backdahl in 1964,[1] and Skoog in 1965[28, 29] reported and recommended bone grafting the alveolar cleft at a much later stage of maxillary development and as a secondary procedure.

Several types of bone grafts are used in correcting cleft palate: (1) the onlay graft, designed primarily to improve the contour of the upper lip and provide support for the alar base, and (2) the inlay graft, accomplished by morticing the graft between the alveolar stumps.

Clinicians have differed regarding appropriate timing for repair of the alveolar defect in patients with unilateral and bilateral clefts.[8, 9, 22, 23, 26, 27] Some prefer to repair the alveolar defect at the time of the primary lip repair. Others prefer to repair the defect as a secondary procedure after lateral growth of the maxilla is complete.[1, 28, 29] Recent literature largely supports the latter approach, and our entire surgical experience has been in performing secondary osteoplasty of the defect in older children (i.e., average age 9 to 11 years), adolescents, and adults. The results of bone grafting of the alveolar defect in infancy have been generally unfavorable, because such grafts tend to inhibit maxillary growth and interfere with the dentition.[12, 13]

Replacement of the missing bone between the alveolar segments is a primary objective. This stabilizes the lateral segments. In bilateral clefts, stability of the premaxilla also is accomplished by bone grafting, and repositioning can be done at the same time if necessary.

Closure of pre-existing oronasal fistulae at the time of secondary repair prevents food from escaping into the nose and restricts oral and nasal secretions to their respective confines. The resulting bony bridge across the cleft provides hygienic and esthetic advantages. The bony base will also provide for orthodontic alignment of proximal teeth and guidance of unerupted teeth into their proper positions. If teeth are congenitally missing or have been removed in the area of the defect, the grafted bone and mucosal covering provide an excellent tissue contour for the prosthetic appliance. A satisfactory graft of the alveolar cleft will add support to the base of the nose on the cleft side and should be completed before secondary nasal revision. Thus, it is apparent to us that bone grafting of the alveolar cleft significantly aids in restoring patients with this defect toward normalcy.

PRESURGICAL CONSIDERATIONS

Timing of the Treatment

Primary osteoplasty is a procedure carried out simultaneously with closure of the lip. The term *secondary osteoplasty* is applied only to those operations in which bone grafting is employed *after* the lip and palate have been repaired. Those using the primary grafting procedure apparently hoped that the bone graft not only would fill the congenital defect but would also become an integral part of the growing alveolus of the developing maxilla. This does not occur, and therefore it is more appropriate to graft bone after the lateral growth of the maxilla is complete, a time that corresponds closely with the eruption of the maxillary first molars at ages 6 to 7.

Chronologic age is not as important in timing of the bone graft as the development of the teeth and their position in relation to the cleft. Perhaps the ideal time for grafting the alveolar defect is when (1) the permanent canine tooth bud is high and its root is not completely formed, and (2) the deciduous canine is firm in the alveolus. Ideally, the canine tooth will erupt through the bone graft and into position.

A retrospective study was done at the University of Minnesota to evaluate unerupted teeth in the area of alveolar clefts. More than 100 patients have undergone grafting for this defect since 1970. Of this group, 33 patients had unerupted canine teeth in the maxillary alveolar cleft area with potential for eruption. It was found that the best age for grafting is based on the eruptive potential of unerupted canine teeth high in the area of the cleft: 9 to 11 years chronologically and 8 to 10 years dentally. These teeth demonstrated the greatest eruptive potential when the root was between one-third and two-thirds formed; 75 per cent of unerupted teeth in this category showed movement into the bone graft. Teeth that are fully formed had little eruptive potential.

Correction of Malocclusions and Malalignments

Any anterior or posterior crossbites should be corrected and the proper overbite and overjet established before grafting is done. If there are crossbites so severe that they cannot be corrected by tooth movement only, expansion of the collapsed segment should be undertaken prior to bone grafting. Rapid expansion techniques are appropriate in selected cases. In other instances, expansion can be obtained by using more conventional modalities, such as a W-arch or similar orthodontic appliances. Surgical repositioning of the maxillary segments also provides very good results. In any event, moving an entire segment or several segments of the maxilla is easier before bone grafting than after.

A malaligned premaxilla can often be corrected orthodontically before bone grafting. In other instances, proper repositioning of the premaxilla preparatory to bone grafting requires a surgical procedure. Expansion or alignment of the maxillary arch would be required in addition to repositioning of the premaxilla.[21]

Oral Hygiene

It is absolutely necessary that the patient institute good oral hygiene before bone grafting is done. This includes brushing and flossing in order to bring the oral tissues to their maximum health. Performing bone grafting under conditions of poor oral hygiene will compromise healing. It is essential that the oral cavity be kept as clean as possible after the bone graft is done to facilitate healing.

Preservation of Supporting Bone

To preserve as much bone as possible in the area of the cleft prior to grafting, we believe that unerupted supernumerary teeth or malpositioned teeth in the region of the cleft should be left in position as long as possible. Their presence may contribute to bone stimulation, and certainly early removal only destroys bone and enlarges the original defect. The orthodontist should be careful not to upright teeth proximal to the defect so that as much bone as possible will be preserved on the cleft side of the tooth surface.

Treatment Planning for Secondary Osteoplasty

In order to plan a secondary osteoplasty to the maxillary alveolus, the surgeon must have several kinds of records. These include the medical history, family interviews, study casts, and radiographic studies (cephalographs and maxillary occlusal and dental periapical views). In many instances, facial deformities and associated dental compensations are so severe that the usual secondary osteoplasty alone is inappropriate, and arch and jaw alignment may be necessary prerequisites, especially if closure of the alveolar defect has been delayed until the teen-age years. In some instances it is possible to accomplish these alignments by presurgical orthodontic treatment. If not, accomplished repositioning of the maxillary segments must be done by Le Fort I osteotomy or segmental osteotomy procedures combined with bone grafts.

TECHNIQUE

Once the overall maxillary arch form is acceptable, final alveolar bone grafting is completed. The usual procedure is first to close the mucosa of the nasal floor on the labial and palatal sides of the defect. Incisions are made along the cleft margins, splitting the labial/nasal and palatal/nasal mucosa. The mucosal layers are sutured together with 4-0 Dexon, with the ties placed on the nasal side. The bone margin should now be adequately exposed and the bone grafts wedged into position.

Various types of bone graft materials that have been suggested over the years include autogenous bone from various sites, allogenic grafts, and alloplastic or synthetic materials. At present, it is generally agreed that autogenous bone is the material of choice. We have found that a combination of cortical bone and particulate medullary bone is most satisfactory.

The donor site for the bone graft material is usually the iliac crest, where large amounts of spongy bone can be obtained. A triangular segment of corticomedullary bone is formed to fill the triangular defect of the alveolus. Particulate bone marrow is packed around and on top of the block of corticomedullary bone once it is in position.

When surgical repositioning of the premaxilla is indicated, Perko's technique permits performing the entire procedure in one operation.[21] Mucoperiosteal sliding palatal flaps are used to cover the palatal defect. A pedicled mucosal flap from the vestibule is used to cover the graft and extend across the ridge to join with the palatal mucosa in extensive defects. Another option for the labial flap is a sliding full-thickness mucoperiosteal flap (see Figure 17–8*J*, page 1343). This technique has the advantage of placing attached mucosa over the crest of the alveolar ridge.

In grafting bilateral clefts, the mucoperiosteum of the palate is raised on both sides of the cleft and joined in the midline to cover the exposed vomer, leaving a small amount of exposed bone near the lateral edge of the palate. This exposed bone is covered by granulation tissue within a few days. The flap is not raised to expose the gingival crest, but approximately 4 mm of tissue is left on the palatal surface, minimizing alveolar crest bone resorption and providing more rapid healing. In grafting unilateral clefts, only the mucoperiosteal flap from the noncleft side is raised to complete the double thickness of mucosal covering.

Using a pedicle flap from the vestibule rarely foreshortens the vestibule, particularly in young patients. Careful mobilization of the flap and appropriate undermining and tissue closure will leave an adequate vestibule. In patients who have either small nasal fistulae or none, the sliding mucoperiosteal flap as described by Boyne works equally well for less extensive defects.[3] Supramid 4–0 sutures are used to close the tissues. Oral irrigation with 1 per cent neomycin solution is used during the operation. All patients are given antibiotics after surgery.

A preconstructed acrylic splint is used postoperatively to cover the palatal tissue for 1 week. The splint protects the tissue from unnecessary patient exploration and aids in maintenance of oral hygiene. Sutures are removed at 10 days. Diet is full liquid for 3 days, semi-soft for 10 days; a normal diet is given thereafter.

POSTSURGICAL OBSERVATIONS AND COMPLICATIONS

Postsurgical orthodontic treatment is often necessary to provide final dental alignment to supplement surgical arch alignment. Unerupted teeth in the region of the cleft may erupt normally through the graft, or they may need surgical and orthodontic assistance. In instances in which teeth are missing, bridge construction can be safely

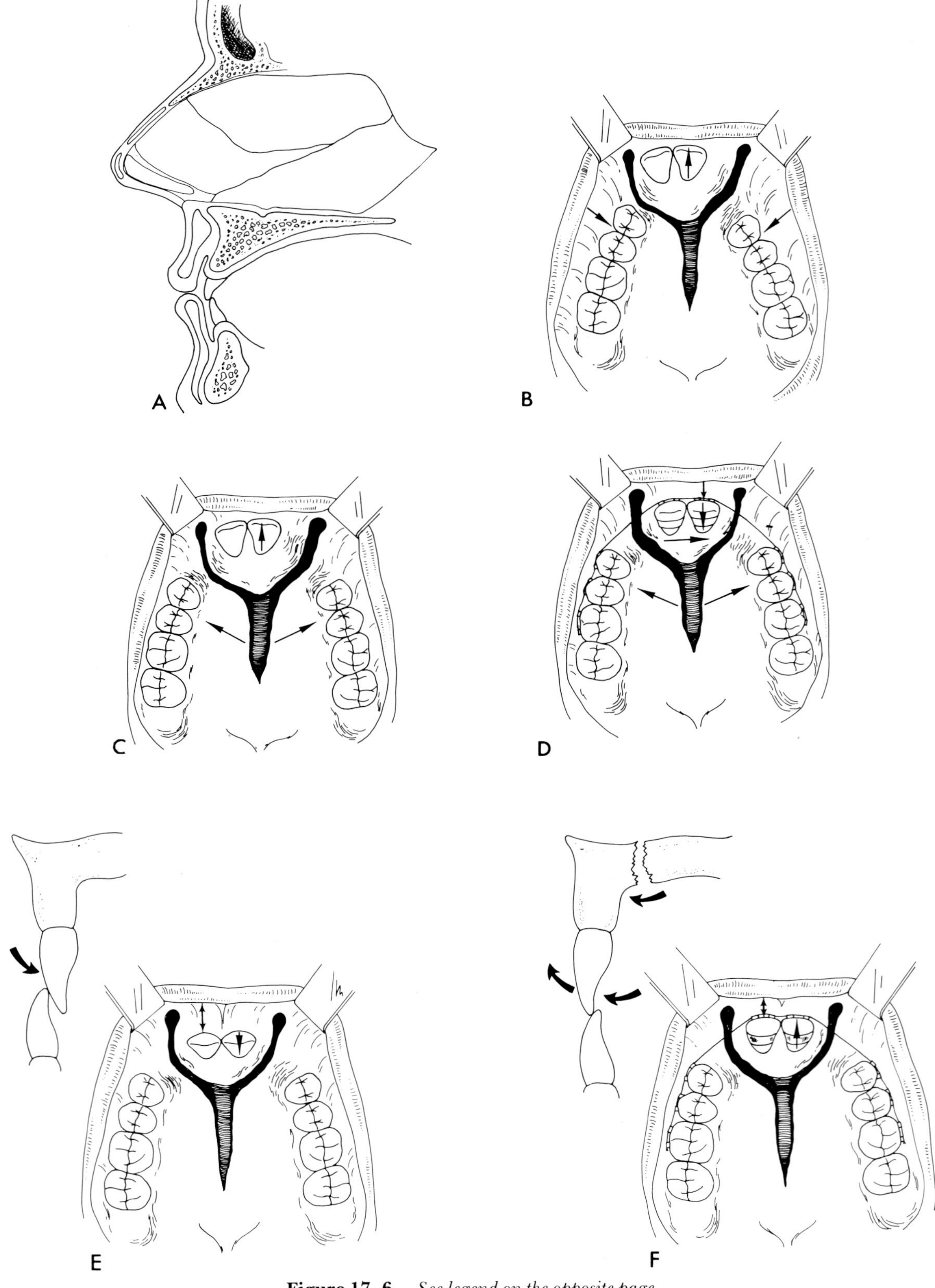

Figure 17–6. *See legend on the opposite page.*

undertaken once the maxillary segments have been immobilized with bone grafts and the pulps of abutment teeth are mature.

Following repair of alveolar defects, some degree of wound dehiscence may occur, although this is rare in our experience. Dehiscence may be related to tension on the pedicle graft or to venous congestion within the flap. Daily "milking" of the pedicle flap toward its base during the early postoperative period may be helpful. When oral wound dehiscence occurs, the presence of mucous discharge is an important warning sign. Discharge is indicative of breakdown of the nasal closure as well and fistulization may reoccur. Antibiotic coverage and nasal decongestants should be administered to these patients until closure occurs or it is evident that refistulization has occurred, necessitating reoperation.

Other complications, such as nasal hemorrhage, can occur. The use of oral endotracheal tubes for anesthesia may help minimize hemorrhage. In patients who have large palatal defects, however, it is difficult to work around the oral tube. Intubation through the contralateral nostril is utilized in patients with unilateral defects. In our experience to date, we have had no complications relating to intubation or extubation.

Breakdown of the nasal flap can be minimized not only by using oral intubation but also by avoiding the use of nasal suction postoperatively — suction on the surgically treated side of the nose can break down the mucosal closure. Adequate humidification during the postoperative period will keep the nasal mucous membranes moist. As soon as primary soft-tissue healing is complete, 10 to 14 days after surgery, an orthodontic retention appliance should be placed. The retainer prevents any undue osseous stress upon the grafted area, ensuring solidification of the graft and minimizing any alteration in the existing occlusion.

On occasion, the healing of the vestibular pedicle flap may leave bulky tissue over the alveolar ridge crest, a shortened vestibule, or a redundant tissue fold. This can be corrected, often on an outpatient basis, utilizing a Z-plasty technique to eliminate the redundant tissue and create an optimal base for a bridge pontic.

Approximately 2 months following uncomplicated surgery, additional orthodontic work can be undertaken or crown and bridge work completed.

Figures 17–6 through 17–10 illustrate surgical technique for treating various cleft lip and palate deformities. The case studies and patient views that follow demonstrate use of the techniques in treating actual patients.

Text continued on page 1366

Figure 17–6. Bilateral clefts of the palate and alveolar process often cause protrusion, rotation, or palatal inclination of the premaxillary segment. *A,* Midsagittal view of normal maxillary alveolus and hard palate. *B,* Typical collapse of the lateral segments, protrusion, and rotation of the premaxilla as seen in the adult dentition. *C,* Lateral segments have been expanded orthodontically. *D,* Sectioning of the vomer has permitted repositioning of the premaxilla. Bone grafting of the alveolar segments can be done simultaneously or as a secondary procedure if their corrected positions are maintained by proper splinting or use of orthodontic appliances. *E,* The premaxillary segment often is tipped lingually and locked in a position lingual to the mandibular incisor teeth. *F,* Sectioning the vomer permits advancement and rotation of the premaxilla to establish proper alignment of the segment and correct overbite and overjet. Postoperative stabilization of the segments can be achieved by a bilateral splint or an orthodontic appliance.

See illustration on the opposite page.

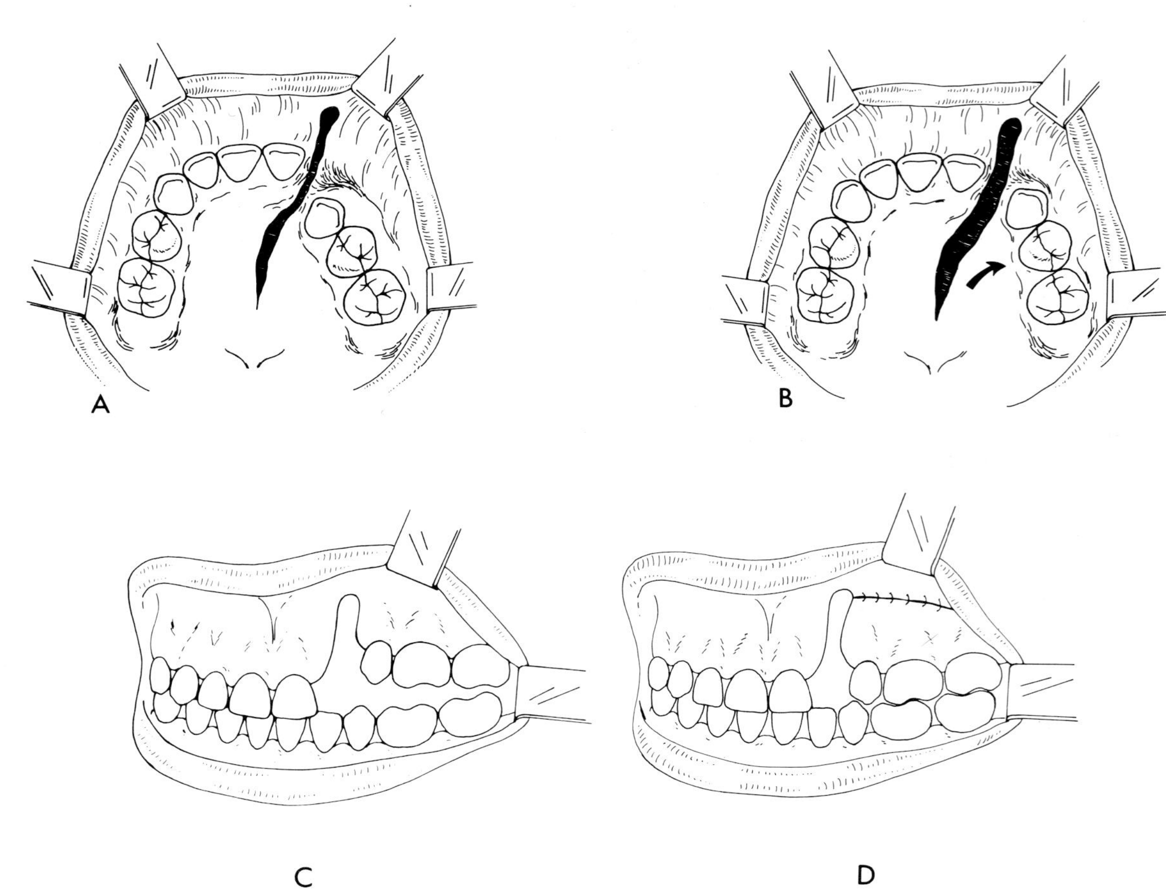

Figure 17–7. Surgical correction of displaced lateral segment in a unilateral cleft of the palate and alveolar process in a child. *A,* Palatal view of unilateral cleft extending through the alveolar process with a typical collapsed lateral segment on the cleft side. *B,* The collapsed lateral segment has been repositioned surgically. Bone grafting to hold the segment in its new position is usually necessary. *C,* Lateral view shows malocclusion of the lateral segment frequently encountered with a unilateral cleft. *D,* Corrected occlusion following surgical repositioning of the lateral segment.

Legend continued on the opposite page

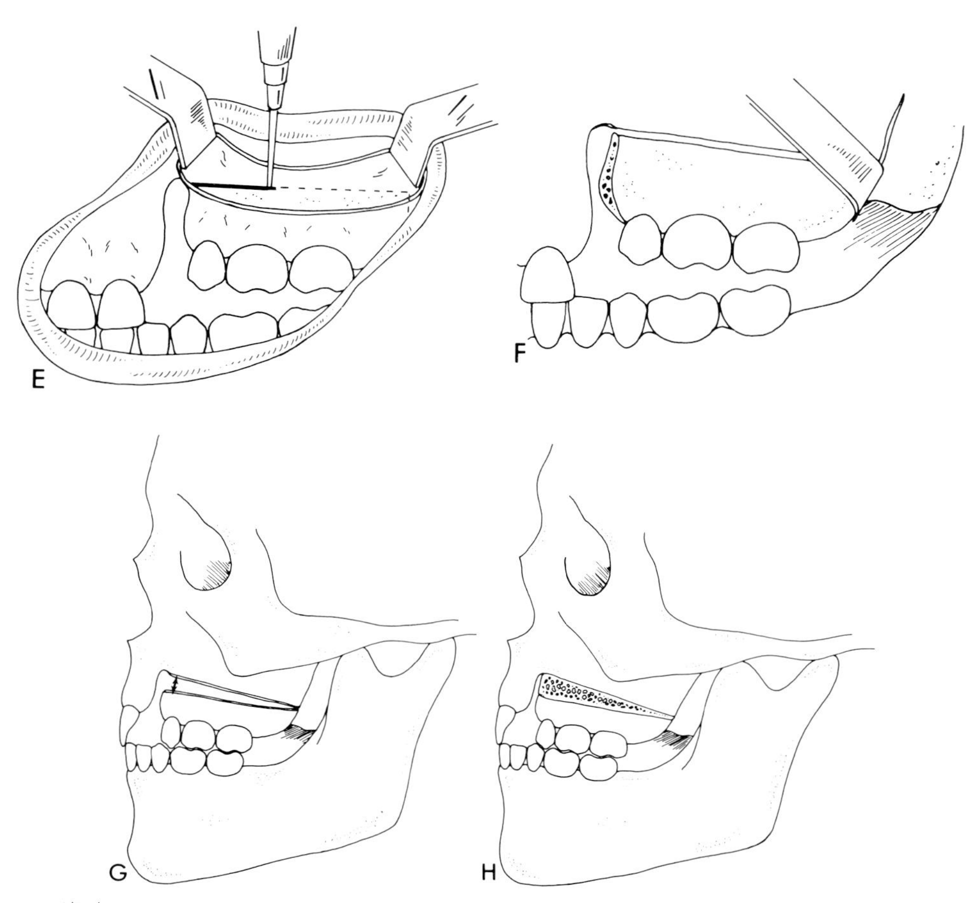

Figure 17–7 *Continued.* *E,* Two bone cuts are made to reposition the lateral segment surgically in order to bring it into proper occlusion. Buccal and palatal cuts are made from buccal aspect. *F,* The posterior cut is made with a broad curved chisel. *G,* Lateral view of the repositioned lateral segment. *H,* Bone graft in place.

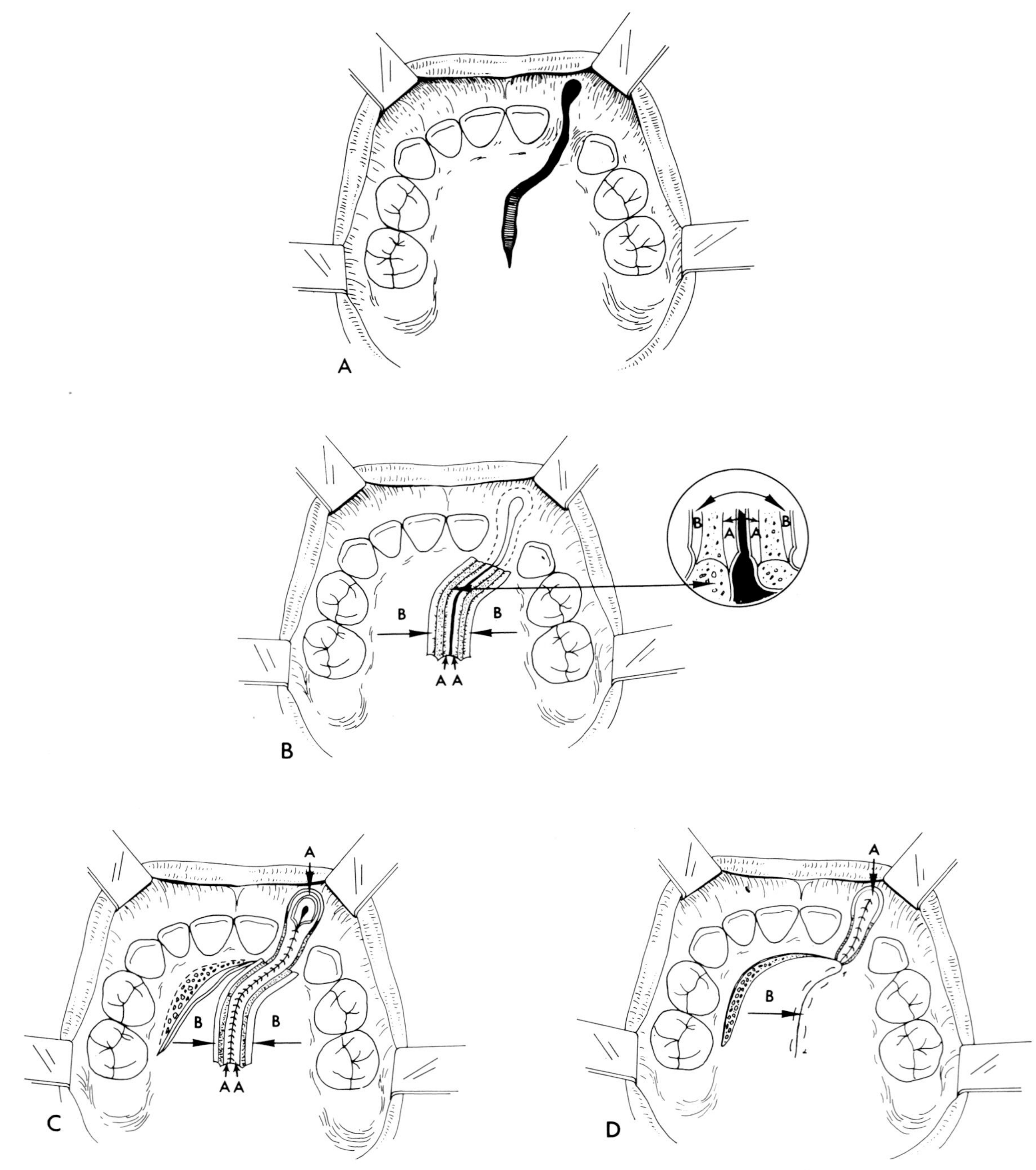

Figure 17–8. *A,* Palatal view of typical unilateral cleft of the palate and alveolar ridge and associated oronasal fistula in the vestibule of a child's mouth. *B,* First step in closure of the palatal defect (closure of the oronasal fistula is shown in *H* and *I*). The mucosal margins on each side of the cleft are split, producing flaps A and B. *Inset* shows close-up view of the bone margins of the cleft and the two flaps resulting from the split of the mucosa. *C,* The A flaps are turned in and sutured together, with the suture knots on the nasal aspect. *Broken line* shows relaxation incision to provide mobility for a palatal mucoperiosteal flap. *D,* Palatal view of completed closure of the palatal defect. The thick palatal mucoperiosteal flap has been raised and sutured with horizontal mattress sutures, leaving some exposed bone, which will be covered by granulation tissue.

Legend continued on the opposite page

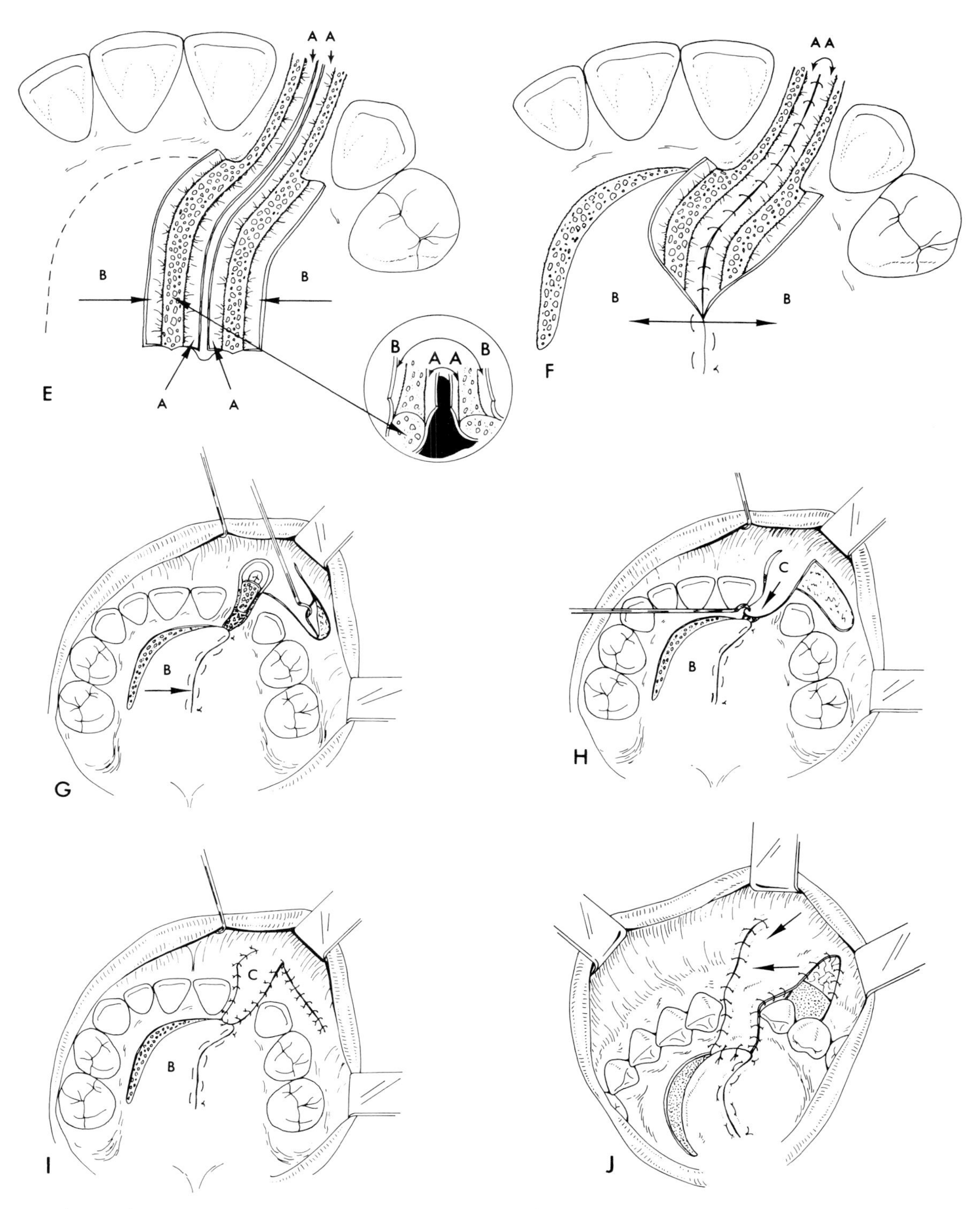

Figure 17–8 *Continued.* *E* and *F*, Close-up view of the creation of the tissue flaps to permit double-layered closure of the defect. *E*, Tissue flaps A and B and the bone edges of the cleft. *F*, Enlarged view of A flaps sutured as shown in *C* to provide closure on the nasal floor. *G*, The palatal defect is closed on both the nasal and oral sides with only the nasal layer closed in the bone graft and fistula area. The initial incision for formation of a pedicle flap from the vestibule is shown. *H*, Pedicle flap has been swung from the vestibule over the bone graft and the oronasal fistula. *I*, Repair completed, with the palatal defect closed with split mucoperiosteal flaps and the fistula and bone graft covered with a pedicle flap. *J*, If the defect is small, the sliding mucoperiosteal flap is advantageous, as attached gingiva is then positioned more closely over the alveolar ridge.

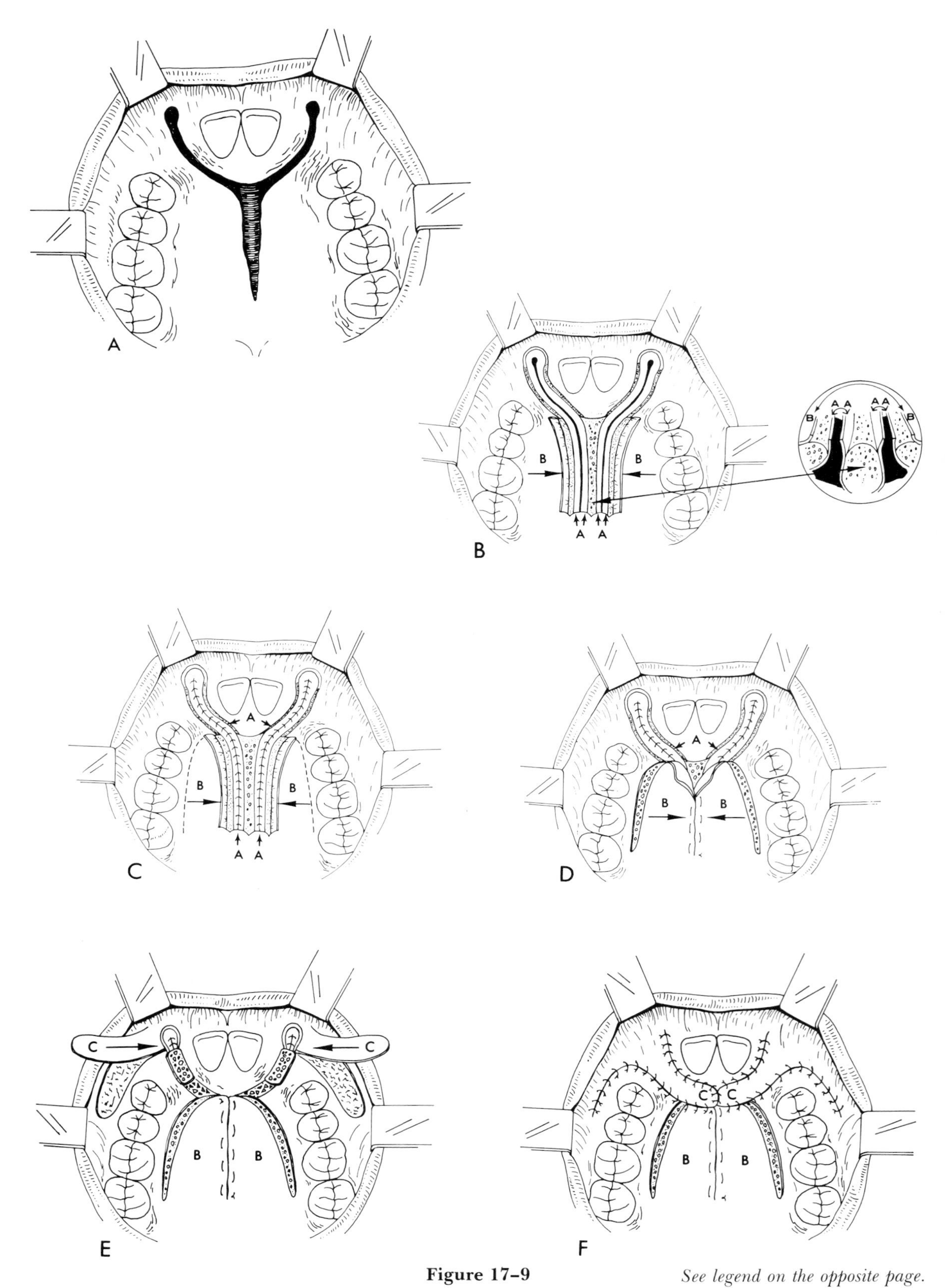

Figure 17–9 *See legend on the opposite page.*

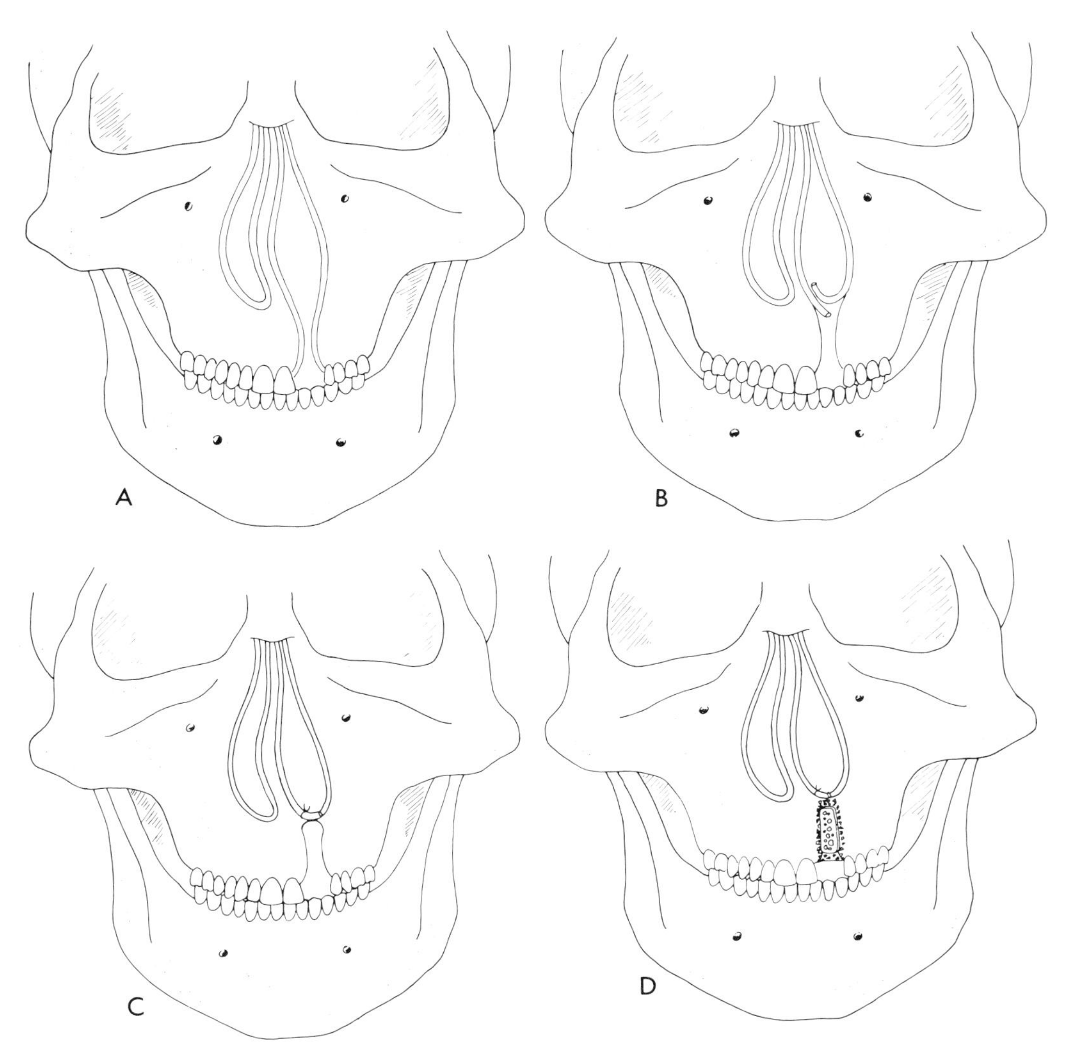

Figure 17–10. Schematic drawings in frontal or coronal section demonstrate steps in the closure of a unilateral cleft and placement of a bone graft. *A*, Original condition. *B*, Establishment of a nasal floor by turning a mucosal flap in on itself. *C*, Nasal floor completely closed. *D*, Bone graft placed in cleft defect.

Figure 17–9. *A*, Palatal view of typical bilateral cleft of the palate and alveolar process and associated oronasal fistula in an adult. *B*, First step in closure of the palatal defect and oronasal fistula. The mucosal margins on each side of the cleft are split, producing A and B flaps. *Inset* shows a close-up view of bone margins on the cleft and the two flaps resulting from the split of the mucosa. *C*, The A flaps are turned in and sutured together with the suture knots on the nasal aspect. *Broken line* shows relaxation incision used to provide mobility of the thick palatal mucoperiosteal flap. *D*, Palatal view of partial closure of the palatal defect and closure of the nasal side of the remaining defect. A thick palatal mucoperiosteal flap is raised, slid over the palatal defect, and sutured with horizontal mattress sutures. *E*, Palatal view shows palatal defect closed on both the nasal and oral aspects and the bone graft in place with only the nasal layer closed in the bone graft and fistula areas. Incisions for pedicle flaps (C) are made in the vestibule. *F*, The pedicle flaps are swung from the vestibule over the bone grafts and oronasal fistulae and sutured. The palatal defect now is closed with split mucoperiosteal flaps and the fistulae and bone grafts are covered with pedicle flaps from the vestibule. See Ch. 9 for further details of simultaneous Le Fort I osteotomy, bone grafting residual alveolar and palatal clefts, and repair of oronasal fistulae.

CASE REPORTS

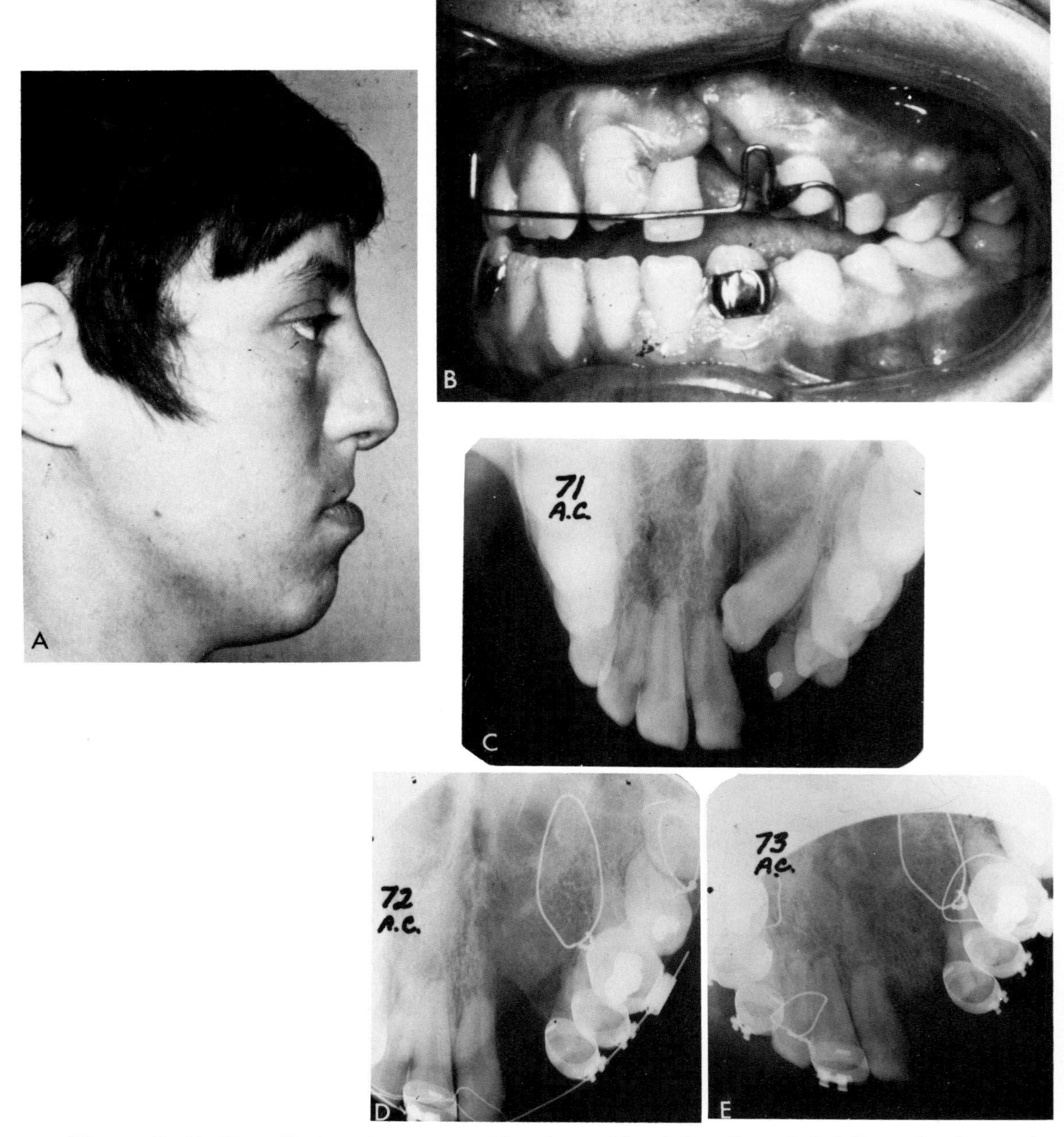

Figure 17–11 (Case 17–1). An 18-year-old patient with a left unilateral cleft lip and palate and a deficient maxilla. *A,* Facial profile. *B,* Close-up view of malocclusion, cleft, and pseudoprognathism. Patient is wearing a Hawley-type appliance that supplies a missing anterior tooth. *C,* Preoperative radiograph shows cleft and canine tooth erupted into the cleft. *D,* Postoperative radiograph following surgical advancement of the maxilla and removal of the canine tooth. Because the defect was treated late, the cuspid tooth had erupted to such an extent that it required removal. Loss of the premolar tooth is a disadvantage of late repair. *E,* Occlusal radiograph taken 1 year following bone grafting of the cleft, which was done 9 months after the maxillary advancement.

Legend continued on the opposite page

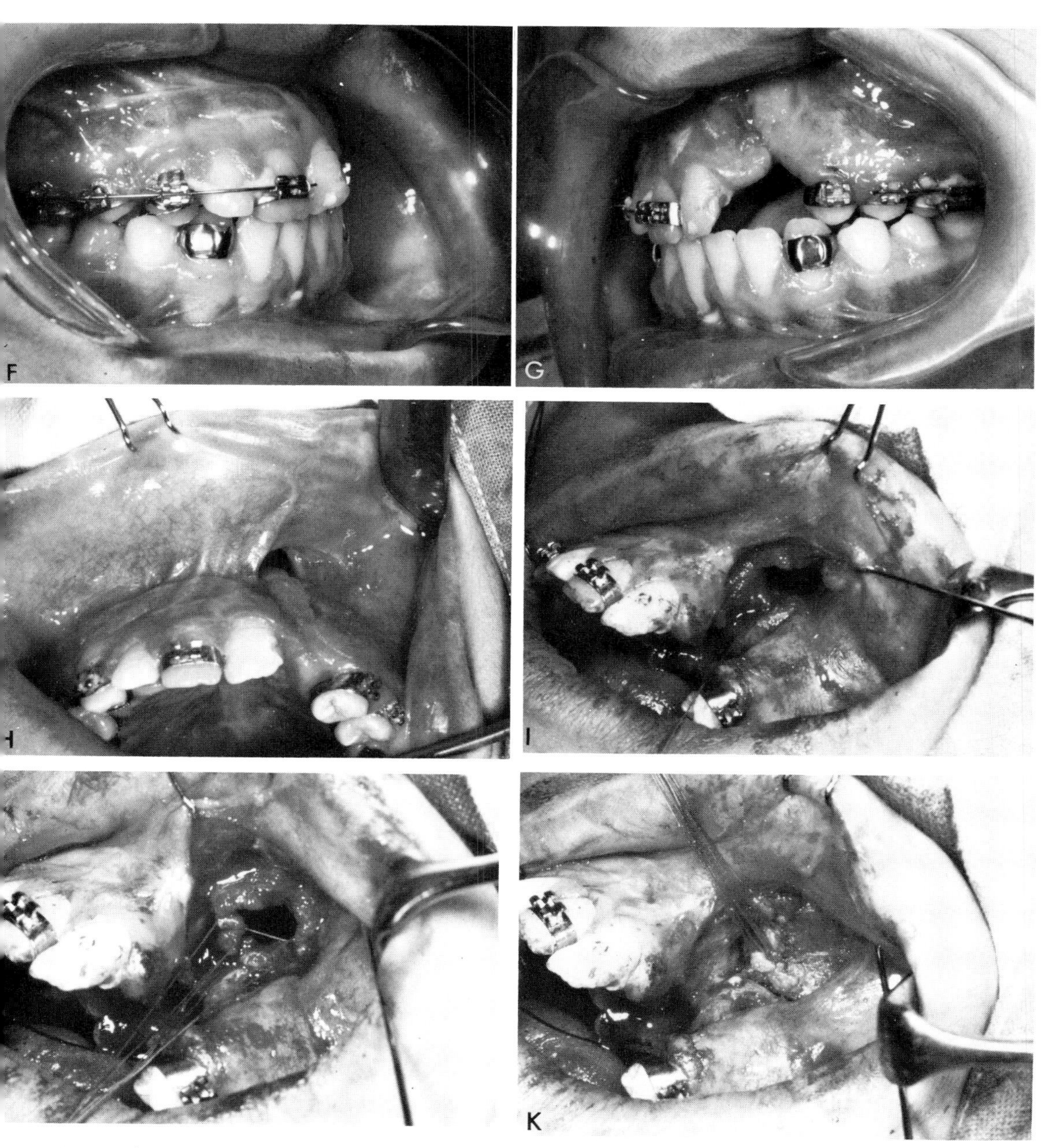

Figure 17–11 *Continued.* *F* and *G*, Postoperative views. *F*, Occlusion of the right side following maxillary advancement. *G*, Cleft side occlusion after the maxillary advancement. Note increase in size of cleft as compared with *B*. *H*, View of cleft area shows labionasal fistula. Steps in closure of the fistula and bone graft of the cleft are shown in following sequence. *I* through *O*, Closure of fistula and bone grafting of cleft. *I*, Initial step in closure of the fistula is creation of tissue flap for forming the nasal side of the vestibule by splitting the rolled edge of the labionasal fistula. *J*, Tissue flaps are inverted to create the nasal floor, extending over the alveolar defect onto the palate if necessary. *K*, Nasal floor is completely closed with suture knots on the nasal aspect.

Illustration continued on the following page

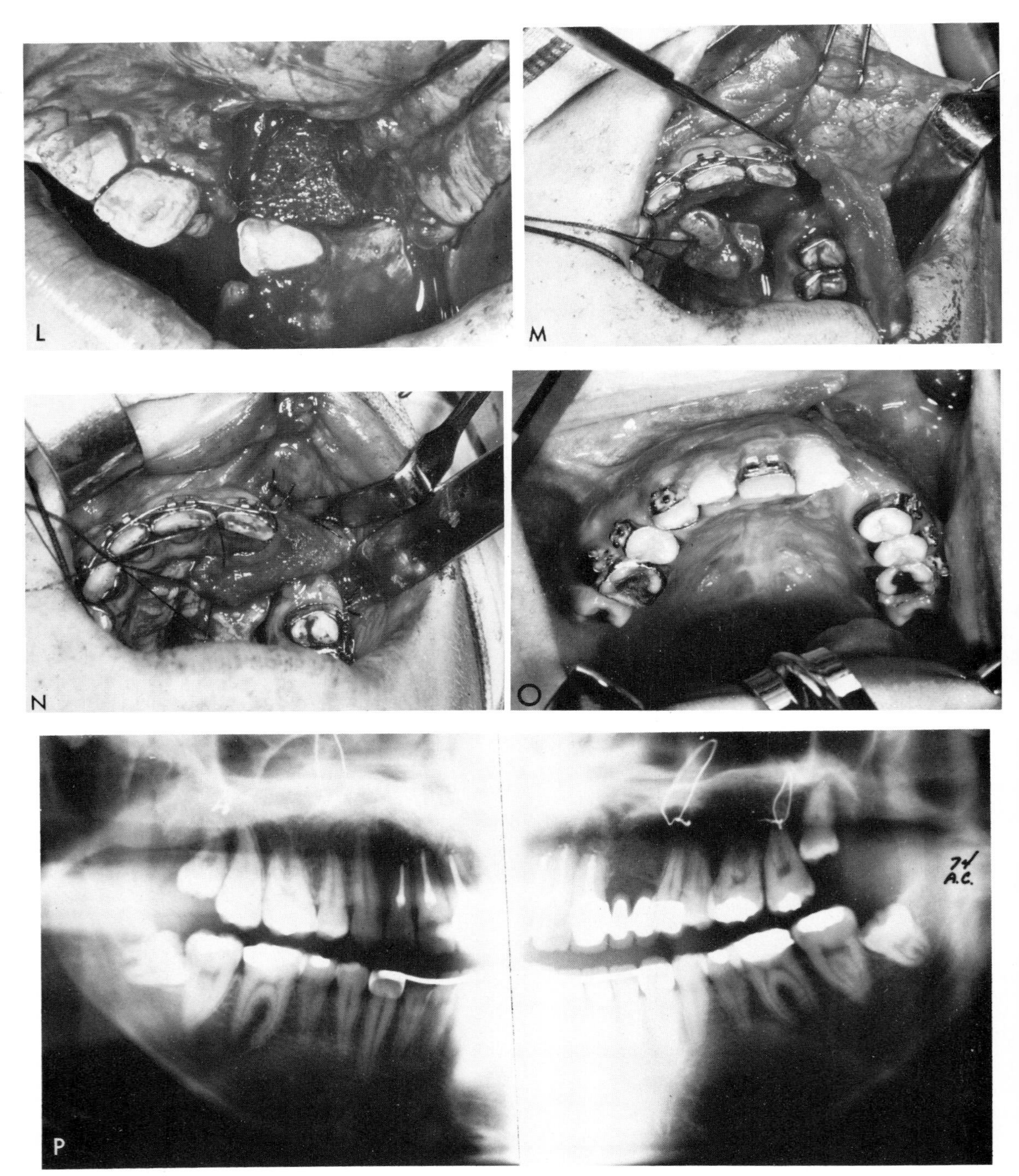

Figure 17–11 *Continued.* *L,* Bone graft is wedged into the alveolar defect with excess of particulate bone marrow packed around the wedge. (Patient is not the same shown in other photographs.) *M,* A full-thickness pedicle flap is taken from the buccal vestibule. *N,* The pedicle is brought across the alveolar ridge over the bone graft and sutured to the palatal mucoperiosteal flap. (Patient not the same as in other photographs.) *O,* A 6-month postoperative view. Note adequate vestibule without vestibuloplasty. Sometimes a secondary vestibuloplasty is required. *P,* Panographic view taken 3 years after initial surgery shows fixed bridgework in place and endodontic treatment provided by the family dentist. Wire sutures present from the maxillary advancement are still evident.

Legend continued on the opposite page

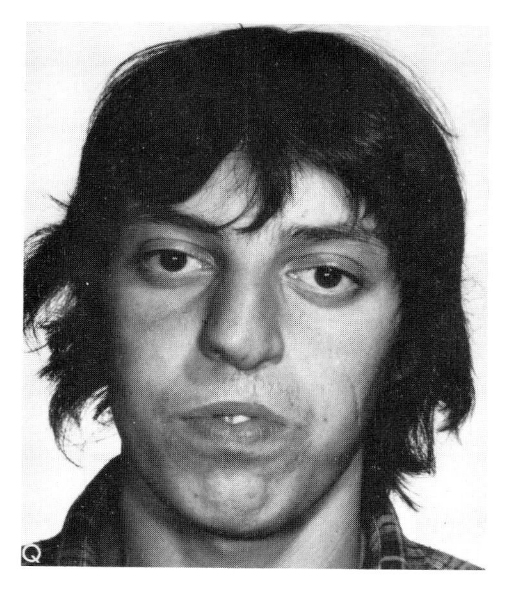

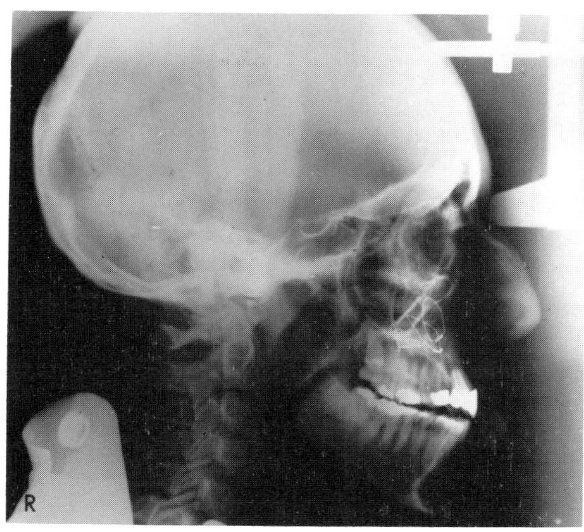

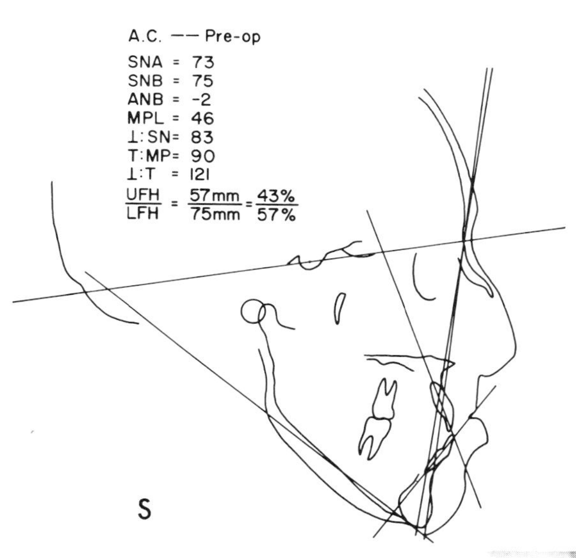

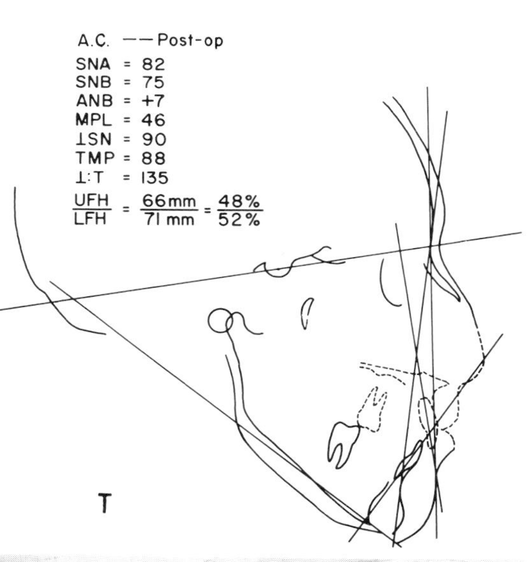

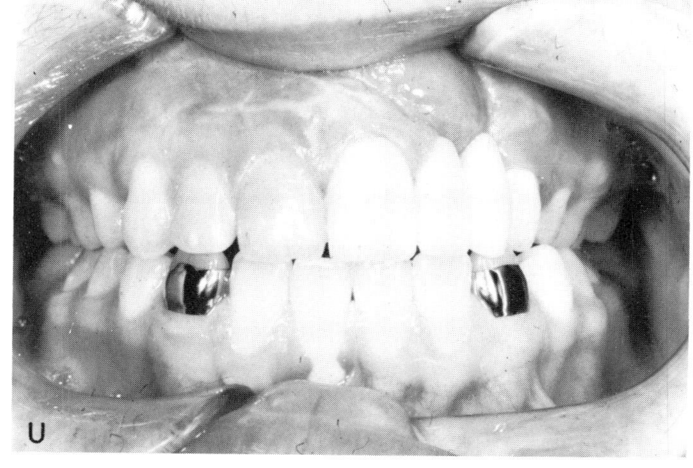

Figure 17–11 *Continued.* *Q*, Anterior photograph of patient 4 years following maxillary surgery. Nose is yet to be repaired. *R*, Lateral cephalogram 4 years post surgery. *S*, Preoperative cephalometric analysis. *T*, Postoperative alveolar cleft repair and maxillary advancement cephalometric analysis. *U*, Final intraoral view. Note: Bridge is in place and there is good arch alignment.

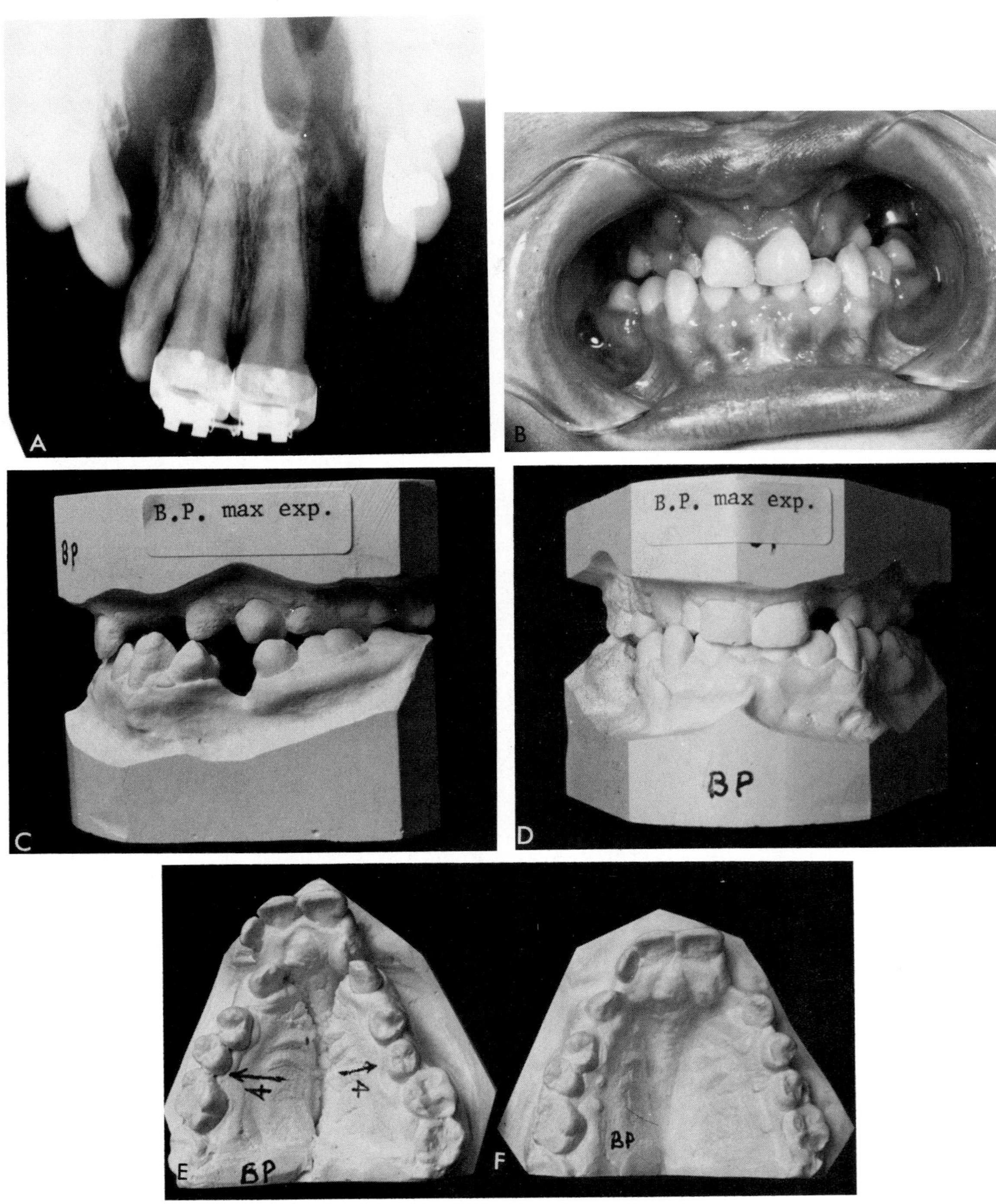

Figure 17–12 (Case 17–2). Treatment of adult with a bilateral alveolar cleft. *A*, Occlusal radiograph. *B*, Intraoral view shows collapse of the lateral segments of the maxilla. *C* through *F*, Casts of patient. *C*, Lateral view of casts made following surgical expansion of the lateral segments but before closure of the alveolar clefts. *D*, Anterior view following surgical expansion of the lateral segments but before closure of the alveolar clefts. *E*, Palatal view of cast made prior to surgery. *F*, Palatal postsurgical cast made 4 months after operation.

Legend continued on the opposite page

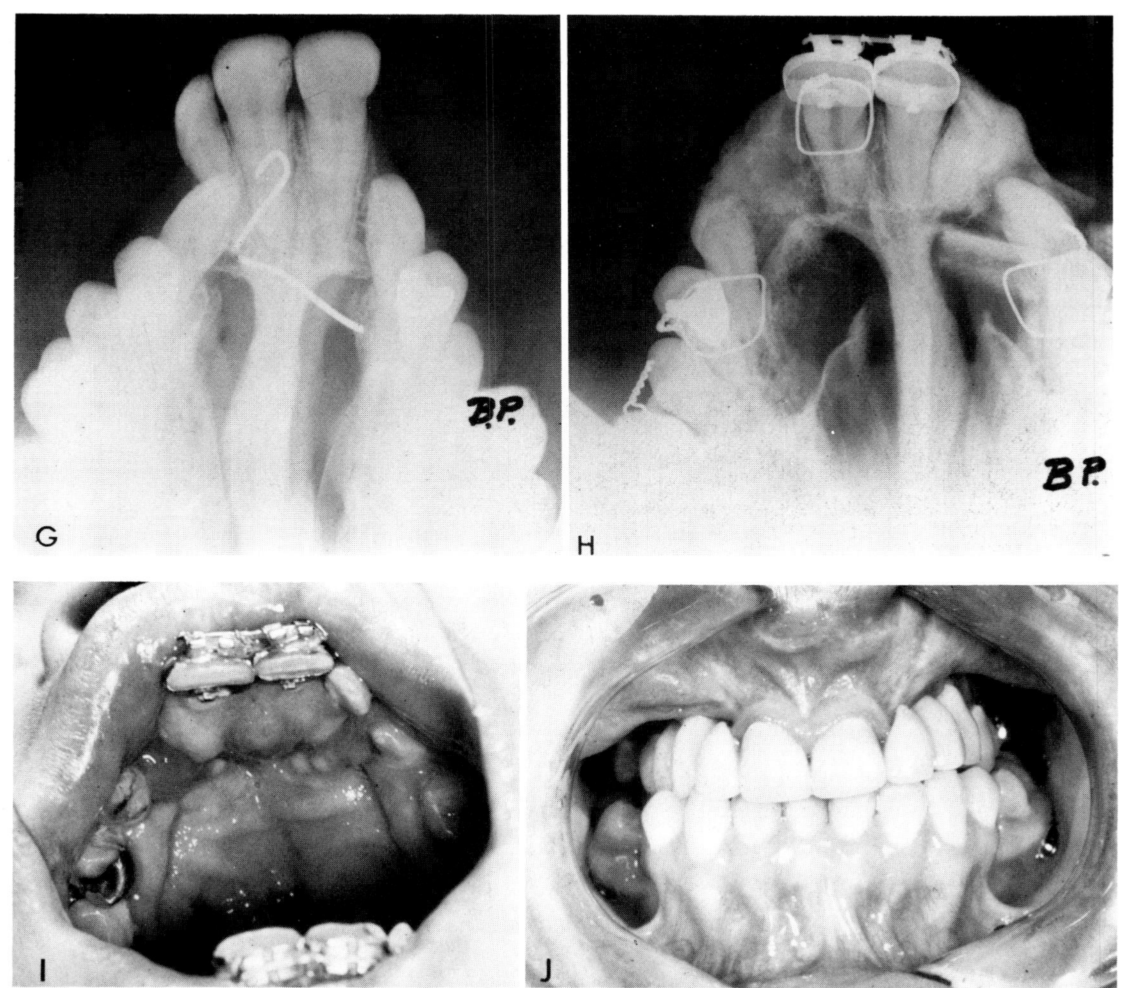

Figure 17-12 *Continued.* *G* and *H*, Occlusal radiographs. *G*, Preoperative. *H*, Postoperative radiograph made 4 months after lateral maxillary segments had been expanded surgically and 10 days after bone grafting of the alveolar clefts (a retainer with wires is in place). *I*, Postoperative palatal view. Note: Arch expansion and closure of defects. *J*, Intraoral view. Note: Prosthesis in place and reasonable occlusion.

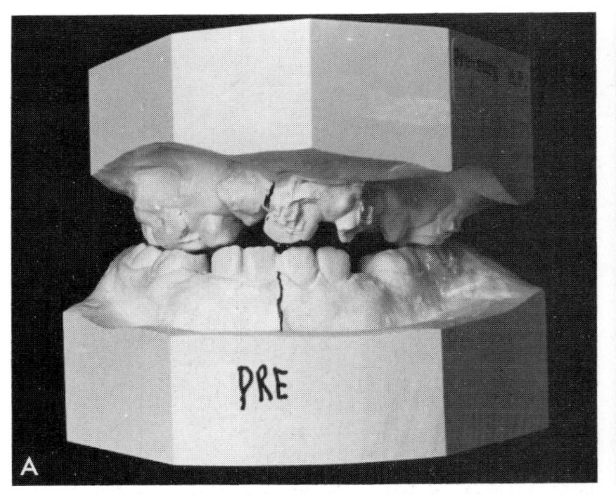

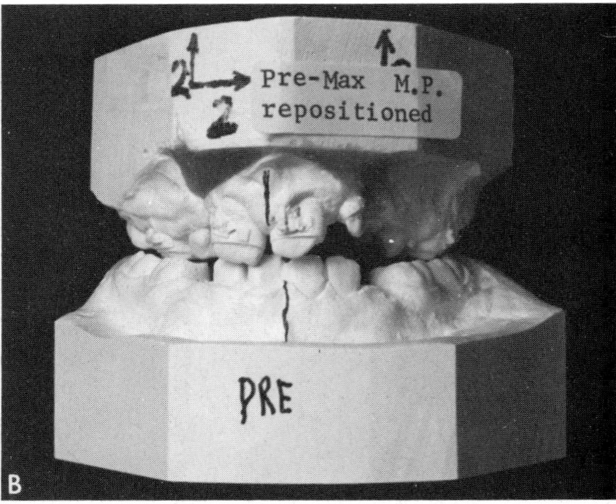

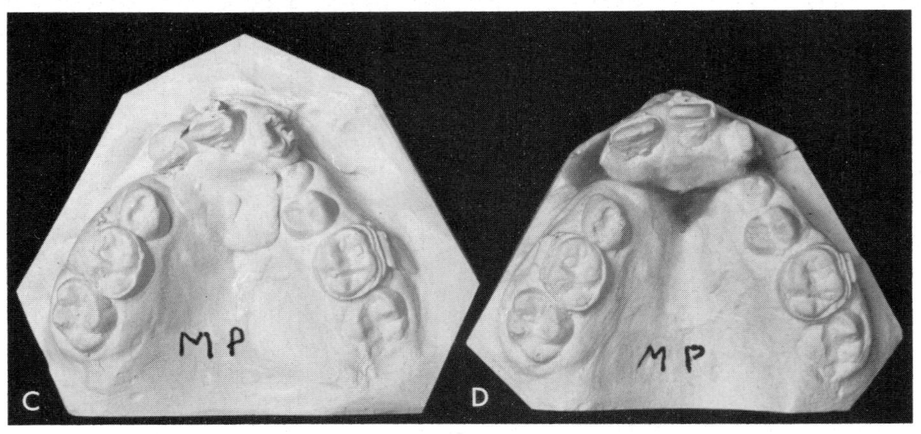

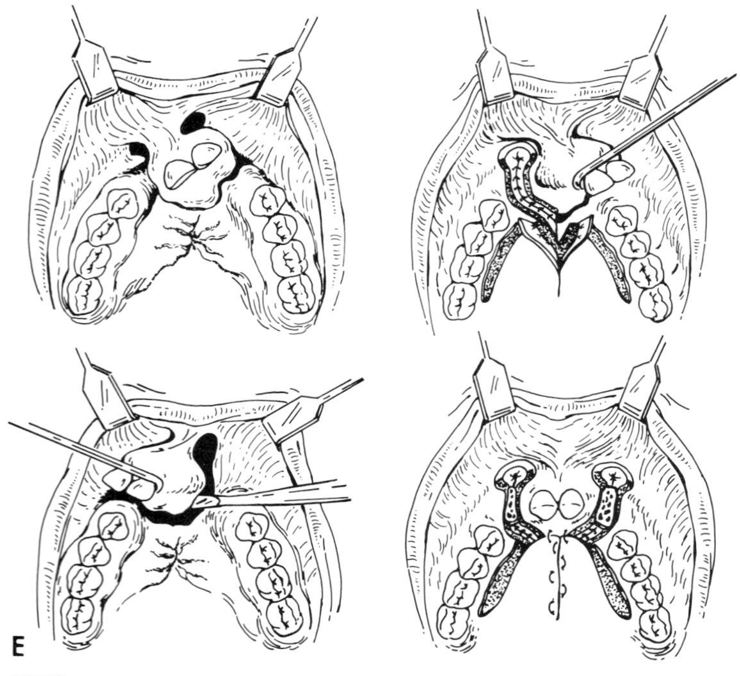

Figure 17–13 *See legend on the opposite page*

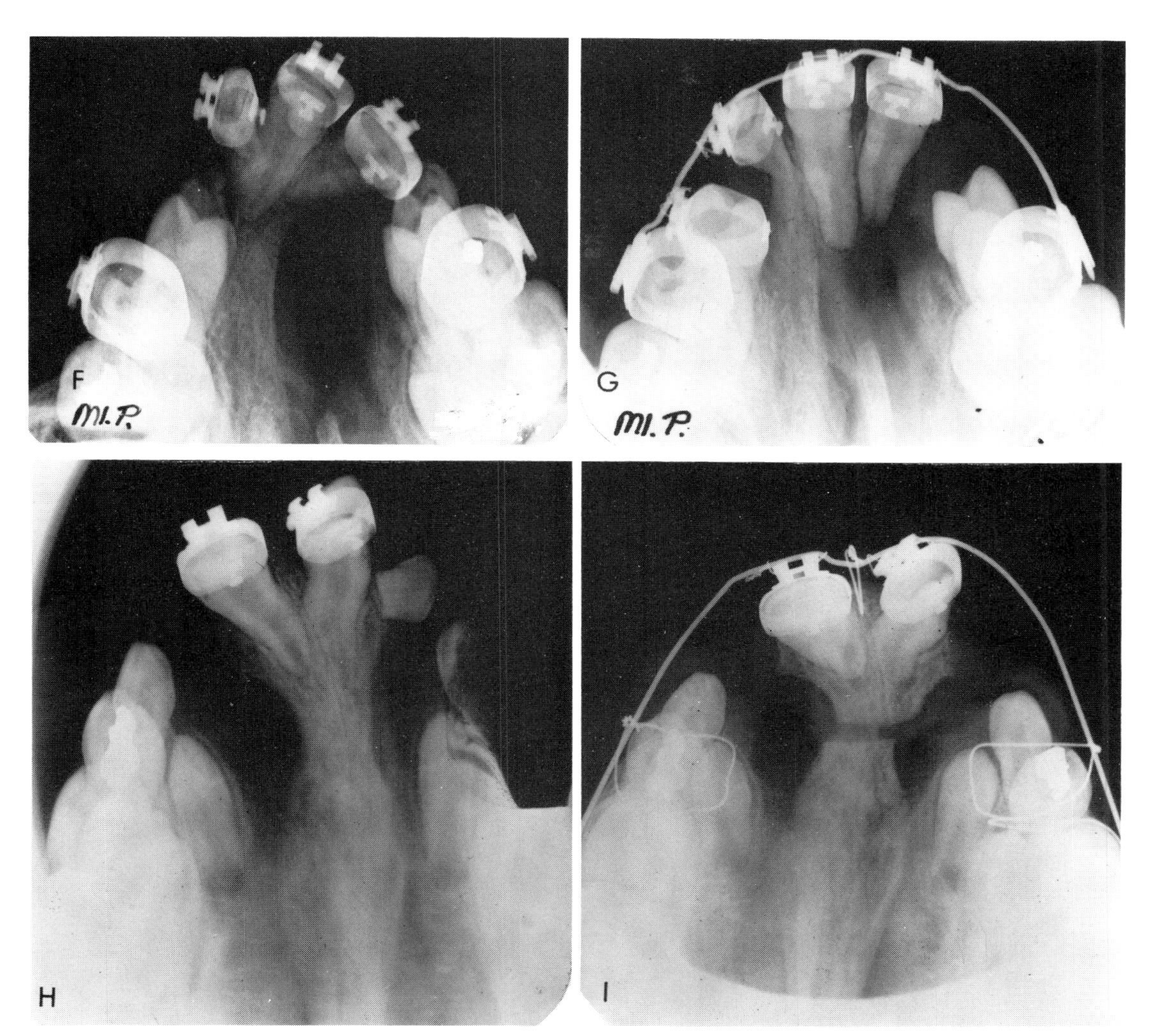

Figure 17–13 (Case 17–3). Treatment of a complete bilateral cleft lip and palate and a deviated premaxilla. *A*, Labial view of preoperative cast. *B*, New position of the premaxilla shown on plaster casts following model surgery. *C* and *D*, Occlusal views of plaster casts. *C*, Preoperative cast. Note obturator that patient wears to occlude an oronasal fistula. *D*, Cast made after model surgery shows premaxilla as it will be positioned following operation. *E*, Schematic drawing of the surgical procedure for repositioning a deviated premaxilla and closing the bilateral alveolar clefts with a bone graft. *F*, Preoperative and *G*, postoperative occlusal radiographs show repositioned premaxilla. *H*, Preoperative, and *I*, 10-day postoperative occlusal radiographs of another patient show repositioning of the deviated premaxilla and sectioning of the vomer.

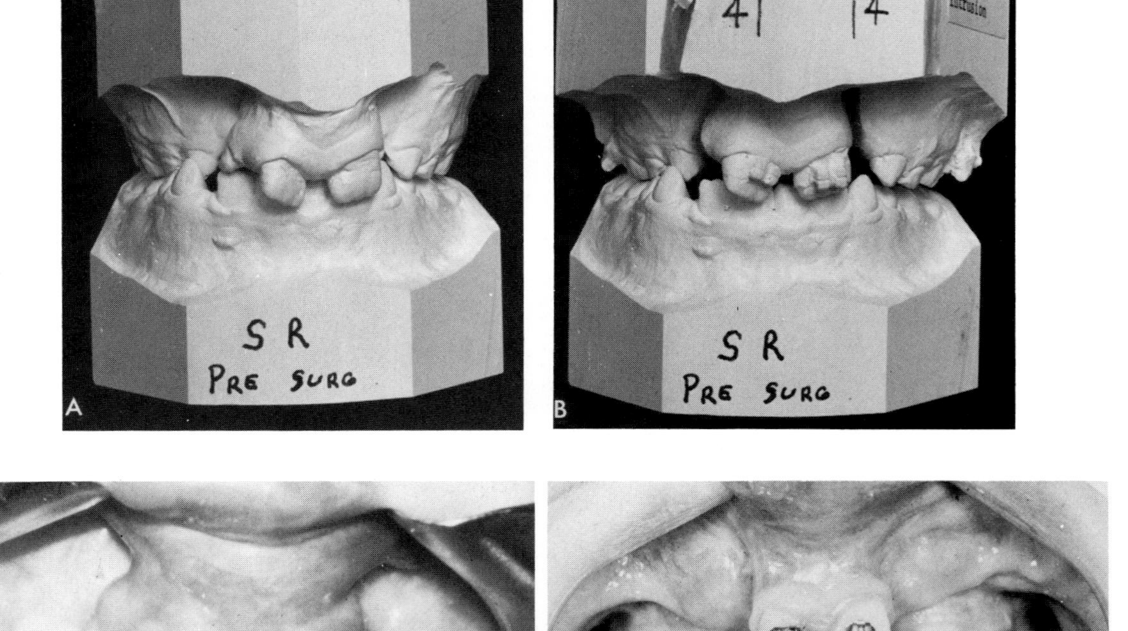

Figure 17–14 (Case 17–4). Treatment of a boy aged 9 years, 6 months, with complete bilateral cleft lip and palate with excessive overbite and protrusion of the premaxilla. *A*, Preoperative cast. *B*, Casts shown after model surgery demonstrating planned repositioning and elevation of the premaxilla. Repositioning can be done concurrently with bone grafting of the alveolar cleft if the lateral segments are in acceptable position. *C*, Preoperative clinical photograph. Note: Deep overbite and bilateral cleft defects. *D*, Postoperative intraoral view. Four years after surgical repositioning of the premaxilla.

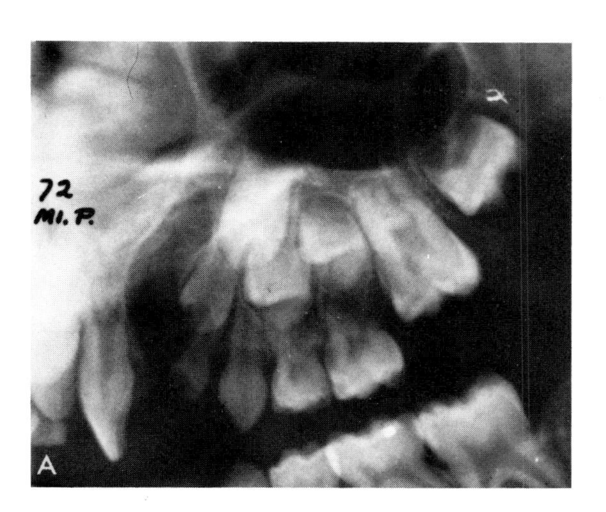

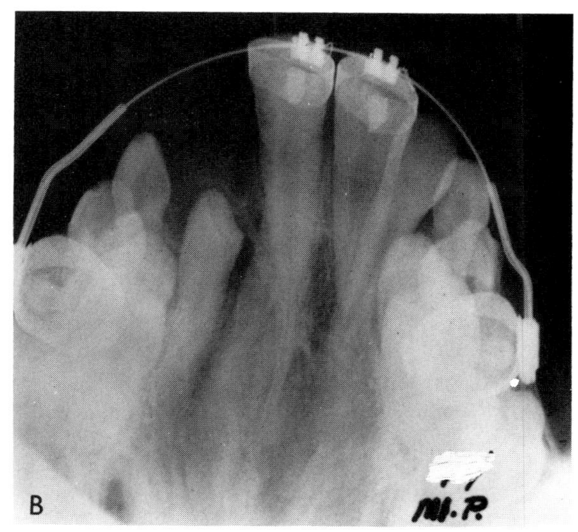

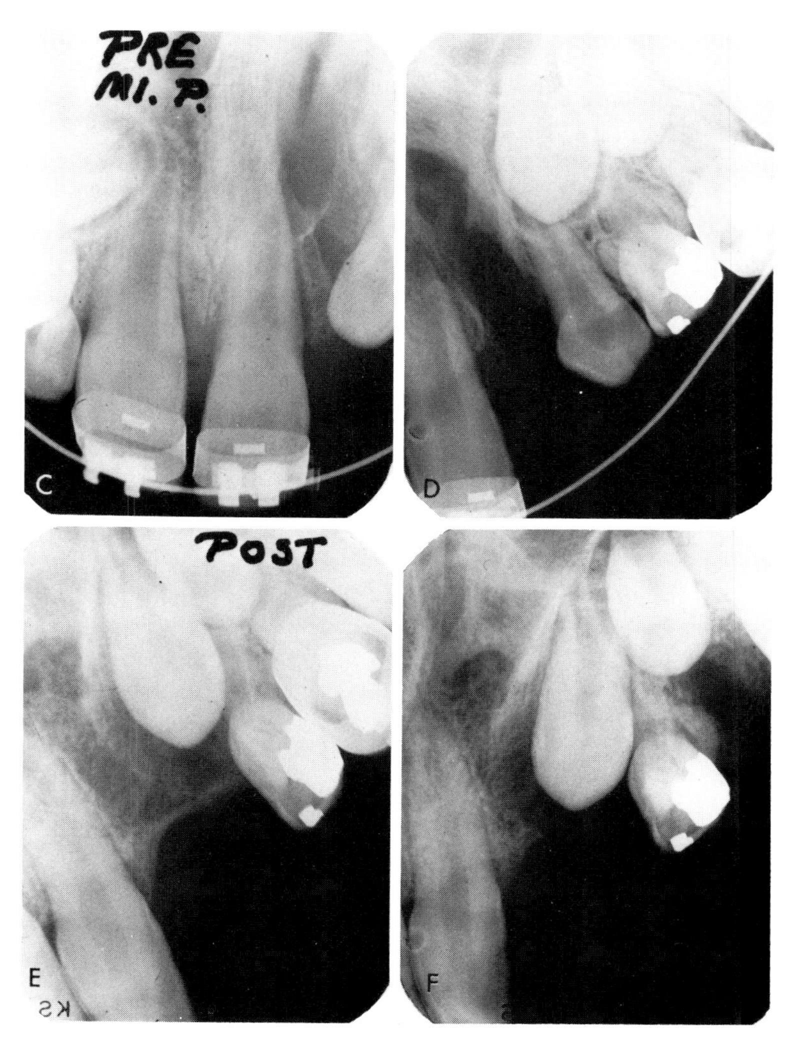

Figure 17–15 (Case 17–5). A unilateral cleft. *A*, Preoperative radiograph. The deciduous lateral incisor was extracted at the time of bone grafting. The malformed lateral incisor was left in place. *B*, Postoperative radiograph 1 year after grafting shows the malformed lateral incisor moving through the graft and the permanent canine erupting. *C* through *F*, Radiographic views. *C* and *D*, Two preoperative views of unilateral alveolar defect in a patient who was treated by bone grafting at 10 years of age. *E*, Postoperative radiograph 18 months after bone grafting shows the canine erupting into the bone graft but not completely erupted. *F*, Surgical exposure of the canine was undertaken to aid in its eruption.

Illustration continued on the following page

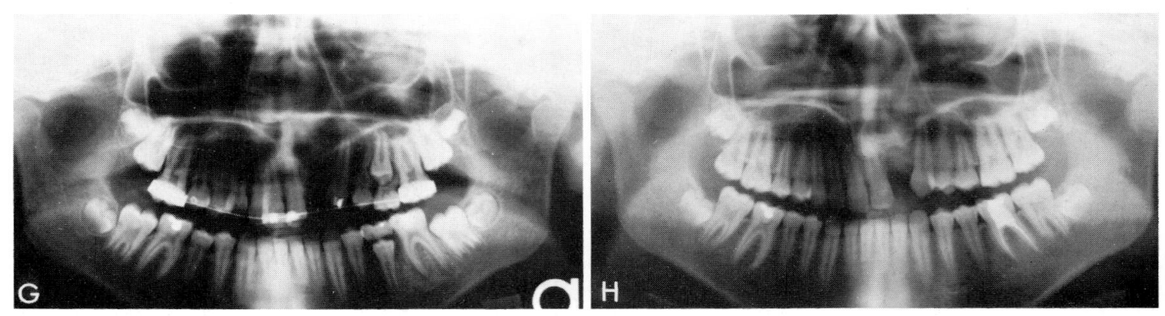

Figure 17–15 *Continued.* *G*, Panogram indicating orthodontic appliance guiding canine into final position 1 year after surgical exposure of the tooth. *H*, Panogram shows good alignment of the teeth after completing the orthodontic treatment and ready for a fixed prosthesis.

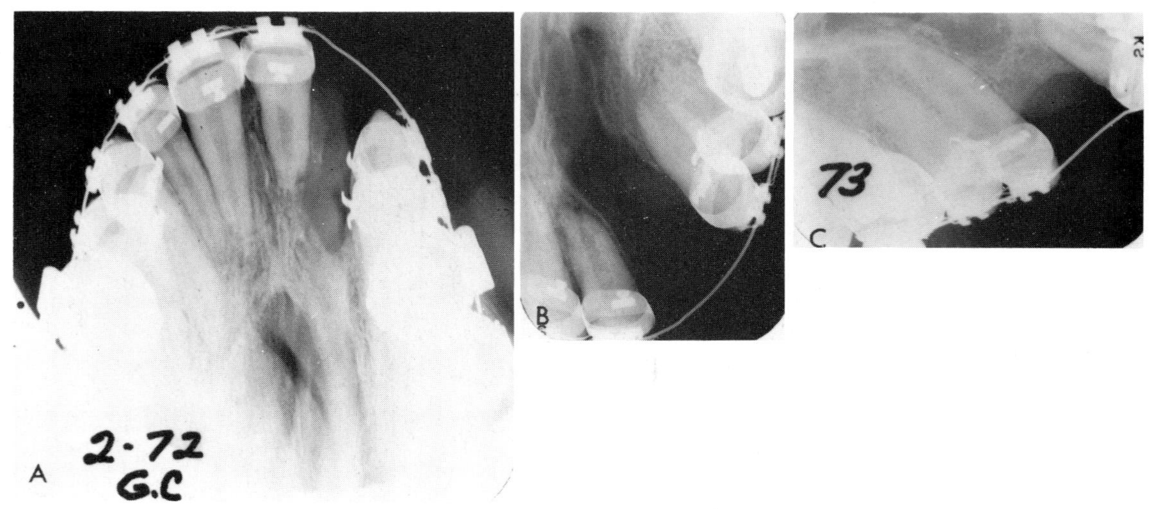

Figure 17–16 (Case 17–6). Unilateral cleft of the alveolus in a 15-year-old patient. *A*, Immediate preoperative occlusal view. Note the near absence of bone distal to the central incisor. *B*, Preoperative periapical view of the same area. *C*, Periapical view of the same area taken 1 year after bone grafting shows good acceptance of the graft at the surfaces of the teeth proximal to the previous cleft area.

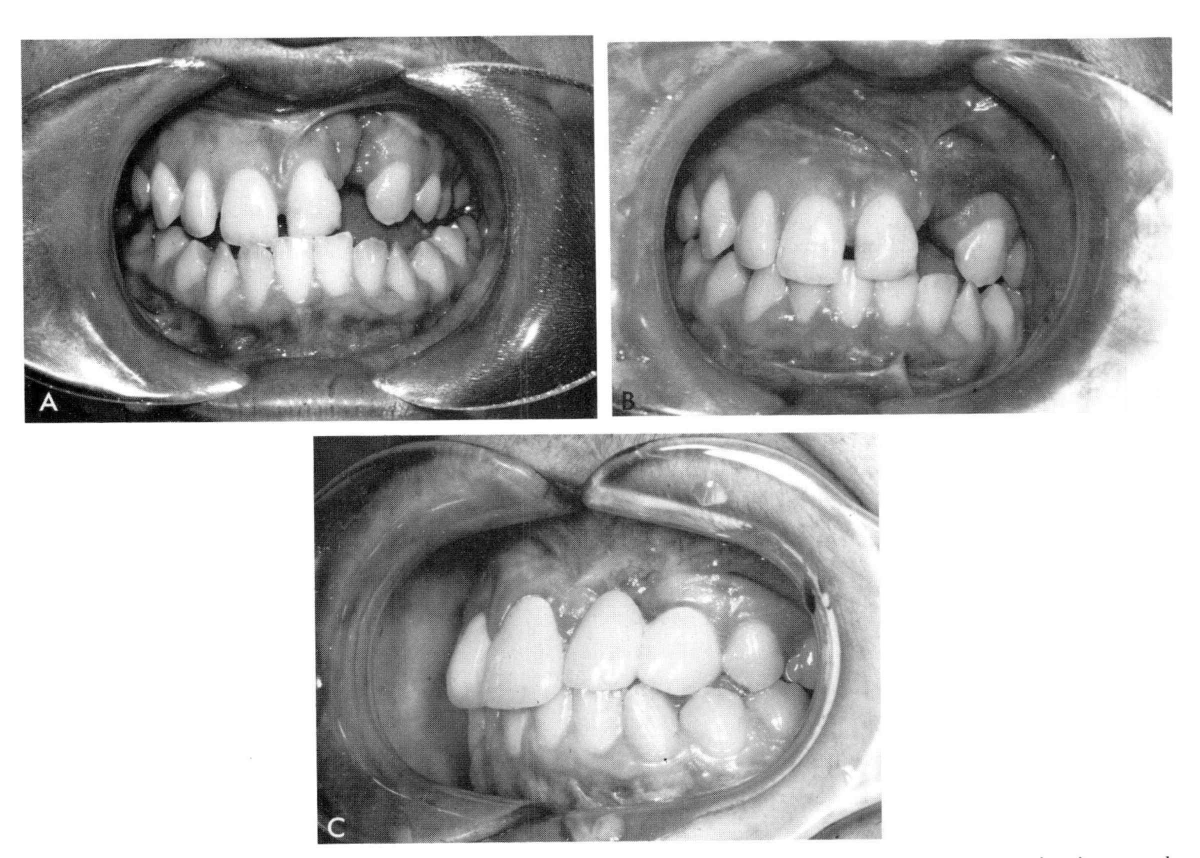

Figure 17–17 (Case 17–7). Patient with malocclusion and alveolar defect. *A*, Preoperative intraoral view. *B*, Postoperative intraoral view shows the alveolar cleft closed following bone grafting. The malocclusion had been corrected orthodontically. *C*, Same area shown in *B* with crown and bridgework in place to complete habilitation of the upper jaw.

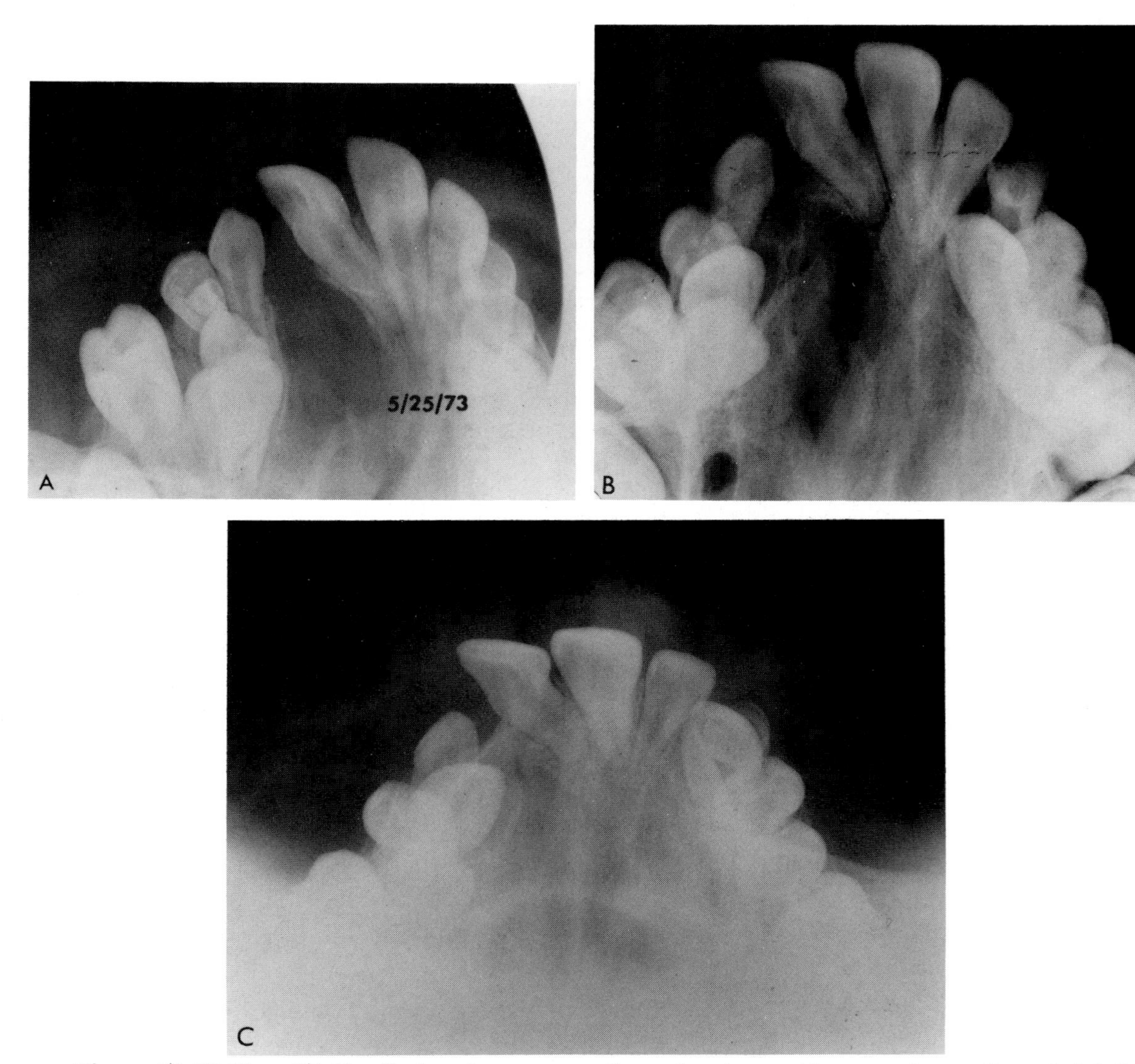

Figure 17–18 (Case 17–8). Series of x-rays are of a patient born with a complete unilateral cleft lip and palate who had a bone graft of the alveolar defect. Lip repair was at age 4 days, palate repair at age 18 months, and bone graft at age 10 years, 7 months. The upper left lateral incisor was congenitally missing. *A*, Preoperative occlusal view of the defect. *B*, Occlusal view taken 6 months postoperatively shows bony bridge. *C*, Occlusal view taken 18 months postoperatively shows canine tooth erupting into the bone graft.

Legend continued on the opposite page

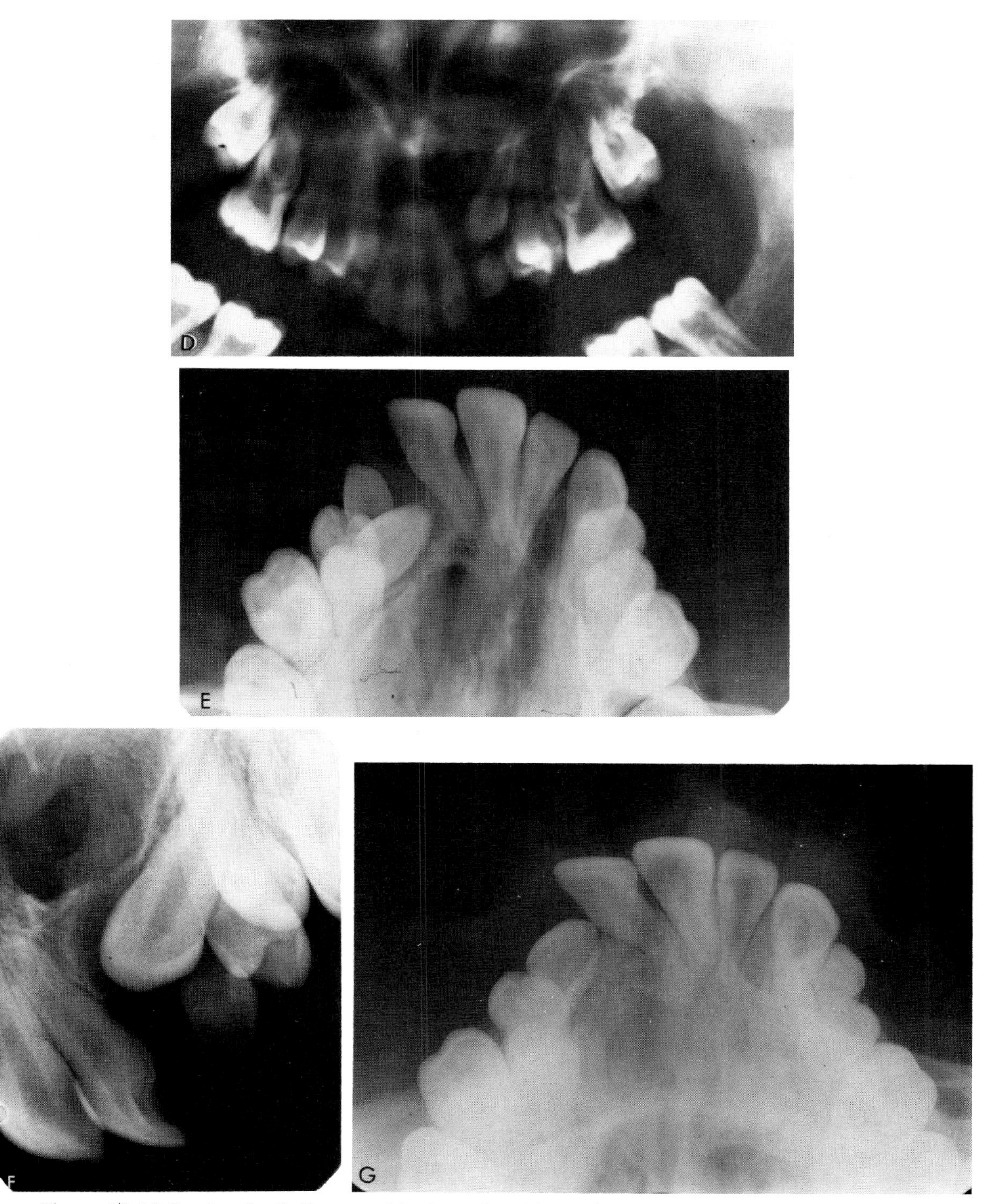

Figure 17–18 *Continued.* *D*, Panographic view taken 19 months postoperatively also shows the canine erupting into the bone graft. *E*, Occlusal view taken 30 months postoperatively shows the canine tooth erupting through the bone graft. *F*, Periapical view taken 30 months postoperatively shows a close-up view of the canine tooth erupting through the bone graft. *G*, Occlusal view taken 48 months postoperatively shows erupted canine through the bone graft.

Illustration continued on the following page

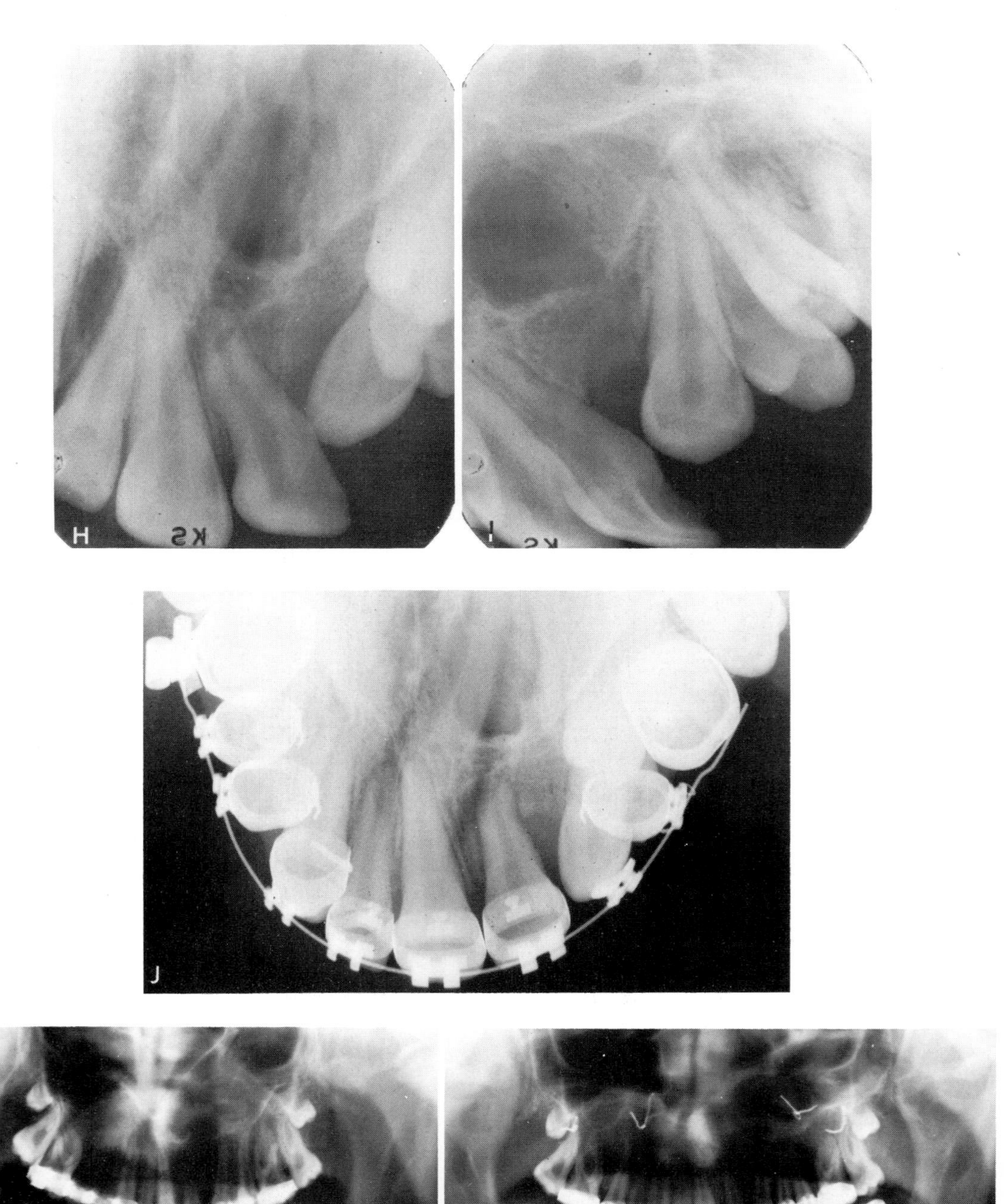

Figure 17–18 *Continued.* *H*, Periapical view taken 48 months postoperatively (at age 14 years) shows good bony bridging between canine and central incisor. *J* and *K*, Orthodontic appliance in position and case nearing completion 5 years after the graft. *L*, Postoperative panograph following maxillary advancement for final treatment.

Illustration continued on the opposite page

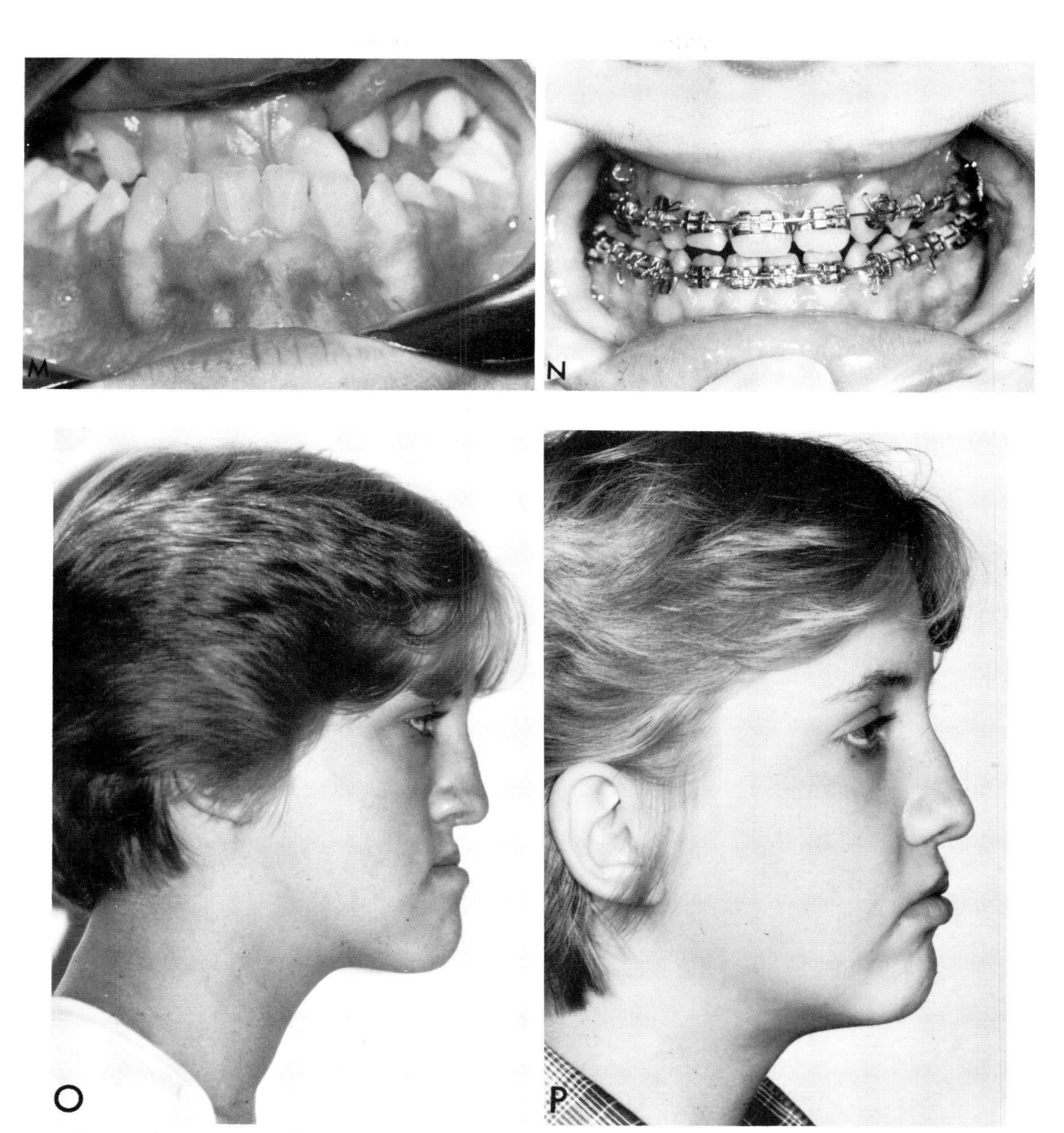

Figure 17–18 *Continued.* *M*, Preoperative intraoral view. Note: significant anterior and posterior crossbite. *N*, Intraoral view after alveolar bone graft and maxillary advancement. Note: Good arch and anterior and posterior teeth alignment. *O*, Preoperative profile shows maxillary collapse. *P*, Final profile after closure and maxillary advancement.

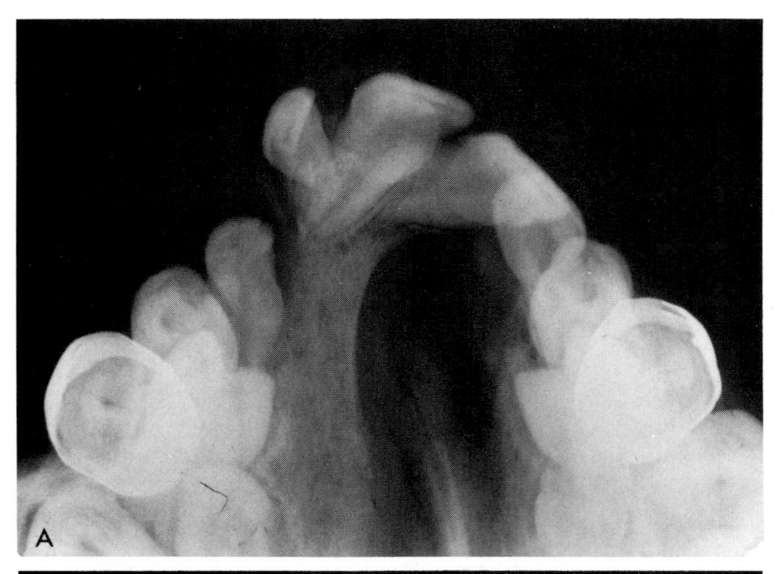

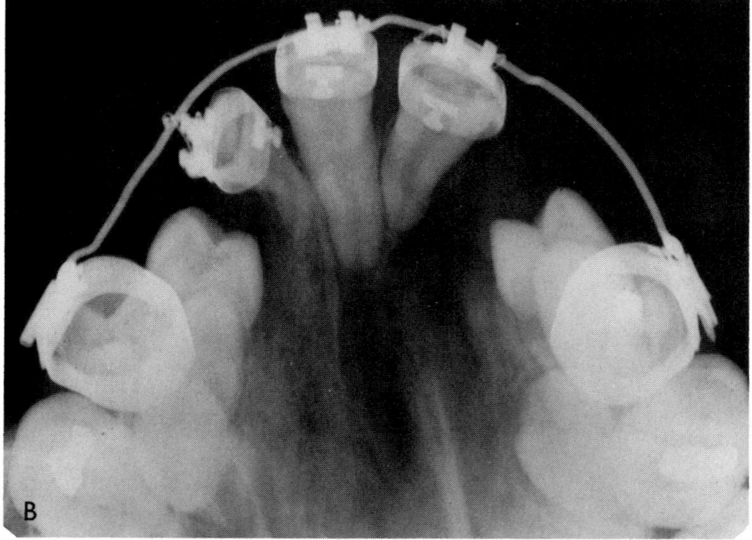

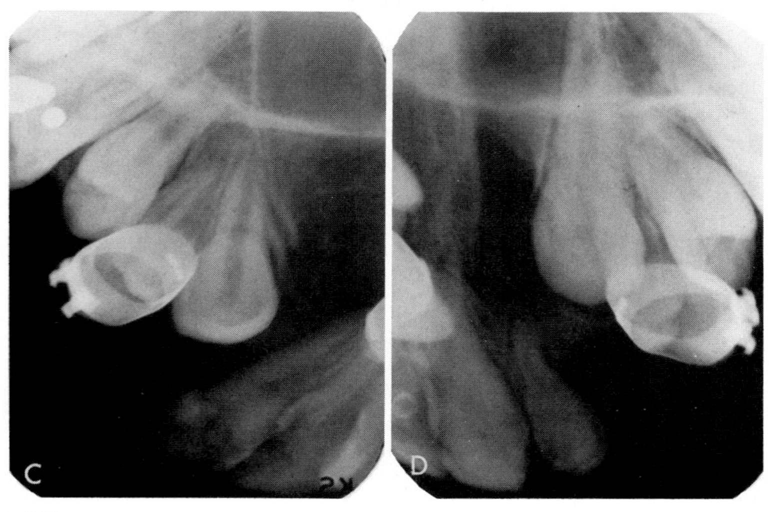

Figure 17–19 (Case 17–9). Repositioning of the premaxilla and subsequent stabilization of the premaxilla with bone grafts in a patient with a congenital bilateral cleft lip and palate as illustrated by radiographs. The lip was repaired at age 6 weeks and the palate at age 18 months. *A*, Preoperative occlusal view taken at age 11 years. The premaxilla was mobile and displaced, and there were bilateral oronasal fistulae. *B*, Postoperative view taken after repositioning of the premaxilla. Six months later, bone grafts were placed to stabilize the premaxilla, and the fistulae were closed. (These measures are now usually accomplished in one stage.) *C* and *D*, X-rays taken 20 months postoperatively show the upper right canine erupting through the bone graft and the upper left canine erupting into the bone graft but not through it. Final adjustment of the canine positions will be done orthodontically.

Legend continued on the opposite page

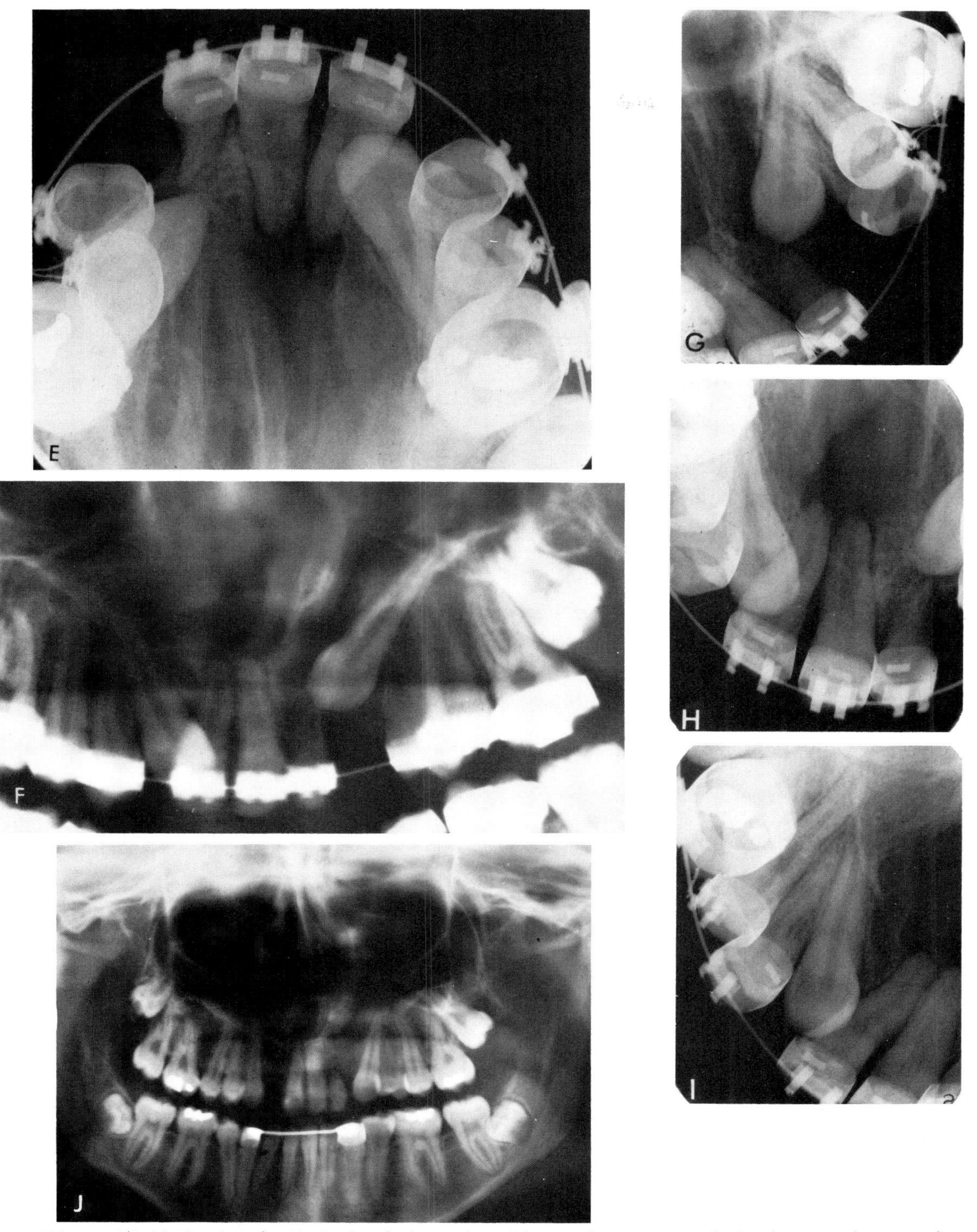

Figure 17–19 *Continued.* *E*, Occlusal view taken 32 months postoperatively shows arch expansion and alignment with the canine erupting through the graft. *F*, Panorex view taken 32 months postoperatively shows erupting canines. *G*, *H*, and *I*, Periapical x-rays taken 32 months postoperatively show erupting right and left canines. *J*, Panogram shows right and left canine teeth in the arch. Note: Good alignment of the teeth ready for fixed bridgework 5 years after original grafting.

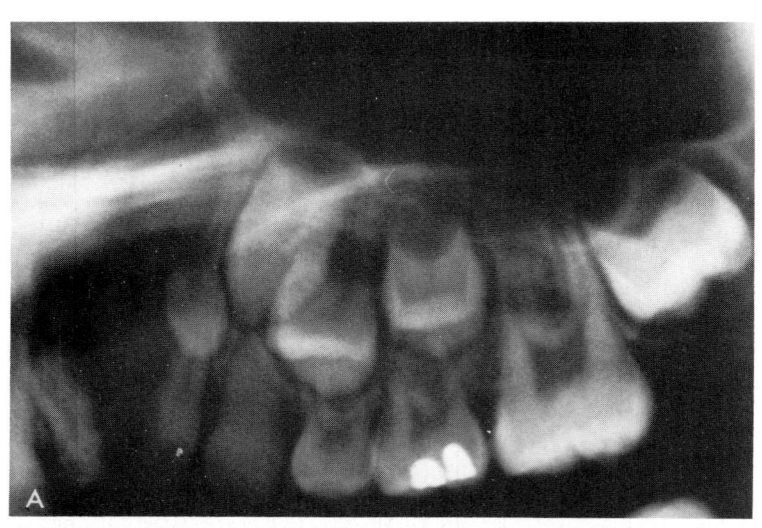

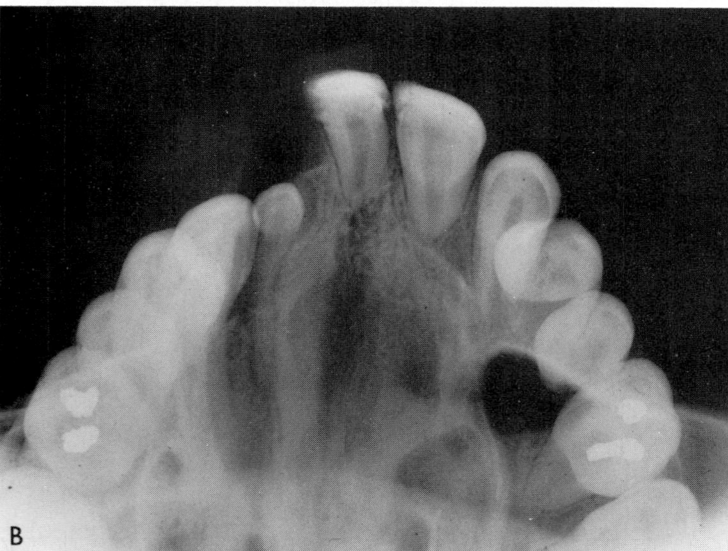

Figure 17–20 (Case 17–10). Results of bone graft of alveolar defect in the presence of a supernumerary tooth in a 10-year-old boy born with a complete unilateral cleft lip and palate, demonstrated by x-rays. *A*, Preoperative view of the defect. Note supernumerary tooth just mesial to the permanent canine. The tooth adjacent to the central incisor has no distal bone coverage and was extracted at the time of bone grafting. The supernumerary tooth was left in place. *B*, Two-year postoperative view of the bone graft site shows excellent bony bridging.

Legend continued on the opposite page

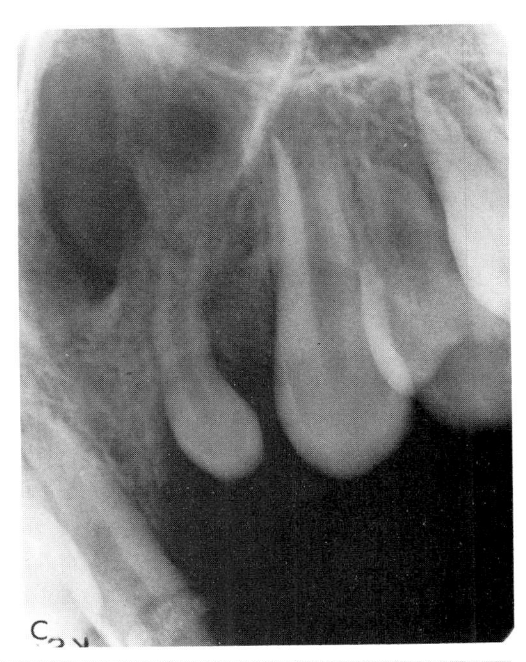

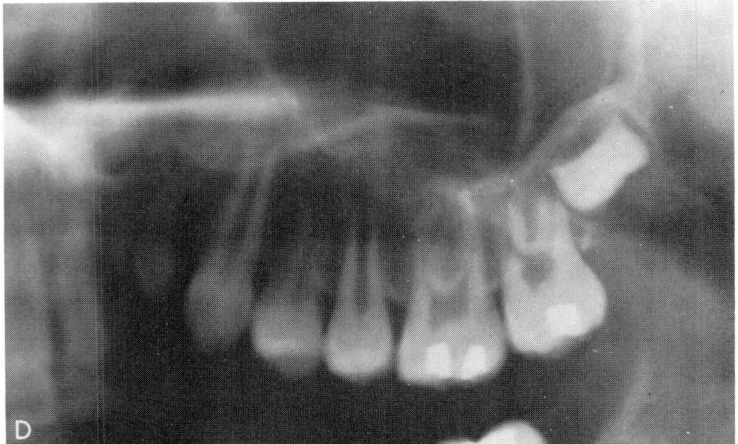

Figure 17–20 *Continued.* *C,* Three-year postoperative view shows both the canine and the supernumerary tooth erupting through the bone graft. *D,* Three-year postoperative Panorex view shows erupting canine and supernumerary tooth.

Illustration continued on the following page

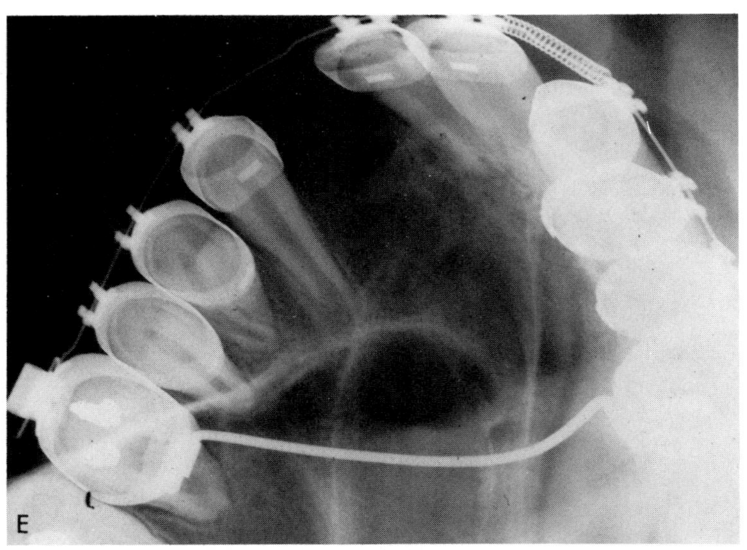

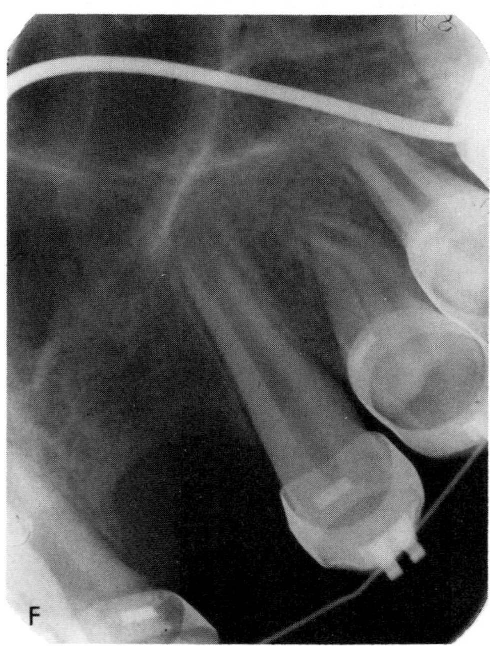

Figure 17–20 *Continued.* *E,* Occlusal view taken 40 months postoperatively shows proper position of canine and extraction of supernumerary tooth. *F,* Close-up view of periapical x-ray taken 40 months postoperatively shows excellent bony bridging. Patient is ready for a final fixed prosthesis.

REFERENCES

1. Backdahl M, Nordin K, Nylen B, Strombeck J: Transactions of the International Society of Plastic Surgeons, 3rd Congress. Amsterdam: Excerpta Medica Foundation, p 193, 1963.
2. Boo-Chai K: An ancient Chinese text on a cleft lip. Plast Reconstr Surg *38*:89, 1966.
3. Boyne PJ, Sand NS: Secondary bone grafting of residual alveolar and palatal defects. J Oral Surg *30*:87, 1972.
4. Brauer RO: Plast Reconstr Surg *35*:148, 1965.
5. Coccaro PJ, Pruzansky S: Cleft Palate J *2*:7, 1965.
6. Dieffenbach JF: Die operative Chirurgie. Leipzig: FA Bockhaus, 1845.
7. Dorrance GM: Lengthening of the soft palate operation. Ann Surg *82*:208, 1925.
8. Epstein LI, Davis BW, Thompson LW: Delayed bone grafting in cleft palate patients. Plast Reconstr Surg *46*:363, 1970.
9. Georgiade NE, Pickrell KL, Quinn GW: Varying concepts in bone grafting of alveolar

palatal defects. Cleft Palate J *1*:43–51, 1964.

10. Hagedorn HC: Über eine Modifikation der Hasenschartenoperation. Centralbl Chir *11*: 756, 1884.
11. Horton CE, Crawford HH, Adamson JE: John Peter Mettauer, America's first plastic surgeon. Plast Reconstr Surg *27*:268–278, 1961.
12. Johanson B: Primary bone grafting in clefts; the Northcroft Memorial Lecture. British Society of the study of orthodontics in the 21st. Biedglass, 1970.
13. Johanson B, Ohlsson A: Bone grafting and dental orthopaedics in primary and secondary cases of cleft lip and palate. Acta Chir Scand *122*:112, 1961.
14. Le Mesurier AB: The treatment of complete unilateral harelip. Surg Gynecol Obstet *95*:17, 1952.
15. Maisels DO: The timing of various operations required for complete alveolar clefts and their influence on facial growth. Br J Plast Surg *20*:230, 1967.
16. Schuchart, K.: Discussion Zum Vortrag Von A. Rehrmann: Ästhetiche Moment in der Lippensplaten Chirurgie (Nase Und Lippe). Fortschr Kiefer Gesichtschir, Bd. 7. Stuttgart: Thieme, 1961.
17. Millard DR: Refinements in rotation-advancement cleft lip technique. Plast Reconstr Surg *33*:26, 1964.
18. Mirault: Letter sur le bec-de lievre. Malgaigne J Chir *2*:257, 1844.
19. Nordin, KD: Treatment of primary total cleft palate deformity. Preoperative orthopaedic correction of the displaced components of the upper jaw in infants followed by bone grafting to the alveolar process clefts. Transactions of the European Orthodontic Society. The Hague, pp 333–339, 1957.
20. Nordin KD, Johanson B: Frei-Knockentransplantation bei Defekten im Alveolarkam nach Kieferortopädischer Einstellung der Maxilla bein Lippen-Kiefer-Gaumen spalten. Fortschr Kiefer Gesichtk. Band I. Stuttgart: Georg Thieme Verlag, 1955.
21. Perko M: Surgical correction of the position of the premaxilla in secondary deformities of cleft lip and palate. Excerpta Medica, International Congress, Rome, Series 174, 1967.
22. Pfeiffer G, Schuchardt K: Transactions of International Society of Plastic Surgeons. 3rd International Congress. Amsterdam: Excerpta Medica Foundation, p 282, 1963.
23. Robinson F, Wood B: Primary bone grafting in the treatment of cleft lip and palate with special reference to alveolar collapse. Br J Plast Surg *22*:336, 1969.
24. Rogers BO: Palate surgery prior to von Graefe's pioneering staphylorrhaphy (1816): an historical review of the early causes of surgical indifference in repairing the cleft palate. Plast Reconstr Surg *39*:1, 1967.
25. Roux J: Observatión sur une divisiόn congenitale du voile du palais et de la luette, guerie au moyen d'une operatiόn analogue a celle du bec de lievre practiquer par M. Roux. J Univers des Sci Med *15*:356, 1819.
26. Schmidt E: Die Annaherung der Kieferstumpfe bie Lippen-Kiefer-Gaumen spalten. Ihre schädlichen Folgen und Vermeidung. Fortschr Kiefer Gesichtk. Band I. Stuttgart: Georg Thieme Verlag, 1955.
27. Schrudde J: Br J Plast Surg *18*:183, 1965.
28. Skoog T: Plast Reconstr Surg *18*:183, 1965.
29. Skoog T: Plast Reconstr Surg *9*:108, 1965.
30. Veau F: Division Palatine. Paris; Masson et Cie, 1931.
31. von Grafe CF: Kurze Nachrichten und Auszuege. J prakt Arneik Wundarztk *44*:116, 1817.
32. von Langenbeck BRK: Operationen der angeborenen totalen Spaltung des harten Gaumens nach einer neuen Methode. Deutsch Arch Klin Med *13*:231, 1861.
33. Wardill WEM: Cleft palate. Br J Surg *16*:127, 1928.
34. Warren JC: On an operation for the cure of natural fissure of the soft palate. Am J Med Sci *3*:1, 1828.

Chapter 18

MANAGEMENT OF SKELETAL AND OCCLUSAL DEFORMITIES OF HEMIFACIAL MICROSOMIA

William H. Ware

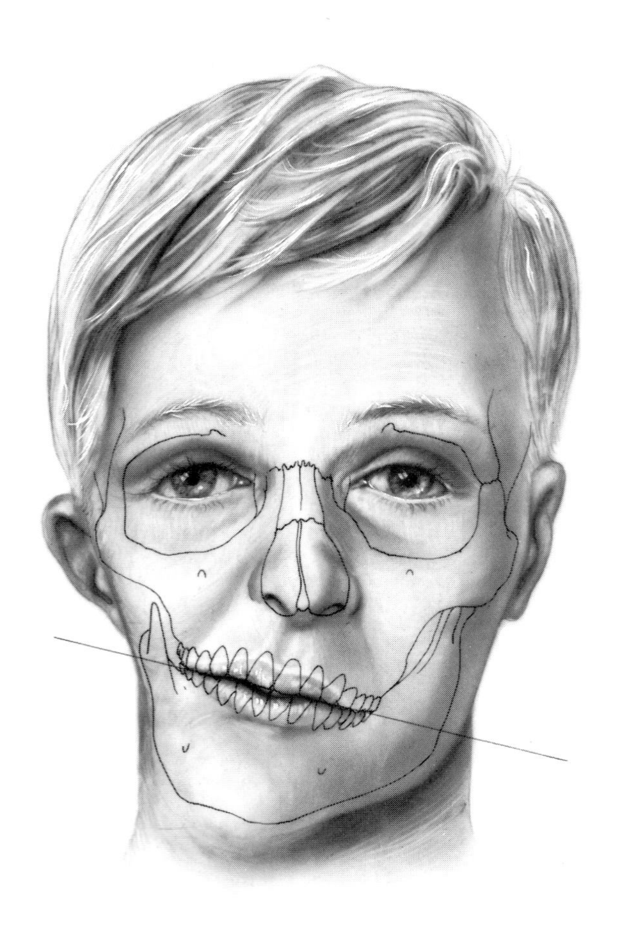

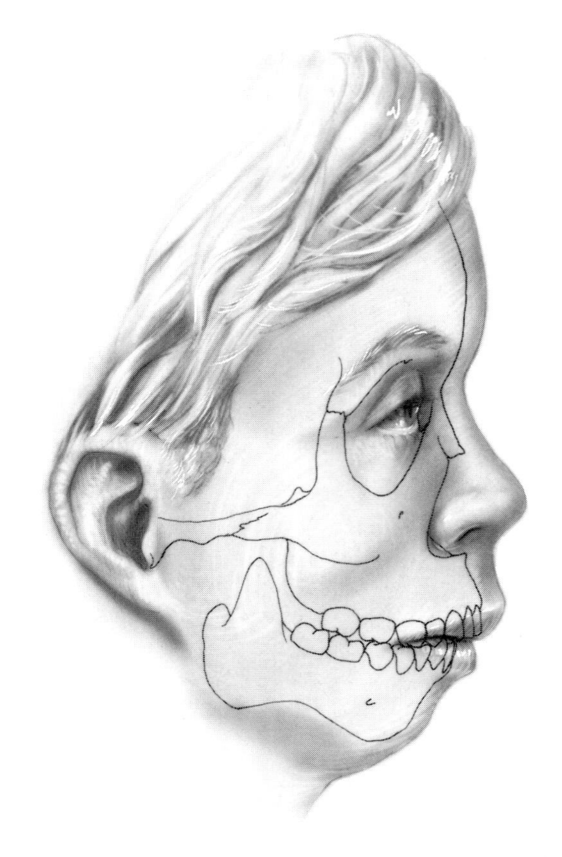

The child with mandibular retrusion, facial asymmetry, and malocclusion may be exhibiting signs of a hemifacial microsomia (first-arch syndrome) (Fig. 18–1). This syndrome is characterized by underdevelopment of the temporomandibular joint, mandibular ramus, and associated muscles of mastication. The maxilla and malar bones on the affected side frequently are underdeveloped. The contiguous parotid gland may be hypoplastic. Preauricular sinus tracts and tags may exist, along with underdevelopment of the associated external ear. Derivatives from the second (hyoid) branchial arch frequently exhibit deformities, and the affected facial nerve and muscles of facial expression may also show dysfunction. The middle ear and its ossicles may be hypoplastic, with resulting reduction in auditory acuity. Occasionally, the deformities are subtle and not apparent for several years. Children exhibiting the more classic signs will be identified at birth. The deformities are more often unilateral. When bilateral defects are found, the "syndrome" is still expressed asymmetrically. One side of the patient's face is more affected than the other.

A variety of descriptive terms are found in the literature to define the distinguishing characteristics of the syndrome. Otomandibular dysostosis, hemignathia and microtia syndrome, oral-mandibular-auricular syndrome, microtia, and unilateral facial agenesis are among the terms used to identify the anomalous conditions. Gorlin and Pindborg[6] reviewed the various names used in describing the syndrome and

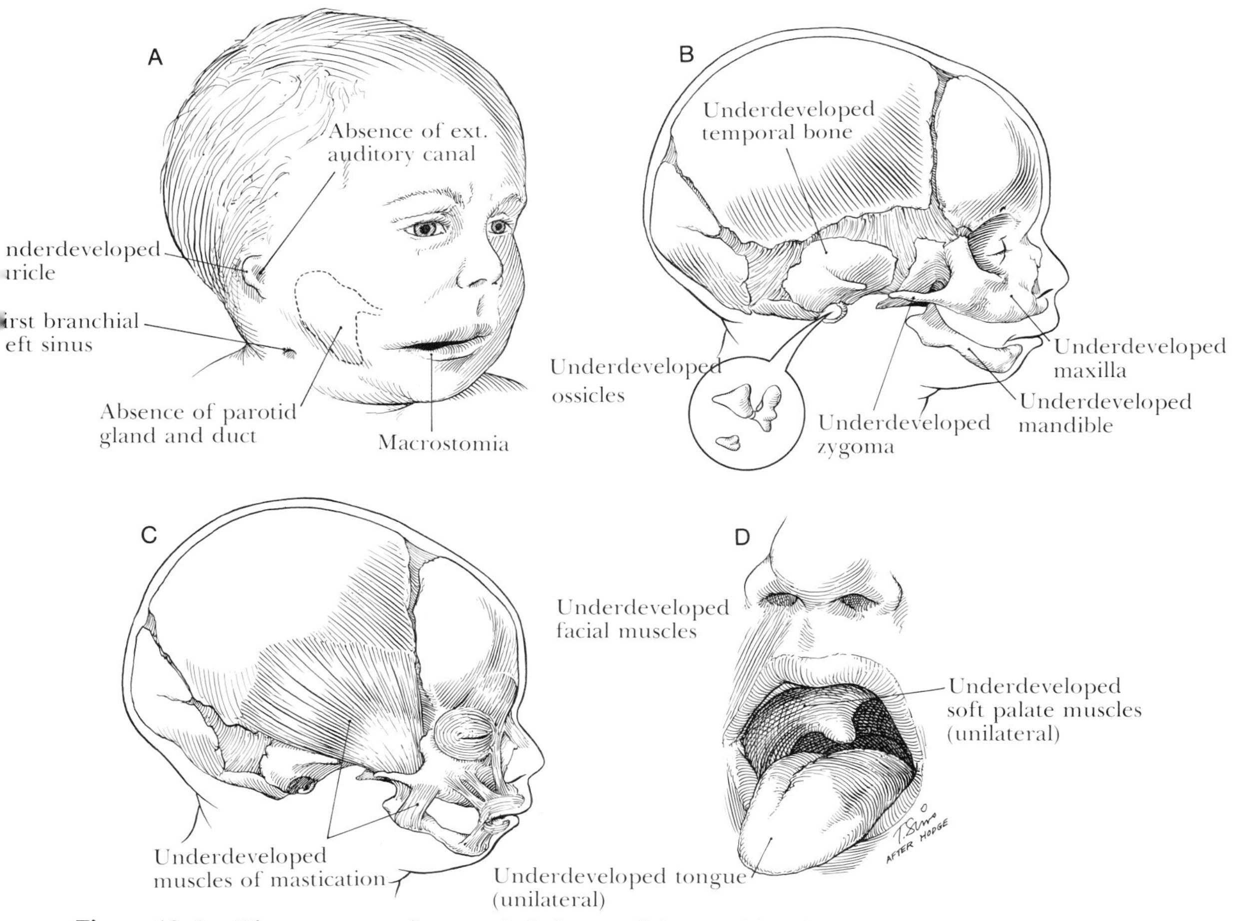

Figure 18–1. The spectrum of congenital abnormalities resulting from hemifacial microsomia (from Grabb[7]).

added their own term, "hemifacial microsomia," emphasizing the unilateral characteristics. The majority of defects can be explained as a maldevelopment of the first (mandibular) and second (hyoid) branchial arches.

Other identifiable craniofacial syndromes have anomalous characteristics similar to hemifacial microsomia. Pierre Robin syndrome (glossoptosis-micrognathia), Treacher Collins syndrome (mandibulofacial dysostosis), Goldenhar's syndrome (oculoauriculovertebral dysplasia), and Hallermann-Streiff syndrome (dyscephalia mandibulo-oculo facialis) all exhibit deformities of the first arch. Other distinguishing characteristics serve to categorize and separate the syndromes from one another and from hemifacial microsomia. To attribute these and other craniofacial anomalies primarily to defective development of the first and second arches would be overly simplistic. Although a unifying explanation for the confusing multitude of terms would be welcome, it is not to be achieved merely by gathering them all under the rubric first-arch syndromes.

SYSTEMATIC DESCRIPTION OF THE DEFORMITY

Esthetic Features

Initially the most disturbing esthetic features of the child with hemifacial microsomia are the deformities of the external ear. The auricle may be missing or grossly misshapen. Accessory tags and sinus tracts may be present along the orotragal line, the area representing the first branchial cleft. The full-face view best demonstrates the asymmetry, with the chin deviated toward the hypoplastic side. Underdevelopment of both the skeletal and soft-tissue components accentuates the asymmetry. The mouth may be enlarged and skewed toward the affected side (macrostomia) as a result of inadequate fusion of the soft-tissue components of the maxillary and mandibular processes. Comparison of the external ears will show the underdeveloped auricle to be set lower on the face than the auricle on the normal side. The maxilla and malar bone may be hypoplastic on the affected side. Although the orbits are less frequently affected, occasionally the eyes will appear to be set at different levels. The profile view emphasizes the mandibular retrusion. The retrusion is primarily the result of the unilateral hypoplasia, but the growth pattern of the opposite, relatively normal hemimandible may contribute to the appearance of retrusion.

Radiographic Features

Oriented head films illustrate the skeletal deformities commonly seen in this "syndrome." The lateral head film demonstrates the mandibular retrusion. Asymmetry is indicated by the differing levels of the lower mandibular borders and the tilting of the occlusal plane. A posteroanterior film exhibits both the asymmetry of the mandible, with the symphysis deviated toward the affected side, and the tilting of the occlusal plane. A panographic jaw film and tomograms of the temporomandibular joints provide more detailed information concerning distortions of the mandibular ramus and condyle. The condyle and ramus may be hypoplastic or even absent. The coronoid process, if present, may appear elongated. The ramus may be broad in an anteroposterior plane and is shortened vertically; antegonial notching can occur. In most cases, temporal bone hypoplasia exists as well. The glenoid fossa of the temporal bone may be absent, and the mandibular condyle, if present, is usually found anterior to its normal location. In some instances, the mastoid process is underdeveloped, and atresia of the external auditory canal may be present (Figs. 18–2 and 18–3).

Occlusal Features

The dental occlusion is altered as a result of the asymmetric growth of the jaws. Insufficient length of the dental arch causes crowding and impaction of teeth, particularly in the mandible. Deficient alveolar bone height in both the mandible and maxilla is evident on the affected side. It is debatable whether this retarded alveolar bone growth is a component of the regional hypoplasia or the product of reduced availability of intermaxillary space for the growth and eruption of teeth. The development of the individual teeth in shape and number is unaffected.

The relative retrusion of the mandible and its asymmetric development contribute significantly to the malocclusion. The maxilla, either as a part of the congenital maldevelopment or as a compensatory response to the mandibular hypoplasia, is less well developed on the affected side. However, suppressed alveolar bone growth and infraeruption of teeth on the affected side, along with the compensatory development of the dentoalveolar elements on the normal side, serve to reduce any occlusal discrepancy. Although the dentition may appear skewed relative to the usual planes of orientation within the skull, the relationship of maxillary and mandibular arches is functional as a result of the compensatory adjustments in the growth of the jaws. Casts of the teeth that do not indicate their orientation to the skull give little indication of the severity of the skeletal discrepancy. In attempting corrective measures (orthodontics or surgery), it is essential to regard the malocclusion as secondary to the more fundamental skeletal deformity.

ETIOLOGY

Little is known about the etiology of hemifacial microsomia. Inferences drawn from descriptive analyses of clinical examples, fetal material, and a small number of animal model studies form the basis for the present theories. Stark and Saunders[21] supported the theory of mesodermal deficiency based on the presence of generalized hypoplasia of the soft and hard tissue. McKenzie,[14] convinced that inadequate blood supply was the key factor, attributed the reduced regional development to a malformation of the external carotid artery system. Pursuing the vascular theory further, Poswillo[19] suggested vessel wall rupture with hematoma formation as the causative agent. Using teratologic agents, Poswillo was able to produce hematomas in the area of the developing stapedial artery in both rodent and primate embryos. Associated with the

Text continued on page 1376.

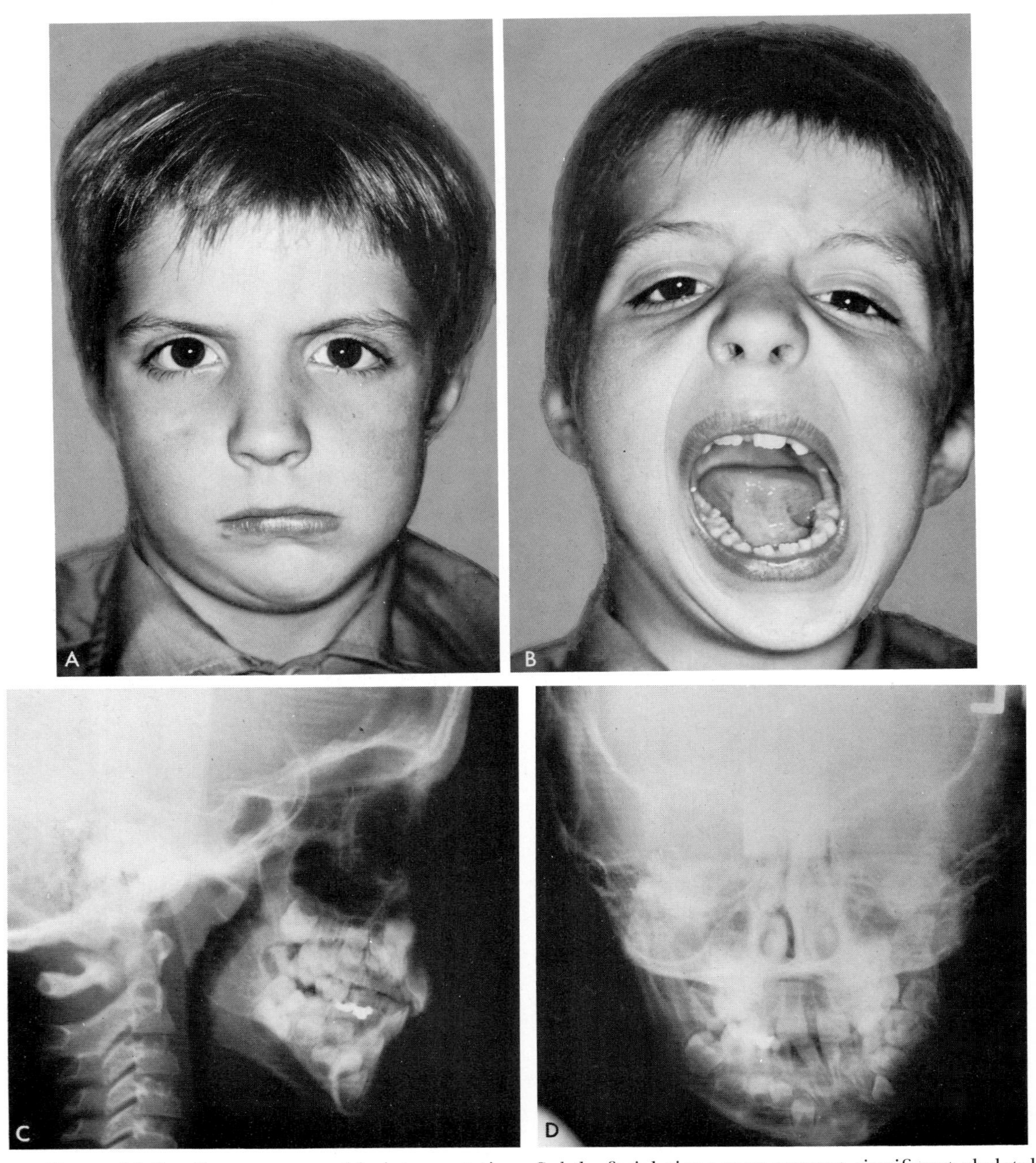

Figure 18–2. Roentgenographic interpretation. Subtle facial signs may suggest significant skeletal hypoplasia observed in hemifacial microsomia. *A* and *B*, Six-year-old boy demonstrates a shift of the chin and mouth to the left side with further deviation upon opening. *C*, Lateral cephalometric film illustrates the asymmetry with the posterior occlusal planes and lower mandibular borders at two levels. *D*, Posteroanterior film more clearly illustrates the mandibular symphysis deviated to the affected side with canting of the occlusal plane.

Legend continued on the opposite page.

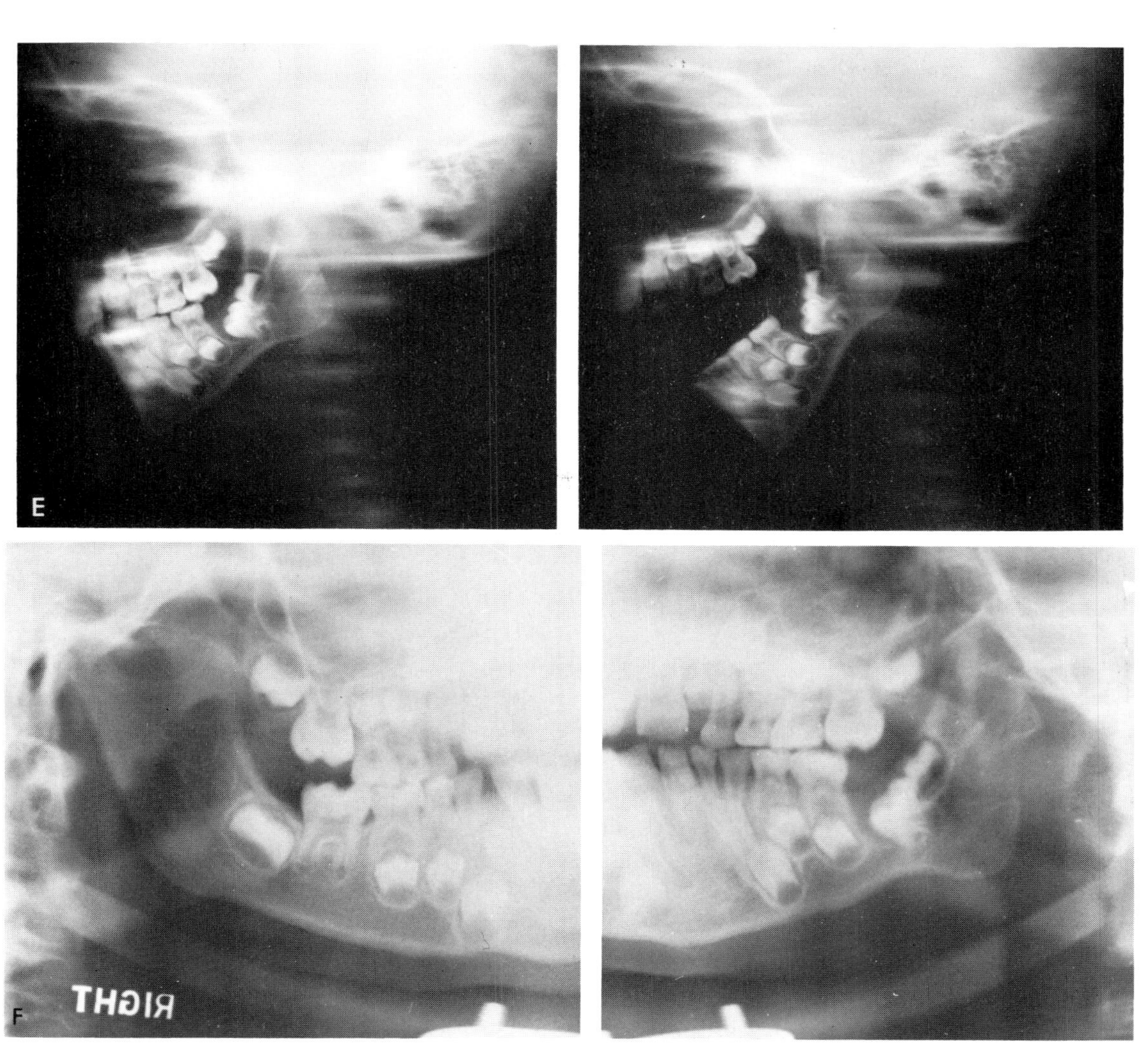

Figure 18–2 *Continued.* *E,* Tomograms of the hypoplastic mandibular ramus demonstrate the dental crowding and impacting of teeth. The acute gonial angle and the antegonial notching are commonly observed when vertical ramus growth is deficient. The ear canal and mastoid air cells appear normal, but the glenoid fossa is not developed. The developmental defect is confined to the ramus and structures of the temporomandibular joint. The open position illustrates the hinge function of the joint. *F,* Comparisons on the panographic film of the normal right side with the underdeveloped left side further demonstrate the hypoplasia of the ramus and the resultant crowding of the teeth.

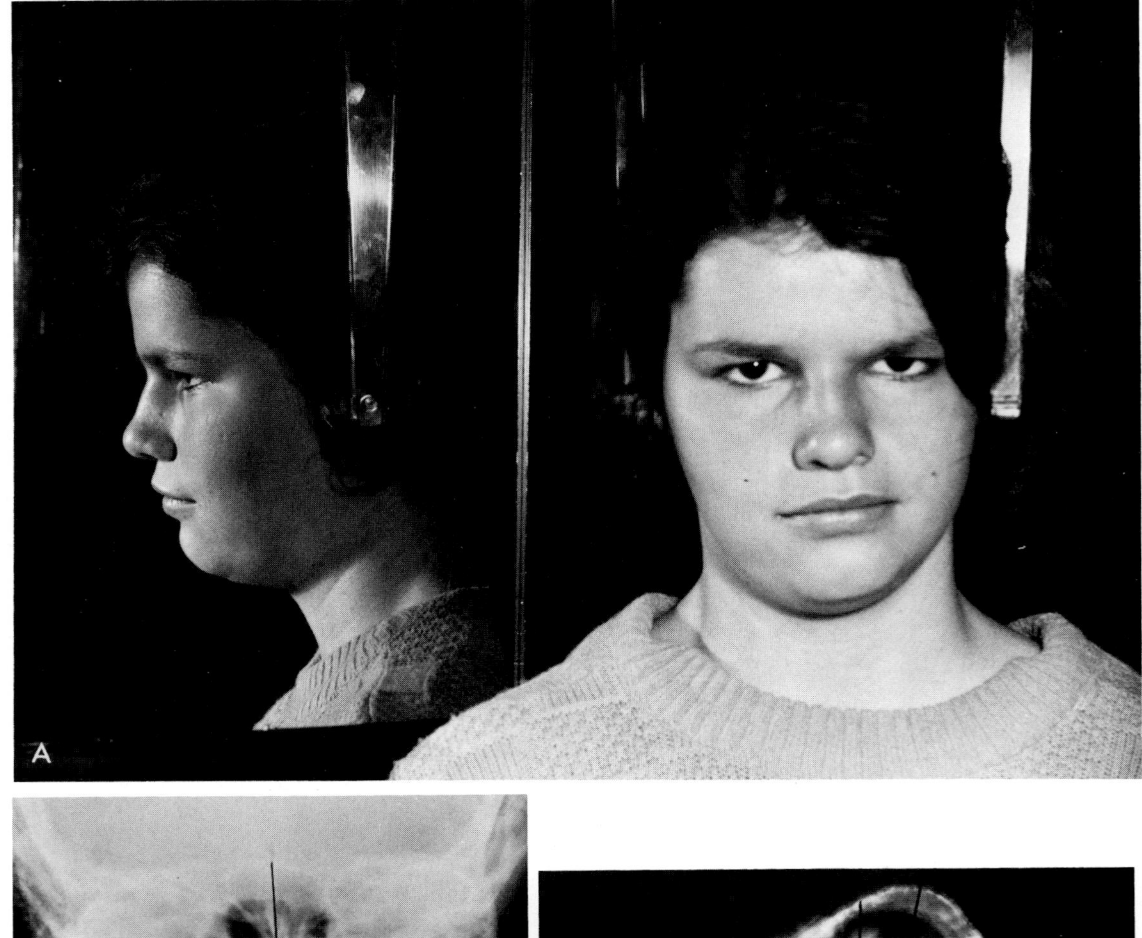

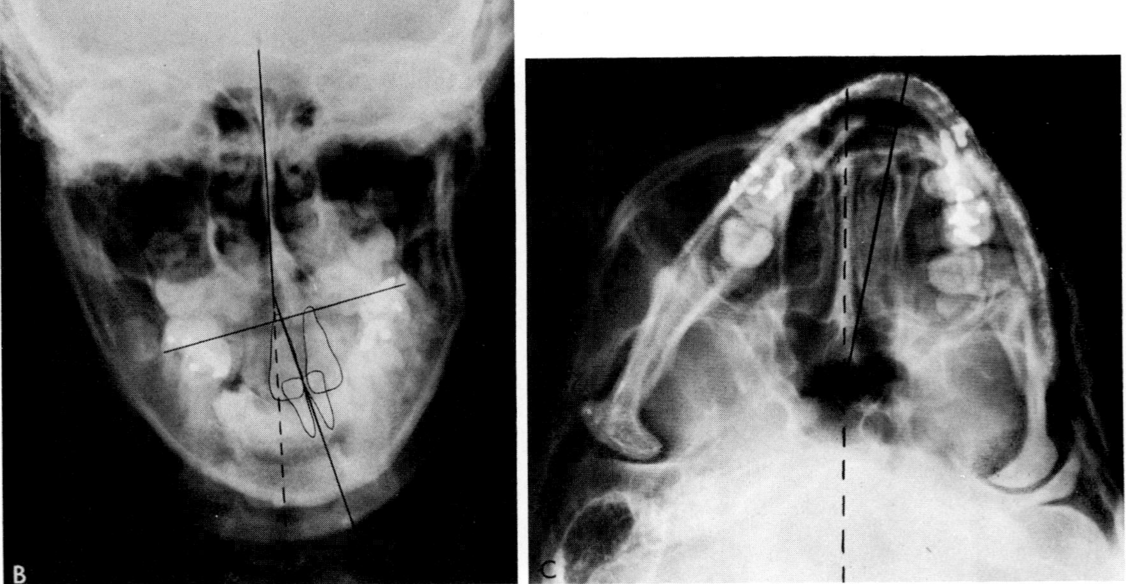

Figure 18–3. *A,* Facial asymmetry in a 13-year-old girl appears as a generalized underdevelopment of the tissues of the left side of the face. *B,* Posteroanterior view demonstrates the skeletal hypoplasia of the left hemimandible, maxillary sinus, and nasal cavity. The dental midline of both the maxilla and mandible is skewed to the affected side with canting of the occlusal plane. *C,* Basivertex view demonstrates condylar development but atresia of the bony ear canal and absence of mastoid air cells on the affected side.

Legend continued on the opposite page.

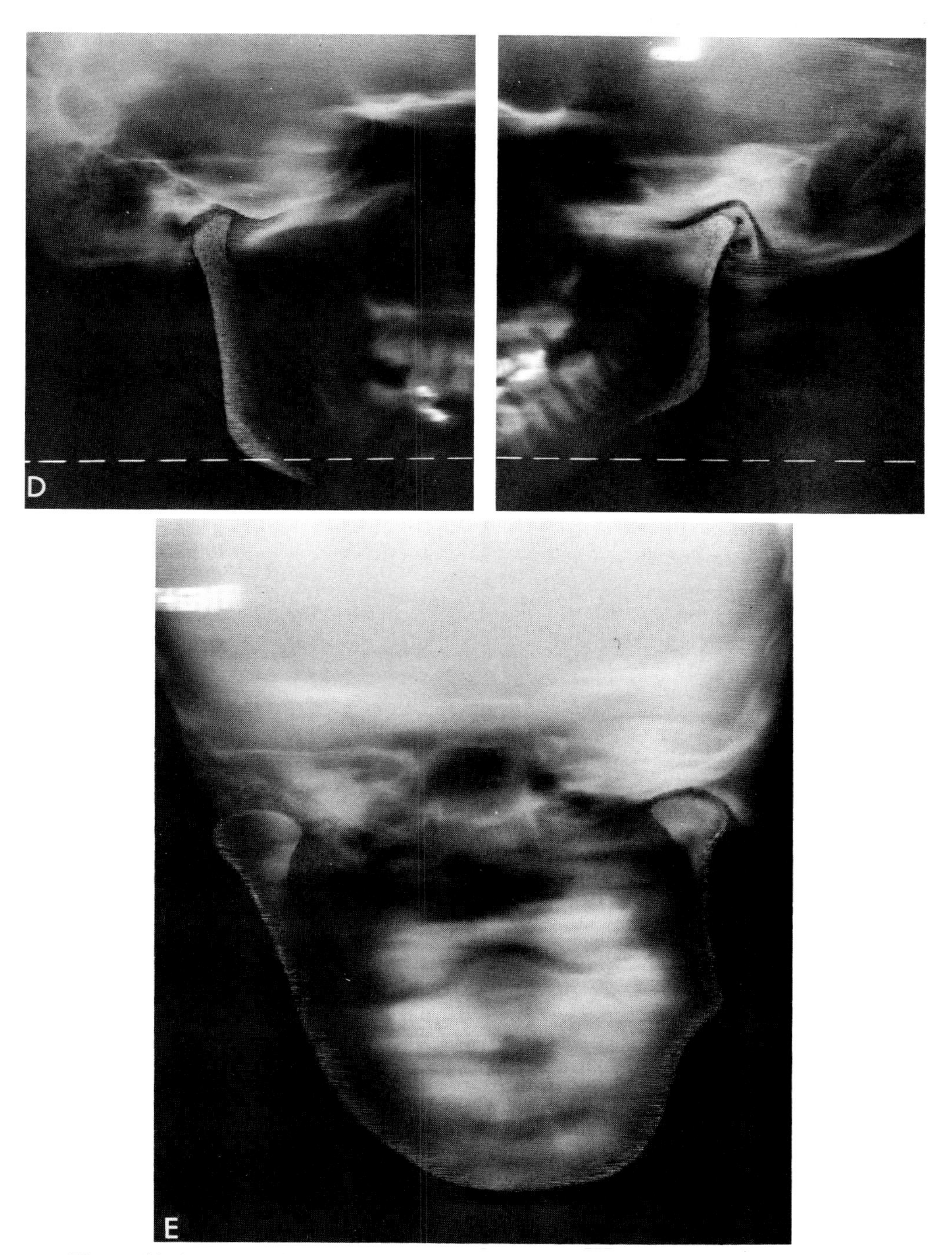

Figure 18–3 *Continued.* *D,* Tomography comparing the normal right side with the left illustrates the hypoplastic mandibular ramus and condyle. Normal development of the temporal bone and middle ear components is lacking on the left side. *E,* Frontal tomogram through the condyles further demonstrates the ramus hypoplasia. (X-rays retouched for clarity.)

hematomas were developmental defects similar to those observed in hemifacial microsomia, the severity of the defects in the animals being proportional to the size of the hematoma that occurred. The resulting hypoplastic tissue was observed to be greatest at the center of the hematoma, with decreasing effects toward the periphery. In light of the wide variety of resulting defects and the fact that tissues contiguous to (but not necessarily derivative of) the first or second arches are often hypoplastic, the hematoma theory seems convincing as a causal mechanism.

Still to be answered is how the embryo comes to be susceptible to such vascular accidents. Genetic propensity has been established in certain animal strains used in teratologic research. Although a familial pattern has been established in several of the craniofacial syndromes, there is as yet no distinct pattern for the development of hemifacial microsomia. Animal studies have shown that a variety of biologic poisons and physical insults will produce similar anomalies. In these studies, the timing and severity of the insult appeared to be more important than the specificity of the causative agent.

Review of the Development of Mandibular and Hyoid Branchial Arches

In order to understand how the deformities of hemifacial microsomia originate, we must look to certain critical stages in the development of the embryo. During ontogenesis the organs of hearing and mastication are related intimately. The ear develops from two distinct anlagen. The inner ear is derived from an ectodermal thickening in the region of the hindbrain, and the elements of the middle and external ear are developed from the dorsal ends of the first two gill arches. Early differentiation and cartilaginous encapsulation of the inner ear may explain the low incidence of neurosensory abnormalities observed in the first- and second-arch syndromes. Differentiation of the branchial structures into their adult derivatives is recognizable between the third and fourth weeks in utero and continues into at least the seventh month. Whereas growth and development of the inner ear are completed during fetal life, maturation of the middle and external ear is not completed until late childhood. As a result of its later maturation, the middle ear apparatus is vulnerable to noxious stimuli during most of fetal life. According to findings based on teratologic experimentation, the middle ear appears to be most susceptible, however, during the period extending from the third to the eighth week in utero.

Just prior to four weeks in utero, the first branchial arches bud bilaterally, giving rise to the maxillary processes. These fuse with the downward-growing frontonasal process to form the fetal mouth and nose. The cartilaginous skeleton of the first arch (Meckel's cartilage) serves as the primary jaw. The rostral ends of this cartilage are eventually incorporated within the region of the symphysis of the mandible. The midportion of the cartilage gives rise to the sphenomandibular ligament, and the proximal ends differentiate into the malleus and incus. The second branchial arch forms a cartilaginous bar (Reichert's cartilage) that gives rise to the hyoid bone and styloid process and contributes to the formation of the stapes (Fig. 18–4). The proximal end of the branchial groove between the first two arches gives rise to the external auditory canal, whereas the corresponding pharyngeal pouch differentiates into the eustachian

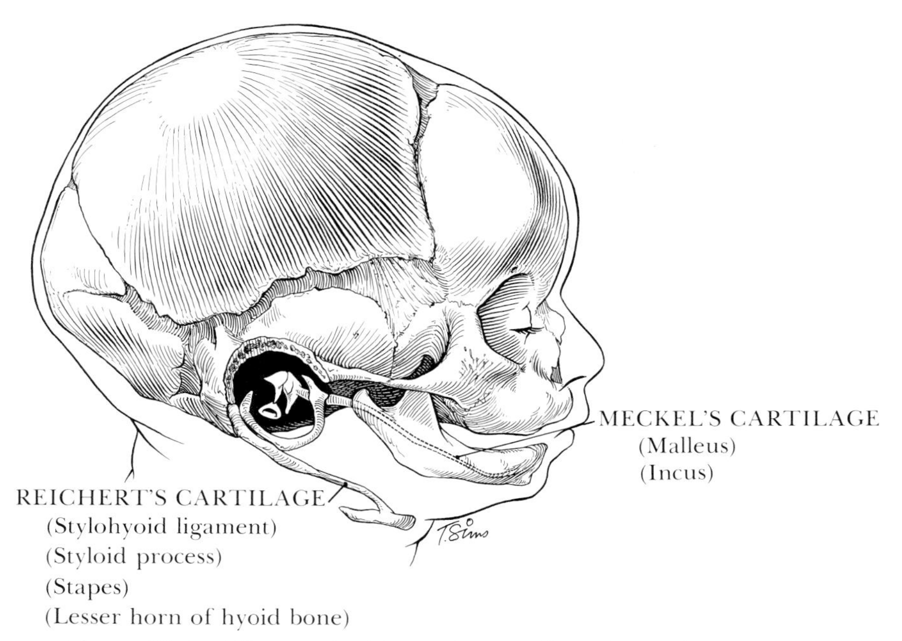

Figure 18–4. The proximal (dorsal) ends of the first and second branchial arch cartilages figure prominently in the development of the ear and temporomandibular joint (from Grabb[7]).

tube and middle ear cavity. The tympanic membrane remains as the adult derivative of the embryonic partition between the proximal parts of the first branchial groove and the pharyngeal pouch. The auricle forms as a result of mesenchymal condensations in the proximal portions of the first and second branchial arches[1] (Fig. 18–5).

Between the third and fifth weeks in utero, the first aortic arch disappears, and the external carotid system develops (Fig. 18–6). This vascular rearrangement from

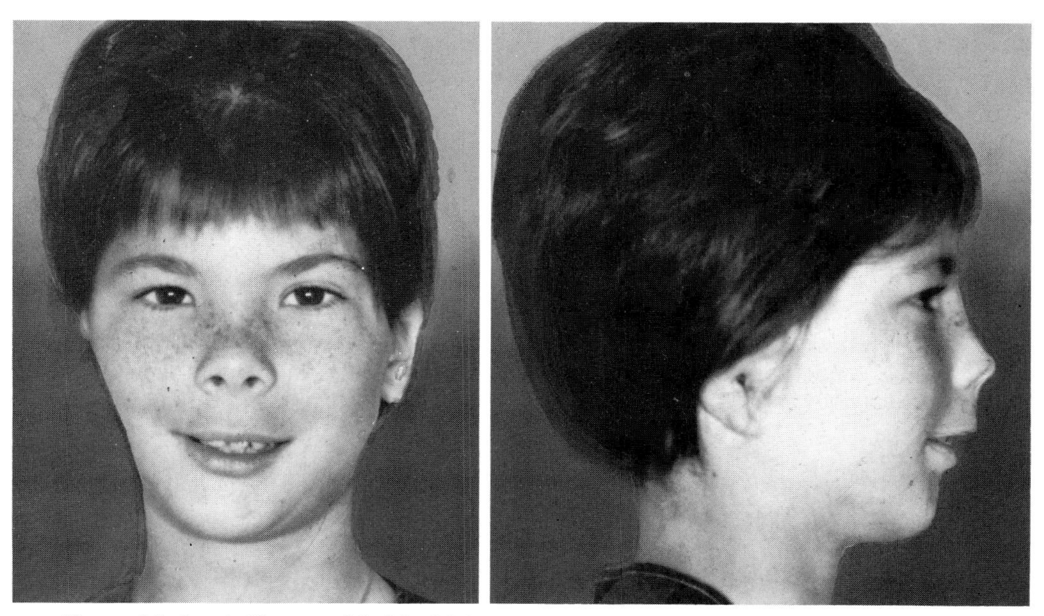

Figure 18–5. A 12-year-old girl with hemifacial microsomia. Microtia of the right auricle is the dominant feature in this instance.

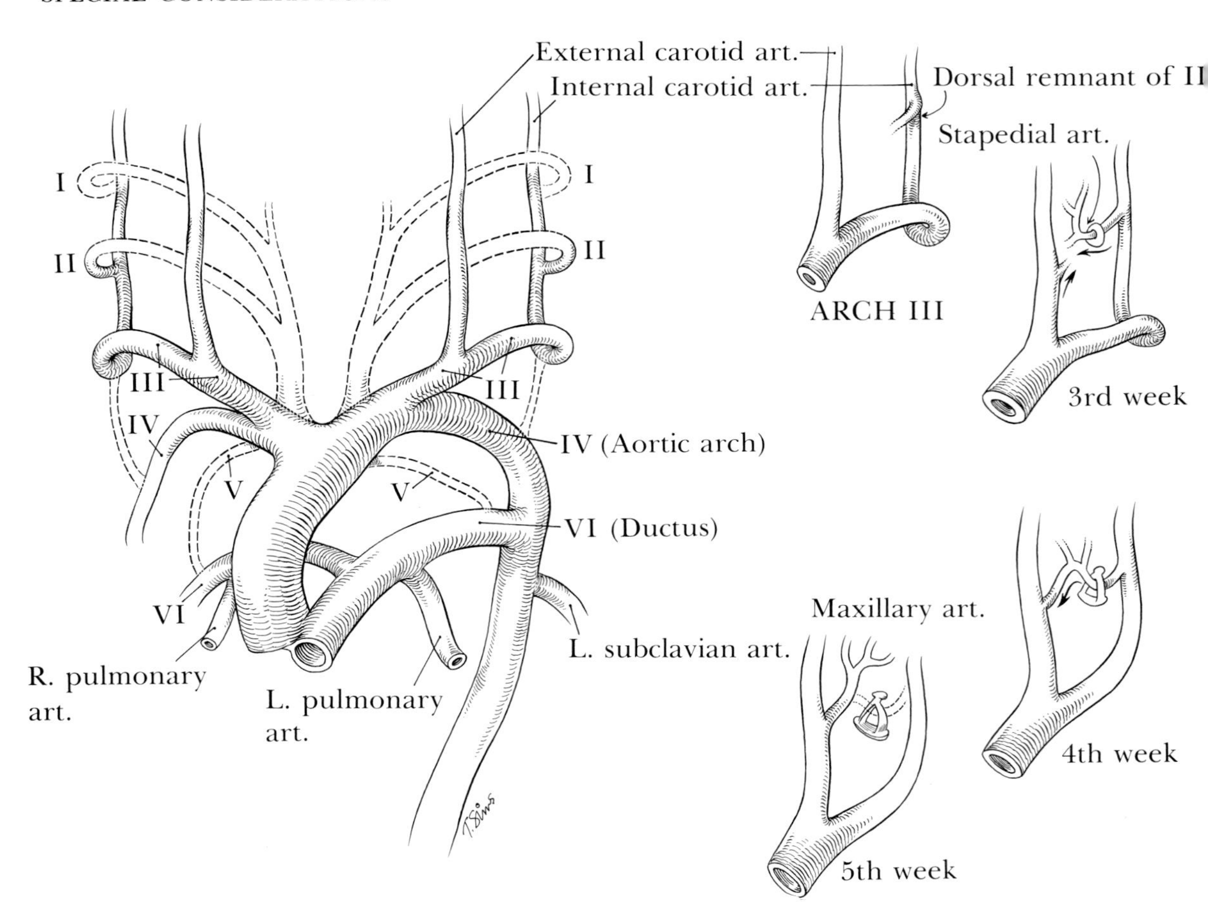

Figure 18–6. The carotid system arises from the embryonic third aortic arch. As the first two aortic arches involute, the third arch becomes dominant, forming the carotid system. The stapedial artery represents a remnant of the second aortic arch and is the main blood supply to the proximal ends of the first and second arches until anastomosis with a branch of the external carotid occurs. The stapedial artery then atrophies, and the external carotid system supplies the structures of the first and second branchial arches. Mishaps in the vascular development may account for the congenital anomalies observed in hemifacial microsomia.

branchial arch vessels to the carotid system forms the weakest link in the developmental chain, since it takes place at a time when an anomalous development is most likely to occur. It is surprising that more anomalies do not occur. As described by McKenzie: "The first branchial arch faces a hazardous existence, dependent for its blood supply during that time on the progression of three successive vessels: (1) the first aortic arch; (2) the stapedial artery; and (3) the external carotid artery. The rapid change requires precise timing as one artery relinquishes and the next provides blood supply to the region."[14] In view of the numerous mishaps that are possible, structures developing during this period would appear to be most vulnerable to any noxious stimuli. When one considers the rapidity with which a mechanism originally designed for gill breathing is transformed into an air-vibration system for hearing, it is surprising that more anomalies do not occur.

Prevention of the deformity will depend on information gathered by researchers in the sciences of teratology and biochemical genetics. In the meantime, children afflicted with this abnormality must depend upon the ingenuity of the surgeon and orthodontic specialist for a small measure of improvement. Esthetic deficiencies in our society can be as handicapping as those of a functional nature. They challenge even those with the strongest personalities, and self-image may be distorted at an early age. In addition to whatever physical adjustment can be accomplished by the clinicians involved, the child and family often require strong psychologic support as well.

BASIC TREATMENT APPROACHES

The earliest treatment ordinarily attempted is the soft-tissue repair of auricular tags and sinus tracts. The benefits derived from early repair are primarily psychologic and are aimed at both the distressed parents and a potentially disturbed child. Repair of auricular deformities is challenging and requires repeated surgery. Achievement of normal appearance is rare. Frequently a prosthesis and appropriate hair styling are used to improve the result.

Optimal management of microtia and middle-ear deformities requires diverse treatment skills. A plastic surgeon, an otologist, and a maxillofacial prosthodontist may all be needed. Despite the close embryologic relationship of auditory defects and deformities of the mandible and teeth, these structures may be repaired independently of one another. Middle and external ear growth is completed by age 10 years, but mandibular and maxillary growth continues to adulthood.

In unilateral defects, the growth pattern of the normal side exaggerates the deformity and contributes to the facial asymmetry. Controversy exists concerning the appropriate timing of reconstructive procedures involving bone in relation to the growth pattern. Opinion is divided among those who advocate delay of surgery until completion of growth and those who support earlier and possibly multiple procedures to achieve "guided growth."

The reasons given for delay are: (1) possible untoward effects of the surgery on subsequent growth and (2) the difficulty in predicting the final facial form. Kazanjian[11] proposed soft-tissue repair during childhood but preferred to delay osseous surgery until after maturity. He emphasized the need for orthodontic management to minimize the mandibular deviation and to maintain a functional occlusion. He was of the opinion that the mandibular deformity increased more because of lack of function than because of the original defect. Obwegeser[15] advocates delay of both the soft-tissue repair and surgery on the facial skeleton until facial growth has ceased. He does not object to early onlay bone grafting to affected parts, but he concurs with Freihofer[4] that osteotomies during childhood interfere with proper growth of the already hypoplastic areas of the facial skeleton. Major spatial rearrangements of the facial skeleton in the adult are accomplished by osteotomies of both the maxilla and mandible and by extensive bone grafting. Obwegeser supports the axiom of "first the bone, then the soft tissues" and delays all soft-tissue repair, including that of the auricles, until skeletal surgery is completed.

Conversely, the reasons for early correction are as follows: (1) creating interocclusal space may promote a more normal eruption pattern of teeth and stimulation of alveolar bone development on the affected side, (2) soft-tissue development on the affected side is stimulated, and (3) there are psychologic advantages to the child and parents in observing esthetic and functional improvement.

Early surgical correction of the facial asymmetry has a number of potential benefits in addition to the positive emotional effect. Longacre[13] stressed early and repeated augmentation of the deficient skeletal areas, using split ribs. The subperiosteal regeneration of ribs in the growing child provides a continual source of bone. Longacre was of the opinion that the grafts provided a stimulus for associated soft-tissue growth. A tendency does exist for progressive resorption of onlay bone grafts when they are not subjected to the stress of function.[17, 22]

Thompson[22] suggested the use of dermal-fat grafts for camouflage purposes in instances of hemifacial underdevelopment in which the defect was primarily of the soft tissue. Although augmentation procedures may occasionally be indicated, they do not improve the occlusal or skeletal disparity. Furthermore, if surgical repositioning of the mandible is contemplated, masking procedures should be delayed until the outcome of the skeletal surgery can be evaluated.

Hovell[10] and Osborne[16] have advocated early and, if necessary, repeated surgery to lengthen the hypoplastic mandible during the time of facial growth. In treatment planning, both advocated creating an open bite on the hypoplastic side in order to establish space for alveolar growth and tooth eruption. Whereas Osborne recommends surgery by age 6 years, Hovell suggests delay until 8 years of age. Converse et al[3] advocate early surgery and suggest the period of mixed dentition (age 8 or 9 years) as the most practical time for the initial surgery. There are usually sufficient permanent teeth by age 9 to provide an aid to intermaxillary fixation. A second surgical stage in late adolescence should be anticipated to correct any disparity of growth following the first operation and to attain adequate facial contour.

Although conventional orthodontic tooth movement is of little value in young patients with hemifacial microsomia, efforts to guide skeletal growth and stimulate the affected areas are indicated. Harvold[9] advocates the use of activators to guide eruption of teeth and prevent midline shift until the time of surgery. This approach may have a stimulatory effect on muscle development and serves to prevent canting of the occlusal plane.

For older patients, the goal of presurgical orthodontics should be to align the teeth as ideally as possible to their own arch in anticipation of surgical realignment of the skeletal parts. This approach usually makes the occlusion worse temporarily. At the time of surgery, it often is advisable to create an open bite posteriorly on the affected side, into which the teeth are extruded orthodontically, afterward.

Basic Surgical Approaches

Mandibular Osteotomies

Bilateral mandibular osteotomies are most often required. The osteotomies allow the repositioning of the tooth-bearing fragment of the mandible without significantly altering temporomandibular articulation. Ordinarily, mandibular repositioning occurs in three planes of space: (1) horizontal repositioning to bring the mandibular symphysis into line with the midsagittal plane of the skull, (2) alignment of the mandibular occlusal plane, and (3) adjustment of anterior and posterior face height in order to attain optimum esthetic results (Fig. 18–7). As a result, the normal hemimandible may be shorter, longer, or the same length, depending on what is required in a given case.

A face-bow is used to position the maxillary cast on a semiadjustable articulator. The traditional pretragal point overlying the lateral pole of the condyle on the normal side is aligned with a comparable point on the affected side that is determined by orienting the face-bow so that the arms are parallel and equidistant from the midsagittal plane of the skull. If the orbits are symmetrical, the interpupillary plane also may be useful for orientation. The method may not be acceptable for accurate recordings of maxillomandibular relations, but it serves to simulate the spatial relationship of the maxillary arch to the skull.

The midpoint between the mandibular central incisors and the midline of the symphysis is determined on the posteroanterior head film and is then marked on the mandibular cast. If the ear is obviously displaced, the head film should be taken in the natural head position rather than with the aid of ear rods. For planning purposes, the mandibular cast is luted temporarily to the mounted maxillary cast in the desired postsurgical position. The midline of the mandible should approximate the midsagittal plane of the skull (not necessarily the midline of the maxillary teeth), and the transverse mandibular occlusal plane should be horizontally corrected. It is not unusual to create a 10- to 15-mm posterior open bite on the affected side and a molar and premolar crossbite on the normal side. The strategy for correcting mandibular retrusion and an alveolar dental arch discrepancy should be considered during this planning process. The relationship of the dental casts, as determined by thorough planning and as established on the articulator, will provide the key for positioning the mandible at surgery (Fig. 18–8). Estimates obtained from positioning acetate cutouts and from prediction tracings, although not exact, serve as additional checks during treatment planning.

Surgical repositioning can be accomplished by either of two approaches: submandibular incisions or intraoral anterior ramus incisions. Submandibular incisions approximately 2 cm inferior to the angle of the mandible and parallel to a neck fold provide an excellent access to the entire ramus. The incision on the hypoplastic side should be placed 3 to 4 cm below the angle of the mandible if significant lengthening of the ramus is anticipated. Anatomic structures encountered during this approach include the marginal mandibular branch of the facial nerve just deep to the platysma muscle, the submandibular gland toward the anterior end of the wound, and the tail of the parotid gland posteriorly and superiorly. The posterior facial vein, with its anterior communicating vessels, may be encountered deep to the platysma muscle. Access to the retromandibular space is afforded by incising the heavy investing fascia that extends from the sternocleidomastoid muscle over the surface of the lower pole of the parotid gland and onto the border of the mandible and the capsule of the submandibular gland. A slightly retromandibular approach affords excellent access to the entire ramus and decreases the potential trauma to the facial nerve. After reflecting the periosteum and posterior attachments of the masseter and medial pterygoid muscles, the bony cut on the normal side is made from the depth of the sigmoid notch to the angle of the mandible. On the hypoplastic side a similar approach is used in exposing the ramus, but nearly always the investing tissues are less developed. Occasionally the parotid gland and masticatory muscles are missing. If there is a functional articulation, it may be anterior and medial to the usual temporomandibular joint. In spite of the aberrant location, no attempt to replace the functioning joint is necessary. An osteotomy below the articulation that is designed to permit lengthening of the ramus is preferable. If the coronoid process with temporal muscle attachment

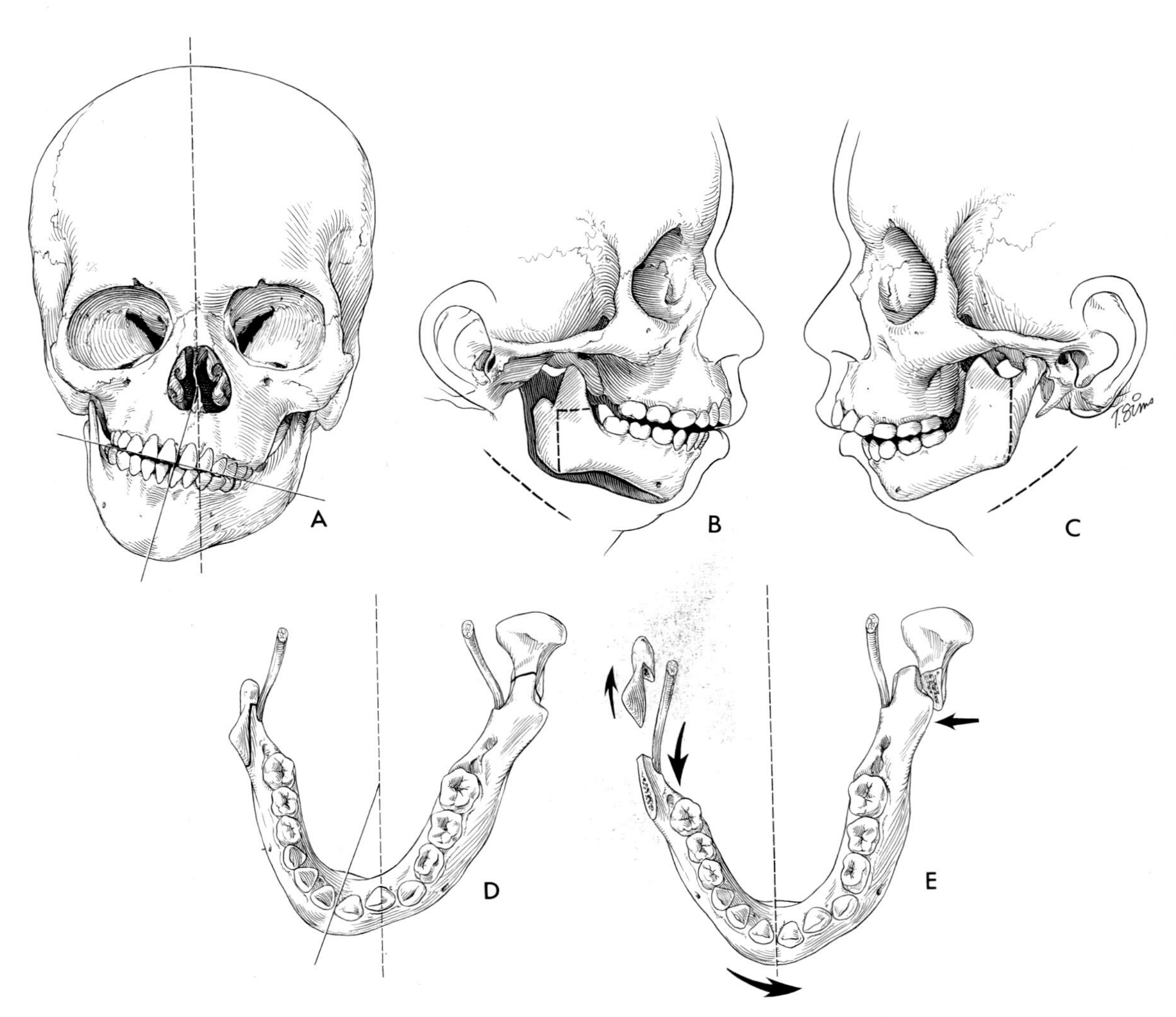

Figure 18–7. Unilateral hypoplasia of the mandibular ramus is the most frequent skeletal deformity observed in hemifacial microsomia. *A,* The mandibular symphysis deviates to the affected side. The occlusion is also shifted and canted upward toward the hypoplastic side. *B,* The condyloid process is ordinarily more affected than other components of the ramus. The articular surface may be anterior on the zygomatic process or medial, approximating the sphenoid bone. Occasionally the entire ramus is missing, with no recognizable articulating area. Mandibular retrusion is obvious on both the hypoplastic (*B*) and normal side (*C*). The heavy dotted lines indicate the position of the skin incisions. The lighter dotted lines outline the osteotomies on the affected (*B*) and normal (*C*) rami. *D* further illustrates the asymmetry and skewed position of the mandible prior to the osteotomies, whereas *E* through *H* emphasize the rotational movements that are required to improve symmetry. An occlusal splint that is fabricated prior to surgery is used to position and stabilize the mandible. The alternative methods of reconstructing the hypoplastic mandible are illustrated in *1* through *3*. When the deformity is only moderately severe, an intraoral approach with sagittal split osteotomy ordinarily works well, as shown in *1*. An alternative method using the reverse "L" type osteotomy with bone grafting is illustrated in *2*. When the entire ramus is missing, a costochondral junction rib graft is advisable, as shown in *3*. The cartilaginous portion of the rib is shaped and butted against the temporal bone anterior to the external auditory meatus. Additional bone may be desirable to reinforce the graft and add bulk to the hypoplastic area.

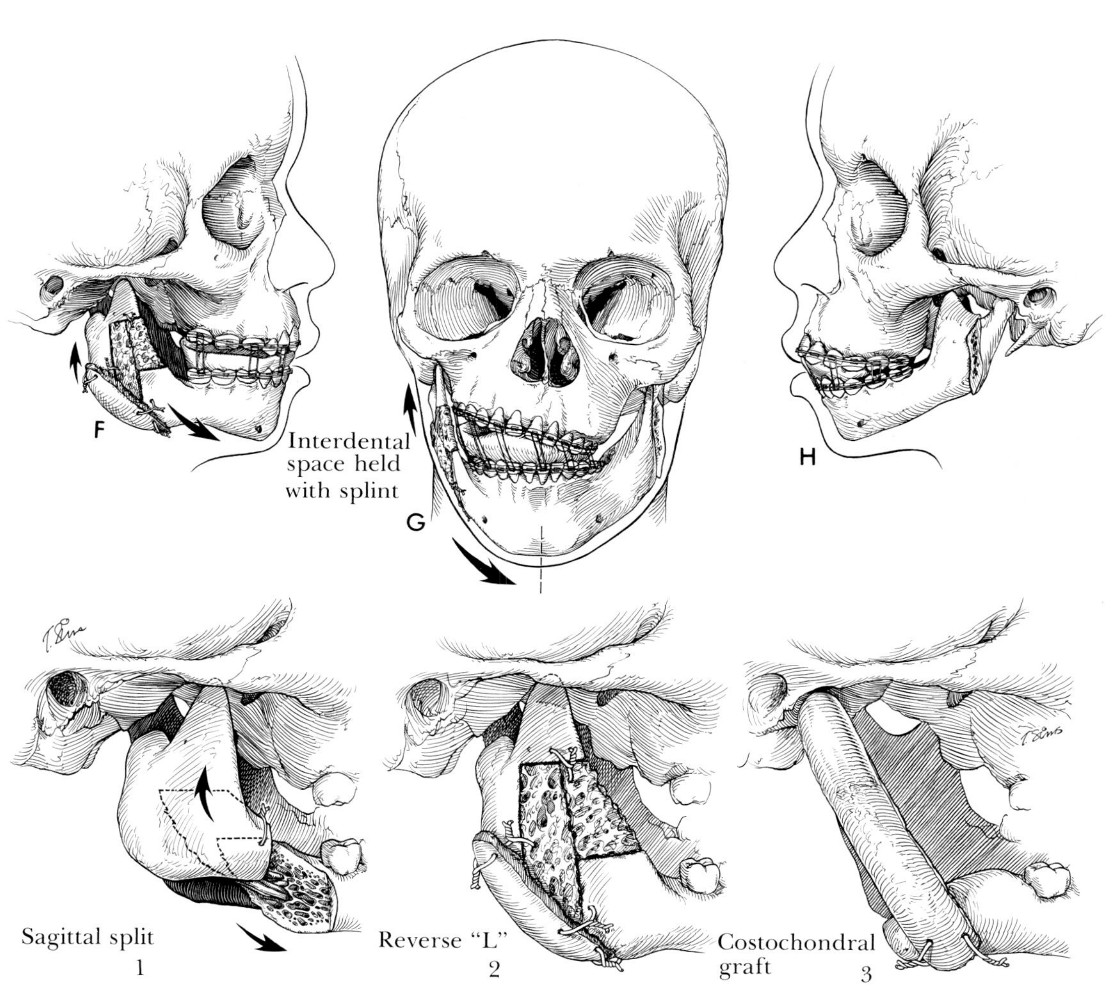

Figure 18–7 *Continued. See legend on the opposite page.*

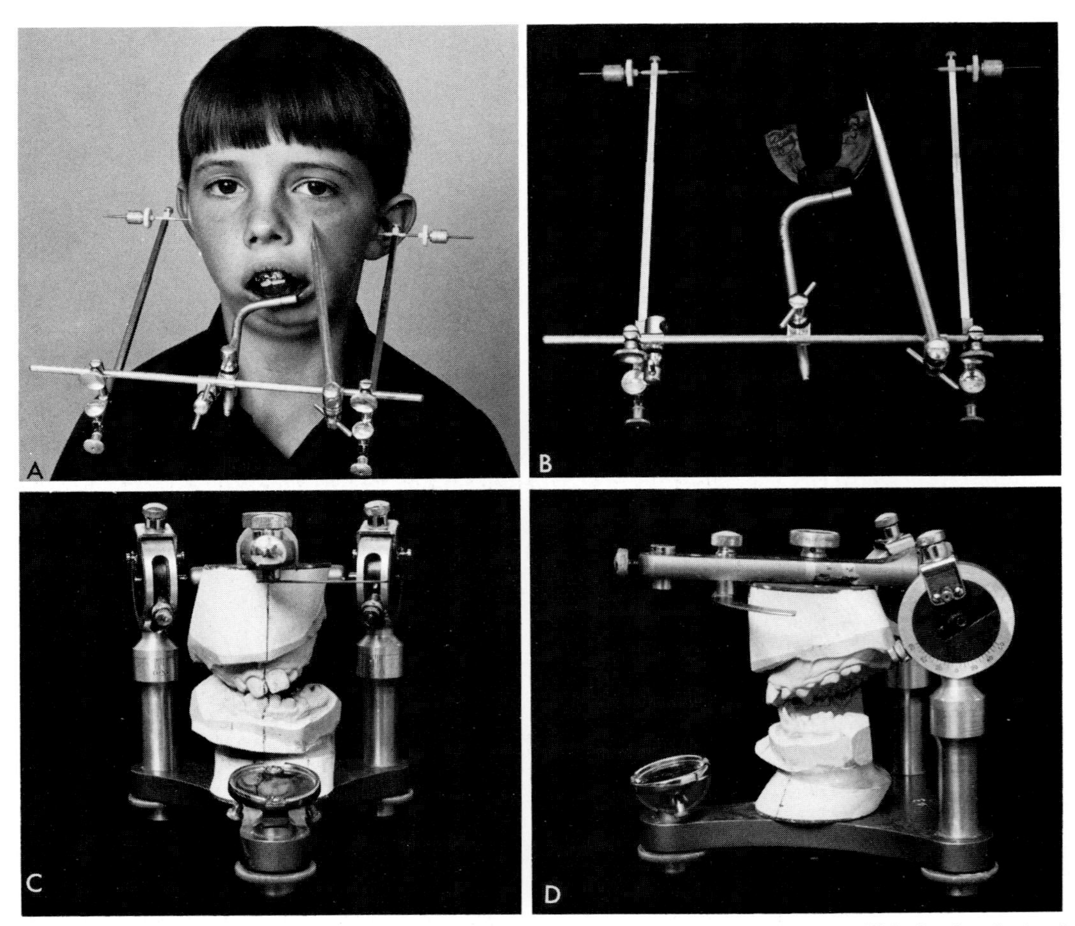

Figure 18–8. An interocclusal splint is used at surgery to place the mandible in the desired relationship to the skull. Construction of the splint is best achieved using the oriented head films and mounted casts of the teeth. *A* and *B* illustrate the face-bow recording of the maxillary occlusion in preparation for the oriented mounting of the model on an articulator. *C* demonstrates the mounting of the maxillary model with the midline oriented to the midsagittal plane. Note that the mandibular model is mounted with the midline of the symphysis in the midsagittal plane and the cant of the occlusal plane is corrected. *D,* An open bite is created on the affected side in order to achieve skeletal symmetry. The interocclusal splint is then constructed on the oriented models.

is present, an osteotomy in the shape of a reverse L works well. Even if there is only minimal bony apposition after the jaw is repositioned, adequate healing can be anticipated. If a large bony defect exists following the repositioning of the mandible, either rib or iliac bone may be grafted to bridge the gap.

An intraoral approach with sagittal split osteotomies in the ramus is possible if the anatomy of the affected side is not overly distorted. With a long sagittal osteotomy, the hypoplastic ramus can be lengthened up to 2 cm without the need for bone grafting. The periosteum along the inferoposterior border of the mandible may have to be split to allow sufficient mobility for lengthening. The sphenomandibular ligament may limit the desired rotation, and the ligament must therefore be dissected free, avoiding the inferior alveolar neurovascular bundle. In exposing the ramus, great care should be taken to perform a subperiosteal dissection, particularly on the medial and posterior aspects of the mandible. If the periosteal envelope must be split in order to attain adequate mandibular mobility, the dissection should be done with great care and under direct vision. Bleeding at the depth of the wound may be hard to control.

The primary advantages of the sagittal split osteotomy are: (1) no external incisions are necessary, (2) risk to the facial nerve is minimal, and (3) significant mandibular lengthening is possible without need for bone grafting. Some disadvantages are: (1) restricted access increases technical difficulties, particularly when the anatomy is distorted; (2) bleeding presents a greater hazard because of potential limited access; (3) risks of trauma to the inferior alveolar neurovascular bundle are increased; and (4) avascular necrosis of the proximal bone fragment is possible.

Grammer et al.[8] showed significant reduction in the blood flow to the proximal bone fragments following sagittal split osteotomies in rhesus monkeys. Bone loss has been reported by Behrman[2] following the operation in adult humans. Trauma to the inferior alveolar neurovascular bundle should be anticipated in the sagittal osteotomy procedure. During the approach to the superior medial surface of the ramus, the bundle may be stretched. Injury may occur within the bony canal. The technique of sagittal osteotomy is fairly straightforward and was described previously in Chapter 10.[15] When the anatomy is distorted, it may prove difficult to preserve the lateral cortical plate intact with the coronoid and condyloid processes, while retaining the neurovascular bundle uninjured in the medial portion of the ramus.

Regardless of the surgical approach, overcorrection may be desirable. The overcorrection may help to compensate for any instability caused by soft tissue (or the lack of it) and continued differential growth rates of the two sides. Intermaxillary fixation is required for six to ten weeks, depending on the amount of rotation, apposition of the fragments, and whether or not a bone graft was part of the surgical procedure. An interocclusal acrylic splint is most helpful as a template for mandibular positioning at surgery and during fixation. The splint is fabricated on the repositioned plaster casts of the dental arches obtained just prior to surgery.

Basic Orthodontic Approach with Mandibular Osteotomies

Prior to surgery, orthodontic treatment consists of banding at least those teeth that will be used for anchorage during fixation. Definitive orthodontic treatment may be deferred until after the mandible has been repositioned surgically. A period of at least three to four months should be allowed following surgery for bony healing and the return of adequate function. It is important that the occlusal splint be worn during this entire time so that the interocclusal space created at surgery (open bite) on the affected side will be preserved. Although intermaxillary fixation is not required for more than six to ten weeks, mild elastic traction is mandatory to maintain proper position of the splint while return of mandibular function is achieved. Orthodontic treatment after surgery consists of: (1) closure of the interocclusal space (open bite) on the affected side, (2) correction of the crossbite on the normal side, (3) alignment of the maxillary midline, and (4) relief of intra-arch crowding. Closure of the interocclusal space on the affected side should be accomplished by extruding the maxillary teeth and developing the alveolar arch rather than by permitting eruption of the mandibular teeth into the space. The extrusion of maxillary teeth corrects the cant of the occlusal plane of the maxilla. A modified Hawley retainer can be used to hold the mandibular teeth in position while the maxillary teeth are being extruded (Fig. 18–9). The splint, supported by the palate, has an occlusal ledge that contacts the mandibular posterior teeth when the jaw is closed, thus preventing eruption of the teeth. The acrylic is trimmed from around the maxillary teeth so that their eruption can occur. Light elastic traction may be used to extrude the posterior maxillary teeth. Closure of the space may take several months. During this period, other aspects of orthodontic arch coordination can be accomplished as well.

Growth Center Transplants

In instances in which the ramus of the mandible is missing and no mandibular articulation is discernible, a reconstruction of the temporomandibular joint may be justified. In children, the donor tissue for the articulation should meet the following criteria: it should (1) be of similar size and shape to a normal mandibular condyle, (2) have growth potential, (3) be relatively easy to obtain with little or no long-term morbidity, and (4) be readily incorporated into the recipient area. At the present time, autogenous grafting is the only practical biologic approach to reconstructing the temporomandibular joint. Possible donor sites include the metatarsal bones, costochondral junctions, head of the fibula, and sternoclavicular joint. Glahn and Winther[5] reported good results with the metatarsal transplant, and Robinson[20] used the costochondral junction to replace the missing condyle and advance the mandible. Although the fibular head and the rib both meet the criteria for condylar replacement, we prefer the rib as a donor site.[23]

In order to establish a suitable articulation, the graft must be fixed securely to the body of the mandible or ramus and placed against the zygomatic portion of the temporal bone. Ordinarily, the bony process anterior to the auditory meatus is flat and lacks any glenoid fossa development. In adults, Obwegeser[15] has advocated reconstruction of the hypoplastic temporal and malar bones prior to mandibular grafting. In children, there is some evidence to suggest that joint function stimulates morphogenesis, and any necessary onlay grafting of the malar and temporal bones would appear best delayed until facial growth is completed.

The submandibular approach provides good surgical access for grafting. An intraoral approach through an anterior ramus incision also may be used. Use of a costochondral junction from the fourth through the eighth ribs has proved satisfactory. All but 1.5 cm of cartilage is trimmed from the osseous portion of the rib. The bony portion of the rib is fixed to the mandibular stump with interosseous wires. The cartilaginous portion of the rib is used as the articular surface against the temporal bone. If satisfactory positioning of the graft cannot be accomplished from either a submandibular or an intraoral approach alone, a preauricular incision can provide additional exposure to the articular surface of the temporal bone. Correction of the facial asymmetry is attempted with the transplant. A ramus osteotomy on the more normal side enhances the opportunity to attain facial symmetry and achieve a more favorable alignment of the alveolar arches.

An interocclusal splint is placed at the time of surgery in order to position the mandible properly. Following the osteotomy on the more normal side and prepara-

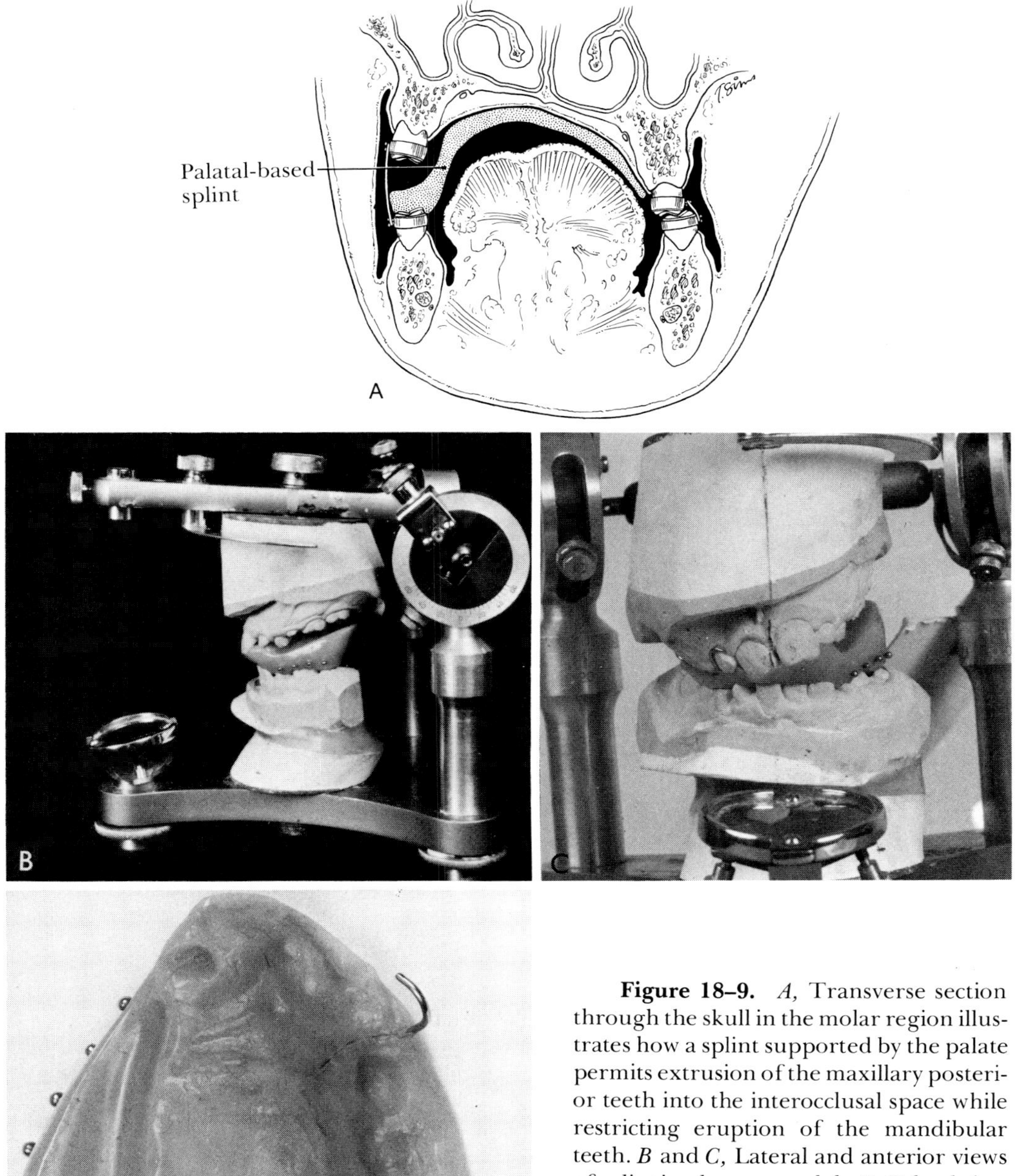

Figure 18–9. *A,* Transverse section through the skull in the molar region illustrates how a splint supported by the palate permits extrusion of the maxillary posterior teeth into the interocclusal space while restricting eruption of the mandibular teeth. *B* and *C,* Lateral and anterior views of splint in place on models. *D,* Palatal view of splint. Relief of posterior maxillary occlusal surface and anchor-knobs to be used for extrusion traction on maxillary teeth.

tion of the graft site, the acrylic splint is placed between the teeth and held in position by intermaxillary fixation. Orthodontic bands, fracture arch bars, cast splints, or preformed arch bars are all acceptable for applying intermaxillary fixation. Following placement of the fixation appliances, attention is returned to the surgical sites. Repositioning of the mandible creates a void between the hypoplastic mandibular stump and the temporal bone. This void must be filled with the graft, which forms a strut that elongates the hemimandible and butts up against the temporal bone. When a costochondral junction is used as the donor, a section of the rib from the patient's contralateral chest provides the best curvature. A 4- to 5-mm wide strip of periosteum-perichondrium bridging the costochondral junction on the lateral surface of the rib is taken with the graft to avoid a separation of the junction. If such a separation does occur, it minimizes the possibility of the transplant's retaining growth potential, and another rib should be obtained. Growth potential of the transplant is unpredictable, and all the critical factors are not known. In order to preserve maximum cellular viability of the graft, an immediate insertion into the recipient site is preferable. If storage of the graft is required during the course of the operation, placement in a physiologic salt solution such as Ringer's lactate has been found useful.

With the development of microvascular surgery, an anastomosis of vessels removed with the graft to those at the recipient site poses interesting possibilities. If a rib transplant is planned, the intercostal vessels might be left attached to the graft

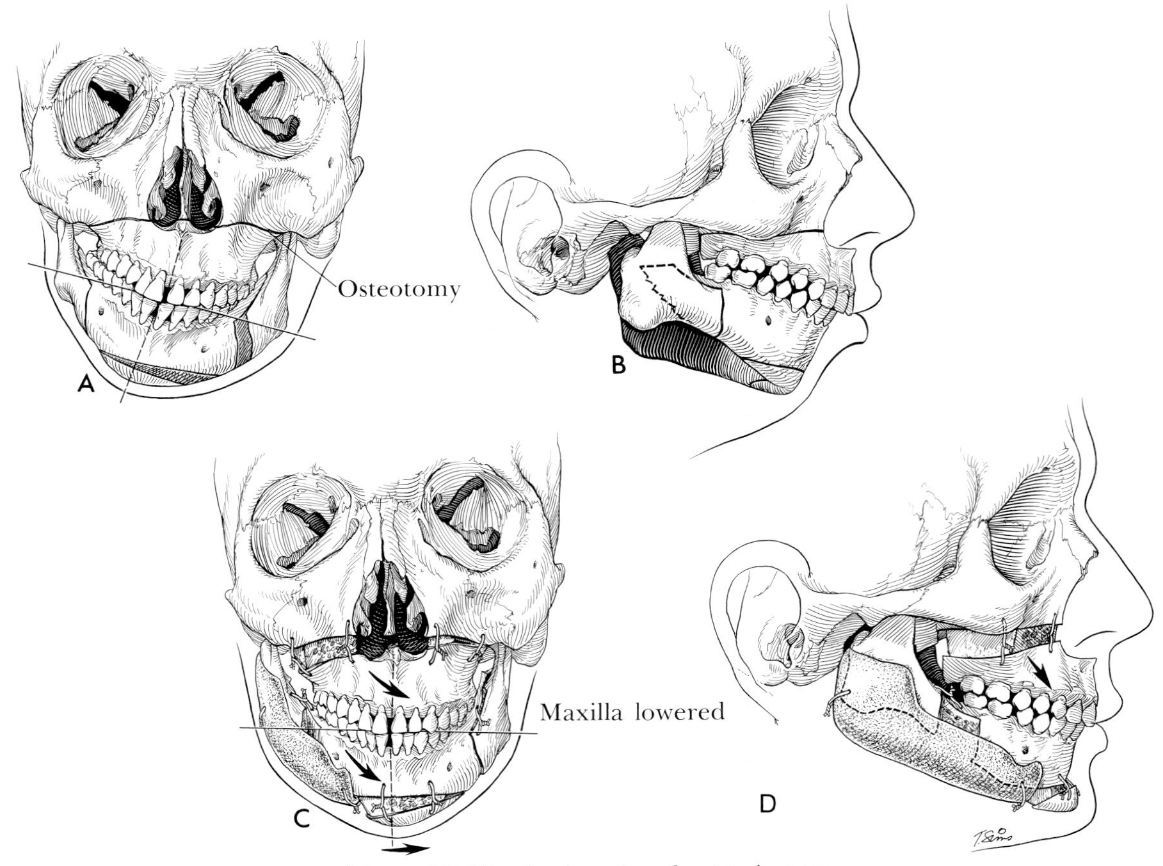

Figure 18–10. *See legend on the opposite page.*

fragment and anastomosed to the anterior facial vessels during transplantation. Technical difficulties would be encountered, but such a maneuver represents a potential method for improving graft viability and maintaining growth potential of the graft. This approach deserves careful investigation.

The orthodontic care is similar to that described earlier in connection with lengthening the affected side by osteotomy in the ramus.

Combined Maxillary and Mandibular Osteotomies

In those instances of moderate-to-severe hemifacial microsomia in which treatment has been delayed until after completion of facial growth, correction of both the facial asymmetry and the malocclusion may require surgery in both the maxilla and mandible (Fig. 18–10). The plan is outlined as follows:

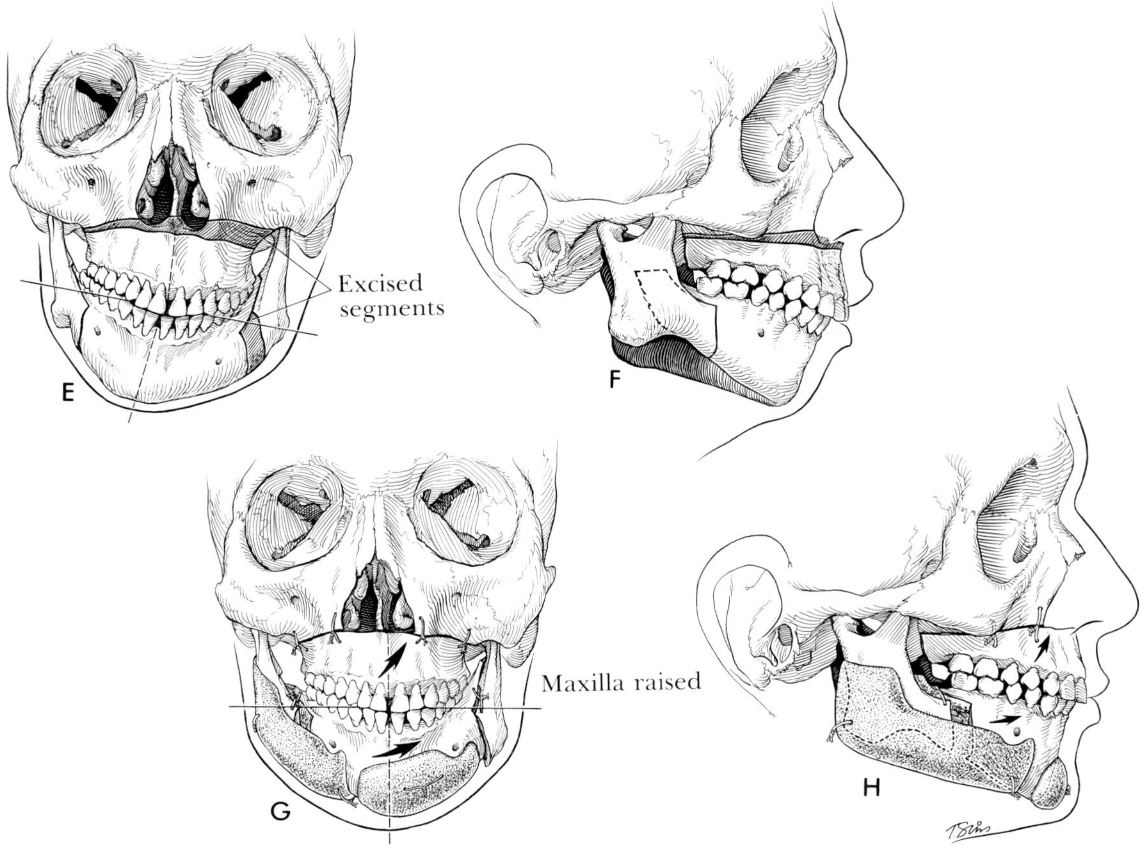

Figure 18–10. In adults with facial asymmetry secondary to hemifacial microsomia, it is necessary to perform an osteotomy on the maxilla, as well as those on the mandible, if both function and esthetics are to be improved. *A* and *B*, Le Fort I type osteotomy permits repositioning of the maxilla. Bilateral sagittal split ramusotomies with an osteotomy of the symphyseal region permit correction of the asymmetry and advancement of the mandible. The entire procedure can be accomplished through intraoral incisions. *C* and *D*, Vertical dimensions of the maxilla on the short side are increased and stabilized by bone grafts. Homogenous bone is acceptable but fresh autogenous bone from the iliac crest or rib is preferable. Occasionally vertical shortening on the normal or long side may be indicated as depicted in *E* and *F*. Following stabilization of the maxilla, the mandible is then repositioned and bone is grafted on the affected side. A genioplasty with additional grafting is usually required to achieve optimum contour and symmetry (*C, D, G, H*).

Preliminary Orthodontic Alignment of Teeth on the Individual Arches

Crowding of the teeth should be eliminated, rotations and tipping of the teeth should be corrected, and the most favorable relation between the teeth and the basal bone should be achieved in each arch. In order to accomplish these objectives, the occlusion will become less functional than before commencing with the orthodontic phase. If possible, the dental arches should be coordinated so that hand-held models of the maxillary and mandibular teeth interdigitate reasonably well prior to surgery.

Surgery

MAXILLA. Maxillary repositioning is the key to correction of the facial asymmetry. The maxilla is realigned to the skull in a symmetrical manner by performing a Le Fort I type osteotomy. The midline of the maxilla should be aligned with the midsagittal plane, and canting of the occlusal plane must be corrected. Since some relapse should be anticipated, overcorrection in both the rotation and tilting of the maxilla is desirable. Some shortening of the normal side may be advisable, but the main adjustment is achieved by interposing bone in the osteotomy space on the hypoplastic side. It is important to carefully consider the occlusal plane angle in an anteroposterior direction as well as correction of the transverse occlusal cant at the time of maxillary repositioning. If the occlusal plane is too steep, the mandibular plane angle will be steep also and the chin will remain retruded. Conversely, if the occlusal plane angle is flattened excessively, the chin may be projected forward more than is desirable. Attention to these details is required during presurgical planning and should not be left to chance at the time of surgery.

Acetate prediction tracings on both posteroanterior and lateral head films, along with proposed surgical cutouts, are helpful in the planning. Perhaps a more useful three-dimensional picture of the positioned relationships of the dental arches to the skull can be developed by the facebow mounting of the dental casts on an articulator. The extent of rotations necessary to properly position both the maxilla and the mandible can be estimated by cutting the plaster bases horizontally and then realigning the models as will be attempted at surgery. The actual distance that the dental casts are moved provides measurements for bone graft requirements and for repositioning the jaws (see Figure 18–13*J*, *K*).

Interosseous fixation of the bone graft with wire at the margin of the piriform aperture and at the base of the zygoma provides the best stability. Occasionally it is advisable to insert bone between the tuberosity of the maxilla and the pterygoid processes of the sphenoid bone on the short side if rotation and advancement create a large void in the pterygomaxillary area. Additional cranial fixation is ordinarily advisable following the mandibular osteotomies. Suspension wires from the zygomatic arches add stability, but the same wires may tend to retract the maxilla. Kufner[12] advocates the use of anterior suspension wires from a pin embedded in the frontal bone just above the frontal sinus. These wires are inserted bilaterally under the periosteum along the bridge of the nose and down to the fixation appliance at the maxillary cuspid region. The direction of the wires is favorable and provides excellent stability for both the maxilla and the mandible during healing. Suspension wires from the nasal buttresses or infraorbital rims are less troublesome to place and also provide satisfactory stability. Stability can be achieved also by the use of a head frame and attachments. No matter what the approach to fixation, it is imperative to have stability during healing in order to decrease the tendency for relapse.

Bone used for grafting may be either homologous or autogenous. Autogenous bone is preferable but has the disadvantage of requiring an additional surgical site and increased operating time for the patient. Either the rib or iliac crest is a satisfactory donor site. Our preference is the iliac crest because of the greater availability of cancellous bone. When placing the bone grafts in the maxillary osteotomy site, the bone is exposed in the cavity of the maxillary sinus without the benefit of a mucosal covering of the medial surface. Revascularization must derive from the vestibular tissues. Supportive measures to prevent infection and to maintain normal nasal and antral physiology enhance the prognosis. Administration of prophylactic antibiotics during and following surgery appears justified. Use of systemic and local decongestants improves aeration of the nasal passages, enhancing sinus drainage and adding to the patient's comfort.

MANDIBLE. Bilateral ramus osteotomies are required to properly position the mandible following realignment and stabilization of the maxilla. Bone grafting on the hypoplastic side is advisable to assure stability and provide adequate tissue bulk. Since the maxillary surgery is performed intraorally, the intraoral approach to the mandible is convenient and provides adequate access. However, if the surgeon prefers approaching the ramus from submandibular incisions, the mandibular osteotomies and grafting can be performed equally well from an extraoral approach. As previously mentioned, the maxilla serves as the guide for mandibular repositioning. When orthodontic arch coordination has been accomplished prior to surgery, the procedure is simplified by placing the teeth in maximum interdigitation at surgery. An occlusal splint is used when function and esthetics indicate the desirability of overcorrection of the mandible. The osteotomy on the normal ramus permits the medial rotation and vertical shortening necessary to accommodate to the maxilla. Freedom to shorten or lengthen the normal hemimandible in a horizontal plane as the situation requires is also assured.

Considerable lengthening of the hypoplastic hemimandible is ordinarily required if facial symmetry is to be achieved. Release of soft tissue restrictions from the distal fragment must be accomplished following the osteotomy. The tissue medial to the ramus often poses the greatest restrictions. Incision of the periosteum and detachment of the sphenomandibular ligaments are necessary. Medial pterygoid and suprahyoid muscle attachments usually must be released from the distal fragment. Judicious dissection is required to avoid injury to the lingual nerve and to preserve the inferior alveolar neurovascular bundle. Adequate exposure and careful control of hemorrhage during dissection are required.

When satisfactory positioning of the mandible is accomplished, intermaxillary fixation in the desired occlusal position is applied. The requirement for bone grafting is determined, and autogenous bone from the iliac crest is preferred. If there is a reliable source of homologous bone, additional surgery to secure donor bone may be avoided.

Camouflage

Improvement of facial symmetry also may be attained by camouflage procedures. Augmentation of contour deficiencies may be indicated in conjunction with the skeletal surgery or as a single procedure in instances in which jaw surgery may not be justified. When surgery is performed for improvement of esthetics only and augmentation alone will suffice, camouflage procedures represent an excellent approach.

Two methods are used to alter contour: (1) biologic materials including both autogenous and homologous tissue may be transplanted to fill in deficiencies or (2) biologically inert materials such as silicone rubber, fluorocarbons, acrylic, or metals may be used. A keen artistic sense as well as knowledge of the various biologic possibilities and restrictions is required to achieve the most pleasing results. Homologous tissues may initiate some degree of host rejection, and autogenous transplants have the advantage of complete biocompatibility. The main disadvantage of autogenous transplants is the requirement of additional surgery to obtain the donor material. Autogenous tissues, particularly cartilage, cancellous bone, and marrow, retain some cellular viability if immediately transplanted following removal from the donor site.[18] Bone, cartilage, and dermal-fat grafts are the tissues most often used for augmentation procedures. If sufficient bone can be obtained from the adjacent facial skeleton to satisfy the requirements for bone grafting, the need for additional surgery at another site is eliminated. A rotational or sliding genioplasty may be all that is required (Fig. 18–11). Transfer of bone from the angle or lower border of the normal or elongated hemimandible to the deficient side may offer a way of improving facial symmetry. Onlay grafting of the deficient mandible, zygoma, or maxilla may be accomplished using rib or iliac crest bone. Longacre[13] advocates the use of split rib grafts to add contour to the facial skeleton, even

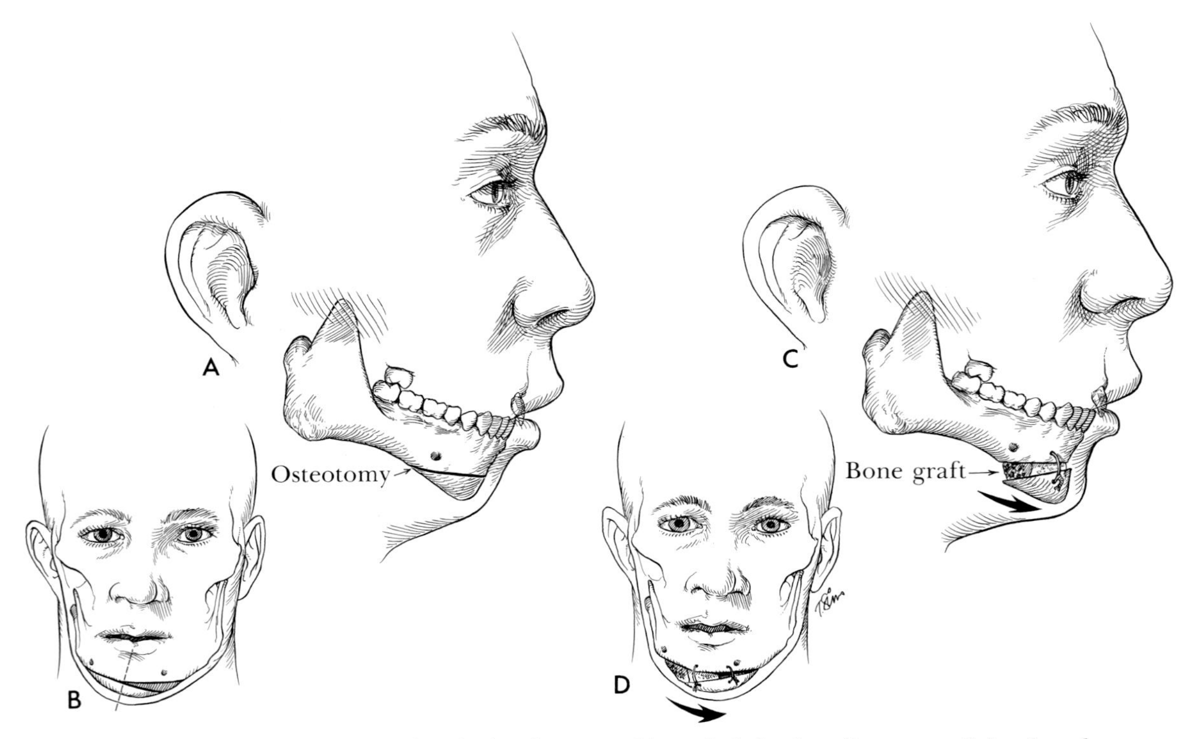

Figure 18–11. Genioplasty. If occlusion is acceptable and skeletal realignment of the dental components is not advisable, facial symmetry may still be improved by shifting the chin point. *A* and *B,* Dotted lines illustrate osteotomy sites for realigning the chin. The shaded portion is used as a free graft to help fill the void and lengthen the short side as depicted in *C* and *D.*

during early childhood, since he feels that the build-up of the skeletal contour aids in soft-tissue development. Remodeling and frequently total resorption of onlay grafts may occur. If fibrous tissue replacement of the graft occurs, some long-term esthetic benefit still may be achieved. Prediction is difficult, and, unfortunately, the immediate postsurgical improvement is often transitory.

In those instances in which there is marked deficiency of soft tissue, bone, or cartilage, onlay grafts will not provide a pleasing, natural contour. A softer, more pliable material is preferred. Subcutaneous insertion of autogenous dermal-fat grafts removed from the buttocks or lower abdomen has been recommended by Thompson.[22] He proposes overcontouring in anticipation of some resorption (approximately 30 per cent). The early revascularization of the free graft primarily through the capillary-rich dermal portion prevents necrosis and the total resorption of the graft. When soft-tissue plumping is indicated, an inert biomaterial such as silicone sponge might be considered. The most obvious advantages are: (1) the accuracy of contour, which may be achieved by shaping of the material prior to surgery and (2) additional surgery to obtain graft material is made unnecessary. Tissue tolerance for the silicone rubber has been demonstrated in patients for more than 15 years. The tendency for the implant to migrate, particularly in an active area such as the face, can be counteracted by perforating the implant to allow tissue ingrowth. Holes of 3 to 5 mm made through the material have been found to stabilize the implant well.

A more recent material developed for use in facial augmentation is a fluorocarbon compound marketed as Proplast.* The material is porous, permitting tissue ingrowth; is relatively easy to shape and carve at surgery; and is essentially biologically inert. However, Proplast is only minimally compressible and black in color. Its greatest use has been in augmenting bone deficits, as the dark color and relative rigidity make it undesirable for soft-tissue augmentation or for placement immediately beneath the skin, where the color may be objectionable.

When planning augmentation surgery, whether with grafts or implants, the use of a facial moulage is frequently helpful. It is neither necessary nor desirable to model and then reproduce at surgery the exact patterns developed from the moulage. Patterns developed by this method invariably have been found to be too large when inserted at surgery. Nevertheless, the moulage, along with oriented photographs and cephalometric films, is a useful aid in formulating the definitive treatment plan.

Incisions

Access to the regions of the zygomatic and mandibular ramus can be accomplished through a preauricular incision. A subcutaneous pocket is developed to conform to the size and shape of the implant. Care should be taken to avoid overdissection, thus creating potential dead space for hematoma formation. If additional exposure is required anteriorly in order to transfix the graft or implant to the zygomatic region, an accessory infraorbital incision is used. A skin fold inferior to the lower eyelid provides a convenient place to make the incision. Use of fine suture material and careful closure will result in a remarkably inconspicuous scar. The mandibular ramus or posterior cheek can be approached through a submandibular incision. If the graft or implant is to be placed

*Smith Kline & French Surgical Specialties, Division of Smith Kline Corporation, 1500 Spring Garden Street, Philadelphia, PA 19101

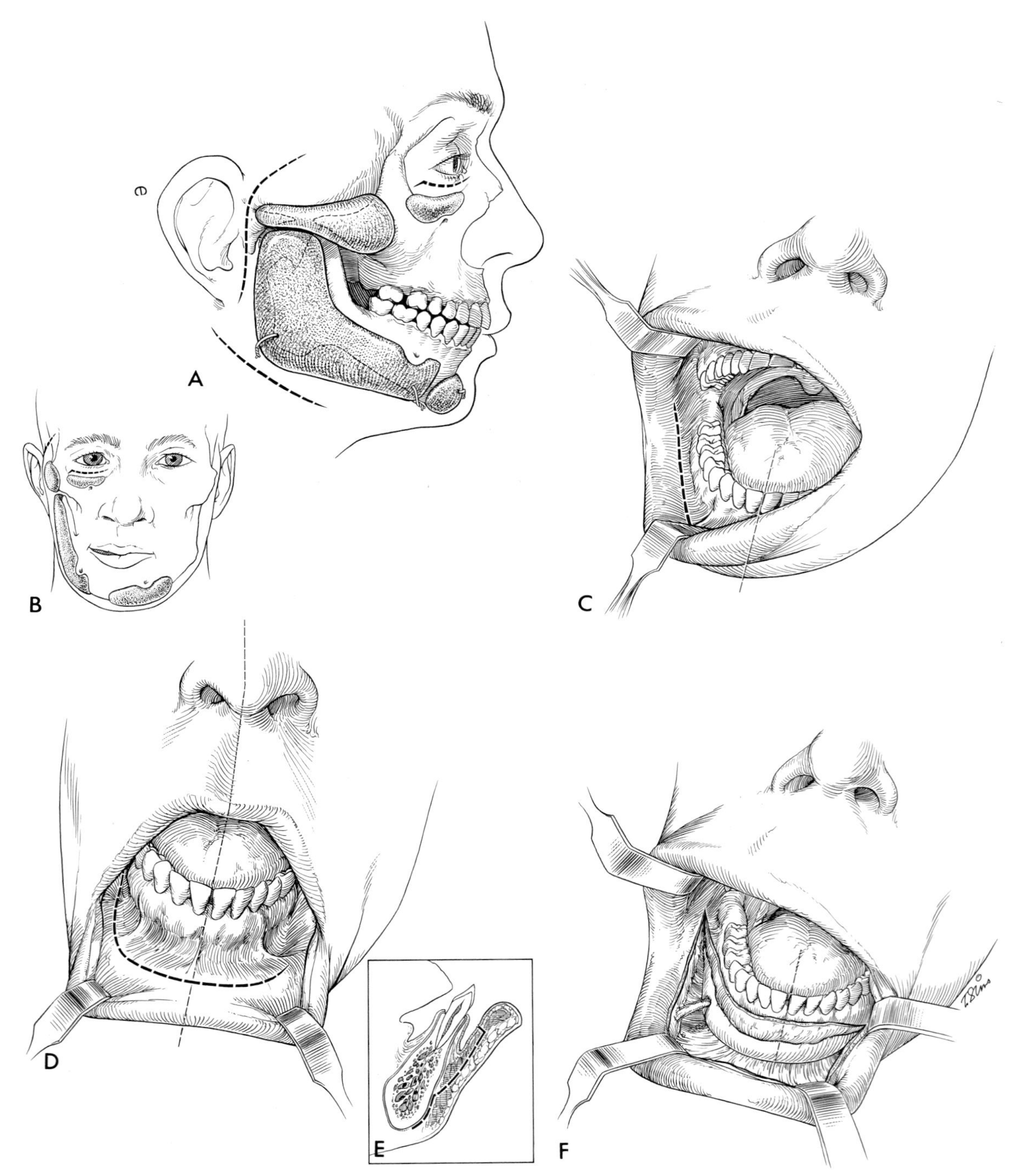

Figure 18–12. *A* and *B,* Insertion of grafts or implants (shaded areas) to augment the zygomatic or ramus regions should be performed through inconspicuous incisions (dotted lines) designed to avoid injury to the branches of the facial nerve. If the procedure can be accomplished entirely through the preauricular incision, the scar can be most inconspicuous; the infraorbital and submandibular incisions occasionally may be required. Careful technique will usually result in an inconsequential scar.

Augmentation of the lateral ramus may also be accomplished through a buccal incision as depicted in *C.* The mandibular symphysis area traditionally has been approached through a submental incision. However, the intraoral approach (*D, E, F*) is preferred for performing either a genioplasty or an augmentation procedure in the anterior mandibular region.

contiguous with the ramus, dissection is similar to that described earlier for ramus osteotomies. If only soft-tissue plumping is planned, a subcutaneous pocket is adequate. Augmentation of the lateral surface of the ramus or lower border of the mandible can be accomplished through an intraoral incision in the buccal mucosa anterior to and paralleling the anterior border of the ramus. The position of the incision and exposure is similar to that used for the sagittal split osteotomy. The region of the anterior mandible and symphysis is conveniently approached through the anterior labial vestibule in the same manner used for performing a genioplasty. The details of these surgical approaches are shown in Figure 18–12 and are also described elsewhere in the book. (See Chapter 14.)

Complications of augmentation include infection, migration, or shifting of the implant and unpredictable resorption of tissue grafts. The incidence of infection can be reduced by obliterating dead space created around the implant. Negative pressure drainage through fine perforated polyethylene catheters for 24 to 48 hours following surgery and a firm pressure dressing for several days are useful in obliterating dead space. Soaking the implants prior to insertion and irrigating the wound during surgery with a broad-spectrum antibiotic solution may be advisable.

Thompson[22] describes cyst formation in dermal-fat grafts that are apparently a result of the entrapped epithelial elements in the dermis. The cysts have been found in biopsies up to 13 years following implantation but reportedly have posed no clinical symptoms.

Migration of transplanted tissue or inert implants, or both, occurs occasionally in response to gravity and the influence of surrounding muscles. Use of nonabsorbable sutures to transfix the transplants to surrounding stable skeletal points will help prevent the dependent settling of the transplanted tissue. Eventually, incorporation with the host tissue and connective tissue encapsulation stabilize the transplant.

Inert nonbiologic implants are stabilized initially by transfixion to adjacent tissue, bone, periosteum, or fascia. Connective tissue ingrowth will rapidly transfix the spongy, porous materials. Solid implants should be perforated to allow tissue ingrowth.

CASE STUDIES

CASE 18–1 (Fig. 18–13)

The following case exemplifies a congenital first-arch defect limited to hypoplasia of the mandibular ramus and condyle. Clinically, the patient's mandibular deviation during extreme opening suggested a unilateral hypoplasia of the lateral pterygoid muscle; otherwise, soft-tissue development appeared normal. No other congenital anomalies were uncovered. There were no known instances of congenital defects in the pedigree. The mother's pregnancy with the patient was uneventful. No abnormalities were noted at birth, and it was not until the patient was 3 years of age that his mother noticed the facial asymmetry. The patient's defect represents a mild and relatively uncomplicated example of the syndrome of hemifacial microsomia. Nevertheless, the principles used in the treatment plan are applicable to the more severe forms of the syndrome, as well as to acquired defects resulting in unilateral underdevelopment of the mandible. For illustrative purposes: (1) clinical features that may be so subtle that they go undetected during neonatal examinations are discussed and (2) a method of treating the skeletal and dental sequelae of the abnormality is presented.

When the patient was 6 years old, his facial asymmetry and relative mandibular retrusion prompted his mother to seek a professional opinion. Referral from a children's dentist to an orthodontist resulted in the patient's appearance at our clinic. Baseline records were obtained, consisting of photographs, cephalometric head films, temporomandibular joint tomographs, and study models of the dentition. The diagnosis was condylar hypoplasia secondary to a congenital defect of the first branchial arch. The head films were repeated at yearly intervals to assess the progress of the deformity. When the patient was 8 years old, it was apparent that the facial asymmetry was increasing. The eruption patterns of both maxillary and mandibular teeth were poor, and the occlusal plane was becoming more severely canted toward the affected side. During the two years of observation, the only treatment had been the placement of a mandibular lingual arch attached to the lower first molar teeth.

PROBLEM LIST

Esthetics

FRONTAL. Lower face with an asymmetry to the left, incompetent lip seal without contracture of inferior labial muscles.

PROFILE. Retrusion of the lower jaw.

Cephalometric Analysis

FRONTAL. Mandibular symphysis 10 mm to left of midsagittal plane. Occlusal plane canted upward to the left side.

LATERAL. Retrusion of mandible; lower border and angle of left hemimandible 12 cm above the right. Occlusal plane at two levels.

TOMOGRAPHIC. Tomography of temporomandibular joints and mandibular rami revealed absence of left glenoid fossa, ramus underdeveloped with hypoplastic condyle.

Occlusal Analysis

DENTAL ARCH FORM. Maxilla: rounded with midline deviation slightly to left. Mandible: midline deviated to left with shortened left side.

DENTAL ALIGNMENT. Crowding of both arches with impaction of lower left second molar.

DENTAL OCCLUSION. Class II molar and canine relationship bilaterally but more severe on left side.

TREATMENT PLAN

Surgical Treatment

1. Advance mandible and correct midline to remedy asymmetry and mandibular retrusion and lip incompetence.
2. Open posterior bite on the left side to level the mandibular occlusal plane and the lower borders of the mandible.
3. Maximally retrude condylar fragment and augment ramus with bone at osteotomy site to correct hypoplastic condyle and underdevelopment of left ramus.

Orthodontic Treatment

1. Maintain level of mandibular occlusal plane with acrylic splint and extrude left maxillary teeth into occlusion to correct posterior open bite.
2. Correct arch crowding postoperatively by extracting the four first premolars and aligning and coordinating the arches.
3. Remove impacted lower left second molar at the time of osseous surgery.

Future Treatment

1. To correct further differential facial growth, perform additional surgery in late adolescence or adulthood—either augmentation or mandibular lengthening coordinated with final orthodontic detailing of occlusion.

COMMENT

This type of planning requires an 8- to 12-year commitment to treatment. Fortunately, much of the time is devoted solely to observation. "Planned neglect" combined with careful observation is often fruitful. The satisfactory skeletal development of this patient following initial treatment illustrates the potential benefits of early surgery and staged orthodontic therapy. Prior to surgery, a cast of the maxillary dental arch was mounted on an articulator using a standard facebow transfer. The cast of the mandibular arch was oriented on the articulator so as to correct the skeletal asymmetry and flatten the occlusal plane. Measurements taken from the head films were used as guides to arrive at the desired position. An interocclusal acrylic splint was constructed and was used at surgery to position the mandible relative to the maxilla. Through an intraoral approach, a modified sagittal split osteotomy was performed on the affected side with a subcondylar vertical osteotomy on the normal side. An 8-cm segment of the right seventh rib was removed, minced, and packed into the periosteal envelope of the hypoplastic side after the mandible was repositioned. At the time, it was thought that there was insufficient bony overlap following the lengthening procedure. In retrospect, the grafting probably was not necessary. More recent experience has demonstrated vigorous subperiosteal bone generation in children without the need for grafting. Preformed arch bars were ligated to the mandibular and maxillary teeth, and intermaxillary fixation was achieved using the interocclusal splint. Immobilization was maintained for eight weeks and was then converted to mild elastic traction with the splint in place for an additional four weeks. During that period the patient could remove the elastics to eat and to exercise the mandible.

At the end of 12 weeks following surgery, the interocclusal splint was replaced with a retainer that would allow eruption of the maxillary teeth while preventing the mandibular teeth from erupting into the interocclusal space on the hypoplastic side. Closure of the open bite, using this technique, required 12 months. During that time, consolidation of the graft and recontouring of the ramus were observed in the periodic roentgenographs. When the deciduous teeth were lost, it was determined that the four first premolar teeth also should be removed to eliminate crowding and permit better arch coordination. The impacted lower second molar bud on the affected side was removed during the original surgery. Otherwise, the orthodontic treatment required no special consideration and was completed when the patient was 14 years old.

During the intervening period (from 8 to 14 years of age), the patient's hypoplastic ramus had undergone remarkable changes. The condyle had elongated and migrated posteriorly, forming a nearly normal-appearing temporomandibular joint anterior to the external auditory meatus. The angle of the mandible had become more obtuse with

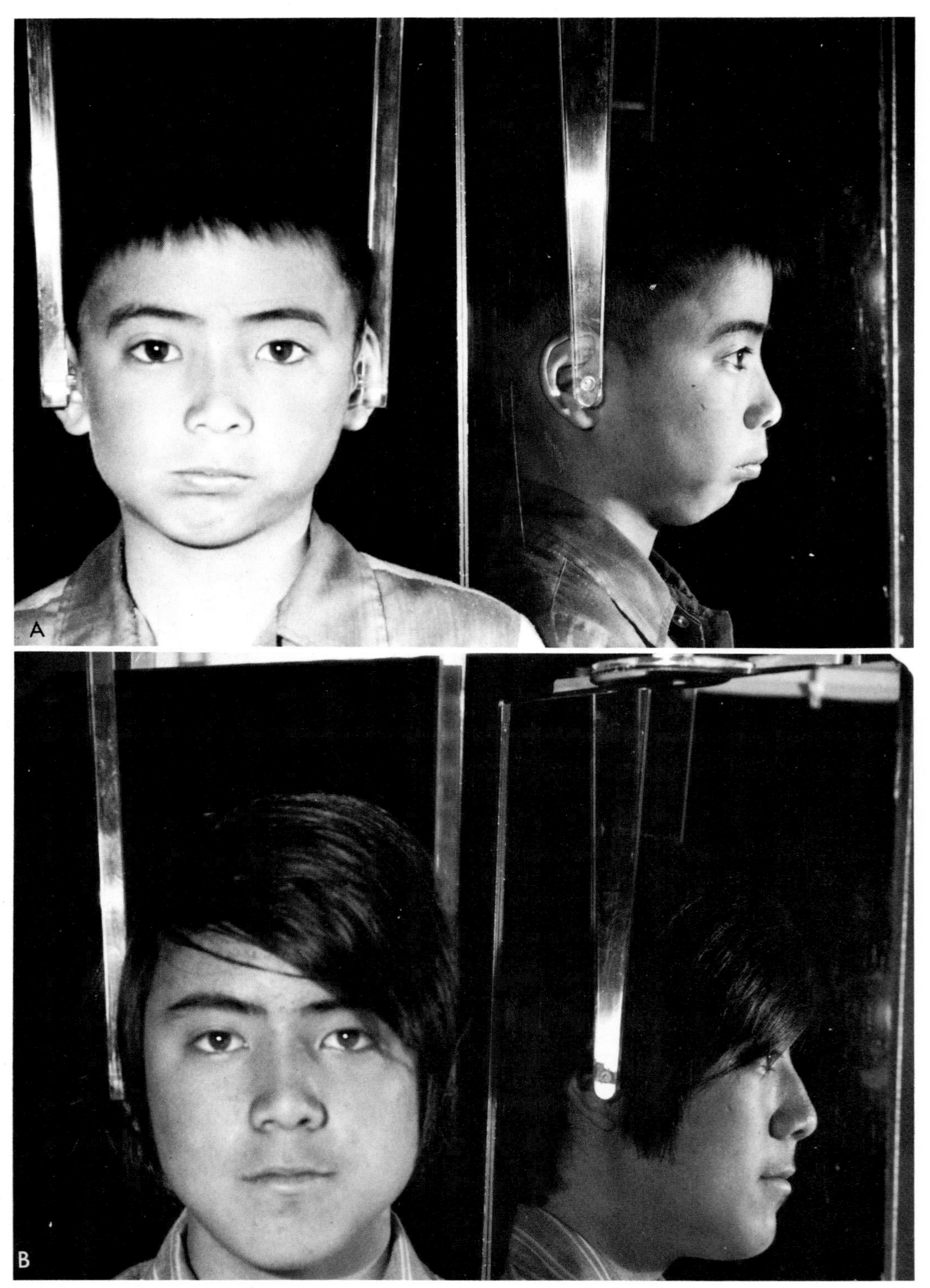

Figure 18–13 (Case 18–1). Eight-year-old boy with facial asymmetry and mandibular retrusion suggestive of hemifacial microsomia. *A*, Pretreatment facial views. *B*, Posttreatment facial views. At age 14 years facial symmetry and mandibular development appear quite normal.

Legend continued on the opposite page.

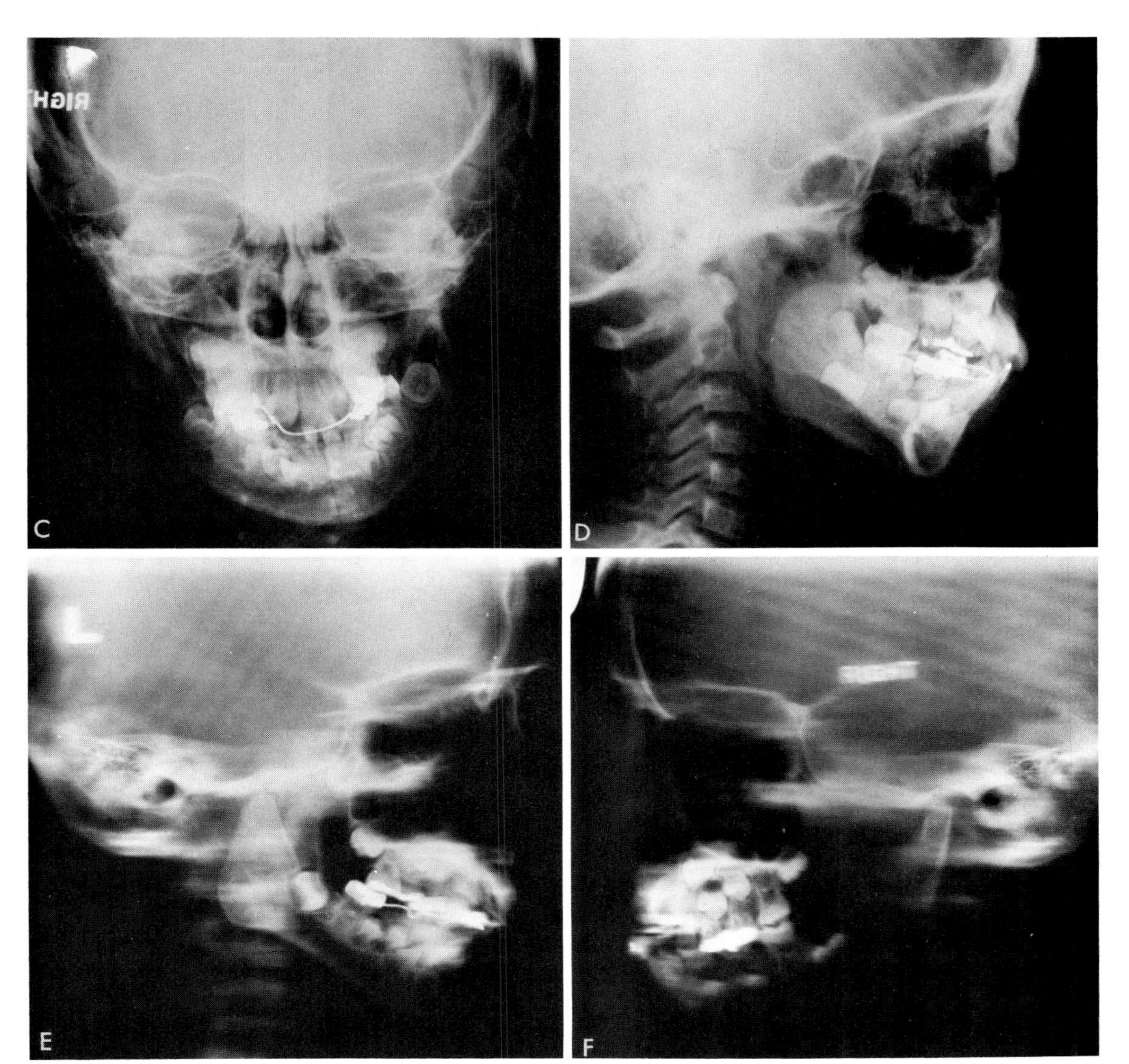

Figure 18–13 *Continued.* *C* and *D*, Posteroanterior (*C*) and lateral cephalometric (*D*) films demonstrate the skeletal asymmetry and mandibular retrusion. *E*, Tomographic film of the left mandibular ramus shows the hypoplasia with the condylar process positioned anteriorly. The glenoid fossa or articular eminence is not developed, as is evident on the normal right side (*F*).

Illustration continued on the following page.

disappearance of the antegonial notch. Growth of the affected side had kept pace with the normal side so that facial symmetry was retained. Function of the mandible was normal except for the continued hypofunction associated with the lateral pterygoid muscle on the affected side. Occlusion and dental health have remained excellent. Except for possible problems related to eruption of the maxillary second molar tooth on the affected side, no further need for treatment is anticipated.

This case illustrates an excellent result that was obtained when early surgery and subsequent orthodontics were coordinated in the treatment plan. Although the remarkable recontouring and growth on the hypoplastic side may not have been the direct result of the surgery, it certainly does not appear that surgery had any deleterious effects upon facial growth.

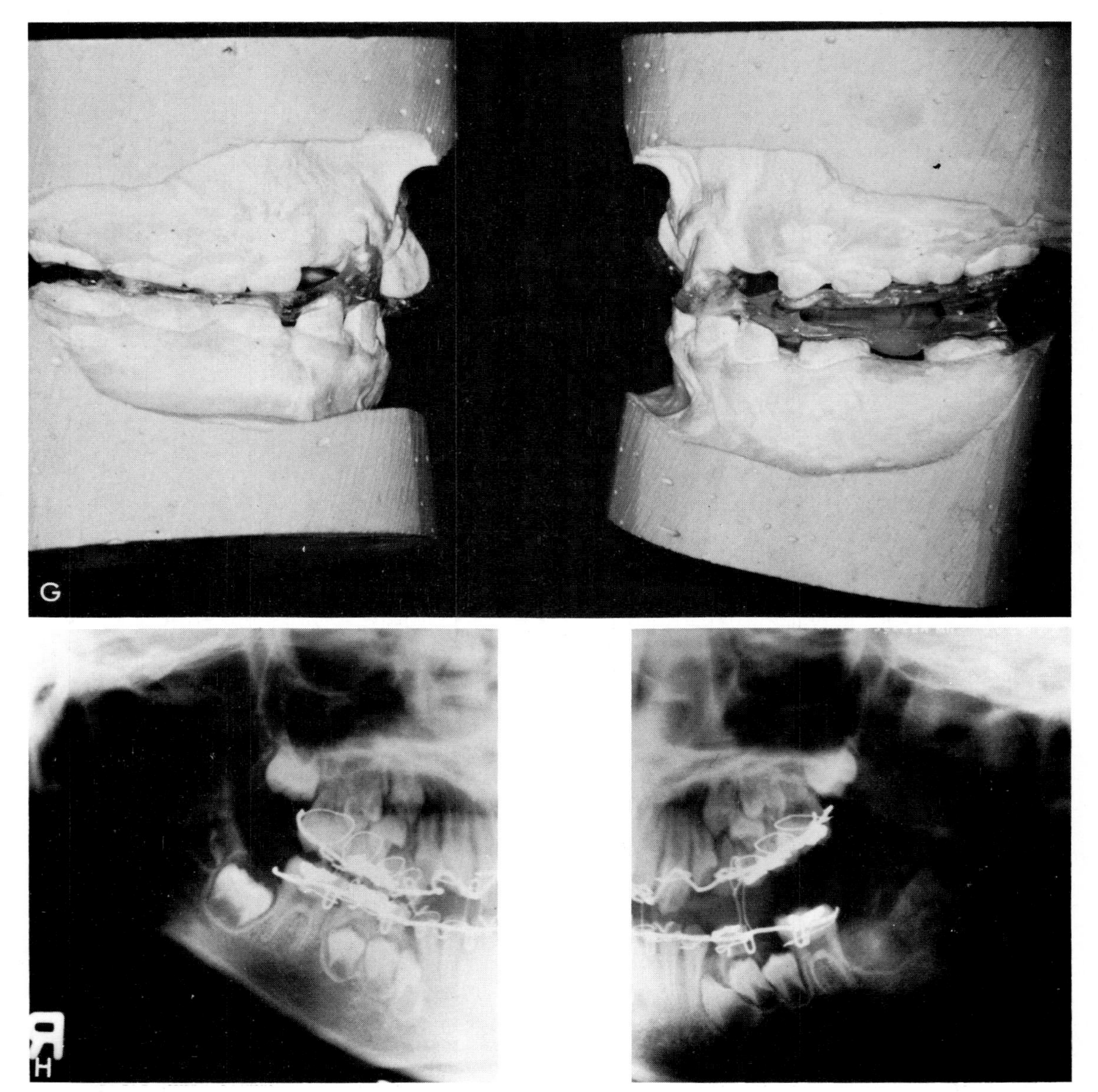

Figure 18–13 *Continued.* *G,* Views of the right and left sides of the dental casts demonstrate the interocclusal splint fabricated prior to surgery. *H,* Panographic film further illustrates the interocclusal space achieved by lengthening the left ramus and grafting with minced rib graft.

Legend continued on the opposite page.

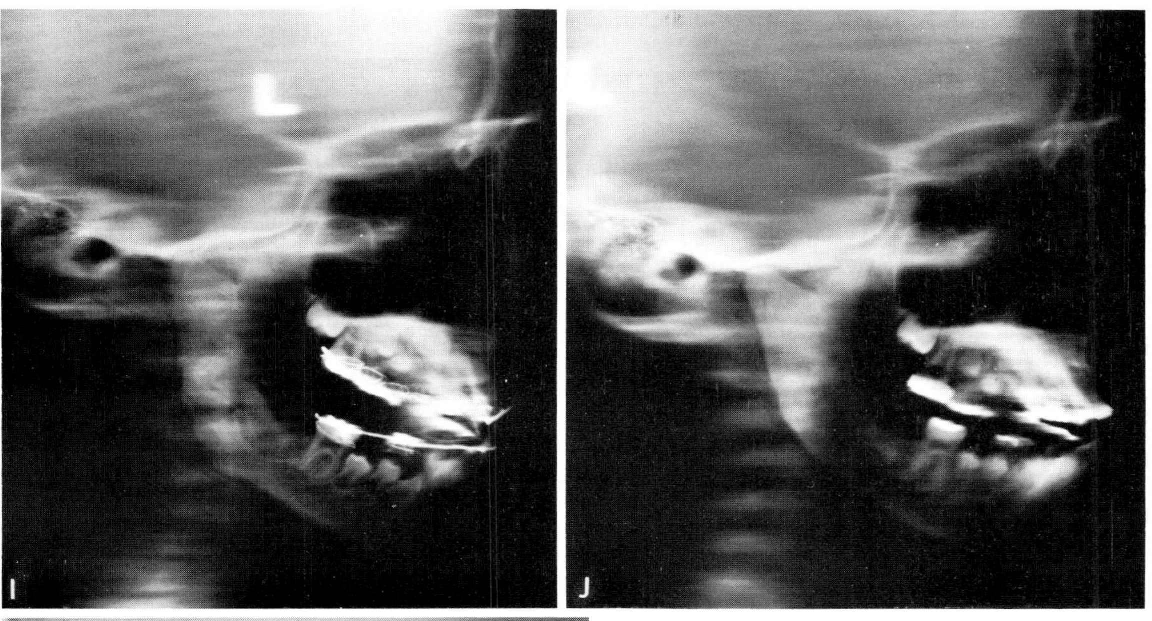

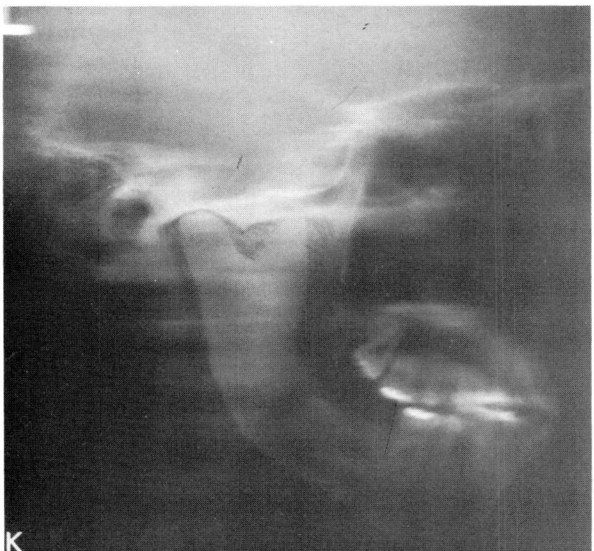

Figure 18–13 *Continued.* *I,* Four months following surgery the ramus with the bone graft shows consolidation occurring. The posterior open bite remains. *J,* Twelve months following surgery further contouring of the ramus is evident, and the condylar process is more distinct and positioned more posteriorly. Extrusion of the maxillary teeth has nearly closed the interocclusal space. *K,* Six years after surgery the ramus contour and condylar position are nearly normal. A glenoid fossa has developed with a small articular eminence evident in the tomogram. A comparison with the presurgical tomogram (*E*) demonstrates remarkable changes.

Illustration continued on the following page.

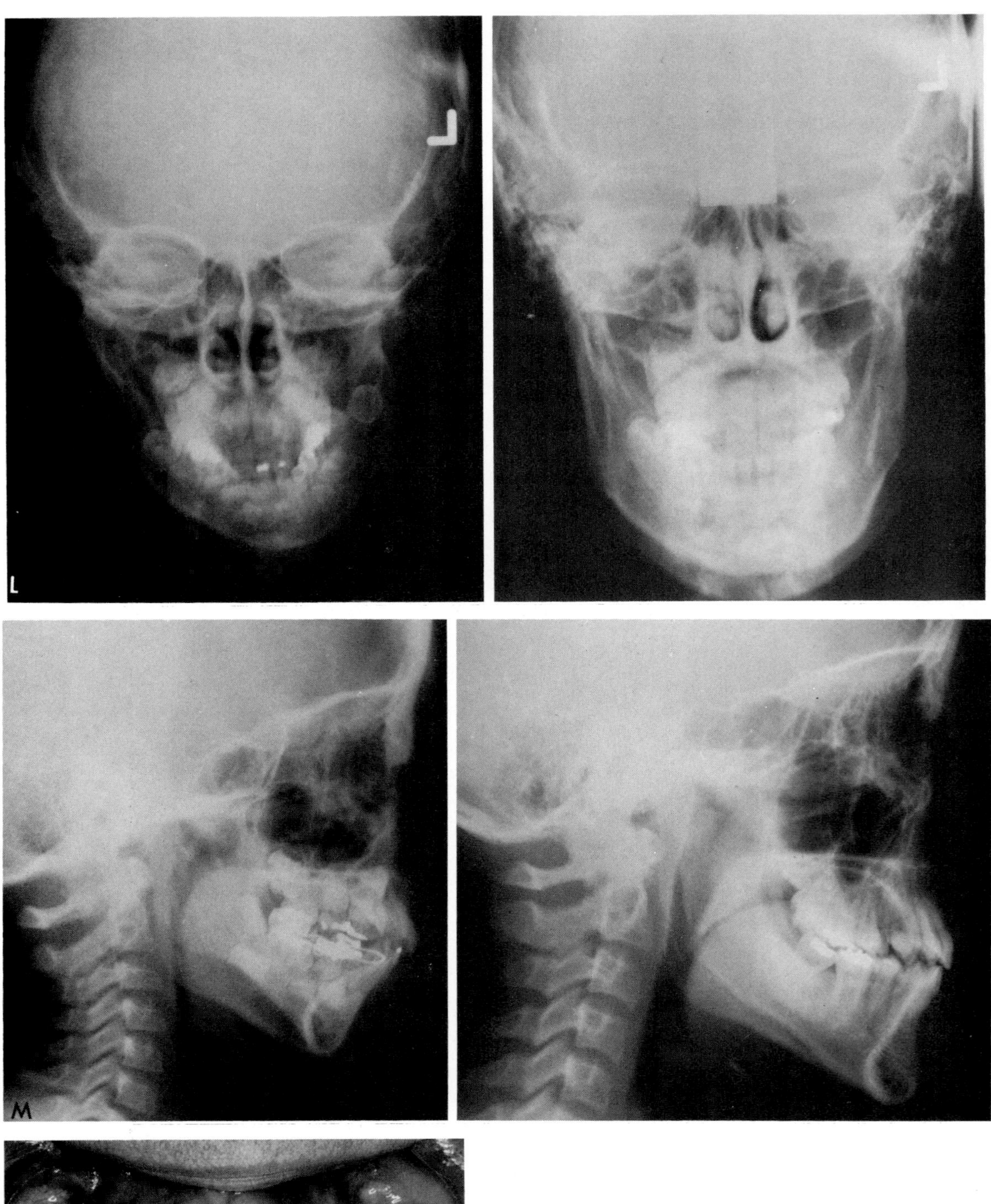

Figure 18–13 *Continued.* *L* and *M*, Comparisons of posteroanterior and lateral cephalometric films between ages 8 and 14 years following completion of orthodontic treatment. *N*, One year following completion of orthodontic treatment, the occlusion is functional and stable. (Orthodontic treatment was performed by Dr. Jack Smithers of Walnut Creek, California.)

CASE 18–2 (Fig. 18–14)

A 19-year-old man requested treatment to improve facial symmetry. At age 6 years he had been diagnosed as having agenesis of the right mandibular condyle (hemifacial microsomia). An autogenous transplant of the left fibular head had been performed with only marginal benefit toward his subsequent facial development. Orthodontic treatment at age 17 years improved the occlusion, but facial asymmetry remained a problem.

PROBLEM LIST

Esthetics

FRONTAL. Facial asymmetry: right side of lower face plump and rounded, left side angular and flattened anteriorly, chin deviated to the right, lip line and occlusal plane tilted upward toward the right.

PROFILE. Contour-deficient chin.

Cephalometric Analysis

FRONTAL. Mandibular symphysis 22 mm to right of midsagittal plane, maxillary incisors 7 mm to right of midsagittal plane, mandibular incisors 12 mm to right of midsagittal plane. Occlusal plane tilted, with right molars 7 mm higher than left. Mandibular gonial angles canted, with the right 20 mm higher than the left. Floor of the right nostril 3 mm higher than the left.

LATERAL. Lower border of the mandible at two levels. Right gonial angle 20 mm superior to the left. Contour-deficient chin.

Occlusal Analysis

DENTAL ARCH FORM. Maxilla and mandible rounded and shortened on right side.

DENTAL ALIGNMENT. Crowding eliminated by removal of maxillary first premolar and right mandibular first molar teeth followed by orthodontic coordination before further surgery was considered.

DENTAL OCCLUSION. Class II molar and canine relationship, midline of mandibular incisors 5 mm to right of maxillary incisor midline.

TREATMENT PLAN

1. To correct facial asymmetry, reposition maxilla to flatten occlusal plane, correct midline. Rotate to left 7 mm, shorten in left molar region 4 mm, lengthen in right molar region 4 mm with iliac crest bone graft on right side. To correct deviated and contour-deficient chin, perform genioplasty with bone graft.

2. To remedy Class II relationship and midline discrepancy, perform anterior positioning of mandible with rotation to improve midline. *Note:* Unfortunately no further surgery was anticipated at the time the orthodontist completed detailing the occlusion. The orthodontic bands were removed. Hand-held casts indicated that rotating the mandible relative to the maxilla would improve the midline relationship and the posterior occlusion. However, it would have been preferable to retain the orthodontic appliances for fixation purposes following surgery and for final detailing of the occlusion later. Both

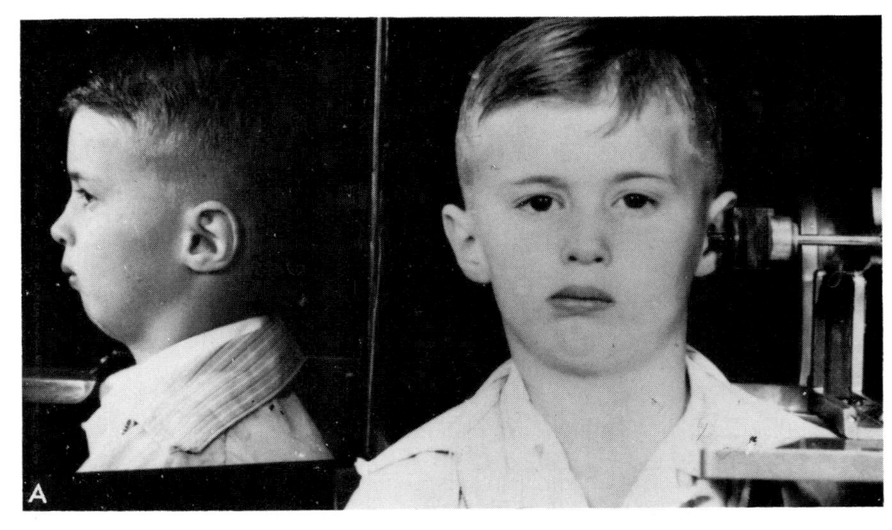

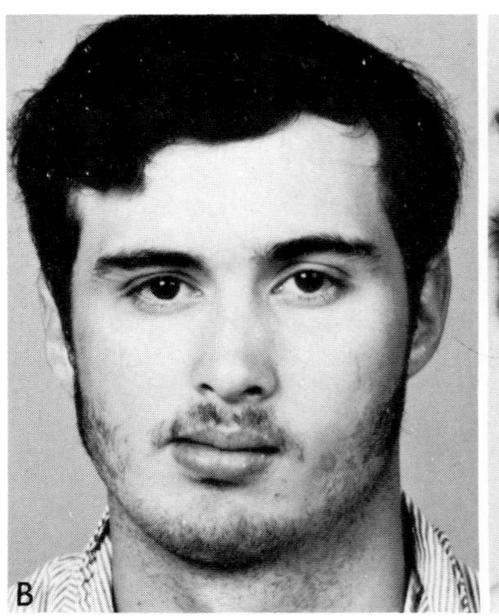

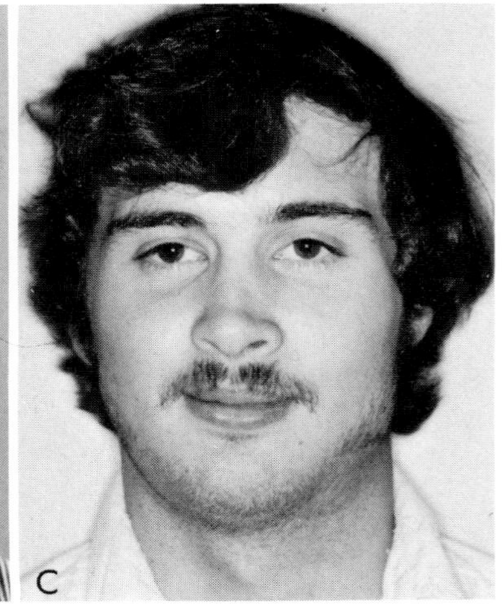

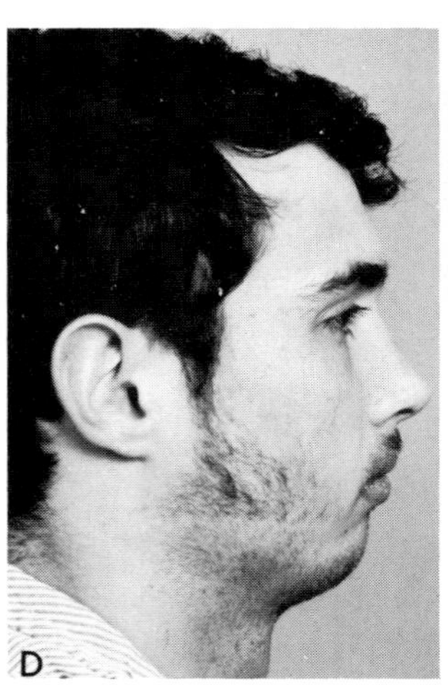

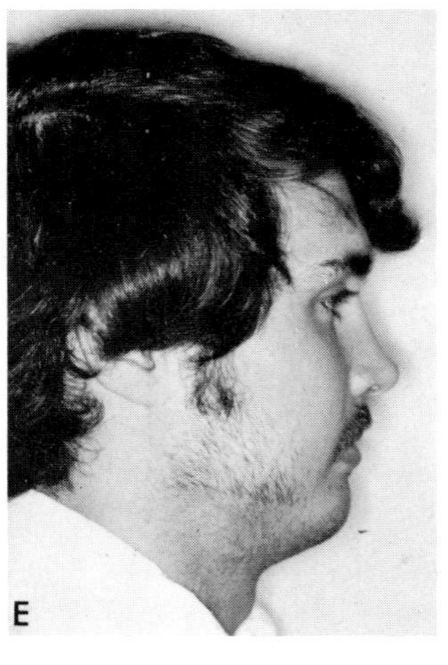

Figure 18–14 (Case 18–2). *A*, Photographs of patient at age 6 show facial asymmetry and agenesis. *B–E*, Profile (*D*) and full face (*B*) photographs at age 19 demonstrate the residual asymmetry and mandibular retrusion. Facial photographs (*C* and *E*) 6 months after surgery illustrate the soft-tissue changes (compare with *B* and *D*) as a result of a Le Fort I maxillary osteotomy with iliac crest bone grafts, bilateral ramus osteotomies, and a genioplasty. Flaring of the nares is an undesired side effect.

Figure 18–14 *Continued.* *F* and *G*, Cephalometric tracings, posteroanterior (*F*) and lateral (*G*), at age 19 further illustrate the skeletal asymmetry. *H* and *I*, Postoperative cephalometric tracings, posteroanterior (*H*) and lateral (*I*), at age 20 demonstrate the postoperative skeletal changes. In *G* the discrepancy in the levels of the lower borders of the mandible is illustrated by the dotted line representing the hypoplastic side. Note the excessive Class II molar relationship. The lower 1st molar had been removed to facilitate orthodontic treatment prior to surgery. After surgery, the lower borders of the mandible

Legend continued on the opposite page.

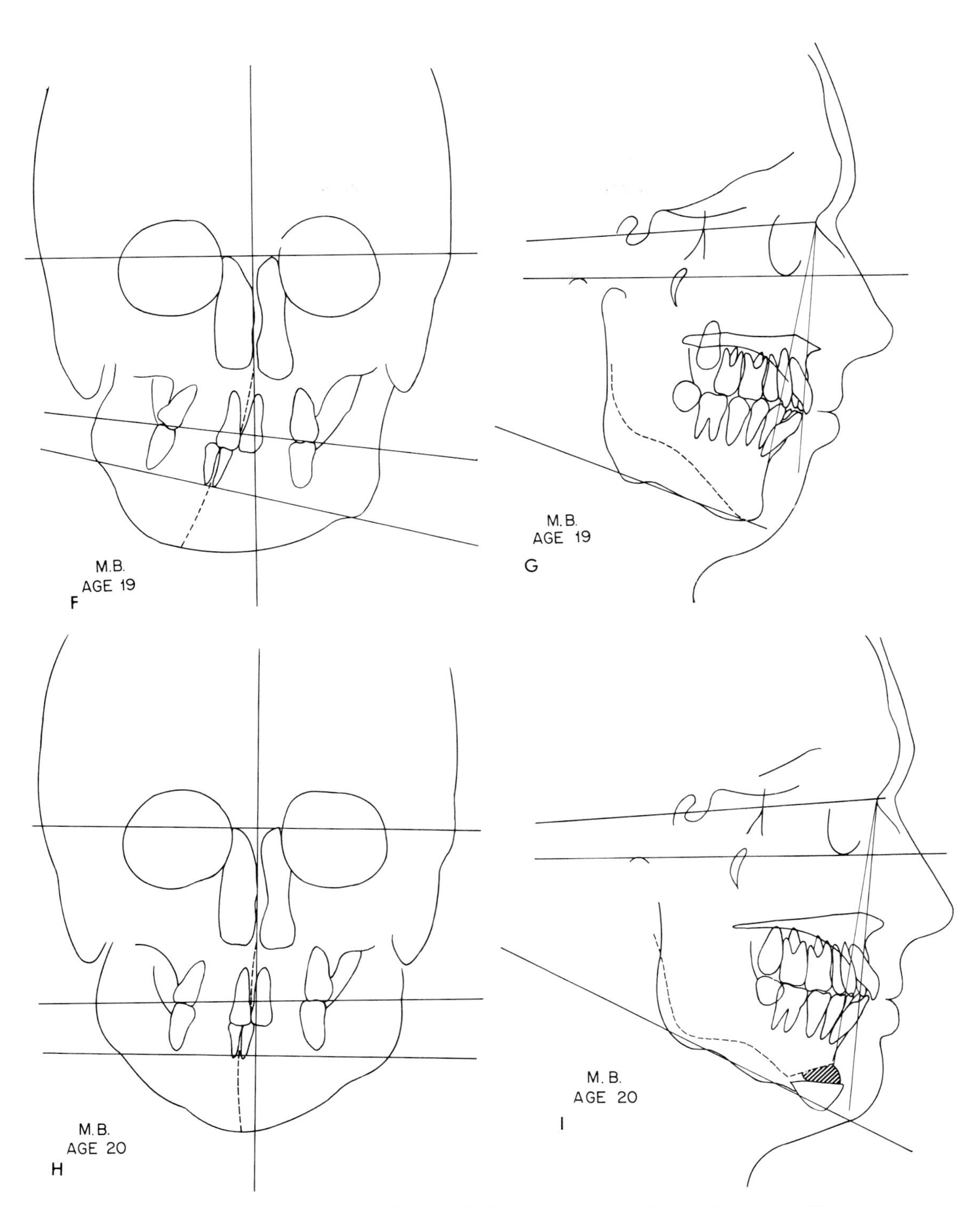

were more closely aligned, as seen in *I*. The facial plane was improved by both the mandibular advancement and the genioplasty. Compared with the tracing in *G* the change in the molar relationship illustrates the result of the anterior horizontal rotation of the hypoplastic mandible relative to the maxilla. The tracing of the PA headfilm (*F*) more graphically depicts the skewing of the lower facial skeleton. Lines are drawn to demonstate the canting of the occlusal plane and angles of the mandible. The maxillary incisor midline is off to the affected side. The mandibular incisor midline is off further with the symphysis skewed to the affected side. After surgery, the canting of the mandibular angles and occlusal plane is significantly improved (*H*). Although the midline of the lower facial structure has not been fully corrected, the improvement is marked and consistent with a more functional occlusion.

Legend continued on page 1407

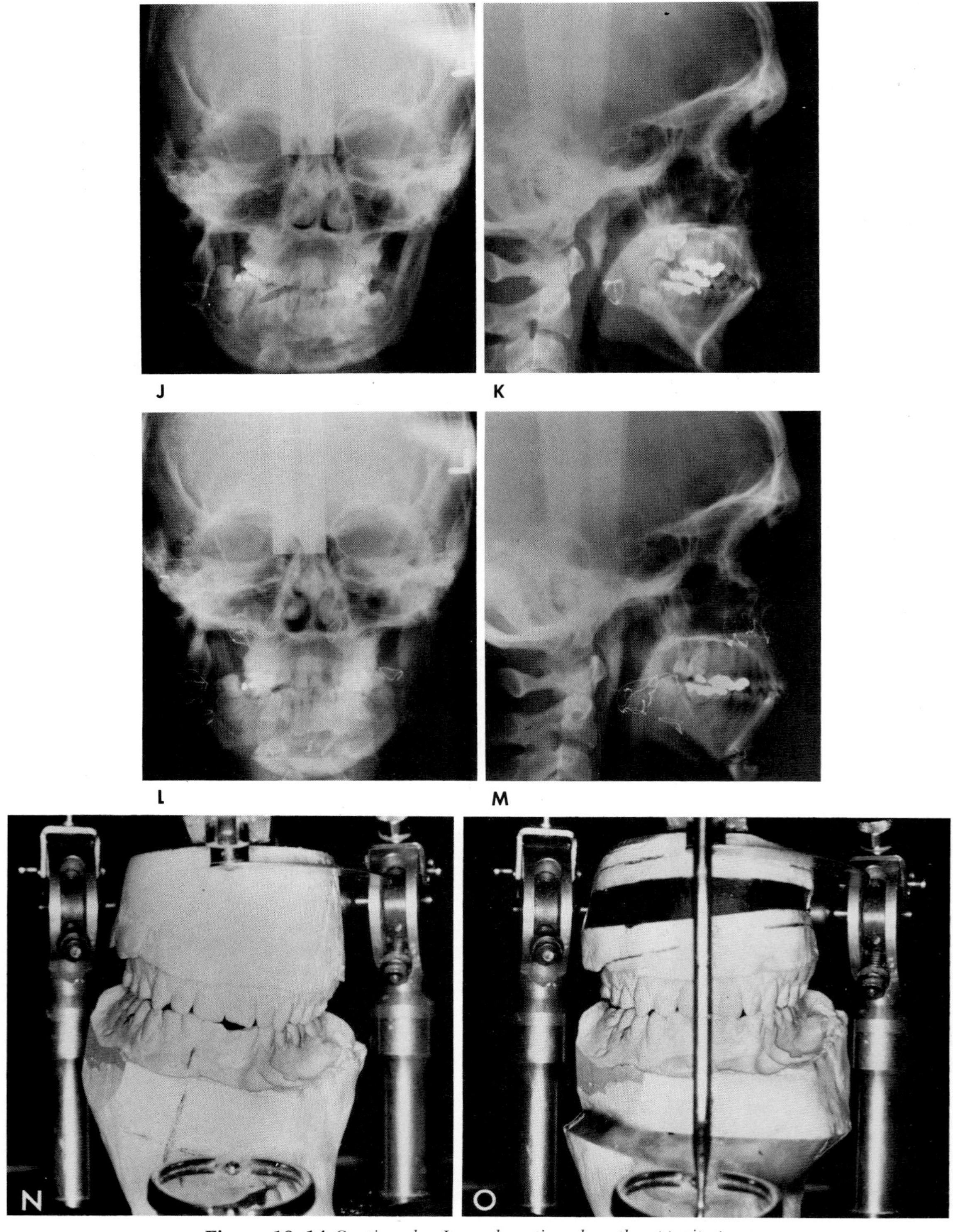

Figure 18–14 *Continued.* *Legend continued on the opposite page.*

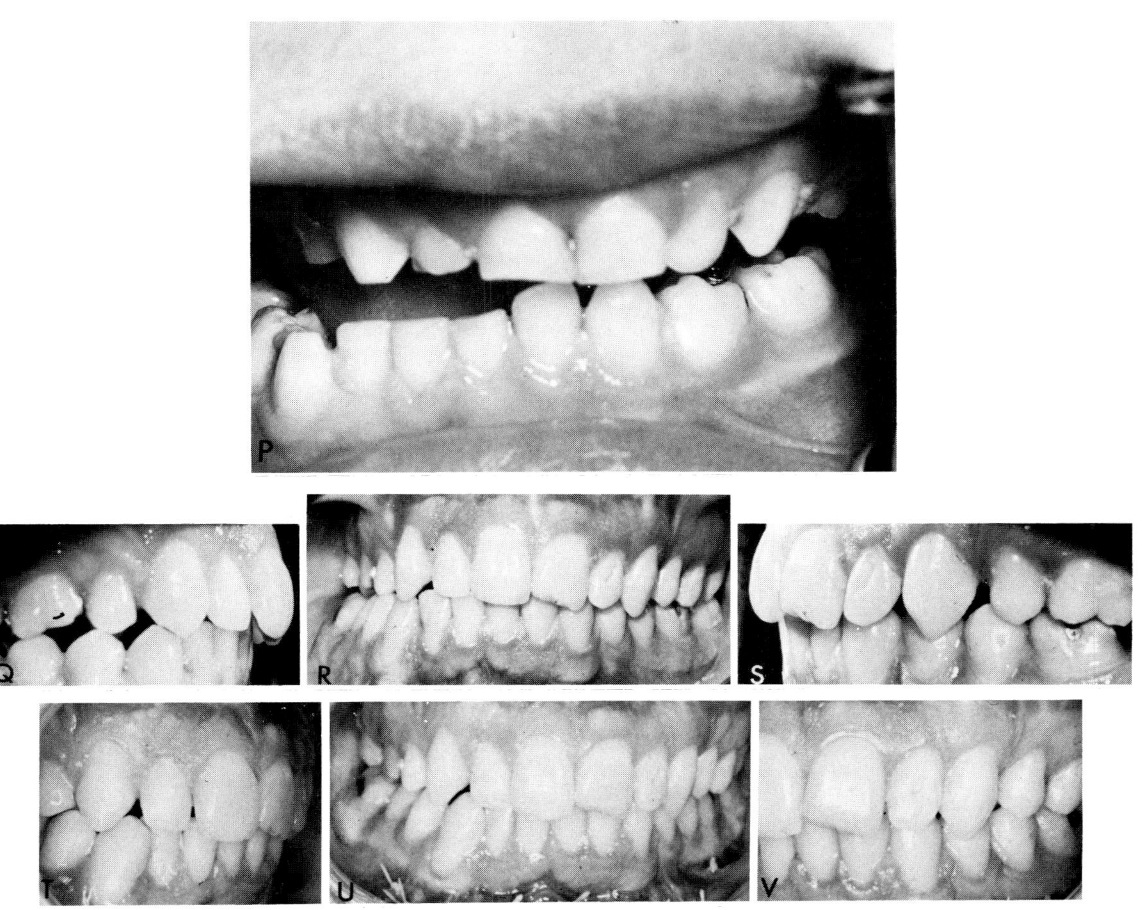

Figure 18–14 *Continued.* *J* and *K*, Cephalograms made prior to surgery. *L* and *M*, Postoperative films. *N* and *O*, Face-bow mounted models are useful in demonstrating the skewed position of the dental arches in relation to the horizontal planes of the skull. Repositioning of the models on the articulator simulates the surgical objectives, i.e., improve occlusion and correct the asymmetry of the facial skeleton (*O*). *P*, Photograph taken with patient in a relaxed posture at the age of 6. The mandibular incisor midline is approximately 8 mm. to the right of the maxillary incisor midline. A fibular head growth center transplant was performed with only marginal beneficial results. *Q–S*, Occlusal views taken after subsequent orthodontic treatment involving removal of maxillary 1st premolar teeth and the lower right 1st molar tooth show that the arch crowding had improved but occlusion was less than desirable. *T–V*, Occlusal changes resulting from surgery.

the orthodontist and the patient preferred not to have the bands replaced, so ligated arch bars were used for fixation.

COMMENTS

A tracheostomy was performed prior to the facial skeletal surgery to insure an airway during the immediate postoperative course. Another method of preventing postoperative airway problems following maxillary and mandibular osteotomies is to leave the nasotracheal tube in place at least 24 hours until normal airway control can be assured. Hypotensive anesthesia with a mean pressure of 60 mm Hg was used to help reduce blood loss. The estimated blood loss during and after the operation was 1200 ml, which was partially replaced with two units of whole blood.

FOLLOW-UP

Subjective

The patient was placed in the intensive care unit for 24 hours following surgery. He received pain medication for three days and prophylactic antibiotics for ten days. Pain and erythema of the heels of both feet occurred for seven days and paresthesia of the left ulnar nerve was present for 2 weeks as a result of improper positioning and excessive pressure during the operation. (During long operations it is advisable to move and reposition the limbs to lessen the chances of pressure necrosis and nerve palsy.) The upper lip and right side of the lower lip and chin were hypoesthetic for six weeks following surgery.

Objective

Intermaxillary fixation was maintained for eight weeks. Single bilateral elastics were placed for two additional weeks while mandibular function was re-established. The occlusion settled during the two months of fixation so that a functional interdigitation of the posterior teeth existed. This was accomplished at the expense of some anterior slippage of the lower right cuspid tooth. If orthodontic appliances had been in place, better control of the individual dental components could have been maintained. Postoperative cephalometric films revealed significant improvement but undercorrection of the deficit.

TREATMENT RESULTS

Skeletal relapse following repositioning of the mandible should be expected. We have observed it particularly in those instances in which lengthening of the bone has significantly stretched muscle groups and accompanying soft tissue. Correction of the facial asymmetry may require lengthening of the normal as well as the hypoplastic side. Relapse appears to be greater in adults than in growing children. Evaluation of the results is more difficult in children because of the variable imposed by growth. Treatment during the growth period is preferred. By taking advantage of alveolar growth potential and by guiding the eruption of teeth, one can achieve occlusal relationships in children that would be impossible in adults. Reports by Converse et al[3] concerning 12 patients with follow-up of up to 12 years suggest that the occlusal relationships remain stable following the surgery and orthodontic therapy. Our experiences with nine children, with follow-up from 3 to 13 years, are similar. Early surgery does not appear to adversely affect subsequent facial growth or function. In fact, it is our impression that early surgery enhances skeletal, dental, and soft-tissue development in children afflicted with the skeletal asymmetry of hemifacial microsomia.

Early recognition of hemifacial microsomia and initiation of definitive treatment have definite psychologic and physiologic benefits for the patient. Although dramatic results can be attained by surgical rearrangement of the adult facial skeleton, a combined surgical-orthodontic treatment program during growth appears preferable to delay of treatment until adulthood.

REFERENCES

1. Arey B: Developmental Anatomy, 7th ed. Philadelphia: WB Saunders Co, 1965.
2. Behrman SJ: Complications of sagittal osteotomy of the mandibular ramus. J Oral Surg *30*:554–561, 1972.
3. Converse JM, Horowitz SL, Coccaro PJ, Wood-Smith D: The corrective treatment of the skeletal asymmetry in hemifacial microsomia. Plast Reconstr Surg *52*:221–231, 1973.
4. Freihofer HP: Results after midface-osteotomies. J Maxillofac Surg *1*:30–36, 1973.
5. Glahn M, Winther JE: Metatarsal transplants as replacement for lost mandibular condyle (3 year followup). Scand J Plast Reconstr Surg *1*:97–100, 1967.
6. Gorlin RJ, Pindborg JJ: Syndromes of the Head and Neck. New York: McGraw Hill, Blakiston Division, 1964.
7. Grabb WC: The first and second branchial arch syndrome. Plast Reconstr Surg *36*:485–508, 1965.
8. Grammer FC, Meyer MW, Rickter KJ: A radioisotope study of the vascular response to sagittal split osteotomy of the mandibular ramus. J Oral Surg *32*:578–582, 1974.
9. Harvold E: (personal communication).
10. Hovell JH: The surgical treatment of some of the less common abnormalities of the facial skeleton. Dent Practit Dent Rec *10*:170–180, 1960.
11. Kazanjian VH: Repair of congenital defects of the mandible. *In* Longacre JJ: Craniofacial Anomalies: Pathogenesis & Repair. Philadelphia: JB Lippincott Co, 1968.
12. Kufner J: A method of craniofacial suspension. J Oral Surg *28*:260–262, 1970.
13. Longacre JJ: The surgical management of first and second branchial arch syndromes. *In* Longacre JJ: Craniofacial Anomalies: Pathogenesis & Repair. Philadelphia: JB Lippincott Co, 1968.
14. McKenzie J: The first arch syndrome. Arch Dis Child *33*:477–486, 1958.
15. Obwegeser HL: Zur Korrektur der Dysostosis otomandibulares. Schweiz Mschr Zahnheilk *80*:331–340, 1970.
16. Osborne R: The treatment of the underdeveloped ascending ramus. Br J Plast Surg *17*:376–388, 1964.
17. Peer LA: Transplantation of Tissues, Vol. 1. Baltimore: Williams and Wilkins, 1955.
18. Peer LA: Cell survival theory versus replacement theory. Plast Reconstr Surg *16*:161–168, 1955.
19. Poswillo D: The pathogenesis of the first and second branchial arch syndrome. Oral Surg *35*:302–328, 1973.
20. Robinson M: Congenital absence of the ramus of the mandible: report of case. J Oral Surg *28*:302–304, 1970.
21. Stark RB, Saunders DE: The first branchial syndrome. Plast Reconstr Surg *29*:229–239, 1962.
22. Thompson N: The surgical camouflage of facial deformities by subcutaneous autogenous tissue transplants. *In* Longacre JJ: Craniofacial Anomalies: Pathogenesis & Repair. Philadelphia: JB Lippincott Co, 1968.
23. Ware WH: Growth Center Transplantation in Temporomandibular Joint Surgery. Transactions of the Third International Conference on Oral Surgery, London, 1970.

Chapter 19

TREATMENT OF THE PROSTHODONTIC PATIENT WITH A DENTOFACIAL DEFORMITY

Roger A. West,
Raymond P. White, Jr., and
William H. Bell

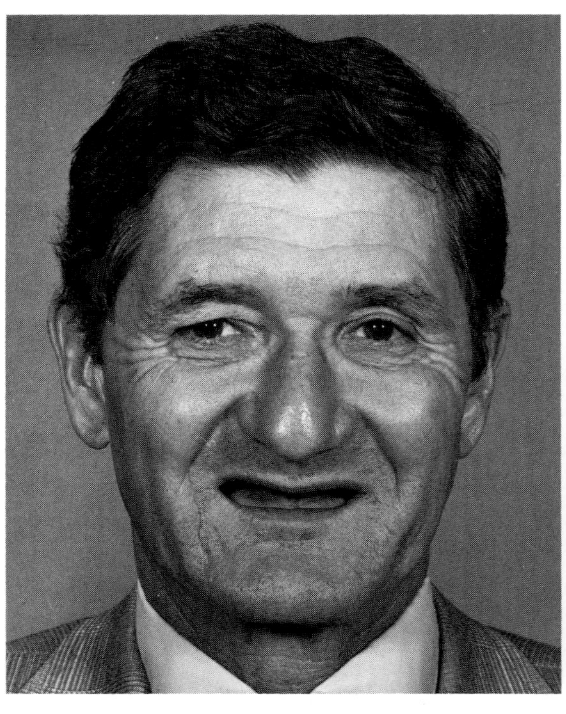

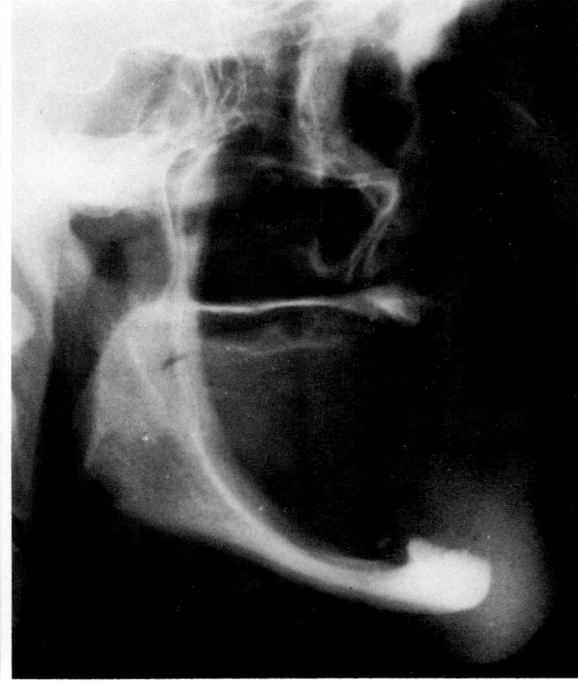

Estimates indicate that 25 to 30 million people in the United States are edentulous in one or both jaws.[3, 4, 29] Periodontal disease, which may lead to tooth loss, afflicts 80 per cent of our adult population. More than half of the population in the United States are edentulous by 60 years of age.[22]

Diagnosis and treatment planning concepts applicable to patients with a natural dentition and a skeletal deformity are applicable also to the management of edentulous patients with a similar problem. Considering the prevalence of dentofacial deformities, one would anticipate that a large number of edentulous patients should benefit from the application of these treatment principles. This chapter is written to review the diagnostic and surgical procedures applicable to the management of the edentulous patient with a dentofacial deformity.

The treatment objectives for the edentulous patient seem little different than those for the patient with a natural dentition. Tallgren,[40] as recently as 1973, stated "the main objective of . . . denture treatment is to re-establish the functional conditions of the masticatory apparatus and to restore the facial proportions and characteristics of the individuals, which are determined by the occlusal jaw relationship and the morphology of the natural dentition." These objectives can be accomplished prosthetically when "normal" skeletal relationships are present, and these same objectives need not be compromised when patients have skeletal jaw discrepancies. As a beginning student, a dentist is taught that any prosthesis is a compromise. Even if all factors seem satisfactory for prosthesis wear, the patient will experience difficulty. When skeletal and alveolar dysplasias are present and accompany the edentulous state, the patient's ability to effectively use complete dentures may be compromised further. Too often, denture treatment for patients with these more difficult problems is approached in the same methodical manner as are the less complex cases. The clinician, because of his previous training, has been conditioned not to expect too much, and he in turn has educated the patient similarly. However, the establishment of proper jaw relationships through surgery can do much to improve the patient's ability to function with complete dentures.

Rehabilitation of the edentulous patient should include (1) maintenance of an optimal functional relationship between the remaining maxillary and mandibular alveolar processes, (2) retention of the maximum amount of supporting structures in a relationship that improves or maintains denture stability, and (3) improvement of the existing esthetics. One objective need not be sacrificed to accomplish another. The surgical techniques described earlier in this text for treating skeletal dysplasias are equally applicable to the edentulous patient. Use of these techniques can aid the clinician in satisfying all three treatment objectives.

In some instances the treatment of dentofacial deformity has come full circle. Patients with an intact natural dentition accompanied by a dentofacial deformity can be treated prosthetically. Sound teeth must be extracted, supporting tissues sacrificed, and prosthetic appliances modified in an attempt to compensate for the deformity. Such treatment techniques can improve facial esthetics but frequently compromise function. For example, a patient with maxillary excess can be treated by extracting the anterior maxillary teeth, performing a radical alveolectomy, and inserting a prosthetic appliance.[1] Today this patient has treatment methods available that can preserve the dentition. An optimal functional relationship between the maxilla and mandible can be obtained, preserving the maximum amount of supporting tissues and improving facial esthetics without rendering the patient partially edentulous.

DIAGNOSTIC EVALUATION AND TREATMENT PLANNING

Facial Changes After Tooth Loss

Facial changes in the edentulous patient are progressive, and problems tend to compound themselves as additional teeth are lost. The clinician must have a good understanding of these changes if facial form and function are to be restored.

Alveolar bone, according to Enlow, "represents a conceptual enigma." It is a tissue that is distinguished customarily from "basal" and "supporting" bone. Alveolar bone is believed to have unusual functional and biologic characteristics. Geometric boundaries between alveolar and basal bone are not distinct anatomically. The physiologic behavior and biologic properties of alveolar bone are difficult to evaluate and explain.[19] Carlsson and Persson,[14] in a longitudinal study, evaluated the changes in jaw morphology that occurred five years following the extraction of all teeth and the use of dentures. During the first six months after extraction of the maxillary incisors, a noticeable reduction in bone continued.[15] Comparing records that were taken two years and five years postsurgically, and after the insertion of the full prosthesis, Carlsson found the following: (1) There was no mean reduction in the alveolar process from the facial, (2) reduction in the height of the alveolar process had occurred, and (3) resorption had occurred on the palatal aspect of the alveolar process. This pattern of resorption may be anticipated and has important clinical implications. For example, in instances of maxillary excess corrected by a "radical alveolectomy," only the palatal cortex may be left intact. With resorption then occurring on the palatal aspect, denture stability may be compromised by having little or no bone at all left in the anterior maxilla.

In a seven-year longitudinal study of patients with complete dentures, Tallgren[38] evaluated the facial changes in relation to ridge reduction and the change of mandibular occlusal position. The study, which was performed using cephalometric roentgenography, indicated that the settling (vertical change) of the mandibular dentures in the anterior region was approximately four times greater than the corresponding vertical change in the maxillary dentures. Owing to the change in mandibular position caused by rotation, the incisal edges of the mandibular denture were brought further forward in relation to the cranial base (Fig. 19–1). With the change in mandibular position and the forward slide of the lower denture on the "basal seat," the horizontal overlap will be reduced and a crossbite may develop. The tendency toward a mandibular prognathism associated with alveolar remodelling may produce a jaw relationship that adds to mandibular denture instability if the reverse horizontal overlap exceeds 5.0 mm. Comparing maxillary and mandibular alveolar bone loss, Atwood and Coy[4] found a marked difference in the magnitude and pattern of resorption between the jaws. The ratio of the vertical reduction of the anterior mandibular to the maxillary ridge gradually increased to 4:1 at the seven-year "stage." Projecting from the findings of Tallgren's study,[39] the reduction in height of the lower ridge during a 25-year period would amount to an average of 10 mm, and that of the upper ridge to 3 mm.

The facial profile changes progressively when teeth are lost in one or both jaws. The loss of dentoalveolar support produces characteristic facial soft-tissue changes around the mouth, the most apparent change being the fallen-in appearance of the

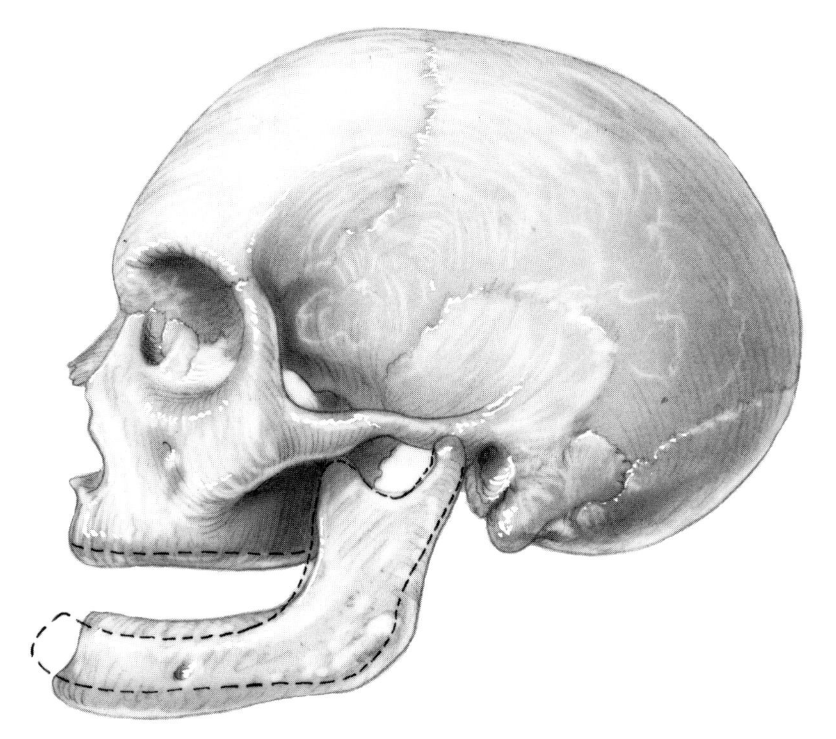

Figure 19–1. Denture base changes associated with alveolar resorption and mandibular rotation.

lower face (Fig. 19–2). The changes in facial contour following extractions and denture treatment have been studied. Martone[28] used physiographic cinematography, whereas Haga et al[21] selected stereophotogrammetry to evaluate these changes. Burstone,[12] Sarnas,[32] and Rudee[31] studied the soft-tissue profile by using cephalometric techniques. The response of the supporting tissues to a prosthesis with unstable load-

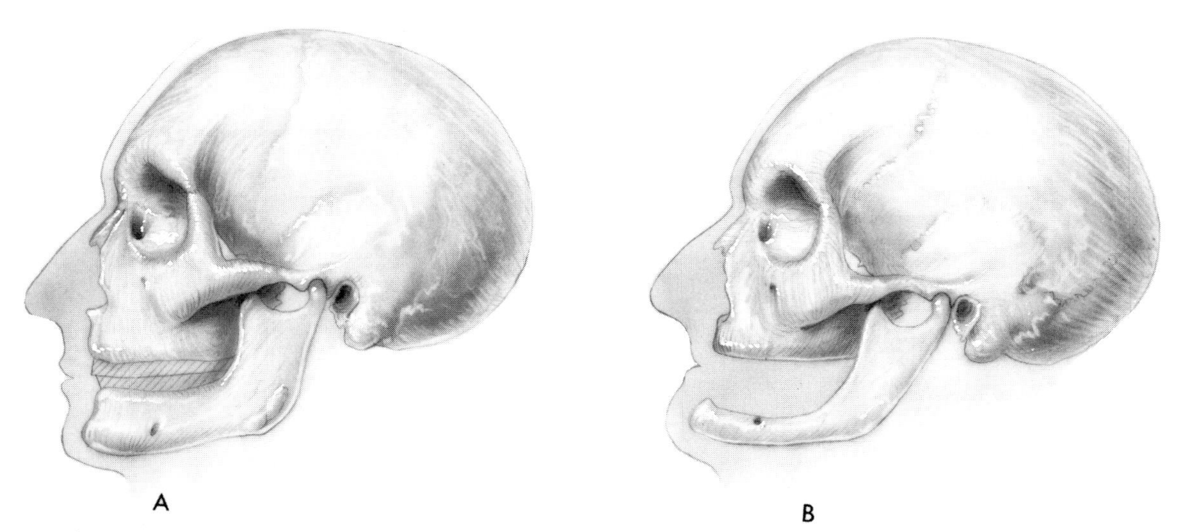

Figure 19–2. Facial profile changes associated with alveolar bone loss. *A,* Proper facial height supported by teeth. *B,* Changes accompanying tooth and alveolar bone loss.

ing, defective fit, and occlusal discrepancy has been documented. This included inflammation of the mucosa, decreased resilience of tissue over the ridges, and extensive bone loss.

The patient with a dentofacial deformity and a progressive pattern of tooth loss must be evaluated carefully. Considering the impact that remodeling changes will have on an already compromised functional relationship, surgically repositioning the remaining supporting bone in the maxilla or mandible must be considered to improve the bony relationships for the present and the future.

Establishing a Correct Facial Height

An evaluation of facial esthetics in a patient who is partially or completely edentulous requires that a proper facial vertical dimension be established. In patients with a full complement of teeth, the evaluation of the full face and profile is conducted with the patient in the natural head position and the teeth in a position of maximum intercuspation. A method of thoroughly evaluating the facial soft tissues has been described in Chapter 5. When teeth are missing, temporary denture record bases must be constructed to establish the proper vertical dimension and to allow for the transfer of jaw records to a semiadjustable articulator. A maxillary occlusion rim must provide for proper support of the upper lip. The maxillary occlusion rim must be modified to include consideration of upper lip length and the anticipated positioning of maxillary anterior teeth in relationship to the edentulous ridge and the lip. The maxillary occlusion rim must also establish an adequate occlusal plane. The mandibular occlusion rim must conform to the maxillary occlusion rim and to the established vertical dimension (Fig. 19–3). If the patient has remaining maxillary and mandibular teeth that contact each other, these teeth may serve as a guide to a proper vertical dimension and facial height. If these remaining teeth had an aberrant position initially or if they have drifted from their original position, other methods such as swallowing patterns and phonetics must be tried to establish a vertical dimension. Standard prosthodontic texts should be consulted for details. Facial photographs and lateral and anteroposterior cephalometric radiographs should be taken, with the facial structures supported by the maxillary and mandibular occlusion rims.

Record Transfer to an Articulator

Dental casts made for diagnostic purposes must be accurate. Periodontal support for the remaining teeth deserves a thorough evaluation. The tissue covering the edentulous ridge should be fixed and free of inflammation and irregularity. Hyperplastic tissue and poorly positioned frena must be modified before impressions are taken for diagnostic casts. Bony exostoses and undercuts should be eliminated to allow for the best support for a prosthetic rehabilitation. Surgery to correct periodontal defects and to increase the amount of attached tissue covering the edentulous ridge must be a part of the plan to correct the patient's problem. After the patient's facial esthetics have been evaluated clinically and adequate photographs and radio-

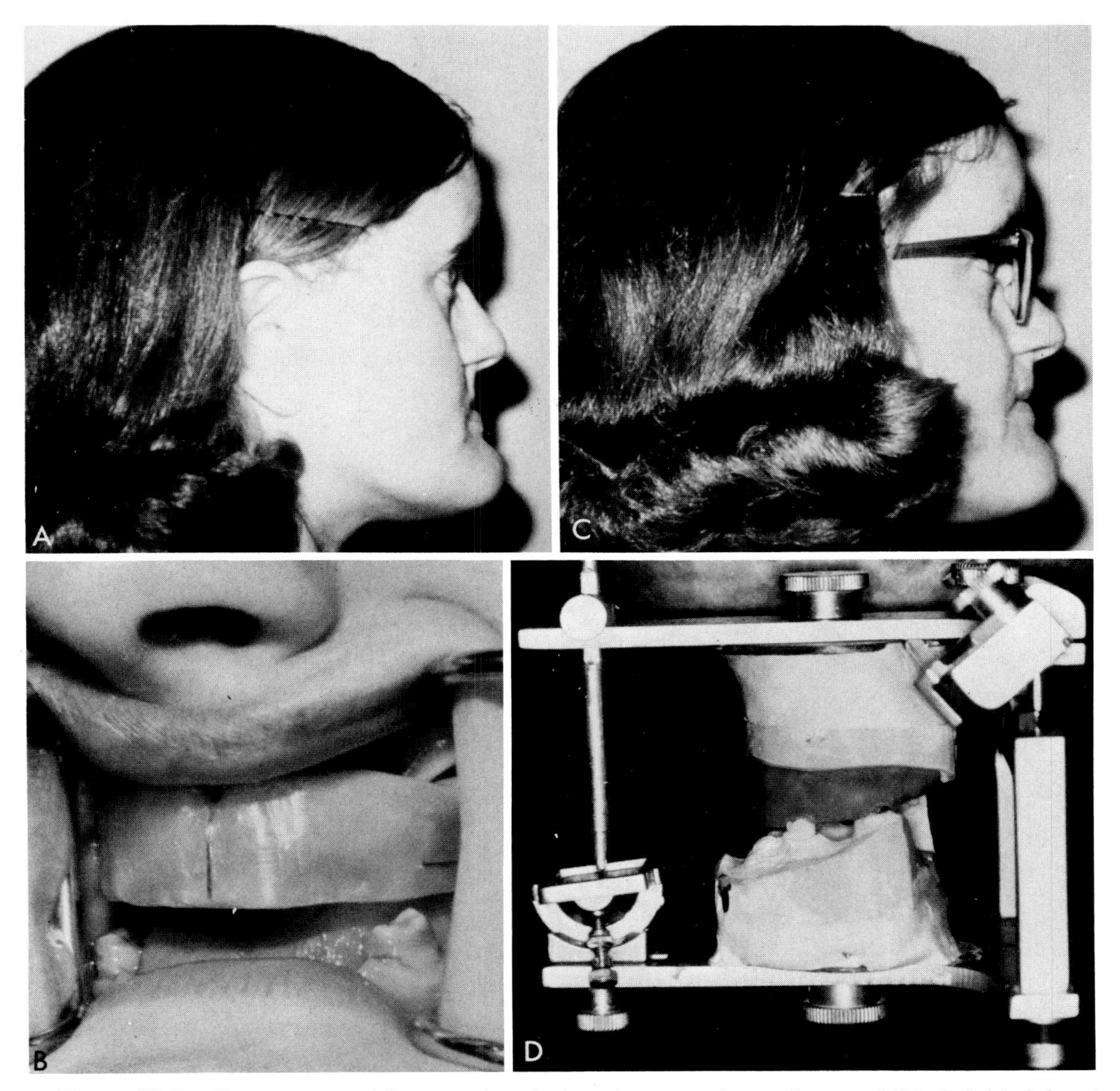

Figure 19–3. Denture record bases and occlusion rims must be used to establish facial height. *A,* Partially edentulous patient without occlusion rim. *B,* Maxillary occlusion rim that supports the lips and establishes the occlusal plane. *C,* Facial height established and lips supported. *D,* Records from the patient transferred to the articulator.

graphs have been taken, jaw relationships must be transferred to a semiadjustable articulator (Class II, Type III, Hartwell and Rahn). The maxillary diagnostic cast is mounted on the articulator with the aid of a facebow transfer; the mandibular diagnostic cast is oriented to the articulator at the vertical dimension established for the patient (Fig. 19–3). Once the mandibular diagnostic cast is fixed to the articulator, an accurate estimate of the patient's jaw function and position is represented on the instrument. Certain semiadjustable articulators may be better than others in planning for the treatment of prosthodontic patients, e.g., the Dentatus instrument has a retrusive adjustment in the condylar mechanism that facilitates estimating a new jaw position without the need for remounting diagnostic casts. Further details regarding dental articulators may be found in Chapter 6 in this text.

Determining a Correct Jaw Position

Planning treatment for the patient with a prosthodontic problem must follow the same approach of rank ordering of problems, establishing tentative solutions, synthesizing a final treatment plan, and predicting a final result as has been discussed in Chapter 6. The prosthodontic problem must be put in the proper perspective among the ranking of the patient's problems. Too often the prosthodontic problem is not considered in the planning stages, and proper input is not provided by the restorative dentist who must complete the final phases of the patient's rehabilitation. The restorative dentist must participate in the rank ordering of the patient's problems. His input is mandatory in establishing a final treatment plan. Missing teeth, poor periodontal supporting tissues, and masticatory stresses that affect a dental prognosis all have a strong bearing on planned changes in jaw position.

Support for both the upper and lower lip is an important determining factor in jaw repositioning for the prosthodontic patient. Once adequate lip support has been assured, the jaws should be realigned to allow for parallel alveolar edentulous ridges and for contact of at least three posterior teeth in each posterior dental quadrant, whether the teeth are natural ones or prosthetic replacements. Remaining natural teeth often are difficult to move orthodontically because of limited anchorage. Prosthetic requirements, fixed and removable, and supporting periodontal tissues limit the options available to the treatment team. After the requirements of masticatory function have been satisfied, the same sequence of the prediction-of-treatment results should be followed as has been described in Chapter 6.

SURGICAL TREATMENT APPROACH

Basis for Surgical Treatment

Both the prosthodontic patient and the patient with a full complement of natural teeth exhibit deformity that may be viewed in three planes of space. Successful treatment must permit correction of anteroposterior deformities as well as vertical and horizontal (transverse) dysplasias. For the purpose of simplification and discussion, treatment approaches, illustrative cases, and treatment results will be considered under three separate classifications: anteroposterior, vertical, and horizontal (transverse) dysplasias. In most instances, changes produced in one plane of space lead to concomitant changes in the other two.

Anteroposterior Dysplasias

Maxillary Excess

Treatment of the prosthodontic patient with maxillary excess has been designed to improve both function and esthetics. To eliminate the oversupported, protruding upper lip associated with maxillary excess, the prosthodontist can modify the denture design. The thickness of the maxillary anterior facial flange has been reduced or, in some instances, the denture flange has been eliminated entirely in hopes of improving lip posture. These modifications have limitations. Eliminating the anterior facial flange of the maxillary denture may compromise denture retention and stability, and a satisfactory esthetic relationship may or may not be achieved. Alveolar bone may be trimmed to allow room for a prosthesis. The amount of bone removed depends upon the severity of the deformity; the more extreme the deformity, the greater the amount of bone that must be removed. In instances of extreme maxillary excess, sufficient alveolar bone cannot be removed to effect good esthetics and a satisfactory bony support for a denture base.

For mild maxillary excess, Dean[18] suggested that alveolar bone be preserved by collapsing the facial cortical plate. Obwegeser and Steinhauser[30] described the intraseptal alveoloplasty for correction of mild protrusion. The approach involves collapsing both facial and palatal cortices of the maxilla following the removal of intraseptal bone. For correction of severe maxillary alveolar protrusion, the literature suggests radical alveolectomy.[1, 25] This technique involves sacrificing the facial cortical plate and intraseptal bone, preserving only the palatal cortical plate. Resorption patterns of palatal bone would make a long-term prognosis for such a patient questionable.

As an alternative to alveolar bone removal, West and Burk suggested an anterior maxillary ostectomy.[44] This procedure can be utilized to correct maxillary excess that is not limited to the alveolus, and an optimal esthetic and functional relationship can be established without sacrificing alveolar bone or its functional longevity. The details of these surgical procedures have been described in Chapter 8. However, additional items must be considered. After completing the maxillary bone cuts, the bony fragments are repositioned to predetermined horizontal and vertical relationships. A previously prepared clear acrylic splint is tried in place over the mobilized bone and soft tissue to determine whether the projected movement is now possible. Occasionally, additional bone must be removed at the ostectomy sites to allow for the planned repositioning of the anterior jaw.

Following repositioning, the anterior maxilla may be stabilized by an acrylic splint or direct interosseous wiring or by using a modified denture. When a splint or denture is used for fixation, it can be removed two to three weeks following the surgical procedure. The immediate use of a splint or denture over the palatal mucosa is probably contraindicated when Le Fort I osteotomy or downfracture technique of anterior maxillary osteotomy is accomplished through a circumvestibular incision. The pressure of such appliances against the palatal mucosa could potentially cause vascular ischemia of the underlying soft tissue pedicle.

Maxillary Deficiency

Maxillary deficiency may be the result of trauma; be associated with congenital deformities, such as cleft lip and cleft palate; or be of developmental origin. Prosthetic goals must provide for optimal esthetic and functional relationships. Modification of the maxillary anterior facial denture flange has been used as a means of masking maxillary deficiency. Additional upper lip support can be provided by increasing the thickness of the denture flange. The extent to which the denture flange can be altered depends upon the overall stability of the denture. A deficient maxilla may be found in conjunction with a shallow anterior facial vestibule and a poor relationship between the maxillary alveolar tubercle and the pterygoid plates of the sphenoid bones. The sum of these factors comprises denture stability and minimizes the thickness of the denture flange that may be used to improve the deficient appearance of the midface and maxilla.

When the height of the residual alveolar ridge is sufficient and a satisfactory ridge-to-soft tissue relationship is present, a maxillary osteotomy should be utilized to establish the desired functional and esthetic relationships. The alveolar arches can be aligned surgically, eliminating the possibility of an end-to-end or crossbite occlusion. The osteotomy can be modified to provide additional soft-tissue support beyond that needed for prosthodontic reasons. When maxillary deficiency exists at the level of the alar region of the nose, the deficiency may be corrected either by advancing the entire maxilla or by advancing only the anterior maxilla. A decision as to which of these two techniques will be used should be based upon the posterior facial or alveolar ridge or transverse ridge relationship. If the alignment of the alveolar ridges in the posterior facial segments is satisfactory, only the anterior maxilla need be advanced. If a crossbite relationship exists posteriorly, advancement of the entire maxilla should be performed. Maxillary advancement will create bony defects, and most surgeons prefer to graft these defects to insure bony union. A minimal amount of bony contact after jaw repositioning at surgery may delay primary union. Grafting provides the chance to correct a vertical discrepancy when it exists. Soft-tissue incisions must be modified to permit grafting of any anticipated defect. Although a horizontal incision placed at the height of the maxillary vestibule will provide sufficient exposure for a total maxillary advancement, such an incision may create an undesirable scar in the region in which a maxillary denture flange will rest subsequently. A splint applied at surgery can help maintain vestibular height and minimize this potential scarring problem. The surgeon may choose an alternative soft-tissue flap design. The lateral wall of the maxilla may be exposed, using vertical incisions and a "tunneling technique." Correction of maxillary deficiency in the prosthodontic patient need not be limited to the height of the nasal alar bases. The osteotomy can, and should, be modified to include all deficient facial areas. If the deficiency involves the infraorbital and/or zygomatic regions, these defects should be corrected by modifications in the surgical technique, or augmentation with alloplastics or bone.

Mandibular Excess

Mandibular excess presents two problems for the prosthodontist or restorative dentist. First, the alveolar ridges may be in an unsatisfactory relationship for denture stability. Second, the pattern of resorption that can be anticipated in both the maxillary and mandibular alveolar ridges will accentuate this already unfavorable relationship (see Figure 19–2).

The success of prosthetic treatment may vary, depending upon the degree of prognathism that is present. When the skeletal disparity is minimal, the prosthodontist may establish an end-to-end occlusion or even a minimal anterior and posterior crossbite. When minimal negative horizontal overlap exists, denture bases are stable. Existing esthetic relationships cannot be improved, but facial form may not be a problem in instances of minimal discrepancy. As has been discussed, alveolar ridge relationships are not static. Loss of vertical dimension and alveolar bone resorption will produce continuing changes, adding to the existing discrepancy in ridge relationships and facial esthetics. Alveolar bone resorption may be accelerated, secondary to the forces that will result from the compromised ridge relationships. These factors must be considered carefully in planning for the young edentulous patient who must wear complete dentures for 15 to 20 or more years. The shape of the mandible that results from severe prognathism may complicate denture wear. The space between the anterior surface of the mandibular vertical ramus and the maxillary alveolar tubercle and tuberosity is reduced and compromises the space available for denture flanges. As a result, proper extension of denture flanges may not be possible without interference during function.[36]

When mandibular prognathism is more extreme, the relationship of the alveolar ridges precludes establishing a stable denture base. Surgical correction of the anteroposterior jaw discrepancy makes it possible to establish an optimal functional relationship between the maxillary and mandibular alveolar ridges. When the mandible is repositioned posteriorly, both function and facial form are enhanced. Numerous surgical procedures can be used to correct mandibular excess (see Chapter 11). A mandibular body ostectomy will improve only the anterior ridge relationships. A surgical procedure in the body of the mandible does not alter the ramus-alveolar tubercle relationship, the posterior horizontal alveolar ridge relationship, or the obliquity of the gonial angle. In most instances, osteotomies in the vertical rami (oblique, vertical, sagittal) are preferable for the prosthodontic patient. A surgical procedure in the ramus of the mandible allows for a correction of alveolar ridge relationships in three planes of space.

Mandibular Deficiency

The edentulous patient with a deficient mandible may not require surgery for successful prosthetic treatment as often as a patient with a protruding lower jaw. When minimal maxillomandibular skeletal disharmonies exist secondary to mandibular deficiency, treatment may be carried out prosthetically, with good function resulting. Facial esthetics will not be improved when the lower face is deficient. If mandibular deficiency is extreme, prosthetic treatment becomes difficult because unfavorable transverse alveolar ridge relationships exist in association with the anteroposterior dysplasias. An unfavorable pattern of alveolar resorption will worsen the transverse discrepancy.

In some instances of mandibular deficiency, the anteroposterior ridge relationships have been improved by performing an anterior maxillary ostectomy to improve the alignment of the arches anteriorly. The balance between the nose, upper lip, and chin must be evaluated carefully. If a prominent nose is not a resulting problem, the anterior maxilla may be repositioned surgically to establish a satisfactory anterior alveolar ridge relationship. The surgical procedures have been described in the section on maxillary excess. Surgical treatment of severe mandibular deficiency will necessitate mandibular lengthening (mandibular advancement). Many surgical procedures have been described for mandibular advancement. Surgical procedures performed in the vertical ramus of the mandible allow for a correction in three planes of space (see

Chapter 13). Skeletal relapse has been documented following mandibular advancement to correct a severe deficiency.[27] The period of fixation may be prolonged and should be continued until cephalometric tracings made from serial roentgenograms demonstrate no evidence of skeletal change. Supplementary extraoral devices such as a "soft cervical collar" have been suggested to minimize relapse. Opinion is divided as to the extent of the problem and the need for the added extraoral devices. Skeletal stability established by serial radiographs is suggested as an added guideline to determine when intermaxillary fixation can be discontinued. This problem is discussed more thoroughly in Chapter 13.

Vertical Dysplasias

Vertical deformities may result from either skeletal or alveolar dysplasias. Reduced vertical dimension can be anticipated as part of the process that accompanies successive loss of teeth. As facial vertical dimension decreases, anteroposterior relationships will change as well. Studies have been conducted concerning the effect on ridge resorption when occlusal vertical dimension is altered prosthetically. Thompson[42] noted that an increase in occlusal vertical dimension of the dentures beyond a resting facial height was accompanied by a subsequent decrease in facial height, presumably by alveolar bone resorption. However, no reduction in bone height was observed when rest vertical dimension was not exceeded. Atwood,[2] studying ridge reduction in complete denture wearers, found no definite association between the increase in facial height and the resorption of alveolar bone. Tallgren,[37] also found no significant correlations between the increase in occlusal vertical dimension and the subsequent reduction in morphologic face height. However, a significant relationship was observed when individuals with complete upper or partial lower dentures were studied. Bone resorption in the maxilla was followed by a decrease in facial height.

The biologic response to surgically increasing lower facial height has not been documented. Whether additional loss of alveolar bone will result when the vertical relationship is modified surgically has not been determined. It has been suggested that since surgery involves detaching the muscles of mastication, the insertion of the muscles will be altered and bone resorption will not follow. No clinical problems have been encountered when facial height is increased in patients with a full complement of teeth.

Vertical deformities can be compensated partially by modifying the dimension of the denture base and teeth. When inadequate inter-ridge space exists in the facial segments, the prosthodontist can reduce the height of the denture teeth or reduce the thickness of the denture base. When an inadequate inter-ridge space exists owing to redundant soft tissue, the problem may be corrected by surgically removing soft tissue without the loss of alveolar bone or perforation into the maxillary antrum. Care must be taken to preserve attached-type mucosa and to maintain the height of the facial sulcus.

Early loss of mandibular posterior teeth may result in supraeruption of the posterior maxillary teeth (Fig. 19–4). In such instances, an ideal inter-ridge space cannot be established by alveolectomy since the maxillary antrum usually accompanies the supraerupted teeth. An ideal inter-ridge relationship can be re-established with a posterior maxillary ostectomy.[44, 45] The maxillary alveolus and any contained teeth can be

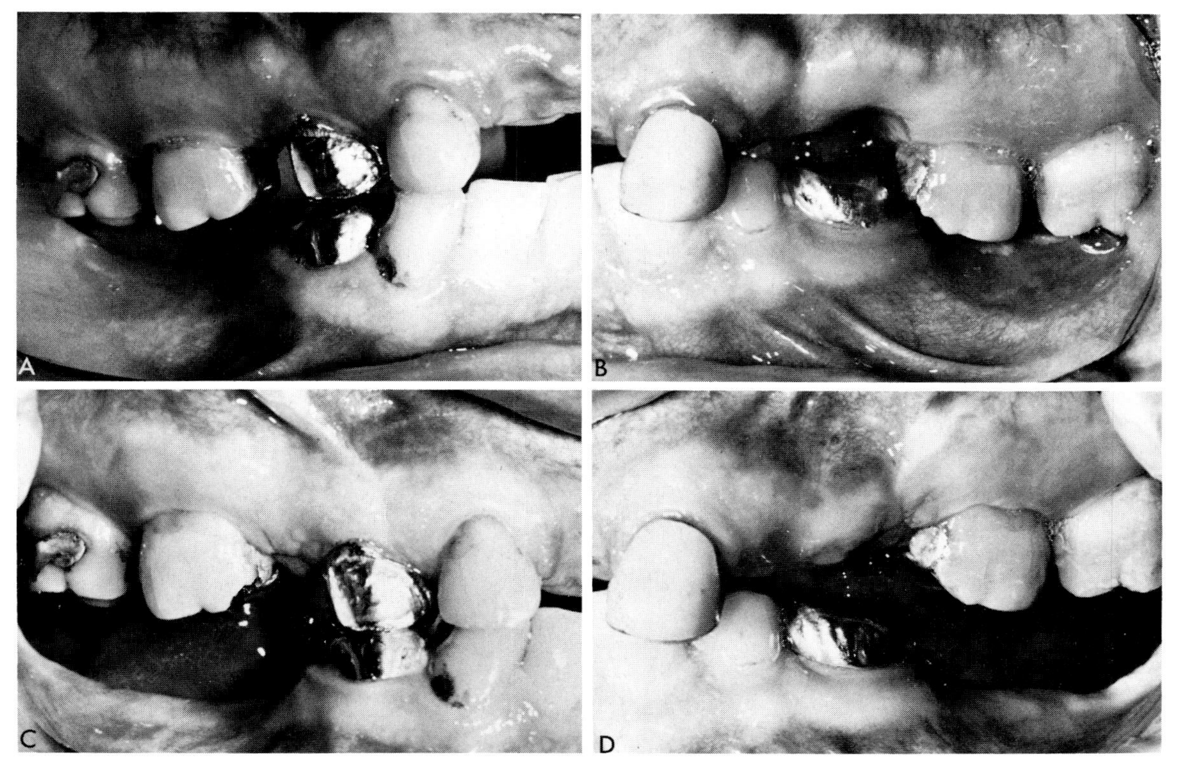

Figure 19–4. Reduced interarch space caused by supraeruption of maxillary molars. *A* and *B*, Preoperative vertical relationships. *C* and *D*, Inter-ridge space following repositioning of posterior maxillary segments to facilitate partial denture construction.

repositioned superiorly to the correct vertical relationship and moved anteriorly if desired, thus preserving alveolar bone. Details of this surgical procedure are described in Chapters 8 and 22.

Anterovertical dysplasia, i.e., increased or decreased anterior inter-ridge space, may complicate prosthetic treatment. For example, prosthetic treatment of the patient with an "open bite" may be accomplished by increasing both the length of the denture teeth and the thickness of the denture bases. Prosthetic treatment alone may be sufficient, depending upon the extent of the open bite and the requirements for lip length and lip support. The anterior maxilla may be repositioned inferiorly by surgery. The extent to which this can be accomplished is limited also by the relationship of the upper lip relative to the maxillary anterior teeth and remaining alveolar bone.

When an increased inter-ridge space exists that is secondary to a "skeletal open bite," the discrepancy is not limited to the vertical plane. Both anterior and posterior relationships are compromised. Generally, prosthetic treatment alone will not be sufficient, nor will "dropping" the anterior maxilla be satisfactory. Neither of these techniques can correct the total problem. Surgical intrusion of the anterior and posterior maxillary fragments permits the mandible to rotate anterosuperiorly. "Closing" the open bite will then improve the anteroposterior ridge relationships. In addition to establishing an optimal functional relationship between the alveolar ridges, facial esthetics will be improved. Lower facial height will also be reduced, eliminating the "long" lower face. Lip incompetency may be improved secondary to the reduction in lower facial height. The relationship of the nose, lips, and chin will be changed because of the increased forward projection of the chin. Additional discussion of the problem may be found in Chapters 8 and 13. The same principles are applicable for the prosthodontic patient as for the patient with a full complement of teeth and an open bite deformity.

Horizontal (Transverse) Dysplasias

Horizontal or transverse dysplasias may be associated with maxillary or mandibular deformity. Posterior facial crossbite may result from a constricted or retruded maxilla. The same horizontal relationships may exist secondary to mandibular prognathism. When the alveolar ridges are in a satisfactory anteroposterior and vertical relationship, horizontal discrepancies may be treated prosthetically by setting the denture teeth in a crossbite. The horizontal relationship of the alveolar segments may become progressively more unsatisfactory with alveolar remodeling and resorption. The crest of the maxillary posterior facial alveolar ridge is remodeled in a medial direction, and the alveolar crest in the mandible is reduced progressively. As a result of this pattern of remodeling, there is a tendency toward a greater and greater posterior facial crossbite (Fig. 19–5). With extreme posterior facial crossbite or with marked resorption, an unfavorable pattern of loading may result. Further loss of alveolar bone support follows. When this problem develops secondary to a markedly constricted maxillary arch, posterior facial segments of the maxillary alveolar ridge

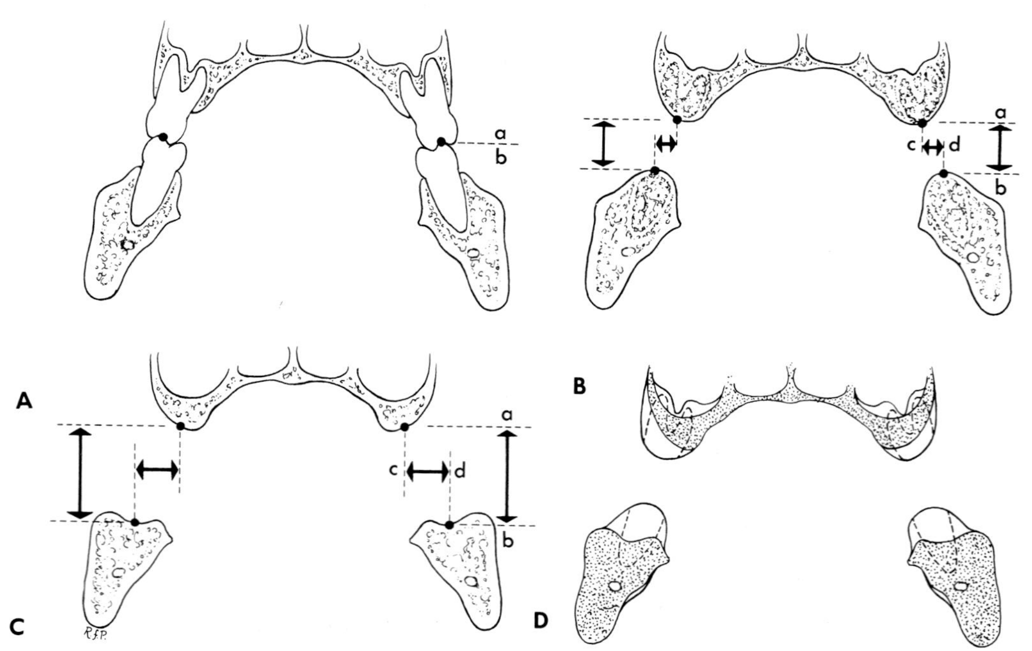

Figure 19–5. Vertical and horizontal alveolar ridge relationships. *A,* Natural dentition. *B,* Early edentulous state. *C,* Chronic edentulous state. *D,* Composite changes that reflect an increased tendency toward a greater posterior facial crossbite. (From Starshak TJ.[36])

can be repositioned surgically to form an optimal functional relationship. Extreme horizontal dysplasias exist in conjunction with anteroposterior and/or vertical deformities as well. The total problem should be evaluated and treated, with a focus extending beyond correcting isolated dentoalveolar segments. For example, in unilateral mandibular hypertrophy, both the horizontal (transverse) and vertical alveolar ridge relationships are affected (see Case Report 19–6). Prosthetic treatment alone would necessitate compensating for both the vertical and horizontal dysplasias by modifying the dimensions and position of the denture teeth and the dimensions of the denture bases. Function would be compromised, and there would be no improvement in facial esthetics. By surgically repositioning the mandible and/or maxilla, the alveolar ridges can be aligned vertically and horizontally, facilitating prosthetic treatment and improving facial symmetry.

The basic treatment approaches to any deformity, whether considering anteroposterior, vertical, or horizontal (transverse) dysplasias, will vary, depending upon the extent of the deformity. The more extreme the problem and the younger the patient, the more likely a combined surgical and prosthetic treatment plan will be required to establish an optimal functional and esthetic relationship.

Intermaxillary Fixation, Splinting, and Occlusion

Healing subsequent to jaw surgery depends on an adequate intermaxillary fixation established at the time of surgery. When a patient has a full complement of natural teeth, intermaxillary fixation can be established with vertical wires or elastics held in place by fracture arch bars, orthodontic bands, or cast splints applied to teeth in the upper and lower jaw. In the partially or completely edentulous patient, any remaining teeth must be splinted to minimize any orthodontic forces from intermaxillary fixation. Splints must also be constructed that will allow the jaws to be fixed firmly in place at the time of surgery. The same splints must function, once the patient's jaws have been mobilized, throughout the period of healing of the jaws and until the restorative dentist can complete the projected prosthetic rehabilitation.

Splints constructed for use in edentulous patients can be made on the dental casts used for diagnostic and planning purposes. Although there are many variations that might be adequate, a separate splint for the upper and lower jaw is suggested. A dental acrylic is the most satisfactory material for splint construction. Acrylic splints can be fabricated easily before surgery and can be modified quickly at the time of surgery. The splints must be adapted closely to the remaining teeth so that orthodontic forces on these teeth will be minimal. The addition of wrought wire clasps to the splint will aid in splint stability during intermaxillary fixation and after the jaws have been mobilized. The flanges of the splints need not be extended as far as in a complete or partial denture, but the splint itself must cover enough mucosal surface area to remain stable on the jaw during the period of intermaxillary fixation and during the subsequent physical therapy associated with mobilization of the jaws.

When natural teeth remain, indentations on the surface of the acrylic that correspond to cusp tips of opposing teeth will provide for an adequate interlocking of the splints. A tongue-and-groove effect may be used when the maxillary and mandibular

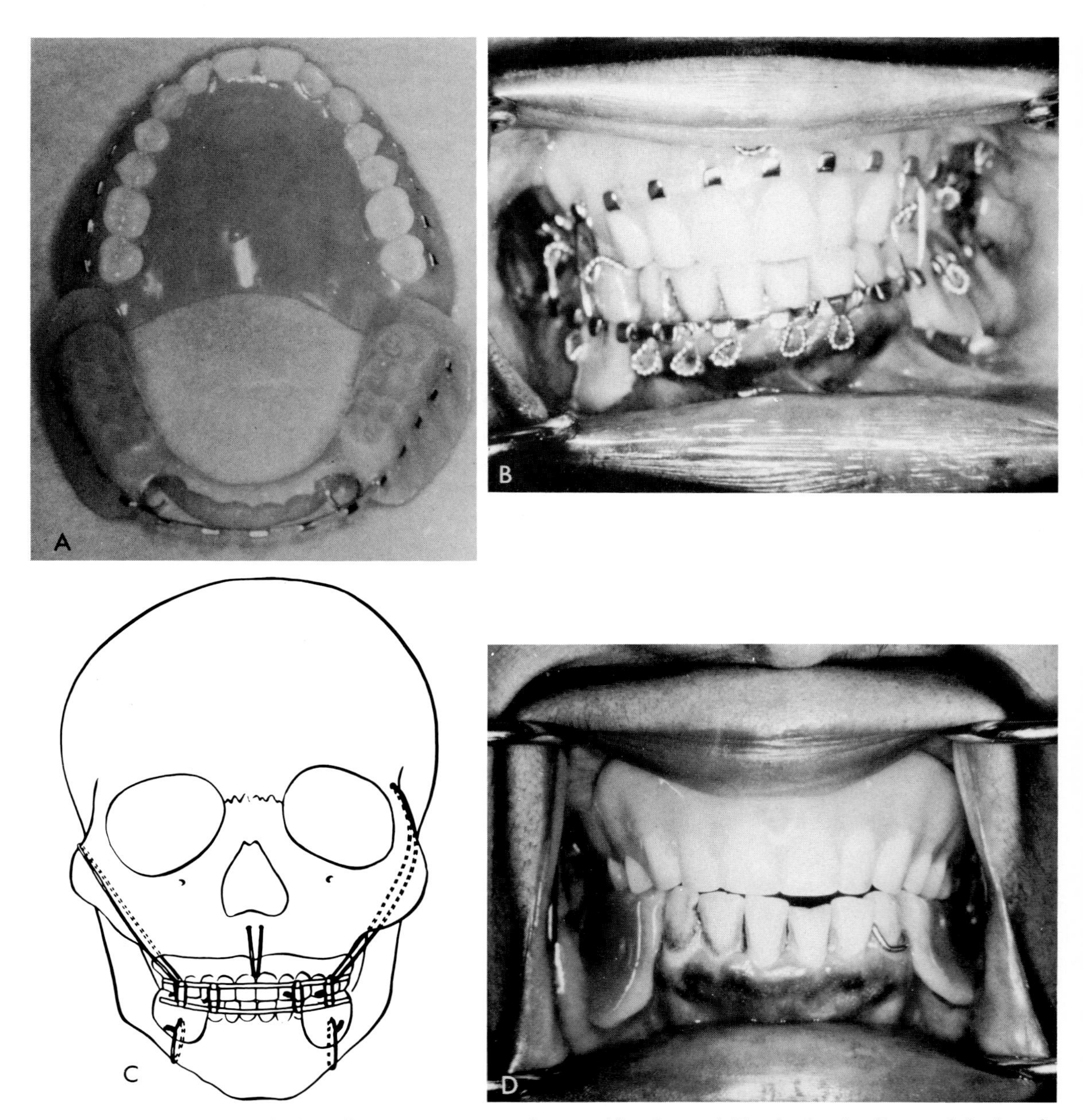

Figure 19–6. Prosthetic splints are constructed as an aid to jaw stability during healing and during the rehabilitative phase. *A,* Intercuspation of maxillary denture teeth into mandibular splint. *B,* Use of splints for jaw stabilization. *C,* Options for fixing splints to the jaws. *D,* Use of splints in the rehabilitative phase.

splints oppose each other. Although this approach is adequate for the management of a patient following facial trauma, the longer period of rehabilitation following surgery during which jaws are repositioned would dictate another approach. The placement of prosthetic teeth in one arch, allowing these teeth to interdigitate into the acrylic surface of the splint in the opposing arch, provides a satisfactory method of splint construction for both the period of intermaxillary fixation and the subsequent period of rehabilitation (Fig. 19–6).

Once constructed, the splints themselves should be held firmly in place on the jaws by a combination of wiring to the remaining teeth and suspension wires or direct wiring to the jaws themselves. Care must be taken to insure that no orthodontic force is applied to the remaining teeth if the splint is to be wired to these teeth. In direct wiring (transalveolar bone) of the splint to the upper or lower jaw, care must be taken to minimize the loss of alveolar bone. Remaining alveolar bone should be protected at all costs. Suspension wires from the nasofrontal, zygomaticofrontal, and zygomatic arch areas provide for stabilization of a maxillary splint. Circum-mandibular wiring will stabilize a mandibular splint. An adequate number of stabilizing wires should be used in each case. However, these wires are uncomfortable to the patient, and the use of each additional wire increases the chance of a localized infection occurring at some time during the period of healing. Wiring to stabilize the splints can be placed under local anesthesia. In elective cases, stabilizing wires are placed most easily during surgery while the patient is under a general anesthetic.

Once intermaxillary fixation has been removed, the edentulous patient must be followed closely during the rehabilitation period. Usually such a patient takes longer to learn the new jaw position established for him. The patient must be seen regularly in the weeks following the removal of intermaxillary fixation, and he should be able to demonstrate that he can repeat the jaw position established at surgery. If adequately constructed, splints utilized for intermaxillary fixation may be worn by the patient for many months, until the final prosthetic procedures can be completed.

Ridge Augmentation as an Aid in Jaw Surgery

William H. Bell

The prosthetic management of the edentulous patient with severe alveolar atrophy is difficult. Increasing the absolute height of the maxillary and mandibular alveolar ridges by free transplantation of bone,[17, 30, 41, 43] cartilage,[11] or alloplastic materials[24] is unpredictable and frequently problematic. The associated problems of resorption of onlay bone grafts and infection with alloplastic materials are common. The results of experiments in animals[8, 10, 34] and clinical studies[9, 20] indicate that the palatal and facial mucoperiosteum in the maxilla and the lingual mucoperiosteum in the mandible provide an adequate nutrient pedicle for single-stage repositioning of the inferior portion of the maxilla or the superior portion of the mandible. Both of these techniques maintain the integrity of the mucosa-periosteum-cortex relationship

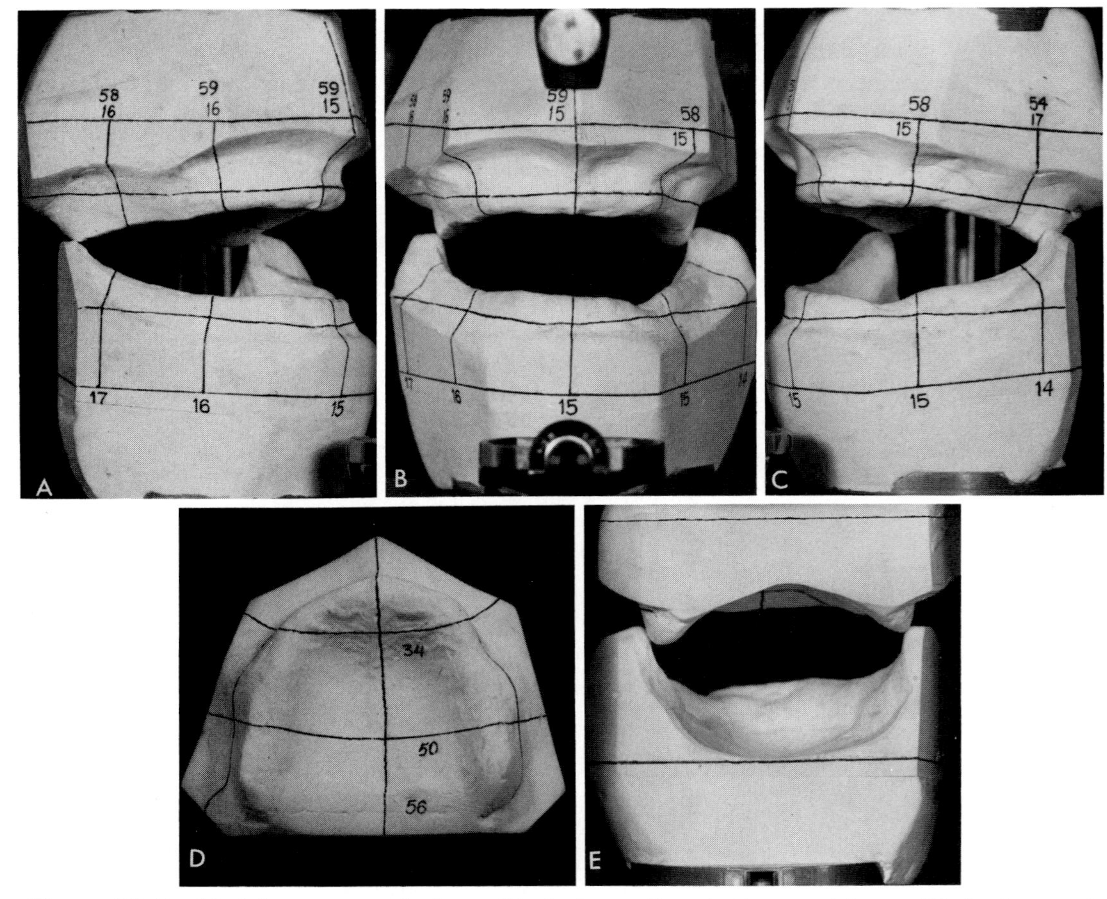

Figure 19–7. Model surgery technique. (Technique of sectioning models modified after method described by Dr. Thomas Hohl at American Society of Oral Surgeons' Clinical Congress on Maxillary Surgery, St. Louis, Mo., 1975.) Edentulous casts mounted on articulator showing inadequate posterior interarch space and anteroposterior and vertical discrepancies in anterior region of atrophic maxillary alveolar ridge. *A–E,* Parallel lines are drawn on the base of the maxillary and mandibular models. Vertical lines are registered perpendicular to the horizontal lines. Magnitude of vertical movements is determined by measuring distance changes between the horizontal base lines and positional changes of the alveolar crests and the horizontal lines preoperatively and postoperatively; anteroposterior movements are determined from positional changes of horizontal lines registered on the maxillary model. *F,* Bite rims used to transfer maxillomandibular relationship to articulator after face-bow transfer. *G–K,* Maxillary model repositioned anteriorly and inferiorly to achieve the desired interarch relationship and increase the amount of alveolar height. The vertical, anteroposterior, and horizontal movements of the maxilla are determined from measured positional changes of the horizontal and vertical reference lines that were registered on the casts before model surgery.

Illustration continued on the opposite page

of the repositioned bone. Preservation of the morphologic form and osseous architecture of the maxilla and mandible may minimize resorption of the transposed basal bone and facilitate early rehabilitation of the patient with a jaw deformity.

If an alveolar ridge must be augmented as part of the treatment for a jaw deformity, the planned movements of the maxilla, determined from clinical and cephalometric studies, are simulated on dental study casts. A facebow transfer is used to mount the edentulous casts on a semiadjustable articulator (Fig. 19–7). The entire

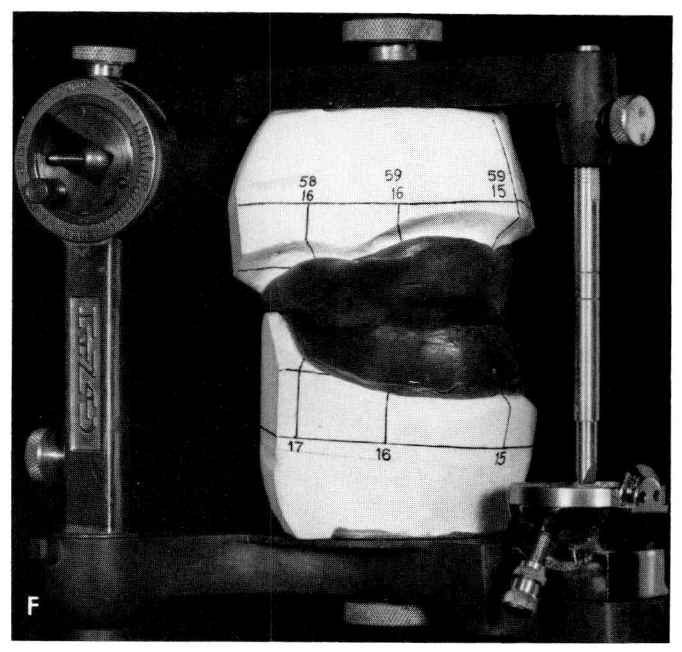

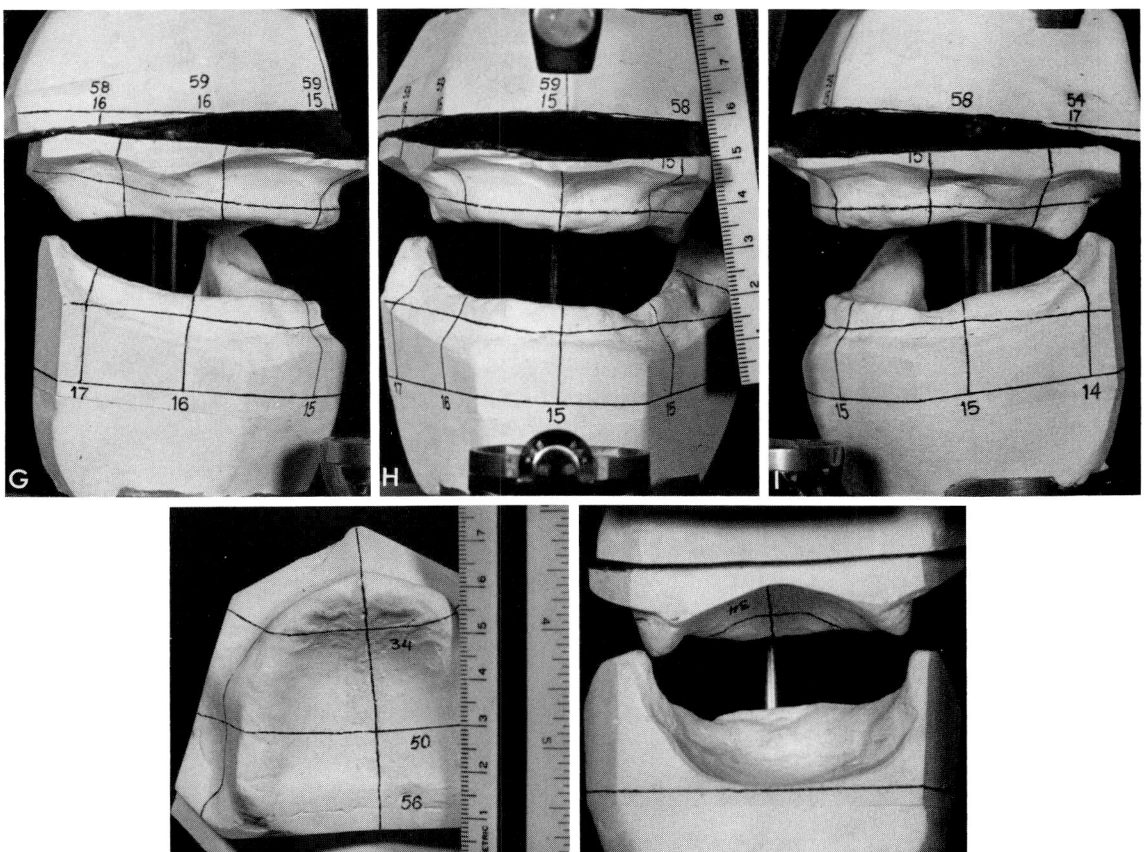

Figure 19–7 *continued.*

See legend on the opposite page

alveolar ridge portion of the maxillary dental cast is sectioned at the approximate level of the nasal floor. Clinical and cephalometric measurements are an aid in determining the magnitude and direction of the maxillary movement. The dental cast can be sectioned into three or four segments to achieve the best objectives. The axial inclination of the future denture teeth, lip posture, interarch relationship, vertical and anteroposterior facial proportions, and upper lip-to-tooth relationship are carefully considered before the sectioned dental cast is repositioned and fixed in its final position to the maxillary model base.

An accurate determination of the three-dimensional changes in the position of the maxilla is made by measuring and comparing the distance between the various horizontal and vertical reference lines on the dental casts before and after the inferior portion of the maxilla is moved into the best possible vertical, anteroposterior, and horizontal relationship with the mandibular ridge. The resultant interarch relationship may indicate the need for concomitant mandibular surgery. The vertical, horizontal, and anteroposterior dimensional changes are recorded on the dental casts. The measurements taken from the repositioned dental casts and the cephalometric measurements serve as a basis for the planned maxillary movements. At surgery the measurements are used to sculpture the bone grafts to the dimensions that will effect the desired esthetic and functional changes. Similar studies are carried out when mandibular surgery is planned.

Maxillary Surgery Technique

The maxillary surgery is performed in the hospital with the patient under hypotensive anesthesia delivered via the nasoendotracheal route. The palatal mucoperiosteum and facial gingiva serve as the vascular pedicle for the mobilized maxilla.[5, 9, 10, 46] A horizontal incision is made in the maxillary vestibule above the mucogingival reflection and is extended from the second molar region of one side to a similar area on the contralateral side (Fig. 19–8*A* and *B*). The margins of the superior flap are raised to expose the lateral walls of the maxilla, zygomatic crests, anterior nasal floor, and piriform apertures. To maximize circulation to the maxilla, the inferior mucoperiosteal tissues are elevated only enough to visualize and palpate the bone that previously encased the apices of the teeth. The posterolateral portion of the maxilla is visualized by subperiosteal tunneling to the pterygomaxillary suture and then positioning the tip of a curved right-angle retractor at the suture. Another retractor is placed anteriorly to facilitate visualization of the anterolateral portion of the maxilla. A horizontal line is etched in the lateral wall maxilla at the base of the piriform aperture and nasal floor. Anterior and posterior vertical reference lines are etched into the bone for anteroposterior orientation after the maxilla is mobilized and downfractured. A horizontal bone cut is made from the lateral part of the piriform rim posteriorly across the canine fossa and through the zygomatic maxillary crest to the pterygomaxillary fissure with a fissure bur in a straight handpiece or a high-speed reciprocating saw (Fig. 19–8*B*).

The mucoperiosteum is detached from the anterior floor of the nose, base of the anterior nasal septum, and lateral nasal walls by subperiosteal tunneling. A nasal septal osteotome is positioned above the anterior nasal spine parallel with the hard plate and is malletted to separate the nasal septum from the maxilla (Fig. 19–8*C*). Next, a periosteal elevator is positioned between the nasal mucoperiosteum and lateral wall to protect the soft tissue, and the anterior lateral nasal wall is sectioned. Sectioning of the posterolateral nasal wall is carried out similarly, using a sharp, thin osteotome. Finally, a sharp pterygoid osteotome is malletted into the pterygomaxillary suture to separate the maxilla from the pterygoid plates (Fig. 19–8*D*), and the maxilla is mobilized in the same manner described in Chapter 8.

Interpositional bone grafts have been placed in two different ways. Originally, dumbbell-shaped blocks of corticocancellous bone from the iliac crest were inlaid between the maxilla and the overlying horizontal bone cuts, with cancellous bone facing the antrum (Fig. 19–8*F*). Additionally, one large slab of corticocancellous bone from the iliac crest has been interposed between the mobilized portion of the maxilla and the medial, lateral, and posterior antral walls and nasal septum to decrease the amount of vertical relapse, provide additional stability to the repositioned maxilla, and obliterate dead space (Fig. 19–8*H* and *I*).[6] The procedure is more difficult technically than placing dumbbell-shaped blocks of corticocancellous bone between the mobilized part of the maxilla and the lateral antral walls only. In such cases, it may be necessary to tap the large reservoir of bone in the posterior iliac crest, as this donor site provides a greater source of bone than does the anterior iliac crest. Freeze-dried homografts have also been used and are sometimes combined with particulate autogenous bone.[23] (See Ch. 20 for bone grafting considerations.)

An acrylic metal template, fashioned preoperatively from a stone cast of the edentulous maxilla, is made to simulate the shape and dimensions of the intended bone graft. A single slab of bone is sculptured to the planned dimensions. If, however, the amount of bone available from the donor site does not allow the entire maxilla to be covered with a single slab of bone, a large block of bone is cut into two triangular sections that are interposed between the mobilized part of the maxilla and the medial, lateral, and posterior antral walls (Fig. 19–8*I*). A separate segment may be placed in the anterior aspect of the maxilla to bridge the gap between the two laterally positioned segments.

The positional changes of the vertical reference lines in the lateral maxilla should closely parallel the measurements taken from the preoperative cephalometric and model studies. The mobile part of the maxilla is suspended to the piriform rims and zygomatic buttresses (Fig. 19–8*F* and *G*). When the bone in these areas is too thin and friable to support interosseous wires, the use of infraorbital rim or circumzygomatic suspension wires attached to the maxillary fixation appliance is preferred.

Thin slabs of corticocancellous bone may be laid along the lines of the osteotomy of the lateral maxilla and in the nasomaxillary or nasolabial areas for additional augmentation of the soft tissues. The soft-tissue wounds are closed by routine techniques. Direct fixation of the repositioned maxilla and stabilization with bone grafts have obviated the need for more complex fixation with conventional denture splints and also facilitate early mandibular function.

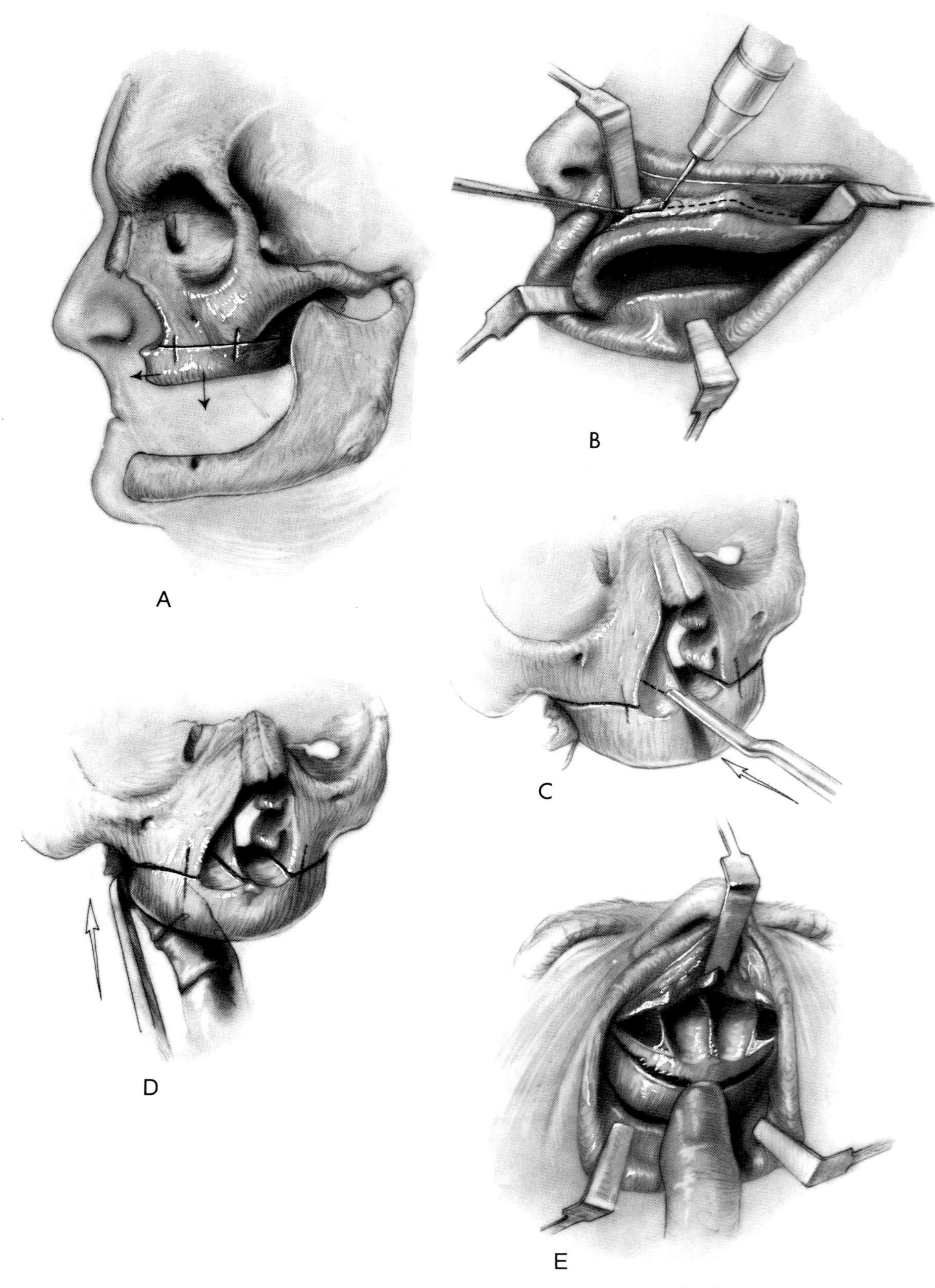

See legend on the opposite page.

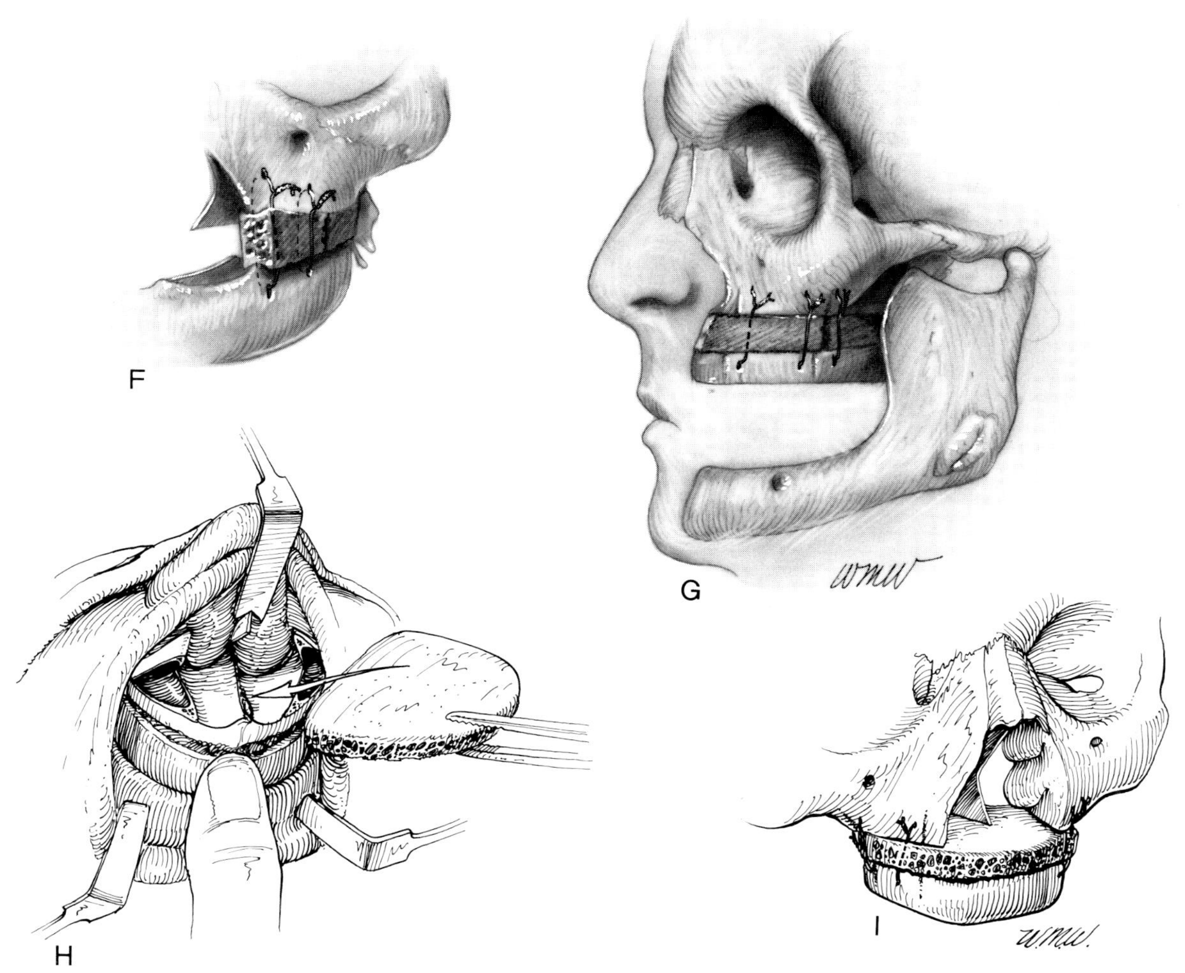

Figure 19–8. Incision of soft tissue and bone for correction of atrophic maxillary alveolar ridge by Le Fort I osteotomy and simultaneous bone grafting. *A,* Facial-skeletal characteristics of edentulous adult with retropositioned atrophic maxillary alveolar ridge. Arrows indicate planned anterior and inferior positional movements of maxilla; horizontal osteotomy of lateral maxilla immediately above the nasal floor extending from piriform rim posteriorly to pterygomaxillary fissure. Anterior and posterior vertical reference lines etched into the lateral maxilla. *B,* Horizontal incision through mucoperiosteum in the maxillary vestibule above the mucogingival reflection from the second molar region on one side to a similar area on the contralateral side; horizontal osteotomy of lateral maxilla immediately above the nasal floor. *C,* Separation of nasal septum from superior part of maxilla, with osteotome placed parallel with hard palate; bone incisions through lateral and medial walls of maxillary antra. *D,* Separation of maxilla from pterygoid plate with osteotome malleted medioanteriorly; surgeon's finger is placed on palatal mucosa to protect vascular pedicle and feel bur as it transects the palatal bone. *E,* Maxilla in down-fractured position; mucoperiosteum has been detached and retracted away from nasal surface of maxilla and horizontal plate of palatine bone. *F,* Dumbbell-shaped blocks of corticocancellous bone inlaid between maxilla and overlying horizontal bone incisions; bone graft fixed with wires placed through and around the graft. *G,* Edentulous maxilla fixed to the piriform rims and zygomatic buttresses with transosseous wires; positional change of vertical reference lines in lateral maxilla after inferior and anterior movements. *H* and *I,* Modified technique: *H,* One large block of corticocancellous bone from iliac crest is interposed between the mobilized portion of the maxilla and both the medial and lateral antral walls and the nasal septum. *I,* Edentulous maxilla fixed to the piriform rims and zygomatic buttresses with transosseous wires; when the amount of bone available from the donor site does not allow the entire maxilla to be covered with a single slab of bone, a large block of bone is cut into two sections that are interposed between the mobilized part of the maxilla and the medial and lateral antral walls.

Mandibular Surgery Technique

As with maxillary surgery, the mandibular surgical procedure is accomplished intraorally in the operating room with the patient under nasoendotracheal anesthesia. Small amounts of a local anesthetic with a vasoconstrictor are injected into the submucosa of the labiobuccal vestibule to aid in hemostasis. The design of the soft-tissue flap for the anterior and posterior mandibular degloving exposure is critical. A mucosal incision is made through the lower lip mucosa midway between the depth of the labial sulcus and the vermilion border of the lower lip (Fig. 19–9). The incision is extended laterally into the mucolabial vestibule and then is angled superiorly to the attached gingiva 1 cm or more distal to the mental foramina (Fig. 19–9*C*). Anteriorly the incision is dissected superficial to the lip muscle and is carried sharply to the chin point. After subperiosteal tunneling to the mental foramina, the mental nerves are identified, dissected free, and retracted posteriorly. The mucoperiosteum is detached minimally from the underlying basal bone to maximize circulation to the repositioned segment. Horizontal and vertical reference marks are etched in the facial bone cortex with a fine rotating fissure bur under constant saline irrigation. A horizontal osteotomy is made with an oscillating sawblade from the mental foramen of the one side to the contralateral foramen to divide the mandibular basal bone into equal superior and inferior parts (Fig. 19–9*C*). Vertical oblique osteotomies are then made to connect the horizontal bone cut with the superior border of the mandibular body at the distal portion of the mental foramina. When the horizontal osteotomy is extended posterior to the mental foramina, the lateral portion of the body of the mandible is decorticated to uncover the inferior alveolar neurovascular bundle. The mental nerves are dissected free and reflected posteriorly and inferiorly to facilitate the planned bony incisions. Alternatively, when feasible, the horizontal bone incision may be extended posteriorly below the inferior alveolar canal.[26] The distal (superior) mandibular segment is carefully upfractured while maintaining a lingual gingival soft-tissue pedicle (Fig. 19–9*D*). Blocks of corticocancellous bone from the iliac crest are sculptured to a predetermined size and shape and interposed between the proximal and distal mandibular segments to maintain the desired vertical dimension (Fig. 19–9*F*). After the segments and bone grafts are stabilized with intraosseous wire fixation, autogenous particulate cancellous bone and cancellous bone slabs are used to fill residual osseous defects. Finally, the soft-tissue incision is closed with interrupted nonresorbable sutures (Fig. 19–9*G*).

Inferior repositioning of the edentulous maxilla by Le Fort I osteotomy and superior repositioning of mandibular bone with simultaneous bone grafting offer new approaches to the management of patients with severe alveolar ridge atrophy. Both the question of stability and resorption of the repositioned bone and the effect of a functional prosthesis on the underlying alveolar ridge must await further postoperative evaluation. Early follow-up studies have demonstrated early consolidation of the grafted bone, minimal resorption of the repositioned osseous segments, and virtually no decrease of alveolar ridge height. The problems of ulceration and exfoliation of bone, commonly associated with free bone grafting to the alveolar ridge, have been minimal, probably because of minimal exposure of the grafted bone to stresses of the denture base. The interpositional type of bone graft receives evenly distributed crushing stresses and is subjected to virtually no shearing stress. Since mandibular basal bone is thought to be relatively resistant to resorption, this method of grafting should afford longer-term stability and resistance to resorption. When such surgery is contemplated with jaw repositioning, the surgical procedures may have to be staged to allow for the best result.

During recent years the design of interpositional grafting techniques has been modified to augment the missing bone mass in the anterior and posterior parts of the mandible, improve the maxillo-mandibular ridge relationship, and restore the sulcus by immediate vestibuloplasty. The versatility of these mandibular surgical techniques is described and illustrated in Figures 19–9 to 19–17.

Figure 19–9*H* (Parts 1 through 12) illustrates the technique of body sagittal osteotomies and anterior horizontal osteotomy with interpositional and onlay bone grafting to the mandible.* This procedure is a further modification of Harle's original mandibular visor operation later altered by Peterson et al., Stoeling et al., and de Koomen et al. (See Selected Readings at the end of this chapter.) The advantages of this modification are as follows: allows improvement of ridge relationships in anteroposterior and lateral dimensions by proximal repositioning of the mobilized segment correcting the pseudoprognathism seen in many edentulous patients with severe mandibular bony deficiency; provides maximum augmentation of total osseous bulk of the mandible by both onlay and interpositional grafts in the body and anterior regions, which is most important in the body areas that usually present the greatest degree of bony deficiency; and results in optimum ridge form with increased width in the body regions for greater support and distribution of forces associated with the prosthesis (Fig. 19–9*H*).

A mouth floor plasty and vestibuloplasty with split-thickness skin grafting is accomplished 12 to 16 weeks following this procedure when autologous bone is used for the graft material. When homologous bone is used this secondary soft-tissue procedure is delayed for at least 6 months to allow for additional healing and revascularization of the graft. This secondary soft-tissue procedure is considered essential to provide as much fixed tissue as possible over the primary denture support area. The mouth floor lowering is very important as the mylohyoid and genioglossus muscles have been raised with the repositioned segment.

The most common complication with this procedure as described is neurovascular bundle injury. In 3 patients in a series of 18 operated, 4 nerves have been severed. Both nerves were transected in the first patient operated during the decompression procedure. They were covered by extremely dense cortical bone and a slow speed rotary instrument rather than the high speed instrument recommended was being used for bone removal. This patient is experiencing neurosensory return after 1 year. In two other patients one nerve was inadvertently parted after decompression by retraction pressure. Both of these nerves were repaired using microsurgical techniques and after 6 months there is beginning neurosensory return.

There is also danger of fracture, as has been discussed previously in this chapter. Fracture of the mobilized segment is not serious and can be simply repaired by a wire suture. Fracture in the host mandible is more serious and occurred at surgery in one of our patients when force was used to mobilize the medial segment. The fracture occurred in the thin posterior body region and it was later noted that the anterior horizontal and sagittal osteotomies were not completely connected by the vertical facial and lingual cortical plate cuts. In this patient, when the medial segment was repositioned, bone grafts

Text continued on page 1458

*Illustrations and text concerning this procedure were supplied by Bill C. Terry, Department of Oral and Maxillofacial Surgery, University of North Carolina School of Dentistry, Chapel Hill, North Carolina.

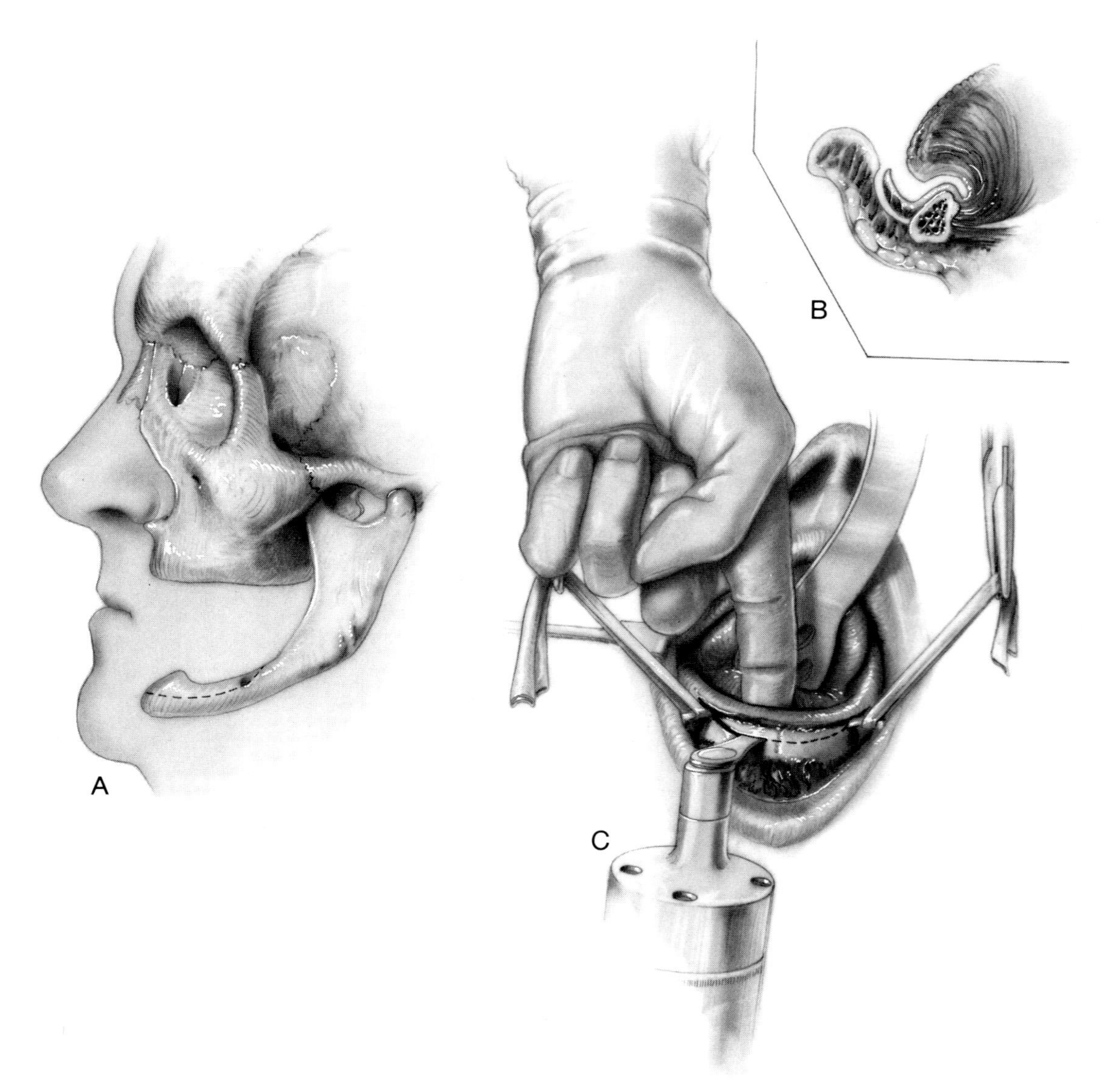

Figure 19–9. Incision of soft tissue and bone for correction of atrophic mandibular alveolar ridge by horizontal mandibular osteotomy and simultaneous bone grafting. *A,* Diagrammatic profile of edentulous patient with atrophic mandible; planned horizontal mandibular osteotomy (*broken line*) extending from mental foramen on one side to opposite mental foramen, dividing the mandible into equal distal (superior) and proximal segments. *B,* View of mandible showing design of soft-tissue incision that is made midway between the depth of the mandibular labial vestibule and the wet line of the lower lip. *C,* Horizontal mandibular osteotomy is made with an oscillating saw; finger is positioned on lingual mucosa to feel saw blade as it transects lingual cortex. The mental nerves are retracted posteriorly to facilitate the bone cut.

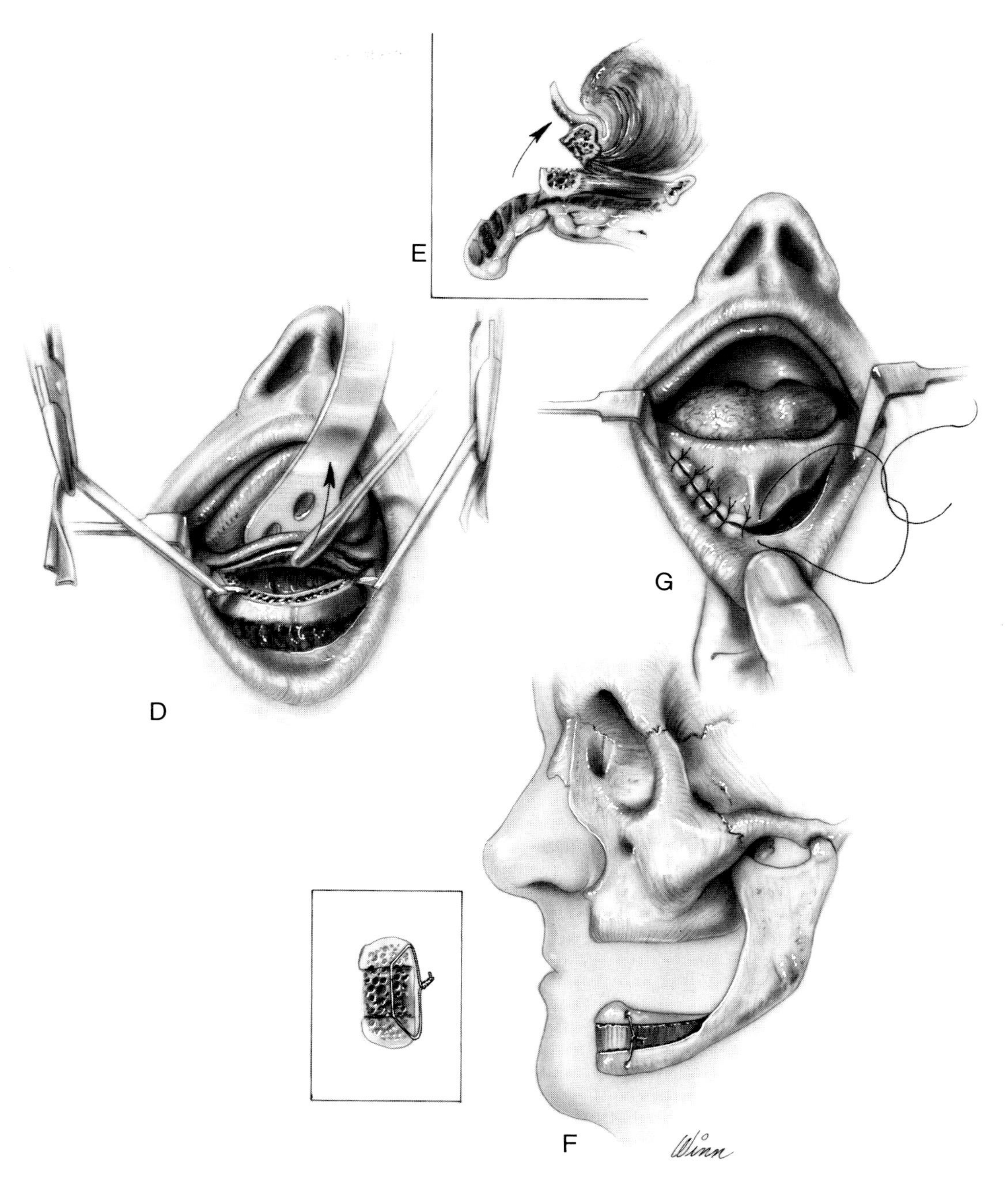

Figure 19–9 *Continued.* *D,* Upfracture of the distal (superior) mandibular segment; care is taken to preserve the gingival and lingual mucosa pedicles. Mental nerves are retracted posteriorly and inferiorly with Penrose drains. *E,* View of the upfractured distal segment of the mandible showing the lingual soft-tissue pedicle consisting of the genioglossus muscle and a portion of the geniohyoid muscle. *F,* Intraosseous wire fixation of interpositional corticocancellous bone graft to the mandible. *G,* Closure of mucosal incision with interrupted resorbable sutures; incision may also be closed with running horizontal mattress suture of #3-0 chromic catgut.

Illustration and legend continued on the following page

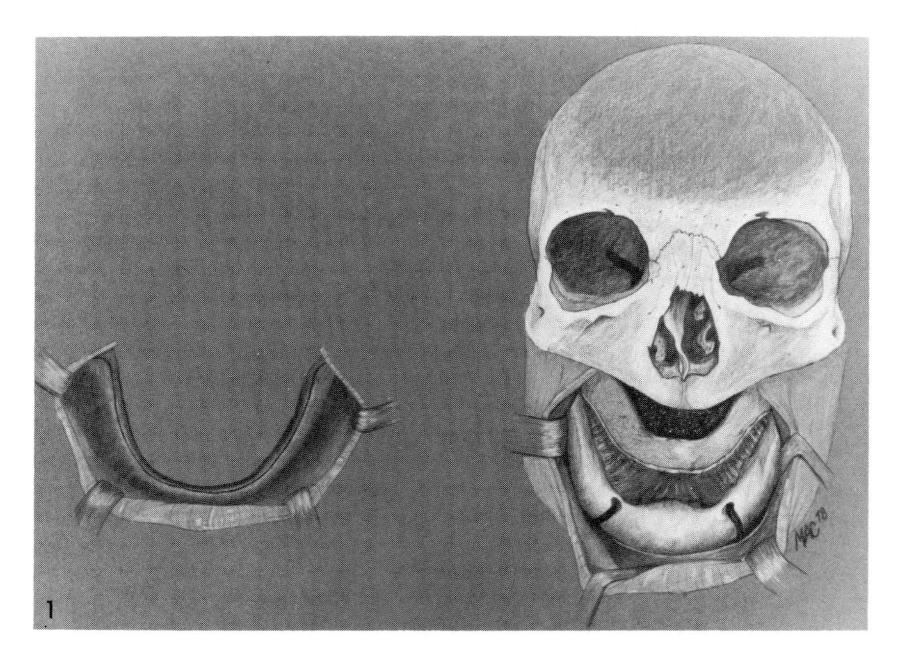

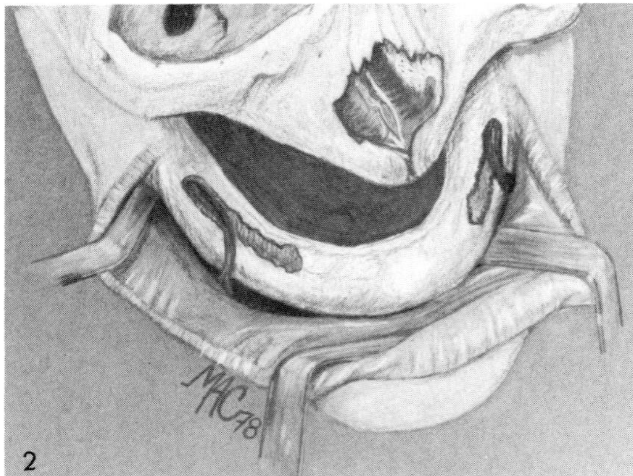

Figure 19–9 *Continued.* *H,* Body sagittal osteotomies and anterior horizontal osteotomy with interpositional and onlay bone grafting to the mandible. (Technique of Bill C. Terry, Chapel Hill, North Carolina.) *1,* An incision is made from the lateral aspects of the anterior ramus splitting the crestal scar tissue to the opposite ramus.[17] A facial mucoperiosteal flap is developed. The mental nerves are identified and dissected free for a few millimeters at their soft-tissue interface. The flap is then raised down to and includes stripping of the periosteum from the inferior border. A full-thickness lingual mucosa flap is developed for several millimeters by reflecting the crestal attachment and separating the tissue from the underlying mylohyoid and genioglossus muscles. *2,* A planned decompression of the mandibular neurovascular bundle is carried out by removing the overlying bone from the mental foramen to the anterior ramus body juncture. This can be accomplished by removing the covering bone along the course of the canal with a round bur revolving at high speed and light brush-like movements. Another method is to outline the course of the nerve with bone cuts through the cortex and then use small osteotomes to deroof the canal. After the neurovascular bundle is exposed the incisal continuation is severed and the bundle is lifted from the canal posteriorly to the ramus body juncture. Careful retraction protects the neurovascular bundle and maintains the integrity of the soft tissue interface and continuation in the ramus.

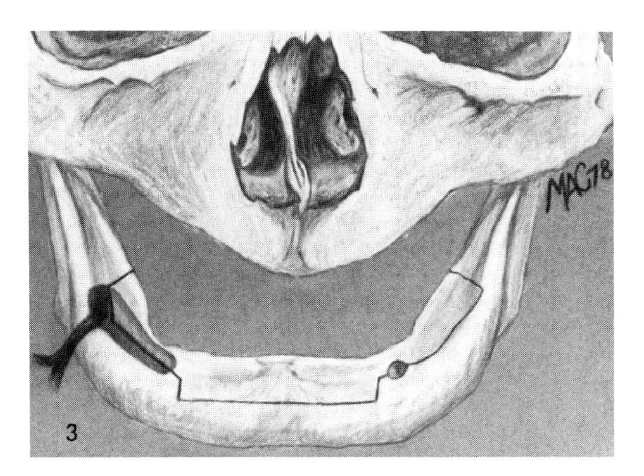

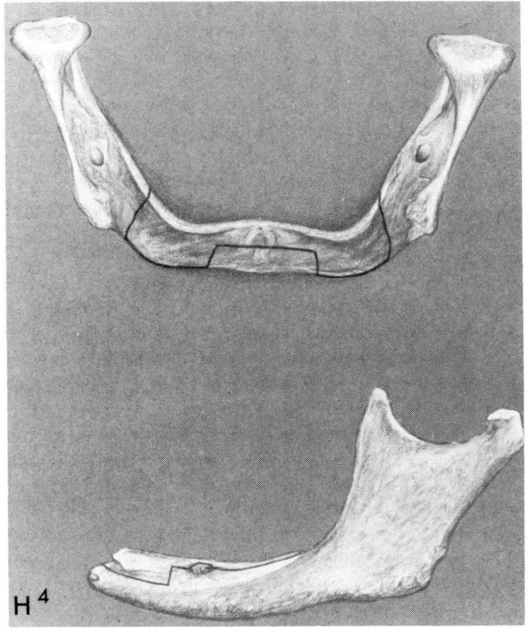

Figure 19–9 *Continued.* *3,* Planned osteotomy lines viewed from the facial. A portion of the mylohyoid muscle is separated from the mandible at the ramus body juncture to allow introduction of a small reciprocating saw. The initial cut through the mylohyoid shelf is at a 30°–40° angle. The osteotomy continues into the residual bony canal depression and a vertical cut is made through the inferior border. This sagittal cut is carried to just past the mental foramen. A flat instrument placed beneath the inferior border protects the adjacent soft tissues. This portion of the osteotomy is completed bilaterally. Next, using a reciprocating or oscillating saw a horizontal osteotomy is made through the anterior mandible about midway between the superior and inferior borders. Using a small fissure bur a vertical cut is made through the facial cortical plate connecting the horizontal and sagittal cuts. *4,* Planned osteotomy lines viewed from lingual and lateral aspects. The periosteum of the degloved anterior mandible is reflected on the linguolateral aspects to the level of the horizontal osteotomy, and again using a fissure bur, cuts are made through the lingual cortical plate connecting the horizontal and sagittal portions of the osteotomy. If the medial segment is not free after completion of all portions of the osteotomy, the anterior area should be checked very carefully to make certain that the horizontal cut and connection to the sagittal cuts on the facial and lingual aspects are complete. Force should never be used to separate the segment to be mobilized as a fracture can easily occur in the freed segment or more seriously in the host mandible.

Illustration and legend continued on the following page

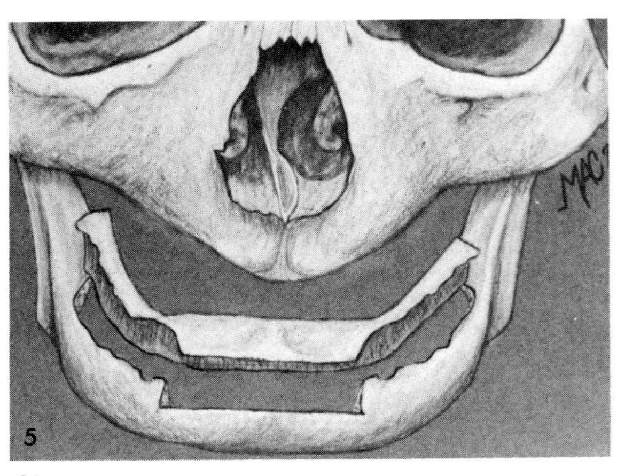

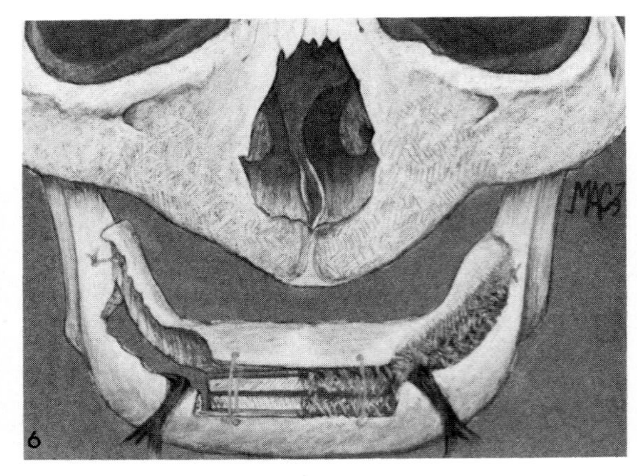

H

Figure 19–9 *Continued.* *5,* The intact medial segment with attached muscles and tissues is displaced superiorly and posteriorly. The proximal ends of this segment are set on the residual mylohyoid shelves and fixed by direct wiring. Anteriorly, the segment is lifted to the desired height. An attempt is made to at least double the vertical dimension of the residual mandible. This height can be increased even more, with a major limiting factor being able to effect a soft-tissue closure without tension. Periosteal relaxing incisions in the facial flap can be made to assist this closure.[17] The superior proximal ends of the repositioned segment may be reduced if the vertical extension in this area is too great. *6,* Wafers of corticocancellous iliac bone are now inserted into the area of the horizontal osteotomy supporting the anterior segment in the desired vertical dimension. A wire is placed on either side of the horizontal osteotomy connecting the repositioned segment and the host mandible. These wire sutures are threaded through the anterior cortical plates and are kept facially compressing the grafts in both vertical and proximal directions. Two circumandibular wires can also be used to achieve the same result. A mixture of cortical and cancellous bone chips are now packed in the created sagittal space in the body regions. Before this space is obliterated, the neurovascular bundles are replaced and bone chips placed over the bundles to completely fill the sagittal space.

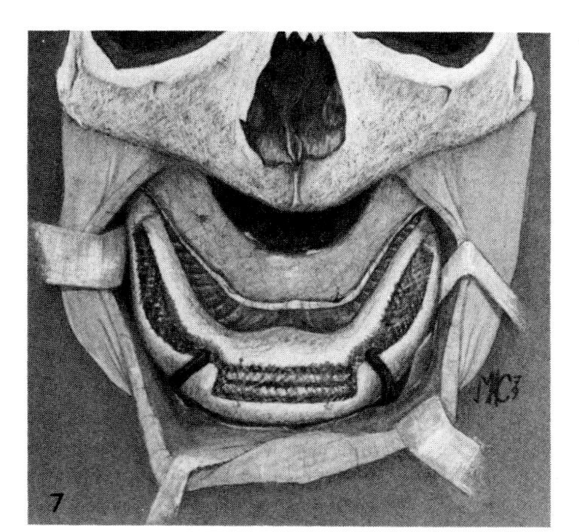

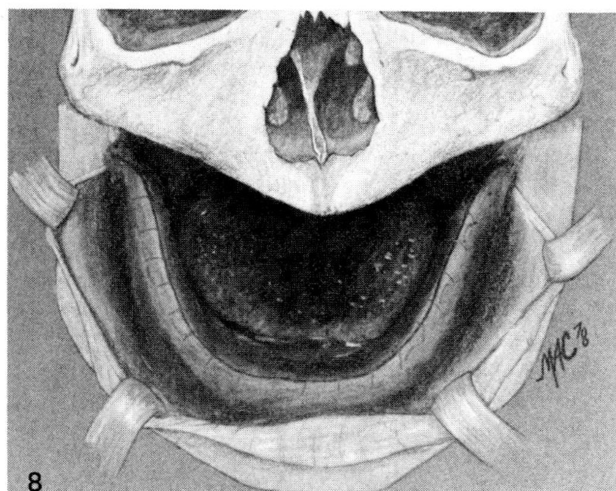

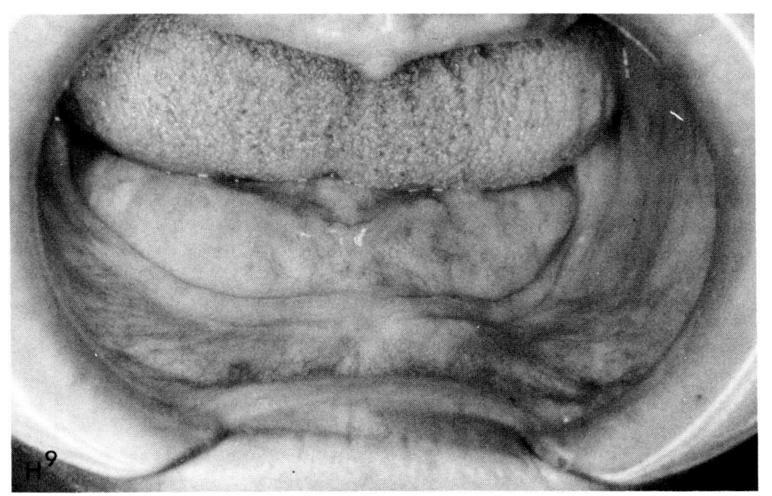

Figure 19–9 *Continued.* *7,* Packing of chips is then continued over the entire superior surface to provide the desired final contour and augmentation. *8,* Soft-tissue closure is accomplished with one primary suture placed in a horizontal mattress fashion from ramus to ramus. This ensures eversion of the flap edges. A second continuous spiral suture reinforces the closure for watertight integrity. Monofilament-type suture material is desired to reduce potential inflammatory response. *9,* Patient with severe mandibular bony deficiency and an inadequate denture support area.

Illustration and legend continued on the following page

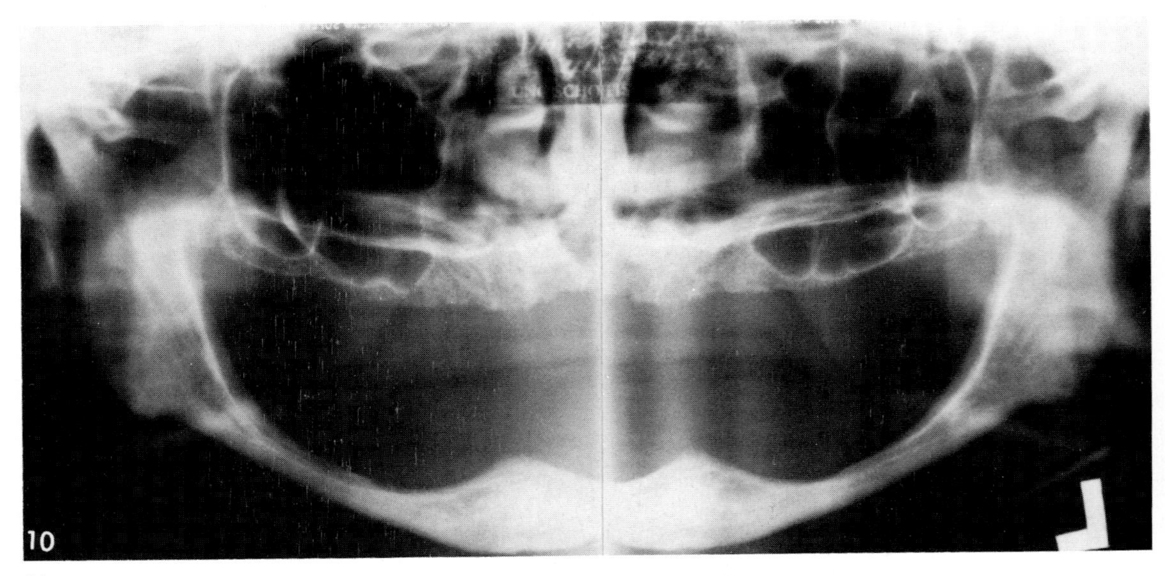

H

Figure 19–9 *Continued.* *10,* Radiograph demonstrating the greatest bony deficiency in the body regions.

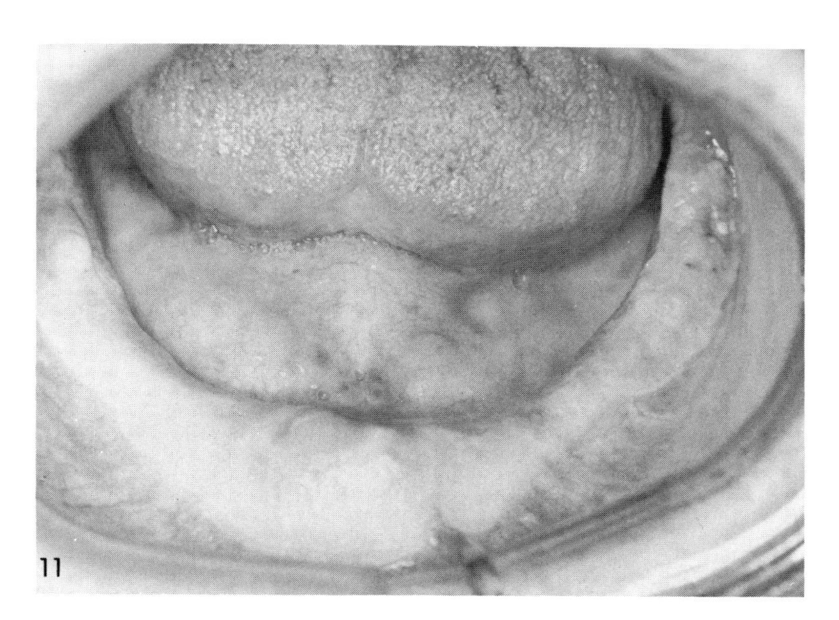

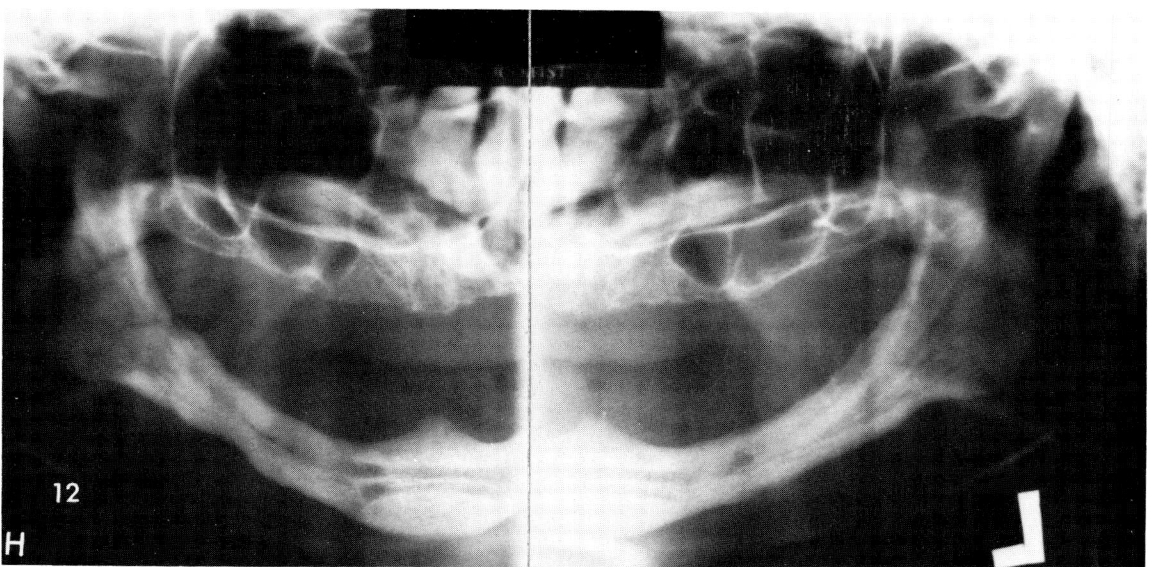

Figure 19–9 *Continued.* *11,* One-year follow-up showing the broad, convex ridge form covered by fixed tissue after bone graft augmentation and a mouth floor plasty and vestibuloplasty with split thickness skin grafting. *12,* One year after bone grafting.

Illustration and legend continued on the following page

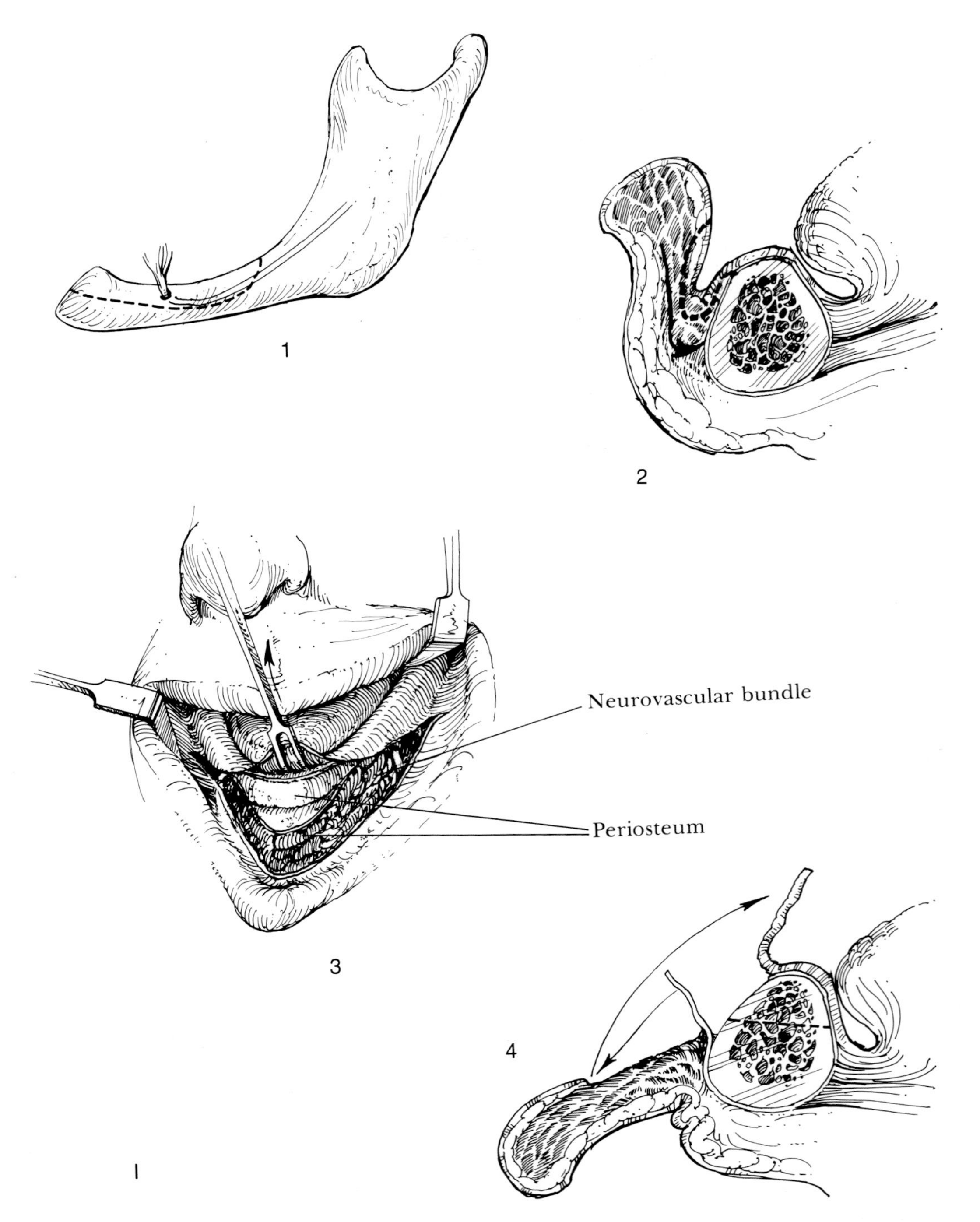

Figure 19–9 *Continued.* *I,* Interpositional bone grafting of atrophic mandible and immediate vestibuloplasty by Edlan technique. (Robert L. Buckles and William H. Bell, Dallas, Texas.) *1,* Diagrammatic illustration of edentulous atrophic mandible with the planned osteotomy represented by a dashed line extending from the 3rd molar region of one side to a similar area on the contralateral side. *2,* Cross section of mandible at symphysis; planned mucosal flap indicated by dashed line. *3,* Soft-tissue flap design anterior to the mental nerves; full-thickness mucoperiosteal flap developed posterior to the mental nerves. *4,* Elevation of mucosal flap and reflection of periosteum starting 2–3 mm. lateral to the attached mucosa.

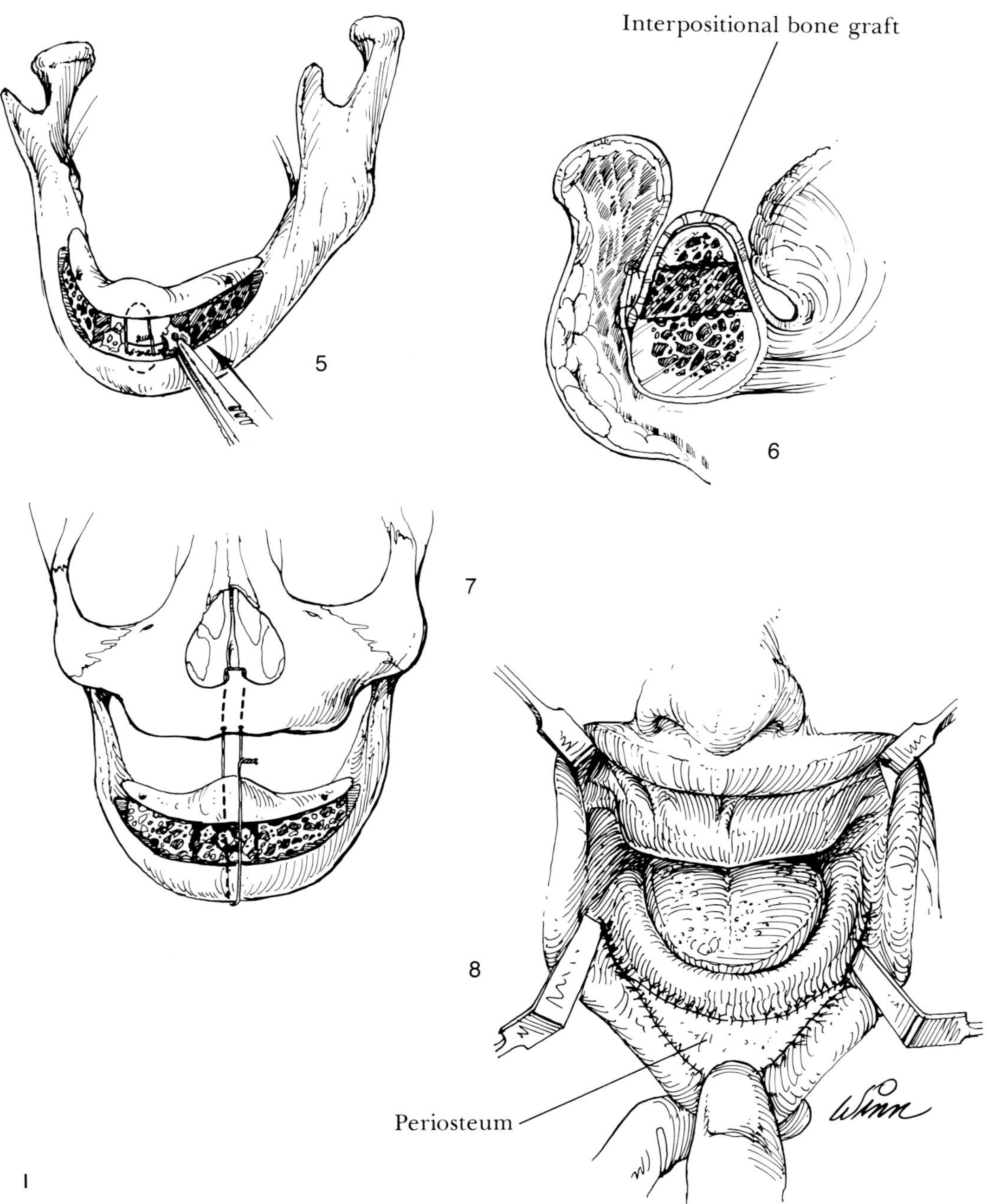

I

Figure 19–9 *Continued.* *5,* Interosseous wire fixation in the symphysis region; the distal and proximal portions of the mandible separated by corticocancellous bone blocks in the premolar–1st molar areas bilaterally. Particulate autogenous marrow grafts are placed between and posterior to the blocks of bone. *6,* Cross section of mental symphysis showing interpositional bone graft; periosteum is sutured to lip mucosa and alveolar mucosa is sutured to periosteum inferiorly. *7,* Anterior mandibular suspension wire extends from the mandibular symphysis to and through the anterior maxillary alveolus and floor of the nose. *8,* The free margin of the periosteal flap is then sutured to the labial mucosal margin of the lip. The mucosal flap is sutured to the inferior aspect of the periosteal flap. Posteriorly, the mucosal wound margins are sutured with continuous absorbable sutures.

Illustration and legend continued on the following page

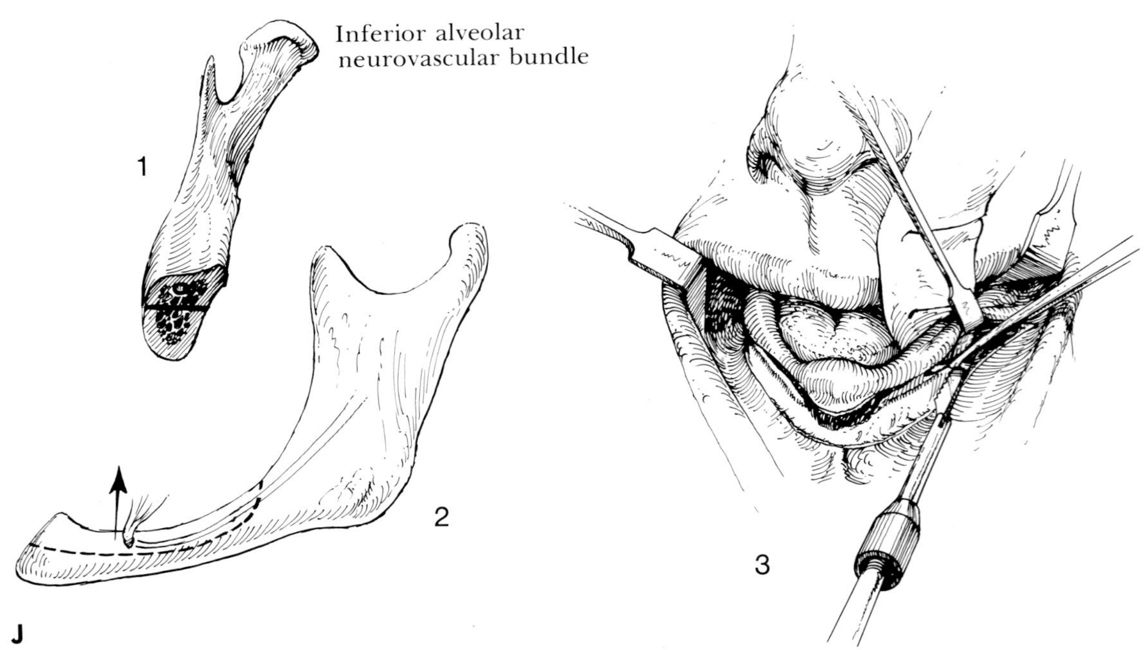

Figure 19–9 *Continued.* *J,* Interpositional bone graft to atrophic mandible without immediate vestibuloplasty. *1* and *2,* Diagrammatic illustration of edentulous atrophic mandible; planned osteotomy represented by a dashed line extending from the 3rd molar region of one side to a similar area on the contralateral side to divide the mandible into equal distal (superior) and proximal segments. Cross-sectional view of posterior region showing the planned horizontal osteotomy below the level of the mandibular nerve canal. *3,* After mental nerves are dissected out of soft tissue, they are retracted with Penrose drains; horizontal osteotomy is made with a reciprocating saw blade below the level of the mandibular canal.

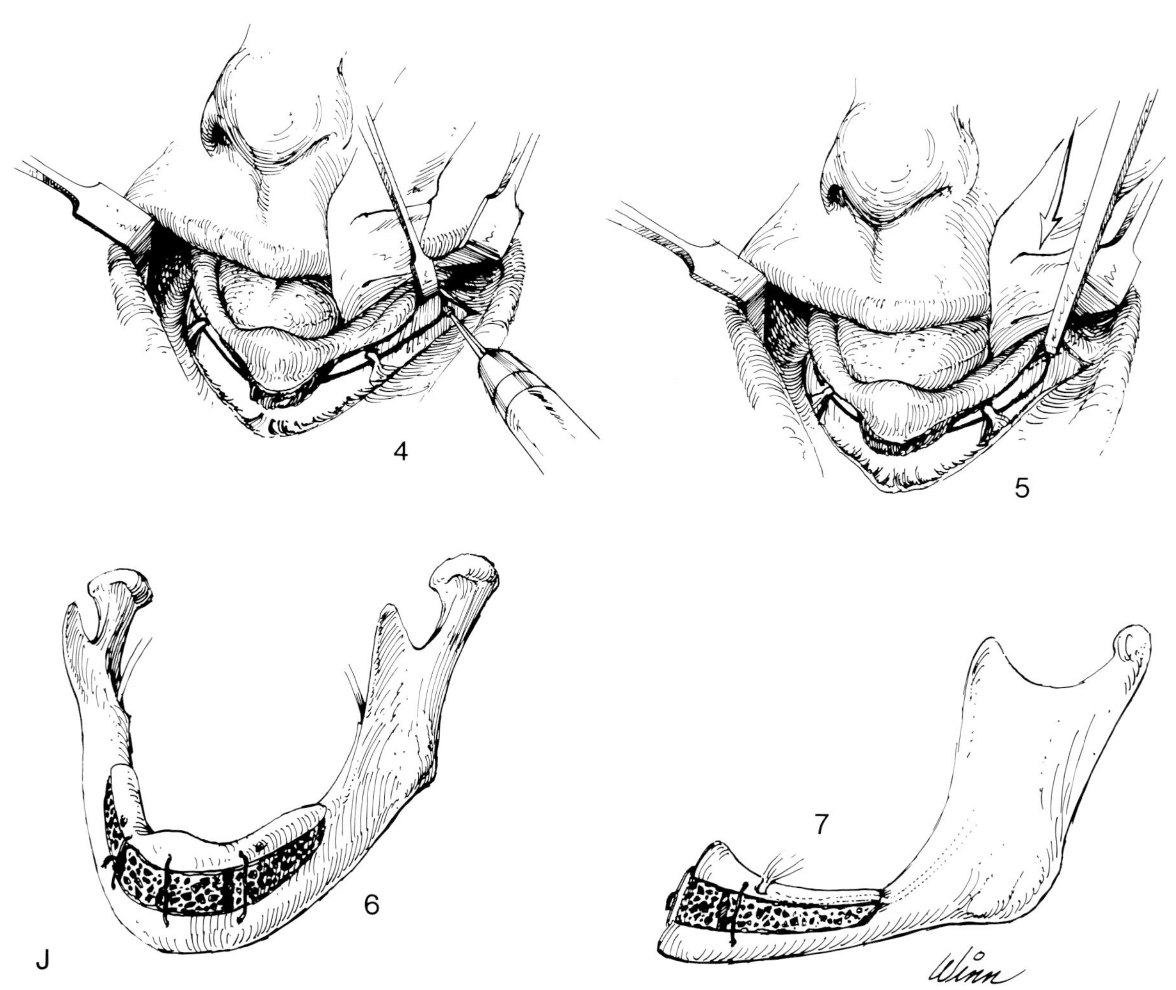

Figure 19–9 *Continued.* *4* and *5,* With the superior margin of the mucosal incision retracted, the posterior lateral and posterior superior aspects of the mandibular body are sectioned with a fissure bur; the segment is mobilized by malleting a spatula osteotome into the incompletely sectioned vertical osteotomy site. *6* and *7,* Interosseous wire fixation of interpositional bone grafts to the mandible.

Illustration and legend continued on the following page

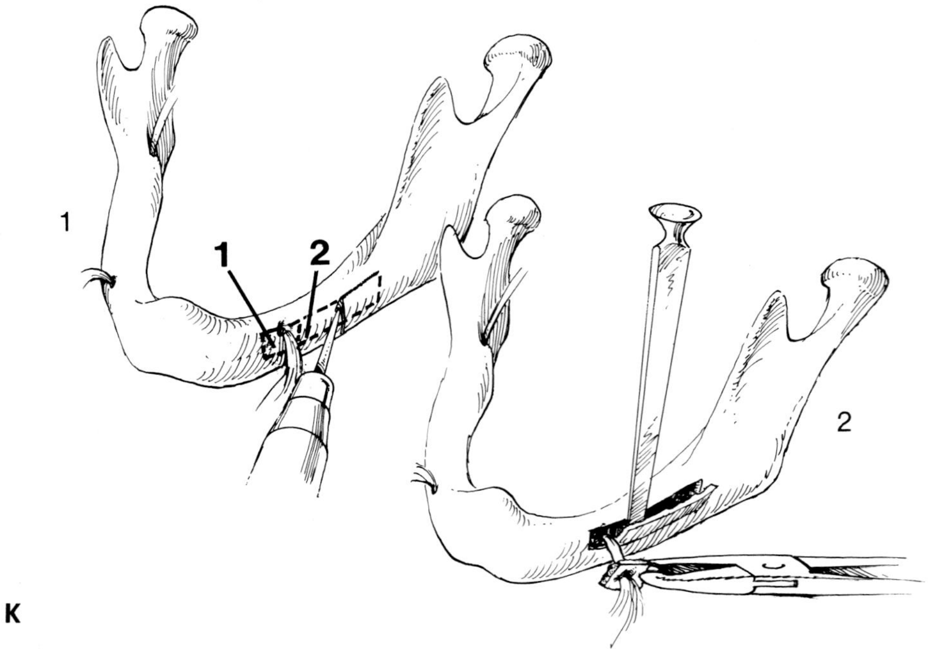

Figure 19–9 *Continued.* *K,* Augmentation of atrophic mandible by interpositional bone graft at level of mandibular nerve canal. *1,* Sequential excision of labial (**1**) and buccal (**2**) cortical plate opposite the mandibular nerve canal. Osteotomy is made through labial and buccal cortical plates to the junction of the cortical and cancellous bones. *2,* Labial and buccal cortical plates opposite the mandibular nerve canal are separated from the subjacent intramedullary bone by malleting an osteotome at the junction of the labial and buccal plates and the intramedullary bone. Bone circumscribing mental nerve is first mobilized and excised with rongeurs.

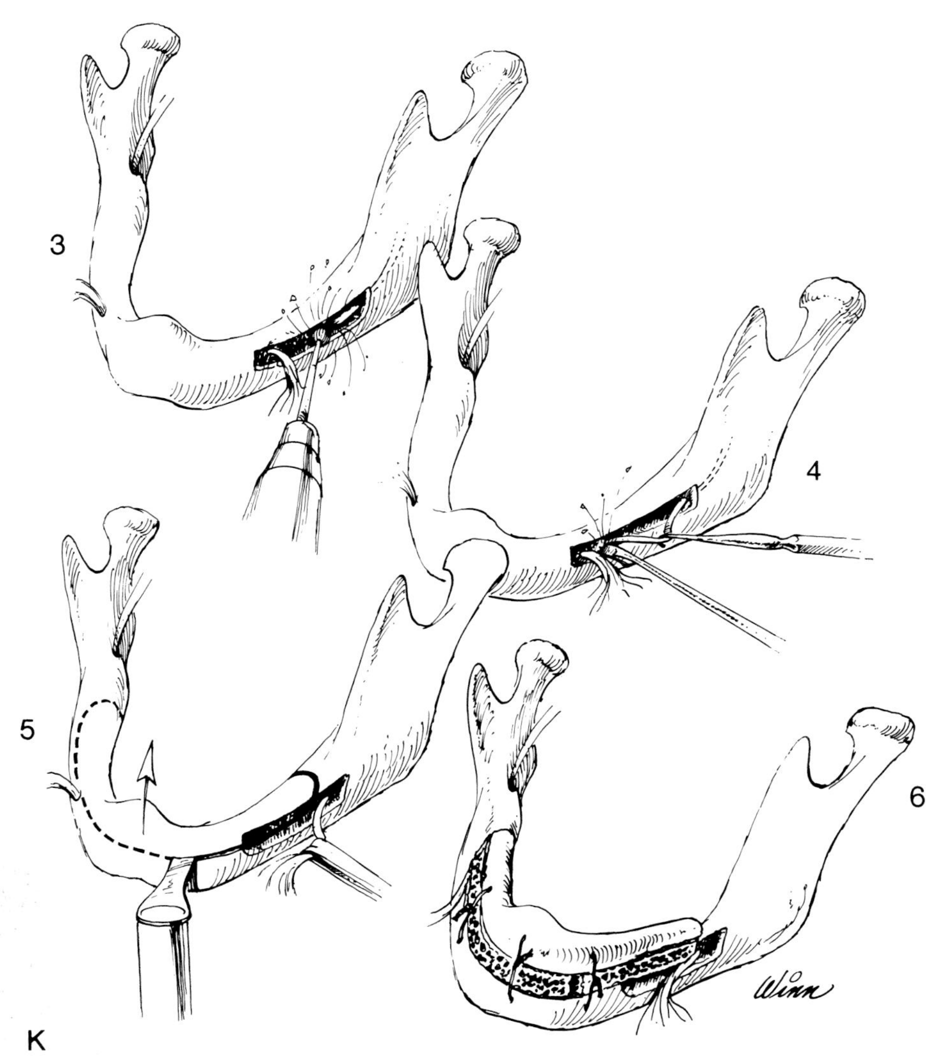

Figure 19–9 *Continued.* *3,* Cancellous bone overlying inferior alveolar neurovascular bundle is carefully removed. *4,* After inferior alveolar nerve is exposed, it is teased from its bony canal with a periosteal elevator and retracted laterally with a nerve hook. *5,* With inferior alveolar nerve retracted laterally, horizontal mandibular osteotomy is made with an oscillating saw blade and fissure bur at the level of the inferior alveolar nerve canal to divide the mandible into equal distal and proximal segments. *6,* Interosseous wire fixation of interpositional bone grafts to the mandible.

Illustration and legend continued on the following page

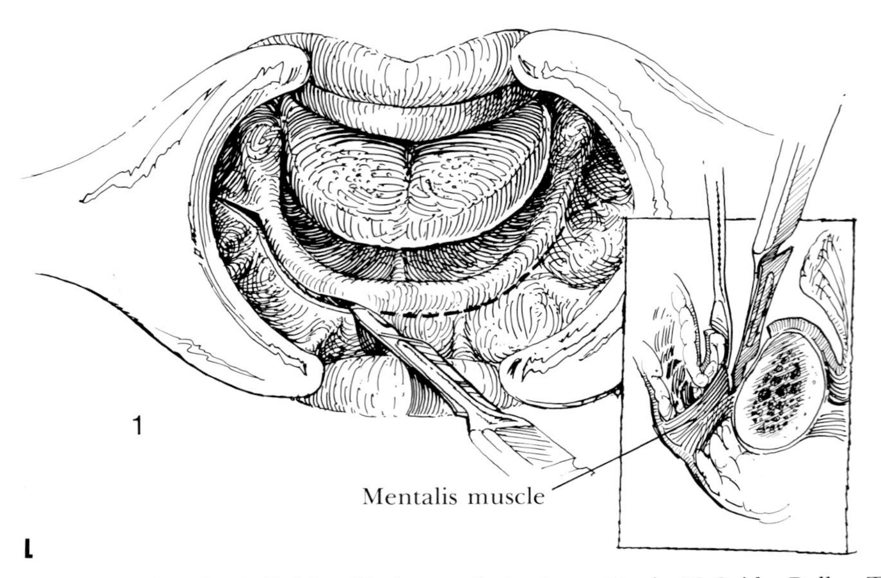

Figure 19–9 *Continued.* *L–N,* Mandibular vestibuloplasty. (Kevin McBride, Dallas, Texas.) *1,* Local anesthetic with vasoconstrictor is injected into the mentalis muscles and supraperiosteally over the labial aspect of the mandible from right 1st molar to left 1st molar. Infiltration of the mylohyoid muscles is performed at this time. An incision is made down to the periosteum from the right 1st molar region to the left 1st molar region approximately 1 mm. lateral to the junction of the free and attached gingiva. (The supraperiosteal dissection is easier to start when the incision is made in the free mucosa rather than in the attached mucosa.) The incision is extended posterolaterally on each side at an angle of about 60° to the mandibular ridge. This angled dissection helps to form a smooth transition from the tissue over the lateral oblique ridge to the deepened anterior vestibule. Improved patient comfort is attained by retention of normal tissue over the lateral oblique ridge that provides a better cushion for the denture flange than does a split-thickness skin graft. Supraperiosteal dissection is performed with a scalpel and facilitated by aggressive retraction of the subcutaneous tissue with a periosteal elevator.

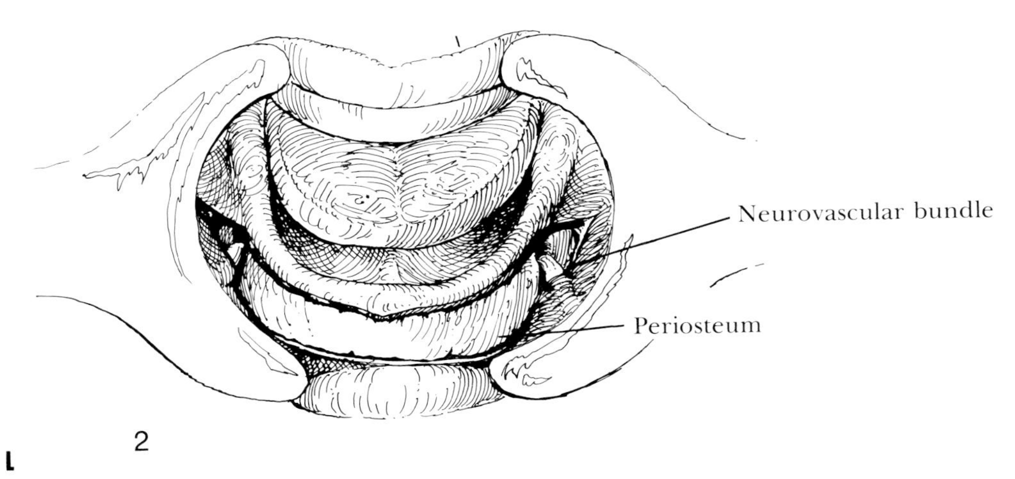

Figure 19–9 *Continued.* *2,* The supraperiosteal dissection is carried 3–5 mm. deeper than the desired position of the mandibular vestibule to provide tissue relaxation at the depth of the vestibule. Maximal soft-tissue attachment is retained around the mental nerves to protect the nerves after healing. Connective tissue and muscle is meticulously removed from the periosteum to ensure an optimal graft bed.

Illustration and legend continued on the following page

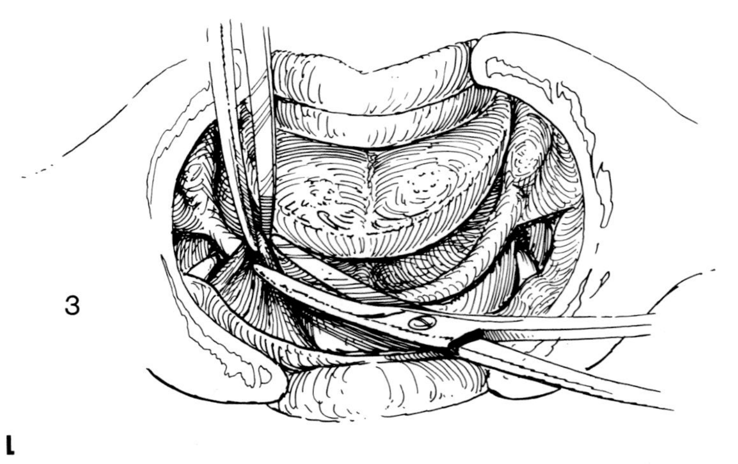

Figure 19–9 *Continued.* *3,* The mentalis muscle and surrounding submucosal tissue is grasped, placed under tension, and partially excised. Tissue approximately 2.5 cm. × 1 cm. × 1 cm., extending from the midline to the mental nerve, is removed bilaterally. This excision reduces the bulk of tissue, which must be repositioned below the newly created mandibular vestibule.

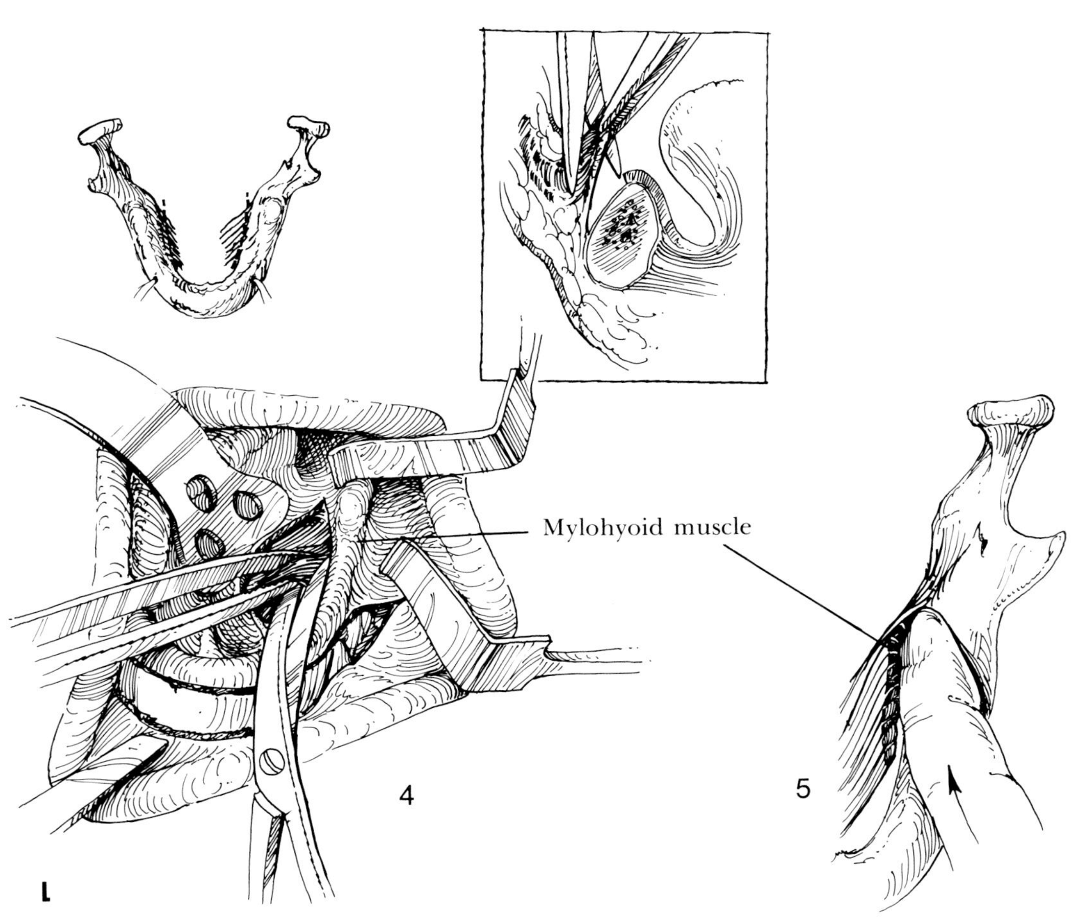

Figure 19–9 *Continued.* *4,* Repositioning of the mylohyoid muscle is initiated by making an incision 2 mm. below the junction of the free and attached lingual mucosa, extending from the posterior edge of the retromolar pad to the 1st bicuspid region. The dissection is carried down to the superior aspect of the mylohyoid muscle. The tongue is retracted in a superomedial direction to elevate the mylohyoid muscle. One blade of a small curved Metzenbaum scissors is forced through the anterior fibers of the mylohyoid muscle. The muscle is then transected along its entire attachment to the mandible. Care is taken to keep the scissors close to the mandible to avoid injury to the lingual nerve. The muscle is pulled superiorly so that it may be cut under tension and direct visualization. *5,* The mylohyoid muscle is palpated to ensure that all posterior fibers have been completely transected.

Illustration and legend continued on the following page

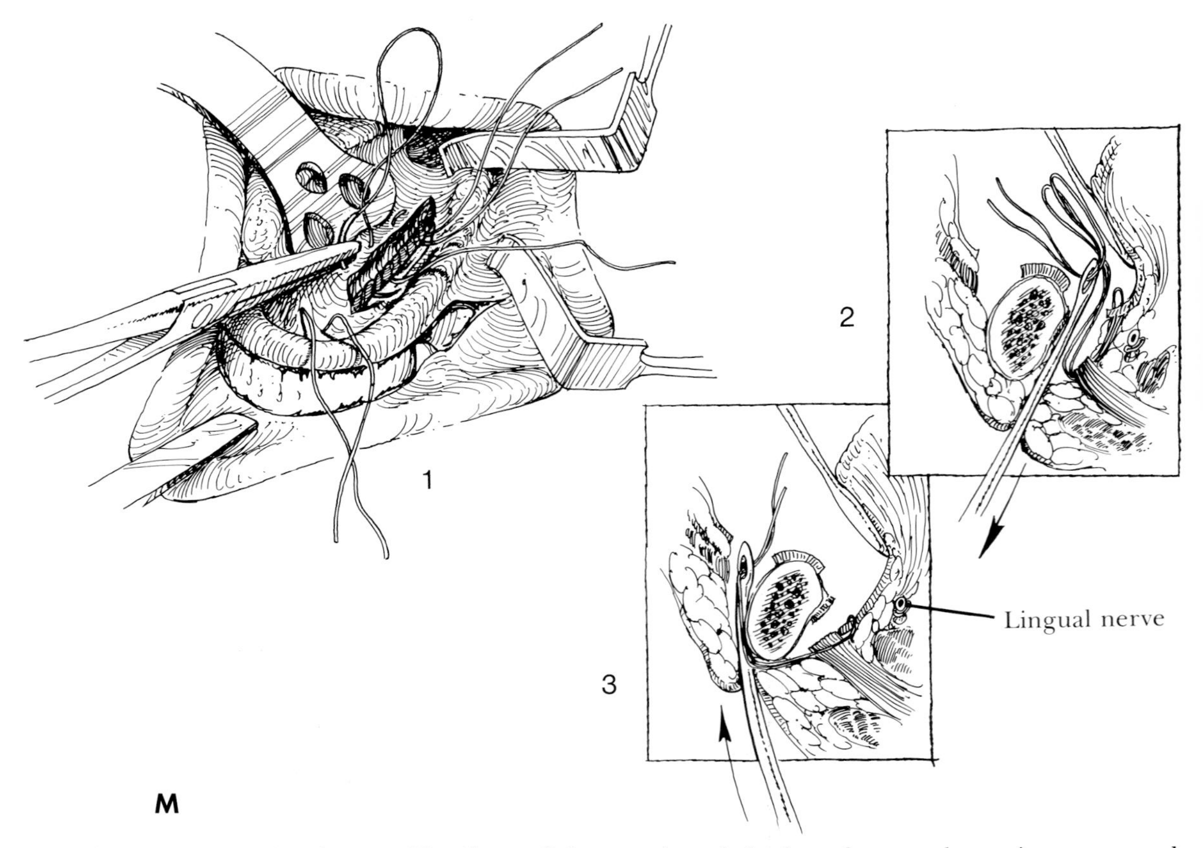

Figure 19–9 *Continued. M1,* The floor of the mouth and the buccal mucosal margin are secured inferiorly with circumandibular sutures. Bilateral horizontal mattress sutures of 0 chromic are passed through the mylohyoid muscle and lingual mucosa at each end of the incision in the floor of the mouth. Two additional sutures, one on either side of the midline, are secured by taking a deep bite of the mucosa and submucosal tissues as close to the mandible as possible. *2,* A passing awl is used to carry the suture around the inferior border of the mandible and into the buccal vestibule. The awl is inserted through the skin of the neck slightly anterior to the location of the suture in the floor of the mouth. The awl is advanced into the dissection between the mandible and the mylohyoid muscle. Both ends of the posterior suture are passed through the eye of the awl. *3,* The awl is then passed around the inferior border of the mandible and brought out into the buccal dissection close to the mandible at a point halfway between the posterior end of the buccal dissection and the mental nerve. The suture ends are freed from the awl, which is then removed.

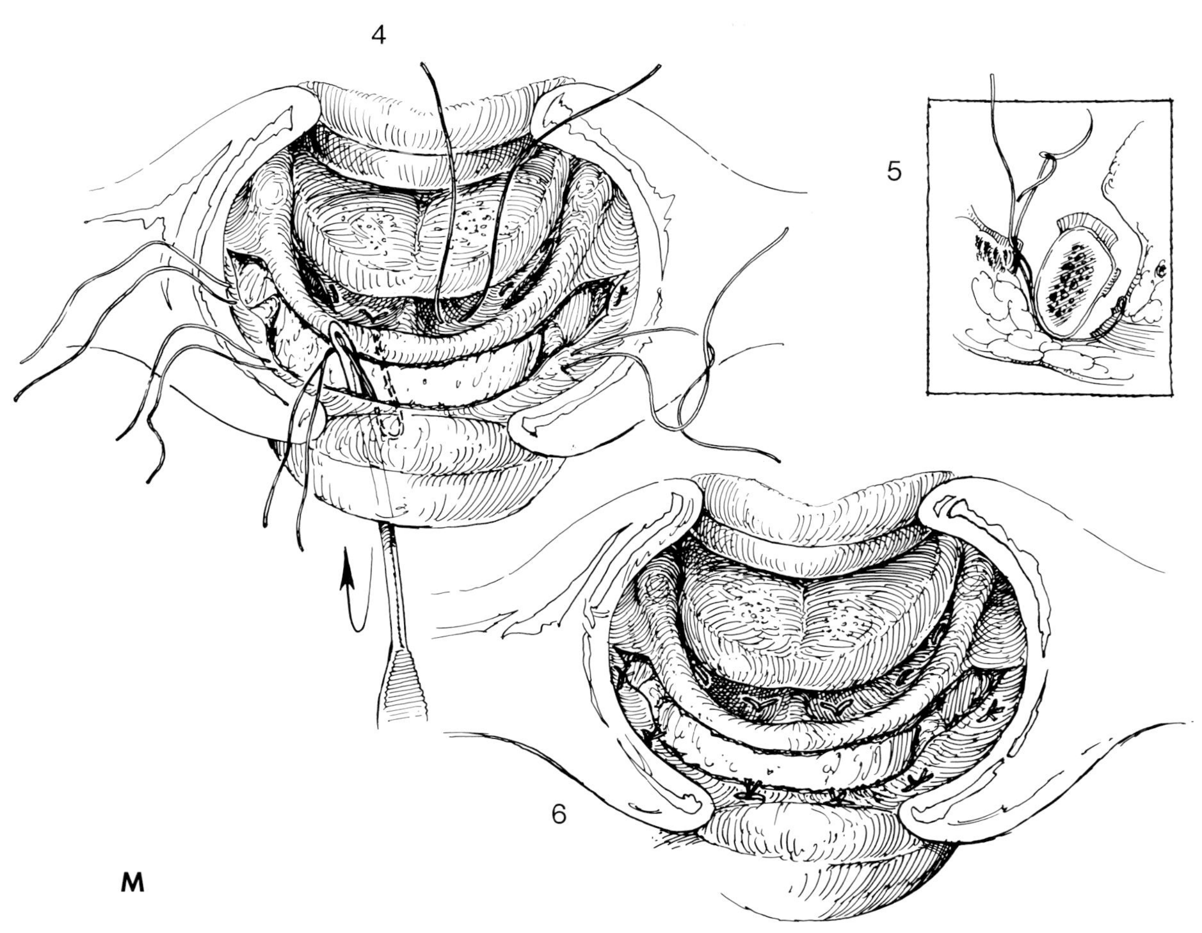

Figure 19–9 *Continued.* *4,* This process is repeated, bringing the suture at the anterior end of the mylohyoid muscle into the buccal dissection at a point approximately 5 mm. anterior to the mental nerve. The sutures adjacent to the midline are carried around to a corresponding point in the buccal vestibule. *5,* A free curved cutting needle is used to pass the sutures through the free mucosal margin in a horizontal mattress fashion. The needle is passed through a bulk of subcutaneous tissue and brought out 1 or 2 mm. from the free mucosal margin. The sutures are passed through subcutaneous tissue to prevent them from being pulled through the mucosal margin. *6,* The most posterior sutures are tightened first. Prior to securing the knot, the sutures must be pulled taut to provide the desired inferior repositioning of the mylohyoid muscle and floor of the mouth. While traction is maintained on the sutures, the knot is advanced to position the mucosal margin at the desired buccal vestibular depth. Due to the anterior angulation of the sutures as they pass from the floor of the mouth into the buccal vestibule the mucosal margin is stretched tightly around the mandible as the sutures are tightened. This provides excellent adaptation of the mucosal margin to the mandible.

Illustration and legend continued on the following page

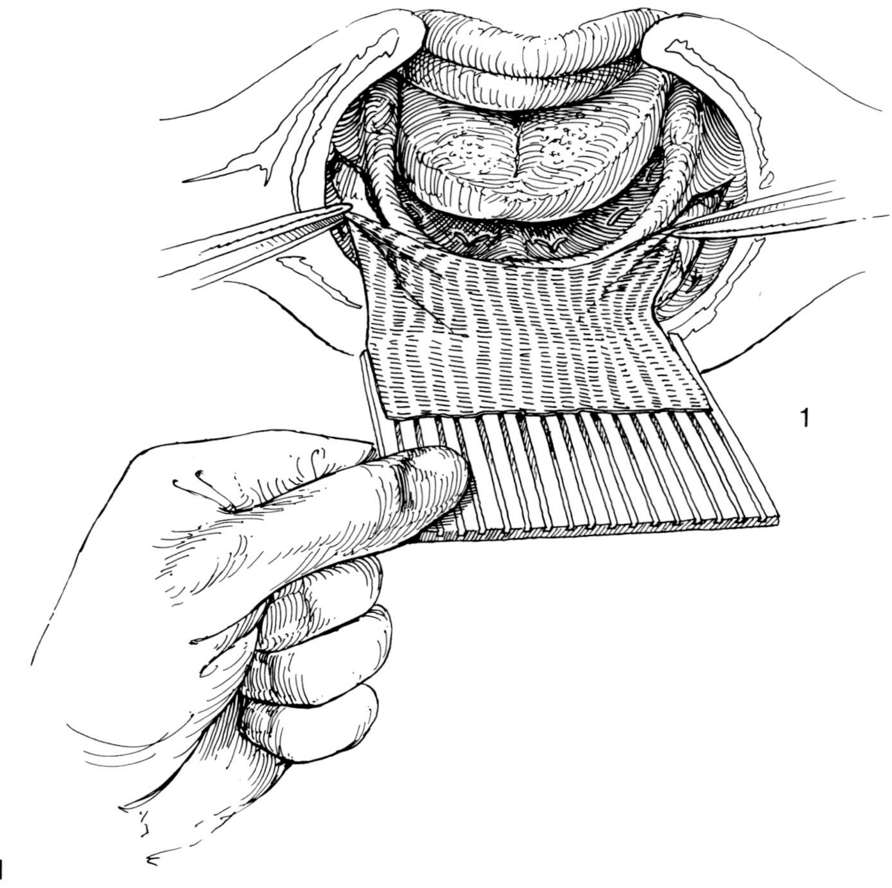

Figure 19–9 *Continued.* *N1,* The derma carrier with the previously meshed skin is held against the moistened lower lip. Utilizing two tissue forceps the skin is pulled across the lower lip and down into the newly created vestibule. A periosteal elevator is utilized to position the skin so that the superior margin is aligned with the cut tissue edge along the mandibular ridge, and one end is aligned with the posterior extent of the newly created vestibule.

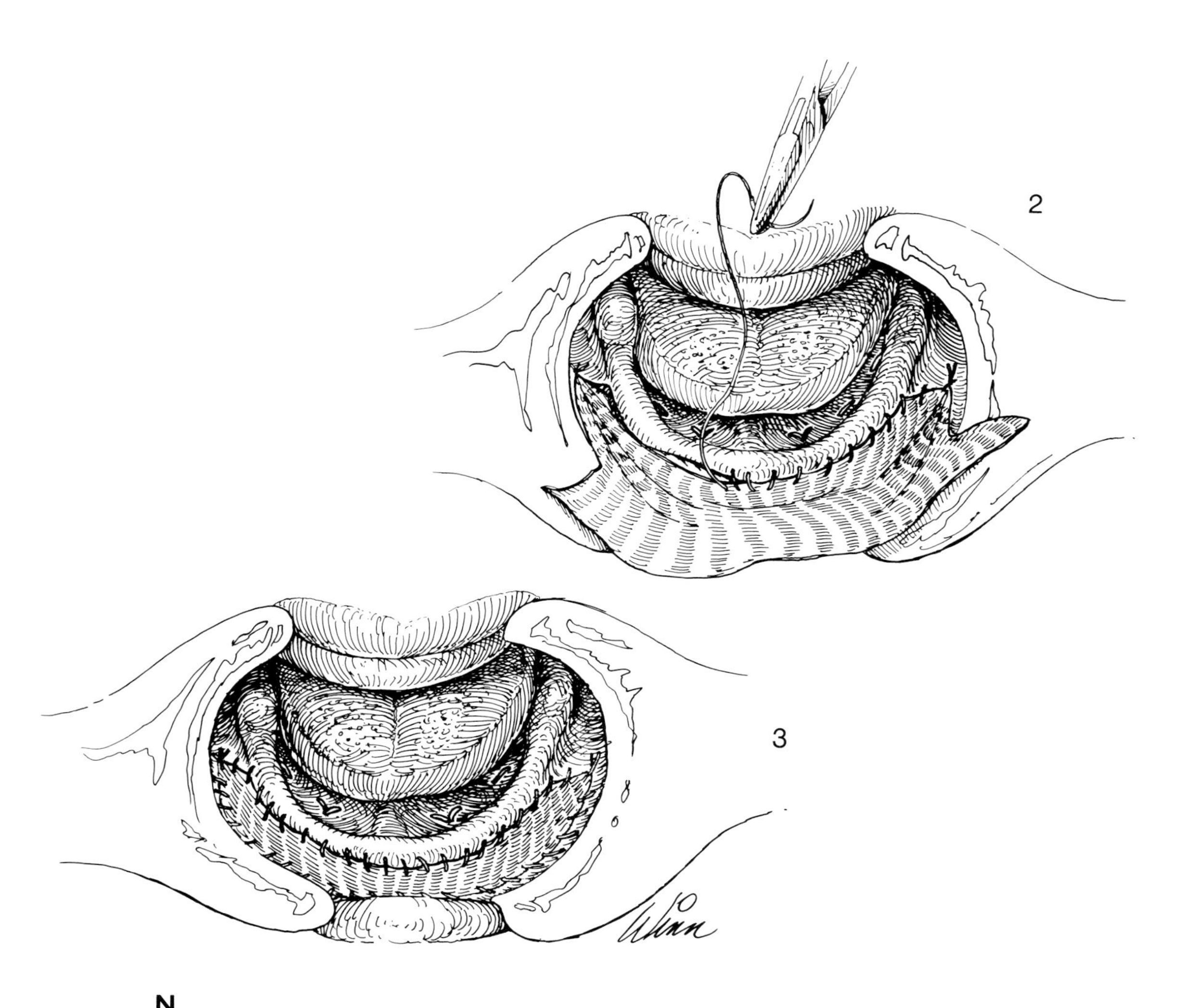

Figure 19–9 *Continued.* *2,* Starting at this posterior alignment point the skin is sutured to the superior mucosal margin utilizing continuous 4–0 plain gut suture. The needle is passed through the slits in the skin graft and the soft tissue at the crest of the ridge without disturbing the graft. The skin graft should be stretched slightly as it is sutured to obtain good adaptation to the ridge. Care is taken to avoid expanding the graft. *3,* The inferior margin of the graft has been trimmed and sutured to the deep mucosal margin. This completes the surgical procedure. A pressure dressing is applied to the lower lip and chin to aid in hemostasis and to pull the lower lip against the skin graft for protection during the first day of healing.

Illustration and legend continued on the following page

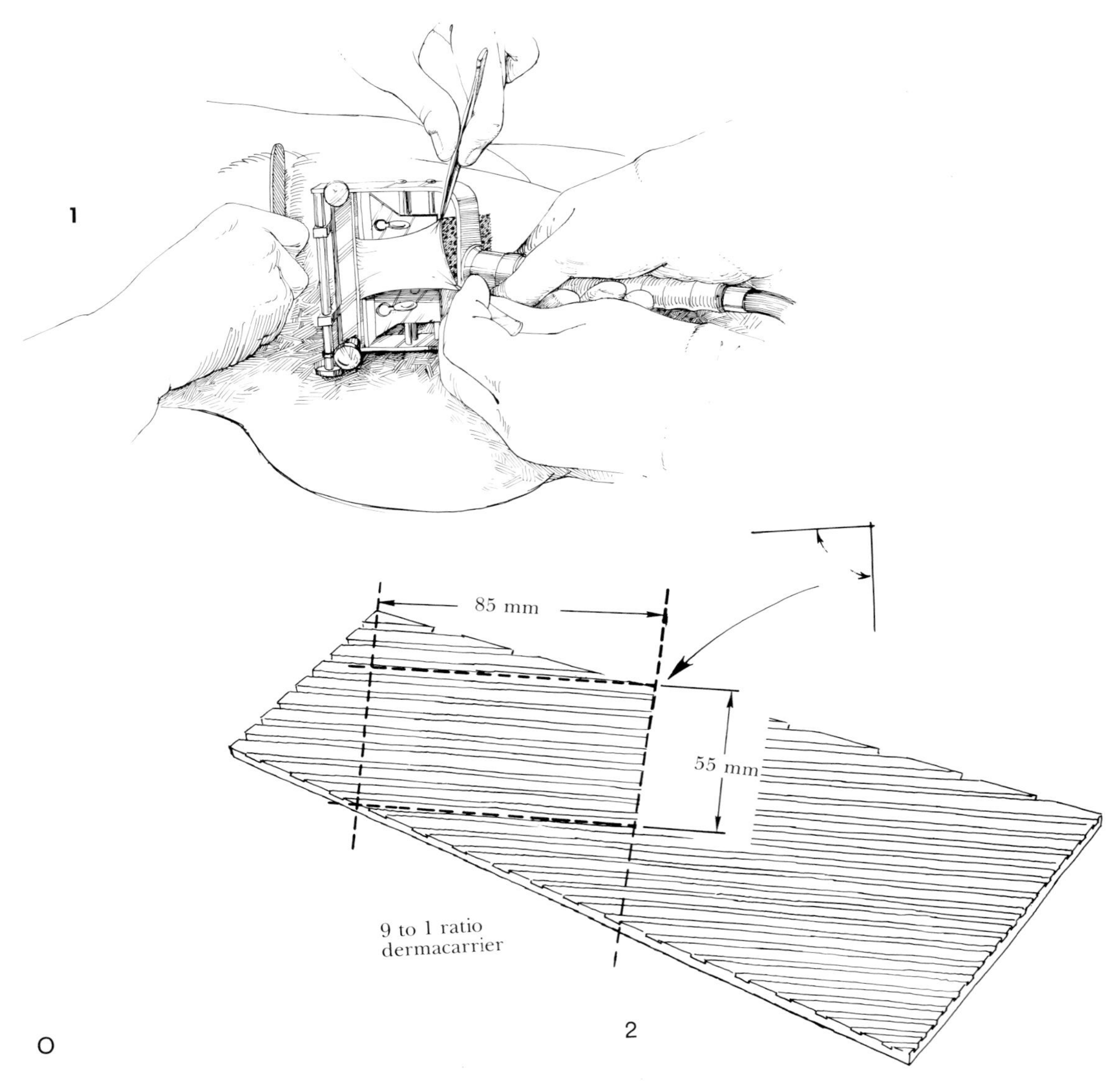

Figure 19–9 *Continued.* *O,* Skin grafting technique. (Kevin McBride, Dallas, Texas.) *1,* The split-thickness skin graft is taken from the anterolateral aspect of the thigh 15 mm. below the iliac crest. Using a mechanical dermatome, a segment of skin 3 cm. × 10 cm. × .0381 cm. thick is removed. Pressure is applied to the donor site with a cold moist compress for a few minutes to aid in hemostasis. The site is then covered with silver sulfadiazine (Silvadene), Telfa, gauze fluffs and a Kerlex bandage. The skin is wrapped in sterile saline soaked until ready for meshing. *2,* A Zimmer meshgraft II dermatome is utilized to fenestrate the skin. A rectangular section 85 mm. × 55 mm. is cut from a 6 to 1 or 9 to 1 plastic dermacarrier. The rectangle is cut with the long edge perpendicular to the grooves in the dermacarrier.

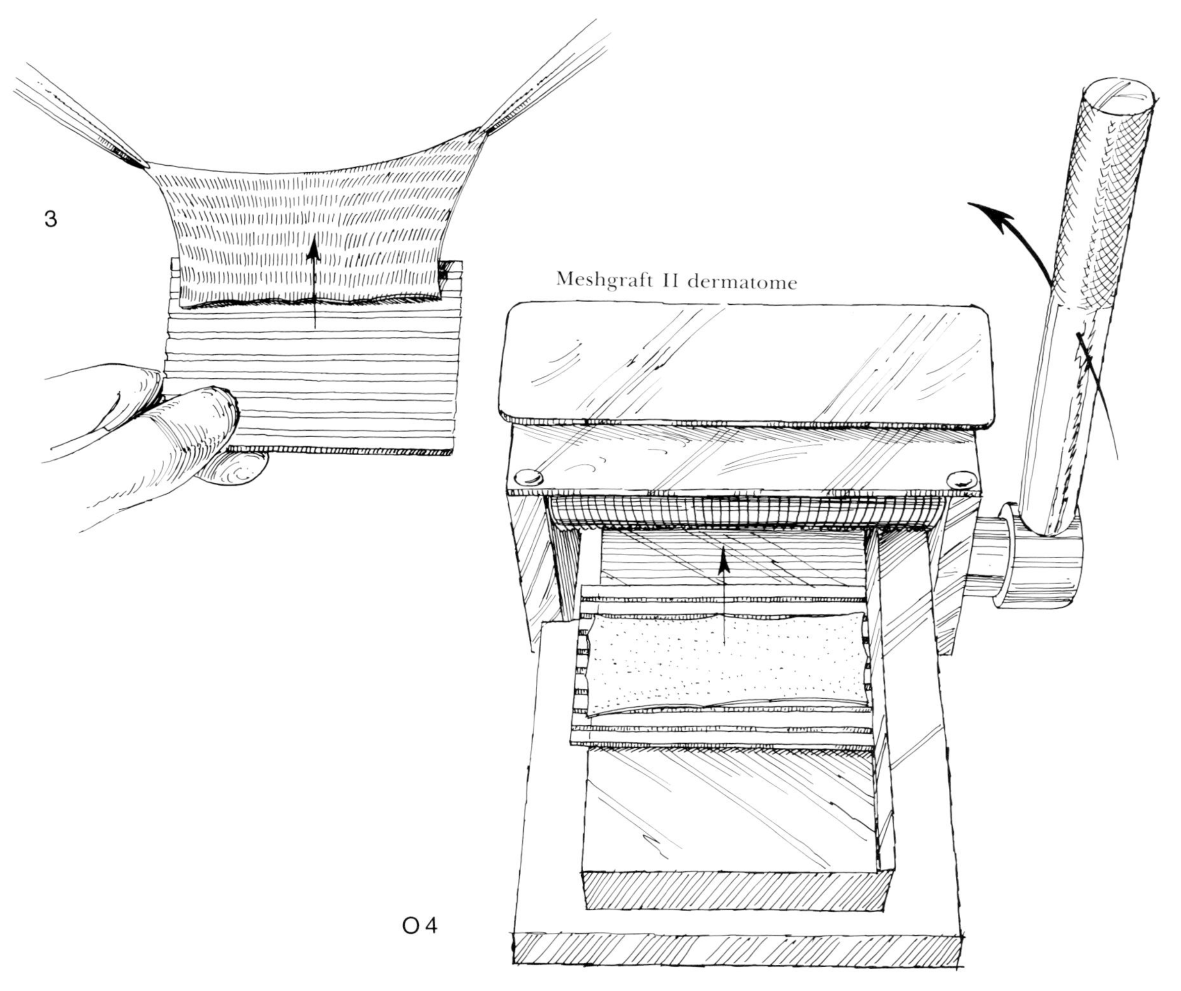

Figure 19–9 *Continued.* *3,* The skin is laid on the grooved surface of the rectangular dermacarrier segment and passed through the dermatome with the grooves perpendicular to the path of insertion. *4,* By cutting the rectangular segment of dermacarrier so that the path of insertion of the grooves might be altered, it is possible to produce a meshed graft that will not expand. Therefore, no gaps are created when the skin is sutured in place. The slits in the graft function to make the skin more manageable for suturing by reducing rolling of the periphery, eliminating hematoma formation by preventing blood from being trapped under the graft, improving adhesion of the graft to the host bed, and simplifying suturing by permitting the surgeon to pass the needle through the slits.

placed, and all wire sutures tightened, the fracture was positively reduced, fixed, and supported. Healing has proceeded uneventfully. A second patient sustained a traumatically induced fracture in the same posterior body area a few weeks post surgery. Because of some displacement of the proximal ramus fragment and continued discomfort, the area was opened via an extraoral approach and an autologous graft from the iliac crest placed, which was supported by a metal crib. The postsurgical recovery has been uneventful.

Although long-term follow-up studies after surgery are not yet available, the 1-year observations are very encouraging. The amount of bone remodeling, resorption, and recontouring should be less than is seen with the onlay bone grafting procedures because of the greater bulk of bone grafted and placement of the majority of the graft between vascularized host mandibular bone. Long-term studies of patients treated with this technique are being conducted.

In Figure 19–9*L* to *N*, the technique for mandibular vestibuloplasty is illustrated.* Mandibular atrophy and bone grafting procedures designed to augment an atrophic mandibular ridge may leave the patient with relatively high buccal and lingual muscles and soft-tissue attachments. Mandibular denture stability may be greatly improved by inferiorly repositioning the muscle and soft-tissue attachments in the buccal vestibule and floor of the mouth. The two muscles primarily responsible for denture instability during speech and mastication are the mentalis and mylohyoid pairs. Surgically repositioning these muscles inferiorly will permit construction of a mandibular denture with longer labial and lingual flanges and will reduce the tendency of these muscles to displace the denture during function. The lengthened labial and lingual flanges contribute to improved denture comfort and stability by distributing stresses applied to the denture over a larger area of the mandible. Mandibular labial vestibuloplasty and lowering of the mylohyoid muscle may be employed after bone graft augmentation of the atrophic mandibular ridge to take full advantage of the newly created mandibular height.

Vestibuloplasty and lowering of the floor of the mouth may be employed in those cases in which the mentalis muscles, mylohyoid muscles, and their associated soft tissues remain attached relatively high on the newly formed mandibular ridge. The mandibular buccal vestibuloplasty and lowering of the mylohyoid muscle permits the surgeon to take full advantage of the increased mandibular height following bone grafting of the edentulous mandibular ridge.

The level of attachment of the mylohyoid muscle may be ascertained by placing the index finger in the floor of the mouth and having the patient protrude his tongue toward the opposite side of the mouth. The level of attachment of the mylohyoid muscle to the mandible may be easily detected with the tip of the index finger. Similarly, the level of attachment of the mentalis muscles can be determined by palpating over the labial aspect of the mandibular ridge while the patient puckers his lips. Puckering or elevation of the lower lip will activate the mentalis muscles, and their level of attachment to the mandible can be readily determined. If it is felt that a satisfactory denture cannot be constructed due to high muscle attachments, a mandibular buccal vestibuloplasty or lowering of the mylohyoid muscle, or both, is indicated.

A technique is described that utilizes suture-immobilized meshed split-thickness skin grafts for the mandibular buccal vestibuloplasty (Fig. 19–9*L-N*). By immobilizing the graft with sutures rather than a stent, it is possible to accomplish all of the goals of the

*Illustrations and text concerning this procedure were supplied by Kevin McBride, Dallas, Texas.

buccal vestibuloplasty while reducing patient discomfort, laboratory procedures, surgical time, and halitosis associated with the fabrication and utilization of stents. By utilizing the suture-immobilized skin graft technique, it is possible to perform the vestibuloplasty within 6 to 8 weeks after bone grafting.

Meshing the skin graft makes it easier to handle, prevents hematoma formation under the graft, simplifies suturing by permitting the needle to be passed through the holes in the graft, and improves the stability of the graft on the periosteum during the suturing phase. Consequently, the few relative disadvantages of suturing intact skin are overcome with the meshing technique. No attempt is actually made to expand the skin by utilizing the meshing technique. Expansion of the graft permits buds of granulation tissue to develop within the holes in the graft. This prolongs healing and produces a somewhat irregular, stippled surface. Consequently, the standard dermacarriers that determine the expansion ratio for the skin after meshing are modified to produce a 1 to 1 ratio that results in no expansion (Fig. 19–90).

Discussion and Complications

Pain, ulceration, and exfoliation of necrotic bone, which are so commonly associated with free bone grafting to the alveolar ridge, have not been observed. In this respect, the relatively small exposure of the grafted bone to stresses of the denture base has probably been significant. The majority of the patients have worn transitional dentures within a relatively short period of time after maxillary and mandibular surgery.

Because the atrophic maxilla is usually small and relatively weak, particular care must be used to properly sequence the planned bone incisions and to completely osteotomize all the segments. Incomplete or incorrect line of sectioning and/or improperly directed forces in downfracturing may predispose the maxilla to an incorrect line of fracture and consequent fragmentation. To date, this complication has occurred twice. In both instances, the posterolateral portion of the tuberosity was probably sectioned incompletely. An undesirable fracture at the junction of the horizontal plate of the palatine bone and posterior part of the maxilla occurred. Despite the fact that mobilization and inferior and anterior movement were more difficult than usual, the repositioned parts of the maxilla were adequately stabilized by multiple blocks of bone.

Based upon our experience with interpositional grafts to the maxilla, secondary vestibuloplasty and skin grafting procedures are usually unnecessary. Secondary re-epithelialization was used for our initial maxillary patient only.

Positional Change and Stability. A retrospective study of postoperative stability and osseous changes was made of nine patients with maxillary or mandibular atrophy who were treated by interpositional bone grafting techniques.[7] A tracing of each preoperative cephalogram was made on acetate paper. The preoperative tracing was then superimposed on the immediate postoperative and the longest available follow-up cephalometric radiograph along the SN plane with registration at sella. Positional changes of the repositioned inferior part of the maxilla and the superior portion of the mandible were determined by recording the change in millimeters before and immediately after surgery. The stability of the procedure was determined by measuring the millimeter change in the values between the initial and the subsequent postoperative radiographs. Table 19–1 shows the linear changes produced by the interpositional grafting procedures and the discernible postoperative changes. There was minimal discernible positional change or resorption of the portion of the maxilla or mandible that was moved by interpositional grafting procedures.

TABLE 19–1. Summary of Linear and Postoperative Changes in Nine Patients Following Interpositional Bone

Other Procedures	*Complications*	*Follow-up (months)*	*Resorption (mm)*	*Patient*	*Age*	*Sex*	*Surgery**	*Amount of Vertical Movement (mm)*	
								ANT.	POST.
Ramus osteotomies Vestibuloplasty and split-thickness skin graft Dentures	–	10	0	M.C.	48	F	2,3	10	–
Submucosal resection Dentures	–	14	1	A.M.	40	M	1,3	10	5
Vestibuloplasty and Split-thickness skin graft Dentures	Asymmetric placement of bone graft	4	0	M.M.	38	F	2,3	12	–
Dentures	–	4	0	R.P.	51	F	1,3	12	–
Mandibular staple Dentures	–	9	1	W.D.	55	M	1,3	11	7
Mandibular subapical osteotomy Partial glossectomy Dentures	Fragmentation of maxilla	8	0	J.D.	36	M	1,3	8	5
–	–	3	0	L.G.	58	F	1,4	8	–
Bilateral ramus osteotomies Vestibuloplasty and split-thickness skin graft	Fragmentation of maxilla	11	1	A.C.	53	M	1,3	10	8
Vestibuloplasty and split-thickness skin graft	Floor of mouth hematoma	3	0	C.A.	62	M	2,3	10	–

*KEY 1. Maxillary interpositional bone graft
2. Mandibular interpositional bone graft
3. Autogenous bone
4. Freeze-dried bone

Sequential radiographic and cephalometric tracings demonstrated early consolidation of the grafted bone, minimal resorption of the repositioned osseous segments, and a very small decrease of alveolar ridge height over an average postoperative follow-up period of seven months.

The distal portion of the maxilla was repositioned inferiorly an average of 9 mm in the anterior region and approximately 6 mm in the posterior region. In the mandible, the average increase of superior ridge height in the premolar region was approximately one-third as much as in the incisor region.

The immediate use of a splint or denture over the palatal mucosa is probably contraindicated when Le Fort I osteotomy is accomplished through a circumvestibular incision. The use of such appliances is deferred at least two weeks to obviate vascular ischemia that could potentially occur because of pressure against the palatal vascular pedicle.

In the maxilla, there is presently no practical "minimum" requirement for the amount of maxillary bone to allow Le Fort I osteotomy and interpositional bone grafting. Several patients have had virtually no alveolar ridge. In the mandible, however, at least 9 to 10 mm of vertical mandibular bone height is necessary for horizontal bisection of the mandibular body and interpositional bone grafting. With this in mind, it is important that dentists "plan ahead" for preprosthetic patients and program surgery so that interpositional grafting is done when the procedure is still feasible. When there is less than 8 or 9 mm of mandibular bone height, onlay bone grafting may indeed be the only recourse.

To date, our animal and clinical results[7, 10] and the experimental results of others[13, 16] support the concept of treating the atrophic maxillary and mandibular alveolar ridge by interpositional bone grafting. Although the short-term stability of this technique has been excellent, most of the patients have worn dentures for less than three years. Long-term follow-up studies are necessary to determine the fate of the repositioned and grafted bone.

Finally, the use of interpositional alloplastics such as hydroxyapatite may be a new frontier.[8] The successful use of such materials would eliminate the greatest problem associated with these procedures, namely the morbidity accompanying procurement of a large block of bone from the hip. The use of bank bone may also be considered.[23] Freeze-dried bone has been used successfully in a limited number of cases and may be combined with autogenous particulate cancellous marrow grafts.

Visor Osteotomy

Franz Härle

The absolute height of an atrophied mandible may be increased by the technique of visor osteotomy. In this procedure the alveolar ridge of the mandible is osteotomized and moved on the principle of a visor. The two parts are fixed together with wires, thus increasing the absolute height of the alveolar ridge. This method avoids the complications of bone transplantation as the risk of infection from the pedicled bone graft attached to the soft tissue is minimal and therefore rejection of the transplant is not a factor.

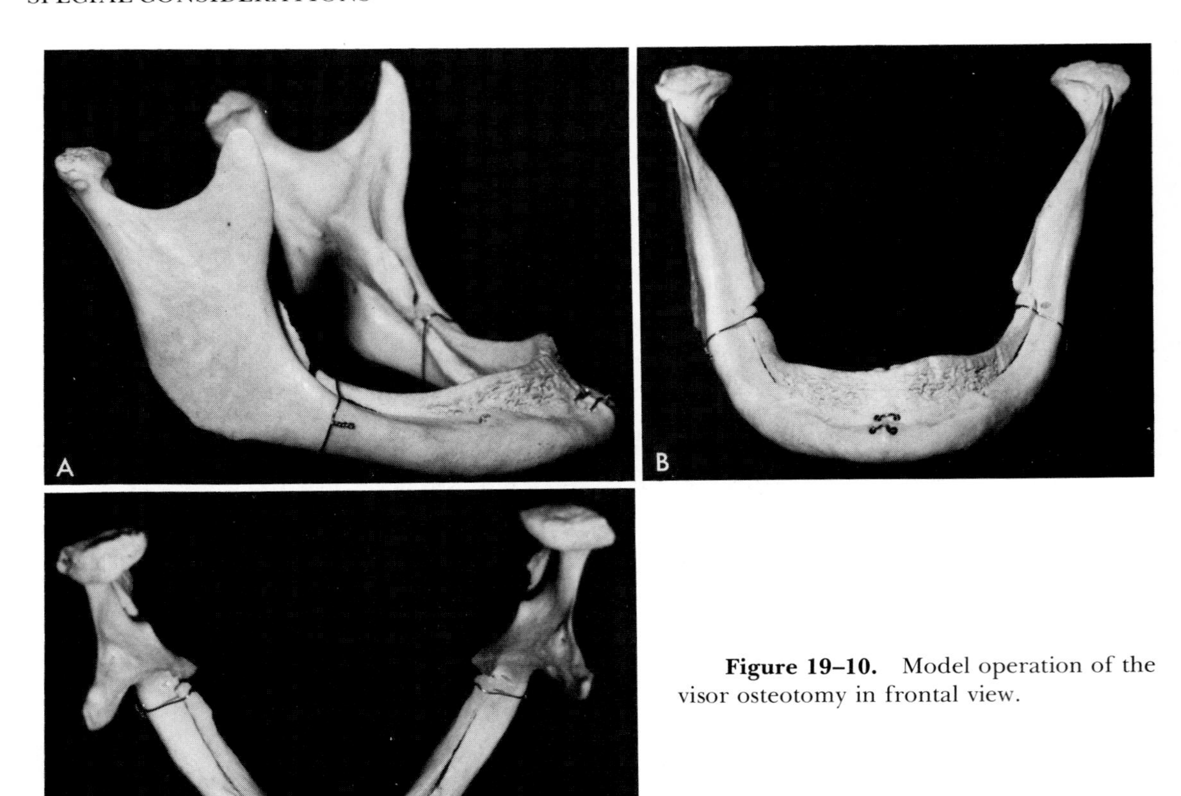

Figure 19–10. Model operation of the visor osteotomy in frontal view.

Mandibular Surgery Technique (Fig. 19–10)

The mandibular surgical procedure is accomplished intraorally in the operating room with the patient under endotracheal anesthesia. A vasoconstrictor is injected into the labiobuccal vestibule and lingual floor to aid in hemostasis. The design of the soft-tissue flap for exposure of the mandible is simple. An incision is made through the mucoperiosteum on the rim of the alveolar ridge in the attached gingiva from retromolar pad to retromolar pad. The mandible is exposed, and the neurovascular bundles at both mandibular foramina are displayed (Fig. 19–11). Reference marks are etched in the occlusal cortex with a fine rotating fissure bur under constant irrigation with saline solution. For further orientation, small holes are drilled with a fissure bur. These holes lie in the lingual third of the horizontal part of the mandible. In the anterior part of the mandible the holes are drilled in the midline. With the use of an extremely fine oscillating sawblade a vertical osteotomy is made from the angle on one side to the contralateral angle in order to divide the mandibular bone into equal lingual and vestibular parts (Figs. 19–12 and 19–17).

The mandible is then split lengthwise, taking care to avoid injury to the neurovascular bundle. The freely movable lingual portion of the split mandible can then be moved upward in the form of a visor, along with adherent soft tissue. The two parts are then fixed together by means of circumferential wiring at the lateral side and intraosseous wiring in the midline area (Figs. 19–13 through 19–15). It is also helpful to reflect the mucoperiosteum from the inferior border of the mandible in order to obtain adequate

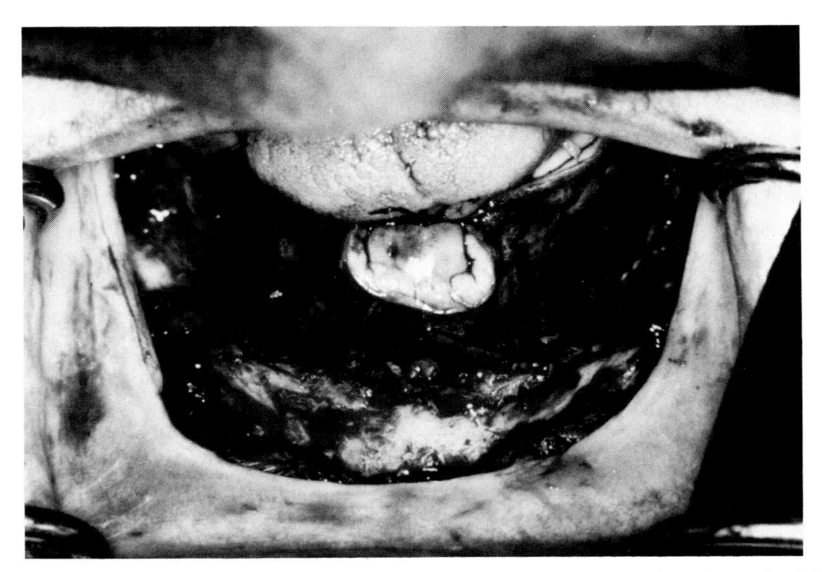

Figure 19–11. Operative view after soft-tissue preparation before bone incision.

tissue to cover the visor-osteotomized mandible with minimal tension. When these maneuvers do not allow adequate relaxation, the periosteum at the inferior border of the mandible is incised longitudinally to improve further relaxation. The mucoperiosteal soft-tissue incision is sutured with continuous nonresorbable sutures.

Discussion and Complications

In one patient the lingual visor-osteotomized bone was broken. The fracture was fixed with wiring, and after consolidation of the bone six months later, a total ves-

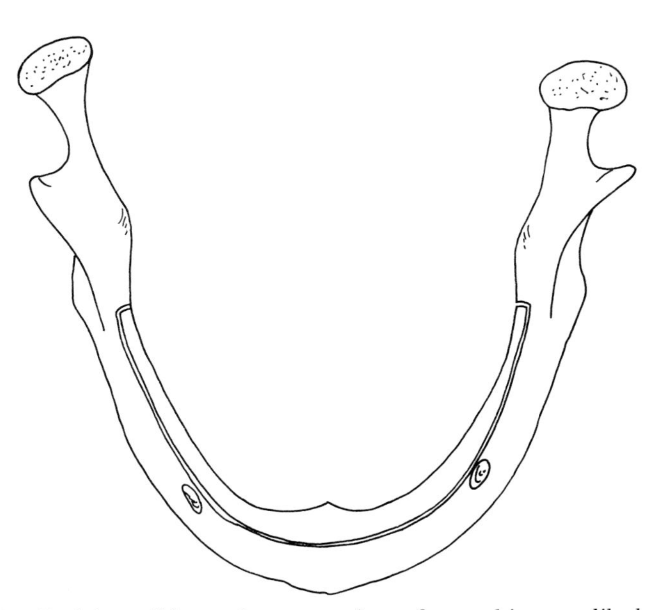

Figure 19–12. Incision of bone for correction of atrophic mandibular alveolar ridge by vertical mandibular osteotomy (visor osteotomy).

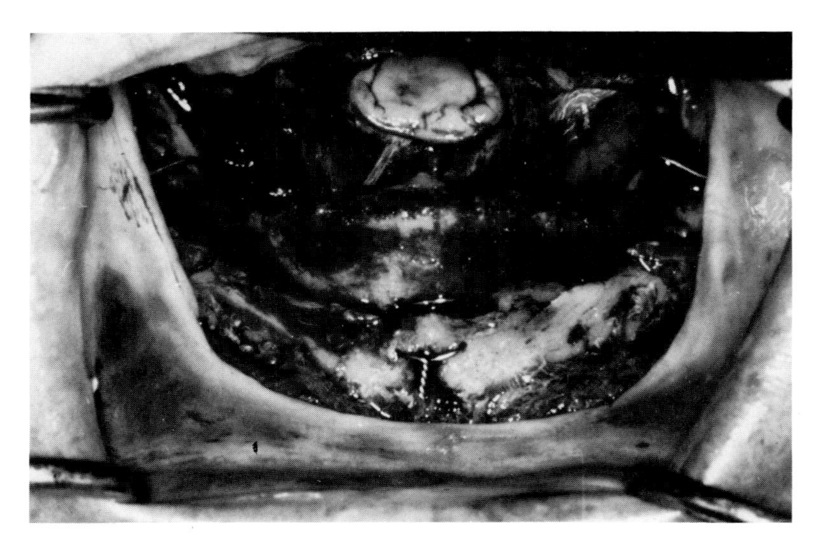

Figure 19–13. Operative view after bone incision, ridge augmentation, and wiring of the visor osteotomized mandible.

tibuloplasty completed the procedure. The wires were removed at this second operation. In all other cases secondary total vestibuloplasty six weeks after visor osteotomy, before denture construction, was necessary. Pain, ulceration, and exfoliation of necrotic bone have not been observed.

A retrospective study of postoperative stability and osseous change was made of ten patients with mandibular atrophy who were treated by the visor-osteotomy technique. The preoperative cephalometric tracing was superimposed on the cephalometric radiographs taken one year and two years postoperatively. At least 8 mm of vertical mandibular bone height is necessary for the visor-osteotomy technique. The resorption of bone was 18 per cent of height in the first year after surgery. In the second year mandibular height resorption was 10 per cent (Fig. 19–16). The visor method of sliding osteotomy improves the pseudoprognathism of the intermaxillary relationship and increases the mandibular height by about 80 per cent. Three of ten patients in the two-year follow-up study were more than 70 years of age.

The principal hazard of the visor osteotomy is injury to the mandibular nerve. Two years after surgery three mandibular nerves were anesthetic, three nerves were hyperesthetic, and fourteen nerves had normal function. Peterson has modified Härle's technique by accomplishing the visor osteotomy and vestibuloplasty simultaneously (Fig. 19–17).

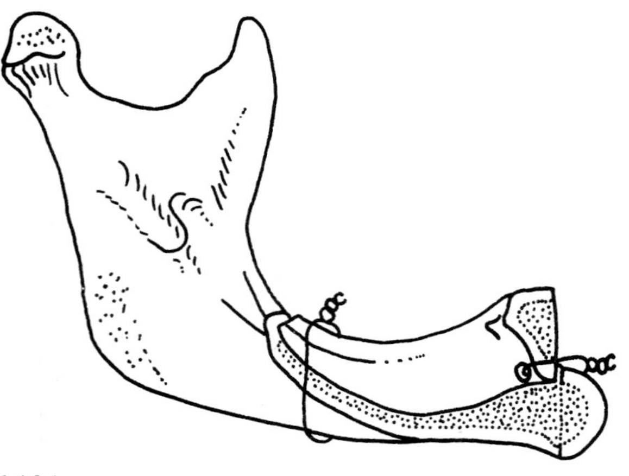

Figure 19–14. Sagittal view of mandible showing design of bone incision.

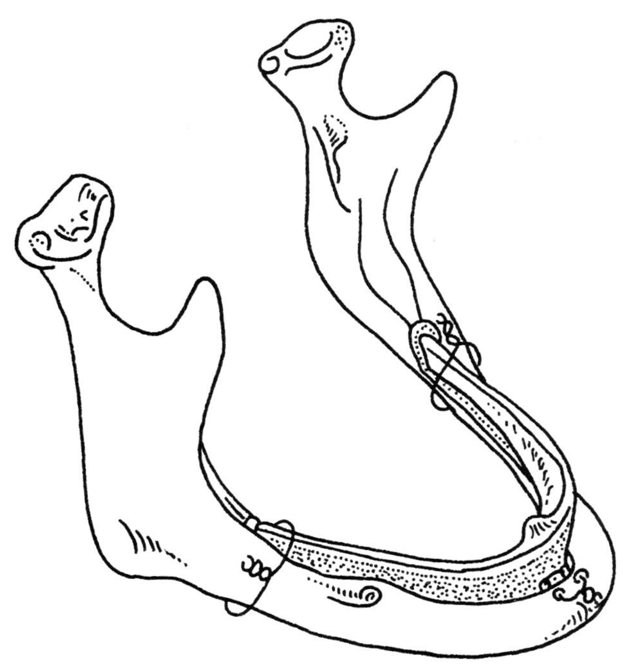

Figure 19–15. Lateral view of mandible showing design of bone incision.

VISOR OSTEOTOMY (10 cases)				
height of mandible	before max 15 mm min 8 mm $\bar{x}$ 12.5 mm	after max 23 mm min 15 mm $\bar{x}$ 20.3 mm	1 year max 22 mm min 14 mm $\bar{x}$ 18.9 mm	2 years max 21 mm min 14 mm $\bar{x}$ 18.1 mm
resorption			1.4 mm = 18 %	0.8 mm = 10 %

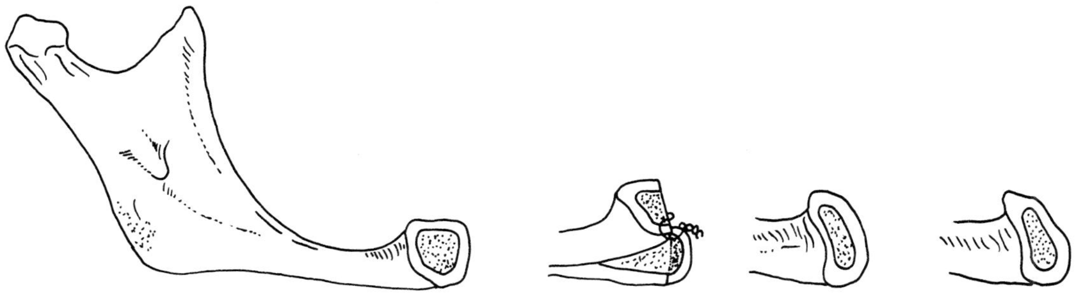

Figure 19–16. Visor osteotomy, 2-year follow-up examination of 10 patients.

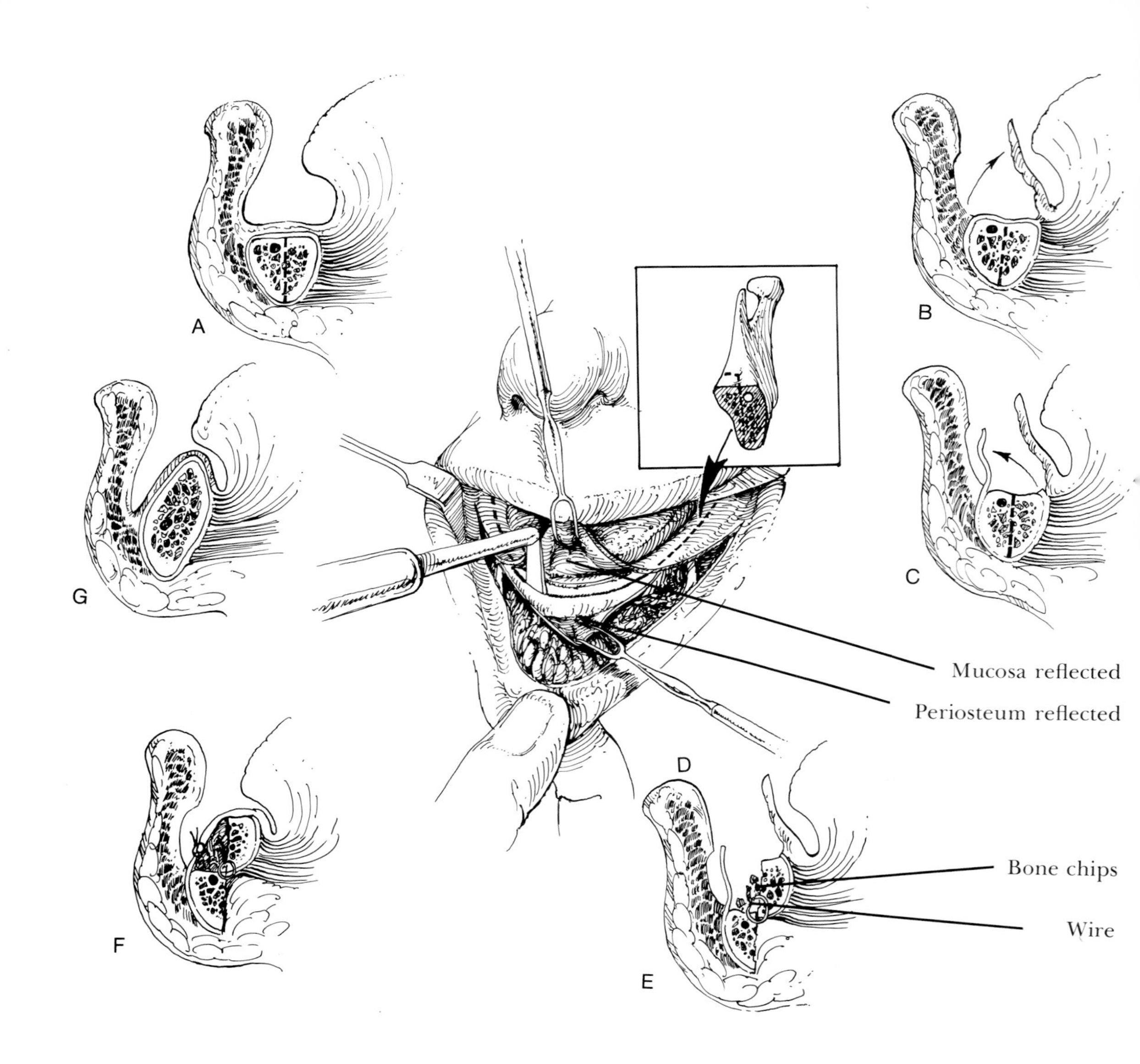

Figure 19–17. *A,* Preoperative cross-sectional view of anterior region of atrophic mandible; the medial-lateral dimension of the mandible is relatively wide. *B,* Sagittal view of the mandible showing design of soft-tissue incision that is made midway between the depth of the mandibular labial vestibule and the wet line of the lower lip; the mucosa is incised to facilitate development of a lingually based mucosal flap. *C,* The periosteum is incised at the lingual aspect of the ridge and reflected buccally; planned vertical osteotomy is represented by a broken line. *D,* With mucosa and periosteum retracted, sagittal mandibular osteotomy is made with a thin oscillating saw blade. The *inset* shows a cross-sectional view of the posterior region of an atrophic mandible; the *broken line* indicates the planned vertical bone incision, which is carefully made by a properly angulated and positioned saw blade. *E,* The lingual segment is pedicled by mylohyoid, genioglossus, geniohyoid, and digastric muscles; the lingual mucosa is repositioned superiorly and fixed with interosseous wire or heavy sutures; the particulate marrow graft is placed on the labial aspect of the repositioned lingual segment. *F,* The wound is closed by suturing the free margin of the lingually based mucosal flap to the free margin of the buccal periosteal flap with running horizontal mattress suture of #3–0 chromic catgut. The particulate marrow graft is packed onto the buccal surface of the repositioned lingual segment. The denuded lip and cheek remain uncovered to re-epithelialize. *G,* Configuration of augmented ridge after healing of mucosal and bony incisions. (Technique of Dr. Larry Peterson, Farmington, Connecticut.)

CASE STUDIES

CASE 19–1 (Fig. 19–18)

A 42-year-old woman was referred for extraction of her remaining teeth, which were severely involved by periodontal disease.

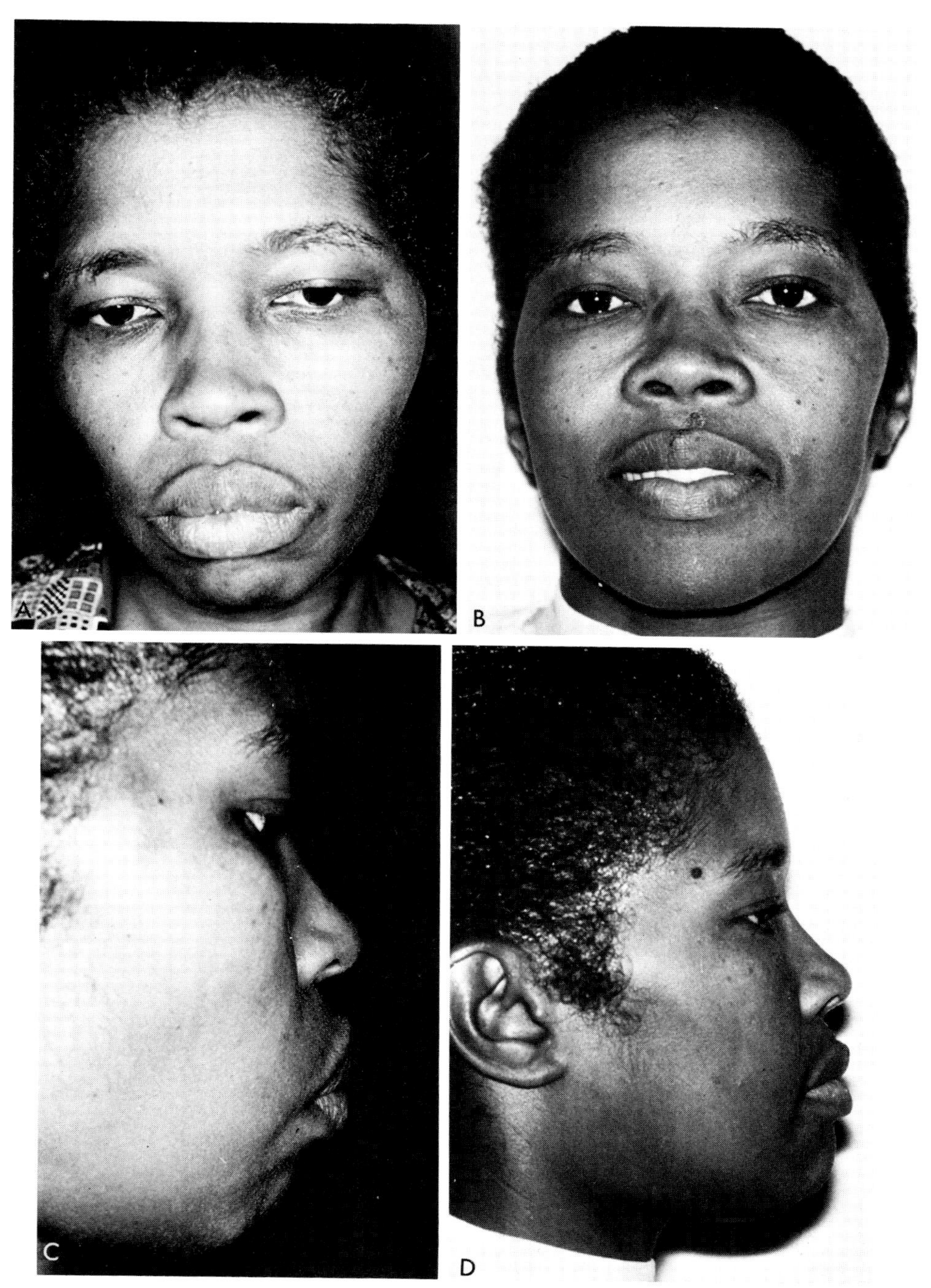

Figure 19–18. *A–D,* Facial appearance of patient. In pretreatment photographs, note procumbent lips and deficient chin (*A* and *C*). Appearance after treatment (*B* and *D*).

Illustration continued on page 1469.

PROBLEM LIST

Esthetics (Figs. 19–18*A* and *C*)

Frontal. Procumbency of the upper and lower lips.
Profile. Protrusive upper and lower lips. Contour-deficient chin.

Cephalometric Analysis (Fig. 19–18*E*)

1. Maxillary excess.
2. Maxillary and mandibular dentoalveolar protrusion.
3. Contour-deficient chin, secondary to numbers 1 and 2.

Occlusal Analysis (Figs. 19–18*G* and *H*)

Dental Arch Form. Maxilla: protrusive and flared dentition. Mandible: procumbant incisors.

Dental Alignment. Multiple missing teeth in mandible and maxilla with diastemas present in anterior maxilla.

Dental Occlusion. Class 1 cuspid relationship with 8-mm horizontal overlap. Reduced vertical space between the left posterior alveolar segments.

TREATMENT PLAN

Surgical Treatment

1. Posteriorly reposition (7.0 mm) anterior maxillary alveolus to correct procumbency of the upper and lower lips.
2. Accomplish relative correction of contour-deficient chin by reduction of dentoalveolar protrusion.
3. Reposition anterior maxilla posteriorly to reduce maxillary excess.
4. Extract dentition and posteriorly reposition anterior maxilla to correct protrusive and flared maxillary dentition.
5. Superiorly reposition (5.0 mm) left posterior maxillary alveolus to correct reduced vertical space between the left buccal alveolar segments.

Nonsurgical Treatment

1. Extract periodontally involved mandibular teeth and replace with complete lower dentures.

FOLLOW-UP (Figs. 19–18*B, D, F, I, J*)

Subjective

Postsurgically, the patient had no complaints of postoperative discomfort.

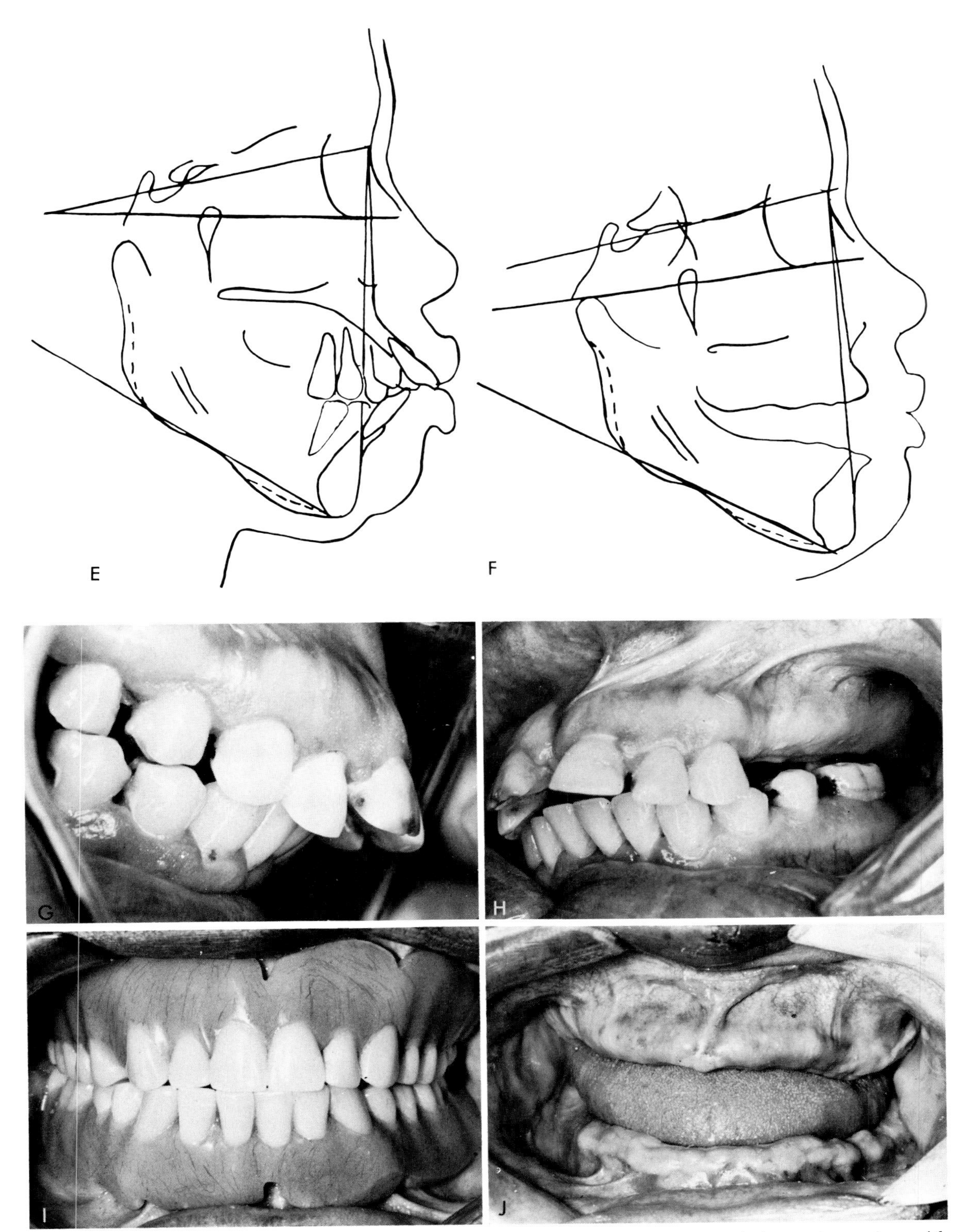

Figure 19–18 *Continued.* *E,* Bimaxillary protrusion. *F,* Post-treatment cephalometric tracing with prosthesis in place. *G* and *H,* Multiple missing teeth, supraeruption posterior teeth. *I,* Occlusal relationship established with combined anterior and posterior maxillary ostectomies with full denture prosthesis. *J,* Interarch space following superior repositioning of posterior maxillary segment.

Objective

The maxillary fragments were stabilized by direct interosseous wiring, and a clear acrylic splint secured by circumzygomatic suspension wires. Three weeks postoperatively, the splint was removed. There was moderate mobility of the anterior maxillary segment; the posterior segment was firm. Two months postsurgery, the bony segments were firm and complete. The upper and lower dentures were fabricated. In addition to the functional improvement, the patient's profile had been improved and bimaxillary dentoalveolar protrusion and the maxillary excess were eliminated. Adequate space was present in the left posterior segment for the maxillary and mandibular dentition.

COMMENT

Maxillary excess could have been eliminated by a radical alveolectomy, necessitating sacrifice of extensive alveolar bone. By using an anterior maxillary ostectomy, alveolar bone was conserved and facial esthetics enhanced.

Inadequate ridge space in the posterior areas would lead to prosthetic compromise unless improved. Even though denture teeth and denture bases can be reduced, this may still be inadequate. When insufficient interarch space exists because of redundant soft tissues, the space may be improved by soft-tissue reduction without loss of alveolar bone or antral perforation. However, reduced posterior space may result from supraeruption of the posterior maxillary teeth following early loss of the opposing mandibular teeth. In this instance, posterior maxillary surgical procedures permit superior repositioning of the posterior alveolus, conserving alveolar bone and establishing an optimal functional relationship.

Surgeon: Roger West, Seattle, Washington. *Prosthodontist:* Joe Ampil, Dallas, Texas.

CASE 19–2 (Fig. 19–19)

A 45-year-old woman was referred for possible improvement of her unstable denture relationship and to "improve her profile." The patient related a history of a Class III occlusal relationship with her natural dentition. A sibling also had a Class III occlusal relationship that had been corrected surgically. The patient had been edentulous in the maxilla for approximately 10 years. A problem list was established:

PROBLEM LIST

Esthetics (Figs. 19–19*A* and *C*)

Frontal. A relative deficiency in the region of the alar bases lateral to the nose. Ptosis of the left upper eyelid, secondary to trauma.

Profile. Maxillary deficiency extending superiorly to the region of the alar bases.

Cephalometric Analysis (Fig. 19–19*E*)

1. Maxillary deficiency.
2. Edentulous maxilla.
3. Relative soft-tissue chin prominence.

Occlusal Analysis (Figs 19–19*G* and *H*)

Dental Arch Form. Maxilla: edentulous. Mandible: normal anteriorly, edentulous bilateral posterior segments.

Dental Alignment. Proclined maxillary denture teeth, satisfactory alignment of the posterior dentition.

Dental Occlusion. Class I molar and cuspid relationship with the maxillary denture teeth set anterior to the denture base.

TREATMENT PLAN

Surgical Treatment

1. Correct relative deficiency in the region of the alar bases by maxillary advancement utilizing a horizontal maxillary osteotomy.
2. Remedy maxillary deficiency extending superiorly to the region of the alar bases by maxillary advancement performed at the level of the alar bases.
3. Reduce maxillary deficiency by maxillary advancement.
4. Improve soft-tissue chin prominence by attempting relative correction using maxillary advancement to provide additional upper lip support.
5. Correct proclined maxillary denture teeth by maxillary advancement with maxillary incisors set over supporting maxillary alveolar bone.

FOLLOW-UP (Figs. 19–19*B, D, F, I, J*)

Subjective

The patient experienced a moderate amount of postoperative discomfort secondary to the bone grafting procedure and the horizontal maxillary osteotomy. The discomfort improved dramatically following the removal of circumzygomatic suspension wires and the surgical splint six weeks following surgical advancement of the maxilla.

Objective

The patient was placed in intermaxillary fixation, bone grafts were inserted, and interosseous wires and suspension wires were placed. Intermaxillary fixation was found to be unnecessary and was removed. This facilitated the patient's ability to communicate, as well as her ability to masticate very soft foods. After the circumzygomatic suspension wires and the circumpalatal wires were removed, the maxillary surgical splint was relined temporarily and within six months of surgery the final prosthesis was constructed.

COMMENT

The unsatisfactory functional relationship that existed between the maxilla and mandible could have been improved by surgically repositioning the mandible posteriorly or advancing the maxilla. However, the discrepancy in the denture bases was determined to be approximately 8 mm. Therefore, it was felt that the magnitude of the mandibular change that would be required would not be esthetically acceptable. In addition, this would not have corrected the deficiency that was present adjacent to the alar bases.

The surgical splints were constructed after the correct vertical skeletal relationships had been determined by the prosthodontist. This would have been necessary had

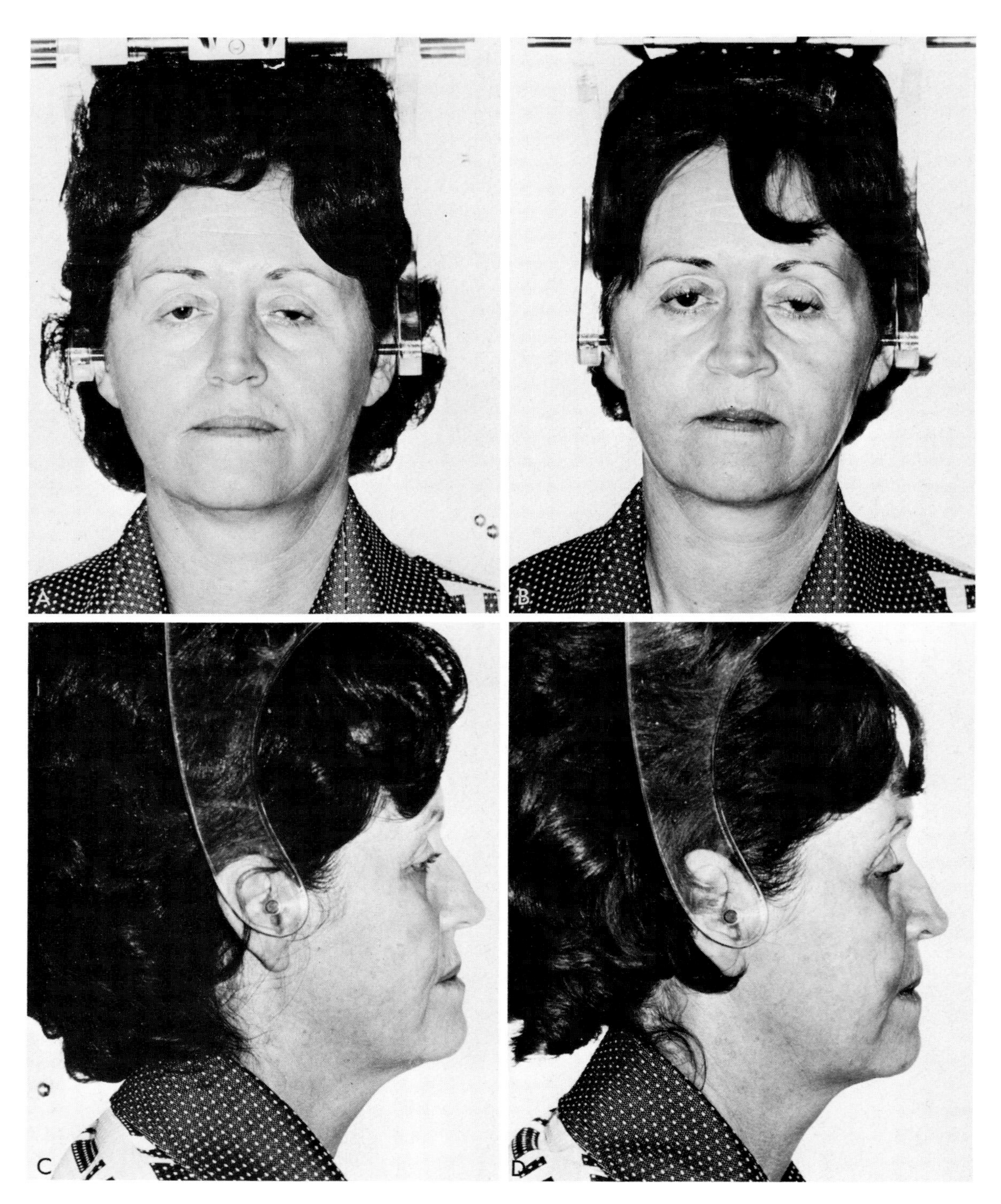

Figure 19–19. *A, C,* and *E,* Maxillary deficiency extending to alar base region, relative chin prominence. *B* and *D,* Post-treatment appearance. *F,* Post-treatment cephalometric tracing with prosthesis in place. *G* and *H,* Pretreatment dental relationship. *I* and *J,* Occlusion following maxillary advancement and insertion of new prosthesis.

Illustration continued on the opposite page

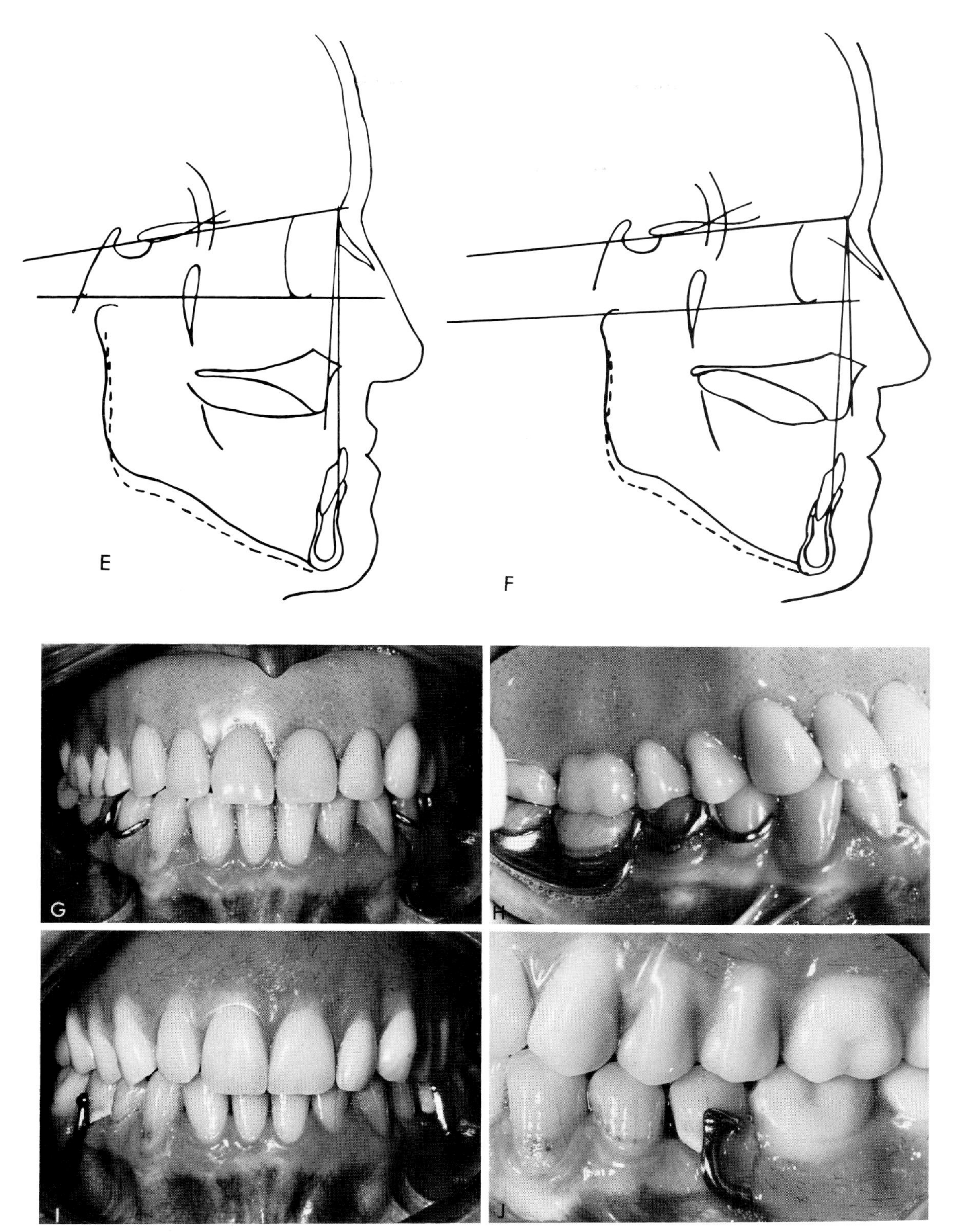

Figure 19–19 *Continued.*

mandibular surgery been selected, as vertical changes would result in anteroposterior changes as well. Maxillary advancement provided a stable correction and, in this instance, was performed without the necessity for intermaxillary fixation, thus minimizing the patient's discomfort.

Surgeon: Roger West, Seattle, Washington. *Prosthodontist:* James Lord, Seattle, Washington.

CASE 19–3 (Fig. 19–20)*

A 42-year-old man was referred by his general dentist for possible improvement in jaw relationship prior to constructing complete dentures.

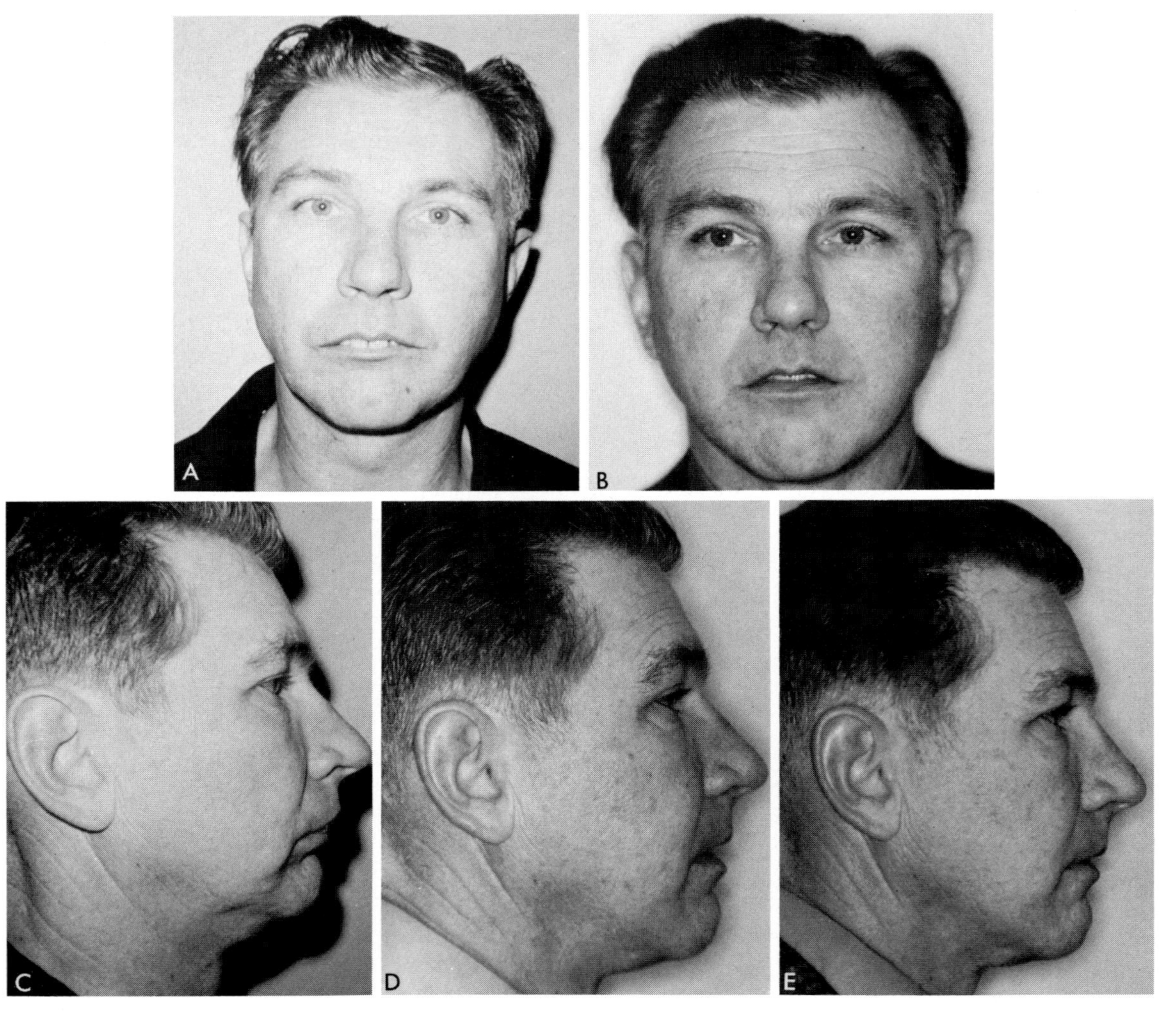

Figure 19–20. *A* and *C*, Deficient lower face. *B* and *E*, Facial appearance 24 months after surgery. *D* and *H*, Improved profile and dental relationship after mandibular advancement. *F*, Excessive horizontal overlap, periodontally involved teeth. *G*, Dental and skeletal Class II relationship. *I*, Dolder bar in place on mandibular canines after palatal mucosal graft to anterior facial vestibule. *J*, Complete dentures in place.

Illustration continued on the opposite page

PROBLEM LIST

Esthetics (Figs. 19–20*A* and *C*)

Frontal. Deficient lower face.
Profile. Lip incompetence, deficient lower face.

Occlusal Analysis (Figs. 19–20*F* and *G*)

Dental Arch Form. Maxilla: protrusive and flared dentition.
Dental Alignment. Multiple missing and periodontally involved teeth.
Dental Occlusion. Dental and skeletal Class II relationship.

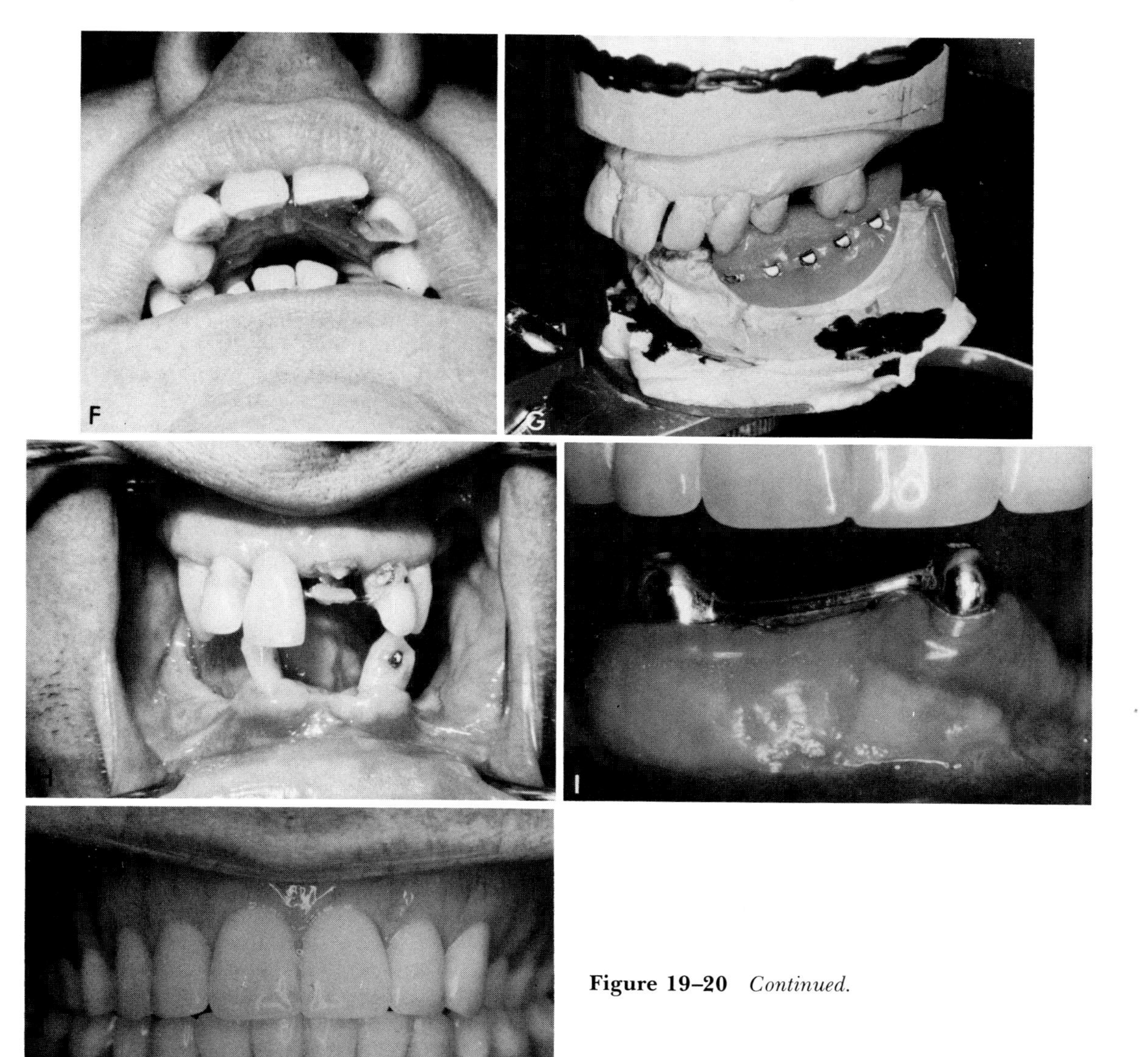

Figure 19–20 *Continued.*

TREATMENT PLAN

Surgical Treatment

1. Reposition mandible in anterior direction to correct deficient lower face.

Nonsurgical Treatment

1. Extract remaining maxillary teeth and mandibular teeth except mandibular canines. Replace teeth with complete dentures.

FOLLOW-UP (Figs. 19–20*B, D, E, H* through *J*)

The mandible was brought forward with a C osteotomy. With the aid of a mandibular denture splint the lower jaw was immobilized for six weeks. At six weeks the jaw was clinically healed and stable. A palatal mucosal graft was placed in the anterior facial vestibule and preparation and fabrication of a Dolder bar for mandibular canine teeth was accomplished. Following insertion of complete dentures, the patient has had a satisfactory esthetic and functional result.

COMMENT

Surgery in the mandible could have been carried out intraorally or extraorally. The extraoral approach was chosen because the patient had a resorbed mandibular posterior alveolar ridge and scarring from an intraoral incision could be eliminated.

Surgeon: Mark Kohn, Lexington, Kentucky.

CASE 19–4 (Fig. 19–21)

A 48-year-old woman sought prosthetic treatment to replace her "loose dentures." The following problem list was established, based upon a review of her records and clinical examination:

PROBLEM LIST

Esthetics (Figs. 19–21*A* and *C*)

Frontal. Significant facial asymmetry with deviation of the chin to the right. Increased vertical dimension on the left side of the face with marked canting of the mandible.

Profile. Concave facial profile with reduced lower facial height.

Cephalometric Analysis (Figs. 19–21*E* and *G*)

1. Marked mandibular and facial asymmetry.

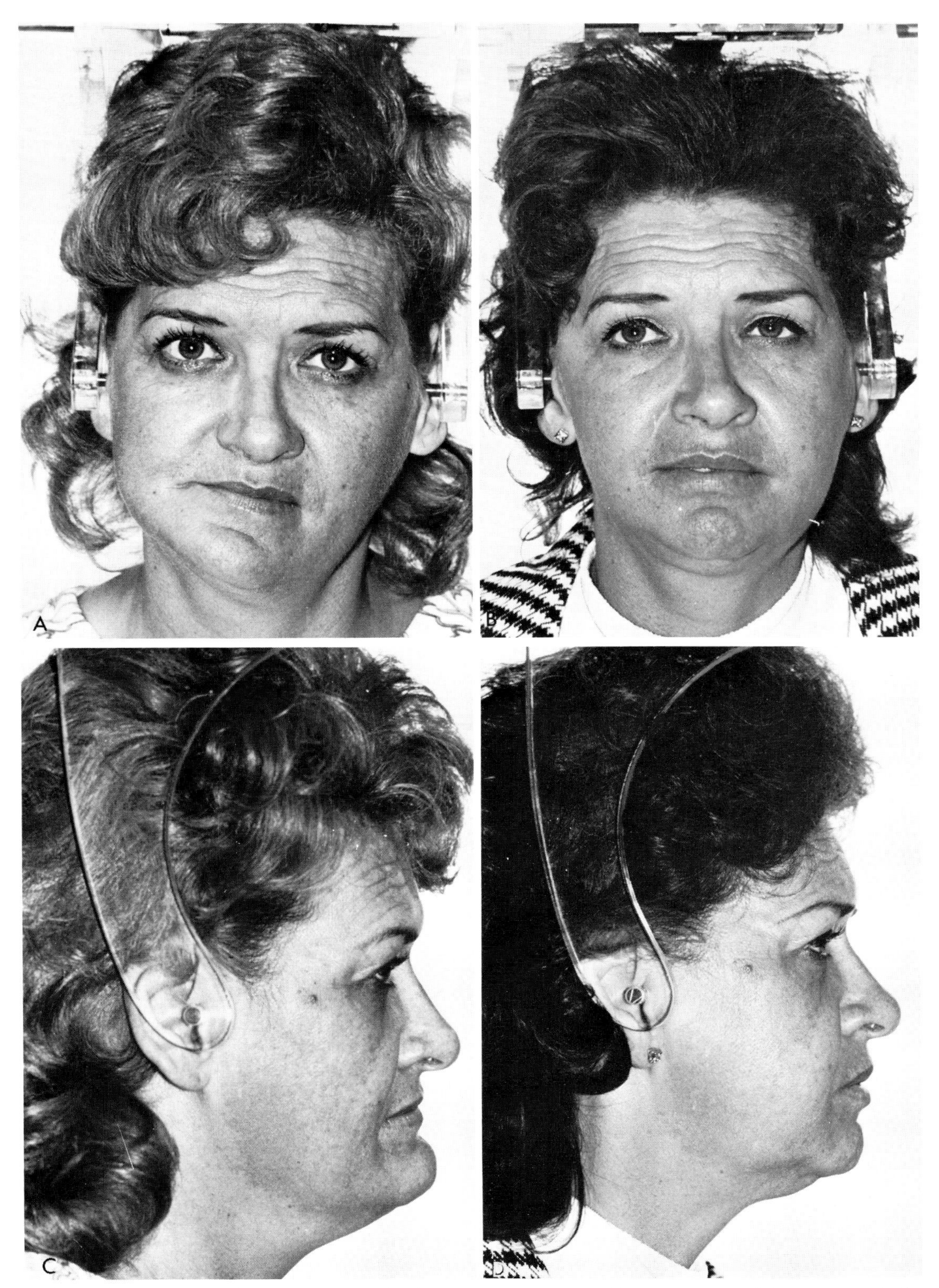

Figure 19–21. *A,* Facial asymmetry, chin deviated to right. *B* and *D,* Appearance following surgical and prosthetic treatment (vertical osteotomy of the right ramus and sagittal osteotomy of the left ramus). *C,* Concave profile.

Illustration and legend continued on the following page

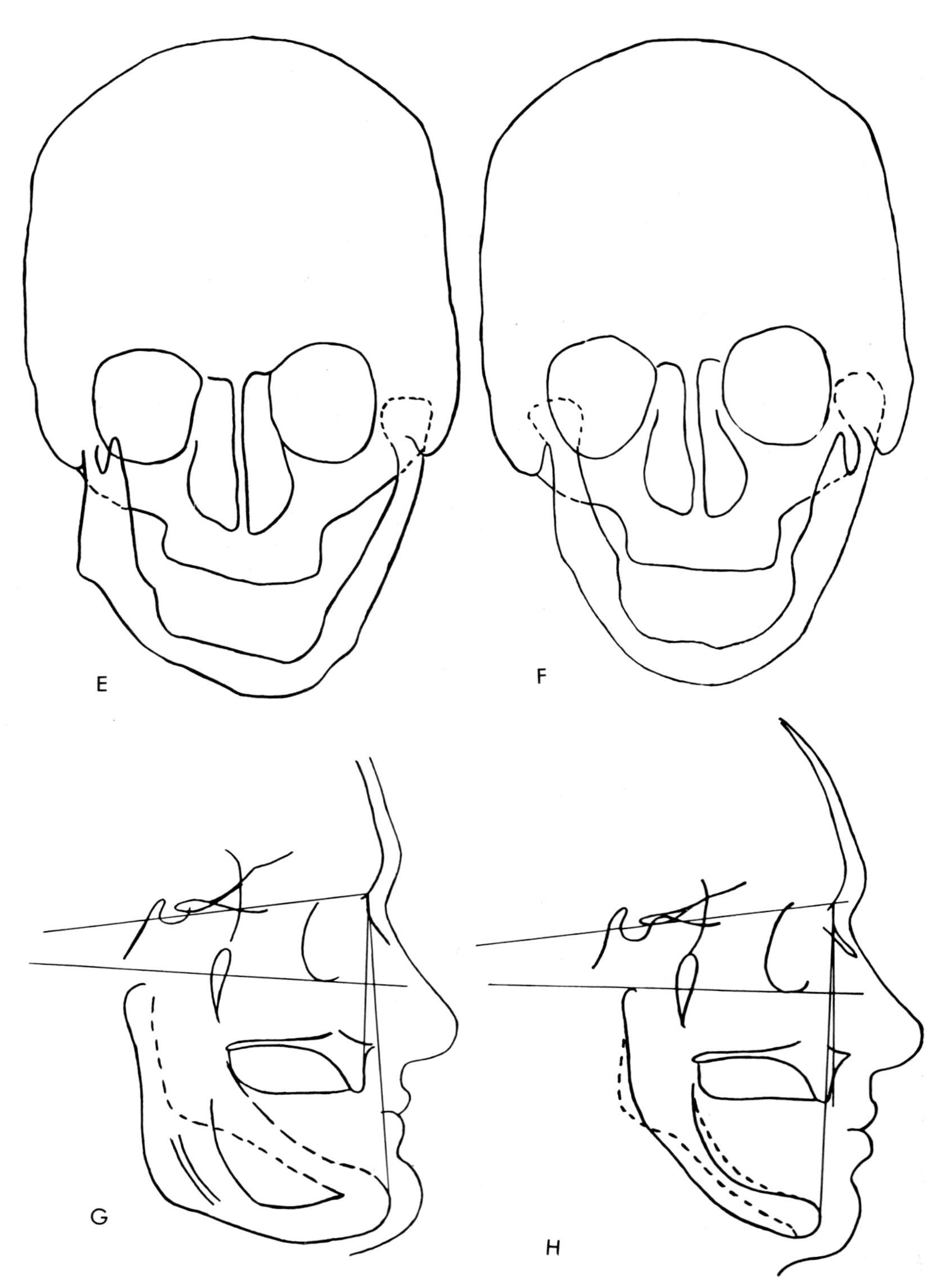

Figure 19–21 *Continued.* *E* and *G,* Marked facial asymmetry. *F* and *H,* Post-treatment lateral and frontal cephalometric tracings with prosthesis in place.

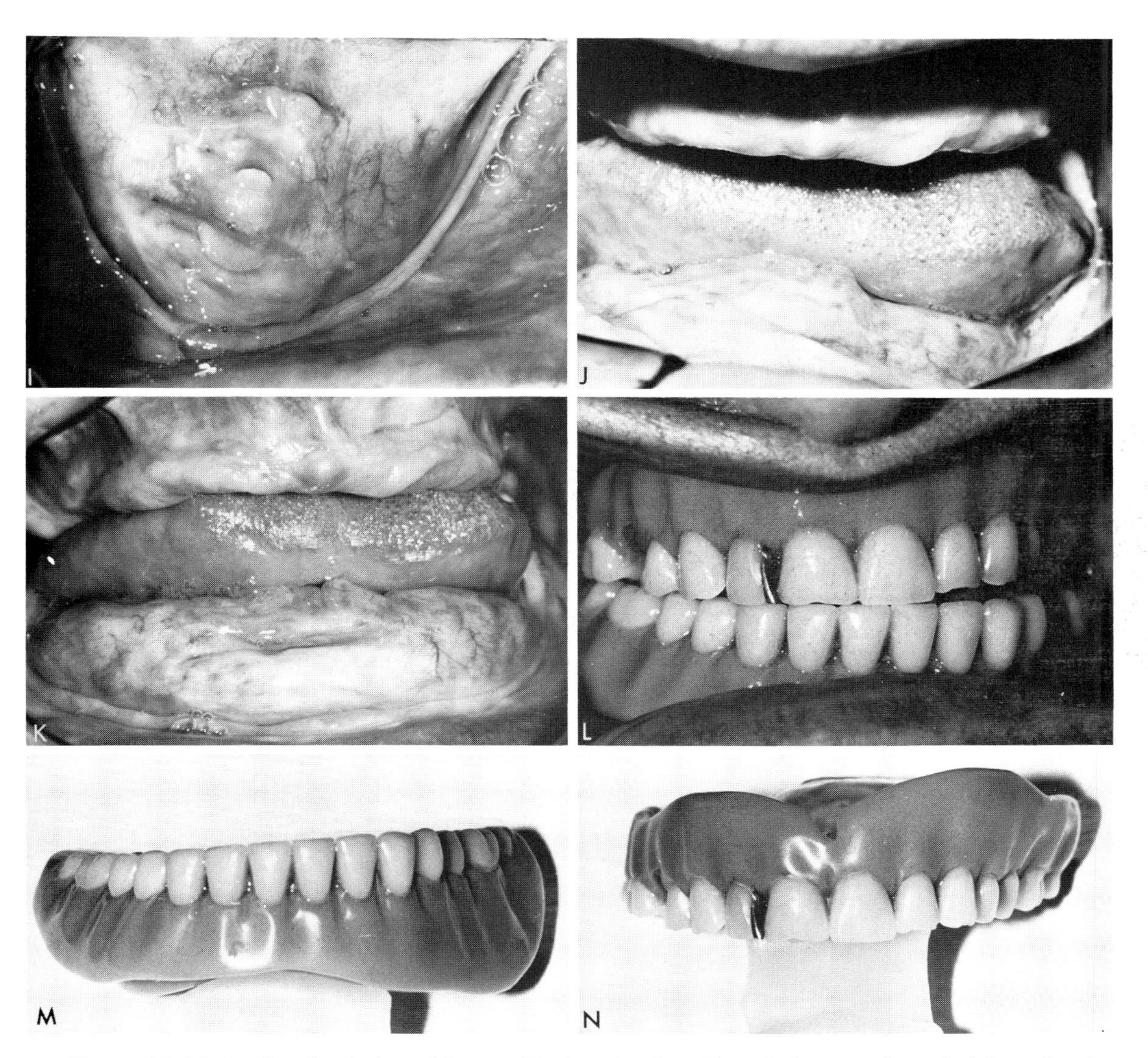

Figure 19–21 *Continued.* *I,* Atrophic mandibular alveolar ridge. *J,* Increased vertical interalveolar distance, left side. *K,* Interalveolar ridge dimension following surgery. *L,* Unilateral open bite. *M* and *N,* Patient's original dentures. Note increased vertical dimension of left side of the dentures to compensate for skeletal asymmetry.

Illustration and legend continued on the following page

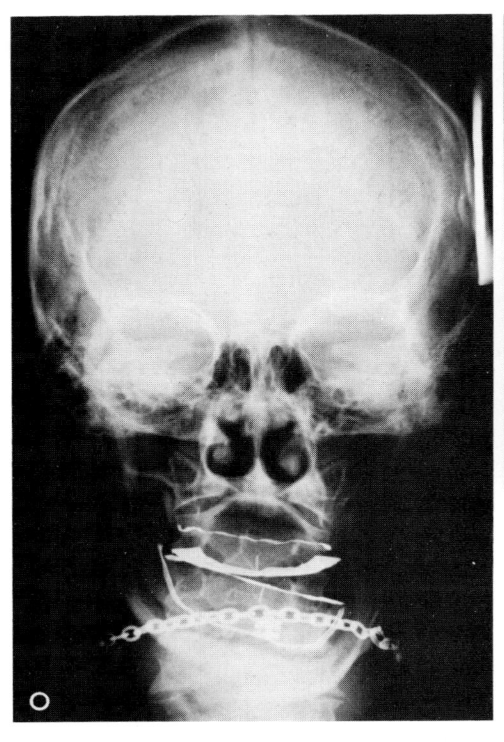

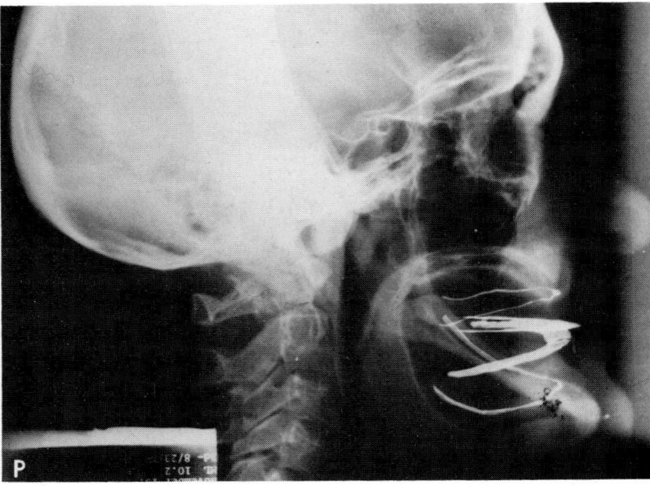

Figure 19–21 *Continued.* *O* and *P*, Frontal and lateral cephalometric radiographs taken with denture bases in place. Radiopaque markers along alveolar ridge, occlusal plane, and skeletal midline facilitate treatment planning.

Occlusal Analysis (Figs. 19–21*I, J, L* through *M*)

1. Edentulous maxillary and mandibular alveolar ridges with increased vertical interalveolar distance on the left side.
2. Crossbite and unilateral open bite on left side.
3. Atrophic mandibular alveolar ridge.

TREATMENT PLAN

Surgical Treatment

1. Correct facial asymmetry with deviation of the chin to the right and increased vertical dimension on the left side with canting of the mandible. This may be done by repositioning the mandible with rotation, reducing vertical dimension on the left, and correcting asymmetry of the chin.
2. Correct left commissure of lip at lower level than right by performing surgical rotation of the mandible, reducing left mandibular vertical dimension.
3. Consider rhinoplasty for deviation of the nose to the left.
4. Remedy concave facial profile with reduced facial height, by surgical repositioning of mandible with increase in lower facial height.
5. Reduce marked mandibular asymmetry by surgical repositioning of the mandible with rotation.
6. Correct edentulous maxilla and mandible with increased vertical interalveolar distance on the left side by surgical repositioning of mandible, establishing symmetric interalveolar dimension.

7. Improve crossbite of left buccal segment with lateral open bite by surgical repositioning of mandible with rotation.

8. To correct atrophic mandibular alveolar ridge, consider possible further preprosthetic surgery, depending upon patient response to surgical realignment of the mandible.

FOLLOW-UP (Figs. 19–21*B, D, F, H, K*)

Subjective

Postoperatively, the patient experienced an unusual and unexplainable pain that resolved approximately five weeks postsurgically. She was happy with the esthetic results that were achieved, even before facial edema subsided completely.

Objective

Three months postsurgery, prosthetic treatment was begun, and final dentures were inserted one month later. In spite of the marked mandibular alveolar atrophy, the patient was able to wear the new dentures without difficulty. An improved functional and esthetic result was accomplished with combined prosthetic and surgical treatment. Postoperative cephalometric tracings, both frontal and lateral, depict the changes.

COMMENT (Figs. 19–21*O* and *P*)

In the edentulous patient with unilateral mandibular hypertrophy, the extent to which mandibular and facial asymmetry may be corrected is limited by the degree of mandibular atrophy. Although recontouring the mandible may be considered when extensive alveolar resorption has occurred, this may not always be possible. To determine the extent to which facial esthetics would be improved by establishing vertical interalveolar symmetry, the following treatment plan was utilized for this specific patient:

1. Symmetric denture bases were constructed. These were lined with radiopaque markers along the alveolar ridge and occlusal plane and in the skeletal midline. These specially prepared denture bases were inserted, and frontal and lateral cephalometric roentgenograms were obtained.

2. A mandibular template, including the prosthesis, was traced from the frontal film and repositioned to achieve the desired functional relationship with the maxillary prosthesis. The tracing revealed that by rotating the mandible to establish coincident maxillary and mandibular skeletal midlines and reducing the left interalveolar dimension, facial asymmetry would be improved and that additional augmentation would not be necessary.

3. The mandibular cast was reoriented to the maxillary cast using the specially prepared denture bases, and a modified type of denture splint was constructed.

Surgeon: Roger West, Seattle, Washington. *Prosthodontist:* Charles Bolender, Seattle, Washington.

CASE 19–5 (Fig. 19–22)

A 55-year-old man was seen in consultation with his general dentist for treatment of advanced atrophy of his maxillary and mandibular alveolar ridges. He had worn complete dentures for 25 years. After clinical examination and analysis of his radiographs and mounted edentulous study casts, the following problem list was developed.

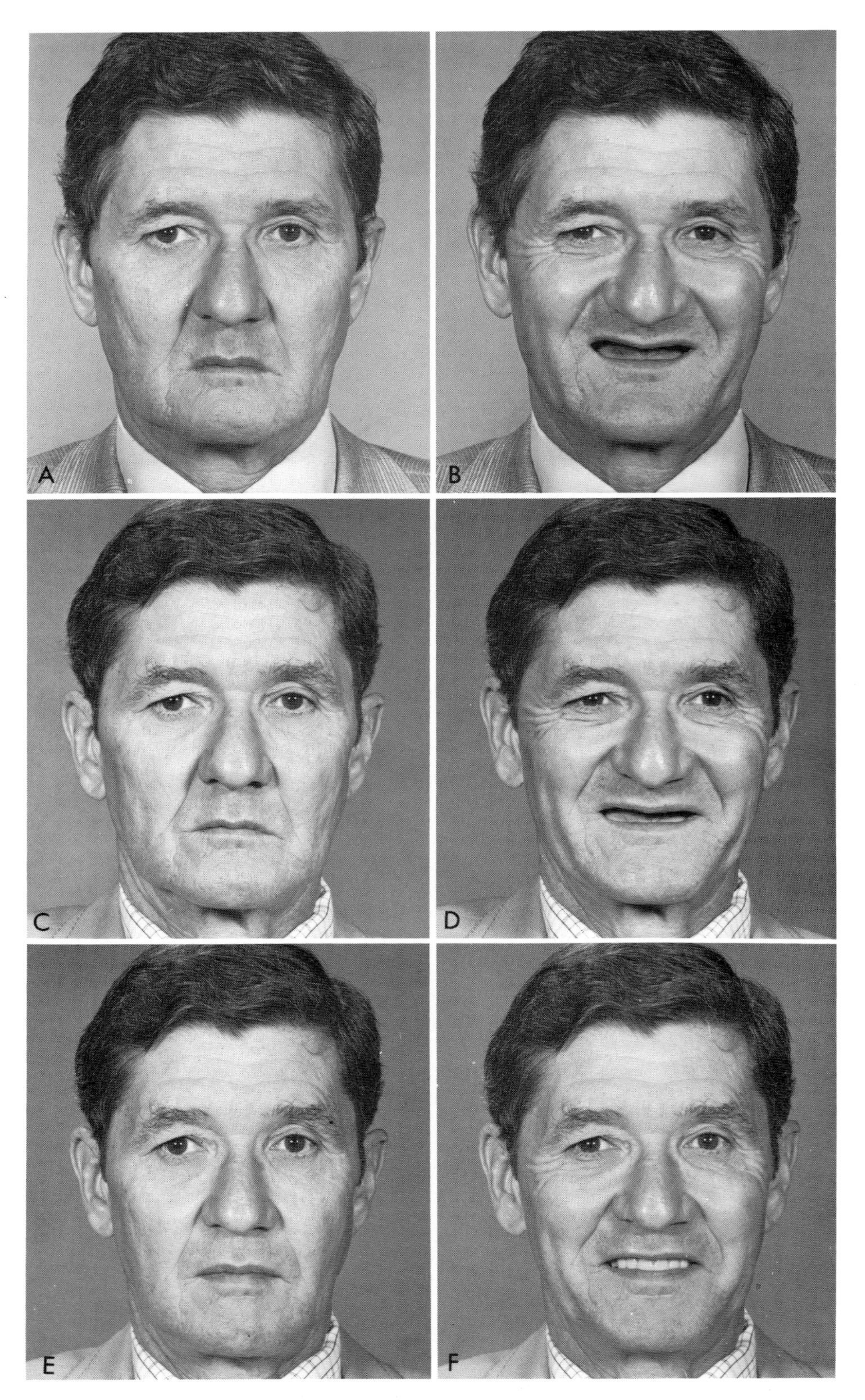

See legend on the opposite page.

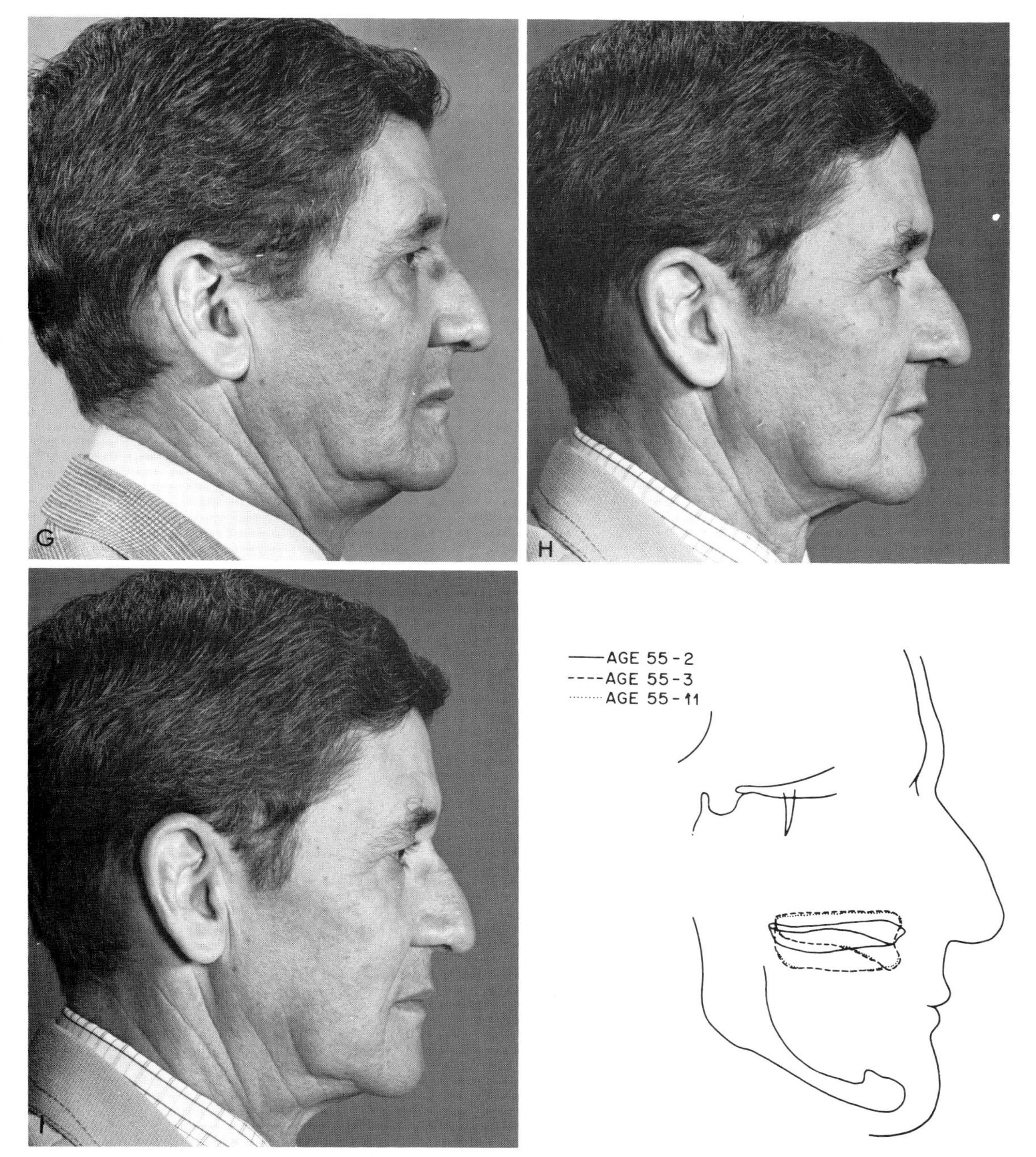

Figure 19–22. *A, B,* and *G,* Typical edentulous appearance before treatment. *C, D,* and *H,* Postsurgical appearance without dentures. *E, F,* and *I,* Post-treatment appearance with dentures in place. *J,* Composite cephalometric tracings before interpositional bone graft (*solid line,* 55 years, 2 months), 1 month after surgery (55 years, 3 months), and 9 months after surgery (55 years, 11 months).

Illustration and legend continued on the following page

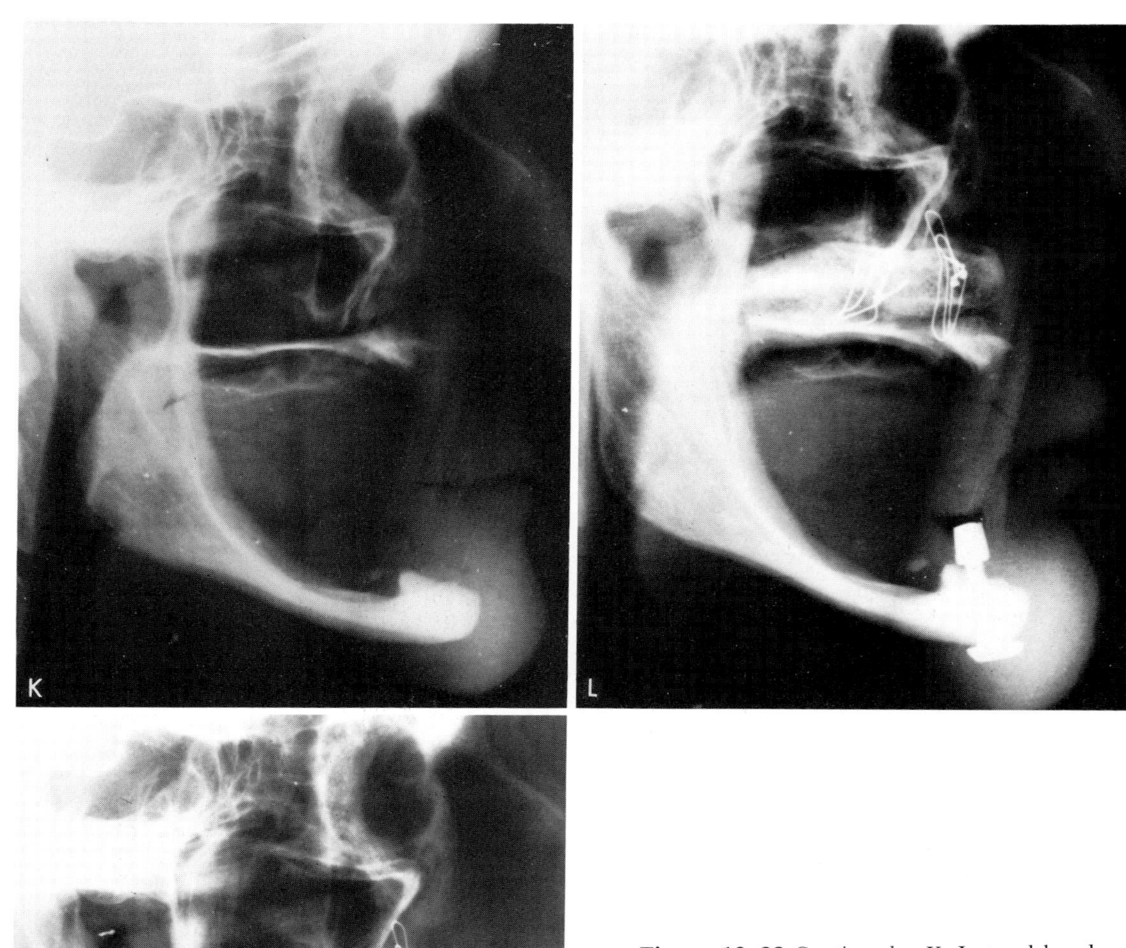

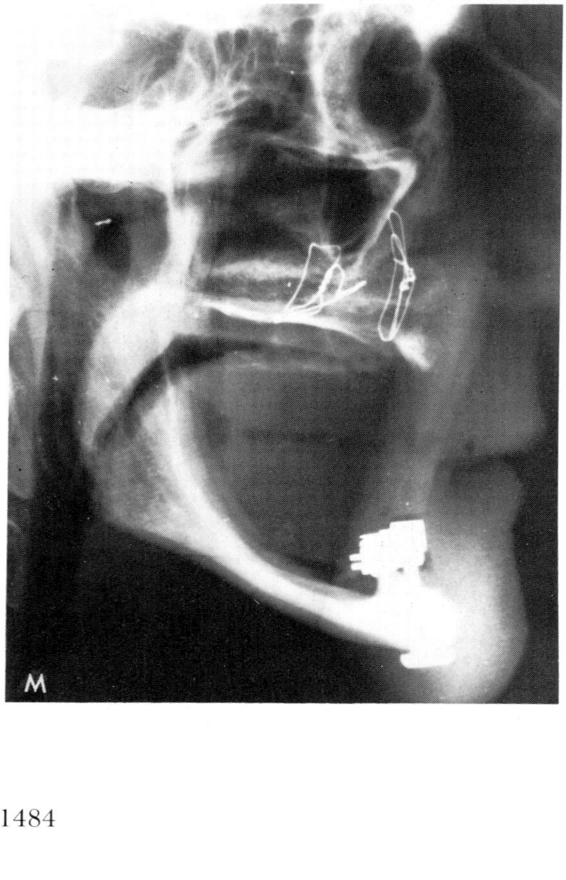

Figure 19–22 *Continued.* *K,* Lateral head radiograph before treatment. *L,* One week after Le Fort I osteotomy and interpositional bone graft and placement of mandibular staple. *M,* Nine months post surgery, showing consolidation of graft to host site without architectural change of mobilized part of maxilla.

Illustration and legend continued on the following page

PROBLEM LIST

Esthetics (Figs. 19–22*A, B, G, J*)

1. Facial symmetry, flattening of the paranasal areas, typical "edentulous look" with retrusion of the upper lip when dentures were out of the mouth.

Cephalometric Analysis (Fig. 19–22*K, N*)

1. Excessive anterior (45 mm) and posterior (35 mm) interarch space, severe atrophy of maxillary and mandibular alveolar ridges, slightly retropositioned edentulous maxilla.

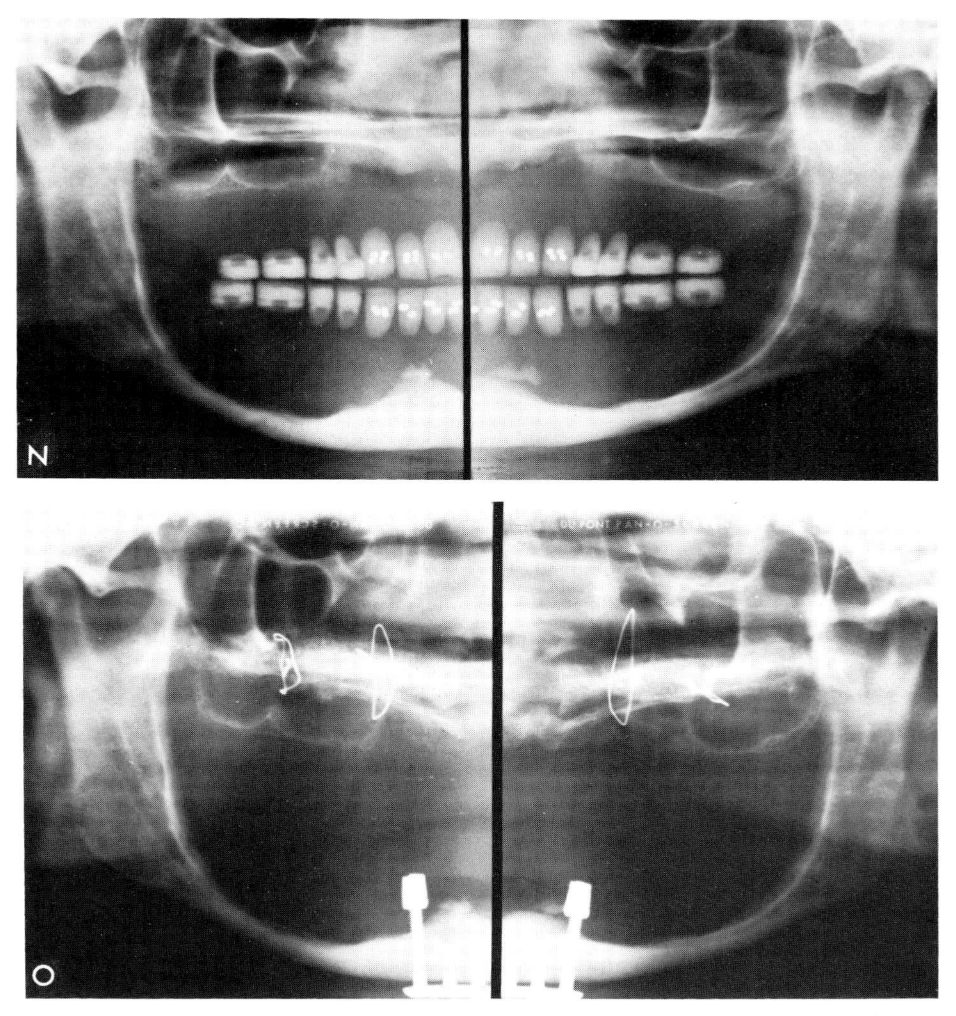

Figure 19–22 *Continued.* *N* and *O*, Panographic view before (*N*) and 10 months after (*O*) treatment.

Illustration and legend continued on the following page

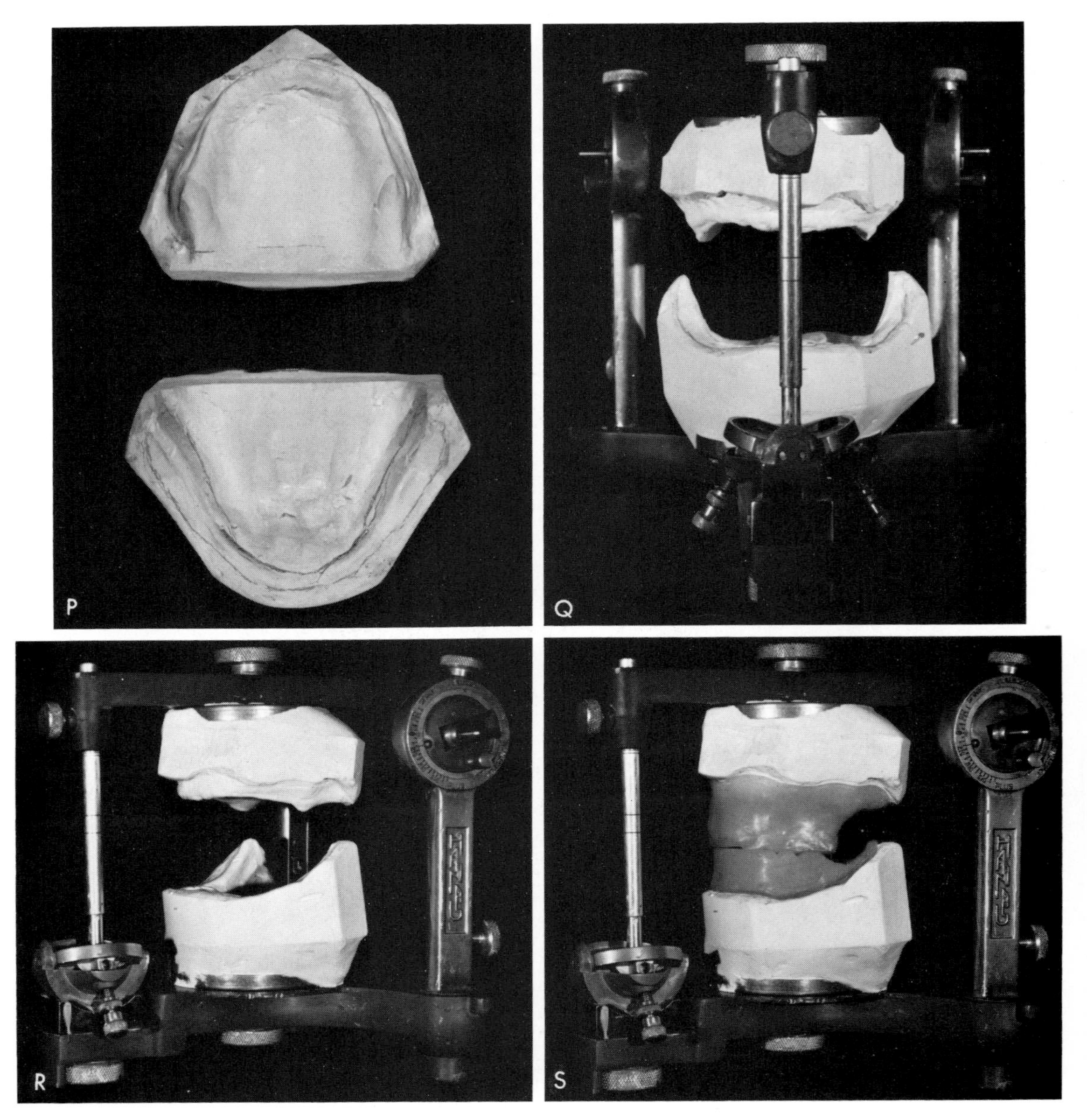

See legend on opposite page.

Occlusal Analysis (Figs. 19–22*P* through *U*)

1. Shallow facial vestibule with high-muscle attachments.
2. Anterior crossbite with small anteroposterior discrepancy.
3. Excessive interarch space secondary to maxillary and mandibular alveolar atrophy, adequate transverse interalveolar relationship.

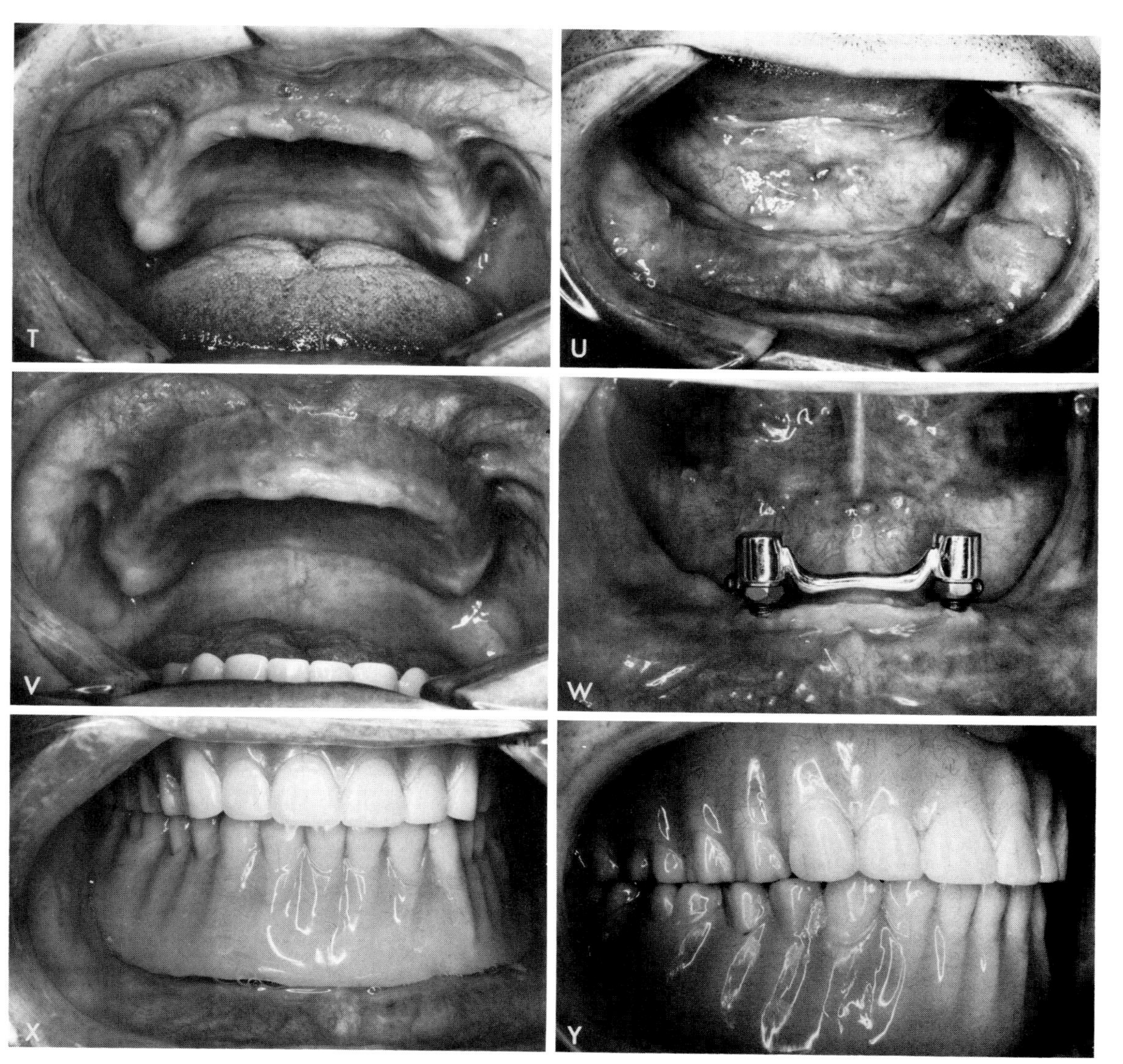

Figure 19–22 *Continued.* *P–R,* Edentulous casts mounted on anatomic articulator in centric relationship after face-bow transfer, showing excessive interarch space and anteroposterior discrepancy in anterior region of atrophic maxilla. *S,* Bite rims used to transfer maxillomandibular relationship to articulator after face-bow transfer. *T* and *U,* Atrophic maxillary and mandibular alveolar ridges before treatment. *V,* Maxillary alveolar ridge 12 months after Le Fort I osteotomy and interpositional bone graft. *W,* Mandibular staple with Dalbo attachments in place. *X* and *Y,* Complete dentures in place.

TREATMENT PLAN

Surgical Treatment

1. Le Fort I osteotomy with interpositional bone graft to:
   a. Surgically reposition maxilla inferiorly (1 cm) and anteriorly.
   b. Decrease excessive interarch space and improve stability of denture.
2. Simultaneous maxillary vestibuloplasty to excise fibrous tissue and high-muscle attachments.

3. Possible interpositional or onlay bone graft to mandible if progressive bone resorption associated with use of mandibular denture has occurred.

Nonsurgical Treatment

1. Restoration of missing teeth with complete upper and lower dentures, 5-pin mandibular staple to improve stability for lower denture.[35]

FOLLOW-UP (Figs. 19–22*C* through *F, H, I, K, L, M, O, W, X, Y*)

Subjective

The patient experienced minimal discomfort throughout the six-month period of treatment. A unilateral maxillary sinusitis two months after maxillary surgery was the sole postoperative problem. This infection (the result of an upper respiratory tract infection or secondary osteomyelitis) cleared rapidly with the use of parenteral antibiotics and a single irrigation of the infected maxillary antrum through the natural ostium of the nose.

Objective

The intraoral wounds healed primarily without dehiscence or infection after surgery and insertion of the mandibular staple, which were accomplished simultaneously under general anesthesia. The patient's old dentures, lined with soft reliner, were used transitionally until the final complete upper and lower dentures were constructed.

The vertical relationship achieved at surgery was based upon plans and priorities that were arrived at jointly by the prosthodontist and oral surgeon. The feasibility of surgery must be carefully weighed against the ideal vertical relationship and the patient's needs and wishes. The principal functional and esthetic objectives were achieved by the surgical and prosthetic treatment.

Although it is still too soon to determine whether or not bone grafting to the mandible will be necessary, there has been minimal discernible resorption of grafted or repositioned bone to date. Secondary vestibuloplasty and skin grafting to the maxilla were unnecessary. To date, this has been our experience with the majority of patients treated by Le Fort I osteotomy and interpositional bone grafting.

Postoperatively the patient's breathing through his nasal passages was much improved when compared with his breathing through his partially obstructed preoperative nasal airway. This is not an uncommon experience for patients who have had Le Fort I osteotomy surgery.

Surgeon: William H. Bell, Dallas, Texas. *Prosthodontist:* Joe Ampil, Dallas, Texas.

CASE 19–6 (Fig. 19–23)

A 48-year-old woman was referred for evaluation and treatment of severe mandibular atrophy that resulted from wearing complete dentures for most of her adult life. Her atrophic and prognathic mandible made construction of a functional mandibular denture difficult and problematic.

PROBLEM LIST

Esthetics (Figs. 19–23*A* and *D*)

Frontal. Protrusive mandible with the lower lip that was prominent and everted in relation to the upper lip and chin, paranasal deficiency.

Profile. Manibular excess, inadequate support for the upper lip.

Cephalometric Analysis (Fig. 19–23*G, H* through *K*)

1. Mandibular excess with Class III ridge relationship, 8-mm negative anterior horizontal overlap.
2. Vertical height of anterior portion of mandible approximately 10 mm.

Occlusal Analysis (Fig. 19–23*L*)

1. Severe atrophy of mandibular alveolar ridge.

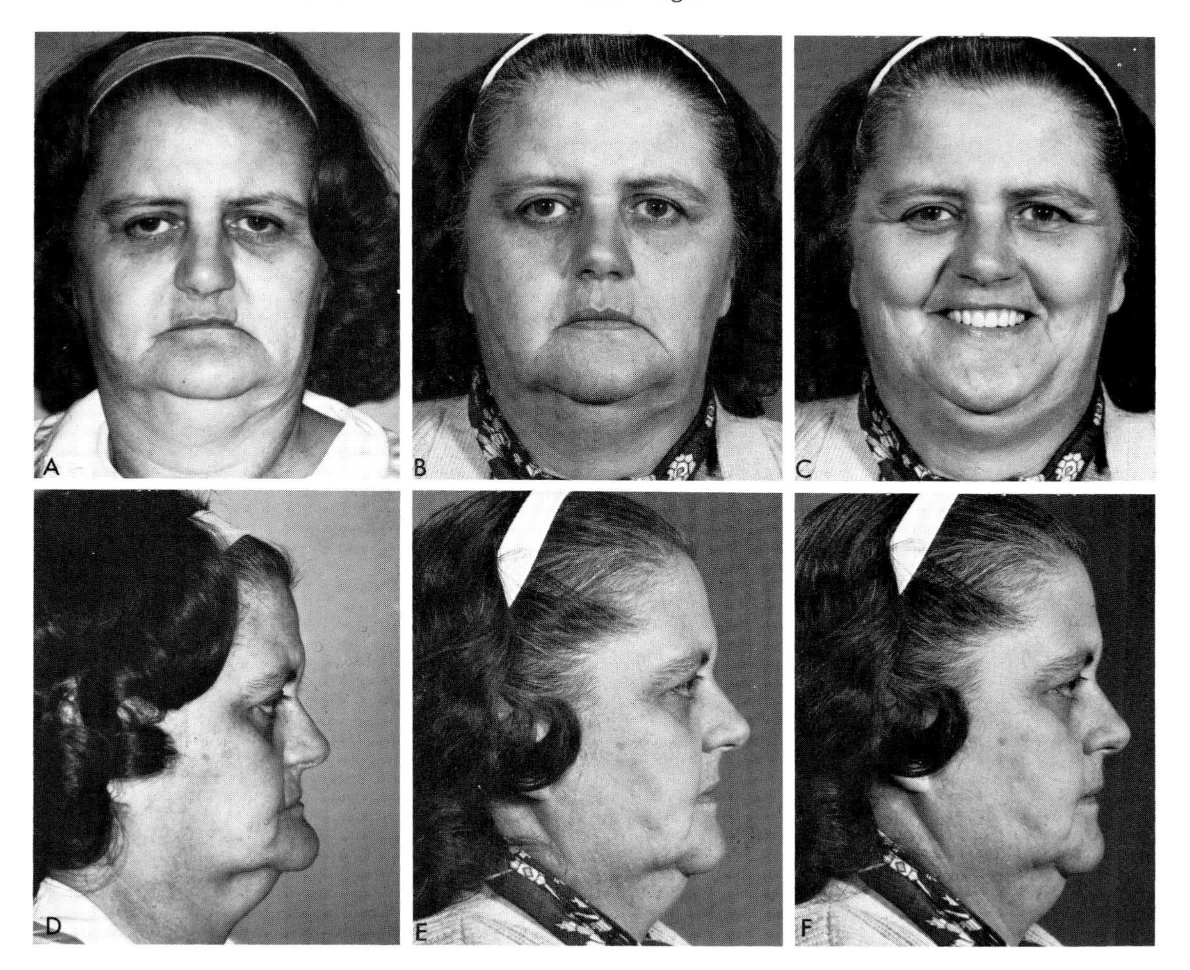

Figure 19–23. *A* and *D,* Pretreatment appearance. *B, C,* and *F,* Post-treatment appearance with dentures in place. *E,* Post-treatment appearance without dentures.

Illustration and legend continued on the following page.

TREATMENT PLAN (Fig. 19–23*M* through *R*)

Surgical Treatment

1. First stage: Correct mandibular excess with Class III relationship by bilateral intraoral oblique ramus osteotomies to reposition mandible posteriorly 8 mm.
2. Second stage: Correct atrophic mandible by horizontal osteotomy of the mandible and interpositional bone graft from iliac crest to increase the vertical height of the anterior portion of the mandible (surgery performed by technique illustrated in Fig. 19–9).
3. Third stage: Correct shallow facial vestibule and high-muscle attachments by secondary vestibuloplasty with split-thickness skin graft.

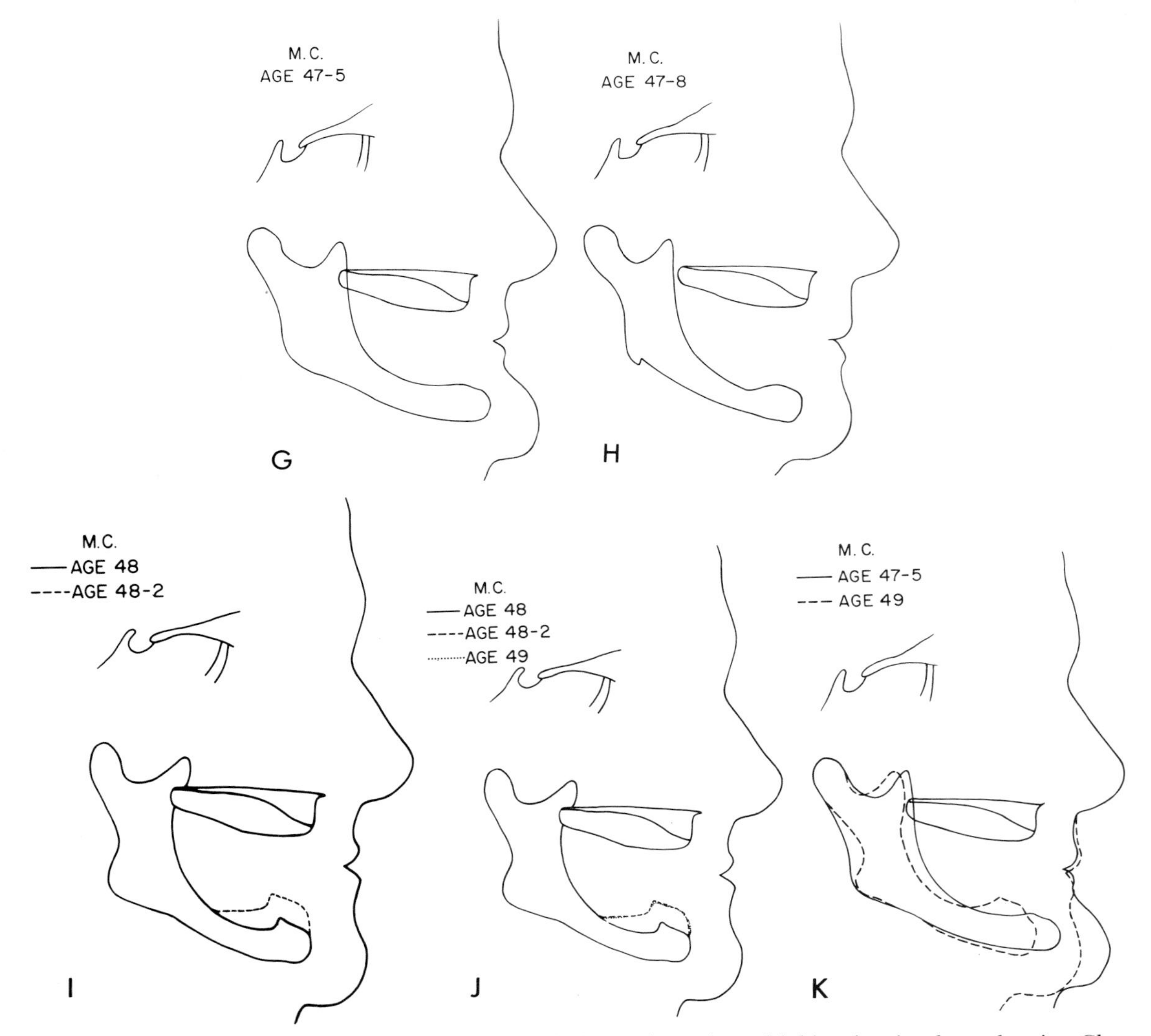

Figure 19–23 *Continued.* *G,* Pretreatment cephalometric tracing with bite rims in place, showing Class III ridge relationship. *H,* Cephalometric tracing after vertical ramus osteotomies to correct mandibular prognathism. *I–K,* Composite cephalometric tracings before interpositional bone graft (*solid line,* age 48 years), 2 months after surgery (*broken line,* age 48 years, 2 months), and 12 months after surgery (*dotted line,* age 49 years).

Nonsurgical Treatment

1. Restore occlusal function with complete dentures.

FOLLOW-UP (Figs. 19–23*S* through *V*)

Subjective

The patient required little postoperative pain medication and experienced an uneventful recovery from the three surgical procedures that were performed in three stages. After vertical ramus surgery to retract the mandible, eating and speech were facilitated by a space in the anterior part of the denture splints.

Objective

The desired interarch relationship was maintained by the use of denture splints and intermaxillary fixation for six weeks after vertical ramus osteotomies. After release from intermaxillary fixation, the splints were used transitionally for another four weeks to maintain the planned jaw relationship and until normal mandibular function was re-established.

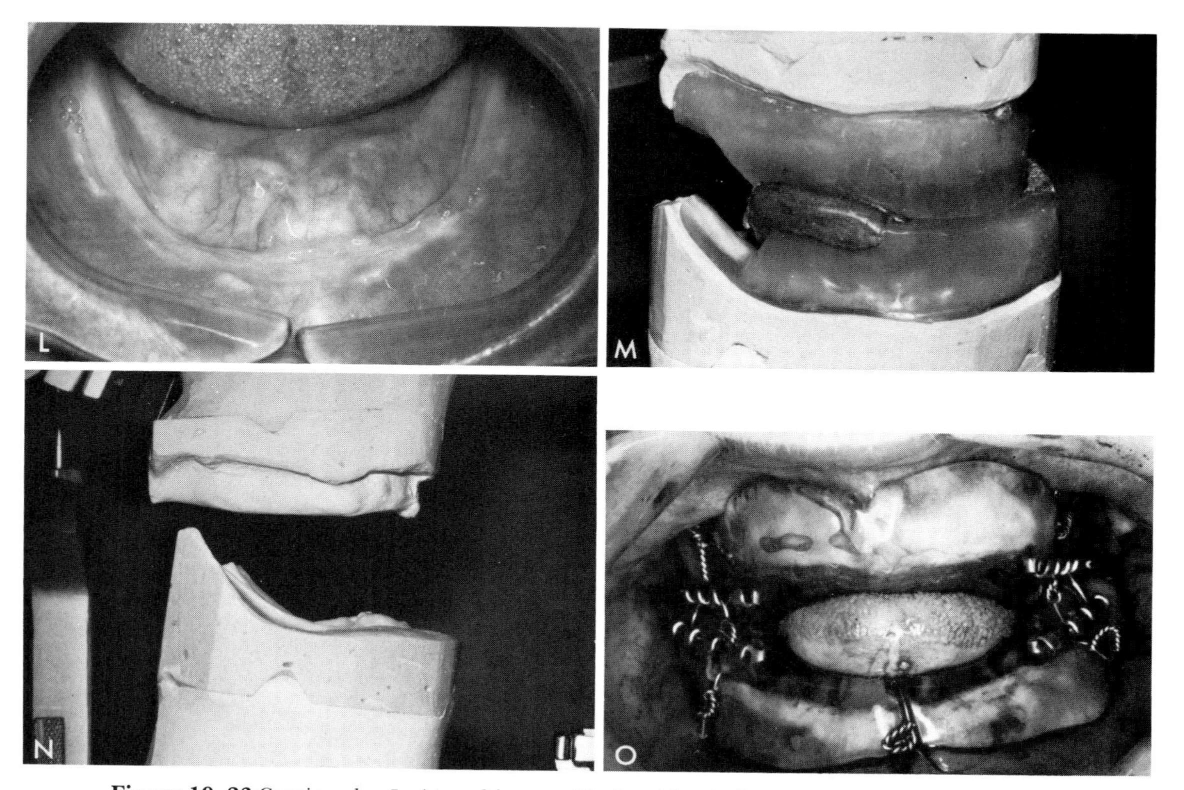

Figure 19–23 *Continued.* *L,* Atrophic mandibular ridge before treatment. *M,* Bite rims used to transfer maxillomandibular relationship to articulator after face-bow transfer. *N,* Edentulous casts mounted on anatomic articulator in centric relationship after face-bow transfer, showing Class III ridge relationship. *O,* Intermaxillary fixation with denture splints.

Illustration and legend continued on the following page

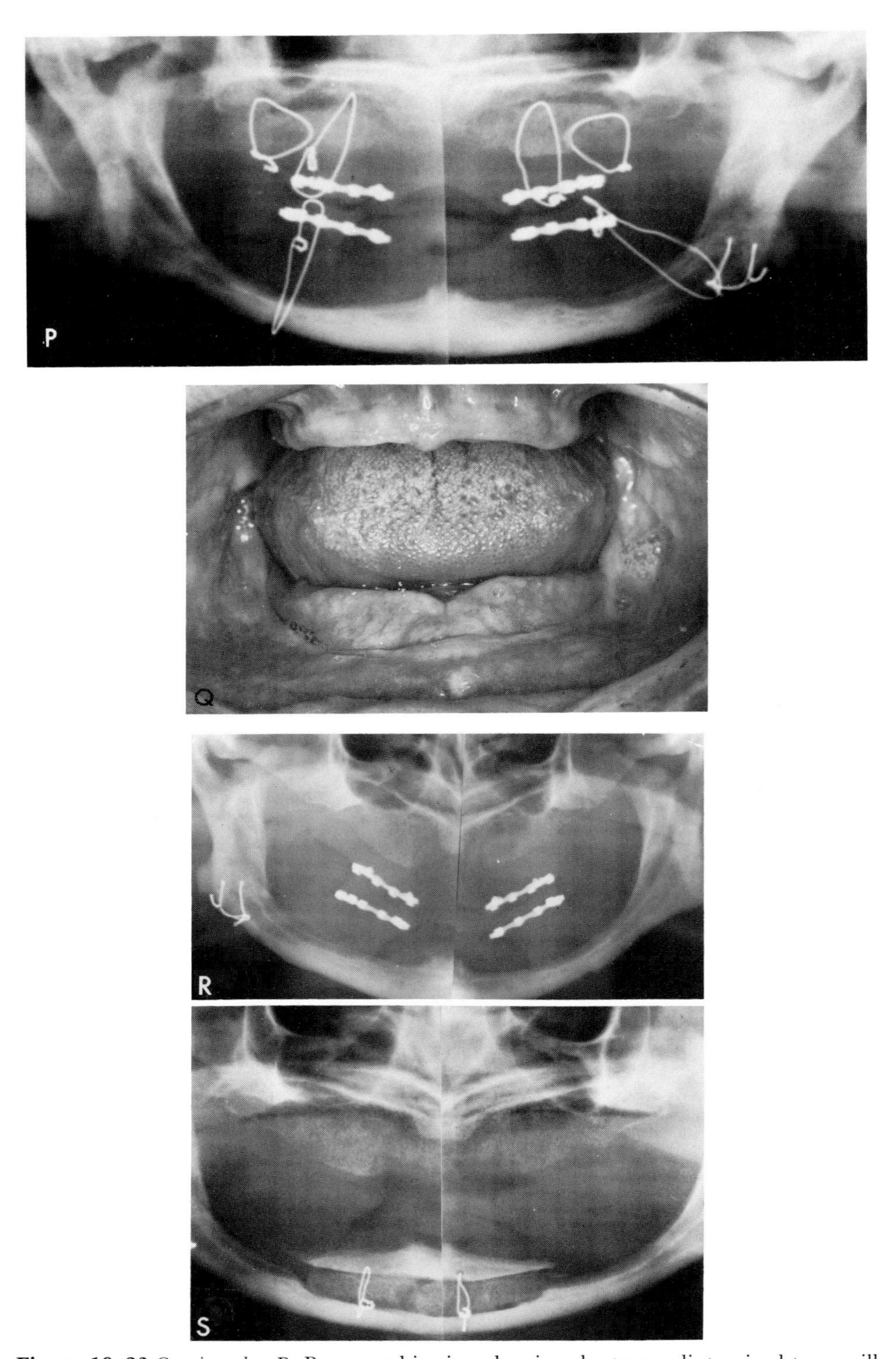

Figure 19–23 *Continued.* *P,* Panographic view showing denture splints wired to maxilla and mandible. *Q,* Interarch relationship after correction of prognathic mandible. *R,* Panographic view of atrophic mandibular alveolar ridge before treatment. *S,* One month after horizontal osteotomy of mandible and simultaneous bone graft between proximal and distal segments to increase mandibular height 1 cm. (Surgery performed by technique illustrated in Fig. 19–9.)

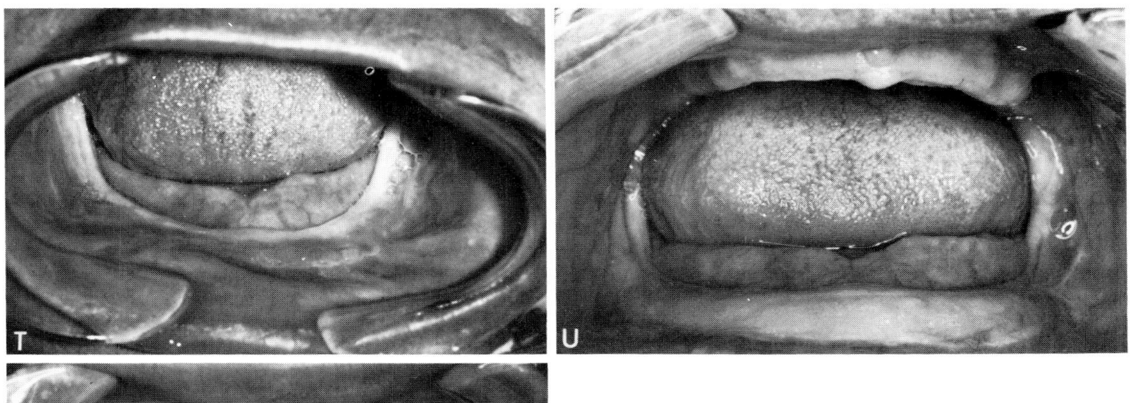

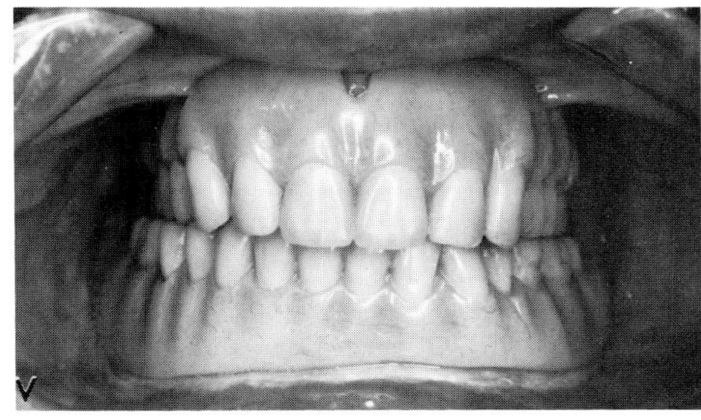

Figure 19–23 *Continued.* *T,* Four weeks after interpositional bone graft. *U,* Postsurgical alveolar ridge relationship 2 months after secondary vestibuloplasty and skin graft. *V,* Complete dentures in place.

The interpositional graft (second stage) was placed approximately three months later. Postoperative radiographs revealed an increase of 1 cm in vertical height of the mandible. Six weeks after surgery, a vestibuloplasty with skin grafting was carried out. Within another six weeks, the patient was rehabilitated with functional complete dentures. There has been virtually no resorption of the bone in the repositioned superior segment. The interpositional graft rapidly became consolidated with the host bone and was remodeled without discernible loss of bone mass or height of the grafted or repositioned bone.

Surgeons: Robert Buckles, James Kennedy, and William H. Bell, Dallas, Texas. *Prosthodontist:* Joe Ampil, Dallas, Texas.

CASE 19–7 (Fig. 19–24)

A completely edentulous 32-year-old man requested treatment to replace his poorly functioning dentures. Anteroposterior disharmony of the maxillary and mandibular denture bases had resulted from his long-term use of ill-fitting prostheses and associated gradual posterior and medial migration of the crest of the anterior portion of the maxillary alveolar ridge. Based upon a clinical examination and review of his prosthetic records, the following problem list was developed:

PROBLEM LIST

Esthetics (Fig. 19–24*A*)

1. Flattening of the nasomaxillary and nasolabial areas; retrusion of the upper lip in relationship to the nose, lower lip, and chin.

Cephalometric Analysis (Fig. 19–24*D*)

1. Anteroposterior maxillary deficiency.

Occlusal Analysis (Fig. 19–24*E*)

1. Class III ridge relationship with 8-mm anteroposterior discrepancy and complete crossbite.

TREATMENT PLAN

Surgical Treatment

1. Correct retrusion of upper lip and flattening of nasomaxillary and nasolabial areas by 8-mm maxillary advancement by Le Fort I osteotomy and bone grafting the pterygomaxillary junction and by augmentation of the nasolabial and nasomaxillary areas.
2. Correct anteroposterior maxillary deficiency by 8-mm advancement of maxilla.
3. Correct Class III ridge relationship with 8-mm anteroposterior discrepancy and complete crossbite by 8-mm maxillary advancement.

Nonsurgical Treatment

1. Complete upper and lower dentures.

FOLLOW-UP (Figs. 19–24*B, C, F*)

Subjective

The patient experienced minimal postoperative pain. The use of Gunning-type splints facilitated eating and speech during the period of intermaxillary fixation.

Objective

A slight widening of the alar bases of the nose and augmentation of the paranasal areas improved the patient's overall facial esthetics. An improved interarch relationship facilitated prosthetic restoration with complete dentures.

COMMENT

A similar interarch relationship could have been attained by vertical ramus osteotomies and surgical retraction of the mandible. Correction of the maxillomandibular disharmony in the maxilla, however, provided a means of simultaneously augmenting the midface, the principal esthetic problematic site. The prosthodontist planned the an-

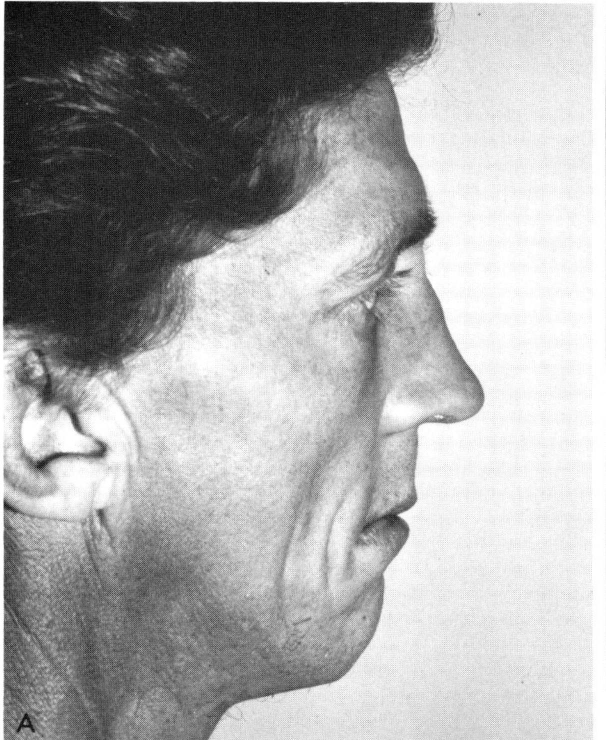

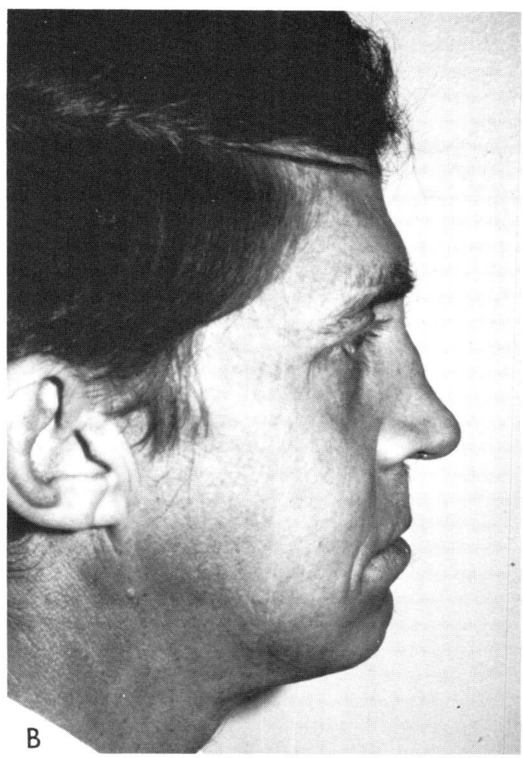

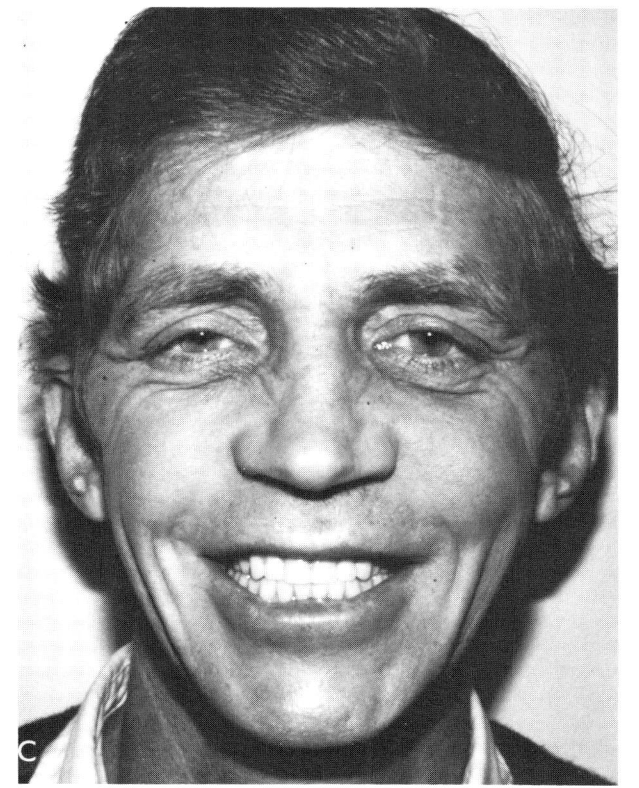

Figure 19–24. *A*, Pretreatment appearance. *B* and *C*, Post-treatment appearance with dentures in place.

Illustration and legend continued on the following page

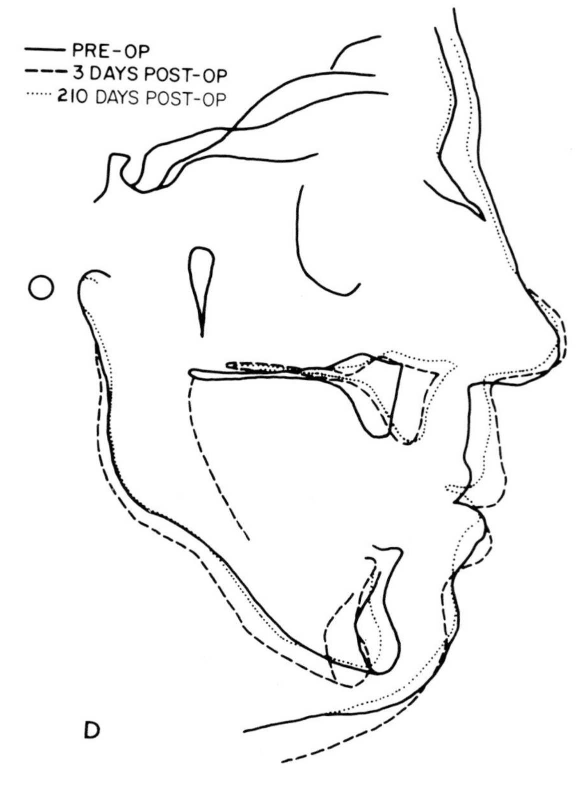

Figure 19–24 *Continued.* *D,* Composite cephalometric tracings showing surgical changes and postoperative stability. *E,* Old dentures in place before treatment. *F,* Complete dentures in place after surgery.

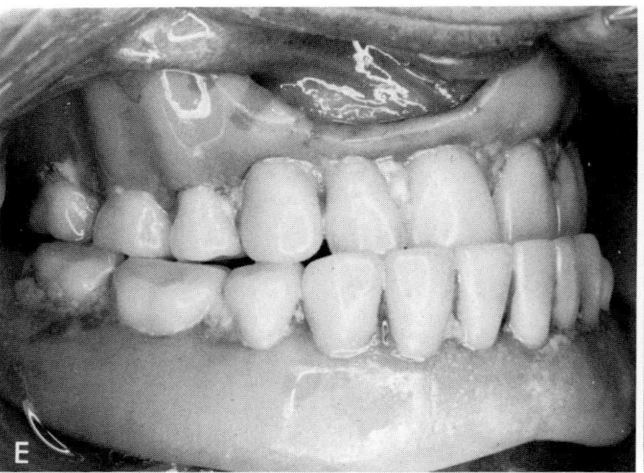

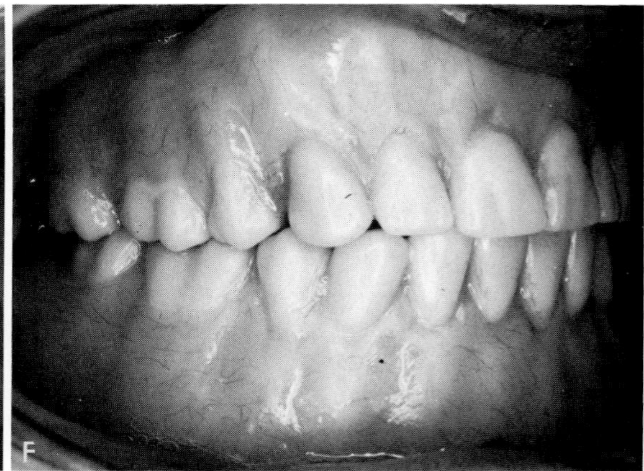

teroposterior and vertical interarch relationship by analysis of articulated edentulous study casts that were mounted in centric relation. The maxillary cast was then repositioned into the best possible interarch relationship.

Surgeons: Ray Fonseca, Iowa City, Iowa; William H. Bell, Dallas, Texas. *Prosthodontist:* Joe Ampil, Dallas, Texas.

CASE 19–8 (Fig. 19–25)

A 75-year-old woman was referred for evaluation and treatment of severe mandibular atrophy that resulted from wearing complete dentures for 35 years. The atrophic

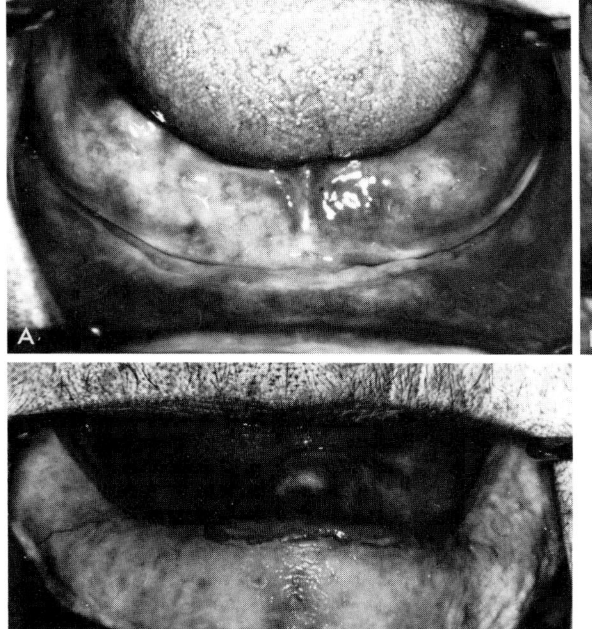

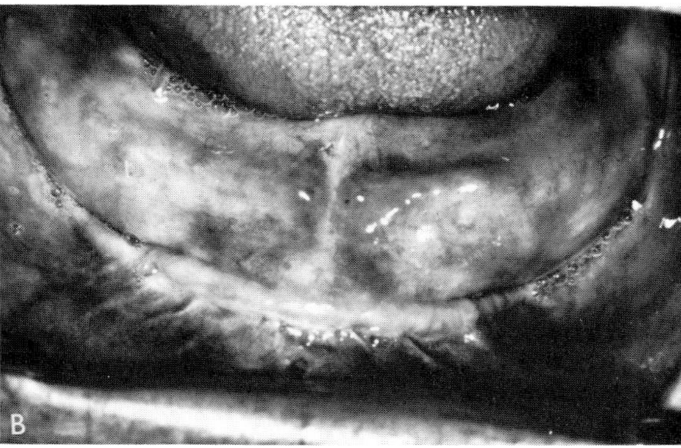

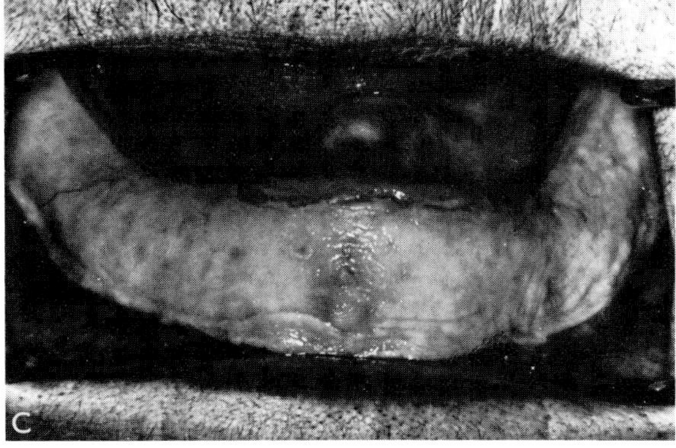

Figure 19–25. *A,* Intraorally, there is inadequate residual ridge to provide denture stability and retention. *B,* Six weeks after visor osteotomy and before total vestibuloplasty. *C,* Two years after visor osteotomy and total vestibuloplasty. *D–F,* Cephalometric radiography before (*D*), after (*E*), and 2 years after (*F*) visor osteotomy. *G,* Denture before and after surgery.

Illustration continued on the following page

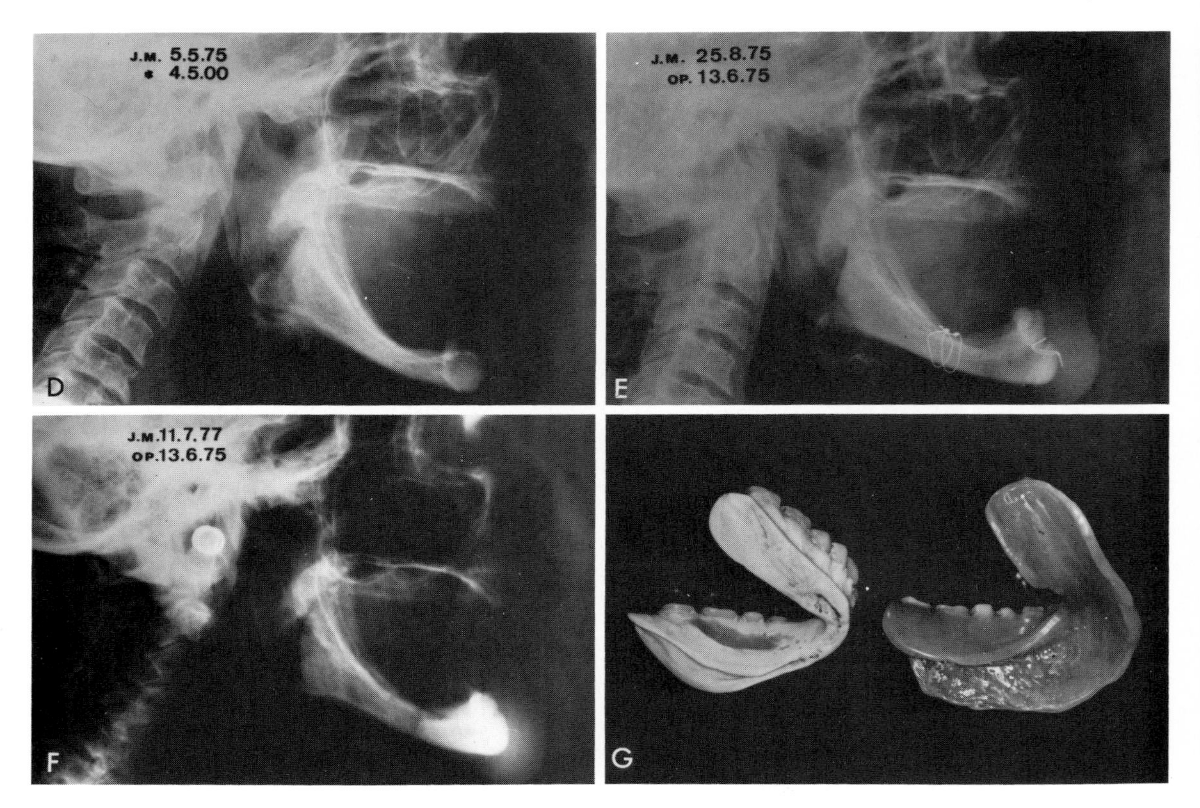

Figure 19–25 *Continued.*

mandible made construction of a functional mandibular denture difficult and problematic (see Figure 19–17).

PROBLEM LIST

Esthetics (Fig. 19–25*A*)

1. Inadequate residual ridge.

Cephalometric Analysis (Fig. 19–25*D*)

1. Height of the mandible in the vertical dimension measured 1.4 cm.

Occlusal Analysis

1. Atrophic mandible with shallow labial and buccal vestibules and high-muscle attachments.

TREATMENT PLAN

Surgical Treatment

1. Correct reduced mandibular vertical dimension (measuring less than 1.5 cm) by vertical osteotomy (visor osteotomy) of the mandibular body.
2. Correct atrophic mandible with shallow labial and buccal vestibules and high-muscle attachments by secondary vestibuloplasty with split-thickness skin grafting.

FOLLOW-UP

Subjective

The patient did not require antibiotics or medication for postoperative pain and experienced a quick recovery. Facial edema was minimal.

Objective (Figs. 19–25*B, C, E, G*)

Postoperative cephalometrics revealed an increase of 0.9 cm in vertical height of the mandible. Six weeks postoperatively a vestibuloplasty with skin grafting was carried out. Within another six weeks, the patient was rehabilitated with functional complete dentures.

Surgeon: Franz Härte, Freiberg, Germany.

REFERENCES

1. Archer WH: Oral Surgery: A Step-by-Step Atlas of Operative Technique, ed 4. Philadelphia: WB Saunders, 1966.
2. Atwood DA: Cephalometric study of the clinical rest position of the mandible. Variability in the rate of bone loss following the removal of occlusal contacts. J Prosthet Dent 7:544, 1957.
3. Atwood DA: Reduction of residual ridges: a major oral disease entity. J Prosthet Dent *26*:266, 1971.
4. Atwood DA, Coy WA: Clinical, cephalometric, and densitometric study of reduction of residual ridges. J Prosthet Dent *26*:280, 1971.
5. Bell WH: Le Fort I osteotomy for correction of maxillary deformities. J Oral Surg *33*:412, 1975.
6. Bell WH: Correction of the short face syndrome — vertical maxillary deficiency. A preliminary report. J Oral Surg *35*:110, 1977.
7. Bell WH, Buckles RL: Correction of the atrophic alveolar ridge by interpositional bone grafting. J Oral Surg *36*:693, 1978.
8. Bell WH, Finn RA: Bone healing and revascularization following horizontal osteotomy of the mandible and interpositional bone grafting — unpublished studies in the dog and monkey.
9. Bell WH, Buche WA, Kennedy JW III, Ampil JP: Surgical correction of the atrophic alveolar ridge. Oral Surg Oral Med Oral Path *43*:485, 1977.
10. Bell WH, Fonesca RJ, et al: Bone healing and revascularization after total maxillary osteotomy. J. Oral Surg *33*:253, 1975.
11. Boyne PJ, Cooksey DE: Use of cartilage and bone implants in restoration of edentulous ridges. J Am Dent Assoc *71*:1426, 1965.
12. Burstone CJ: Integumental profile. Am J Orthod *44*:1, 1961.
13. Canzona JE, Grand NG, Waterhouse JP, Laskin DM: Autogenous bone grafts in augmentation of the edentulous canine mandible. J Oral Surg *34*:897, 1976.
14. Carlsson GE, Persson GT: Morphologic changes in the mandible after extraction and wearing of dentures: a longitudinal, clinical, and x-ray cephalometric study covering 5 years. Odontol Rev *18*:27, 1967.
15. Carlsson GE, Bergman B, Hedegard B: Changes in contour of the maxillary alveolar process under immediate dentures; a longitudinal, clinical and x-ray cephalometric study covering 5 years. Acta Odontol Scand *25*:45, 1967.
16. Danielson PA, Nemarich AN: Subcortical bone grafting for ridge augmentation. J Oral Surg *34*:887, 1976.
17. Davis WH, Delo RI, et al: Transoral bone graft for atrophy of the mandible. J Oral Surg *28*:760, 1970.
18. Dean OT: Surgery for the denture patient. J Am Dent Assoc *23*:2124, 1936.
19. Enlow DH: Alveolar bone. *In* Lang BR et al (eds): International Prosthodontic Workshop on Complete Denture Occlusion. Ann Arbor: Univ of Mich School of Dentistry, 1973, pp 3–41.
20. Farrel CD, Kent JN, Guerra, LR: One stage interpositional bone grafting and vestibuloplasty of the atrophic maxilla. J Oral Surg *34*:901, 1976.
21. Haga M, Ukiya M, et al: Stereophogrammetric study of the face. Bull Tokyo Med Dent Univ *5*:10, 1964.
22. Israel H: Loss of bone and remodeling-redistribution in the craniofacial skeleton with age. Fed Proc *26*:1723, 1967.
23. Kelly JF, Freidlander GE: Preprosthetic bone graft augmentation with allogeneic bone: A preliminary report. J. Oral Surg *35*:268, 1977.
24. Kent JN, Homsey CA et al: Pilot studies of a porous implant in dentistry and oral surgery. J Oral Surg *30*:608, 1972.
25. Kruger GO: Textbook of Oral Surgery, ed 3, St Louis: CV Mosby, 1968.
26. Lekkas, K.: Absolute augmentation of the mandible. Int J Oral Surg *6*:147, 1977.
27. McNeill RW, Hooley JR, et al: Skeletal relapse during intermaxillary fixation. J. Oral Surg *31*:212, 1973.
28. Martone AL: Physiographic cinematography studies of a prosthodontic patient: an initial report. J. Prosthet Dent *14*:1069, 1964.
29. Nakamoto RY: Bony defects on the crest of the residual alveolar ridge. J Prosthet Dent *19*:111, 1968.
30. Obwegeser H, Steinhauser E: Rebuilding the alveolar ridge with bone and cartilage autografts. *In* Husted E et al (eds): Transactions of the Second International Conference on Oral Surgery. Copenhagen, Munksgaard, 1967, pp 203–208.
31. Rudee DA: Proportional profile changes concurrent with orthodontic therapy. Am J Orthod *50*:421, 1964.
32. Sarnas KV: Inter- and intra-family variations in the facial profile. Odontol Revy (Malmo) *10*(Supp 4), 1959.
33. Schuchardt K, Scheunemann H., Schwenzer N.: Transplantationen im Mund-, Kiefer- und Gesichtsbereich. Stuttgart: Georg Thieme, 1976.
34. Shepherd N, Maloney P, et al: Subcortical ceramic implants for elevation of alveolar ridges. IADR abstract #729. J Dent Res, Feb 1976.
35. Small IA: Metal implants and the mandibular staple bone plate. J Oral Surg *33*:571, 1975.
36. Starshak TJ: Preprosthetic Oral Surgery. St Louis: CV Mosby, 1971.
37. Tallgren A: The reduction in face height of edentulous and partially edentulous subjects during long-term denture wear, a longitudinal roentgenographic cephalometric study. Acta Odontol Scand *24*:195, 1966.
38. Tallgren A: Positional changes of complete dentures; a 7 year longitudinal study. Acta Odontol Scand *27*:539, 1969.

39. Tallgren A: The continuing reduction of the residual alveolar ridges in complete denture wearers: A mixed-longitudinal study covering 25 years. J Prosthet Dent *27*:120, 1972.
40. Tallgren A: Changes in the relationship of complete dentures to the supporting tissues. *In* Lang BR et al (eds): International Prosthodontic Workshop on Complete Denture Occlusion. Ann Arbor: Univ of Mich School of Dentistry, 1973, pp 260–270.
41. Terry BC, Albright JE, et al: Alveolar ridge augmentation in the edentulous maxilla using autogenous ribs. J Oral Surg *32*:429, 1972.
42. Thompson JR: The rest position of the mandible and its significance to dental science. J Am Dent Assoc *33*:151, 1946.
43. Wang JH, Waite DE, et al: Ridge augmentation: an evaluation and follow-up report. J Oral Surg *34*:600, 1976.
44. West RA, Burk JL: Maxillary ostectomies for preprosthetic surgery. J Oral Surg *32*:13, 1974.
45. West RA, Epker BN: Posterior maxillary surgery: its place in the treatment of dentofacial deformities. J Oral Surg *30*:562, 1972.
46. Wilmar, K.: On Le Fort I osteotomy. Scand J Plast Reconstr Surg Suppl 12, 1974.

SELECTED READINGS

1. Barrow-St. Pasteur J: Plastia reconstructiva del Reborde alveolar. Nuestra investigacion clinico-quirurgica. Acta Odont Venez *8*:168, 1970.
2. de Koomen, HA: A prosthetic view on vestibuloplasty with free mucosal graft. Int J Oral Surg *6*:38–41, 1977.
3. de Koomen, HA, Stoelinga, PJW, et al.: Interposed bone-graft augmentation of the atrophic mandible. J Maxillofac Surg *7*:129–135, 1979.
4. Peterson, LJ, and Slade, EW: Mandibular ridge augmentation by a modified visor osteotomy. J Oral Surg *35*:999–1004, 1977.
5. Schettler, D: Sandwichtechnik mit Knorpeltransplantat zur Alveolar-Kammererhohung in Unterkiefer. *In* Schuchardt, K: Fortschr Kiefer Gesichtschir *20*:61, 1976.
6. Stoelinga, PJW, Tideman, H, Berger, JS, et al.: Interpositional bone-graft augmentation of the atrophic mandible: a preliminary report. J Oral Surg *36*:30, 1978.

Chapter 20

BONE GRAFTING IN DENTOFACIAL DEFECTS

Dale S. Bloomquist

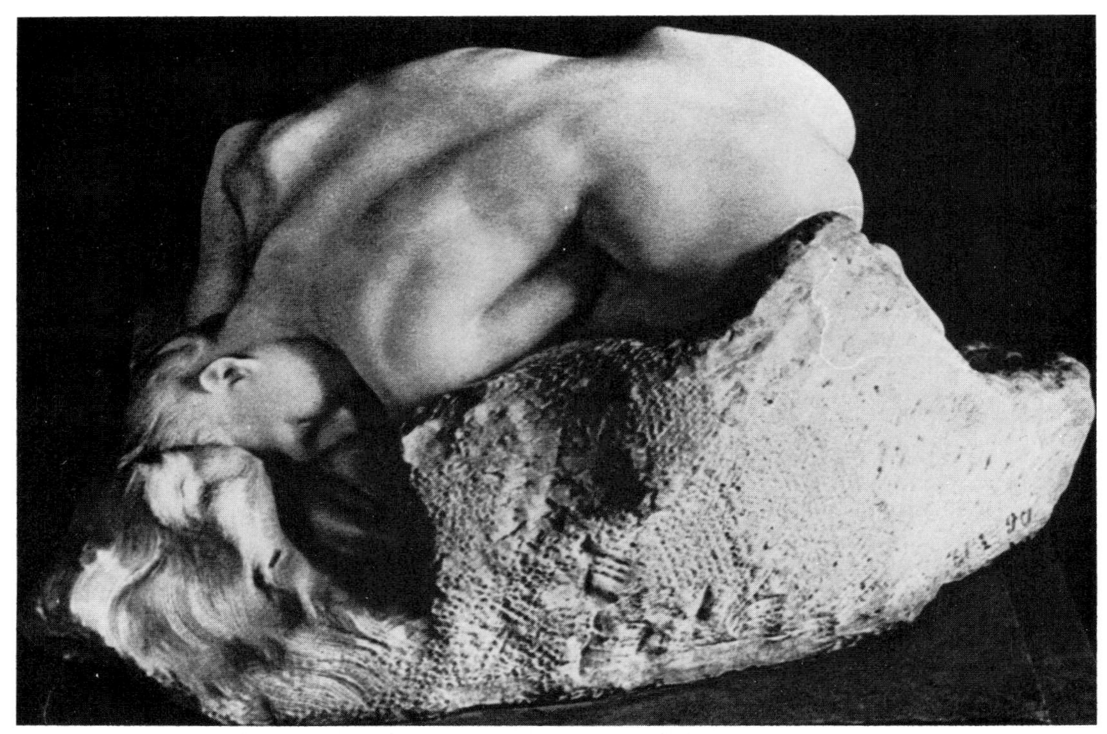

ESTABLISHING CRITERIA

Bone grafting has always played an important role in the correction of craniofacial defects. The recent proliferation of successful maxillofacial surgical procedures has resulted in more careful scrutiny of materials and techniques that can be used in bone grafting. Unfortunately, clinicians have received little help from researchers in establishing criteria by which appropriate grafting methods can be chosen for a particular surgical procedure. Most clinical and animal research is primarily concerned with whether the material will be tolerated by the host and whether it will be replaced by new bone. Although these criteria are extremely important, this information is not sufficient to determine whether a particular technique will obtain the best possible results in a particular situation. For a proper perspective to be achieved, the following properties should also be considered: (1) whether increased osteogenesis will result, (2) whether a matrix for new bone formation will be provided, and (3) whether mechanical stability will be obtained. When considering a graft for a particular surgical procedure, the surgeon must establish priorities for these properties, since no graft technique meets all of the objectives equally well.

Increasing Osteogenesis

The ability of bone grafts to increase osteogenesis is especially important in maxillofacial surgery, since an increase in the healing rate can decrease the time of intermaxillary fixation.[19, 39, 69] Unfortunately, many surgeons don't realize that only a few graft materials actually do increase osteogenesis. This can be done in two ways: (1) by providing viable cells that are either osteoblasts or can differentiate to osteoblasts and (2) by inducing the host tissue to increase the number of osteoblasts.

Clinicians have traditionally attributed the success of autogenous grafts to their ability to provide viable osteoblasts. Therefore, surgeons initially often included periosteum with the grafts, simply to provide more osteoblasts.[35, 49, 79] It has now been shown that few osteoblasts survive this type of transplant; thus, including periosteum with the graft is not generally recommended.[7, 36, 60] Autogenous cortical grafts are also weak in this ability to provide viable osteoblasts. In fact, it has been suggested that this method offers very little advantage as compared with some homogenous grafts.[17, 38, 68] Autogenous cancellous bone and marrow appear to be the only graft material that has a significant cell survival.[4, 59]

Urist[73, 74] has been instrumental in promoting an increased interest in osteogenic induction by bone grafts. Although first discussed by Levander in 1938,[45] the osteogenic induction ability of grafted bone has been poorly understood, and the ability of different graft materials to provide osteogenic induction has only recently been studied in detail. Since only autogenous cancellous bone and marrow have the ability to transfer a significant number of viable cells, clinicians should be more cognizant of those materials that appear to stimulate the formation of osteoblasts at the recipient site.

Providing a Matrix for New Bone Formation

The role of bone graft in providing a matrix is described by Burwell as having two parts.[16] The first, or passive, part is the ability of the graft to permit vascular and cellular invasion by tissue. This basically is dependent upon the size and number of "channels" through the graft. This aspect is important, both in the rate of graft stabilization and in the rate of graft replacement. Therefore, certain materials, such as freeze-dried cartilage, cannot be relied upon to provide stabilization between bone fragments[40] and remain unresorbed for years[68] because of minimal porosity.[16]

The second, or active, part of the matrix role overlaps with the first, in that it is defined as the ability of the graft to stimulate the invading tissue to produce bone. Awareness of this ability is important for the clinician, as some materials have a limited capacity to induce new bone formation while the graft is being resorbed. This results in the clinical effect of graft shrinkage that is frequently noticed on sequential radiographs. Heterogenous grafts most commonly undergo this resorption without replacement, but it is also noted in autogenous cortical grafts.[21, 53]

Providing Mechanical Stability

This is a practical consideration and is important in some types of orthognathic surgery in which bone is placed in osteotomy sites to assist holding the bone fragments in the correct position. Grafts used for this property only have to have a cortical component to allow for the required rigidity.[29, 76]

TYPES OF GRAFTS AVAILABLE

When considering the type of graft to be used for a particular surgical procedure, a ranking of the desired properties should be made before deciding on a specific graft. For example, when deciding on the graft material to be used along the osteotomy sites in an advancement of the maxilla at the Le Fort I level, the ability of the graft to increase osteogenesis would be a prime requirement and the matrix and mechanical properties would be of less importance. On the other hand, the material to be used between the tuberosity and the pterygoid plates in this procedure should have the ability to provide a long-term mechanical block. This material, therefore, should be replaced very slowly, in order that immediate relapse can be prevented until the osteotomy sites are healed. Thus, in the Le Fort I maxillary osteotomy, an iliac crest donor site could be considered because it would provide both autogenous cancellous bone and marrow for the osteotomy site and a block of cortical bone for the pterygoid plate.

In the following sections, various materials that either have been suggested for or have been utilized in maxillofacial surgery will be discussed. Unfortunately, good objective evaluation has not been made for many graft materials used in maxillofacial surgery. Therefore, the clinical impressions and recommendations of many authors will be used for the evaluation of the materials. The reader should be aware of the limitations of such evaluations.

Autogenous Bone Grafts

Autogenous bone has always been used as the standard against which other graft materials are judged. Most clinicians who first performed bone grafting used autogenous cortical bone taken from long bones, such as the femur or tibia, to graft skeletal defects.[79] However, ribs and the cortical portion of the iliac crest were commonly used for maxillofacial defects prior to World War II.[7, 76] Mowlem was the first to realize that cancellous bone offered advantages over cortical bone in craniofacial grafting and, in particular, noted two specific improvements.[53, 54] First, an apparent increase in healing rate was observed, and second, a relatively high tolerance to infection of the graft was noted. Since that time, numerous authors have supported Mowlem's observations concerning autogenous cancellous bone and have developed greater possible uses of this material.[1, 9, 19, 31, 59]

As pointed out by Mowlem, a differentiation should be made between cortical and cancellous bone when discussing autogenous bone grafts.[53] A third form of autogenous graft, the corticocancellous graft, should also be considered separately, since it offers different possibilities for the clinician.[20]

As mentioned previously, autogenous cortical grafts are of importance historically but at the present time are rarely utilized in maxillofacial surgery. This stems primarily from both clinical and research experience, which indicates that autogenous cortical grafts probably offer very little advantage over homogenous frozen or freeze-dried grafts.[4, 17, 38] Because of this limitation, autogenous cortical grafts should be used only when there is a readily available source that does not require a significant increase in surgery for the patient. Such a source would be the mandible, such as the chin, as suggested by Köle and others. Cortical grafts from the long bones should be considered impractical in maxillofacial surgical procedures.

Use of autogenous cancellous bone and marrow for patients undergoing maxillofacial surgery recently have received a significant amount of attenton. This is due mainly to Boyne, whose early work showed the practicality of using this material to repair facial-skeletal defects.[12, 62] The primary advantage of cancellous bone and marrow grafts is their ability to significantly increase osteogenesis. This appears to result from an osteogenic inductive capacity,[73] as well as the ability to provide viable cells that differentiate into osteoblasts.[59] The success of utilizing cancellous bone and marrow grafts in facial-skeletal surgery has also been enhanced by their almost unique ability to survive oral contamination or even infections, either of which would cause the failure of other types of grafts. The only apparent disadvantage to grafts using autogenous cancellous bone and marrow is their inability to provide mechanical stability.

The combination of cortical and cancellous bone in maxillofacial surgery has been popular,[21] but no attempt has been made to differentiate this form of autogenous graft from either a cortical or cancellous bone graft. This differentiation is important, as corticocancellous grafts do not simply combine the strong properties of the other two grafts. For example, corticocancellous grafts will not have the ability to increase osteogenesis as much as simple cancellous grafts because of the layer of relatively nonporous cortical bone. This layer of cortex prevents all cells but those close to the cancellous margin from receiving the nourishment needed for survival after the graft is transplanted.[81]

The advantages of corticocancellous grafts, however, are their ability to provide some mechanical stability similar to cortical grafts and at the same time provide for some increase in osteogenesis.[1, 76] The two commonly used sources of corticocancellous grafts are the ribs and ilium. The method of obtaining these types of grafts will be discussed later in this chapter. It should be emphasized, however, that the type of corticocancellous graft obtained varies greatly between these two sources. The rib, for example, contains relatively less cancellous bone than the ilium. There is even a wide variation within the ilium in the amount of cancellous bone available for this type of graft.

Surgical Techniques for Removing Autogenous Bone Grafts

As mentioned previously, cortical grafts have historically been obtained from long bones, such as the femur, tibia, or fibula. Because of the limitations of this type of autogenous graft, these sources are rarely used in maxillofacial surgery. A more practical source of cortical graft is the facial skeleton, most commonly the mandible.[2, 42, 72, 80] As previously discussed, this source has certain advantages in that it does not require a separate donor site. Köle[63] and Meyer[50] have suggested techniques using the symphysis for a block cortical graft to correct an anterior open bite (Figs. 20–1 and 20–2). This particular problem may be better managed by other procedures, but this source of bone should be kept in mind. Cortical bone removed during the correction of mandibular asymmetry has also been suggested as a potential graft material.

Aufricht has suggested that autogenous cartilage removed from the dorsum of the nose is valuable in augmentation of the chin.[3] This is a widely used technique,[18] although reports of long-term follow-up have never been published.

RIB

There are two primary methods by which rib grafts can be used in maxillofacial surgery. First, the corticocancellous rib graft may be used for augmentations or spanning osteotomy defects.[47] Second, rib may be used to provide a costochondral graft for condyle replacement, especially when further mandibular growth is expected.[77, 78]

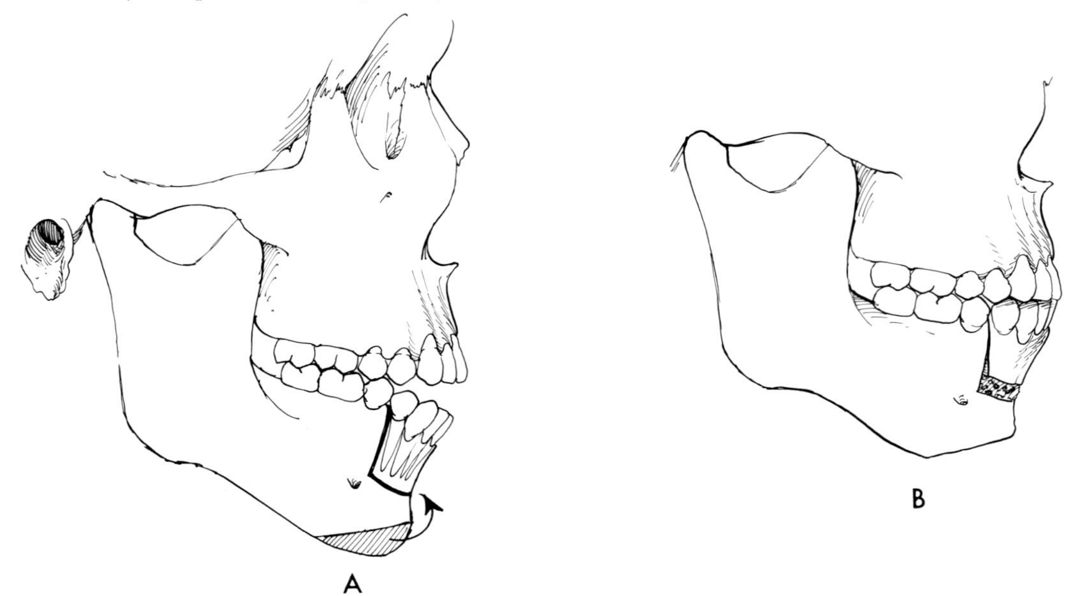

Figure 20–1. Köle technique for using cortical bone from chin in closing anterior open bite.

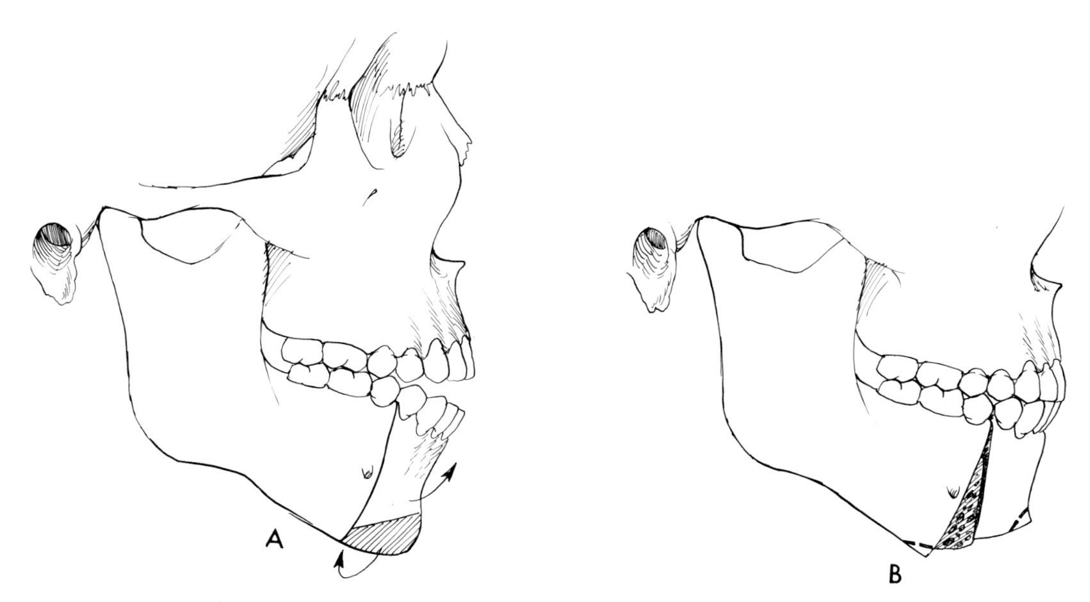

Figure 20–2. Meyer technique for closing anterior open bite.

The approach in obtaining both grafts is basically the same, with the fifth, sixth, or seventh rib generally chosen as a donor.[46] Most commonly, maxillofacial surgeons prefer to use general or thoracic surgeons to obtain the graft because few maxillofacial surgeons have the specific surgical experience and training in postoperative management required.

The rib graft procedure starts with the patient in a lateral position. The incision is made over the rib or ribs chosen for removal. If more than one rib is required, alternate ribs are taken to decrease postoperative morbidity.[46] Longacre has stressed the importance of closing the periosteum after the rib is removed, which will allow regeneration of a new rib. This technique allows a renewable source of graft material when multiple-staged procedures are planned.[46, 47, 48]

After removal, the rib is split, exposing the cancellous portion of the graft. These corticocancellous rib grafts can be shaped as desired to adapt to the recipient site. Various shapes can be produced by scoring the cortical plate of the rib graft (Fig. 20–3). Split rib can also be curved simply by forceful bending, but care must be exercised to prevent a complete fracture.

Removal of the costrochondral joint is similar to excision of the rib graft alone, except that a strip of periosteum should be retained at the cartilage-bone junction to prevent separation at this point. When transplanting this joint, part of the cancellous bone should be exposed to increase the possibility of union of the graft.

ILIUM

The ilium has been the most consistently utilized source of autogenous bone graft, as all three types of graft (cortical, cancellous, and corticocancellous) may be obtained.[7, 26, 76] Two limitations to using the ilium as a donor site have been mentioned in the literature. The first is that the iliac crest is one of the growth centers of the ilium,[39, 40] and the second is the morbidity associated with the surgery.[7, 39]

The concern of many surgeons about the possibility of disturbing iliac growth by

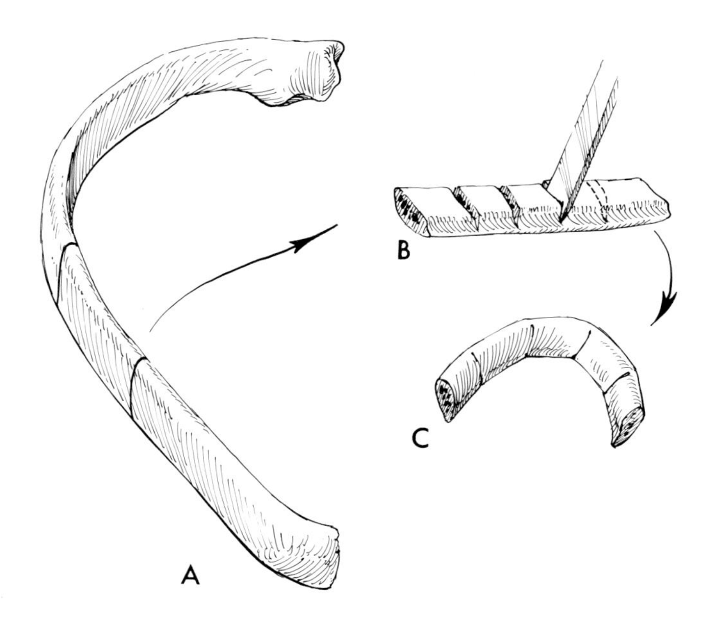

Figure 20–3. Design of bone cuts in rib needed to obtain curvature. *A,* Anterior view, *B,* superior view, and *C,* superior view after curvature.

taking grafts from the area has not been borne out clinically.[21] This does not mean that grafts can be obtained indiscriminately from this area, however, and care should be taken through the second decade of the patient's life, since the epiphyseal cartilage tends to persist beyond puberty. A method of removing bone from the ilium in children will be described later in this chapter. The problem of morbidity in removal of iliac bone grafts is due primarily to damage to either the gluteus medius or the gluteus maximus muscle.[1, 21] Subsequently, the patient will experience discomfort and difficulty with ambulation for a prolonged period after the surgery. Fortunately, this morbidity can be kept to a minimum in most cases.[26]

Although some surgeons claim that any portion of the iliac crest can be used as a donor source,[7,26] the most commonly used areas are the anterior and posterior iliac crests.[1,25] The major difference between the two areas is the amount of cancellous bone available.[25] Figure 20–4 compares sagittal sections through various portions of the ilium, illustrating differences in cancellous bone availability. This figure demonstrates the advantage of the posterior ilium as an excellent donor source for large amounts of cancellous bone. This amount of cancellous bone is necessary in grafting large mandibular continuity defects when a "crib" is used as discussed by Boyne.[11] Thick cancellous blocks that are extremely helpful in preprosthetic "sandwich" grafting of the maxilla[5a, 29a] or mandible[68a] can only be obtained from this site.

The anterior ilium is the popular and most practical source of bone for most surgical-orthognathic procedures. These procedures use relatively small amounts of bone such as the thin corticocancellous grafts that are placed along osteotomy cuts. Cortical or corticocancellous block grafts sometimes used in maxillary advancements can also be easily obtained from this region. The obvious advantage of this donor site is the ease with which grafts can be taken especially if two surgical teams are used.

Surgical Approach to the Anterior Iliac Crest

A wide variety of techniques have been recommended for obtaining bone from the ilium.[1, 7, 21, 31, 54, 66, 78] However, the soft-tissue approaches are basically similar, and

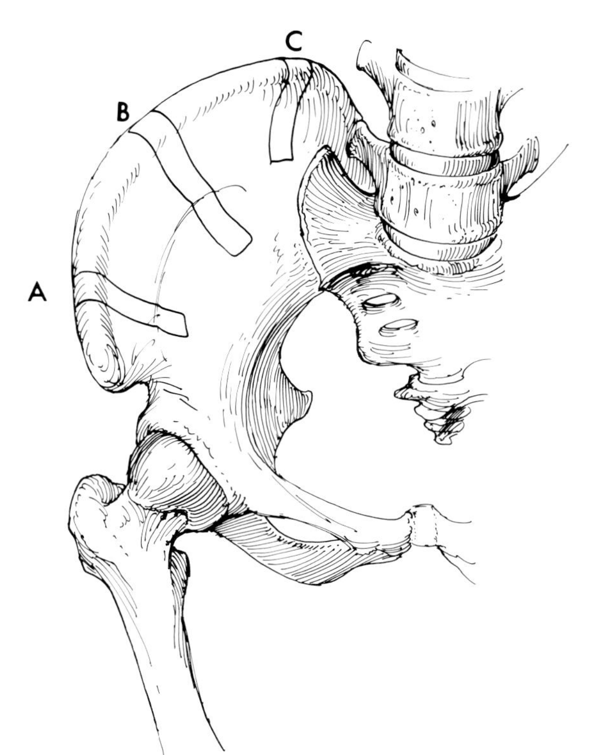

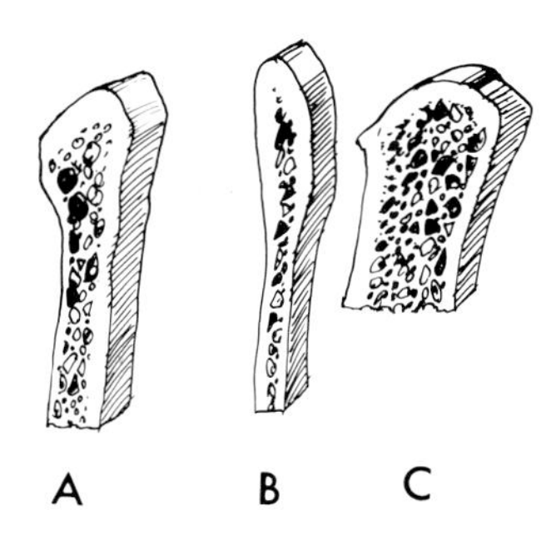

Figure 20–4. Comparison of section through the ilium at different parts of the crest. Section *A* is through the anterior crest and *C* is through the posterior crest.

the differences occur in the method of bone graft removal. Generally, it is recommended that the iliac crest itself be maintained in order to decrease surgical morbidity. Retaining the crest preserves the shape of the ilium and decreases the possibility of a "landslide" hernia. Another concern, as previously mentioned, is that trauma to the gluteal muscles attaching to the lateral portion of the crest causes a significant amount of discomfort as well as difficulty with ambulation.[1, 21] Therefore, it is generally recommended that the bone be obtained from the medial surface of the ilium to avoid damage to the gluteus medius, gluteus minimus, and tensor fasciae latae muscles.[21] These gluteal muscles may be spared by "trap-dooring" the iliac crest, as discussed in the following section. Unfortunately, elevating the periosteum with the attachment of these gluteal muscles from the lateral surface of the ilium is necessary when obtaining large grafts or grafts in children, in whom the epiphysis has to be preserved.[1, 21]

Technique. The patient is placed in the supine position, with anesthesia being administered as dictated by the maxillofacial procedure. A sandbag or rolled towel is placed beneath the buttocks to elevate and slightly rotate the anterior iliac crest. The surgical area is prepped in a routine fashion and draped with towels, and a sterile Vi-drape is placed. The face can then be prepped, taking care not to contaminate the donor area. Additional draping is done in a routine fashion for the specific maxillofacial procedure. The iliac donor site can then be re-exposed by cutting an opening through the drapes. This approach is used for either one or two operating teams and does not necessarily result in cross-contamination of the wounds. However, if simultaneous surgical procedures are undertaken, care must be exercised to avoid contamination of the donor site from the oral cavity.

The landmarks for the anterior iliac crest surgery include the anterosuperior iliac spine and the iliac crest as it curves superiorly and posteriorly from the spine. The relationship of significant anatomic structures to these bony landmarks is illustrated in Figure 20–5*A*. The anterior iliac spine should be considered the surgical boundary medially because of the potential for damaging nerves and vessels medial to the spine, such as the lateral femoral cutaneous nerve. An incision is made through the skin, starting approximately 1 cm lateral and inferior to the anterior iliac spine and continuing in the "hollow" below the iliac crest for 6 to 8 cm. It has been our experience that a 6-cm incision is the minimal length required for good exposure and does not

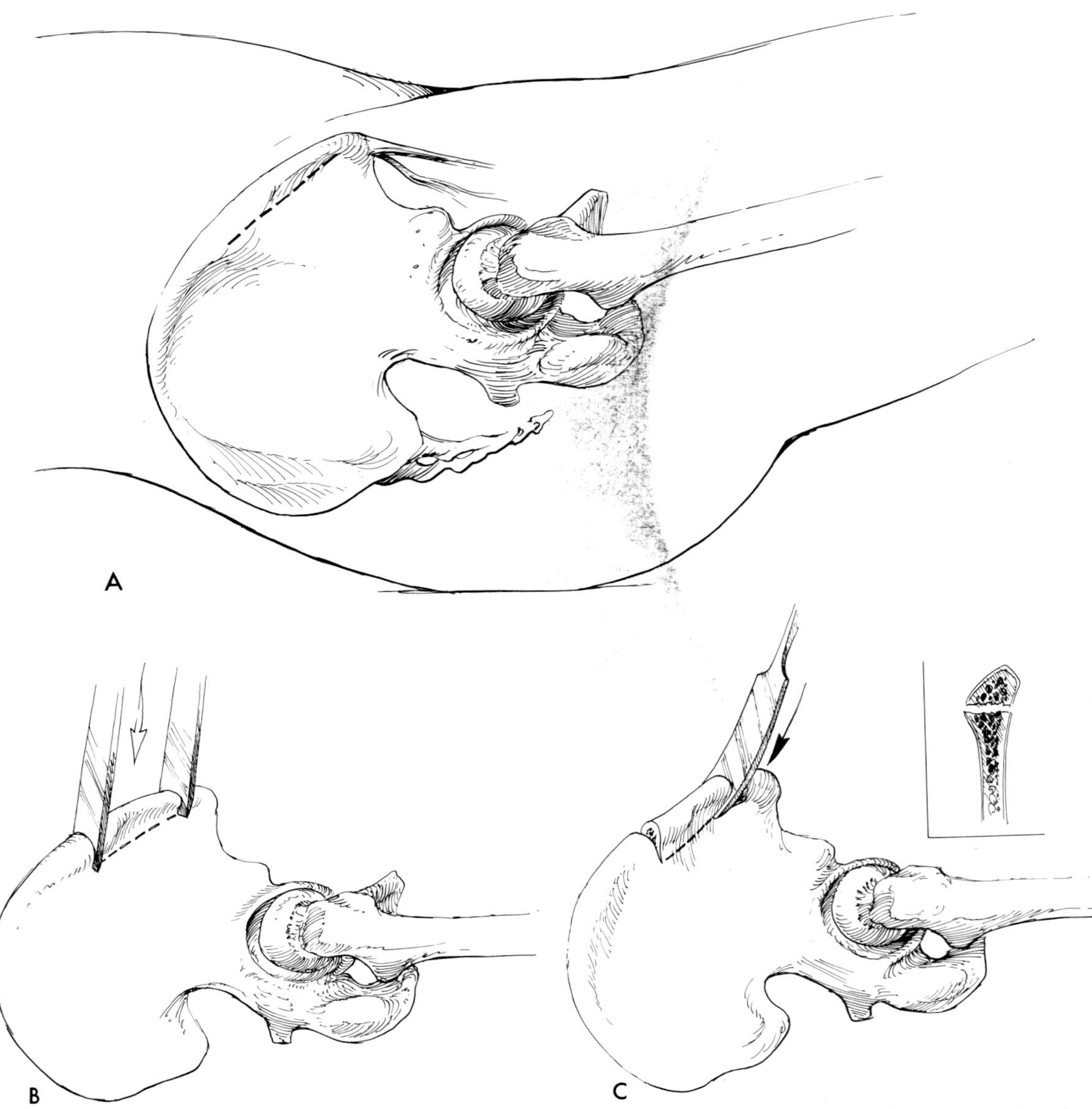

Figure 20–5. Steps in obtaining anterior crest grafts. *A,* Line of incision in relation to crest, inguinal ligament, and lateral femoral cutaneous nerve. *B,* Vertical cuts with straight osteotomy. *C,* Medial cut with curved osteotome. *D,* "Trap-door" of iliac crest fractured laterally. *E,* Cancellous bone removed with bone curette.

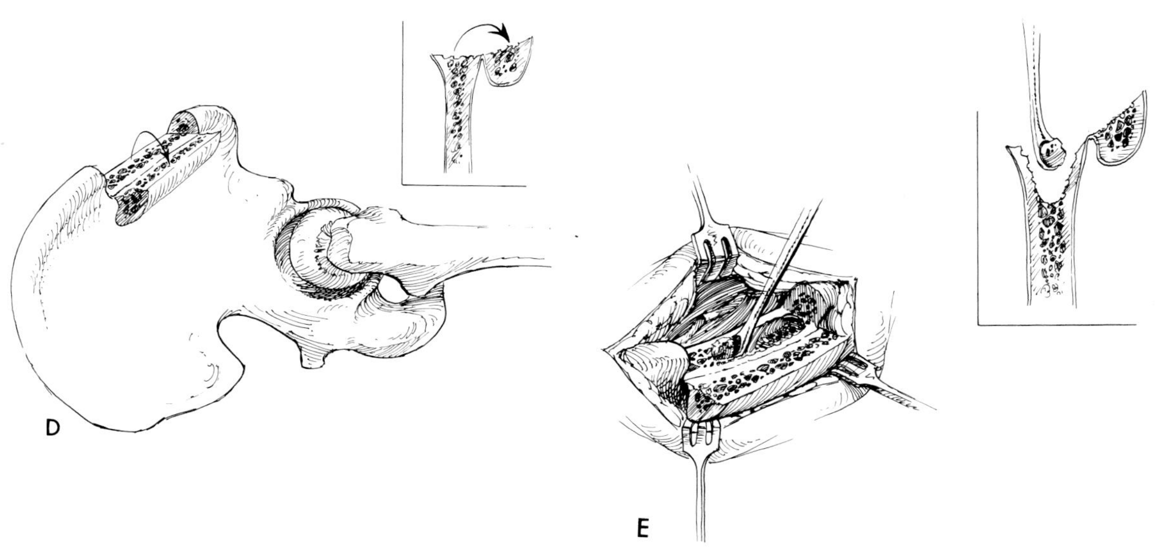

Figure 20–5 *Continued.* *See legend on the opposite page.*

cause any significant increase in morbidity compared with the smaller incisions that have been recommended. After passing through the skin, the superior edge of the incision can be retracted superiorly and the top of the iliac crest identified. A white line of periosteum between the gluteal and abdominal muscles is identified, and an incision is made down to bone through this area. This incision should be no closer than 1 cm from the anterior iliac spine to prevent damaging the inguinal ligament. A large orthopedic periosteal elevator is then used to carefully strip the periosteum medially from the crest. The removal of this periosteum can be difficult because of the attachments of the abdominal musculature. Below this point, in the iliac fossa, the stripping of the periosteum is easier and is accomplished with moist gauze. The iliacus muscle is stripped from the medial wall to a depth of about 8 cm. Moist gauze is placed at the depth of this wound, and a Taylor retractor is used to expose the donor site. This blood-soaked gauze is changed midway through the procedure and is used for the storage of the bone graft.

A "trap-door" is created by making two vertical cuts about 1 to 2 cm through the cortex with a 1-inch straight osteotome (Fig. 20–5*B*). These two cuts are connected along the medial surface with a half-inch curved osteotome (Fig. 20–5*C*). The iliac crest is then fractured laterally, hinging on the lateral periosteum and gluteal musculature (Fig. 20–5*D*). At this point, different approaches are employed, depending on the type of material needed.

Cancellous Grafts. Cancellous bone can be easily removed in strips by using orthopedic gouges, taking care to preserve the lateral cortex (Fig. 20–5*E*). Fractures through the medial cortex will often occur, however, and are not of any concern. In most cases, bone can only be taken to a depth of approximately 8 cm, since below this depth, the cortices come together and very little cancellous bone is available. An antral curette can be used to remove any remaining cancellous bone that is located under the crest, either medial or lateral to the trap-door. This bone should be stored in blood-soaked gauze, since the viability of the cells will be decreased if left exposed to room air or even if stored in saline-soaked gauze.[4, 61]

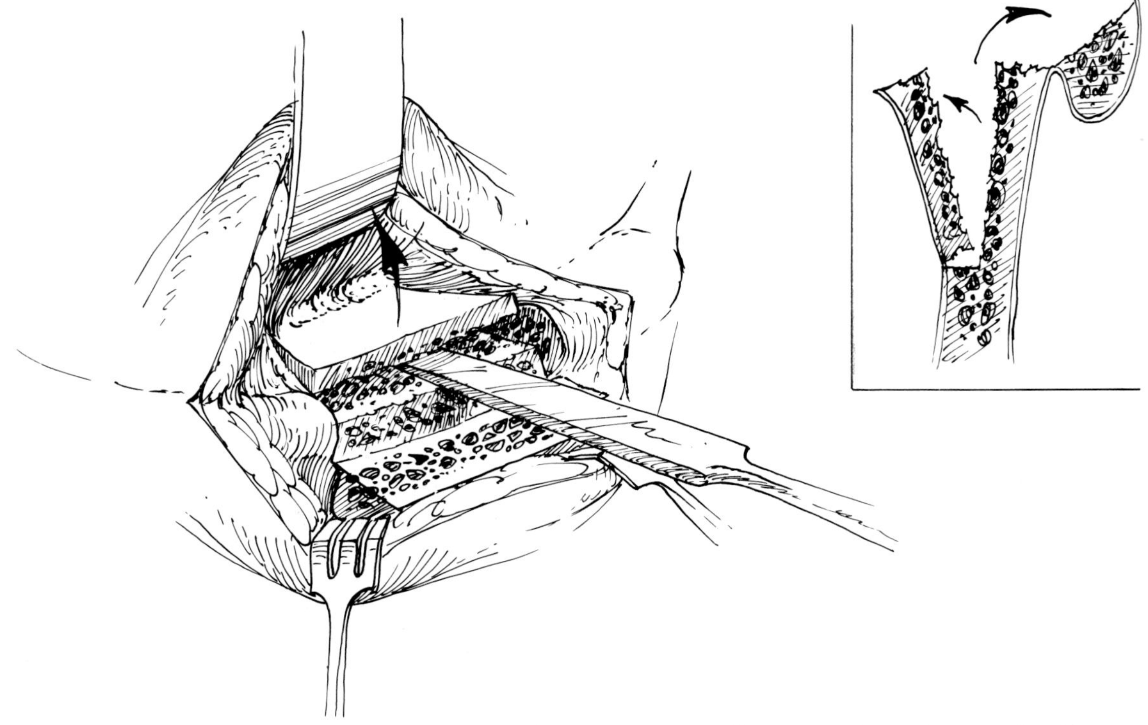

Figure 20–6. Superior views of the removal of a corticocancellous block from the anterior ilium.

Corticocancellous Grafts. A block of corticocancellous bone may be taken from the medial surface of the iliac crest by first making two parallel 6- to 8-cm vertical cuts with either a chisel, a bur or a reciprocating saw. The inferior portion of these vertical cuts is connected by an oscillating saw. A straight chisel is next used to separate the graft from the lateral cortex (Fig. 20–6). This large corticocancellous graft can then be shaped for use in the maxillofacial procedure and is then stored in blood-soaked gauze.

Following the removal of either the cancellous or corticocancellous graft, the basic procedure is resumed. All bone bleeding is stopped with bone wax, and external drains will not be required if hemostasis is achieved at this point. The gauze sponge is removed and the trap-door replaced. The abdominal muscles are sutured to the periosteum on the iliac crest with 2-0 chromic gut (Fig. 20–7). Care should be taken to insure tight closure so that the trap-door is held in position. The remaining portion of the wound is closed in layers, first with 2-0 chromic sutures for the superficial fascia and fat and then with 3-0 plain sutures for the subcutaneous tissues. Skin can be closed in a number of ways, but we prefer 3-0 nylon in a running fashion. Following application of a fine mesh dressing, fluff and Elastoplast are utilized to insure constant pressure over the wound and to prevent superficial hematoma formation. The patient is confined to bed for at least 12 hours and then is encouraged to ambulate. The patient is usually discharged by the second postoperative day and by then should be able to walk with only minor assistance, such as use of a cane. Skin sutures are removed on the tenth postoperative day.

Alternative Methods of Anterior Iliac Surgery. Full-thickness grafts from

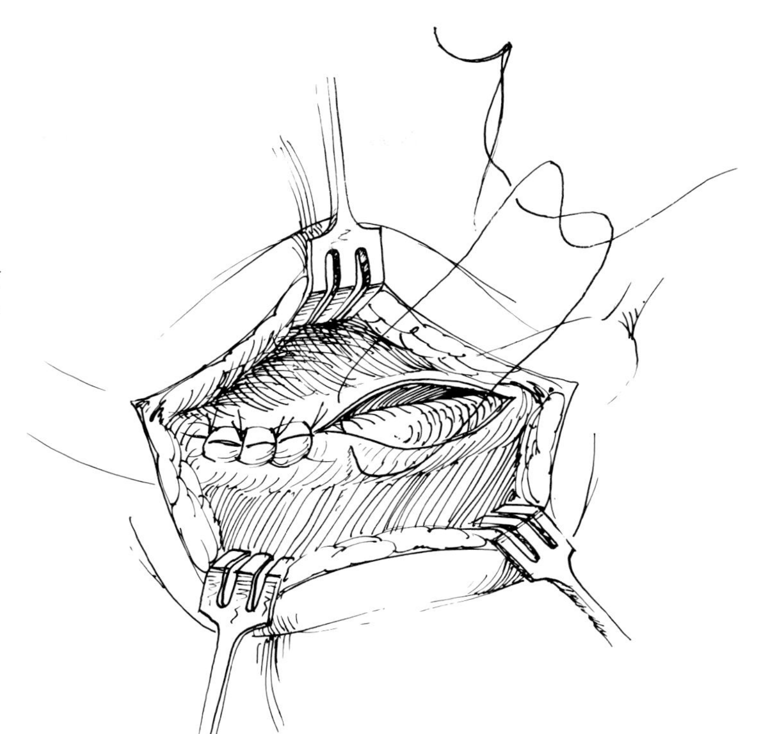

Figure 20–7. Superior view of suturing the muscle periosteal flap over the replaced "trap-door."

the anterior ilium are sometimes needed, and the approach utilized differs only in that the periosteum and gluteal muscles are stripped from the lateral cortex. An attempt should still be made to preserve the iliac crest, and therefore it is best to remove the graft from the gluteal fossa (Fig. 20–8).[21] The closure is similar except that the gluteal muscles are sutured directly to the iliacus muscle to prevent hematoma formation.[26] Thus, ambulation following this extensive procedure will be more difficult for the patient.[21]

Removing a graft from the ilium in children requires that only the lateral cortex

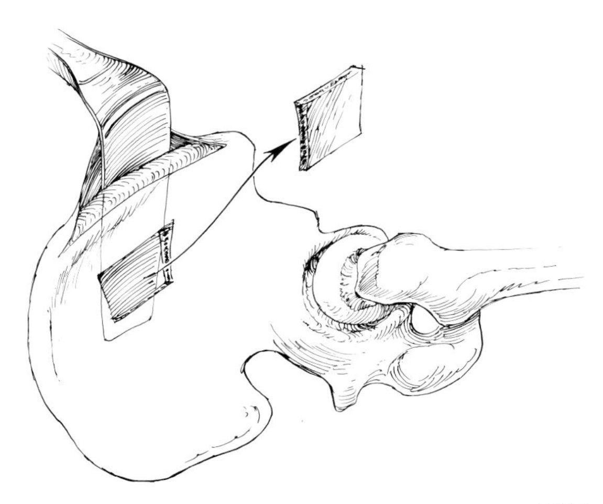

Figure 20–8. Removal of entire block of ilium without disturbing the crest.

be approached, with the epiphyseal trap-door hinged on the medial periosteum and abdominal muscles.[1] Cancellous and corticocancellous grafts can then be obtained in a fashion similar to the adult procedure. Although there is more pain caused by this approach than would be expected following the adult approach, the ilium is still the best source of cancellous bone in children.

Since periodontal bone surgery is primarily done on an outpatient basis, periodontists have developed methods by which cancellous bone can be removed from the anterior iliac crest with modified trephine biopsy needles.[51] This method is useful because only local anesthesia and sedation are required. The trephine technique usually requires a simple small incision down to the iliac crest, with the needle and stylet punctured through the cortex. The biopsy needle is then used to obtain the cancellous bone. As many as 20 cores of bone can be obtained in this manner. This technique, however, has little usefulness if the patient is under general anesthesia, since larger amounts of bone can be obtained more rapidly with the previously discussed procedures.

Surgical Approach to the Posterior Iliac Crest

As with the anterior iliac crest procedure, the surgeon should be thoroughly familiar with the local anatomy before approaching the posterior iliac crest. The success of the surgical procedures, with resultant minimal morbidity, depends upon this knowledge and expertise. In the posterior approach, the surgeon must be aware of the position of the stabilizing ligaments of the sacroiliac joint, as well as the position of the sciatic notch. Damage to these areas should not occur if thorough knowledge and proper technique are utilized.

TECHNIQUE. Anesthesia is first established, and the patient is rotated to a prone position. A large sandbag is placed under both anterior iliac crests to support the pelvis and also to provide room for respiration. For female patients, towels can also be placed along the lateral portions of the thorax to allow for respiration and prevent excessive pressure on the breasts. Before prepping the area, the surgeon should locate the landmarks, including the vertebrae, posterior iliac crest, and posterosuperior iliac spine. The area is then prepped and draped in a routine fashion with the Vi-drape covering the skin. Unlike the anterior iliac crest, the posterior crest usually cannot be visualized. It is therefore preferable to mark the position of the crest, vertebrae, and posterior iliac spine before making an incision. Multiple incisions have been suggested for the approach to the posterior ilium. However, we prefer a vertical incision extending superiorly from the posterior iliac spine and approximately 2 cm lateral to the vertical portion of the iliac crest to insure that damage to the cutaneous nerve supply is minimal (Fig. 20–9*A*). The incision is usually about 10 cm long to allow for proper access. The sharp dissection is extended down through fat to the gluteal fascia (Fig. 20–9*B*). At this point, the landmarks should be reidentified and an incision made along the posterior iliac crest between the attachments of the abdominal and gluteal muscles. The posterosuperior iliac spine is the inferior limit of this incision to prevent damage to the sacroiliac ligaments. The periosteum and the attachment of the gluteus maximus muscle are then carefully stripped laterally with a periosteal elevator. As is true for surgery on the anterior ilium, the stripping of the muscles from the crest is difficult. However, below the crest the periosteum can be

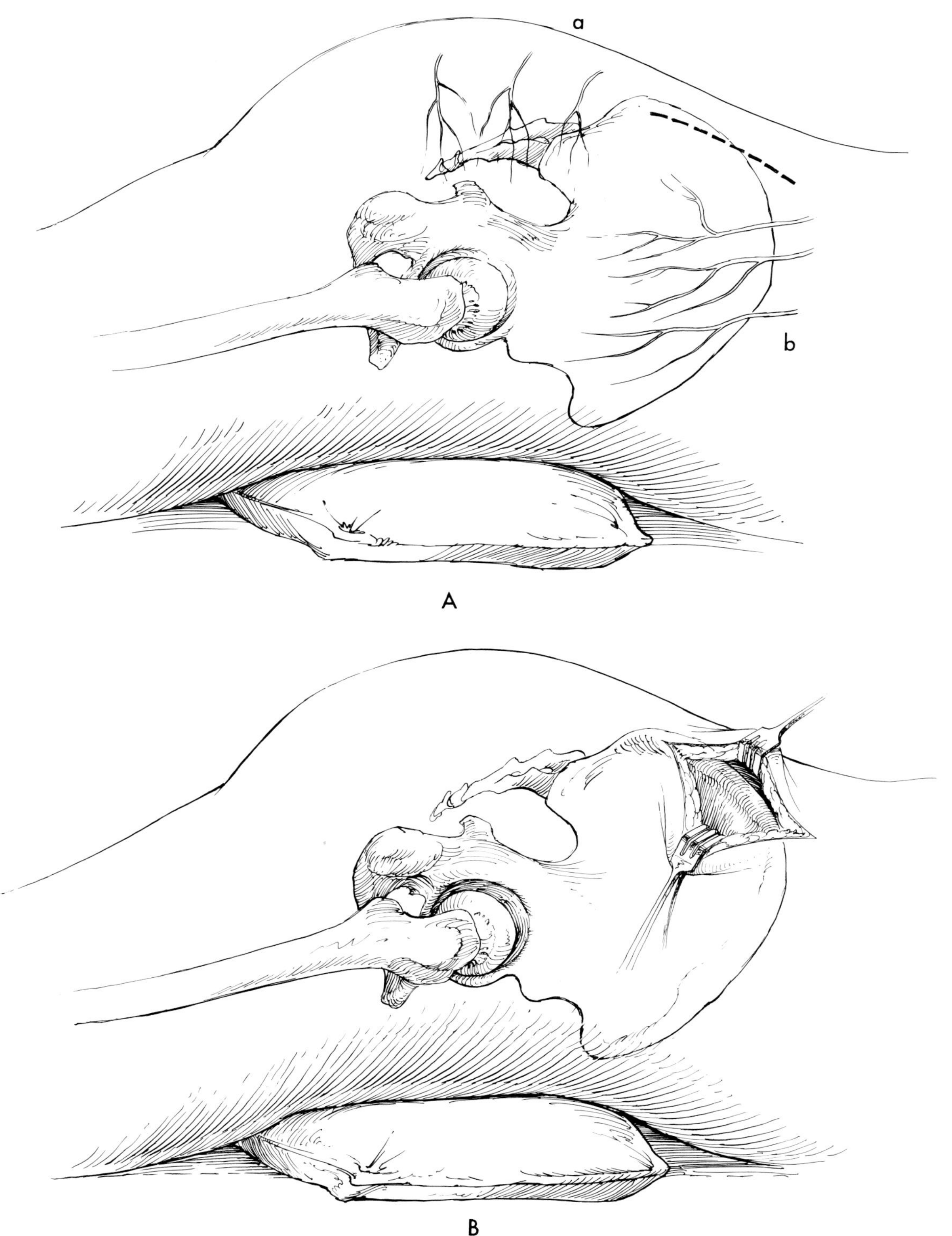

Figure 20–9. Steps in obtaining grafts from the posterior ilium. *A*, Incision from a labial view in relation to the crest and the middle cluneal nerves (*a*) and superior cluneal nerves (*b*). *B*, Exposure of the lateral crest.

Illustration continued on the following page

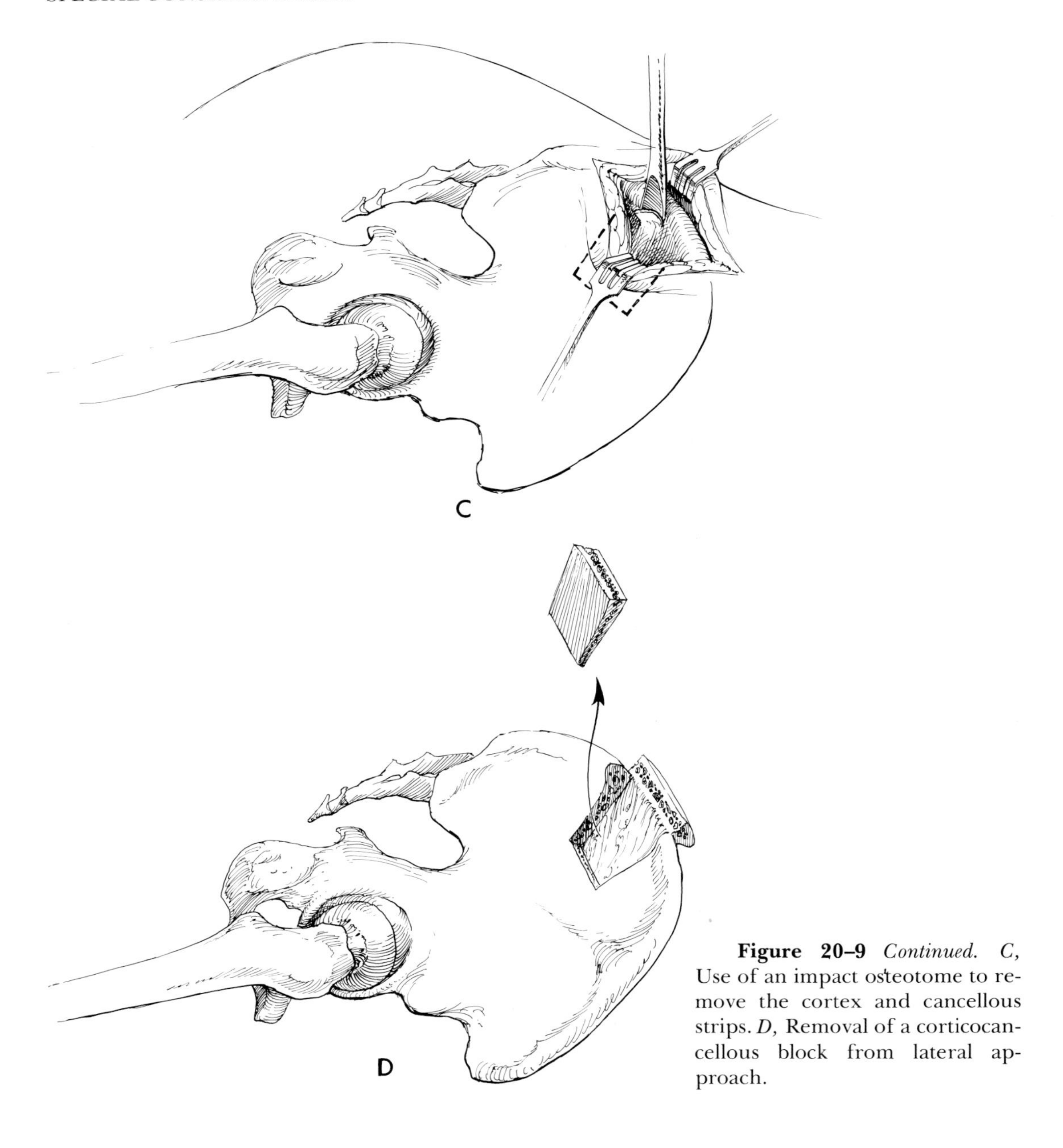

Figure 20–9 *Continued. C,* Use of an impact osteotome to remove the cortex and cancellous strips. *D,* Removal of a corticocancellous block from lateral approach.

elevated with moistened gauze. Before placing any deep retractors, the sciatic notch should be identified. Moist gauze is then placed in the depth of the wound, followed by placement of the Taylor retractor. At this point different approaches can be used, depending upon whether cancellous or corticocancellous grafts are desired.

Cancellous Grafts. A Stryker impact osteotome is used to remove all the cortical bone from the lateral portion of the ilium in an area of about 8 sq cm. The lateral cortex is thin and may easily be removed with the gouge attachment on the impact osteotome (Fig. 20–9*C*). The cancellous bone is then removed in long, thin strips with this instrument and is stored in blood-soaked gauze. Since the cancellous bone is approximately 2 cm thick in this area, a large amount of bone can be removed. Care should be taken not to penetrate the medial cortex to prevent entering the sacroiliac joint.

Corticocancellous Grafts. The posterior iliac crest is trap-doored, similar to the trap-door created for the anterior crest, except that the hinge is based on the medial periosteum and abdominal muscles. The posterosuperior iliac spine is preserved by keeping the trap-door at least 2 cm away from this structure. The remainder of the procedure is similar to the procedure discussed for the anterior ilium (Fig. 20–9*D*). It should be remembered that cancellous bone in the posterior ilium is approximately two times thicker than cancellous bone in the anterior crest. Therefore, a thicker graft can be removed. The graft is then cut to size and stored in blood-soaked gauze.

After removing either the cancellous or corticocancellous graft, the bleeding is controlled with bone wax and the gluteus maximus muscle and periosteum are tightly sutured to the periosteum of the crest and abdominal musculature. Tight closure is usually more difficult than in the anterior crest procedure, and it is preferable to use a near-far suturing technique, as illustrated in Figure 20–10. Following closure of the muscle and periosteum, the fascial and fat layers are closed with 2-0 chromic sutures, and the subcutaneous layer and skin are closed in any preferred manner. Dressings are placed similar to those for the anterior crest procedure, with care being taken to insure pressure to prevent superficial hematoma formation.

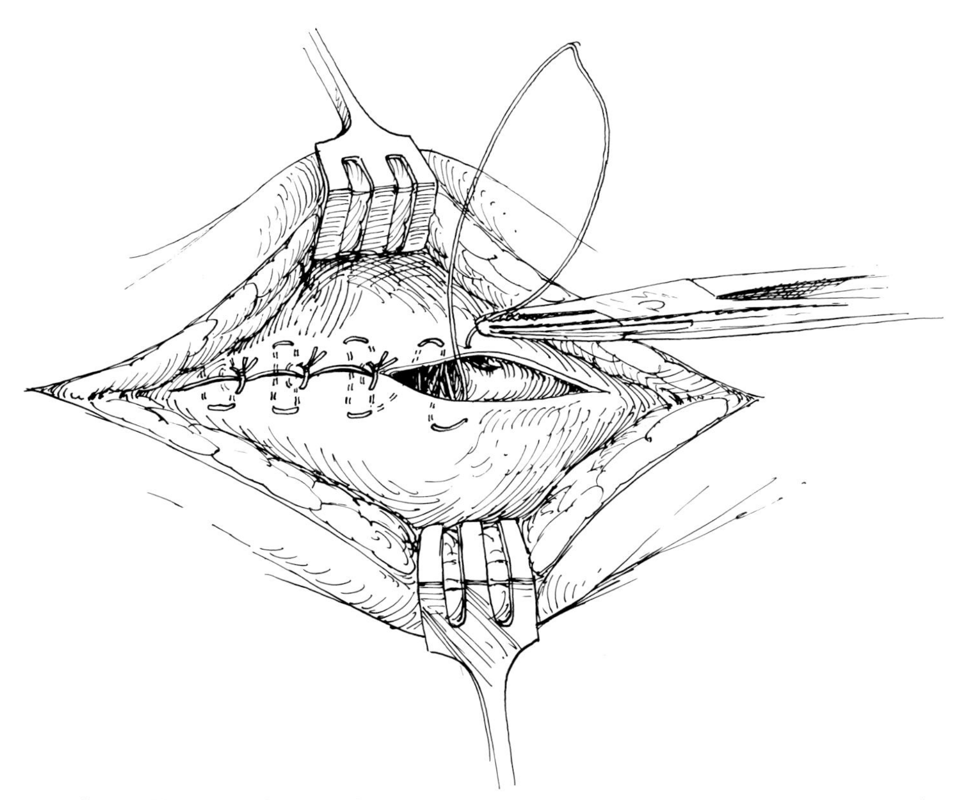

Figure 20–10. The use of the near-far suturing technique in closing the muscle-periosteal flap.

Morbidity and Complications of the Iliac Crest Surgery

The significant difference between anterior and posterior iliac crest surgery is in the amount of cancellous bone available from the posterior crest, as has been noted previously. Usually about three times as much bone can be removed from the posterior crest. Postoperative morbidity following the two procedures is similar, except when the lateral periosteum is stripped from the anterior ilium. Patients having anterior iliac crest surgery usually have a noticeable postoperative limp, whereas those with posterior iliac crest surgery have a minimal limp but have difficulty climbing stairs and rising from a sitting to a standing position. Although almost all patients complain initially of having more pain from the hip procedure than from the maxillofacial procedure, the patients retrospectively have stated that the overall discomfort from both areas is about the same.

The most frequently mentioned complication from either surgical procedure is damage to the cutaneous nerve supply. In anterior iliac crest surgery, care should be taken to avoid damaging the lateral cutaneous nerve that runs medial to the anterosuperior iliac spine.[21] This nerve is sometimes traumatized by excessive retraction. However, this is a transient problem and sensation normally returns.

The superior and medial clunial nerves are sometimes damaged during the posterior iliac surgery, but we have not had this problem when using the vertical incision, as previously described. Some surgeons claim that this is a minor complication and is not of any significance to the patient.

Other problems, such as the landslide hernia of the anterior ilium and damage to the sacroiliac joint or the contents of the sciatic notch in the posterior surgery, are extremely rare complications and are most commonly due to poor surgical technique. Infections to the donor areas are also rare, and in our experience with more than 100 cases, we have not noted this complication, probably because prophylactic antibiotic therapy is routinely begun prior to the surgical procedure.

The removal of large segments of bone from the anterior iliac crest can result in a "sartorius rupture." This loss of the insertion of the sartorius muscle usually occurs in the immediate postoperative period and can be disconcerting to the patient. The problem can be prevented by preserving the lateral cortex, especially in the area of the anterosuperior iliac spine.

The blood loss is usually slightly greater with the posterior iliac crest procedure, ranging from 200 to 500 ml. This loss can be kept down if the surgeon works rapidly after the bone is exposed, since most blood loss occurs at this time, and the bleeding cannot be controlled until the bone wax is in place. Postoperative bleeding is potentially a significant problem because large amounts of blood can be lost in this area without noticeable swelling. Therefore, other signs of significant blood loss must be watched for.

In general, the morbidity following the iliac procedures is minimal if the tissues are treated gently and care is taken during surgery. This minimal amount of postoperative discomfort has led us to a freer use of the ilium as a source of bone graft materials, and, therefore, less reliance has been placed on other forms of grafting.

Homogenous Bone Grafts

Homogenous bone grafts, like autogenous grafts, have been utilized clinically for more than a hundred years. However, because of its immunogenic potential, this source of bone graft did not become popular until World War II, when the development of newer methods of preservation led to the establishment of bone banks.[21, 44] At the present time three types of bank bone have achieved enough clinical success to make their use in maxillofacial surgery practical. Two of the three types, freeze-dried[8, 10, 41] and decalcified homogenous bone,[17, 56] have received extensive investigation and support in the United States. The third, frozen bone, is not presently as popular in this country, but has been used extensively in the Eastern European countries with apparent significant success.[19, 43]

There has been debate concerning the ability of homogenous bone to stimulate or induce osteogenesis. Urist and Burwell have provided the most extensive investigations in this area, and they generally conclude that decalcified bone produced by a weak hydrochloric acid solution has some potential for inducing osteogenesis.[16, 17, 74] This ability appears to be very fragile, however, and can be decreased by sterilization methods, such as radiation[75] and antibiotics.[17] Whether or not freeze-dried bone provides any increase in osteogenesis is still being debated, and any induction potential that may exist is apparently very weak and sensitive to sterilization methods.[17] For the best results, it has been suggested that homogenous bone be taken from fresh cadavers under sterile conditions. The bone should then be prepared (decalcified or freeze-dried) and repeated checks made for sterility.[28]

The immunogenicity of homografts that are treated by one of the three methods of preparation appears to be very minimal, and although immunogenicity can be demonstrated,[71] its clinical significance is minor.[58, 64] There seems to be no advantage to any of the three methods in this respect.[15]

Clinically, frozen and freeze-dried bone should therefore be considered valuable in providing both a matrix for new bone growth and some ability for mechanical stability with little osteogenesis.[8, 21] Decalcified bone, however, is a relatively soft material. This prevents any mechanical support but does provide a good matrix and has a definite advantage over other homografts in its potential to stimulate osteogenesis.[17]

Clinical Use of Freeze-Dried Bone

The common source of freeze-dried material in the United States is the Bethesda Bone Bank in Bethesda, Maryland. Bone to be used in maxillofacial surgery is usually provided by freeze-dried rib or corticocancellous strips. The bone bank should be contacted approximately four weeks before planning a procedure in which the use of freeze-dried material is being considered. The quantity and type of material needed should be specified, and information about the patient will also be required. Bone will then be sent in sealed glass containers. This material is sterile within the containers and can be used directly in the operating room. The bone can be reconstituted by placing it in a saline solution for the specific time period recommended by the bone bank. Many surgeons, however, have found that a time period that is shorter than recommended can be used. At the present time penicillin and streptomycin are added to the material used by the Bethesda Bone Bank, and the surgeon should therefore check the patient for possible allergies to these drugs. The addition of the antibiotics is probably a desirable safety factor, even though a loss in whatever osteogenic inductive capacity this kind of bone may have probably occurs.

As mentioned previously, homogenous bone can be used for surface augmentation or as a matrix in osteotomy gaps.[21] When used in augmentation surgery, it should be realized that the graft is replaced very slowly and that the final result of this technique may not be known for a significant period of time. A decrease in the graft size can be expected because of freeze-dried bone's lack of osteogenic induction, which results in some replacement with fibrous tissue during its resorption. Although not well studied, the amount of bone loss from this process can probably be equated to the loss with autogenous cortical bone, since the materials seem to be comparable in most experimental situations. Therefore, it should be anticipated that at least a 50 per cent loss of bone will occur after the graft is completely replaced.

The use of freeze-dried bone appears to be more practical for spanning gaps created during facial skeletal osteotomies. In these situations, mechanical stability and the ability to provide a matrix for bone growth are the two most important properties required of the graft. For example, when performing midface osteotomies in young, healthy individuals for whom a good osteogenic response would be expected, this material may provide a more practical solution when the additional surgery necessary for autogenous bone grafting is undesirable.[21]

Use of other homogenous materials such as dentin[57] and cartilage has been suggested in maxillofacial surgery, but in most cases any advantage over bone has not been demonstrated.[21, 26] Freeze-dried cartilage has been used successfully in Europe for facial skeletal augmentation.[68, 70]

Heterogenous Bone Grafts

Heterogenous bone grafts in humans have been utilized since the seventeenth century, but only recently have these materials have been considered for correction of defects in the maxillofacial region. Originally, heterogenous bone grafts were suggested as material to fill small defects in the jaw,[13, 23, 30] and most clinicians emphasized that these grafts did not provide any osteogenic potential but instead formed the matrix for growth of new bone. During early clinical use of these materials, however, it was suggested that heterogenous materials may, in fact, slow normal healing processes.[5]

Calf bone, which has generally been treated by some organic solvent, is the most common source of heterogenous grafts.[30] During its processing much of the immunogenicity of the graft is removed.

Only individual cases of the use of heterogenous bone grafts in the treatment of craniofacial deformities have been reported,[34] and, therefore, extensive evaluation of these grafts has not been made. It is generally accepted, however, that heterogenous material is not, at present, a viable alternative in maxillofacial grafting.[10]

Alloplastic Implants

Many types of alloplastic materials have been used in correcting facial skeletal defects, but at best these provide only a temporary replacement for bone. Biodegradable alloplasts have recently received some attention because of their obvious potential advantages in bone grafting. At this time, the calcium triphosphate ceramics appear to offer the greatest potential in this area, since animal studies and early clinical trials demonstrate that the material is replaced by bone.[6, 27, 33, 52] This material is replaced very slowly, and some studies suggest that the process can take up to six months. Clinical experience has been limited, although there has been some success in treating alveolar clefts. If the initial experience with this ceramic is supported by further trials, it can be considered as a material that would provide a matrix for bone formation as well as some mechanical stability. The alloplast would have the additional benefit of not requiring much care in handling, since it can be re-autoclaved if necessary. Other biodegradable alloplasts that have been suggested for maxillofacial surgery have been the polylactic acid materials.[24, 33] The suggested use of these materials is limited to fixation plates and cribs for autogenous cancellous bone,[65] and no claim has been made that the material can be used as a graft that will be replaced by bone.

REFERENCES

1. Abbott LC et al: The evaluation of cortical and cancellous bone as grafting material. J. Bone Joint Surg. *29*:381, 1947.
2. Aslanian RA et al: Use of mandibular bone for revision of malunion of the maxilla: report of case. J Oral Surg *29*:825, 1971.
3. Aufricht G: Combined nasal plastic and chin plastic correction of microgenia by osteocartilaginous transplant from large hump nose. Am J Surg *25*:292, 1954.
4. Bassett CAL: Clinical implications of cell function in bone grafting. Clin Orthop Research, *87*:49, 1972.
5. Bell WH: Use of heterogenous bone in oral surgery. J Oral Surg *19*:459, 1961.
5a. Bell WH, et al: Correction of the atrophic alveolar ridge by interpositional bone grafting: A progress report. J Oral Surg *36*: 693, 1978.
6. Biggs A et al: Inducing osseous proliferation with biodegradable ceramic implants. IADR Abst 1974.
7. Billington W et al: Bone-grafting in gunshot fractures of the jaw. Proc Royal Soc Med *12*:41, 1919.
8. Blackstone CH: Freeze-dried bank bone and its application in clinical oral surgery. Milit Surg *114*:437, 1954.
9. Blocker TG et al: Use of cancellous bone in the repair of defects about the jaws. Ann Surg *123*:622, 1946.
10. Boyne PJ: Treatment of extravasation cysts with freeze-dried homogenous bone grafts. J Oral Surg *14*:206, 1956.
11. Boyne PJ: Implants and transplants: review of recent research in this area of oral surgery. JADA *87*:1074, 1973.
12. Boyne PJ: Osseous grafts and implants in the restoration of large oral defects. J Periodontol *45*:378, 1974.
13. Boyne PJ et al: Use of an organic heterogenous bone in oral bony defects. US Armed Forces Med J *8*:789, 1957.
14. Burwell RG: Studies in the transplantation of bone. VII. The fresh composite homograft-autograft of cancellous bone. An analysis of factors leading to osteogenesis in marrow transplants and in marrow-containing bone grafts. J Bone Joint Surg *46*(B):110, 1964.
15. Burwell RG: The scientific basis of bone homotransplantation. The Scientific Basis of Medicine, Annual Reviews. New York: Oxford Univ Press, 1968, p 147.
16. Burwell RG: The fate of bone grafts. *In* Apley AG (ed): Recent Advances in Orthopaedics. London: Churchill, 1969, p 115.
17. Burwell RG: The fate of freeze-dried bone alloplasts. Transplant Proc *8*(Suppl 1):95, 1976.
18. Converse JM: Restoration of facial contour by bone grafts introduced through the oral cavity. Plast Reconstr Surg *6*:295, 1950.
19. Converse JM: Technique of bone grafting for contour restoration of the face. Plast Reconstr Surg *14*:332, 1954.
20. Converse JM et al: Experiences with a bone bank in plastic surgery. Plast Reconstr Surg *5*:258, 1950.
21. Converse JM et al: Bone grafts in surgery of the face. Surg Clin North Am *34*:375, 1954.
22. Cooksey DE: Application of freeze-dried bone

grafts in cysts of the jaws. J Dent Res *33*:655, 1954.
23. Costich ER et al: Heterogenous "anorganic" bone grafts in humans. Transplant Bull *4*:130, 1957.
24. Cutright DE et al: Degradation rates of polymers and copolymers of polylactic and polyglycolic acids. Oral Surg *37*:142, 1974.
25. Dick IL: Iliac-bone transplantation. J Bone Joint Surg *28*:1, 1946.
26. Dingman RO: The use of iliac bone in the repair of facial and cranial defects. Plast Reconstr Surg *6*:179, 1950.
27. Driskell TD et al: Calcium phosphate resorbable ceramics: A potential alternative to bone grafting. IADR Abst 1973.
28. Egydi P: Sterilization of infected bone by lyophilization and rehydration with antibiotic solutions. J Maxillofac Surg *4*:65, 1976.
29. Enneking WF et al: Human autologous cortical bone transplants. Clin Orthop *87*:28, 1972.
29a. Farrell CD, et al: One-stage interpositional bone grafting and vestibuloplasty of the atrophic maxilla. J Oral Surg *34*:901, 1976.
30. Gardner AF: Use of anorganic bone in dentistry. J Oral Surg *22*:332, 1964.
31. Gerrie J et al: Carved cancellous bone grafts in rhinoplasty. Plast Reconstr Surg *6*:196, 1950.
32. Getter L et al: A biodegradable intraosseous appliance in the treatment of mandibular fractures. J Oral Surg *30*:344, 1972.
33. Getter L et al: Three biodegradable calcium phosphate slurry implants in bone. J Oral Surg *30*:263, 1972.
34. Gimenez EJ: Subtotal transbuccal osteotomy of the face. Int J Orthod *10*:93, 1972.
35. Haldeman KO: The influence of periosteum on the survival of bone grafts. J Bone Joint Surg *15*:302, 1933.
36. Hayward JR et al: Iliac autoplasty for repair of mandibular defects. J Oral Surg *13*:44, 1955.
37. Heiple KG et al: Healing process following bone transplantation. J Bone Joint Surg *45*:1593, 1963.
38. Holmstrand K: Biophysical investigations of bone transplants and bone implants. An experimental study. Acta Orthop Scand *26*(Suppl):1–46, 1957.
39. Hovell JH: Bone-grafting procedures in the mandible. Oral Surg *15*:1281, 1962.
40. Ivy RH: The repair of bony and contour deformities of the face. Am J Orthod *30*:76, 1944.
41. Khosia VM: Reconstruction of a mandibular defect with a homogeneous bone graft: report of case. J Can Dent Assoc *1*:35, 1971.
42. Kline SN et al: Use of autogenous bone from the symphysis for treatment of delayed union of the mandible: report of case. J Oral Surg *28*:540, 1970.
43. Kolesov AA et al: Reconstructive operations on mandible in children (clinico-experimental study). Acta Chir Plast *13*:4, 1971.
44. Kreuz FP et al: The preservation and clinical use of freeze-dried bone. J Bone Joint Surg *33*(A):863, 1954.
45. Levander G: A study of bone regeneration. Surg Gynecol Obstet *67*:705, 1938.
46. Longacre JJ et al: Further observations of the behavior of autogenous split-rib grafts in reconstruction of extensive defects of the cranium and face. Plast Reconstr Surg *20*:281, 1957.
47. Longacre JJ et al: Reconstruction of extensive defects of the skull with split rib grafts. Plast Reconstr Surg *19*:86, 1957.
48. Longacre JJ et al: The early versus the late reconstruction of congenital hypoplasias of the facial skeleton and skull. Plast Reconstr Surg *27*:489, 1961.
49. McWilliams CA: The periosteum in bone transplantations. JAMA *62*:346, 1914.
50. Meyer RA: Mandibular symphysis as donor site in bone grafting for surgical correction of open bite: report of case. J Oral Surg *30*:125, 1972.
51. Midda M: Hip marrow implants in periodontal surgery. Br J Oral Surg *12*:40, 1974.
52. Mors W et al: Resorbable ceramic implants in surgically created cleft palates in dogs. IADR Abst, 1974.
53. Mowlem R: Bone and cartilage transplants, their use and behaviour. Br J Surg *29*:182, 1941.
54. Mowlem R: Cancellous chip bone-grafts. Report of 75 cases. Lancet, (*ii*):746, 1944.
55. Narang R et al: Improved healing of experimental defects in the canine mandible by grafts of decalcified allogenic bone. Oral Surg *30*:142, 1970.
56. Narang R et al: Experimental osteogenesis with decalcified allogenic bone matrix in palatal defects. Oral Surg *37*:153, 1974.
57. Nordenram A et al: A clinical-radiographic study of allogenic demineralized dentin implants in cystic jaw cavities. Int J Oral Surg *4*:61, 1975.
58. Pappas AM et al: Bone transplantation: correlation of physical and histologic aspects of graft incorporation. Clin Ortho *61*:179, 1968.
59. Peer LA: The fate of autogenous human bone grafts. Br J Plast Surg *3*:233, 1950.
60. Pollock GA et al: The value of periosteum in bone grafting operation. Mayo Clin Proc *15*:443, 1940.
61. Puranen J: Reorganization of fresh and preserved bone transplants. An experimental study in rabbits using tetracycline labelling. Acta Orthop Scand *92* (Suppl): 9, 1966.
62. Rappaport I et al: The particulate graft in tumor surgery. Am J Oral Surg *122*:748, 1971.
63. Reichenbach E et al: Chirurgische Kieferorthopadie. Leipzig: Johana Ambrosins Barth Verlag, 1965, p 152.

64. Reynolds FC et al: Experimental evaluation of homogenous bone grafts. J Bone Joint Surg 32(A):283, 1950.
65. Riley RW et al: Cancellous bone grafting with collagen stents. Int J Oral Surg *5*:29, 1976.
66. Robertson IM et al: A method of treatment of chronic infective osteitis. J Bone Joint Surg *28*:19, 1946.
67. Robinson M et al: Surgical-orthodontic treatment of a case of hemifacial microsomia. Am J Orthod *57*:287, 1970.
68. Sailer HF: Experiences with the use of lyophilized bank cartilage for facial contour correction. J Maxillofac Surg *4*:149, 1976.
68a. Schettler, et al: Clinical and experimental results of a sandwich technique for mandibular alveolar ridge augmentation. J Oral Surg *5*:199, 1977.
69. Scheurmann HA: Osteoplasty and its application in oral surgery. Oral Surg *20*:436, 1965.
70. Schofield AL: A preliminary report on the use of preserved homogenous cartilage implants. Br J Plast Surg, *6*:26, 1953.
71. Smith RT: The mechanism of graft rejection. Clin Orthop *87*:15, 1972.
72. Szmyd L et al: Anterior ramus graft of the mandible: report of case. J Oral Surg *27*:132, 1969.
73. Urist MR et al: Genetic potency and new-bone formation by induction transplants to the anterior chamber of the eye. J Bone Joint Surg *36*(A): 443, 1952.
74. Urist MR et al: Inductive substrates for bone formation. Clin Orthop *59*:59, 1968.
75. Urist MR et al: Excitation transfer in bone. Arch Surg, *109*:486, 1974.
76. Waldron CW et al: Mandibular bone-grafts. Proc Soc Med *12*:11, 1919.
77. Ware WM: Growth center transplantation in temporomandibular joint surgery. Trans Cong Int Assoc Oral Surg 1970, p 148–57.
78. Weinstein IR: Bone grafting after mandibular resection. J Oral Surg *26*:17, 1968.
79. West CE: Experiences with transplant grafts in ununited fracture of the mandible. Proc R Soc Med *12*:26, 1919.
80. Youmans RD et al: The coronoid process: A new donor source for autogenous bone grafts. Oral Surg *27*:422, 1969.
81. Zeiss IM et al: Studies of transference of bone. II. Vascularization of autologous and homologous implants of cortical bone in rats. Br J Exp Path *41*:315, 1960.

Chapter 21

MAXILLARY ASYMMETRY

Richard R. Bevis and Daniel E. Waite

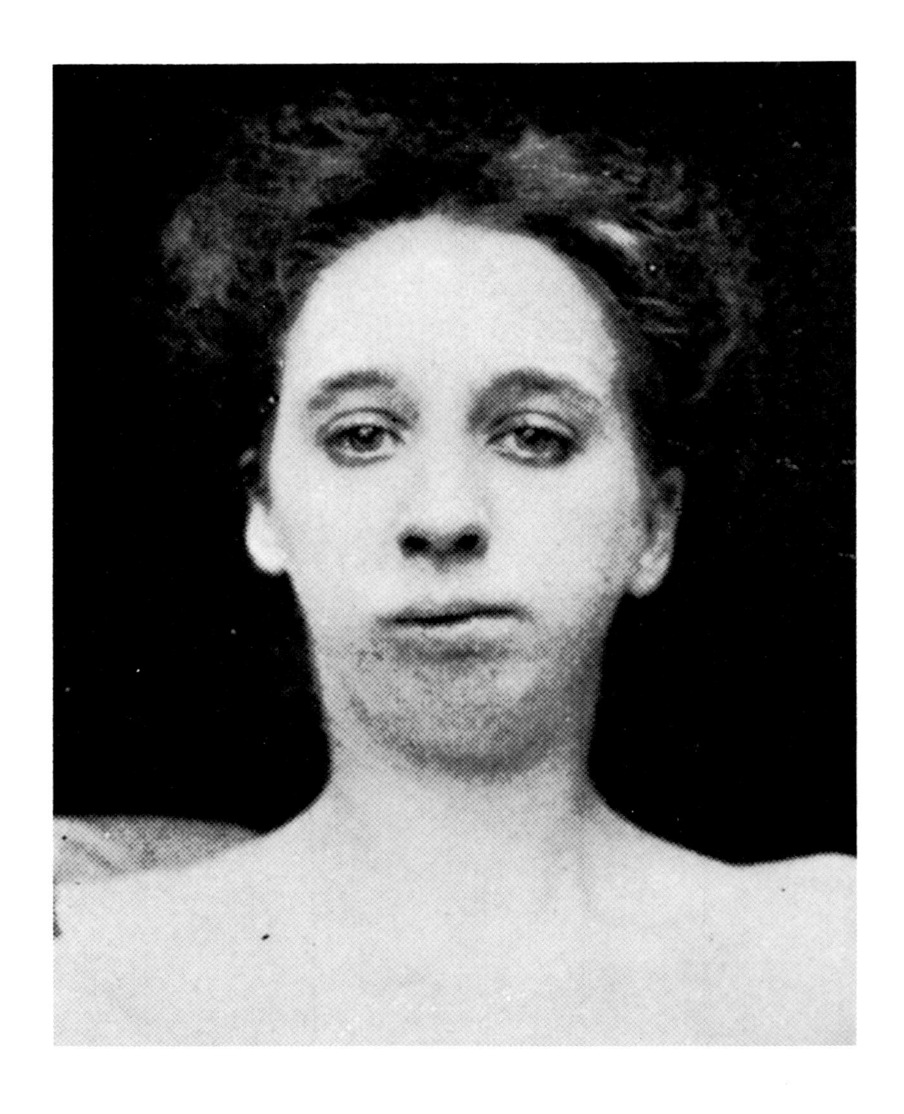

Maxillary asymmetry is not an uncommon entity. For many years, however, its correction has not received significant attention, in part because of the technical difficulty of maxillary surgery and insufficient understanding regarding the etiology of the disorder. The surgical techniques that have been developed more recently have made correction of this deformity somewhat easier, although the etiology and the classification of asymmetries is still not fully understood, except for the asymmetries that are obviously caused by trauma, tumors, or ablative surgery.

For purposes of this discussion, maxillary asymmetry is defined as an obvious disproportion of the right and left maxillae. This disproportion can occur in any one or all three planes of space (i.e., vertical, horizontal, or sagittal) and can involve the skeleton, the dentition, the soft tissue, or any combination of the three. The underlying skeletal deformity responsible for the deviation is the main subject of this chapter.

Esthetically, even the best-looking faces have some small asymmetries, as can be seen on a frontal photograph or upon clinical examination. When the asymmetry becomes severe enough to cause functional or psychologic problems or both, correction should be considered. In many instances, asymmetries of the dentition are correctable by orthodontic treatment alone, whereas asymmetries of the skeleton may require both surgery and orthodontic management. Current total or segmental surgery of the maxilla or surgical-orthodontic treatments of both maxilla and mandible provide new approaches to the management of facial asymmetry. Patients who would not have been treated in the past can now undertake a treatment plan not only to correct their facial asymmetry and the canted occlusal planes esthetically but also to achieve good functional correction.

EVALUATION OF MAXILLARY ASYMMETRY

Careful evaluation of the patient with facial asymmetry is crucial to a good result. The degree of the bony, dental, and soft-tissue deformity must be determined. Included in a thorough clinical examination is the careful examination and evaluation of normal facial components as well as the abnormal structures. To accomplish this, a number of special records *must* be obtained.

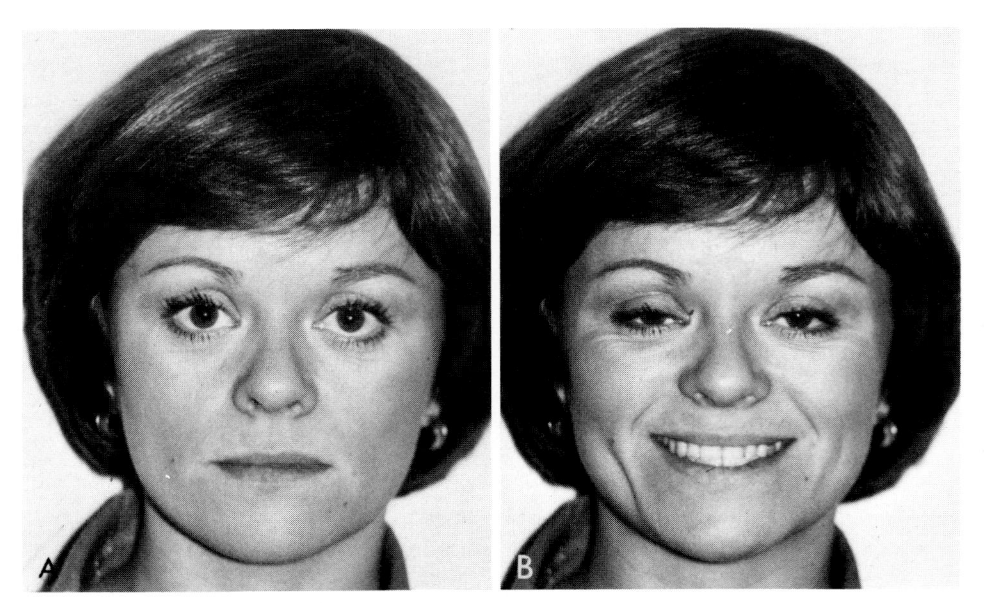

Figure 21–1. *A,* A carefully oriented photograph taken with the patient's lips at rest to show natural lip posture. *B,* A "full smile" photograph is taken to verify lip position in relation to the teeth and gingivae and to show muscle action.

1. *Well-oriented photographs.* Full-face photographs should be taken with patient's head in natural head position, i.e., true horizontal plane parallel to the floor. Photographs should be taken both with the patient smiling and with the lips relaxed. Profile photographs taken with the lips touching and relaxed will often show important soft-tissue postural positions (Fig. 21–1). Occasionally photographs taken from an oblique position or with a tongue blade indicating the occlusal plane may be useful. Adequate views of the dentition should include the anterior occlusion, the posterior occlusion, centric relation and centric occlusion views if warranted, and possibly a freeway space view if lengthening of the maxilla is being considered.

2. *Posteroanterior and lateral cephalograms.* These two radiographic views are well known to both oral surgeons and orthodontists. Proper exposure to show soft-tissue registration and as near true orientation as possible are absolutely necessary. The need for follow-up radiographs for treatment evaluation makes the cephalogram especially significant.

The lateral cephalometric radiograph is evaluated in the standard manner utilizing Reidel's analysis of skeletal and dental landmarks. Relative maxillomandibular anteroposterior positions can be determined. Soft-tissue evaluation using the Minnesota integument analysis can be done from the lateral radiograph.

The posteroanterior cephalogram is most important in the evaluation of maxillary asymmetry in the horizontal and vertical planes as well as in evaluating cants of the occlusal plane. Measurement reference lines are drawn vertically through stable structures like the crista galli–cribriform plate area and bisecting the nasal cavity (Figs. 21–4 and 21–5). A horizontal reference line is drawn perpendicular to the vertical line at the level of the occlusal plane to measure the deficiencies or excesses in the maxillary alveolus. These measurements can be either vertical or horizontal.

3. *Properly related and mounted study models.* A facebow transfer is needed for accurate model mounting and is done in accordance with the type of articulator used, i.e.,

Whip-Mix or Hanau (see Case 21–2, Figure 21–15). Asymmetries involving abnormal external auditory canals or abnormal condyle-fossa relationships are best mounted on the Hanau-type facebow, which allows for digitally palpating the point of condylar rotation. Relating to Frankfort horizontal plane is also helpful in asymmetry cases and can be done with the facebow according to its manufacturer's instructions. A wax bite is used to relate the maxillary and mandibular teeth in centric relation. (Cases involving only small segmental repositioning may require mounting in centric occlusion.)

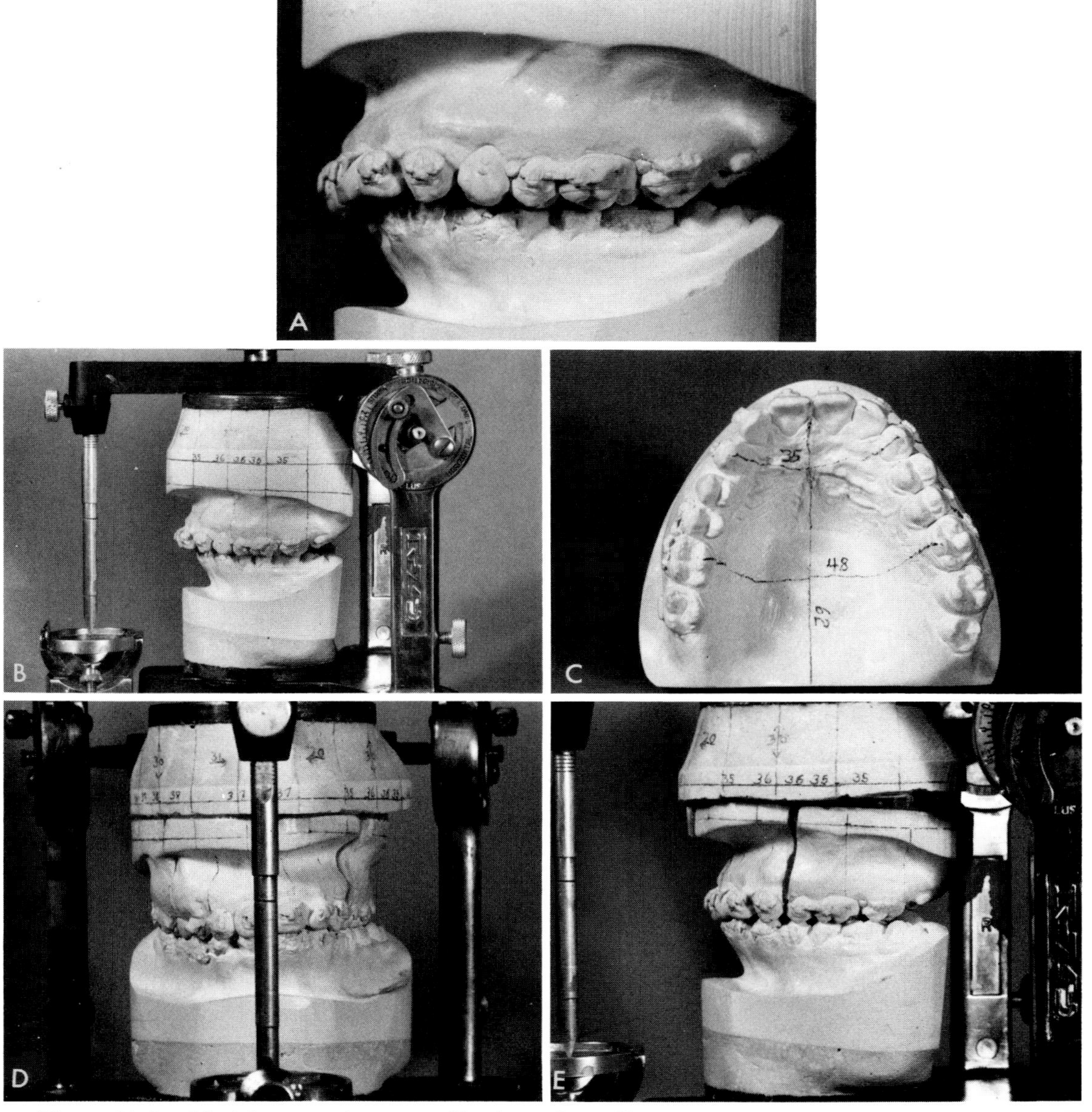

Figure 21–2. Model surgery in a case of horizontal maxillary asymmetry. *A,* This cast demonstrates the amount of discrepancy between the maxillary and mandibular arches in a horizontal plane. *B,* The models are mounted in a fully adjustable articulator utilizing a face-bow transfer. Marks are made on the cast in the vertical, horizontal, and anteroposterior dimensions. *C,* This occlusal view of the maxillary model shows the intercuspid, intermolar, and anteroposterior dimension recordings. *D* and *E,* These two views show the model surgery cuts in frontal and left lateral views. Accurate measurements in model surgery are essential for excellent surgical results.

4. *Facial moulage.* This technique may be useful for accurate assessment in patients who require extraoral prosthodontic treatment and rehabilitation.

5. *Model surgery.* Accurate model surgery simulating the planned bone movements is essential for the well-planned maxillary asymmetry correction. The models are mounted on an anatomic articulator as described in Chapters 6 and 8. Vertical and horizontal reference lines are drawn on both the maxillary and the mandibular model bases and on the palatal aspect of the maxillary cast. The appropriate reference numbers, as they relate the mandible and the maxilla to one another and to the articulator, are then recorded. All appropriate dento-osseous segments of the maxilla are then sectioned from the model as previously determined by clinical and cephalometric measurements and prediction tracings, in the same manner as that planned for the actual surgery. If the anterior segment is to be included in the surgery, this segment is the first to be repositioned. This allows for the proper axial inclination, anteroposterior relation, and vertical positioning of this vital segment. The planned lip position, maxillary and mandibular incisor relationship, and vertical tooth position (to attain the best functional and esthetic result) are thus accomplished. The posterior segment or segments are then moved into the planned occlusion. The various horizontal and vertical reference lines are again measured and an accurate three-dimensional prediction of the planned surgery is established (Fig. 21–2).

CLASSIFICATION OF MAXILLARY ASYMMETRY

Most asymmetries involve both the maxilla and mandible, with the severity of involvement depending upon the growth stage at which the asymmetry manifests itself. Head and neck syndromes or trauma are usually responsible for the very severe facial asymmetric deformities.

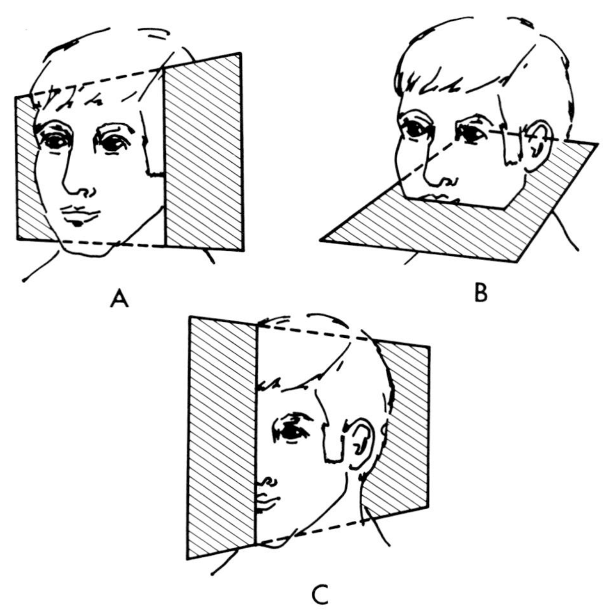

Figure 21–3. Schematic representation of the three planes in which maxillary, mandibular, or combined maxillary-mandibular asymmetry may be described. *A,* vertical; *B,* horizontal; *C,* sagittal.

Attempts to classify maxillary asymmetries have described the vertical, horizontal, or sagittal planes (Fig. 21–3). Since a combination of planes will be involved in most asymmetries, they are best categorized by their primary plane of asymmetry. There may also be additional combinations such as an asymmetric segment of the occlusion and a bony abnormality at the same location. The problem may be further compounded by soft-tissue deficiency in the same anatomic area.

VERTICAL MAXILLARY ASYMMETRY (DEVIATION FROM THE HORIZONTAL PLANE) (Fig. 21–4)

Vertical asymmetry is present when the right and left halves of the maxilla are at different levels when related to the horizontal plane. The asymmetry may involve the entire maxilla or a portion of it, i.e. one or more teeth, half the arch, or the entire arch (Fig. 21–4*A*).

Esthetic Features

A frontal examination of the patient may show noticeable right-left facial asymmetry (Fig. 21–4*A*). This of course will vary with the severity of the deformity. At rest, the lips may be canted and asymmetry of the alar bases and nasolabial folds may be noted. The midline of the upper lip and the midpoint of the chin and the mandible are generally deviated. The discrepancies are accentuated when the patient smiles and exposes the teeth and associated occlusal plane. For further detail, refer to Case 21–2.

Cephalometric Features

Conventional lateral cephalograms can be helpful in confirming certain aspects of vertical asymmetric deformities. The vertical discrepancy of the maxillary dentition may be noted as well as a coexisting mandibular asymmetry if a discrepancy of the inferior border is present (Fig. 21–4*C*).

The posteroanterior radiograph is the most useful in treatment planning. Maxillary and mandibular occlusal cants, maxillary and mandibular bony and dental midline deviations, and mandibular gonial angle deviations can all be measured from this view. Coexisting orbital or malar asymmetries may also be noted, although if these occur, they are usually minimal. In patients with hemifacial microsomia or certain other congenital abnormalities, severe asymmetry may be noted in this region.

Occlusal Analysis

The most noticeable characteristic in the occlusal disharmony is alveolar enlargement. The magnitude of the discrepancy is best seen in properly mounted models and posteroanterior radiographs.

Alignment of the Arch

Although the major discrepancy is in the vertical dimension, study of the models will help to reveal any associated right-left arch alignment discrepancy.

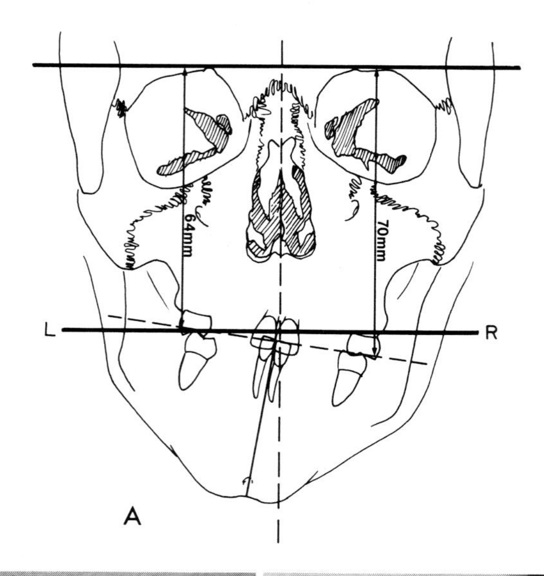

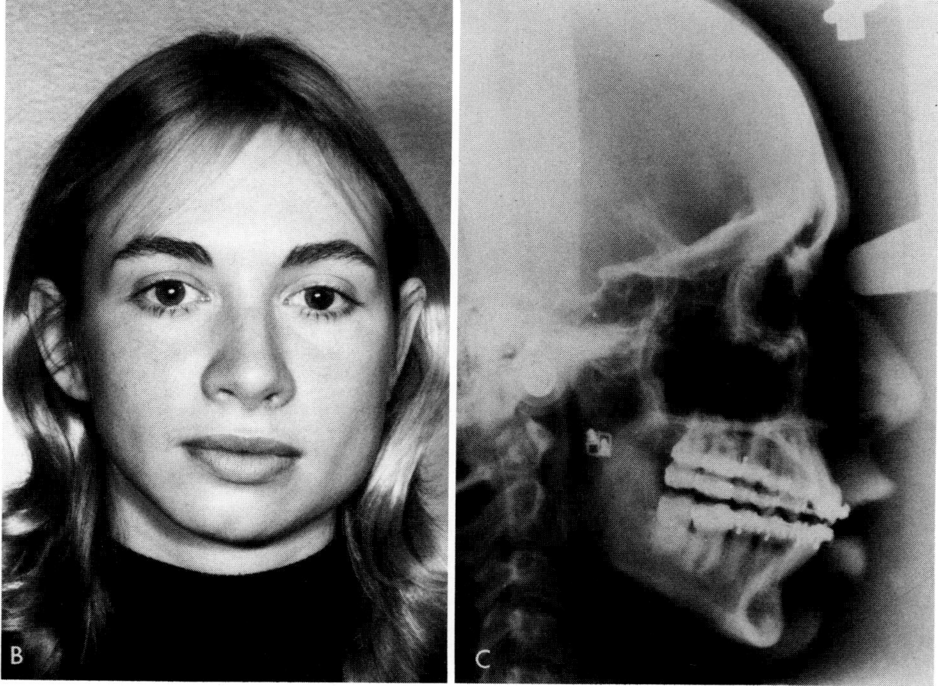

Figure 21–4. Vertical maxillary asymmetry (deviation from the horizontal plane). *A,* Schematic representation of the deformity. *B,* This patient demonstrates maxillary asymmetry of the vertical classification. Childhood injury to the left condylar head has caused asymmetric growth of the maxilla and mandible (see Case 21–2). *C,* A lateral cephalometric radiograph demonstrating maxillary occlusal cant.

Interarch Relations

Properly trimmed models mounted on an anatomic articulator (e.g., Whip-Mix or Hanau) by means of a facebow transfer and an interocclusal wax checkbite in centric relation will provide valuable information. Since the mounting reflects true horizontal, accurate determinations of right-left vertical discrepancies are possible. The facebow mounting and evaluation of the bite relation of the maxilla and mandible to the mandibular condyle (the point of mandibular autorotation) allow accurate assessment of the autorotation that will occur during the proposed operations.

Treatment of Vertical Maxillary Asymmetry

The decision of which side of the face or maxilla is more pleasing is the key to treatment planning. Full life-size photos are cut and reassembled to help determine which side is most esthetically pleasing (see Case 21–2). Tooth to lip relationships are established from lateral cephalometric radiographs, clinical photos, or direct observation of the patient smiling and unsmiling. Midline relationships can be carefully assessed using an imaginary line down the center of the face. All deviations from this line can be observed and recorded.

Once the clinician has decided which side of the maxilla is more pleasing, model surgery is used as a guide in determining the extent of surgical movements needed. It is usually necessary to combine mandibular surgery with maxillary surgery to obtain an acceptable result. Movement of the maxilla to correct vertical asymmetries can be managed by total or segmental maxillary osteotomy. With either of these techniques, the segment(s) can be moved superiorly or inferiorly as well as laterally, medially, anteriorly, or posteriorly. Timing of maxillary and mandibular surgery is discussed later in this chapter.

HORIZONTAL MAXILLARY ASYMMETRY (DEVIATION FROM THE SAGITTAL PLANE) (Fig. 21–5)

Horizontal asymmetry is present when the right and left sides of the maxilla are at different widths when related to the sagittal plane (Fig. 21–5*A*).

Esthetic Features

Maxillary asymmetry in the horizontal plane does not usually produce significant facial disharmony unless the deformity is great or is combined with canted asymmetries (Fig. 21–5*B*). The maxillary dental midline may be displaced, but the primary deviation usually exists in the posterior maxilla. This deformity is not generally associated with a mandibular asymmetry.

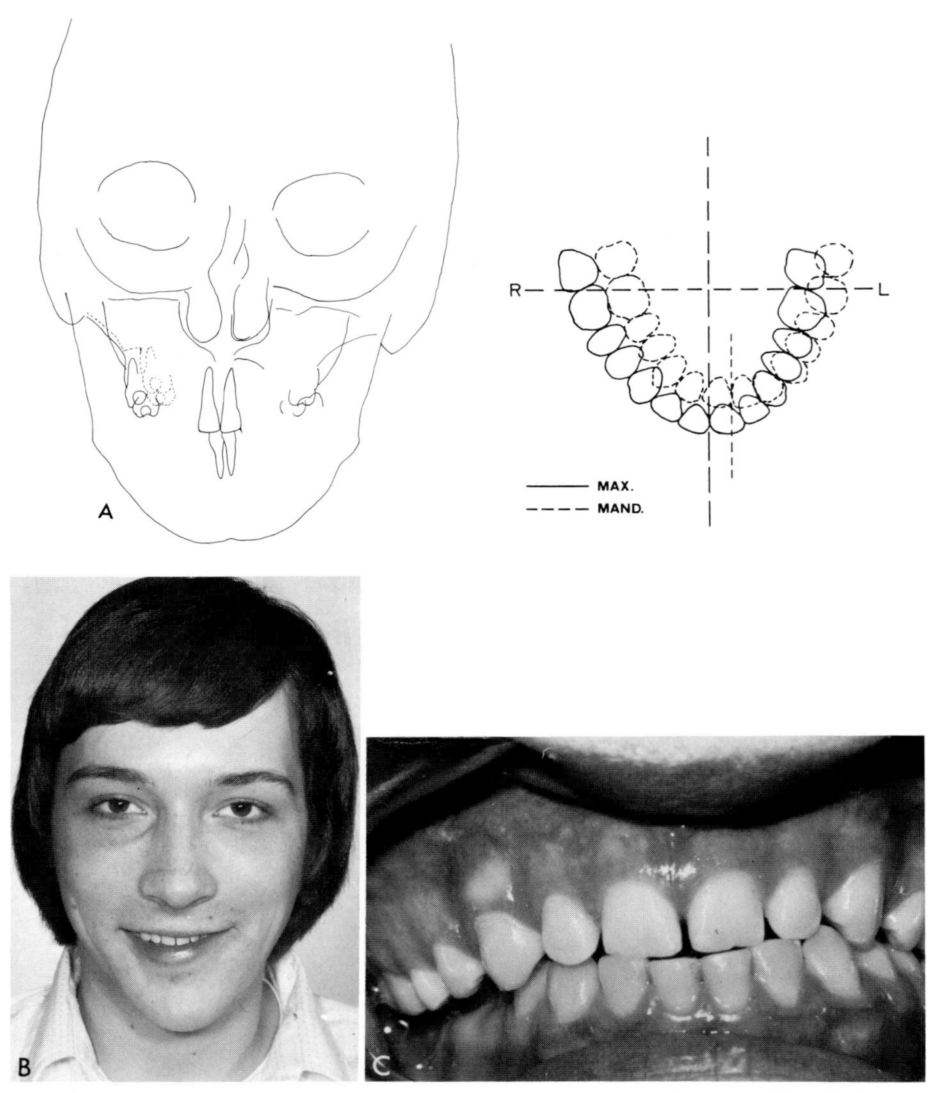

Figure 21–5. *Horizontal maxillary asymmetry.* *A,* Schematic view of the deformity. *B,* Patient R. R. demonstrates horizontal maxillary asymmetry of unknown etiology. Note that facial asymmetry is slight, but the occlusal arch asymmetry (*C*) is extreme. *C,* Upper left buccal segment demonstrates a complete overbite.

Legend continued on the opposite page

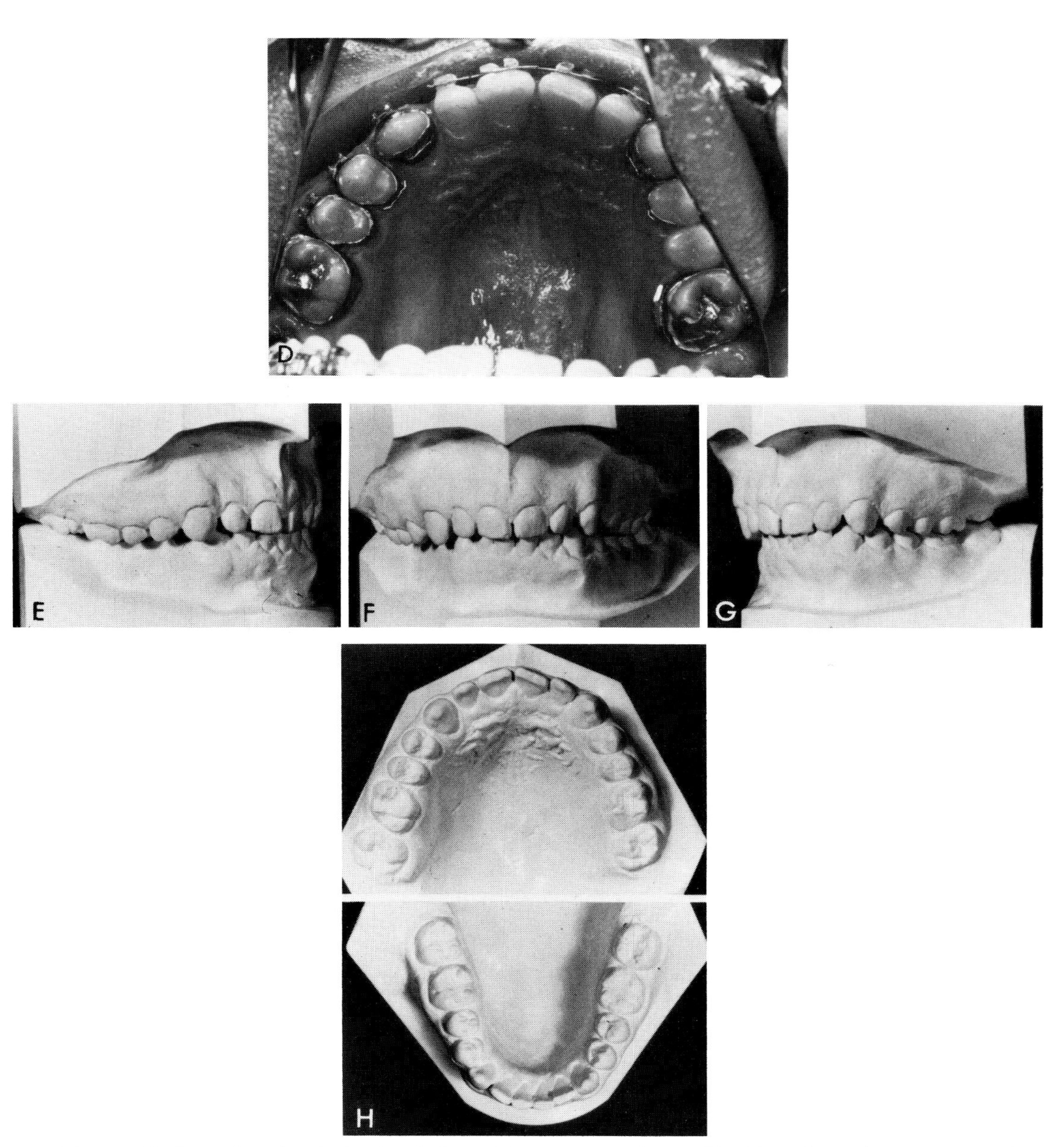

Figure 21–5 *Continued.* *D,* Occlusal view of the asymmetric maxilla. Note the right arch expansion. *E* through *H,* Lateral anterior and occlusal views of the preoperative models.

Cephalometric Features

The nature of the deformity may be revealed by measuring the distance of the right and left molars from the sagittal midline on the posteroanterior cephalogram.

Occlusal Features

Alignment of the Arch

When the maxillary model is examined, the palatal aspect will usually reveal the right-left asymmetry. A line drawn on the midline of the palate of the model permits measurement of the right-left discrepancy.

Occlusion

The patient with a primary horizontal maxillary asymmetry will exhibit some form of posterior crossbite (Fig. 21–5*C*). It involves either constriction or overexpansion of the maxillary segment and is *usually* unilateral. The articulated models should be studied in centric occlusion or centric relation, depending on the nature of the discrepancy and on whether the treatment will involve unilateral or bilateral surgery. Articulated models are checked for occlusal discrepancies in right-left lateral and protrusive jaw movements in order to avoid placing teeth in traumatic occlusal relationships and/or torquing of the segmental osteotomy sections. Following unilateral surgery, an occlusal adjustment is often necessary.

Treatment of Horizontal Maxillary Asymmetry

Horizontal maxillary asymmetries can be corrected with segmental procedures (e.g., posterior maxillary osteotomy) or during a total maxillary or total alveolar osteotomy. The size and type of segment to be mobilized is determined according to the degree of malocclusion and the esthetic asymmetry that exists. In most instances, however, because the asymmetry involves more than one dimension, it is necessary to mobilize the total maxilla and divide it into multiple segments. The downfracture technique for total maxillary osteotomy has been discussed and illustrated by Bell[1] (Fig. 21–6). (See also Chapter 8.) In some patients, particularly those with cleft palates, the rapid maxillary expansion method employing orthodontic-surgical procedures has been used with good results. Some patients with borderline maxillary asymmetry or crossbite also benefit from this technique (Fig. 21–7).

POSTERIOR MAXILLARY ALVEOLAR SEGMENTAL OSTEOTOMY (Figs. 21–8 and 21–9)

A horizontal incision is made in the maxillary vestibule above the apices of the teeth, extending from the tuberosity to the anticipated anterior limit of the osteotomy. The mucoperiosteal flap is reflected superiorly only enough to permit access for the horizontal osteotomy. The flap is also reflected gingivally near the anterior limit

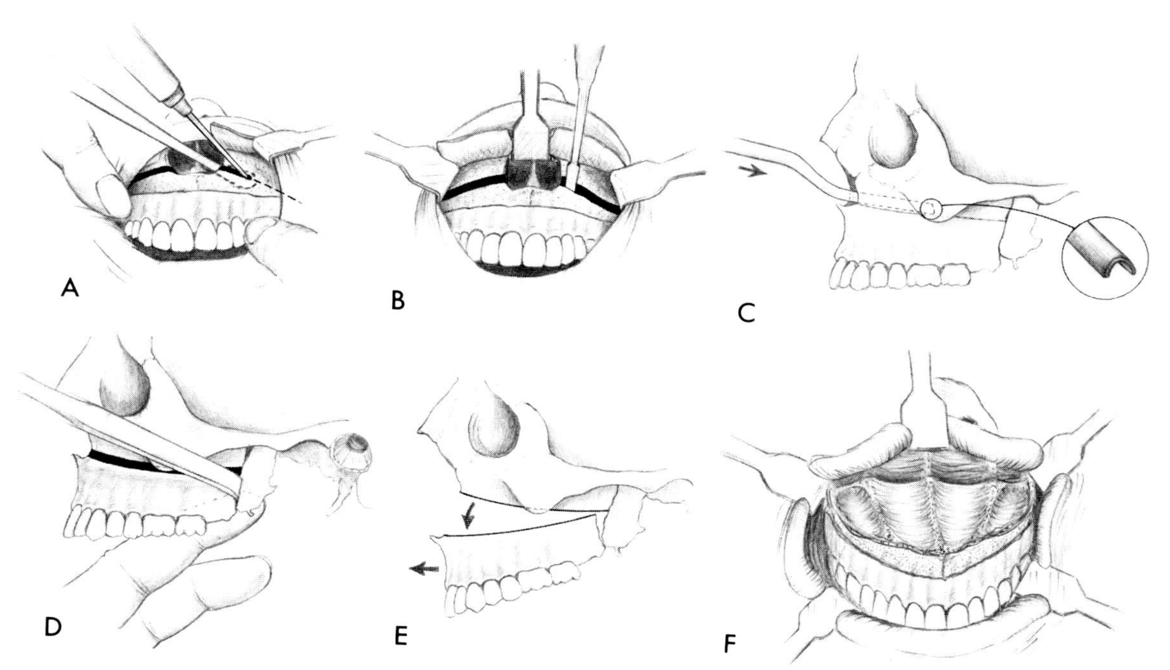

Figure 21–6. Schematic of Le Fort I (downfracture) osteotomy. Incision and flap reflection in the vestibular mucosa from the area of the zygomatic buttress bilaterally. *A,* While an instrument protects the nasal mucosa, the first bone cut is made in the lateral wall. *B,* The medial wall of maxilla is cut with osteotome. *C,* A nasal septal chisel is used to separate the cartilaginous septum from the nasal crest of maxilla. *D,* Separation of the pterygoid plates. *E,* Downfractures of entire maxilla. *F,* View of floor of nose following downfracture. (See also Chapter 8.)

of the planned osteotomy to permit access for the vertical bone cut between the roots of the indicated teeth (a vertical incision is not necessary). The vertical bone cut is first scored with a bur on the buccal bone and then completed with fine osteotomes to avoid injury to the roots of the adjacent teeth. The horizontal buccal osteotomy and ostectomy are then completed with the surgical bur.

The transantral approach is used to reach the palatal alveolar bone with a fine curved osteotome directed against the palate, inferior to the palatal process and the maxillary nasal wall but superior to the tooth roots. A finger should be placed on the palatal mucosa during sectioning to avoid mucosal perforations. In some instances, it is possible to make this palatal cut with a rotating bur in patients with high palates in whom an ostectomy of the lateral antral wall has been performed.

The pterygomaxillary sutures are then sectioned with a curved osteotome to permit complete mobilization of the maxillary segment, which can then be moved into its desired position and secured by ligation to the stable portion of the maxilla and a suspension wire to an interocclusal splint. In some cases, the splint will be unnecessary and wiring directly to bone will be sufficient. Closure of the incision is done in the usual manner with 4–0 Supramid or Dexon sutures.

Bone grafting should be considered in cases of extensive expansion where minimal bony interface occurs, in segmental lengthening procedures, and in cleft cases, as it affords greater stability and faster bone union. If considerable buccal movement is necessary to correct the crossbite, the palatal mucosa may be a limiting factor, and a palatal relaxing incision may be necessary to relieve tension and permit greater movement. If expansion of the arch is intended and the palatal vault is high, the buccal

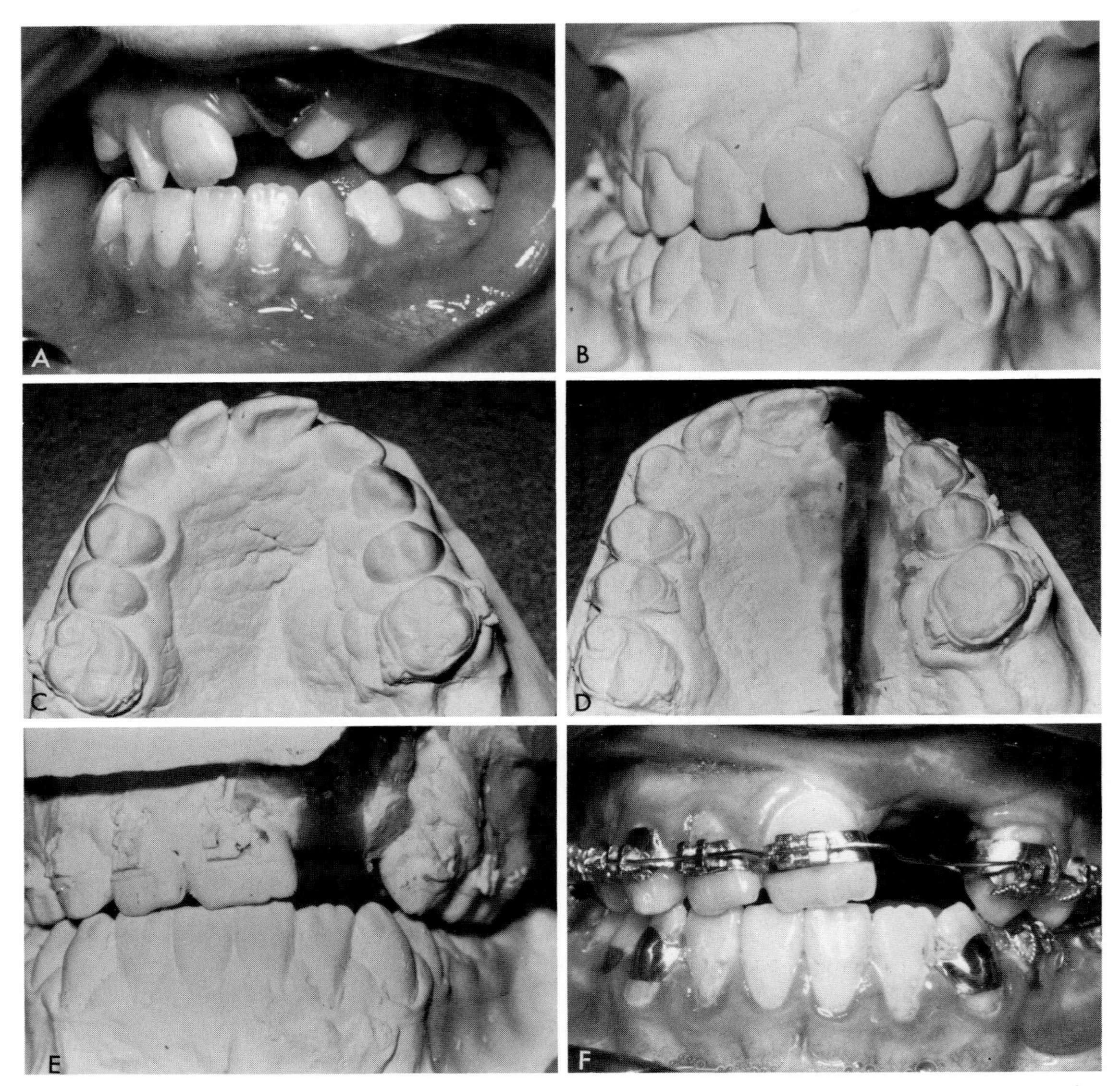

Figure 21–7. Rapid maxillary expansion. In selected cases, such as patients with cleft palate, the technique of rapid maxillary expansion is useful. *A–C,* Collapsed maxillary arch form. *D* and *E,* Model surgery. *F,* Final occlusal relations after rapid maxillary expansion.

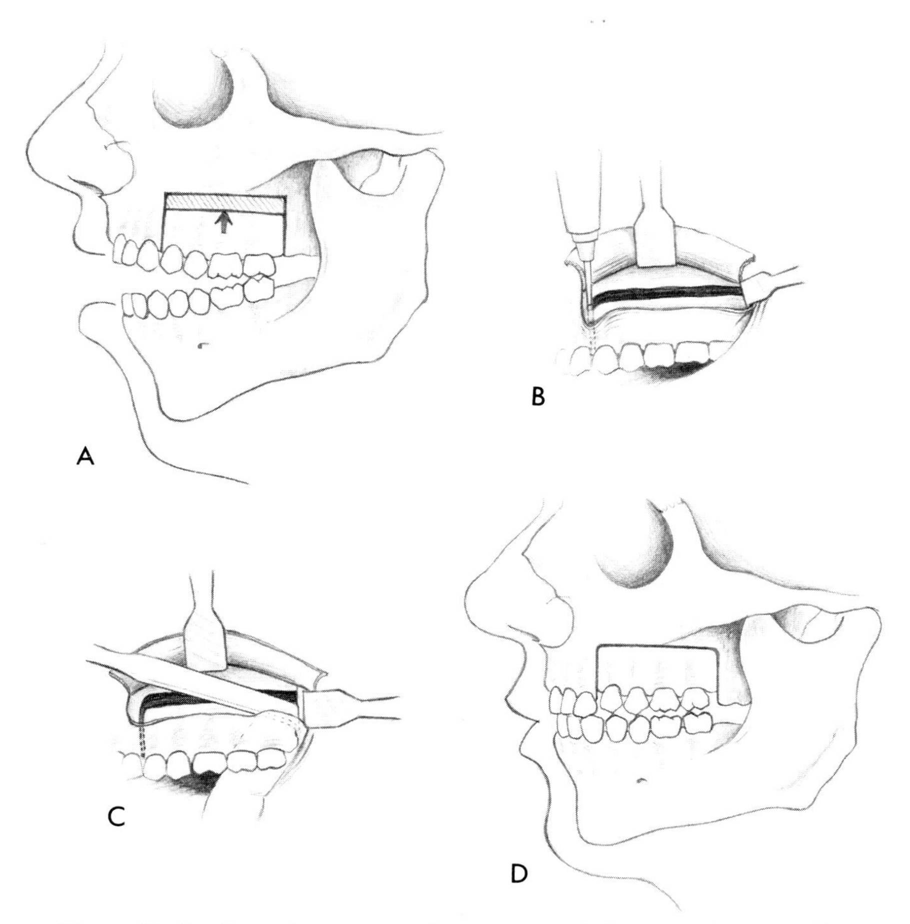

Figure 21–8. Posterior segmental osteotomy. *A*, Preoperative open bite and design of maxillary bone cuts. *B*, Buccal flap elevated and bone cuts made in lateral wall of maxilla removing measured bone sufficient for the correction. *C*, The palatal wall of the alveolus is cut with burs or fine osteotomes using a finger on the palatal mucosa as a guide. The pterygoid plates are separated with an Obwegeser or similar type of chisel. *D*, The maxillary posterior segment has been superiorly repositioned, allowing the mandible to autorotate giving the desired occlusion and increased chin prominence.

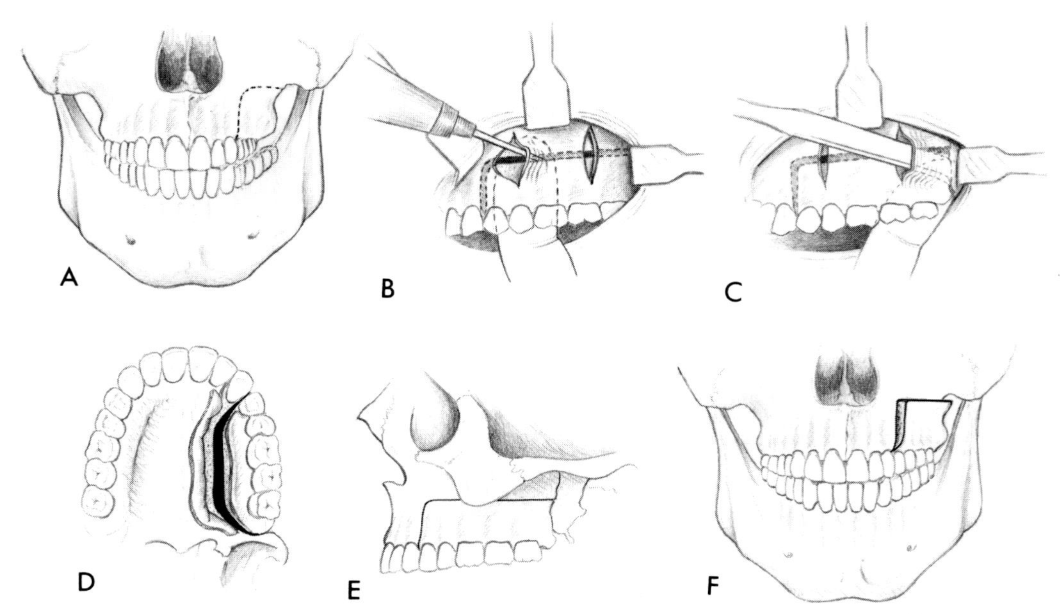

Figure 21–9. Alternative incisions and bone cuts for segmental posterior maxillary osteotomy for correction of crossbite and/or maxillary asymmetry. *A,* Preoperative crossbite. *B,* Bone cuts through vertical incisions; note palatal digital guide. *C,* Pterygoid plate separation. *D,* Palatal flap and bone cuts. *E,* Segment repositioned, lateral view. *F,* Frontal view of postoperative result.

approach is excellent. Occasionally, however, a dual approach combining the buccal incision with a palatal incision, as described by Bell and Turvey,[4] may be necessary, if the palatal vault is low. Alternate incisions that are especially useful when palatal surgery is also indicated are shown in Figure 21–9.

SAGITTAL MAXILLARY ASYMMETRY (DEVIATION FROM THE VERTICAL PLANE) (Fig. 21–10)

Sagittal asymmetry is present when one half of the maxilla is positioned farther forward than the other (Fig. 21–10). Pure maxillary sagittal asymmetry will exist in syndromes such as hemifacial microsomia, for example. Some patients with cleft palate have sagittal asymmetries because of disturbed growth.

Esthetic Features

In facial asymmetry involving only the sagittal plane, one side of the maxilla appears more prominent than the other, the columella is displaced to the less prominent side, and the dental midline may or may not be in the proper position. In the majority of patients with sagittal asymmetries of the maxilla, however, the horizontal

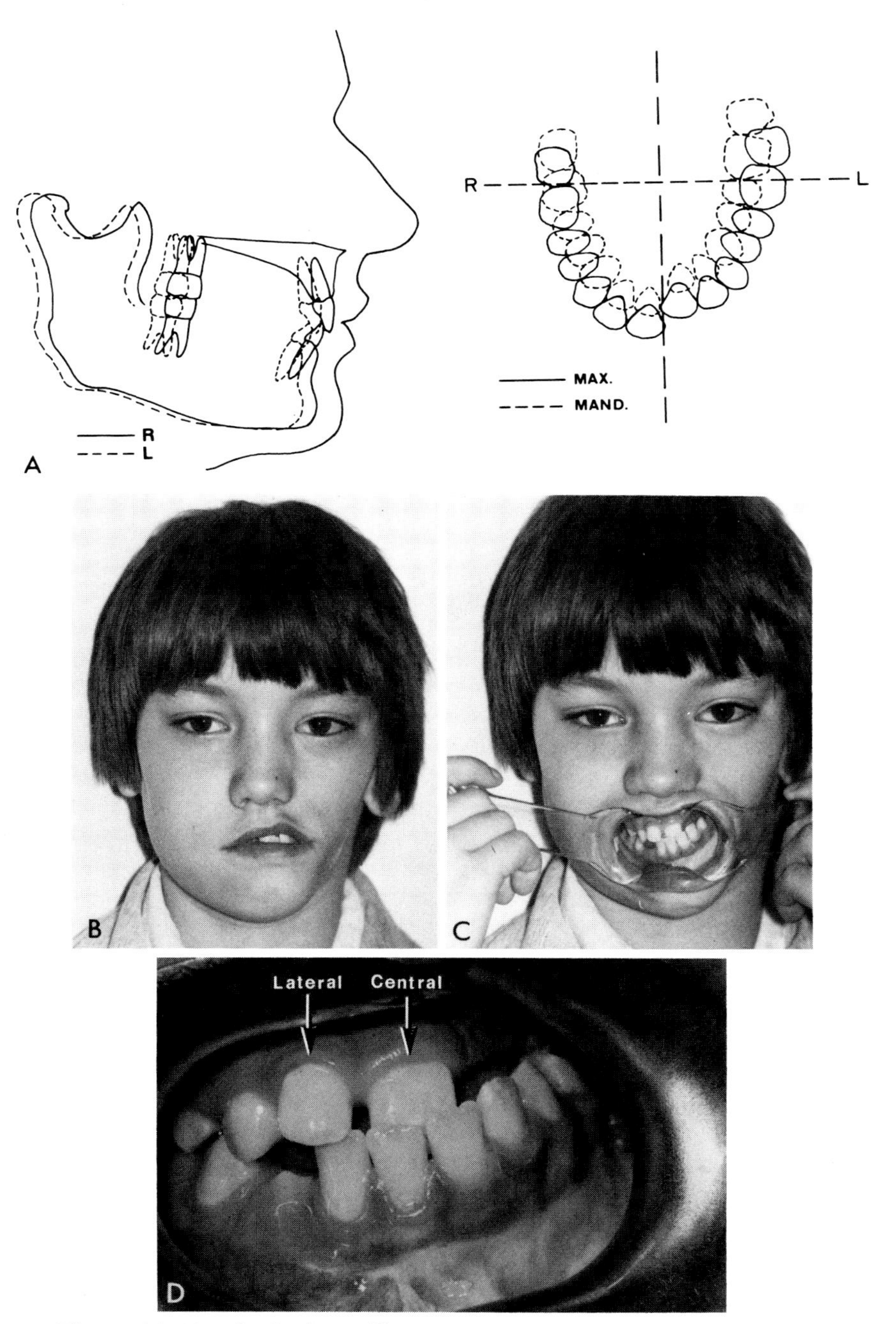

Figure 21–10. Sagittal maxillary asymmetry. *A*, Schematic representation of the deformity. *B* and *C*, Twelve-year-old patient with hemifacial microsomia causing a sagittal maxillary asymmetry. *D*, Note the large upper right lateral can be mistaken as a central incisor. Canted occlusal plane and midline deviation are severe.

and vertical planes will be involved (e.g., hemifacial microsomia or hemifacial hypertrophy). These deformities may also involve the mandible and the zygoma or both and thus appear as total facial malformations.

Cephalometric Features

Posteroanterior cephalometric findings are not diagnostic in cases of purely sagittal asymmetry, although their importance in vertical and horizontal asymmetries necessitates their inclusion in a thorough evaluation of the defect. The lateral cephalogram may show that the anteroposterior position of the left and right central incisors and first molars differs. Placing radiopaque markers (i.e., silver points temporarily cemented on the buccal surfaces of the maxillary first molars) helps to identify a discrepancy that otherwise may be difficult to evaluate owing to superimposition of the left and right teeth.

Occlusal Features

Alignment of the Arch

Examination of the arch alignment will usually reveal one side anterior to the other with dental compensation in the incisor region that allows the central incisors to make contact.

Occlusion

In pure sagittal asymmetry, there will be malocclusion on the abnormal side unless the mandible has also compensated, in which case adequate occlusion is possible.

Interarch Relation

Properly mounted and related study models help identify which side is abnormal and what other planes of asymmetry are involved.

Treatment of Sagittal Maxillary Asymmetry

Surgical treatment of pure (i.e., traumatic) sagittal asymmetry involves segmental maxillary osteotomy (half-arch) to reposition the abnormal side. Total maxillary osteotomies in multiple segments, however, are more commonly used in cases involving the sagittal plane since the other planes are usually also involved. In patients with hemifacial microsomia, all three planes are affected along with the mandible and the soft tissues, and the treatment usually involves correcting the mandibular asymmetry first. The excess interocclusal distance on the involved side is maintained with an acrylic splint until adequate healing has occurred, and then the total maxillary procedure is performed, utilizing an interpositional bone graft. These cases may also involve soft-tissue reconstruction to allow for adequate lengthening of the involved side. Current techniques allow simultaneous correction of both maxilla and mandible for asymmetric deformities.

TOTAL MAXILLARY ANTEROPOSTERIOR MALRELATIONSHIP

This deviation, like sagittal asymmetry, is not a discrete maxillary deformity. Examples of this deviation include anterior maxillary alveolar hypoplasias and posterior maxillary hyperplasias. The anterior teeth, in essence, are on a different horizontal plane than the posterior teeth, and therefore the problem usually presents as an anterior open bite. Satisfactory surgical correction of the various maxillary asymmetries with an associated total maxillary vertical malrelationship usually involves multiple segmental maxillary osteotomies.

DISCUSSION

The various asymmetries of the maxilla can be treated surgically by the segmental maxillary osteotomy, the total maxillary osteotomy, or a combined maxillary and mandibular procedure. Selection of the specific technique is based on a combination of factors such as the anatomic location of the asymmetry, the presence or absence of crossbite, the degree of exposure of anterior teeth, the cant of the occlusal plane, and similar considerations. No single combination is routinely used, and therefore treatment of each patient must be planned individually. Several segmental surgical procedures for asymmetries involving the anterior portion of the maxilla are available: the Wunderer technique, which is a direct palatal approach with an anterior labial pedicle (Fig. 21–11);[10] the Wassmund technique, which is more conservative and largely consists of tunneling on the palate (Fig. 21–3),[12] and the anterior maxillary downfracture as described by Bell (Fig. 21–13).[2] Any of these techniques when applied to an appropriate situation will yield good results, and all have been well supported by biologic studies relating to feasibility, revascularization, and healing.[5, 8] For extensive posterior movement of the anterior maxilla, the Wunderer method gives better vision for the ostectomy, and precision work can be done. If superior repositioning is the dominant requirement, the downfracture method is preferred.

Depending upon whether the asymmetry is clinically manifested in the form of excess palatal height, improper arch contour, maxillary excess, or some other deformity, several surgical methods are available for correction.[2] For asymmetries involving the entire maxilla, the treatment of choice is the maxillary osteotomy, of which there are two important variations: total maxillary osteotomy[3] and total maxillary alveolar osteotomy.[6]

The total maxillary Le Fort I downfracture osteotomy gives stable results. It permits sectioning of the entire maxilla into segments if necessary. Other advantages of the total maxillary osteotomy are:

1. It provides excellent exposure and access to the principal problematic areas (the perpendicular process of the palatine bone and the pterygoid plates of the sphenoid bone and maxilla interface).

2. Any inadvertently transected vessels in the region of the posterior maxilla are readily accessible, and hemorrhage is easily controlled with pressure.

3. Bony interferences in any area can be readily identified and removed under direct visualization by using a bur, rongeur forceps, or osteotome.

4. Transverse, sagittal, interdental, or circumpalatal sectioning of the maxilla is easily accomplished from the superior aspect.

5. Widening of the maxilla can be accomplished by a horseshoe palatal osteotomy and by narrowing a palatal ostectomy of the appropriate width.

6. Should superior repositioning be sufficiently extensive to compromise the nasal structure, the horseshoe palatal osteotomy can be done from the superior maxillary

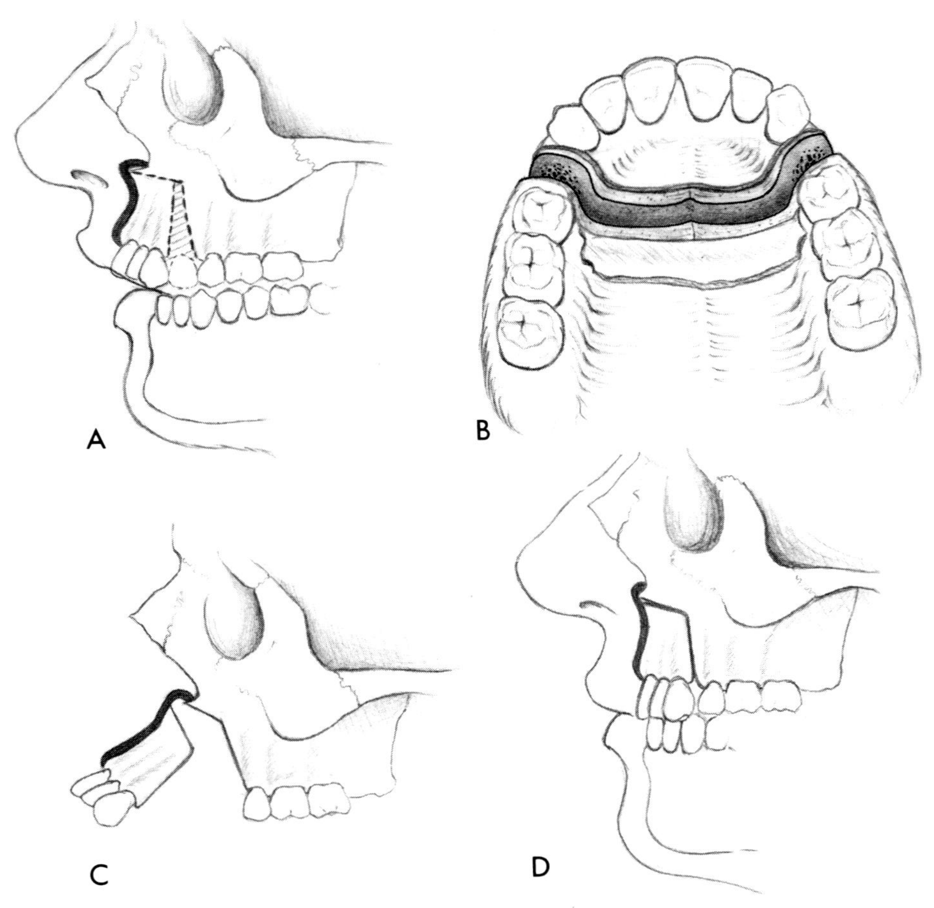

Figure 21–11. Wunderer technique of premaxillary osteotomy. *A,* Outline of planned cuts for setting back protrusive anterior maxillary segment. Note bone to be removed in area of extracted 1st premolar (*B*) palatal flap; and palatal osteotomies (*C*). Following separation of anterior maxilla the segment remains pedicled to the labial mucosa. *D,* Postoperative result. Note improved upper lip relationships and proximity of teeth and bone.

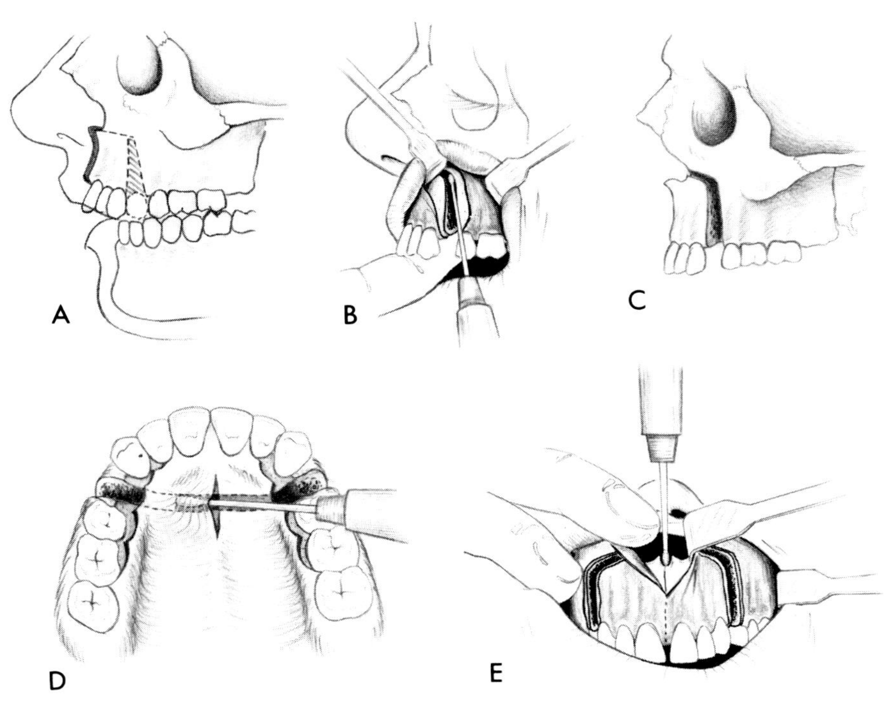

Figure 21–12. Modified Wassmund technique of premaxillary osteotomy. *A,* Outline of planned osteotomies. Note segment of bone to be removed in area of extracted 1st premolar. *D,* Palatal cuts utilizing tunneling technique through a midpalatal incision. *E,* Repositioning of anterior maxillary segment.

surface with the maxilla in the downfracture position. This permits the midline structure of the palate and nose to remain unaltered. Surgical access for this procedure is excellent. Inferior turbinectomy and submucous resection of the cartilaginous nasal space may also need to be done to allow increased superior repositioning.

The maxillary alveolar osteotomy technique involves mobilizing the entire alveolar portion of the maxilla in a unit or in segments, permitting anterior or superior movement, tilting, or similar maneuvers with the distinct advantage of no surgical manipulations of the midline structure of the nasal cavity.[7] The major disadvantages of this procedure are technical difficulty and the more limited movements possible.

Maxillary asymmetries with associated mandibular asymmetry present multiple treatment planning options. These deformities have a maxillary vertical asymmetry component and therefore require repositioning of both the maxilla and the mandible. Maxillomandibular asymmetries involving differential superior repositioning of the maxilla may be done in one stage, or the maxillary surgery may be done first. The preoperative decision of whether to do the surgery in one or two stages depends upon the amount and direction of movement needed and the growth potential of the patient. Positional appliances can be effective for redirecting asymmetric growth in the younger patient. The one-stage maxillomandibular procedure requires adequate maxillary bony interface to provide sufficient stabilization during the healing phase.

Asymmetries involving inferior repositioning of a maxillary segment, and therefore requiring an interpositional bone graft, may be treated in one or two stages. If two operations are done, the mandibular surgery is accomplished first. The interoc-

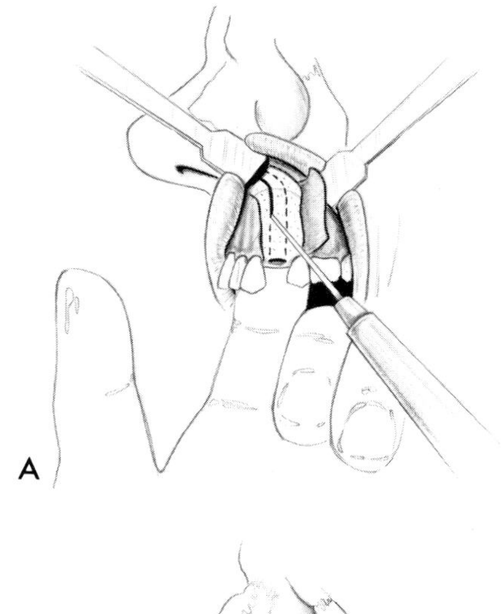

Figure 21–13. Bell technique of anterior maxillary downfracture. *A,* Lateral maxillary bone cuts to the anterior nasal margin. *B,* Midline palatal bone transected from the anterior and lateral position to permit downfracture. *C,* In the downfracture position, the bone is freed to permit superior repositioning. Technique modified after Epker.

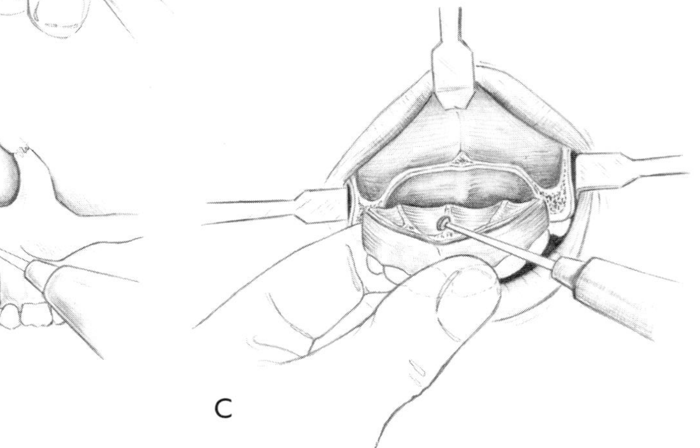

clusal space created by the surgery is maintained during the healing period with an acrylic splint. Once the mandible has healed adequately, the maxillary surgery or orthodontic closure of the surgically created open bite may be performed. Simultaneous maxillary and mandibular surgery is preferred whenever possible.

Asymmetries in the growing patient that have a maxillary vertical component and associated mandibular asymmetry (e.g., hemifacial microsomia or restricted growth secondary to unilateral ankylosis of the temporomandibular joint) are treated by performing the mandibular surgery first. In such cases, however, after adequate mandibular healing and removal of intermaxillary fixation, the acrylic splint can be periodically thinned on the affected side to allow for potential maxillary growth. With this treatment, maxillary growth may be sufficient to make maxillary surgery unnecessary.

It should be noted that no set treatment plan is suitable for all types of maxillary asymmetry. Most maxillary asymmetries occur in all three planes of space. Comprehensive preoperative study and thorough understanding of the numerous maxillary and mandibular surgical procedures and the indications for their use are therefore essential to adequate treatment.

ORTHODONTIC TREATMENT

Most orthodontic approaches to maxillary asymmetry are concerned with correction of the dental compensations associated the maxillary deformity. Both upper and lower dental arches are banded, and light arch wires are used to achieve preliminary alignment. The angular compensations so common in asymmetry problems are righted in the anterior region with light wires, but posterior torquing with transpalatal arches and edgewise mechanics must be introduced before posterior dental asymmetric compensations can be corrected. Posterior cross-elastics can be used during round-wire stages to begin molar and premolar decompensation while the anterior teeth are being righted.

Presurgical Orthodontic Treatment

The presurgical orthodontic phase of any combination treatment involves various treatment goals depending on the patient's age, the surgical options chosen, and the tooth movement required. It is very important that the patient understand the treatment time involved in each phase. The shortest presurgical orthodontic treatment period are those of patients who: (1) have already had preliminary alignment of their teeth, (2) have a good molar and cuspid width before treatment, and (3) have segmental maxillary surgery. Longer presurgical orthodontic treatment periods are sometimes necessary if the result of combination treatment is to be adequate.

In cases of maxillary asymmetry, the orthodontic presurgical phase of combination treatment involves either continuous arch wire or segmented arch wire techniques.

CONTINUOUS ARCH WIRE TECHNIQUES

The use of continuous arch wire techniques is common in presurgical orthodontic preparation for total maxillary surgical procedures. The presurgical phase involves progressively increasing the size of the arch wires to achieve final stability in the post-surgical occlusion. If .018 edgewise brackets are used, the minimum size of arch wire for a total maxillary surgical splint is .016 x .022 without palatal splinting and .016 x .016 if acrylic or metal palatal splinting is used. The rationale for using a large arch wire prior to total maxillary surgery involves the immediate post-surgical stability of the posterior segments. They should be well stabilized prior to surgery by large wires so that they will withstand the pull of the suspension wires placed during surgery and retained during healing. When tightened, a surgical suspension wire will place torque on the posterior segments of the maxilla and this can cause buccal overjet in the posterior region and eventually result in anterior open bite if the posterior segments are not well stabilized during the actual surgery.

When surgical palatal splinting of either cast chrome cobalt or heavy acrylic-reinforced wire is used, we have found that tying the wire to the acrylic prior to the postfixation phase and then using lighter arch wires is acceptable for the postsurgical healing period. Also, transpalatal orthodontic wires will add stability to posterior segments, where circumzygomatic wires may be needed.

SEGMENTED ARCH TECHNIQUE

The segmented orthodontic arch technique is very commonly used in preparation for a segmented surgical procedure. The recent use of segmented maxillary surgery in treating maxillary asymmetries has allowed a shortening of the orthodontic treatment because the orthodontist can align each segment without being concerned about the relationship of the segments to each other. The surgeon will perform final alignment of the segments.

The disadvantage of the segmented techniques is the possibility that when surgical suspension wires have to be used on the segments, inadequate fixation will allow the crowns of the segments to be buccally torqued, causing posterior buccal overjet and open bite due to lingual cusp interference. If interocclusal splinting is used during the first week or two postoperatively, buccal torquing of the segment is minimized.

The preliminary clinical and cephalometric evaluations and the model surgery give a good indication of whether the segmented technique or the total maxillary technique will be the more advantageous. The case studies presented at the end of this chapter demonstrate the use of both techniques.

DIRECT BONDING

The technique of directly bonding metal brackets to the teeth has been found to be extremely reliable in providing orthodontic fixation for patients who do not have adequate interproximal space prior to surgery or in whom the upper arch and its relationship to the lower arch are extremely important as far as interproximal band space is concerned. In any patient who does not need lower banding or in those cases in which lower banding is needed only for fixation, molar bands plus anterior brackets directly bonded to the premolars and anterior teeth will provide adequate presurgical orthodontic treatment preparation for any surgical technique. Directly bonded brackets provide a reliable fixation for heavy .016 x .022 arch wire, for intermaxillary fixation and for segmented maxillary surgery as long as the cuspids and other posterior teeth are banded with conventional orthodontic bands.

Postsurgical Orthodontic Treatment

The postsurgical phase of orthodontic treatment involves various final adjustments in the occlusal relationships and the final tooth alignment. This final phase usually lasts from 3 to 4 months, but this time can be increased dramatically if:

1. The preoperative evaluation of the patient has been inaccurate and the final occlusion is not adequate.

2. Problems were encountered during the placement of the fixation device and the maxillary segments or the entire maxilla is not held in its proper predesignated position.

The team that works the best together is the team that is not rushed in the presurgical orthodontic phase. The maxillary segments or the entire maxilla can then be properly aligned and the surgery can be accomplished expeditiously with a stable result and very little postsurgical orthodontic correction. Postsurgical adjustments with either wire suspension or elastics is often necessary to establish the final occlusion. Postsurgical orthodontic treatment can become very lengthy when the presurgical orthodontic phase is compromised.

CASE STUDIES

CASE 21–1 (FIG. 21–14)

A female patient, K. N., age 18 years, 2 months arrived at the maxillofacial clinic with complaints of "face dropping" and temporomandibular joint pain. Previous orthodontic history was recorded at age 11 years, 6 months. The full-banded orthodontic appliance was removed at 13 years, 11 months. The orthodontic treatment records revealed a long history of Class II elastic wear on the right buccal segments. At age 15 years, 7 months the patient was dismissed from further orthodontic recalls. Six years later the patient entered the maxillofacial clinic complaining of temporomandibular joint pain and facial disproportions. A complete history revealed that at age 7 her right condyle was fractured in a fall from a second story window. The medical records reveal a subcondylar fracture. Maxillofacial records taken at 18 years, 2 months confirmed a diagnosis of right unilateral condylar hypoplasia.

PROBLEM LIST

The examination revealed a right-sided maxillary and mandibular asymmetry, verified by cephalometric radiographs and tracings. The deficient right condyle contributed to the concomitant growth malformation and functional malocclusion.

TREATMENT PLAN

The proposed treatment included maxillary and mandibular orthodontic appliances for tooth alignment and later an intermaxillary fixation. The surgical plan included maxillary Le Fort I osteotomy lengthening the right side of the maxilla and shortening the left. Mandibular osteotomy (intraoral sagittal split) was utilized to level the mandible and position it into the new maxillary position. Genioplasty was also done for final facial symmetry. Although this patient was treated in two surgical stages with an interpositional splint, we prefer, when possible, to treat similar cases in one surgical stage.

Text continued on page 1551

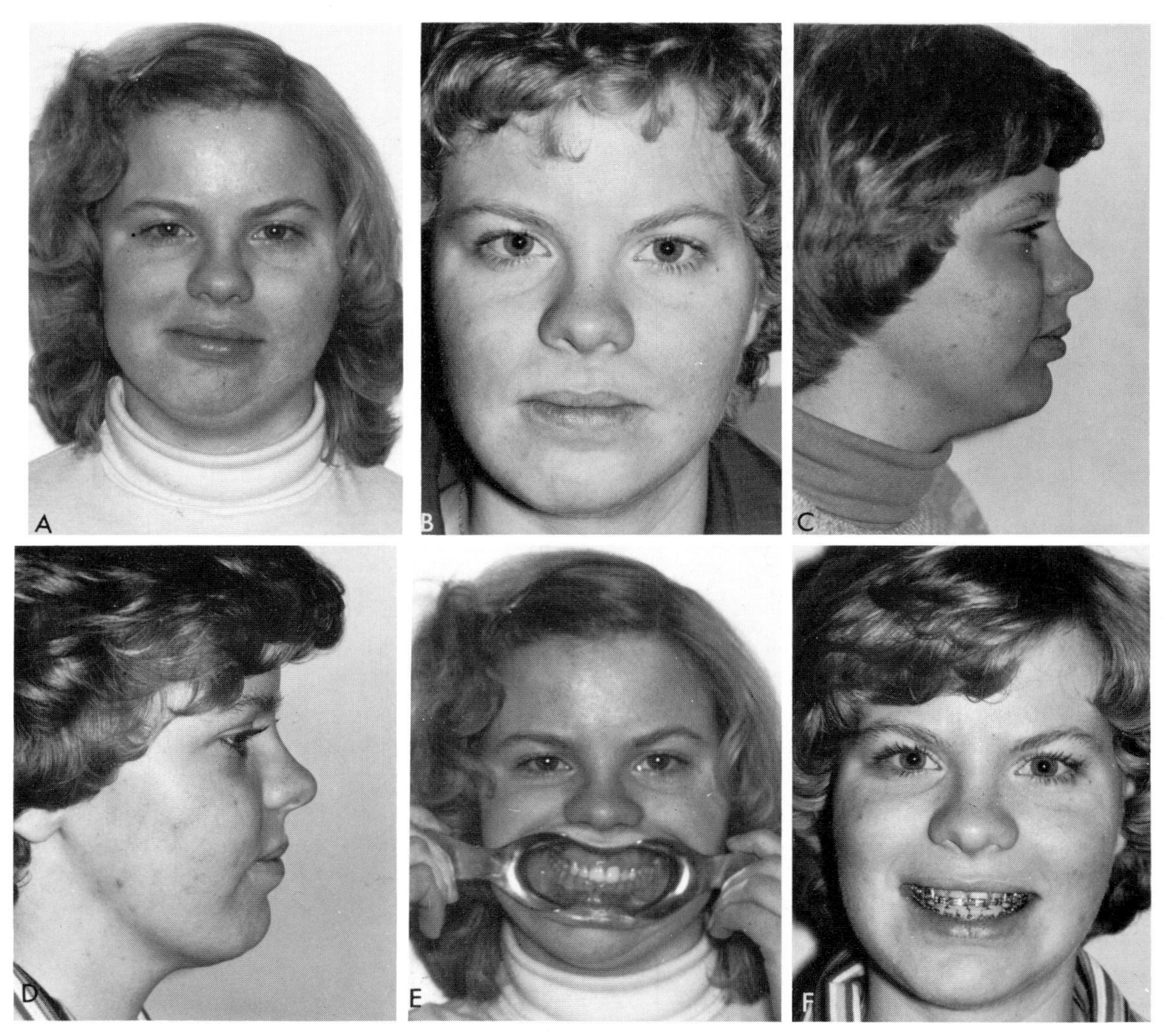

Figure 21–14 (Case 21–1). *A,* K.N., an 18-year-old woman, sought maxillofacial surgery owing to "face dropping" and temporomandibular joint pain. Previous orthodontics did not correct her facial asymmetry. History of condylar fracture due to fall at age 7 years. *B,* Postsurgical and orthodontic results after a double procedure designed to level both the maxilla and the mandible. The maxillary osteotomy consisted of a two-piece inferior positioning of the right maxilla and a superior positioning of the left side. An iliac crestal augmentation was made to the superior aspect of the osteotomized right maxillary segment. *C,* Lateral facial aspect demonstrating the "short" right mandible and maxillary complex. Age 17 years. *D,* Completed right facial profile demonstrating the postsurgical-orthodontic result. Note the more favorable anterior position to the chin. *E,* Pretreatment anterior face and dentition demonstrating the canted occlusal plane. *F,* Postsurgical smile demonstrating a more favorable symmetry to face, smile line, and occlusal plane.

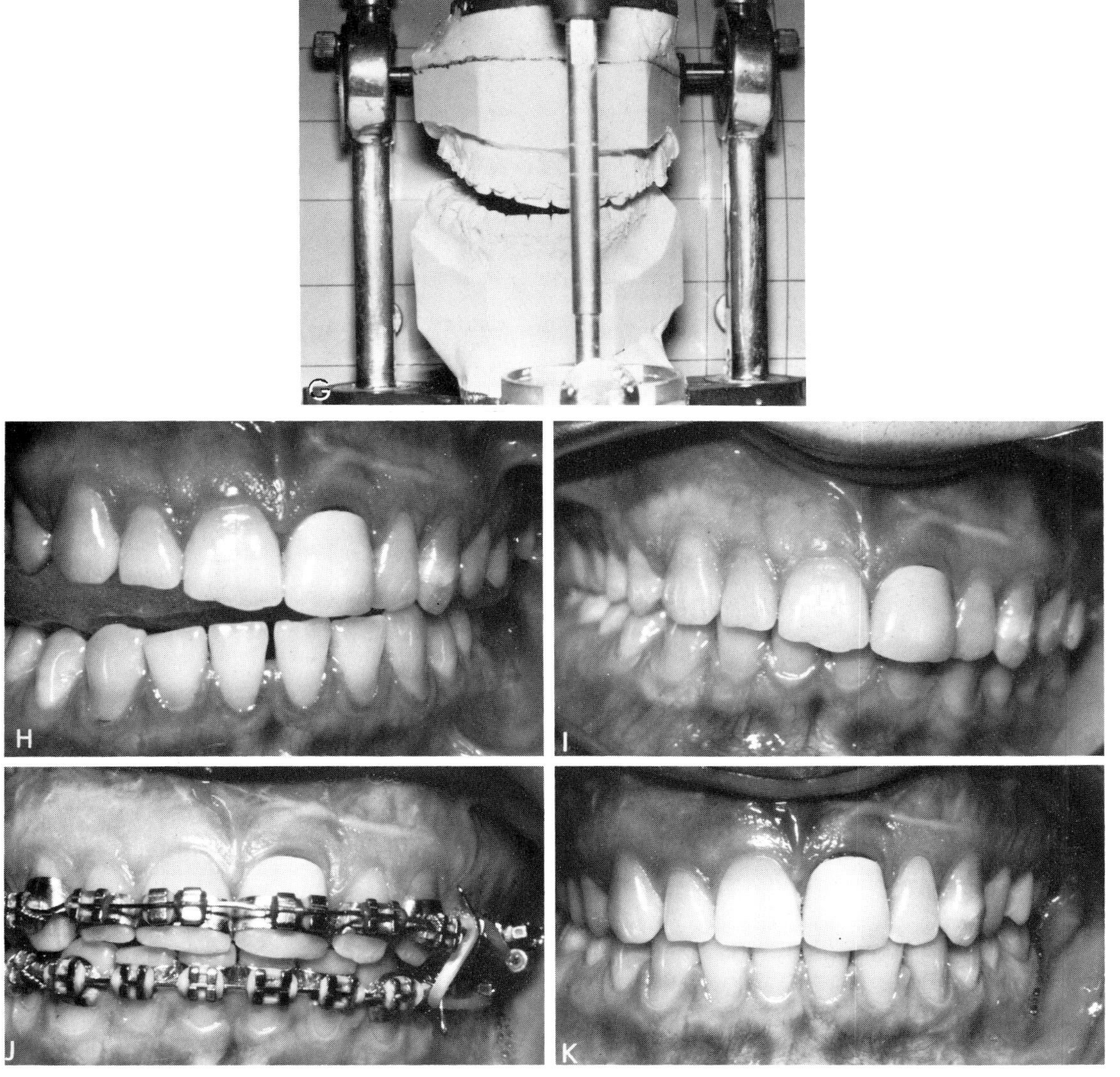

Figure 21–14 (Case 21–1) *Continued.* *G,* Intermediate mounting of surgery casts demonstrating the opening necessary in the right buccal occlusion to establish a level lower occlusal plane. *H,* Intermediate postmandibular surgery following the interocclusal splint designed to maintain the new interdental maxillary relationship to the "level" lower dentition. *I,* Pretreatment anterior dental view demonstrating the starting midline of the dentition. Note the cant of the occlusal plane and the midline deviation of 80 per cent of the lower incisor. *J,* Postsurgical photo demonstrating the maxillary repositioning achieved to the previously leveled mandible. Note a slight overcorrection in the dental midline. *K,* Anterior view demonstrating post-treatment result.

Illustration continued on the following page

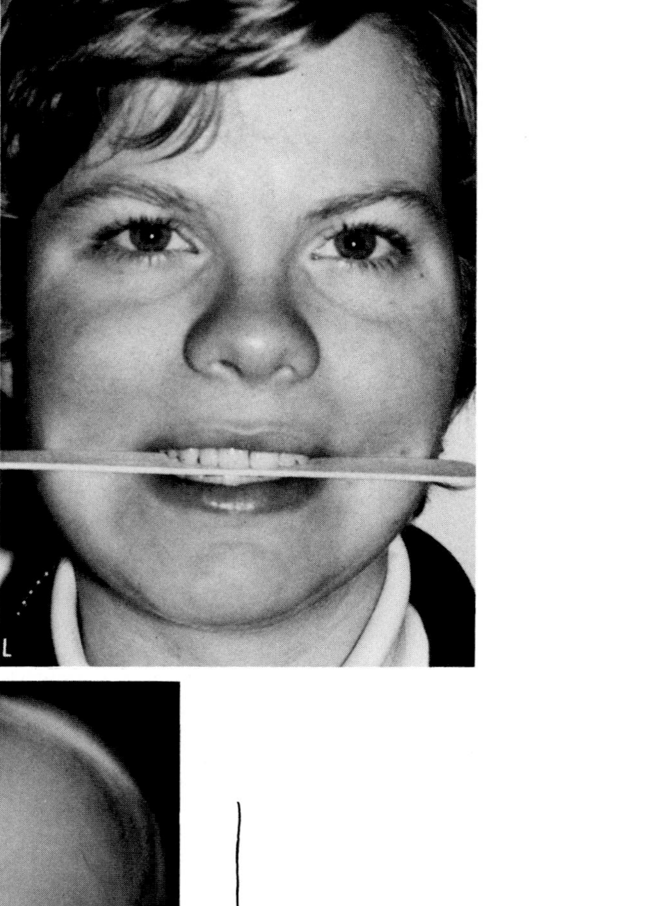

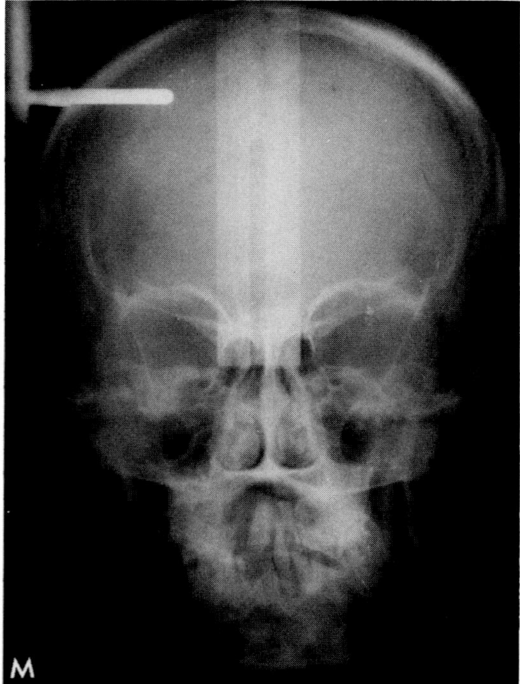

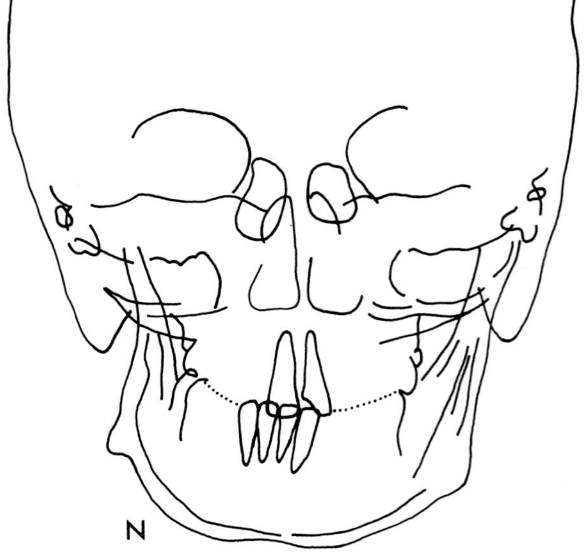

Figure 21–14 (Case 21–1) *Continued.* *L,* Photograph demonstrating the correction achieved in the occlusal plane. *M,* Pretreatment P-A cephalogram. *N,* P-A cephalometric tracing pretreatment.

CASE 21–2 (FIG. 21–15)

Before consulting our clinic, patient L. H., a 23-year-old woman, had consulted an oral surgeon and an orthodontist in her home state for evaluation of her occlusal and facial deformities. The oral surgeon advised her that surgical correction was possible, but she moved before treatment could be initiated.

During her interview at our institution, the patient complained of both facial asymmetry and temporomandibular joint pain and was of the opinion that these two complaints were equally important to her. The joint pain seemed to be bilateral and was usually initiated by extensive jaw activity, such as "eating a big steak" or "laughing a lot at a party." The pain was initially sharp and localized specifically to the temporomandibular joint. At times, the pain in the left joint extended into the left temporal region. The pain persisted for approximately 2 hours after onset, but the patient did not notice stiffness in the jaw or limitations in movement during this period. She did feel a persistence of possible subluxation on opening the jaw wide, but she was always able to close her jaw.

The patient's other complaint concerned the enlarged, bulky appearance of the left side of her jaw, which gave her face asymmetric proportions. The patient also complained of a canted or "cockeyed" appearance of her lip line and, to a lesser extent, of her occlusal plane. Moreover, her chin appeared off-center to the right. The patient stated that she was particularly concerned about correcting the facial asymmetry; she felt that leveling the plane of occlusion would also be desirable since the canting was very noticeable to her when she opened her mouth. She was considering a career as a professional singer at the time of the initial examination.

CLINICAL EXAMINATION

The patient's dentition was intact and her overall occlusal relationship was very good. Both the maxillary and mandibular dentition were in good repair with moderate upper and lower anterior crowding of the teeth. On closing, there was a slight premature contact in the left posterior regions that produced a slight slide into centric relation. The occlusal plane was extremely canted being higher on the right side than on the left. The lip line was also canted, in the same direction and to the same extent as the occlusal plane. The chin point appeared to be 8 to 10 mm deviated toward the right. The left side of the face was definitely longer than the right in the area over the body of the mandible and the ramus. During clinical examination, both mandibular condyles moved symmetrically, and there was no clicking felt or heard.

The patient remembered that during childhood she had experienced a number of blows to the jaw during athletic activities and falls from gymnastic and play apparatus. The patient remembered one instance when she had experienced severe pain and swelling in the left side of the face over the ramus of the mandible after falling while swinging upside down from a tree limb. The inferior soft-tissue gnathion demonstrated a one-inch scar resulting from this fall.

EVALUATION OF INITIAL RECORDS

The original full-face view shown in Figure 21–15*A* reveals the asymmetry. Split-image photography was used to show the patient the expected results of a left maxillary impaction or a right maxillary elongation to level the occlusal plane.

Text continued on page 1559

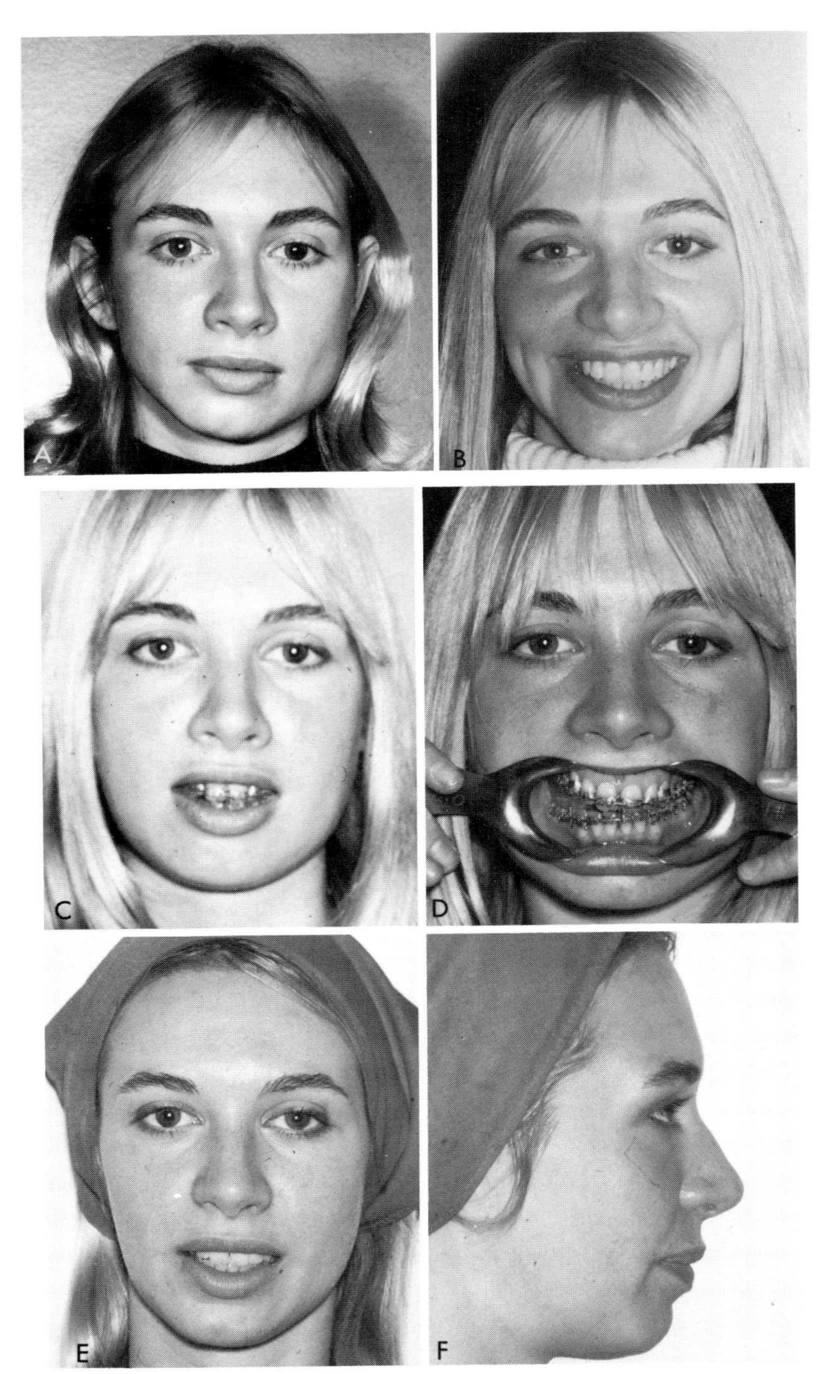

Figure 21–15 (Case 21–2). *A*, Patient photographed 2 years earlier in another state. The canted lower border of the mandible is clearly apparent. Canted lip line gives some indication of similar cant of the occlusal plane: Soft-tissue midline of the chin is 10 mm. to one side of the midline of the face. *B*, Patient as she presented to the orthosurgery clinic of the University of Minnesota. She had changed her hair style to cover the asymmetric mandibular gonial angles. Smile line of lips demonstrates horizontal canting of the occlusal plane of the maxilla and the short right mandibular ramus. *C*, Postoperative facial view (swelling apparent) demonstrating the symmetry achieved by the bilateral vertical osteotomy of the mandibular rami and insertion of the acrylic splint. *D*, Postoperative facial view demonstrating the midline correction and level lower occlusal plane. Note the correct midline position of the chin. *E*, Post-treatment anterior facial view. Comparison with *A* demonstrates the horizontal correction accomplished by the bilateral surgery and orthodontic correction. *F*, Post-treatment view of elongated right face. Six-month postoperative scar visible in cervical crease.

Legend continued on the opposite page

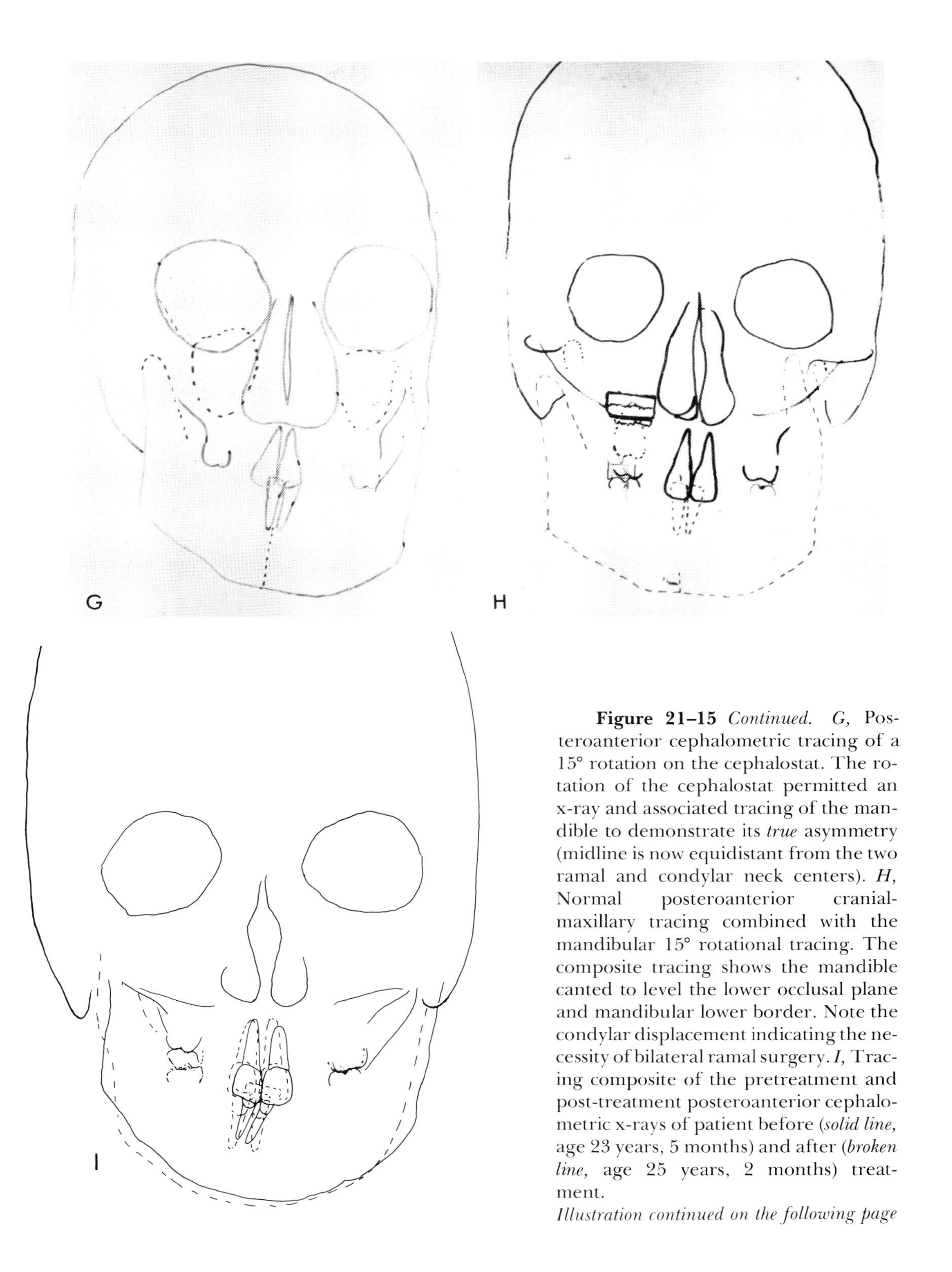

Figure 21–15 *Continued. G,* Posteroanterior cephalometric tracing of a 15° rotation on the cephalostat. The rotation of the cephalostat permitted an x-ray and associated tracing of the mandible to demonstrate its *true* asymmetry (midline is now equidistant from the two ramal and condylar neck centers). *H,* Normal posteroanterior cranial-maxillary tracing combined with the mandibular 15° rotational tracing. The composite tracing shows the mandible canted to level the lower occlusal plane and mandibular lower border. Note the condylar displacement indicating the necessity of bilateral ramal surgery. *I,* Tracing composite of the pretreatment and post-treatment posteroanterior cephalometric x-rays of patient before (*solid line,* age 23 years, 5 months) and after (*broken line,* age 25 years, 2 months) treatment.

Illustration continued on the following page

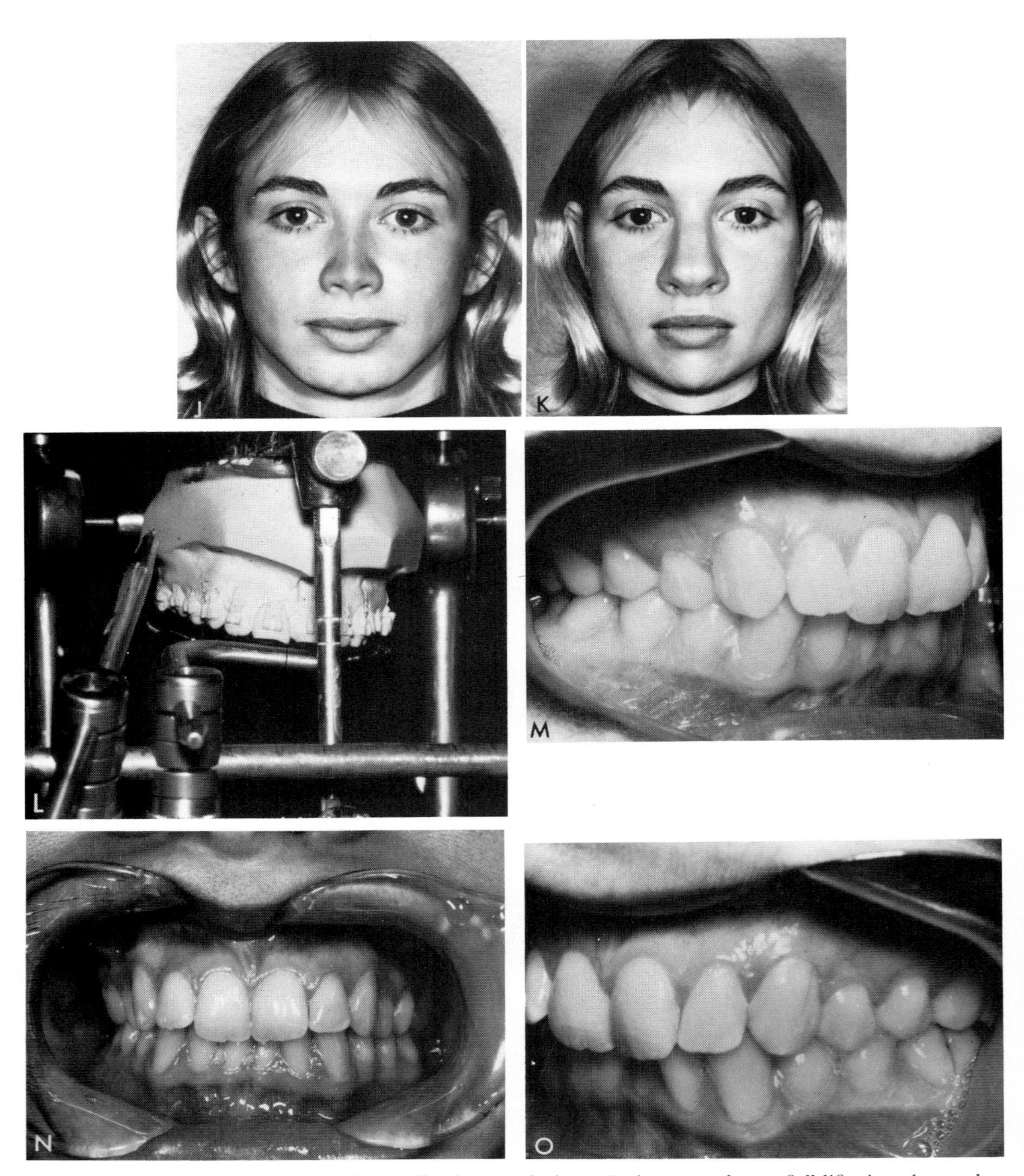

Figure 21–15 *Continued.* *J* and *K,* Split-photo technique. Patient was shown full life-size photos that were cut and reassembled to help determine which side is more esthetically pleasing. *L,* Face-bow transfer of maxillary cast demonstrating the canted occlusal plane. Note increasing cant toward posterior in right occlusal plane. *M–O,* Preoperative occlusions. *M,* Right buccal view demonstrating end-to-end Class II molar occlusion. *N,* Anterior view of occlusion demonstrating 50 per cent overbite. Lower incisal inclination demonstrates the dental compensations. *O,* Left buccal view demonstrates a normal Class I molar and cuspid relationship.

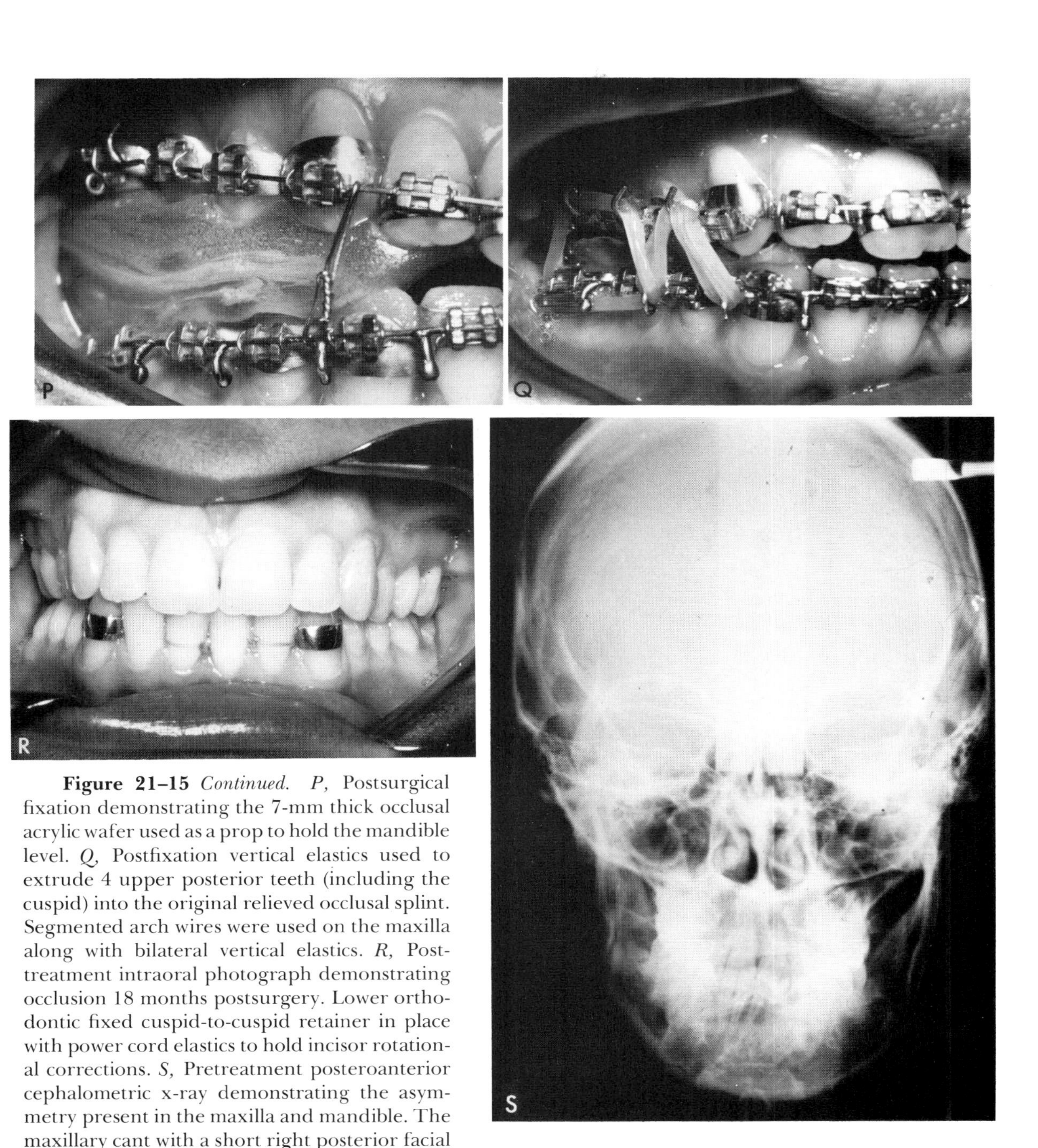

Figure 21–15 *Continued. P,* Postsurgical fixation demonstrating the 7-mm thick occlusal acrylic wafer used as a prop to hold the mandible level. *Q,* Postfixation vertical elastics used to extrude 4 upper posterior teeth (including the cuspid) into the original relieved occlusal splint. Segmented arch wires were used on the maxilla along with bilateral vertical elastics. *R,* Posttreatment intraoral photograph demonstrating occlusion 18 months postsurgery. Lower orthodontic fixed cuspid-to-cuspid retainer in place with power cord elastics to hold incisor rotational corrections. *S,* Pretreatment posteroanterior cephalometric x-ray demonstrating the asymmetry present in the maxilla and mandible. The maxillary cant with a short right posterior facial height is clearly recognizable.

Illustration continued on the following page

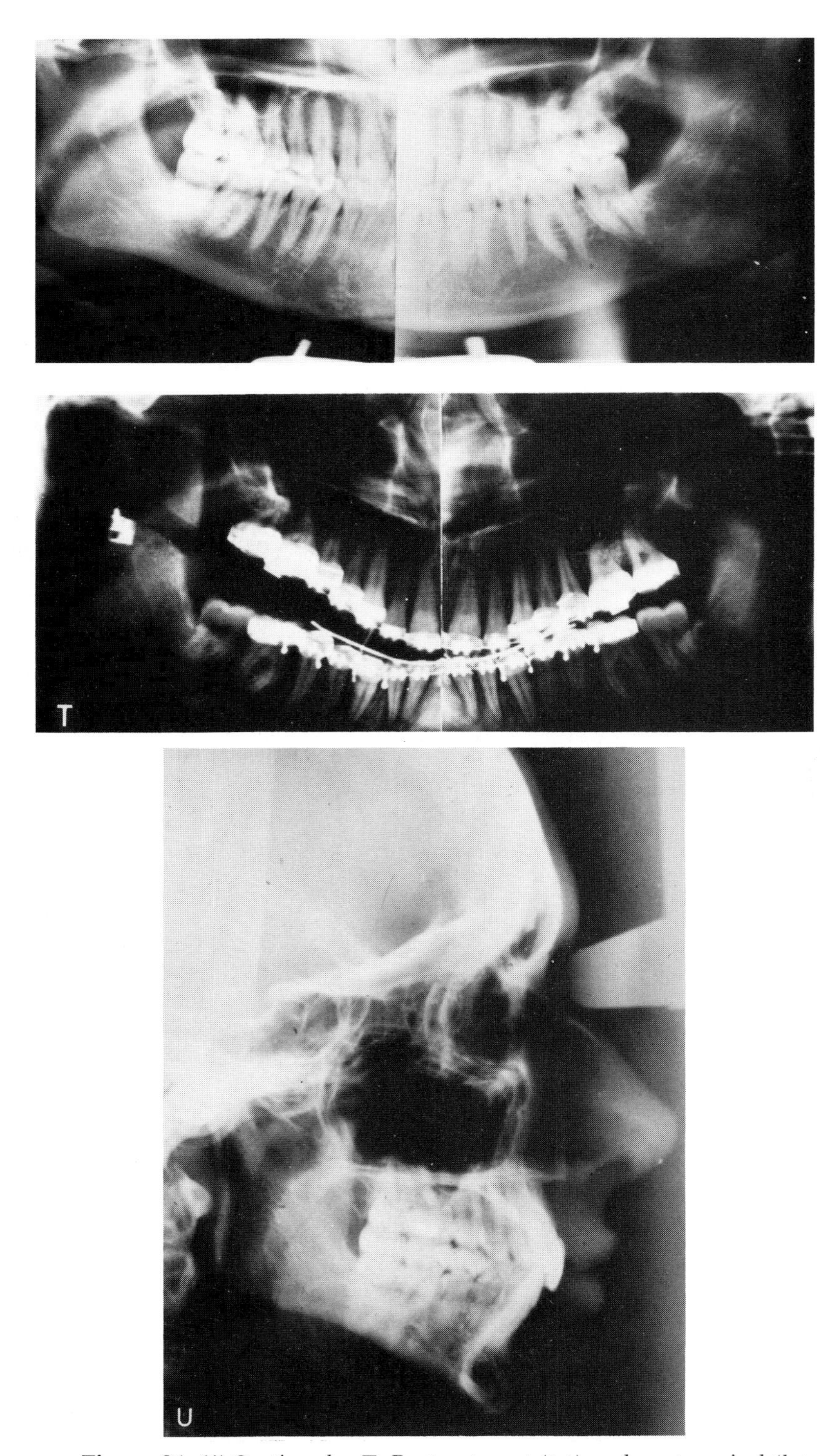

Figure 21–15 *Continued.* *T,* Pretreatment (*top*) and postsurgical (*bottom*) comparison of panoramic x-rays demonstrating the right ramus lengthening and associated right buccal open bite of 7 to 8 mm. *U,* Pretreatment lateral cephalogram demonstrating severe asymmetry of the right and left occlusal planes. Also note the discrepancy between the right and left lower borders of the mandible.

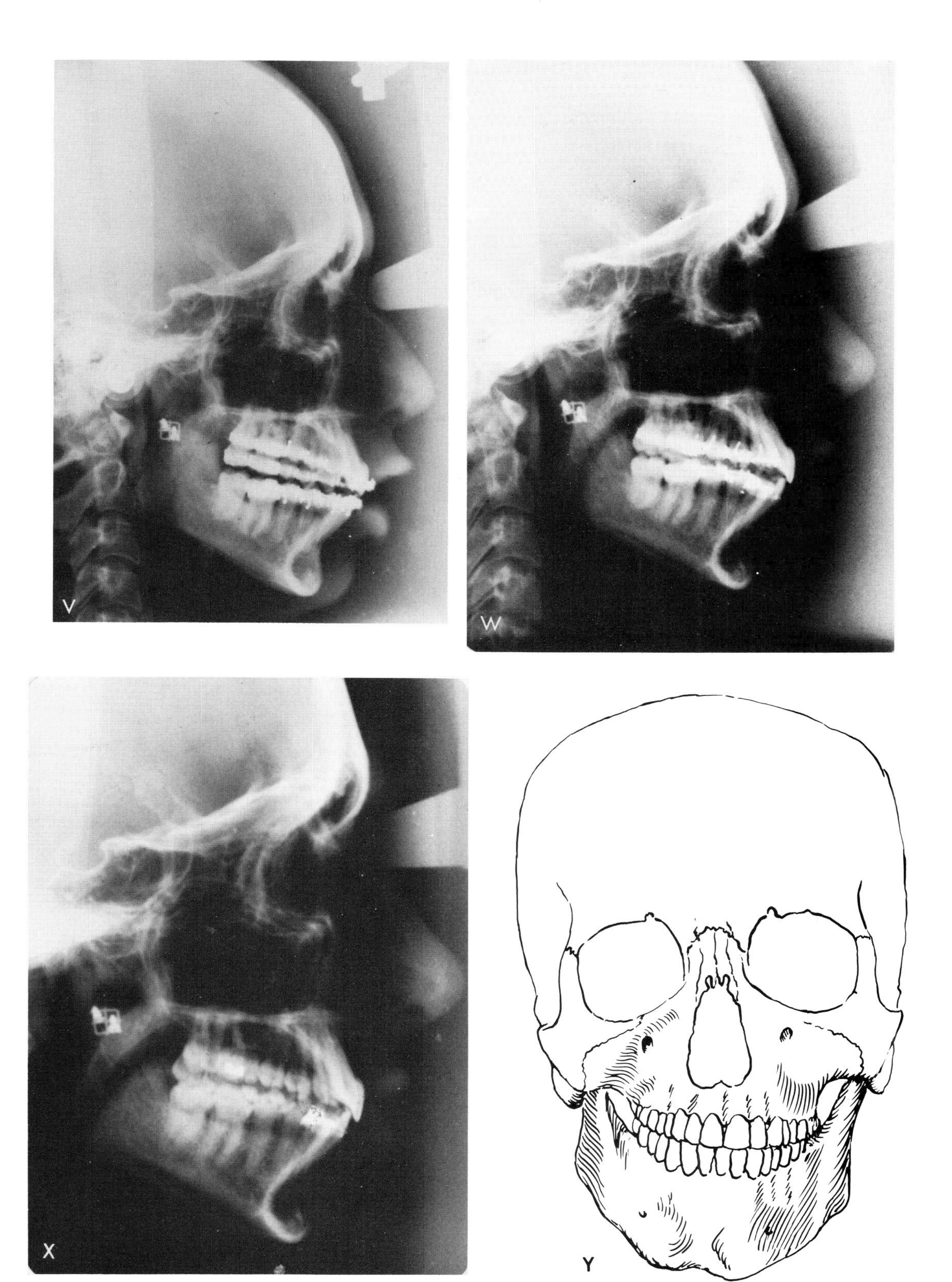

Figure 21–15 *Continued.* *V–Y,* Composite lateral cephalographic series demonstrating the four stages of surgical-orthodontic combination treatment. The series encompasses about 2 years of treatment time. *V,* Postsurgical opening of mandible (leveling). *W,* Postorthodontic movement (maxillary); 6 months post surgery. *X,* Post-treatment; 18 months after surgery. *Y,* Facial asymmetry at the start of treatment.

Illustration continued on the following page

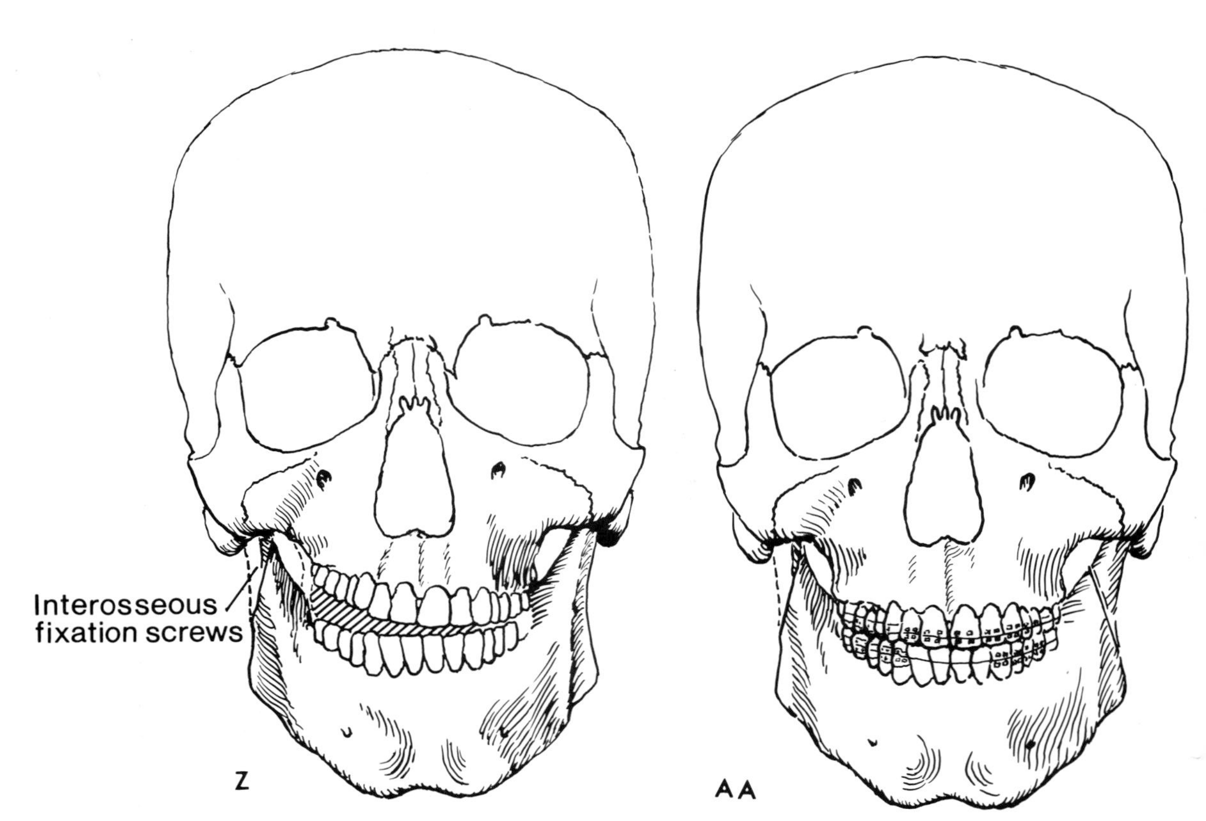

Figure 21–15 *Continued.* *Z,* After bilateral vertical mandibular surgery, before orthodontic segmental right extrusion. Cross-hatched area shows splint used to maintain surgical leveling of mandible. *AA,* Interarch vertical elastics to close right posterior open bite following a bilateral vertical osteotomy.

Evaluation of the posteroanterior and lateral cephalometric head films, laminagraphs of the temporomandibular joint, and the panoramic x-rays revealed the following:

1. The posteroanterior cephalometric film demonstrated marked asymmetry of the mandible with associated canted maxillary asymmetry and a shift of the maxillary dental midline approximately 3 mm to the right.
2. The left mandibular ramus appeared hypoplastic, as did the condylar neck and the left condyle itself.
3. The right mandibular ramus and condyle appeared anatomically normal but enlarged in proportion to the contralateral ramus and condyle.
4. The left body of the mandible was bulkier than the right body. Lateral cephalometric evaluation demonstrated and confirmed the different high levels of the occlusal plane along with different levels of the lower border of the right and left mandibular body.
5. The upper portion of the neck and the posterior border of the mandibular rami were closely approximated on superimposition of the lateral cephalometric films and laminagraphs.
6. Films of the temporomandibular joint showed equal bilateral condylar movement.

DIAGNOSIS

1. Hypoplasia of the right mandibular ramus and condyles secondary to childhood trauma.
2. Facial asymmetry secondary to hypoplasia of the right mandibular ramus and condyle.

TREATMENT PLAN

The clinical and radiographic findings were discussed with the patient, and she was advised that surgical contouring of the mandible could give her a more pleasing facial appearance but could not correct the canted occlusal plane and lip lines. The patient stated that she wanted maximal correction of her deformity and that she was willing to undergo combined orthodontic and oral surgical treatment if necessary. At a treatment conference between orthodontists and oral surgeons at the University of Minnesota, it was decided that the following treatment plan could meet the patient's expectations:

1. Orthodontic alignment of the upper and lower teeth, maintaining the original posterior occlusion. Torquing and cross-elastic wear on the upper and lower anterior teeth to "overcorrect" the dental compensations induced by asymmetric growth.
2. Initial surgery consisting of bilateral vertical osteotomies of the mandibular rami to lengthen the short ramus without placing undue stress on the left condyle. (The patient had stated during her case presentation that she definitely liked "the longer left face" better than the "shorter right face.")
3. The next phase of treatment could involve either:
   A. Surgical repositioning of the entire maxilla, or
   B. Orthodontic movement of the entire upper right posterior segment to the new mandibular (previously surgically leveled) occlusal plane.
4. Since final treatment could be decided on later, presurgical orthodontic treat-

ment was initiated to align the teeth and correct the dental compensations induced by the dentofacial asymmetry.

ACTIVE TREATMENT

During 8 months of presurgical orthodontic treatment, the upper and lower arches were aligned and most of the anterior dental inclination compensations were corrected with anterior uprighting of the roots. When orthodontic alignment reached the stage of .016 x .022 arch wires, the patient was admitted to the University of Minnesota Hospital for bilateral vertical osteotomies.

The right distal segment was lowered along the proximal segment as far as possible without losing overlap of the segments. A tantalum mesh was fastened with tantalum screws over the approximation of the right distal and proximal ramal segments. Further fixation of the mandible was achieved with an acrylic surgical splint and four intermaxillary wires in the buccal segments. Final right buccal opening of the posterior bite was measured as 6.5 mm between the upper and lower right first molars and 3.5 mm between the right cuspids.

After 8 weeks of fixation, the intermaxillary wires were removed and the upper right occlusal plane of the splint was reduced to allow vertical elastic closure of the right buccal open bite. The surgically created right posterior open bite was closed by extruding the segment including the upper right cuspid, the two premolars, and the first molar. The upper right second molar was used as a prop to extrude the upper posterior teeth as much as possible without affecting the surgical correction of the lower occlusal plane. Some movement of the lower occlusal plane did in fact occur, causing a 10 per cent relapse of the surgical correction.

Leveling of the lower occlusal plane and lower border of the mandible surgically followed by the orthodontic correction of the canted maxillary occlusal plane resulted in an esthetically pleasing and functional correction of a severe maxillary and mandibular asymmetry.

CASE 21–3 (FIG. 21–16)

This 20-year-old woman was referred to the University of Minnesota School of Dentistry for evaluation of her congenital asymmetric facial deformity. As a result of consultation with the Department of Human and Oral Genetics, her condition was diagnosed as a variant of the first brachial arch syndrome.

CLINICAL EXAMINATION

The patient's left-sided maxillomandibular asymmetry was evaluated by cephalometric radiographs and tracings as seen in Figure 21–16*E* and *M*. The deficiency in the left mandibular ramus and concomitant growth disturbance in the maxilla resulted in a canted occlusal plane as well as soft-tissue manifestations in the ocular, aural, and other areas.

RECORD EVALUATION AND TREATMENT PLAN

This case was presented at a surgical-orthodontic conference, where it was decided to use bilateral vertical subcondylar osteotomies or sagittal split osteotomies to

Text continued on page 1564

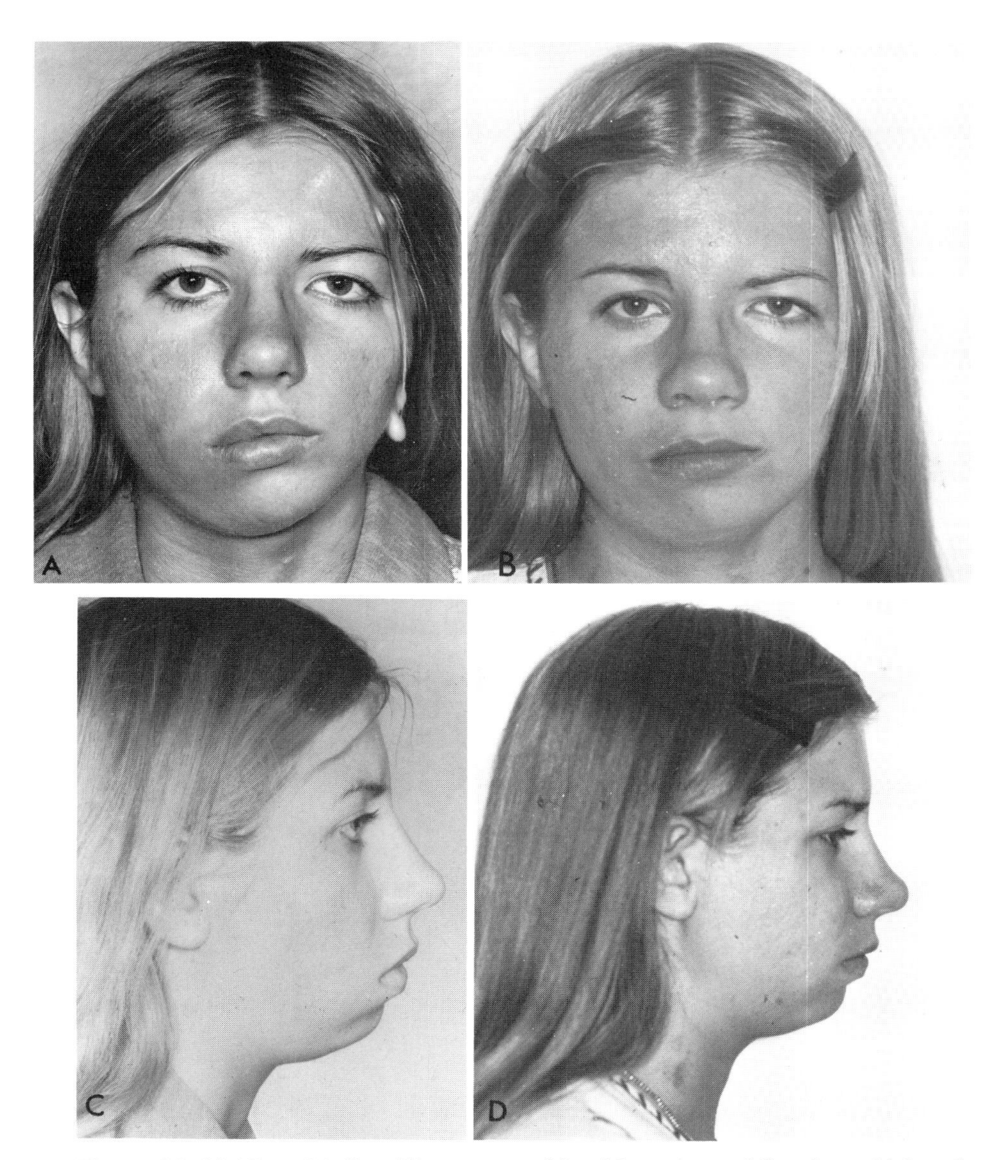

Figure 21–16 (Case 21–3). Woman, age 20, with variant of first branchial arch syndrome. *A–D,* Facial views. *A* and *C,* Pretreatment views. *B* and *D,* Facial views 4 years after treatment consisting of bilateral vertical osteotomy, Le Fort I maxillary osteotomy, and orthodontic correction.

Illustration continued on the following page

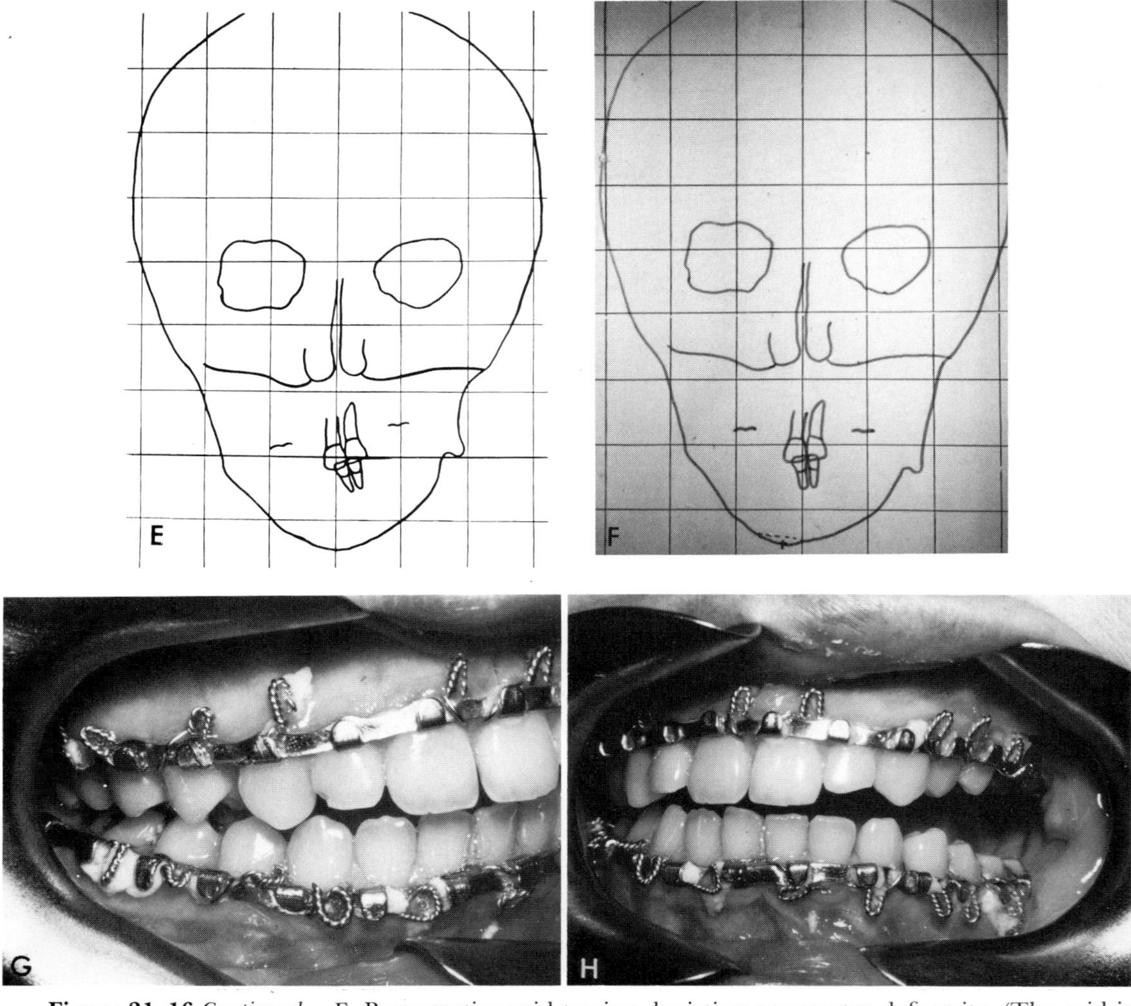

Figure 21–16 *Continued.* *E,* Preoperative grid tracing depicting asymmetry deformity. (The grid is used to line up known anatomic landmarks in order to note areas of deficiency and deviation from the norm.) *F,* Postoperative prediction grid tracing showing anticipated results of surgical procedure and orthodontic treatment. *G* and *H,* Interim occlusion. *G,* Right lateral view. *H,* Left lateral view. Note the left-sided open bite after vertical osteotomies and before Le Fort I osteotomy. (An interim interarch splint was maintained until the second procedure.)

Legend continued on opposite page.

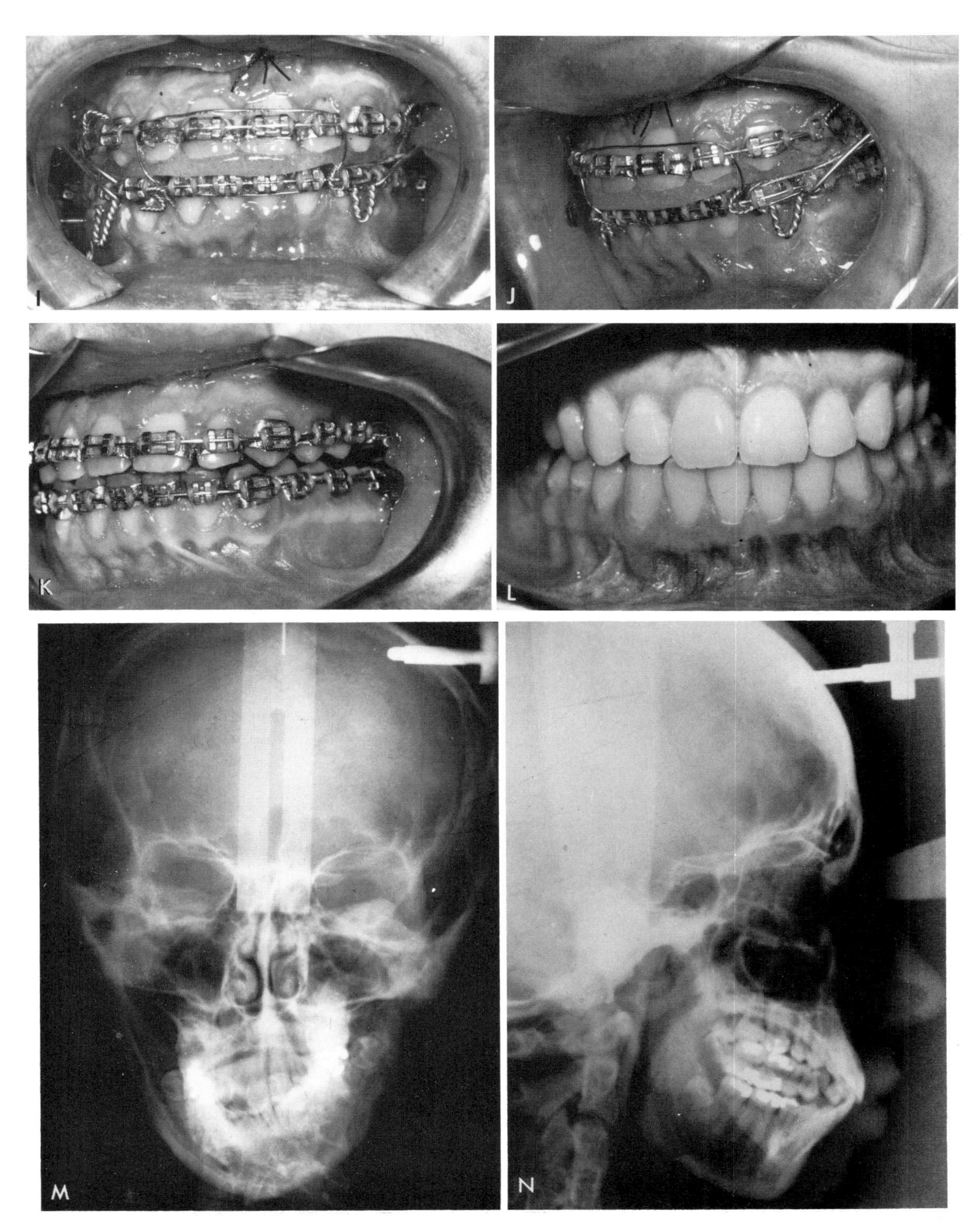

Figure 21–16 *Continued.* *I* and *J*, Occlusion immediately following Le Fort I osteotomy. *I*, Frontal view. *J*, Left lateral view. (In this case orthodontic management was done post surgically.) *K*, Occlusion after surgical and orthodontic treatments just prior to removal of bands. *L*, Frontal view 4 years after surgical leveling of the maxilla. Patient wearing tooth positioner two nights per week. *M* and *N*, Preoperative cephalograms. *M*, Posteroanterior view. Note left-sided asymmetry manifested by left mandibular ramus deformity and cant of occlusal plane. *N*, Lateral view. Note lack of superimposition of teeth and mandibular inferior border.

Illustration continued on the following page.

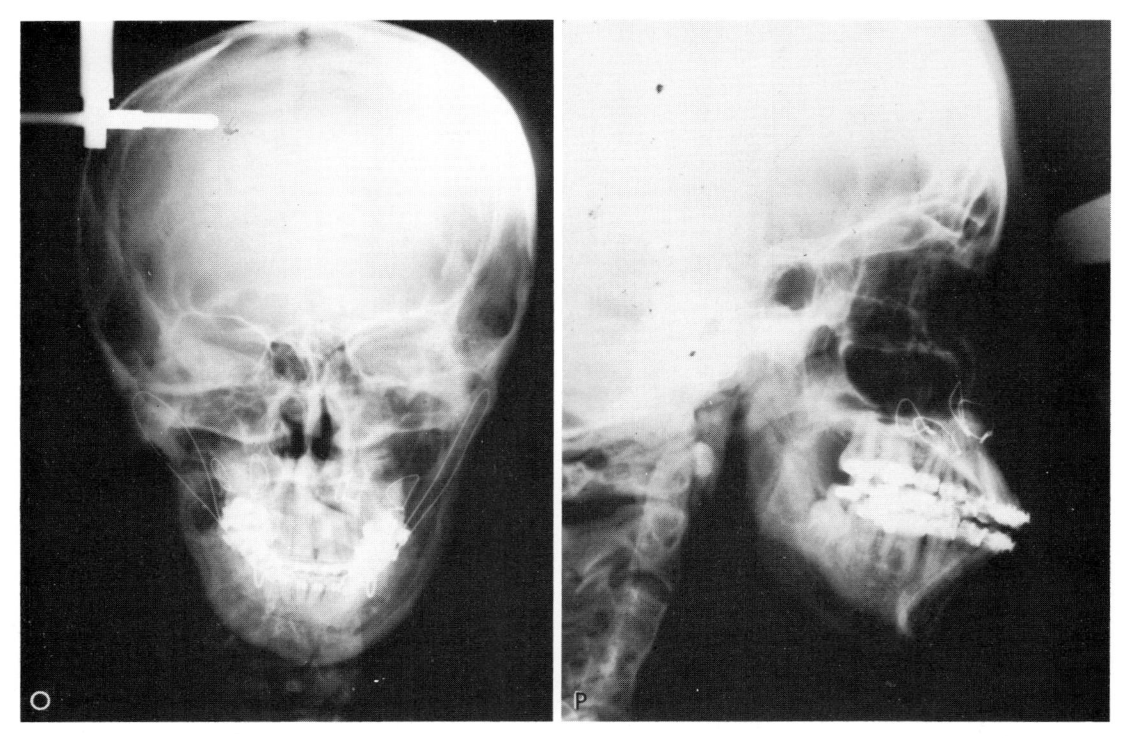

Figure 21–16 *Continued.* *O* and *P*, Postoperative cephalograms following bilateral vertical osteotomies and Le Fort I maxillary osteotomy. *O*, Posteroanterior view. *P*, Lateral view. Note improvement of inferior border superimposition compared with preoperative view.

correct the mandibular component of the deformity. This would leave an interim open bite that would be corrected by a total maxillary osteotomy. Orthodontic treatment would consist of minor tooth alignments before and after the maxillary osteotomy.

SURGICAL AND ORTHODONTIC TREATMENT

Treatment was initiated with bilateral vertical subcondylar osteotomies, which were followed by segmental orthodontic treatment and a total maxillary osteotomy. A stability splint was used to maintain the difference in occlusion between the two procedures.

CASE 21–4 (FIG. 21–17)

R. R., a young man, aged 19 years, 5 months, presented with unilateral maxillary hypertrophy. The history was noncontributory.

CLINICAL EXAMINATION

Hypertrophy of the maxilla was noted at the right malar eminence. Oral examination revealed complete buccal overbite from the upper right cuspid to the second molar. The overbite was more severe in the posterior portion of the segment.

Text continued on page 1568

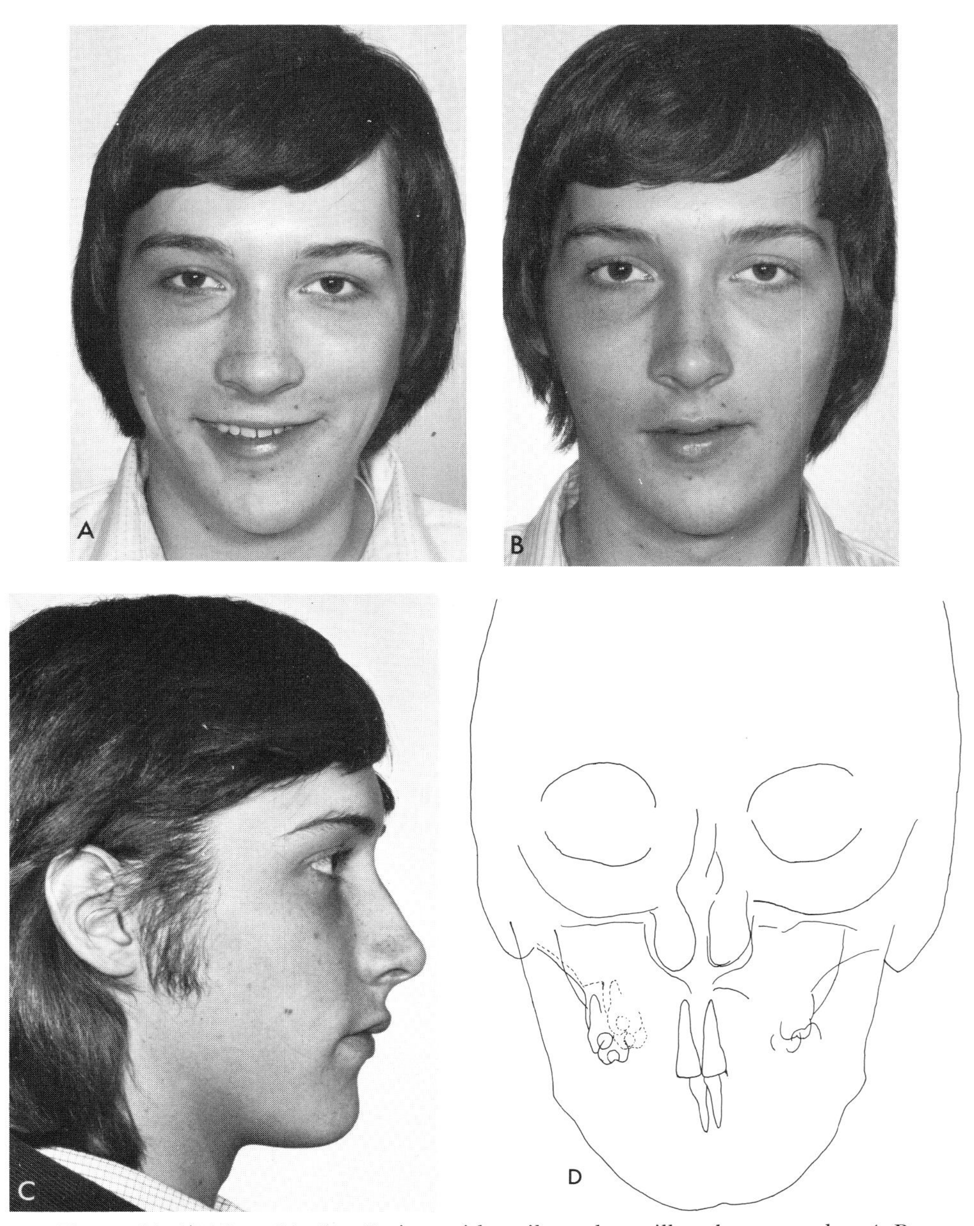

Figure 21–17 (Case 21–4). Patient with unilateral maxillary hypertrophy. *A*, Preoperative frontal view. Note facial asymmetry due to large cant and increased buccal overjet in the right upper posterior occlusion. Smile line of lips also demonstrates the asymmetry. *B*, Postoperative frontal view. *C*, Postoperative lateral view demonstrating soft-tissue changes associated with the intraoral medial movement of the right upper posterior segment. *D*, Pre- and post-treatment tracing demonstrates the unilateral repositioning of the upper right maxillary quadrant. Before (*solid line*, age 19 years, 5 months) and after (*broken line*, age 20 years, 6 months) treatment.

Illustration continued on the following page

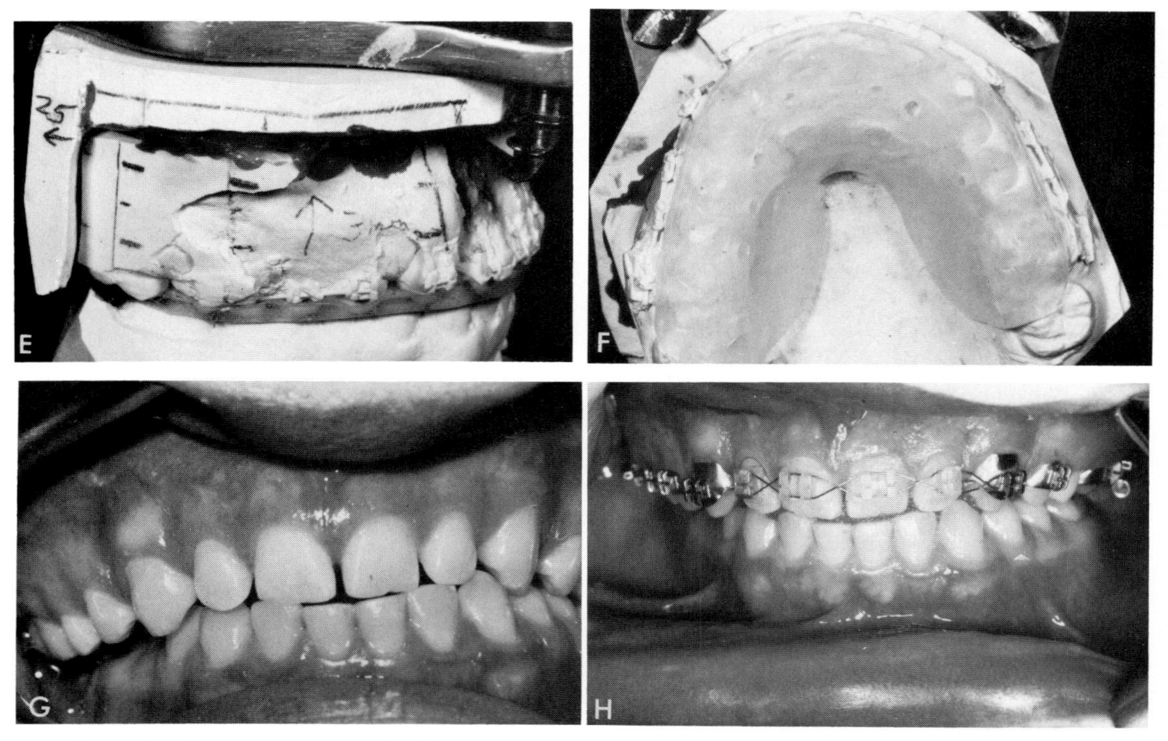

Figure 21–17 *Continued.* *E,* Model surgery. Segment moved posteriorly 2.5 mm and superiorly 3 mm. in the cuspid region and 6 mm in the molar region. There was a 3-mm. (medial) rotation of entire segment. *F,* Palatal view of acrylic splint used in fixation after segmental maxillary procedure. *G–L,* Occlusal views. *G,* Preoperative anterior intraoral view. Note right maxillary posterior excess and crossbite with associated buccal overbite. *H,* Preoperative view of dentition with orthodontic appliance in place.

Legend continued on the opposite page

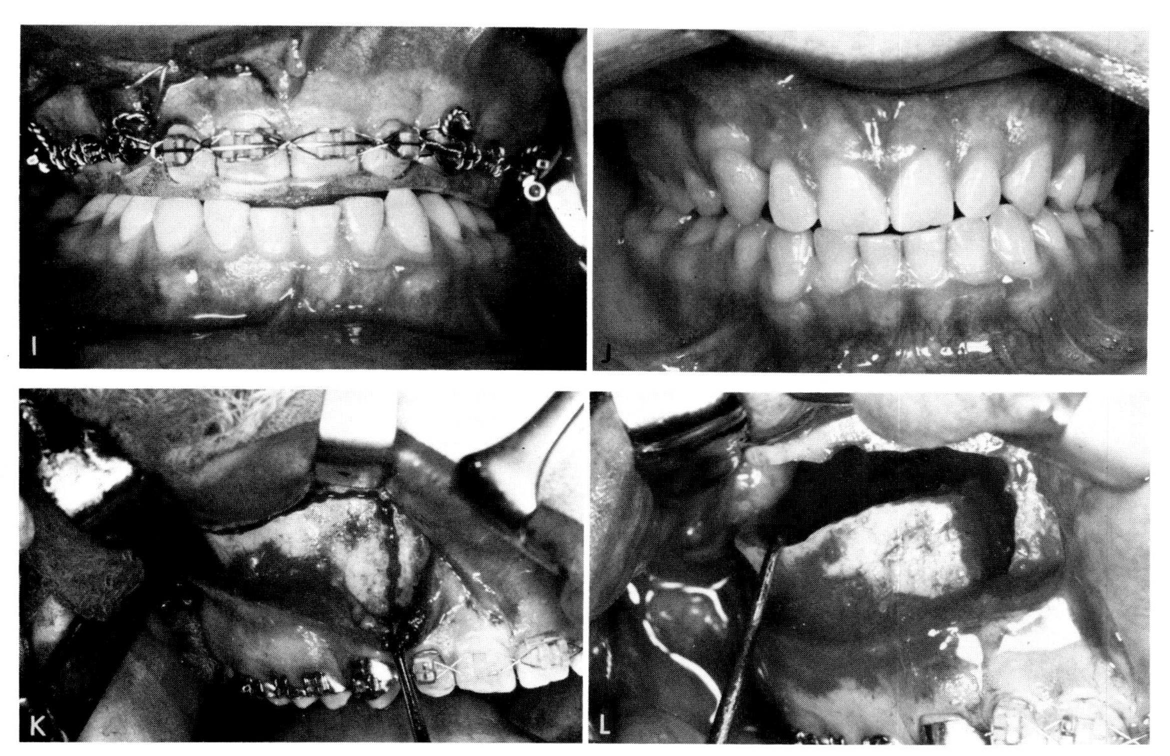

Figure 21–17 *Continued.* *I*, Postoperation view following segmental surgical procedure with fixation. *J*, Postoperative anterior intraoral view. Note orthodontic correction of anterior diastema. The surgical-orthodontic correction of the right posterior segment was accomplished without changing the anterior dental midlines. *K*, Flap design and surgical section for correction of posterior maxillary segment for treatment of unilateral maxillary asymmetry. *L*, Transantral approach for sectioning of the hard palate to reposition the maxillary segment.

Illustration continued on the following page

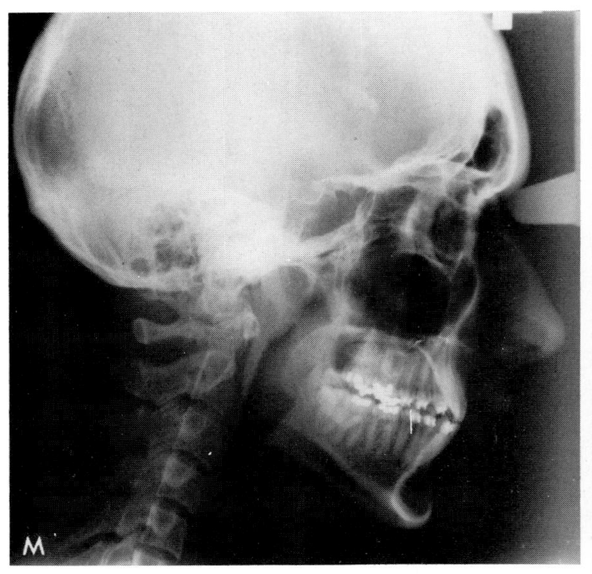

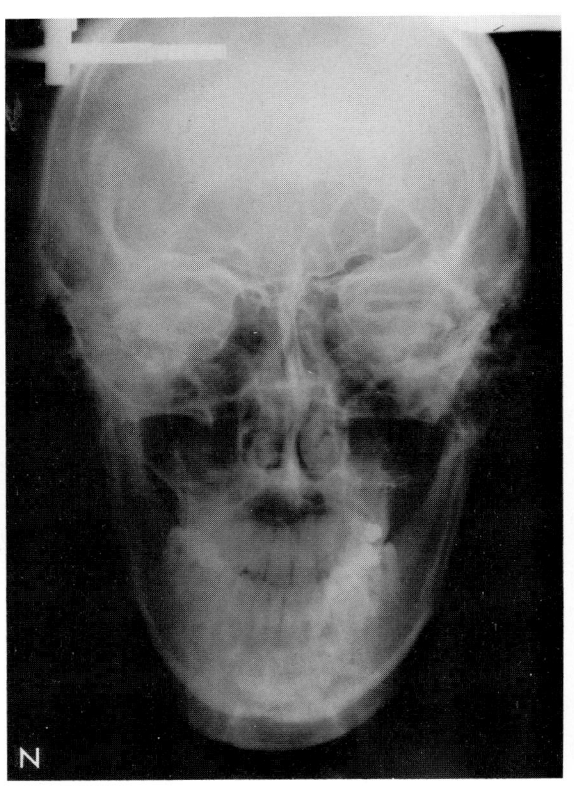

Figure 21–17 *Continued.* *M* and *N*, Postoperative cephalograms. *M*, Lateral view demonstrates the correction achieved on the maxillary occlusal plane. Note the intraosseous wires. *N*, Posteroanterior view showing the buccal overjet correction achieved by the unilateral segmented combination treatment. Note the intraosseous wires.

RECORD EVALUATION AND TREATMENT PLANNING

Complete records were taken including lateral and posteroanterior cephalometric x-rays and two sets of accurate models with a centric relation posterior trim on the backs of the models. Following facebow transfer on the Hanau articulator, model surgery determined that a wedge of bone 3 mm thick at the anterior and 6 mm at the posterior end was to be removed from the right posterior maxilla between the right cuspid and the right second molar. During the orthodontic stage of treatment, the impacted upper third molars were removed to make sectioning of the surgical site easier. Following 3 months of segmental orthodontic treatment, surgery in the right upper buccal quadrant was planned. Impressions were taken for final model surgery and a palatal acrylic splint was constructed.

ACTIVE TREATMENT

A posterior maxillary segmental osteotomy was performed as shown in Figure 21–17. The bone cuts used allowed the segment to move vertically, 3 mm anteriorly and 6 mm posteriorly. The segment was rotated 3 to 4 mm medially. Postsurgical orthodontics involved only minor tooth movements to improve cuspid interdigitation.

REFERENCES

1. Bell WH: Le Fort I osteotomy for correction of maxillary deformities. J Oral Surg *33*:412–426, 1975.
2. Bell WH: Correction of maxillary excess by anterior maxillary osteotomy. Oral Surg Med Pathol *43*:3, 1977.
3. Bell WH, McBride KL: Correction of the long face syndrome by Le Fort I osteotomy. J Oral Surg *44*:493–520, 1977.
4. Bell WH, Turvey TA: Surgical correction of posterior crossbite. J Oral Surg *32*:811–822, 1974.
5. Bell WH et al: Bone healing and revascularization after total maxillary osteotomy. J Oral Surg *33*:253–260, 1975.
6. Hall, HD, Roddy SC Jr: Treatment of maxillary alveolar hyperplasia by total maxillary alveolar osteotomy. J Oral Surg *33*:180–188, 1975.
7. Hall HD, West RA: Combined anterior and posterior maxillary osteotomy. J Oral Surg *34*:126–141, 1976.
8. Nelson RL et al: Quantitation of blood flow following anterior maxillary osteotomy: investigation of three surgical approaches. J Oral Surg *33*:106–111, 1978.
9. Wassmund M: Lehrbuch der Praktischen Chirurgie des Mundes und der Kiefer, vol. 1, Leipzig: JA Barth, pp 260–282, 1935.
10. Wunderer S: Die prognathi Operation mittels frontal gestieltem maxilla Fragment. Osterr Zeitschr Stomat *59*:98–102, 1962.

RECOMMENDED READING

1. Bell WH: Correction of the short face syndrome — vertical maxillary deficiency, a preliminary report. J Oral Surg *33*:110–120, 1977.
2. Hullihen SP: Case of elongation of the under jaw and distortion of the face and neck, caused by a burn, successfully treated. Am J Dent Sci *9*:157–165, 1849.
3. Knowles CC: Cephalometric treatment planning and analysis of maxillary growth following bone grafting to the ramus in hemifacial microsomia. Dent Practit *17*:28–38, 1966.
4. Osborne R: The treatment of the underdeveloped ascending ramus. Br J Plast Surg *17*:376–388, 1964.
5. West RA: McNeill RW: Maxillary alveolar hyperplasia — diagnosis and treatment planning. J Max Surg *3*(4):239–250, 1975.
6. Willmar K: On Le Fort I Oosteotomy. Scand J Plast Reconst Surg *12*[Suppl], 1974.

Chapter 22

SURGICAL-PROSTHETIC REHABILITATION OF ADULT DENTOFACIAL DEFORMITIES

William H. Bell and Kevin McBride

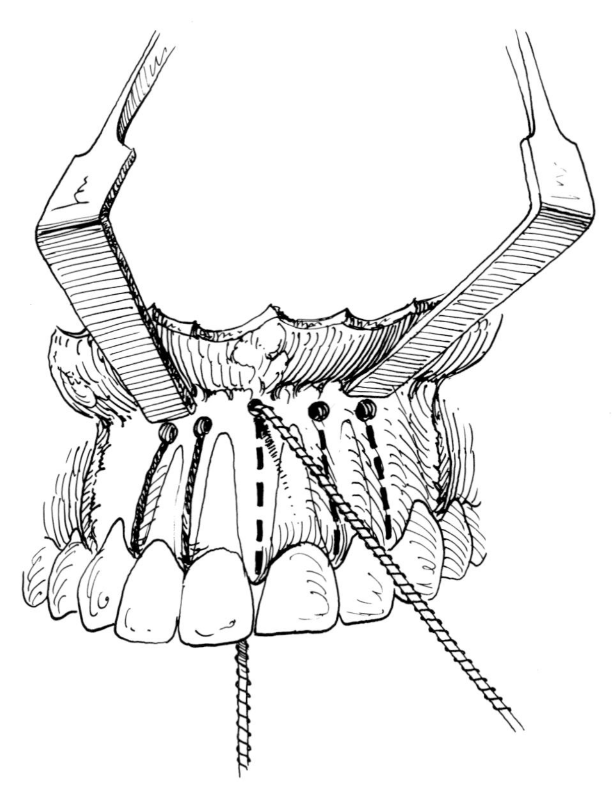

Method of Kretz to immediately reposition the incisor teeth. After the maxillary alveolar process was exposed, holes were drilled in the apical region of the teeth. A thin Gigli's wire saw was then passed into the holes and was used to section the inter-radicular septa. He also excised a "wedge-shaped trough" on the palatal aspect of the maxilla at the apical level. Then, with the use of dental forceps, the dento-osseous segments were repositioned palatally. The mobilized segment was then fixed in the planned position by ligating a labial arch wire to the previously banded teeth.

"A tooth in its normal position without vitality is more valuable than a vital tooth in an abnormal relationship. Since the ability of bone to repair itself is well known, as seen in fractures, it is better to divide the alveolar process in its entirety. The procedure is ideally suited for adult patients."[20] Cunningham (1893)

Those who treat adults with dentofacial deformities must become involved in a new spectrum of challenging prosthetic, occlusal, and esthetic problems over and beyond the ones they routinely manage in adolescents. A constellation of surgical, prosthetic, and orthodontic factors must be considered when planning treatment for adults with dentofacial deformities. The condition of the periodontium, missing posterior anchorage teeth, buccal and palatal crossbites, supererupted teeth, and lack of interarch space may preclude treatment by conventional orthodontic or prosthetic methods. Severely tipped, rotated, ankylosed, spaced, or crowded teeth are some of the other common problems associated with the treatment of adult malocclusions.

The reservoir of adult orthodontic patients is vast. Adults seeking correction of their dentofacial deformities constitute a significant proportion of patients treated by orthodontists. With the predicted four-fold increase in the number of adults over age 40 within the next decade, some estimate that approximately 50 per cent of patients treated by orthodontists in the future will be adults.

Many adults, however, object to wearing orthodontic appliances for prolonged periods of time, when the results of such treatment will be compromised in terms of esthetics, function, and stability. Patients' careers, the geographic unavailability of specialty care, socioeconomic factors, and cessation of jaw growth and development are additional considerations which compound the problems of conventional orthodontic management of adult patients.

Principles of Treatment

Treatment of jaw dysplasias in partially edentulous adults should follow the same therapeutic principles used to manage patients with a full dentition. Classically, however, these patients have frequently received compromised treatment. Supererupted, rotated, tipped, ankylosed, and crowded teeth have all too frequently been summarily extracted. Radical alveolectomies at the expense of the denture base and facial esthetics have been performed all too frequently. The consequences of modifying the position of the denture teeth on the alveolar ridge to compensate for skeletal crossbites is well known to all dental practitioners. Denture instability and undesirable resorption of the alveolar ridges are the hallmarks of such therapy.

A compromised alveolar ridge relationship not only compounds the difficulties associated with prosthetic management of the partially edentulous adult but also accelerates alveolar ridge resorption. Anterior-posterior changes, manifest clinically as the development of a Class III ridge relationship, may occur as a consequence of the reduction in vertical alveolar ridge height.

Orthognathic surgery refers to surgical procedures that deal with repositioning the maxilla, mandible, and dentoalveolar segments to achieve facial and occlusal balance. One, two, or multiple dental-osseous segments of the maxilla or mandible can be simultaneously repositioned superiorly, inferiorly, anteriorly, posteriorly, laterally, or medially to treat various types of malocclusions and jaw dysplasias and facilitate orthodontic and prosthetic management of the partially edentulous adult. An optimal functional occlusal relationship and balanced facial esthetics can usually be attained by surgically repositioning the maxilla or mandible in single or multiple segments. In this chapter we describe how orthognathic surgery, in concert with prosthetic and orthodontic treatment, can be used to rehabilitate virtually all dentulous or partially edentulous adults with dentofacial deformities.

SURGICAL-PROSTHETIC REHABILITATION OF THE PARTIALLY EDENTULOUS PATIENT

The general dentist or prosthodontist plays a vital role in planning treatment to produce an ideal tooth-to-ridge and ridge-to-ridge relationship in the vertical, anteroposterior, and transverse planes of space. With carefully coordinated, planned, and executed surgery and prosthetic treatment, improved function, esthetics, and stability can be achieved in most adults with dentofacial deformities.

The restorative dentist has great latitude in planning treatment because of the many surgical procedures that can be used to alter the spatial relationship of the jaws, the tooth-to-bone relationship, and the jaw-to-jaw relationship (See Fig. 22–1.)

Clinical Analysis

The clinician must determine where the deformity is primarily manifest by a correlative clinical, cephalometric, and occlusal analysis. Treatment is planned to achieve optimal esthetics, function, and stability. The key to achieving treatment objectives is to examine the patient carefully to determine the principal functional and esthetic problematic areas and then coordinate the results of these studies with the cephalometric and model analyses.[9]

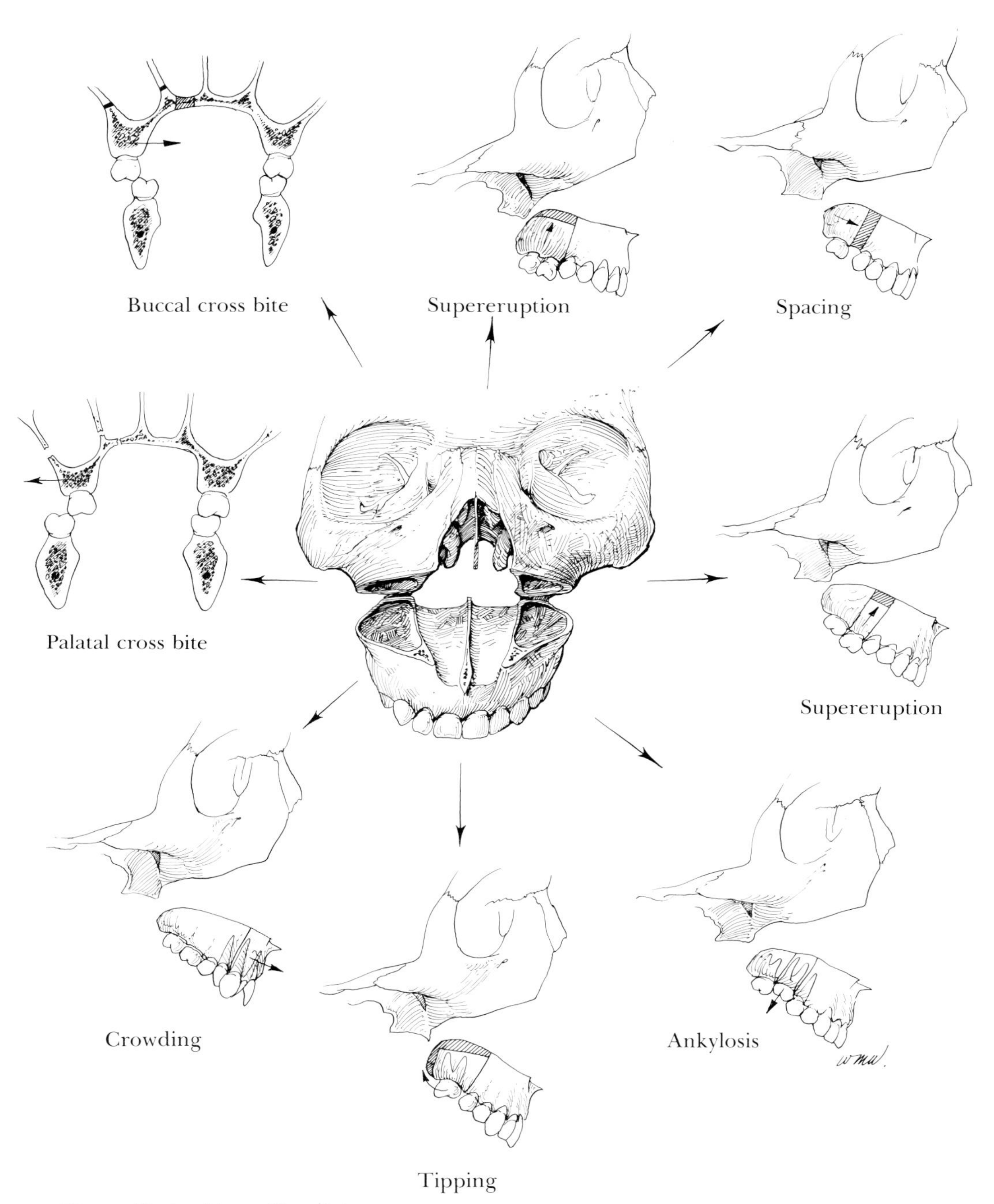

Figure 22–1. Versatility of the Le Fort I osteotomy to treat variable dentofacial deformities in adults.

Clinical analysis of the patient with a preprosthetic problem should determine whether there is a skeletal discrepancy and if it is primarily the result of maxillary or mandibular deficiency or excess in the vertical, horizontal, or anteroposterior plane of space. Frequently there will be a combination of all three at fault. Full-face and profile evaluations are made with the head in the natural position to assess facial proportions and balance and identify the patient's principal esthetic problems.

In analyzing adult facial esthetics, compensations must be made for partially or completely edentulous jaws; this is accomplished with bite splints or prostheses which support the lips. To accurately simulate the existing situation, full-face and profile analyses are performed with the jaws in centric relationship and the head in natural position.

Cephalometric Analysis

Cephalometric analysis will confirm or revise initial impressions formulated during the clinical examination. An accurate simulation of the operative procedure is essential to determine the magnitude and direction of movement required. Cephalometric films which delineate both soft and hard tissues are taken in a natural head position with the lips relaxed. The first exposure is made with the teeth in centric relation; if vertical deficiency is suspected, a second exposure is made with the mandible in rest position and the teeth disoccluded to obviate superimposition of the maxillary and mandibular occlusal planes. When anteroposterior mandibular deficiency is manifest, a radiograph is obtained with the mandible protruded into the desired overjet relationship to simulate the osseous, tooth, and soft tissue changes associated with mandibular advancement.

All of the maxillary and mandibular teeth, bony landmarks, enveloping soft tissue, and the mandibular and mental canals are traced. Then the maxillary or mandibular dentoskeletal structures and their enveloping soft tissues are traced with a different-colored pencil onto a second piece of overlaid tracing paper. An acetate overlay of the portion of the maxilla or mandible to be moved (with or without teeth) is used as a template and is now repositioned to the degree and direction necessary to achieve the desired esthetic and prosthetic objectives. Movement of the templates simulates the projected jaw movements and the resultant occlusion. After a third piece of acetate tracing paper is overlaid, a soft-tissue profile is traced and serves as the basis for simulating additional profile changes by genioplasty or rhinoplasty. (See Maxillary Excess for additional details.) The need for combined maxillary-mandibular surgical procedures is relatively common because many adults with dentofacial deformities manifest problems in both jaws.

Prosthetic and orthodontic treatment objectives dictate positioning of the dental arches in the most stable position over their respective osseous bases. Considerable orthodontic leveling and arch alignment can usually be accomplished after surgery. (See Mandibular Deficiencies, Chapter 10.)

If it is determined diagnostically that maxillary or mandibular incisors must be repositioned during closure of extraction spaces and flaring or consolidation of excess interdental spaces, then the prediction cephalometric tracing must be altered accordingly to represent the anticipated position of the incisors prior to surgery. A tracing is made with the incisors in the anticipated position and the skeletal units are repositioned as part of the overall cephalometric prediction study.

The cephalometric radiograph provides a means of assessing both the vertical and anteroposterior relationship between the jaws. Based upon a correlative study of the cephalometric tracing and the patient's occluded study casts (edentulous or partially edentulous), treatment is planned to reposition either one or both of the jaws to achieve an optimal vertical and anteroposterior relationship.

If the increased interarch space is secondary to jaw atrophy, surgery is programmed to restore the missing bone mass by interpositional or onlay bone grafting. (See Roger West et al., Chapter 19.) An ideal tooth-to-lip relationship can thereby be achieved in edentulous or partially edentulous patients.

Occlusal Analysis

The three-dimensional spatial relationship of the edentulous or partially edentulous jaws should be transferred to an anatomic articulator. A functional analysis is best achieved after a face bow transfer of the vertical, anteroposterior, and horizontal jaw relationship. These findings are subsequently coordinated with the cephalometric and clinical studies. Most of the problems which have previously been considered untreatable and accepted as functional compromises can be managed by carefully planned and executed orthognathic surgical procedures in concert with prosthetic restoration and orthodontic treatment.

Treatment Planning

A coordinated study of the patient's periodontium will frequently reveal that certain teeth must ultimately be extracted. Many of these teeth, however, should be maintained transitionally to stabilize the repositioned mandible or maxilla. Temporary dental restorations may be necessary before surgery. Reconstruction with permanent dental restorations and definitive fixed or removable prosthetic appliances, however, must be deferred until after surgery has achieved a stable maxillo-mandibular relationship. Functional transitional splints or prostheses are important adjuncts to achieve skeletal stability and to guard against postoperative relapse between the time of release from intermaxillary fixation and the time when permanent fixed or removable prostheses are placed.

Much of the definitive periodontal care may likewise be deferred until after orthognathic surgical procedures are completed. The ultimate success achieved in treating adults depends on careful analysis and treatment planning. If long-term success is to be achieved and compromised periodontal healing avoided, periodontal problems must be evaluated and treated appropriately. The majority of definitive periodontal treatment can usually be postponed until after surgery. Acute periodontitis and significant gingival stripping secondary to a lack of attached gingiva are two of the primary indications for periodontal treatment before surgery.

Orthognathic surgery can spare the fate of complete dentures for many partially edentulous patients with mutilated malocclusions.[15] The general dentist and prosthodontist must be involved in the case analysis and are the keystones around which a meaningful plan of treatment is evolved. Generally speaking, the more severe the malocclusion is, the greater need there is for simultaneous movement of the anterior and posterior parts of the maxilla and mandible to correct the malocclusion and to achieve optimal esthetics, function, and stability. Isolated parts of the maxilla and mandible are usually repositioned independently only when these objectives can be accomplished. Nevertheless, surgical repositioning of small dento-osseous segments plays a vital role in rehabilitating adults with dentofacial deformities.

Text continued on page 1580.

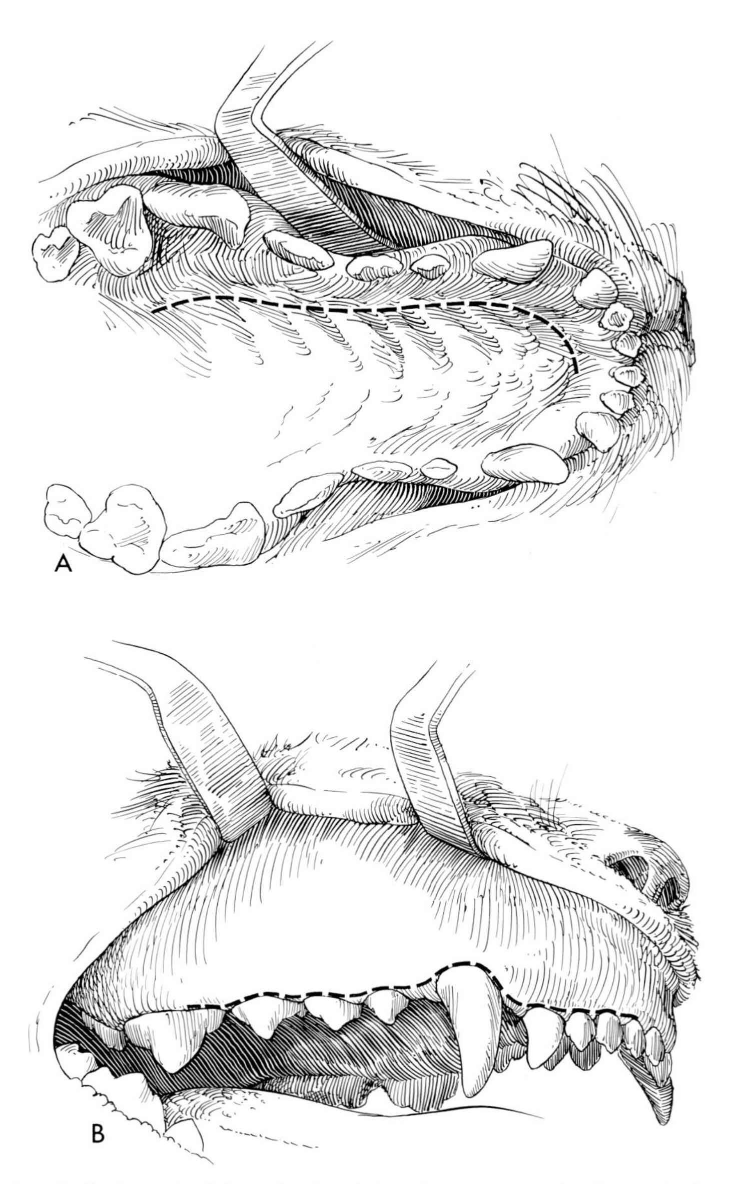

Figure 22–2. Soft-tissue incisions in the delayed two-stage single-tooth dento-osseous technique. The two-stage surgical procedures were separated by five weeks. *A,* Initial palatal mucogingival incision. The palatal mucoperiosteum was incised along the mucogingival sulcus from the 4th premolar to the central incisor. The mucoperiosteum was then elevated medially as a full thickness flap, maintaining the greater palatine vessels intact. *B,* Second-stage buccogingival sulcus incision.

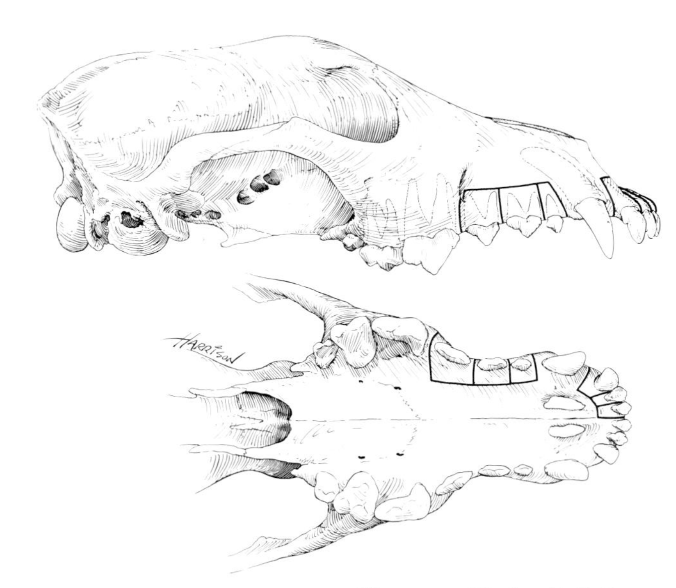

Figure 22–3. Interdental and subapical osteotomies used in both surgical techniques. Small finely tapered osteotomes were used interdentally to connect the buccal and palatal osteotomies. All the single-tooth dento-osseous segments were then fully mobilized and repositioned medially and inferiorly the width of the osteotomies. Fixation was accomplished with Erich arch bars, 24 gauge SSW, and direct bonding acrylic. The 2nd cuspid was not mobilized in any animal and was used for fixation with the molars. Intermaxillary fixation was not used.

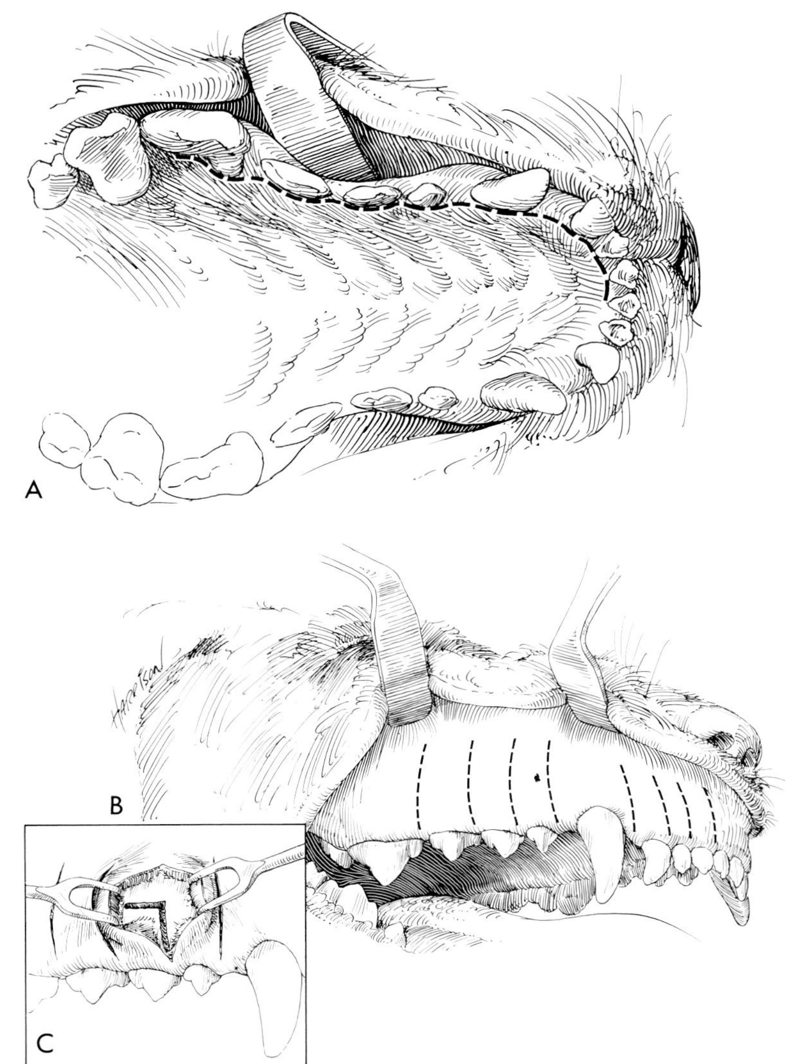

Figure 22–4. Soft-tissue incisions in the immediate one-stage single-tooth dento-osseous surgical technique. *A,* Initial palatal mucogingival incision. The mucoperiosteum was elevated as a full-thickness flap 5 mm. medially and laterally to this incision. The greater palatine vessels were ligated at the distal aspect of the incision. *B,* Multiple buccal vertical mucoperiosteal incisions. The soft-tissue incisions were connected by subperiosteal tunneling superiorly only under the free alveolar mucosa. Corresponding interdental vertical osteotomies were made ending several millimeters short of the crestal bone. Careful attention was directed to the attached mucosa around the vertical soft-tissue incisions so that only enough was reflected to complete the osteotomies (approximately 1 mm. on either side of the incision). A horizontal osteotomy was made at least 5 mm. above the root apices that connected the multiple buccal vertical osteotomies. A small osteotome was then used to complete the palatal and buccal interdental osteotomies and fully mobilize each single-tooth dento-osseous segment. *C,* Insert showing soft-tissue reflection and buccal osteotomies.

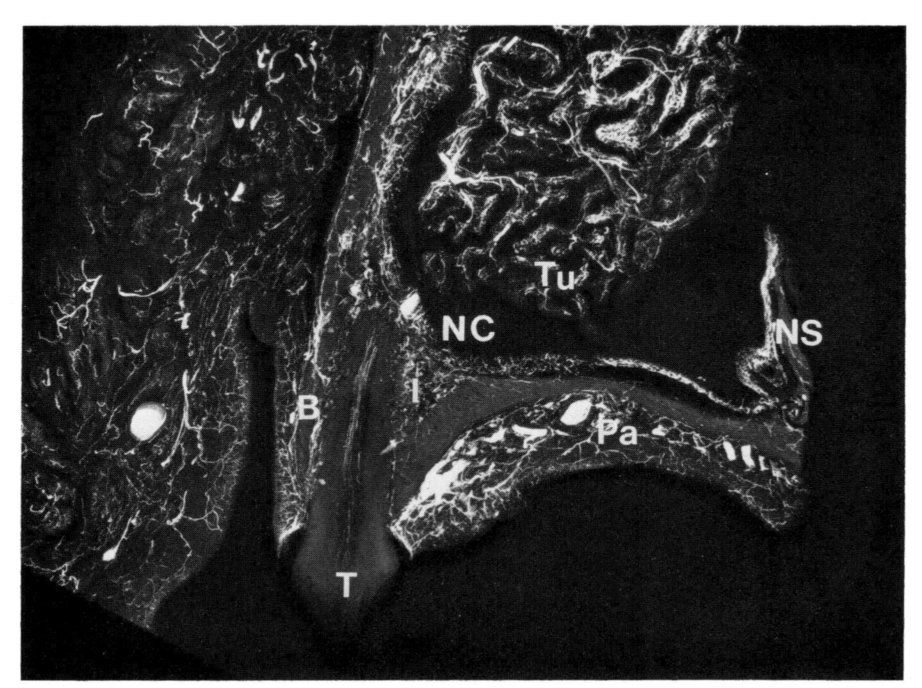

Figure 22–5. Microangiogram of 1 mm. transverse tissue slice from premolar region of control animal: buccal (B), palatal (Pa), and nasal cavity (NC) blood vessels penetrating bone and anastomosing with intramedullary blood vessels (I) and periodontal vascular plexus; premolar tooth (T); turbinate (Tu), and nasal septum (NS).

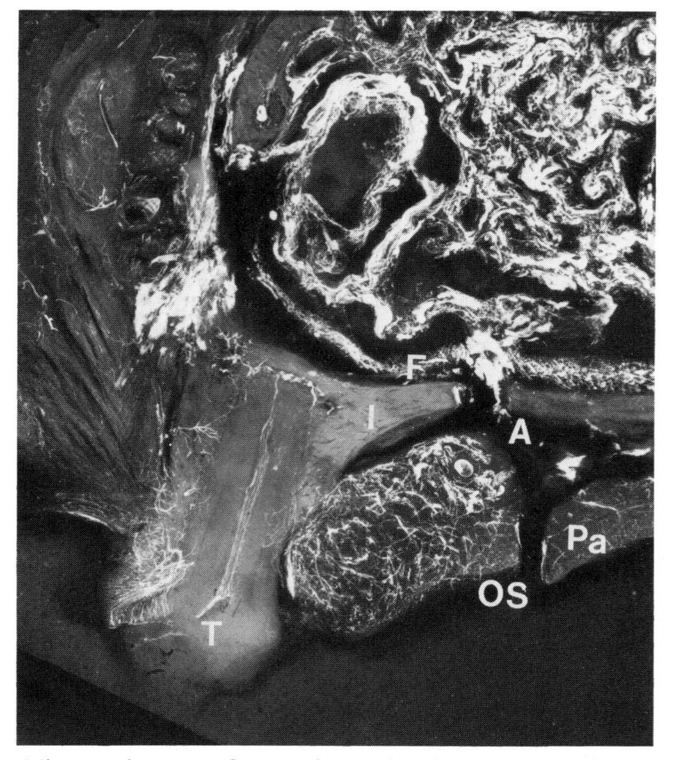

Figure 22–6. Microangiogram of premolar region immediately after one-stage interdental and subapical osteotomies shows intraosseous ischemia (I), avascular zone (A) below palatal and nasal mucosal flaps (F), vascularized premolar (T), palate (Pa), and osteotomy site (OS).

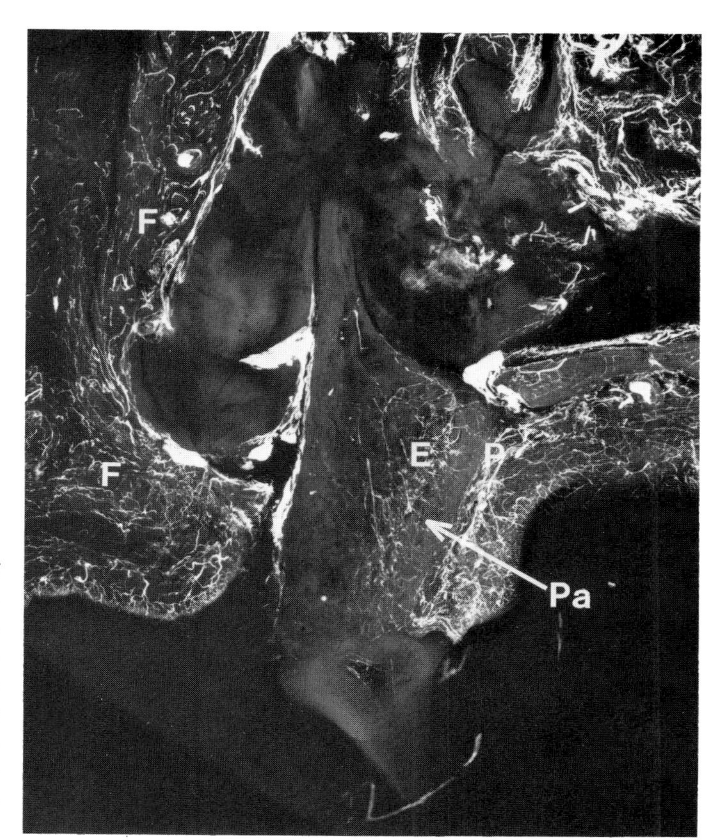

Figure 22–7. Microangiogram of premolar region immediately after two-stage interdental and subapical osteotomies shows intraosseous ischemia of buccal aspect of dento-osseous segment subjacent to raised buccal mucoperiosteal flap (F); periosteal (P) and endosteal (E) vascular beds in the palatal aspect (Pa) of dento-osseous segment are filled with Micropaque.

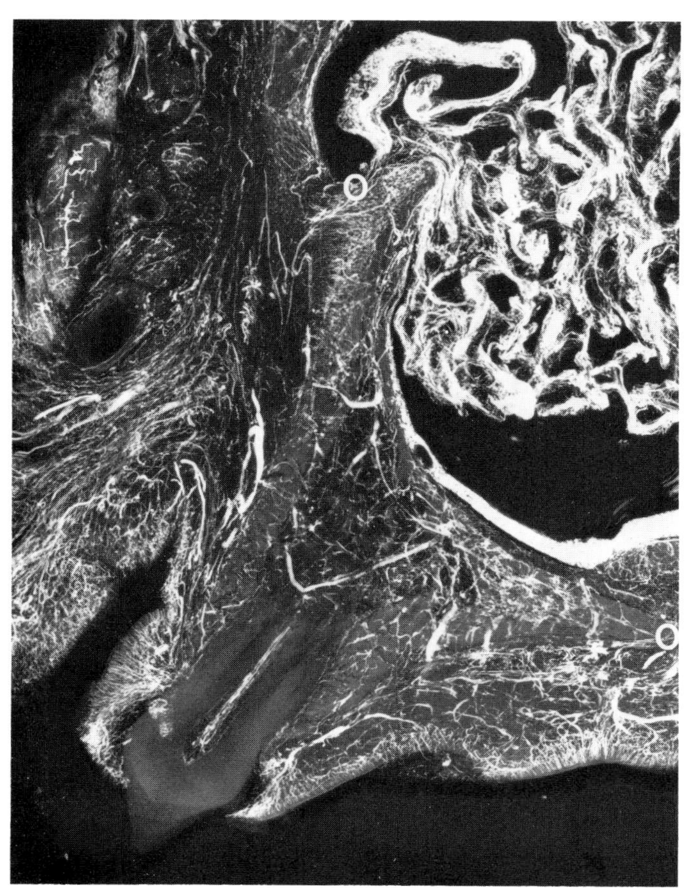

Figure 22–8. Microangiogram of premolar region three weeks after two-stage technique demonstrating revascularization of dento-osseous segment, malalignment of buccal and palatal bone margins, and reconstitution of circulation between osteotomized segments by proliferating vessels. O = osteotomy sites.

BIOLOGIC BASIS FOR SURGICAL REPOSITIONING OF SMALL DENTO-OSSEOUS SEGMENTS

The delivery of an adequate amount of blood to the tissue capillaries for normal function of the organ is the primary purpose of the vascular system. The ability of the arterial circulation in the maxillofacial region to meet the physiologic demands imposed by a surgical intervention is directly related to the anatomy and physical characteristics of the system. A knowledge of the anatomic, morphologic, and physiologic features of the arterial circulation is essential for the orthognathic surgeon.

After surgeons developed predictable, biologically based techniques for immediate repositioning of the anterior and posterior maxillary dentoalveolar segments, which usually contained between three and six teeth[3, 5, 8, 12, 31, 35, 38] (see Chapter 8), the challenge remained to determine whether even smaller dento-osseous segments containing only one or two teeth could be repositioned similarly. Because pedicling the segment to a relatively small amount of soft tissue could presumably imperil circulation to the mobilized dento-osseous segment, many surgeons have avoided such procedures. The results of our animal studies indicate that small dento-osseous segments can be mobilized with only a transient effect on their viability and healing capacity.[16] Depending on the objectives of surgery, the dentoalveolar segment to be repositioned may be pedicled primarily either to the labial-buccal gingiva and mucoperiosteum or to the palatal mucoperiosteum.

Successful transposition of dento-osseous segments depends on preservation of viability of the segment by proper design of the soft-tissue and bony incisions. The collateral circulation within the maxilla and its enveloping soft tissues and the many vascular anastomoses in the maxilla permit technical modifications of both one- and two-stage techniques.[3] For example, when an interdental osteotomy between closely spaced teeth is necessary to reposition a small dento-osseous segment, the surgery may be accomplished in two stages.[13] Palatal osteotomies can be accomplished initially, and four to five weeks later the labiobuccal vertical interdental and subapical bone cuts are made through the retracted wound margins of vertical incisions through the mucoperiosteum opposite the planned vertical interdental osteotomy sites. The reverse procedure is also possible — for example, the labiobuccal bone cuts can be made in the first stage; four or five weeks later the palatal bone cuts are made and the dento-osseous segment is mobilized and moved into the planned position. Although it is theoretically possible to wait only three weeks between the first and second stages of surgery, it is usually advisable for the clinician to wait four or five weeks to allow greater soft-tissue reattachment to the dento-osseous segment being moved. By so doing, there is less chance of stripping the reattached soft-tissue pedicle from the segment by digital manipulation of the segment when the second stage of surgery is accomplished. The immature bone and fibrous connective tissue in the initial osteotomy sites are easily transsected by malleting finely tapered osteotomes into the incompletely sectioned interdental osteotomy sites.

The excessive removal of interseptal and interradicular bone may cause protracted bone healing and have a destructive effect upon the periodontium.[13] The postoperative study parameters (clinical, radiographic, microangiographic, and histologic) revealed that this actually occurred in a few of the interdental osteotomy sites. Surgical technique, and not vascular ischemia, was the probable cause of this problem. The relatively

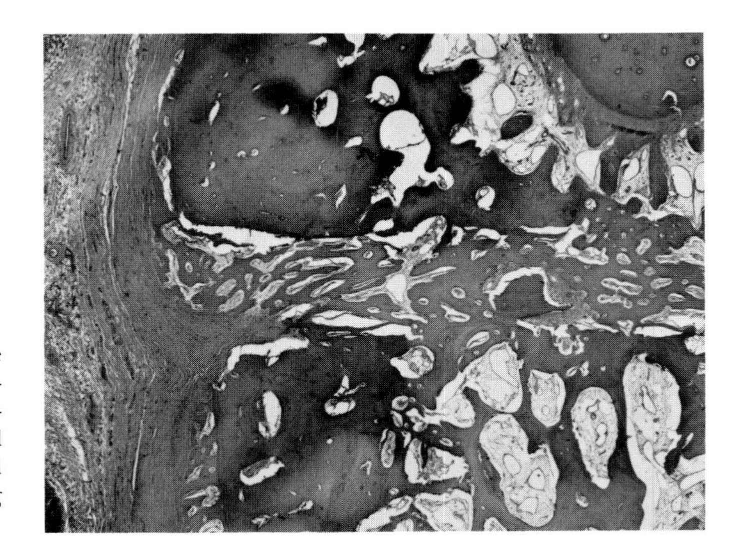

Figure 22–9. Histologic appearance of osteotomy site three weeks after two-stage technique (from buccal subapical osteotomy site). Margins of osteotomized segments are united by viable vascularized osteophytic new bone, osteoid, and young fibrous connective tissue.

short-term animal investigations were not designed to study these effects as such, but they are a calculated risk of any interdental osteotomy.

Histologic studies revealed a disparity in the healing rate of the buccal and palatal osteotomy sites (Figs. 22–9 to 22–11).[16] The reason for this difference was not always

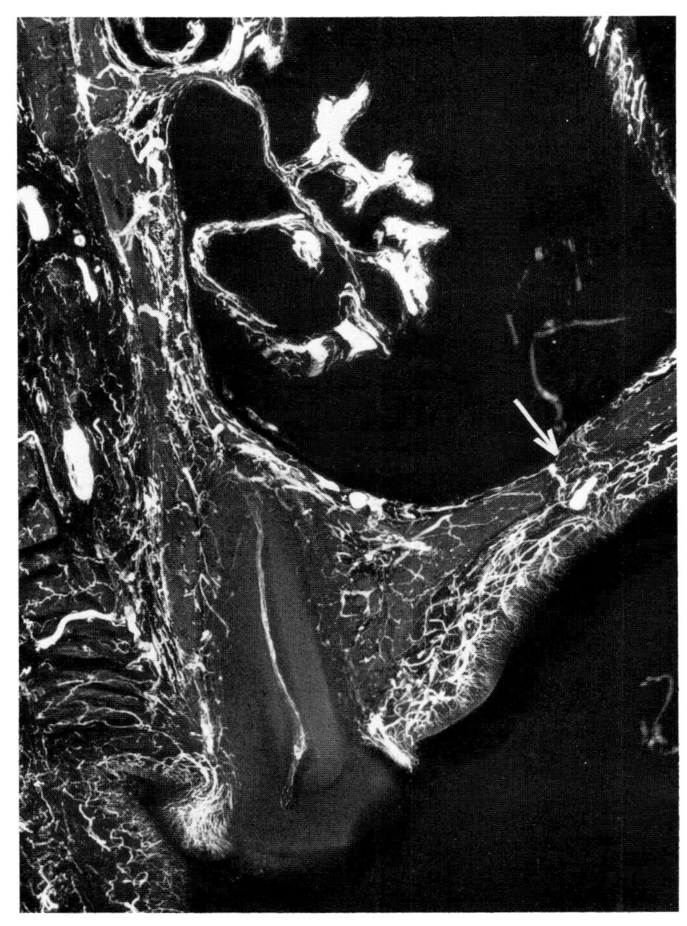

Figure 22–10. Microangiogram of premolar region eight weeks after one-stage technique demonstrating generalized distribution of Micropaque throughout the dento-osseous segment without vascular ischemia.

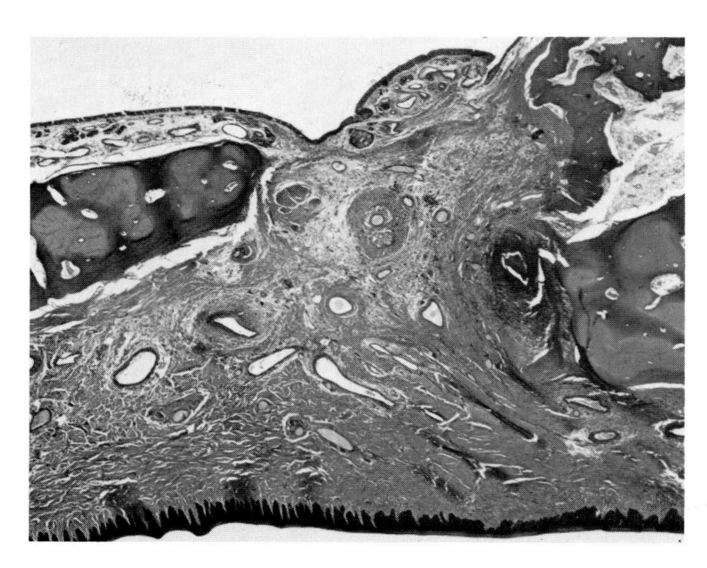

Figure 22–11. Histologic appearance of palatal osteotomy site eight weeks after one-stage technique (from area of microangiogram in Figure 22–10 indicated by arrow) showing lack of any bony bridging between the margins of the osteotomized segments.

clear. In some instances the margins of the segments were not placed into close appositon when the dento-osseous segments were fixated — an obvious healing lag was usually noted. In other instances, there was no bony bridging between the margins of the palatal bone cuts (Fig. 22–11) — this was in sharp contrast to the labial buccal osteotomy sites where there was bony bridging between the margins of the osteotomized segments (Fig. 22–9). Despite this lag in healing, the mobilized segments were "stable" when fixation appliances were removed after six weeks. Such incomplete healing helps to explain gradual postoperative relapse that is occasionally observed clinically after the patient begins to function with an unstable occlusal relationship. These findings give support to bone grafting large gaps between the osseous margins of dentoalveolar segments.

The quality of the histologic material used in our investigations was inadequate to allow a critical analysis of intrapulpal changes. Progressive pulpal fibrosis has been reported by other investigators without any discernible clinical effect.[1, 31] The significance of such changes must yet be determined from long-term animal and clinical studies. Clinical experience with surgical movement of single-tooth and small dento-osseous segments over a period of ten years has failed to demonstrate progressive ankylosis and root resorption, periapical abscess, or idiopathic resorption, the hallmarks of ischemia.[4, 7, 14] Despite the fact that subapical osteotomies may denervate teeth, pulp vitality is primarily a function of an intact blood supply.

Microangiographic and histologic studies of both one-stage and two-stage techniques for immediate surgical repositioning of single-tooth dento-osseous segments showed early but transient vascular ischemia, minimal osteonecrosis, and osseous union between most of the osteotomized segments.[16, 32] The attached soft tissue provided an adequate nutrient pedicle for immediate repositioning of single-tooth dento-osseous segments by interdental and subapical osteotomies when the bone cuts were made away from the apices of the teeth and the mobilized segments remained pedicled to mucoperiosteum and gingiva. The results of these clinically analogous studies support the clinical use of techniques which maximize the attachment of the gingiva to the mobilized dento-osseous segment.

Planning for Segmental Surgery

The use of alveolar osteotomies for movement of one, two, or more teeth opens many imaginative possibilities for treating adults, but presents certain technical problems in planning and design.[2, 4, 7, 19, 21, 22, 27, 29] The feasibility of surgery is determined by a careful correlative study of the clinical condition, high-definition periapical and cephalometric radiographs, and sectioned articulated dental study casts. Periapical radiographs are used to delineate potential osteotomy or ostectomy sites in the interdental spaces and in the area between the apices of the maxillary teeth and the anterior nasal aperture and maxillary sinus, or between the mandibular teeth and the subjacent mental or inferior alveolar nerves. Dental study casts are trial-sectioned in the proposed osteotomy sites to determine three-dimensional movements of the segments and to predict the results of treatment. Model surgery may indicate that there is a need to bone-graft certain osseous defects that occur as a consequence of segmental surgery. After the feasibility of surgery has been determined by trial sectioning of articulated study casts, an arch wire or arch bar is contoured to the sectioned casts for postsurgical fixation of the mobilized dental-osseous segments. A cast metal splint, Gunning-type splint, transitional prosthetic appliance or a permanent fixed or removable appliance can be used to fix and stabilize the repositioned dento-osseous segment. An acrylic interocclusal splint is routinely made to key the mobilized segment or segments into the desired position at the time of surgery. An orthodontic arch wire is an effective and efficient means of stabilizing the repositioned dento-osseous segment and usually obviates the need for intermaxillary fixation.

The majority of independent segmental surgical procedures are accomplished in a single stage without intermaxillary fixation. When dentoalveolar surgery is accomplished in concert with ramus surgery or Le Fort I osteotomy, intermaxillary fixation for six to eight weeks is generally necessary. When segmental surgery is accomplished as an independent procedure or in concert with orthodontics, the arch wire may be changed and activated three or four weeks after surgery when the interocclusal splint is removed and the segment is clinically stable.

CORRECTION OF ADULT MALOCCLUSIONS

Prosthetic Considerations — Intra-Arch Relationships

Interdental Spaces

Interdental spaces due to congenitally missing teeth or secondary to loss of teeth for any reason are prosthetic problems when they are either too large or too small to accommodate the crown size that would normally fit in that space and harmonize with the other crown forms in the arch. When interdental spaces in the natural dentition are to be closed for esthetic reasons, a good prosthetic result can be achieved only if the space to be closed is less than 1 to 1.5 mm, or when the interdental spacing involves multiple teeth so that symmetrical harmonious crown forms may be developed. Excessive interdental spaces create problems for the prosthodontist not only with regard to esthetics but also because the contours of oversized crowns produce a poor anatomic relationship with the gingiva. As a result, good oral hygiene is made more difficult and this predisposes the adjacent teeth to periodontitis. Since interdental spaces of 1 mm or less may create periodontal problems because of their predilection to food impaction, they should usually be closed prosthetically, orthodontically, or surgically. If the space is greater than 1.5 to 2 mm, the potential for food impaction is relatively small and the space is usually self-cleaning. When the space is closed to improve esthetics, correct a malocclusion, or prevent migration and tipping of teeth, it can generally be accomplished by orthodontics or surgery.

In adults, the orthodontic closure of interdental spaces which have been present for a long time may be difficult if not impossible due to the density and bulk of cortical bone in the interdental space. The labiolingual narrowing of the alveolus in the interdental space reduces the relative amount of cancellous bone and increases the amount of cortical bone in the path of root movement. Cases of this type are handled expeditiously by excising the appropriate amount of interdental bone and moving the teeth surgically as small dento-osseous segments. Preoperative or postoperative orthodontics may be necessary to correct minor rotational and alignment discrepancies. In most cases intermaxillary fixation is unnecessary because adequate stability is obtained by ligating the mobilized dento-osseous segment to the adjacent teeth with an arch bar, heavy arch wires and acrylated arch bar, or a cast metal splint. The excellent bony contact that is usually obtained between segments with this type of surgery promotes early union.

Intra-arch Space Deficiency Secondary to Extraction of Posterior Teeth

Posterior bite collapse as a result of premature loss of first molar teeth is one of the most common problems encountered by dentists. Interdental spacing secondary to the extraction of a posterior tooth frequently leads to mesial migration with tipping of the tooth or teeth distal to the space. With the loss of arch integrity, the second and third molar teeth drift mesially and their axial inclination is altered. Tipping of the posterior teeth tends to produce an anatomic relationship resulting in difficulty in cleaning and contributing to periodontal pocket formations on the mesial aspect of the tooth. As a consequence of mesial tipping there is concomitant altered distribution of occlusal forces, supereruption, and occlusal traumatism of the opposing teeth. To correct this malocclusion prosthetically without considering the position of the teeth may invite periodontal problems. The compromised pontic design, inadequate embrasure spaces, nonaxial distribution of forces, and abnormal bone–marginal ridge height produce an ideal environment for the progression of periodontal pocket formation on the mesial aspect of the second molar.

Prosthetic restoration of the tipped tooth may create the appearance of improved occlusal relationships; however, the periodontal pocket remains. As a result, particular attention should be directed toward restoring proper axial inclination to the tipped tooth prior to prosthetic restoration. Attainment of correct arch form and proper axial inclination may be achieved by orthodontic or surgical uprighting of the second and third molar teeth. After such treatment adequate embrasure on the mesial and distal

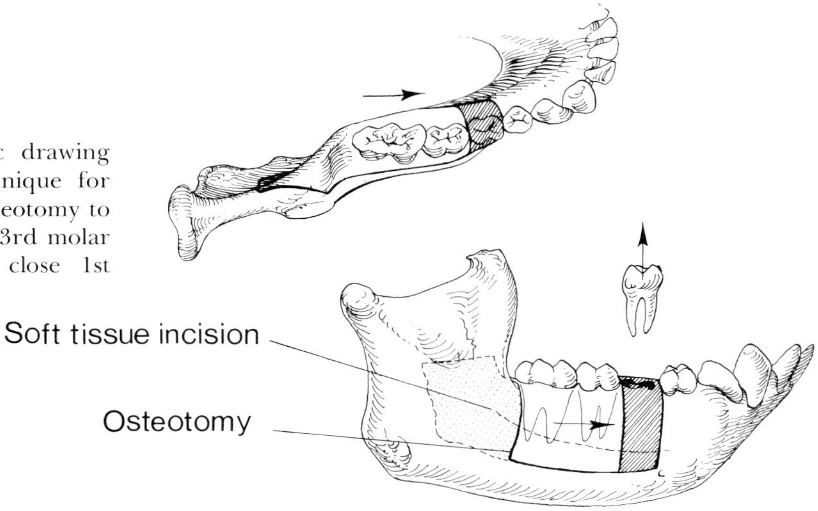

Figure 22–12. Schematic drawing of experimental surgical technique for combined sagittal-subapical osteotomy to advance mandibular 2nd and 3rd molar dentoalveolar segments and close 1st molar extraction space.

Soft tissue incision

Osteotomy

aspects of the pontic can be achieved. In the adult, considerable time can be saved by uprighting the teeth surgically. Not only does this produce a more rapid repositioning of the teeth but it avoids the need for orthopedic forces (i.e., cervical traction, which is not acceptable to many adults).

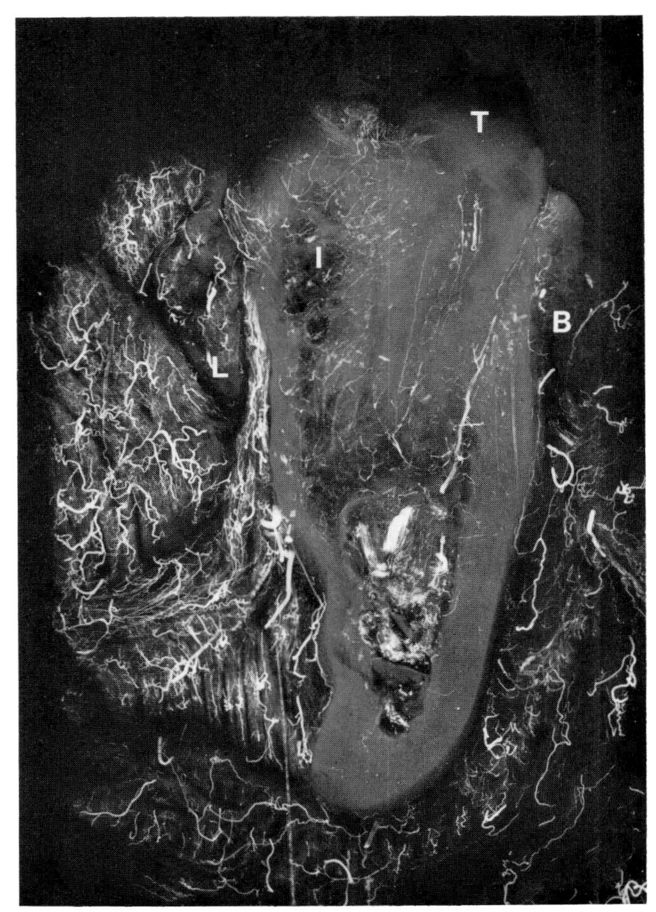

Figure 22–13. Microangiogram of 1 mm. transverse tissue slice from molar region of control animal: buccal (B) and lingual (L) blood vessels anastomosing with intramedullary blood vessels (I); molar tooth (T).

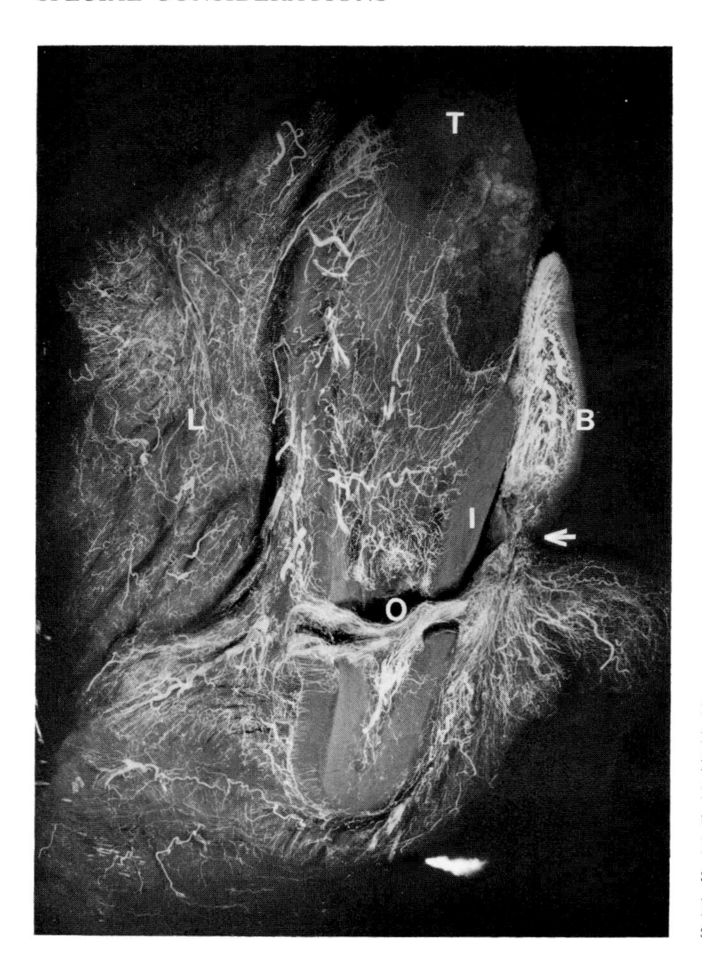

Figure 22–14. Microangiogram of molar region three weeks after surgical technique depicted in Figure 22–12 demonstrating generalized distribution of Micropaque in soft tissues, bone, and pulp canals of molar tooth (T); O = osteotomy site; L = lingual; B = buccal; I = ischemia of alveolar bone subjacent to previously raised buccal mucoperiosteal flap, healing buccal mucoperiosteal flap (*arrow*).

Correction by Surgery

The results of analogous animal studies indicate that immediate surgical repositioning of mandibular molar teeth is biologically sound (Figs. 22–12, 22–13, and 22–14). Several anatomic factors, however, make such procedures in the molar region more difficult and problematic than similar procedures in the anterior part of the mandible. Firstly, because there is virtually no muscle attachment above the level of the mylohyoid muscle, the lingual mucosa can become detached and compromise blood supply to the dento-osseous segment. Secondly, the proximity of the apices of the molar teeth to the inferior alveolar neurovascular bundle may complicate subapical bone cuts.

ANATOMIC PRINCIPLES ASSOCIATED WITH MOVING POSTERIOR MANDIBULAR SEGMENTS

Surgical repositioning of posterior mandibular dentoalveolar segments is potentially problematic because of a tenuous vascular pedicle in the posterior mandibular area.

During surgery the soft-tissue pedicle is easily traumatized and may become detached from the mobilized dentoalveolar segment. In addition, the subapical bone cuts are potentially problematic because of the close proximity of the tooth apices to the inferior alveolar nerve. Consequently, great care must be exercised in case selection and execution. Several anatomic factors must be evaluated when considering uprighting tipped posterior teeth.[26]

As a tooth in one arch tips anteriorly into a space, the mesial edge of the tooth may rotate apically so that it is positioned below the occlusal plane. The opposing dentition usually supererupts to compound the problem in the opposite arch. Thus, therapy is complicated by the fact that both arches must be leveled rather than simply uprighting the tipped tooth. In selected cases, when the only therapy necessary is uprighting of the tipped tooth, it may be accomplished fairly simply.

Specific anatomic considerations which determine the feasibility of uprighting mandibular posterior teeth include: (1) The number and position of the teeth to be moved; (2) the amount of bone between the apex of the tooth or teeth and the mandibular canal; (3) the amount and quality of attached gingiva, particularly on the lingual aspect; and (4) the desired distance and direction that the segment is to be moved.

Ideally, 4 to 5 mm of bone should be present between the apex of the tooth to be uprighted and the superior aspect of the mandibular canal. With careful dissection, the horizontal bone cut can be made without traumatizing the tooth or the inferior alveolar nerve (Fig. 22–15). Furthermore, many teeth to be uprighted must have the distal root inferiorly repositioned to bring the tooth's occlusal surface level with the occlusal plane of the arch. In such cases more than 5 mm of bone must be available between the apex of the tooth and the inferior alveolar canal to permit an ostectomy equal to the desired inferior repositioning of the tooth. In clinical practice, however, the amount of bone between the tooth apices and the mandibular nerve canal is less than 2 or 3 millimeters and precludes conventional subapical osteotomy. When there is inadequate bone between the nerve canal and the apices of the teeth, an optional technique for decorticating the nerve and retracting the nerve from the subapical bone cut site is used (Fig. 22–16 *A* to *F*). Clinical application of this technique is shown in Figure 22–16 *G* to *N* (Case Report 22–1).

CASE 22–1 (Fig. 22–16)

S.J., a 22-year-old gentleman, was referred by his restorative dentist for surgical closure of his posterior open bite.

EVALUATION

Esthetics

Frontal. Good facial balance and symmetry.

Profile. Slight anteroposterior deficiency of upper lip projection and prominent nose.

Cephalometric Evaulation

1. Relative maxillary deficiency (SNA = 77°, SNB = 77°).

Text continued on page 1593

Figure 22–15. Edentulous space closure via posterior mandibular subapical osteotomy without repositioning of neurovascular bundle. *A,* Closure of posterior mandibular edentulous space with simultaneous uprighting of a mesially tipped molar tooth is accomplished with a posterior mandibular subapical osteotomy. The amount of movement anteriorly and inferiorly may be determined from cephalometric and model studies. If sufficient space exists between the inferior alveolar neurovascular canal and the apices of the tooth to be moved, the procedure may be carried out without repositioning the neurovascular bundle. A horizontal incision is made in the depth of the buccal vestibule starting approximately 1 cm. posterior to the planned posterior vertical osteotomy and extending anteriorly approximately 1 cm. in front of the anterior ostectomy. The dissection is carried down to bone on the lateral aspect of the mandible and a mucoperiosteal flap is elevated over the site of the proposed horizontal and vertical osteotomies. Maximum soft-tissue pedicle is maintained on the segment to be mobilized. The dotted lines represent the area of the planned horizontal and vertical osteotomies. *B,* The diagram depicts the direction and amount of movement necessary to close the edentulous space and upright the molar tooth. The cross-hatched area represents the shape and location of the planned ostectomies and the posterior line represents the location of the posterior osteotomy. Note that the posterior osteotomy is carried out as far posteriorly as possible to maintain the largest possible dentoalveolar segment. This permits retention of a large soft-tissue pedicle. The stippled area represents the area of subperiosteal dissection that is needed for free movement of the tissue without tension. Generally it is necessary to incise the lingual periosteum along the inferior edge of the horizontal osteotomy and the posterior edge of the vertical osteotomy so that adequate mobilization may be accomplished. *C,* The osteotomy sites are approached through the horizontal incision. The length of the tooth to be moved is ascertained from well-oriented periapical radiographs. Five mm. are added to the tooth length and this measurement is scribed in the buccal cortex to mark the level of the horizontal osteotomy. The osteotomy is performed with an oscillating saw, taking care to curve the posterior end of the cut superiorly to follow the course of the inferior alveolar canal. A finger is placed on the lingual aspect of the mandible to detect perforation of the cortex by the saw blade. Both cuts of the ostectomy may be completed before mobilization of the segment, or the vertical osteotomies may be completed, the segment mobilized, and the ostectomies performed with a large bur under direct visualization. After the osteotomies have been completed, the segment is mobilized and an attempt is made to move the segment to the previously planned position. Compression of the soft tissue over the edentulous space may prevent adequate advancement of the tooth. If this is the case, a small elliptical segment of attached gingiva is excised over the crest of the edentulous ridge. Care is taken to maintain the marginal tissue around the adjacent teeth. With the tissue excised, the segment is moved to the planned position. If undue tension on the soft-tissue pedicle cannot be relieved by undermining the buccal and lingual mucoperiosteum, it may be necessary to incise the lingual periosteum, as previously described, along the lines of the horizontal and posterior vertical osteotomies. *D,* The segment is stabilized in its new position with a heavy arch wire, arch bar, circumdental wires, or occlusal acrylic stent. Direct transosseous wires are placed through the buccal cortex along the anterior vertical and horizontal osteotomies. The horizontal and elliptical incisions are closed with continuous resorbable sutures.

See illustration on the opposite page.

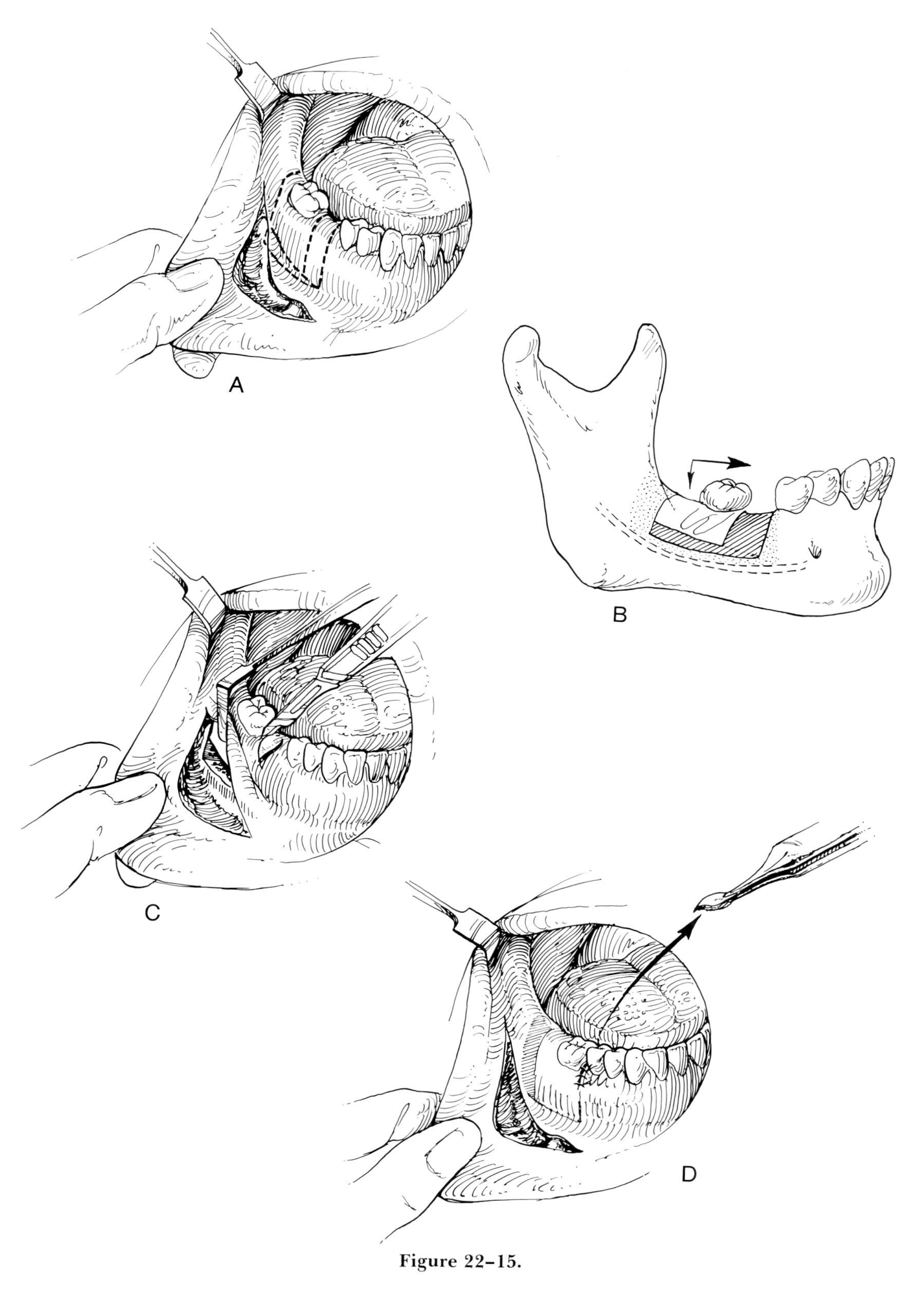

Figure 22–15.

Figure 22–16 (Case 22–1). Schematic illustration of surgical treatment plan: Le Fort I osteotomy in two pieces with advancement and closure of diastema; left posterior mandibular subapical osteotomy with repositioning of neurovascular bundle to close open bite, close interdental spaces, and upright 2nd molar. *A,* Posterior open bite due to undererupted mandibular posterior segments is a typical deformity requiring posterior mandibular subapical osteotomy. In this instance, the mandibular 1st molar tooth has been lost with subsequent mesial tipping of the 2nd and 3rd molar teeth. This is associated with a bilateral Class III malocclusion. The surgical plan includes Le Fort I osteotomy with advancement to correct the Class III malocclusion and mandibular posterior subapical osteotomy to close the posterior open bite. Extraction of the 3rd molar tooth from the posterior segment permits easier uprighting of the 1st molar tooth and provides balanced occlusion owing to the lack of a maxillary 2nd molar. A vertical wedge ostectomy is performed between the 2nd premolar and 2nd molar tooth to permit uprighting of the 2nd molar. Uprighting of a molar tooth in the absence of a posterior open bite necessitates a horizontal wedge ostectomy with excision of bone at the posterior end of the segment to permit inferior repositioning of the posterior aspect of the segment rather than superior repositioning of the anterior aspect. *B,* With the inferior alveolar neurovascular bundle retracted, the horizontal subapical osteotomy is completed utilizing an oscillating saw. A finger is placed on the lingual aspect of the mandible to detect perforation of the lingual cortical plate by the oscillating saw blade. The mucoperiosteum over the planned vertical osteotomy sites is reflected with minimal dissection. The soft tissue is retracted and the vertical osteotomies are completed utilizing an oscillating saw or straight handpiece. Sufficient bone is removed along the lines of the vertical osteotomies to permit repositioning of the segments into the previously prepared occlusal acrylic stent without the application of pressure or traction on the associated soft tissues. When the segments are superiorly repositioned, the periosteum on the lingual aspect of the mandible must be incised along the path of the horizontal osteotomy. It is generally necessary to incise periosteum along the posterior vertical osteotomy to permit advancement of these segments. During all phases of the procedure, particular care is taken to preserve maximal soft-tissue pedicle on the labial and lingual aspects of the mobilized segments. Elevation of soft tissue for access to the surgical sites is preferentially performed on the nonmobilized segments. *C,* A horizontal incision is performed at the depth of the labial vestibule extending from the mandibular 3rd molar to the lateral incisor tooth. Mucoperiosteum is reflected inferiorly to a point below the inferior alveolar canal. Minimal elevation of the superior margin of the incision is performed so that maximal soft-tissue pedicle to the mobilized segments may be maintained. Utilizing a 6-mm. diameter mastoid bur, bone is removed from the lateral cortex of the mandible along the anticipated path of the inferior alveolar neurovascular bundle. The mastoid bur permits rapid removal of bone, provides good exposure of the corticated neurovascular canal, and minimizes the chance of injury to the neurovascular bundle owing to the broad surface contact area. After the cortical plate of the neurovascular canal has been identified, a small curette may be utilized to decorticate the lateral aspect of the canal and expose the neurovascular bundle, which is then gently teased from the canal and retracted with nerve retractors or umbilical tape. *D,* With the nerve retracted and protected, the horizontal osteotomy is performed with the oscillating saw. By performing the osteotomy through the neurovascular canal, it is possible to complete sectioning of the lingual plate below the level of attachment of the mylohyoid muscle. This permits retention of this excellent soft-tissue pedicle. The vertical osteotomies and ostectomies are then performed and these segments are mobilized. *E,* The segments are superiorly repositioned and advanced with appropriate relaxation of the lingual soft-tissue pedicle by incision of the periosteum along the posterior vertical osteotomy and the horizontal osteotomy. *F,* The segments are positioned in the desired occlusal relationship with the occlusal acrylic stent and stabilized with direct transosseous wires and intermaxillary fixation. The neurovascular bundle is permitted to retract into its normal location below the mobilized segments. The soft tissue is closed with a continuous horizontal mattress suture.

See illustration on the opposite page.

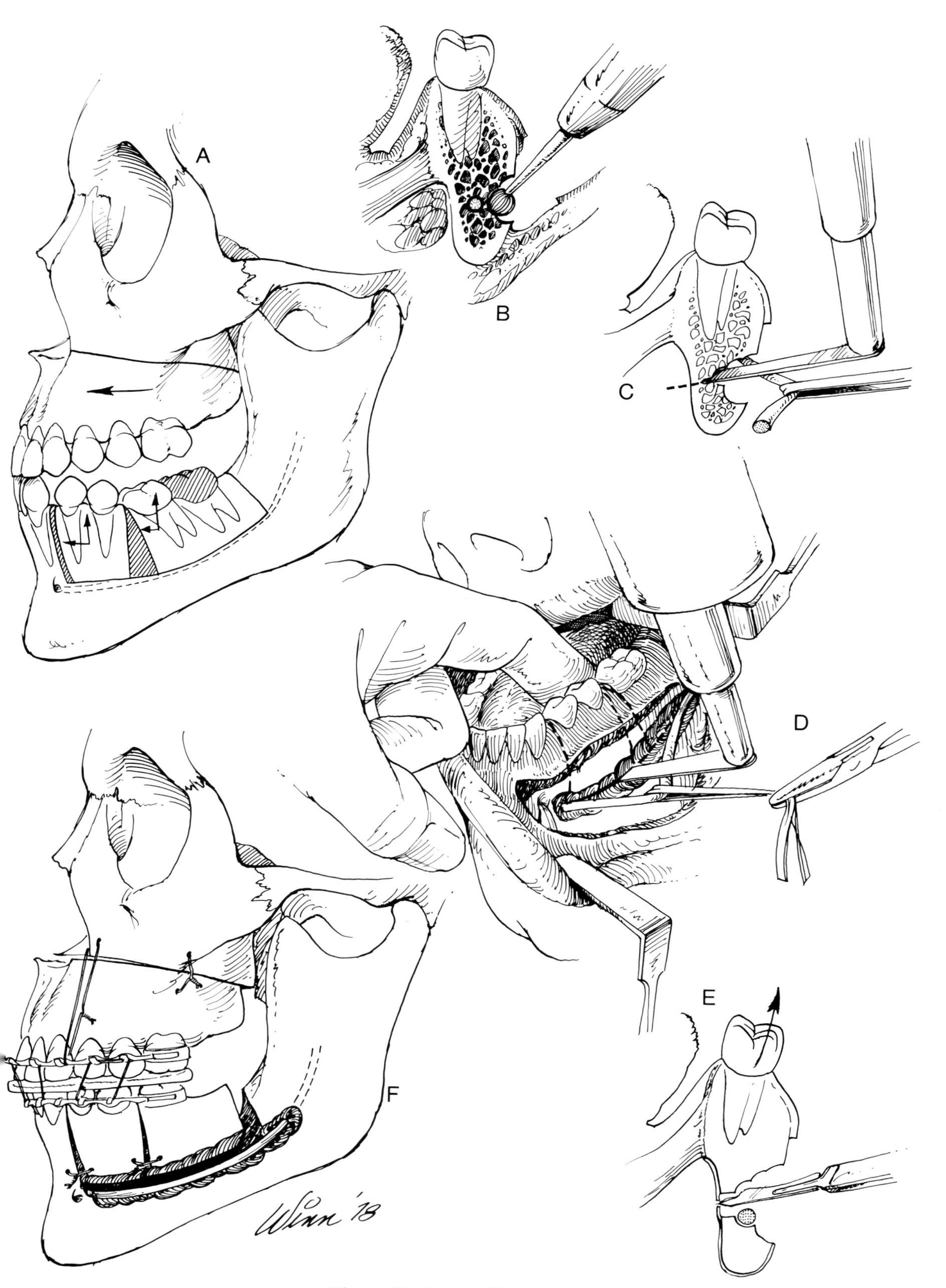

Figure 22–16. *Illustration and legend continued on the following page.*

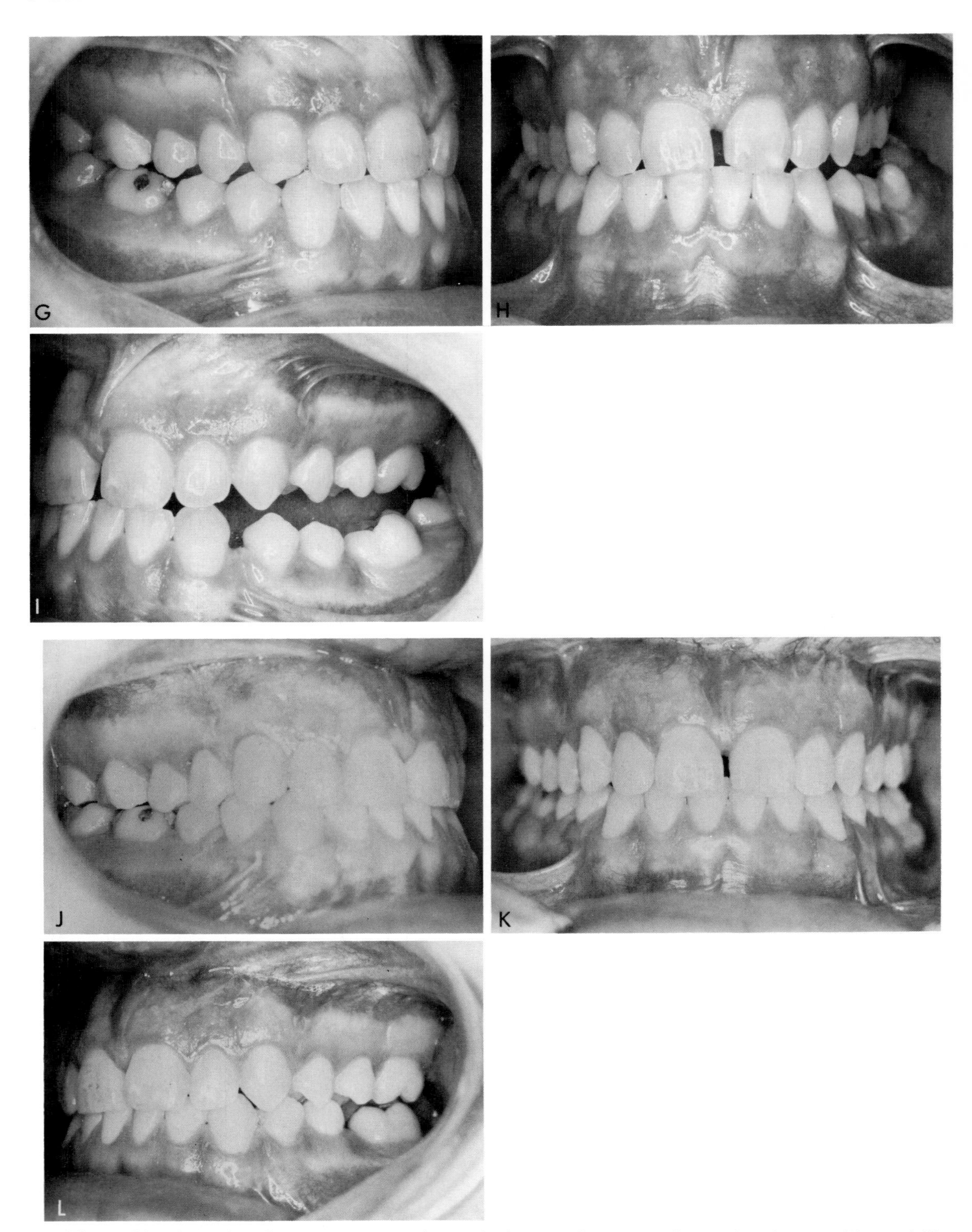

Figure 22–16 *Continued.* *G–I,* Preoperative occlusion — Class III canine and molar, maxillary midline diastema, posterior left open bite, missing mandibular left 1st molar, tipped mandibular left 2nd and 3rd molars. *J–L,* Postoperative occlusion after surgical procedure illustrated in *A* to *F.*

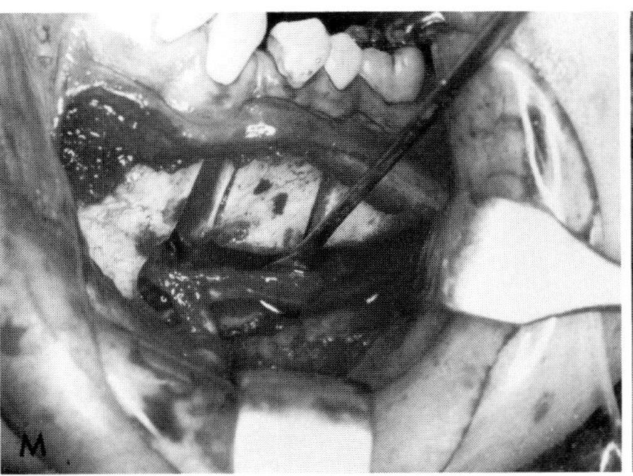

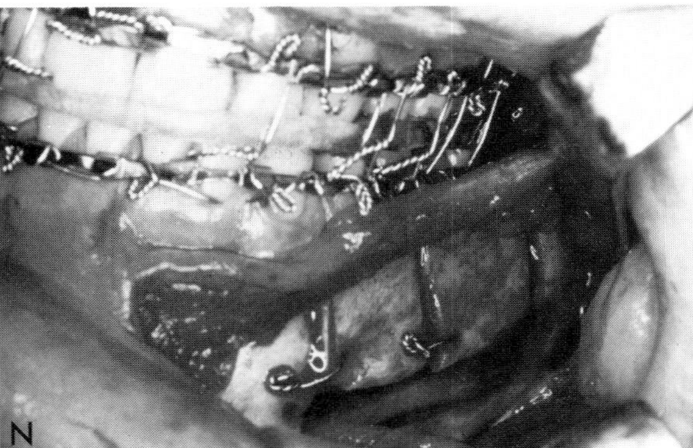

Figure 22–16 *Continued.* *M* and *N*, Surgical exposure of neurovascular bundle, maintenance of integrity of incisive branch; stabilization of dento-osseous segments with transosseous wires, and retraction of neurovascular bundle under segments prior to suturing incision.

Occlusal Analysis (Fig. 22–16, G, H, and I)

Dental Arch Form. Constricted maxillary arch.

Dental Alignment. Left posterior mandibular interdental spaces with second molar tooth tipped into first molar extraction site.

Dental Occlusion. Class 3 malocclusion bilaterally; end-to-end bite in anterior and right posterior, maxillary palatal crossbite in left posterior quadrant, missing mandibular left first molar tooth, left posterior open bite (6 mm) and maxillary midline diastema.

TREATMENT PLAN (Fig. 22–16, *A* to *F*)

Le Fort I osteotomy in two segments with advancement (3 mm), expansion (3 mm), and midline ostectomy to:

a. Correct Class III malocclusion
b. Close midline diastema
c. Correct posterior crossbite

2. Left posterior mandibular subapical osteotomies between the canine-first premolar, second premolar-second molar, and third molar interdental spaces with advancement and superior repositioning of the posterior segment and advancement, posterior rotation, and superior repositioning of the posterior segment to:

a. Close the canine-first premolar interspace.
b. Upright the mandibular second molar tooth.
c. Close the space between the second bicuspid and second molar tooth.
d. Close the posterior open bite.

FOLLOW-UP

Subjective

Patient experienced minimal postoperative pain and edema.

Objective

The posterior mandibular segments were stabilized with an arch bar and direct transosseous wires. The maxilla was stabilized with direct transosseous wires and anterior suspension wires. Intermaxillary fixation was removed three weeks postoperatively. Elastic intermaxillary fixation was maintained during the night for three weeks after removal of wire intermaxillary fixation. Good clinical union without mobility was present eight weeks postoperatively. Satisfactory bilateral class I canine and molar relationship was established, the posterior open bite was eliminated and the midline diastema closed. As a result of the patient's failure to wear his maxilllary retainer, he experienced some relapse with opening of the midline diastema to approximately 1 mm. Eight months postoperatively the occlusion has remained stable.

COMMENTS

Owing to the close approximation of the mandibular posterior root apices and the inferior alveolar canal, it was elected to reposition the inferior alveolar neurovascular bundle to prevent damage while completing the horizontal osteotomy (Fig. 22–16, *M* and *N*). The patient experienced transient left lower lip paresthesia for three weeks. Complete return to normal sensation was noted at the three-week postoperative check-up. Extraction of the mandibular left third molar tooth facilitated completion of the posterior osteotomy through the extraction site.

Surgeons: Kevin L. McBride, Dallas, Texas and Barry Acker, Tyler, Texas.

The surgeon should take advantage of any excess bone by placing the horizontal osteotomy or ostectomy as close to the inferior alveolar canal as feasible to ensure the largest possible dento-osseous segment with the maximal lingual and buccal mucoperiosteal pedicle. The lingual mucoperiosteal vascular pedicle provides the majority of the blood supply to the mobilized mandibular dento-osseous segment. The degree of dependence upon the lingual supply to the mobilized segments will vary with the length and position of incisions and the extent to which the mucoperiosteum is stripped from the buccal bone. In general, the lingual mucoperiosteum is thin and friable and great care must be taken to maintain its integrity when moving posterior segments. Attached gingiva has considerably more strength and resilience than free lingual mucosa. Therefore, the more attached gingiva available on the lingual aspect of the segment to be mobilized, the less danger there is in compromising the circulation to the segment during manipulation. When sufficient bone is present below the apex of the mobilized teeth, the horizontal osteotomy is angled medially and inferiorly so that the lingual bone cut is inferior to the level of the mylohyoid muscle attachment. This muscle provides additional blood supply to the mobilized segment and helps to preserve the integrity of the lingual mucoperiosteum, the principal vascular pedicle.

The direction in which a dento-osseous segment must be moved to achieve an optimal position must be considered in case planning. It is generally easier to reposition a segment superiorly than it is to reposition it inferiorly because, with superior repositioning, it is not necessary to perform an ostectomy along the horizontal cut. The segment may simply be raised into the desired position and stabilized with an appropriate appliance. An edentulous space may be reduced in size more readily than it may be expanded because expansion requires mobilization of the attached gingiva over the

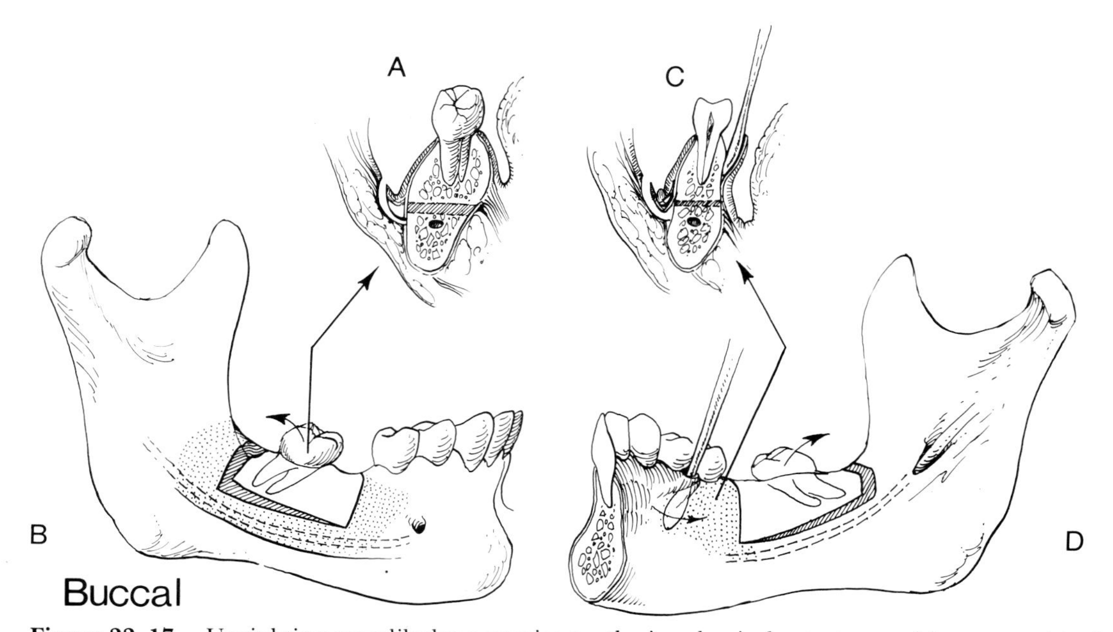

Figure 22–17. Uprighting mandibular posterior tooth via subapical osteotomy without repositioning of neurovascular bundle. *A,* Uprighting of mesially tipped posterior mandibular teeth when partial closure of the edentulous space has taken place necessitates posterior repositioning of the tipped tooth to re-establish the normal edentulous space or anterior repositioning of the segment to close the edentulous space. In either case, sufficient relaxation of the associated soft tissues must be achieved to permit repositioning without tension while maintaining adequate soft-tissue pedicle to assure vascularity of the mobilized segment. The lines of osteotomy are approached through a horizontal incision a few millimeters lateral to the depth of the buccal vestibular fold. Care is taken to direct the anterior end of the incision superior to the mental nerve. The incision is extended 1 cm. beyond the proposed vertical osteotomies at each end of the segment. The mucoperiosteum is elevated from the stable segment in all directions. Sufficient mucoperiosteum is elevated from the mobilized segment to permit adequate visualization of the proposed osteotomy sites. When edentulous space exists adjacent to the tooth to be mobilized, the vertical osteotomies should be made as far from the tooth as possible to create the largest possible segment. This permits retention of a relatively larger soft-tissue pedicle. Superior or inferior repositioning of the segment must be considered in selecting the vertical osteotomy sites to prevent formation of a level discrepancy in the alveolar bone adjacent to a tooth. When sufficient space exists between the apices of the teeth to be mobilized and the inferior alveolar canal, the horizontal osteotomy may be completed without repositioning the neurovascular bundle. The length of the tooth is ascertained from well-oriented periapical radiographs. Five mm. are added to the tooth length and this measurement is scribed in the buccal cortex to mark the level of the horizontal osteotomy. The osteotomy is performed with an oscillating saw, taking care to curve the posterior end of the cut superiorly to follow the course of the inferior alveolar canal. A finger may be placed on the lingual aspect of the mandible to detect perforation of the cortex by the saw blade. Both cuts of the osteotomy may be completed before mobilization of the segment, or the vertical osteotomies may be completed, the segment mobilized, and the ostectomies performed with a large bur under direct visualization. *B,* The amount and shape of osteotomy needed to upright and posteriorly reposition the mandibular 2nd molar tooth is demonstrated. The stippled area represents the amount of buccal subperiosteal dissection that must be performed to permit adequate mobilization of the segment. This dissection is easily performed through the horizontal incision. *C,* The relationship between the horizontal osteotomy and the position of the molar apices, inferior alveolar canal, and mylohyoid muscle is demonstrated. *D,* Adequate mobilization of the lingual soft tissues on the stable segment must be accomplished in order to permit appropriate repositioning of the segment. A periosteal elevator is inserted at the free gingival margin and directed subperiosteally to a level below the horizontal osteotomy.

Illustration and legend continued on the following page.

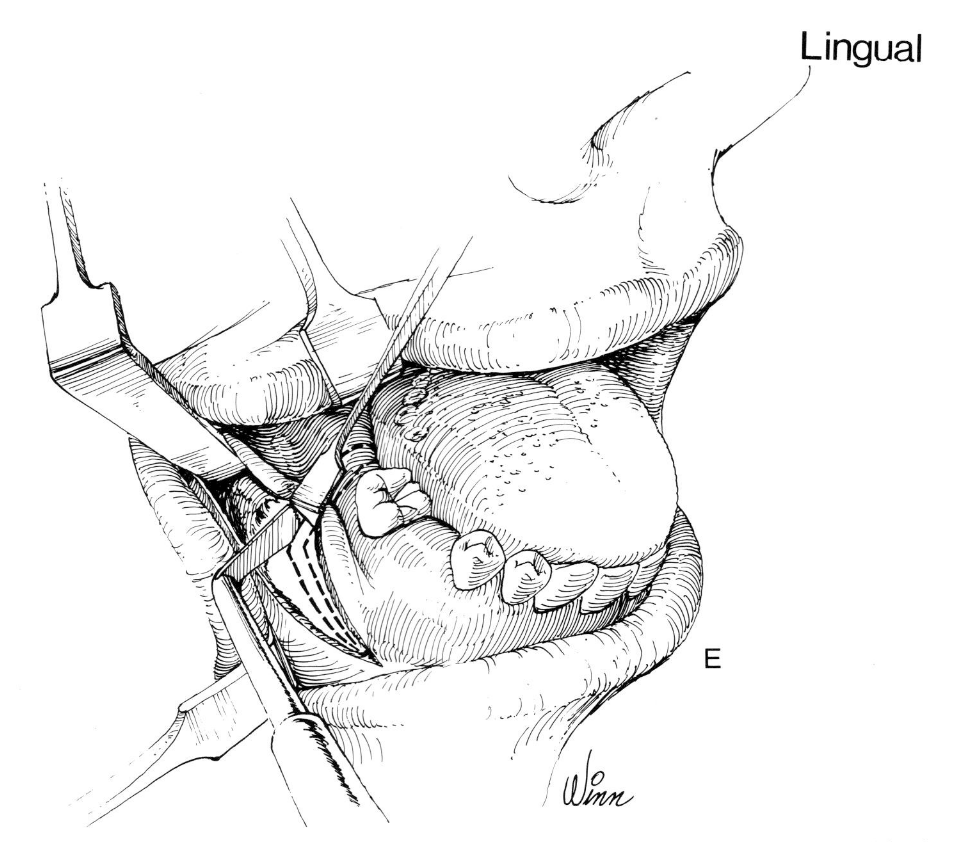

Figure 22–17 *Continued.* *E,* The tip of the periosteal elevator is moved back and forth to free the deep subperiosteal tissues without mobilizing an excessive length of the free gingival margin. Care is taken not to mobilize any of the soft-tissue pedicle from the mobilized segment. Owing to the difficulty of mobilizing the lingual mucoperiosteum below the level of the horizontal osteotomy, the periosteum is sharply incised as low as possible along the line of the osteotomy.

edentulous space and around adjacent teeth. An edentulous space may be expanded an amount equal to approximately 50 to 75 per cent of the pre-expansion dimension. If the desired expansion exceeds this amount, it may be necessary to mobilize the attached gingiva around teeth in the nonmobilized segment to obtain sufficient soft-tissue relaxation. If excessive expansion is attempted, marginal periodontal defects may develop following extensive mobilization of attached gingiva. Such problems can be avoided by oblique incisions through the lingual mucosa. If an edentulous space in excess of 5 mm is to be closed, it may be necessary to excise some attached gingiva from the center of the edentulous space, taking care not to disturb the marginal gingiva on either side of the space. This prevents the excess soft tissue from folding down into the osteotomy site, thereby creating a periodontal defect.

The number and relative position of the teeth to be uprighted significantly affect the difficulty of the surgical procedure. The simplest case is one involving a single tooth with a large edentulous space on either side of it. This configuration provides an optimal flexibility with regard to direction and magnitude of movement, and selection of osteotomy sites. A frequently encountered problem is the mandibular second molar tooth which has tipped anteriorly into the space created by the early extraction of the first molar. The simplest surgical solution to this problem involves uprighting the second molar tooth with slight posterior repositioning to permit restoration of the first molar space with a fixed partial denture (Fig. 22–17). If the third molar tooth is present, it usually has tipped forward with the second molar, creating periodontal defects between the second and third molars as a single segment. Therefore, the third molar may be extracted at the time of surgery to facilitate the posterior vertical osteotomy through the extraction site (Fig. 22–18 *I*). Clinical application of this technique is illustrated in Figure 22–18 *A* to *M* in Case Report 22–2.[26]

CASE 22–2 (Fig. 22–18)

L. W., a 28-year-old gentleman, was referred by his general dentist for surgical repositioning of several teeth prior to fabrication of crown and bridge restorations.

EVALUATION

Esthetics

Frontal. Good facial balance and symmetry.

Profile. Anteroposterior chin deficiency and relative prominence of the upper and lower lips.

CEPHALOMETRIC EVALUATION

1. Relative mandibular anteroposterior deficiency — SNA = 85°, SNB = 79°.

OCCLUSAL ANALYSIS (Fig. 22–18, *A* to *H*)

1. Missing right mandibular second premolar and second and third molar teeth. Supereruption of maxillary right second and third molars into mandibular edentulous second and third molar space. Missing maxillary right first molar tooth. Unrestorable maxillary right second premolar tooth.
2. Missing mandibular left first molar tooth with tipping of second and third molar teeth into the edentulous space. Missing maxillary left first molar tooth.

TREATMENT PLAN (Fig. 22–18 *I*)

1. Right posterior maxillary subapical osteotomy to advance (5 mm) and superiorly reposition (4 mm) the second and third molar teeth to:
   a. Partially close the edentulous space between the first premolar and the second molar teeth.
   b. Establish occlusion between the maxillary second molar and mandibular first molar teeth.
   c. Level the maxillary occlusal plane to permit restoration of the remaining edentulous space with a fixed bridge.

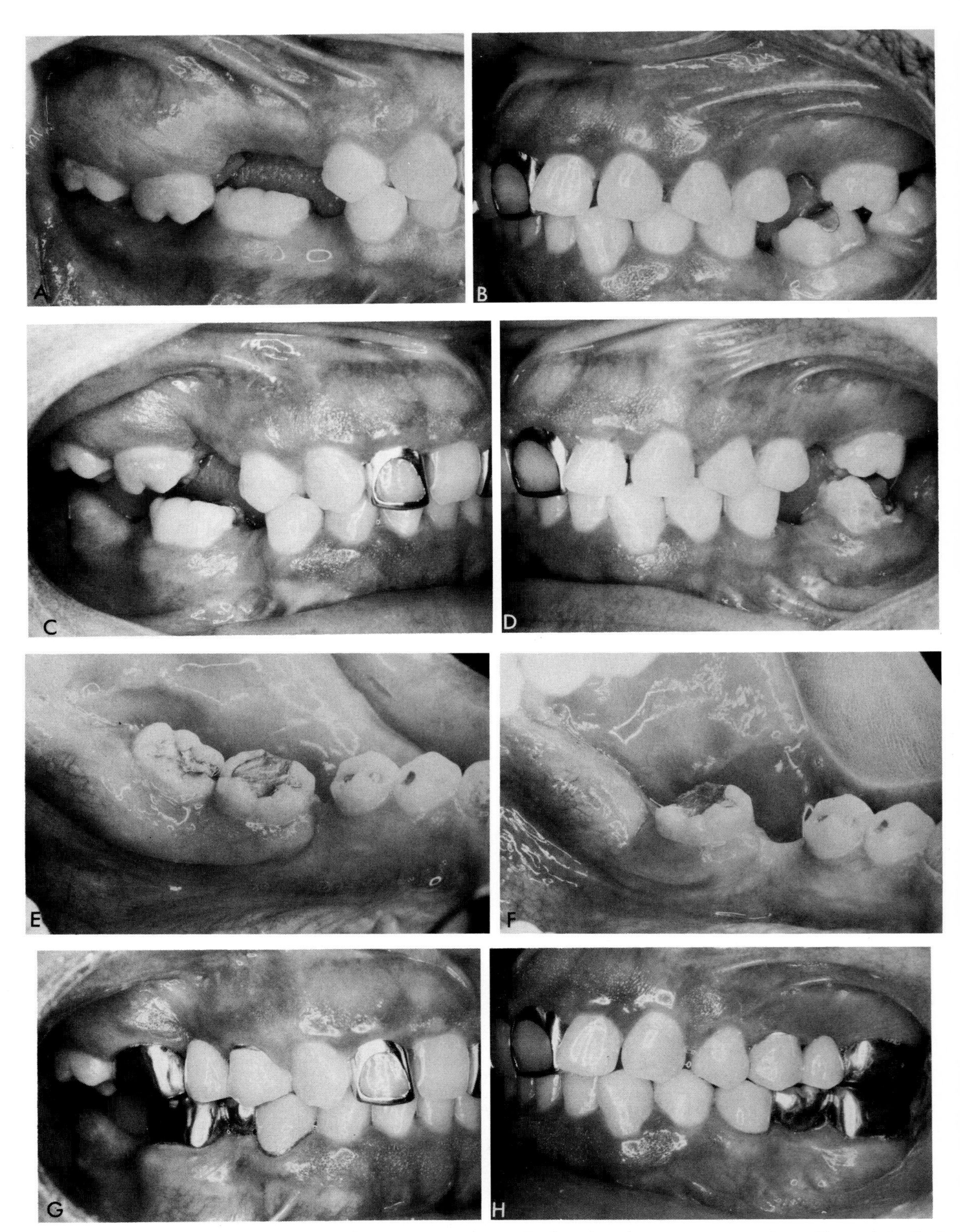

Figure 22–18 (Case 22–2). *A* and *B,* Preoperative occlusion showing supererupted maxillary right 2nd and 3rd molar teeth and mesially tipped mandibular left 2nd and 3rd molar teeth. *C* and *D,* Six weeks postoperatively after removal of stabilizing appliances. *E* and *F,* Lingual view of left mandibular 2nd molar tooth before and after repositioning showing the leveled occlusal surface, increased interdental space, and improved periodontal contour. *G* and *H,* Two-year postoperative occlusal views showing final restorations and stability of occlusion.

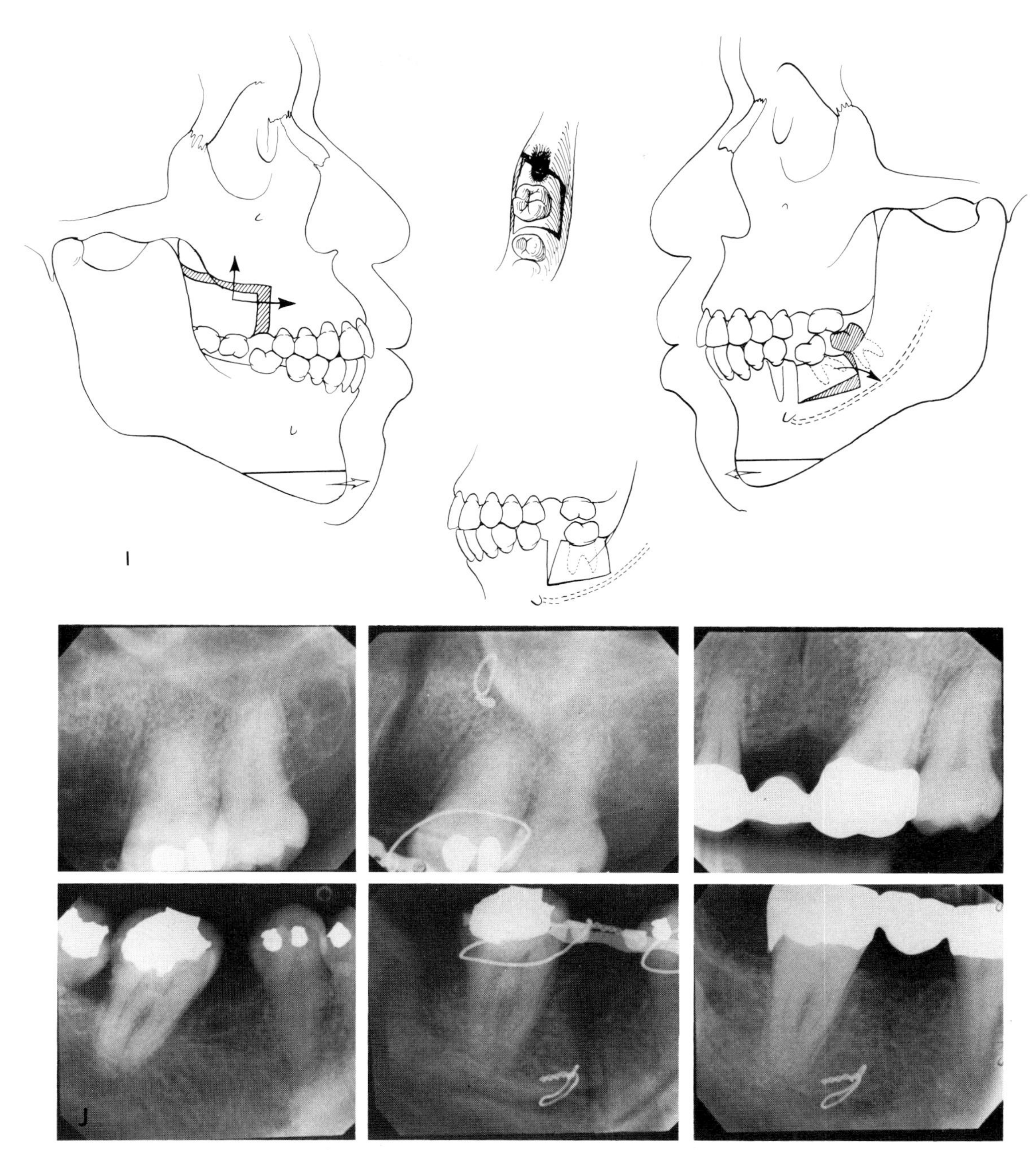

Figure 22–18 *Continued.* *I,* Schematic illustration of surgical plan: maxillary right subapical osteotomy and augmentation genioplasty; arrows indicate positional changes. *J,* Periapical radiographs showing the right posterior maxillary segment preoperatively (top left), the osteotomy site immediately postoperatively (top center), and consolidation of the osteotomy site 1 year postoperatively (top right); the left mandibular 2nd molar preoperatively (bottom left), the osteotomy sites immediately postoperatively (bottom center), and consolidation of the osteotomy sites 1 year postoperatively (bottom right).

Illustration and legend continued on the following page

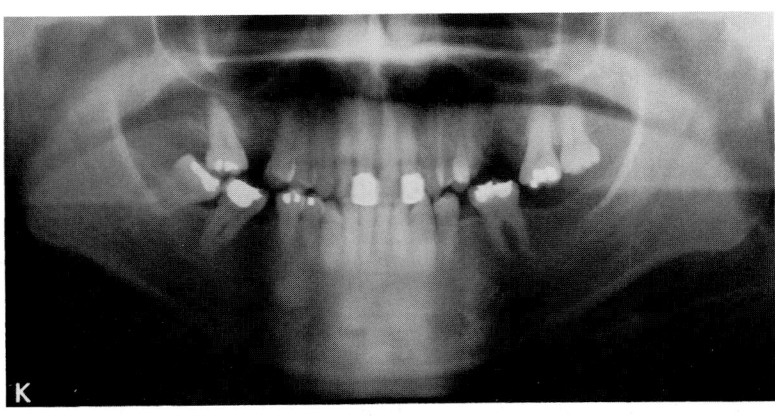

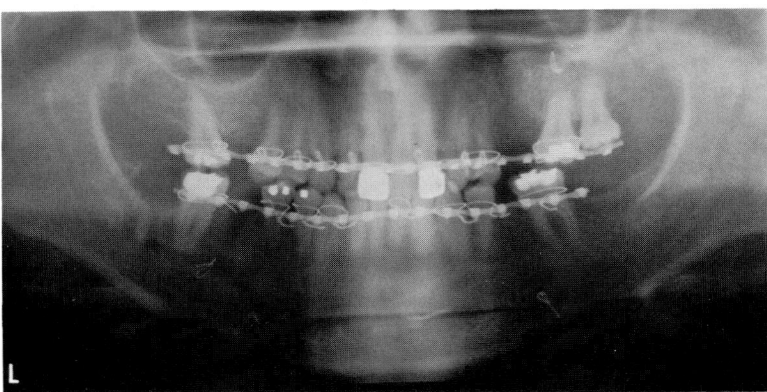

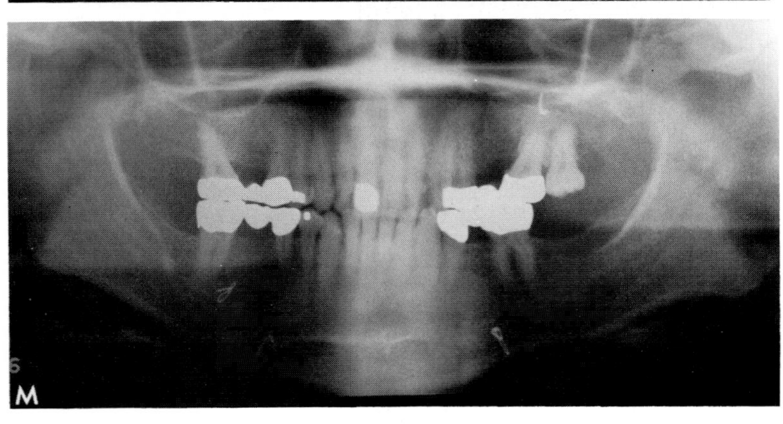

Figure 22–18 *Continued. K,* Preoperative panoramic radiograph showing supererupted maxillary right 2nd and 3rd molar teeth and tipped mandibular left 2nd and 3rd molar teeth. *L,* Immediate postoperative panoramic radiograph showing superior and anterior repositioning of right maxillary and posterior repositioning of left mandibular molar segment. *M,* Two-year postoperative panoramic radiograph showing stability of occlusal relationship, consolidation of bone, and final restorations.

2. Left posterior mandibular subapical osteotomy to inferiorly (2 mm) and posteriorly (5 mm) reposition the second molar tooth. Extract the tipped mandibular left third molar tooth to permit appropriate repositioning of the second molar. This procedure would accomplish the following:
    a. Upright the second molar tooth to establish normal periodontal tooth-to-bone relationship.
    b. Establish edentulous space in the mandible equivalent to the edentulous space in the maxilla to permit restoration of the occlusion with fixed bridge work.
    c. Level the occlusal plane of the second molar to permit restoration of normal crown contour in the fixed bridge.
3. Restoration of edentulous spaces with fixed bridges.
4. Augmentation genioplasty with horizontal sliding osteotomy.

FOLLOW-UP

The patient experienced minimal postoperative discomfort and only slight impairment of masticatory function.

Objective

The segments were stabilized with arch bars and direct transosseous wires, which eliminated the need for intermaxillary fixation. Consequently the patient was able to eat relatively normally in the immediate postoperative period. Good clinical union without mobility was present six weeks postoperatively. Restoration of the edentulous spaces was started eight weeks postoperatively (Fig. 22–18, *J* to *M*).

COMMENTS

Posterior maxillary and mandibular subapical osteotomies provided a rapid means to improve the occlusal curve, establish more prosthetically manageable interdental spaces, and establish normal axial inclination of the teeth.

Profile esthetics was improved by the augmentation genioplasty.

Surgeons: Kevin L. McBride, Dallas, Texas and Michael Zide, New Orleans, Louisiana. *Restorative dentistry:* Claude Ricks, Loma Linda, California.

When first and second molar teeth are missing from the mandibular arch, the remaining posteriorly positioned third molar tooth may be moved anteriorly and uprighted into a functional relationship by the technique illustrated in Figure 22–19. The principal advantages of this combined sagittal-subapical osteotomy procedure are that it creates a relatively large segment with a greater soft-tissue pedicle. Furthermore, a greater and more versatile positional change of the dento-osseous segment is probably more achievable with this method than with the conventional subapical osteotomy techniques because of the extensibility of the surrounding soft tissues.

When there is a minimal edentulous space adjacent to the teeth to be uprighted, the roots of the adjacent teeth may limit the surgeon's ability to establish ideal positioning and inclination of the tipped tooth. Multiple tooth segments may also be uprighted. In general, latitude in moving these segments is not equal to that of repositioning a single tooth segment. Decortication of the inferior alveolar nerve and retraction of the nerve from the surgical site will facilitate the planned subapical osteotomy and movement of multiple dento-osseous segments.

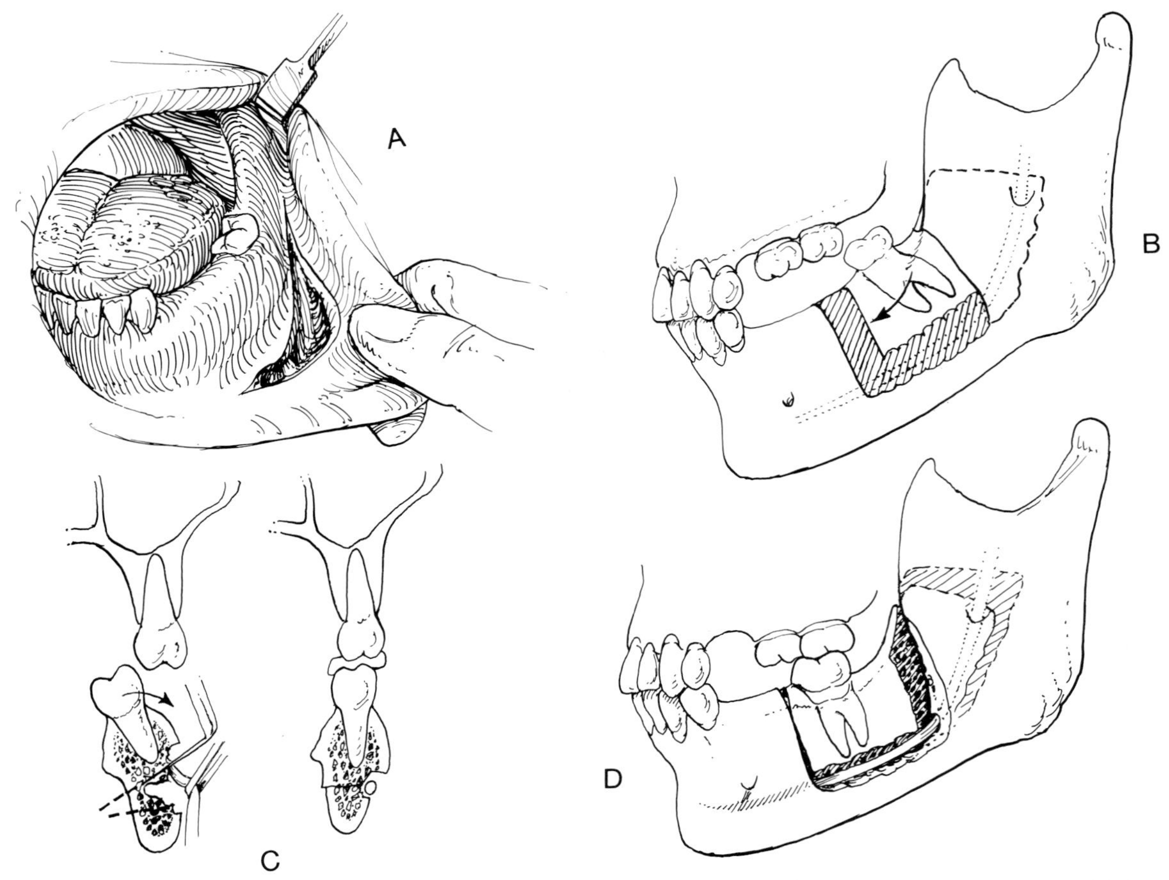

Figure 22–19. *A–D,* The sagittal-subapical osteotomy technique to reposition a malposed mandibular 3rd molar tooth. Extreme care must be exercised to maximize the attachment of the mucoperiosteum to the repositioned dento-osseous segment. Buccal ostectomy and careful decortication opposite the inferior alveolar nerve are essential to facilitate inferior movement of the segment. (See Chapter 10 for additional details of combined sagittal-subapical osteotomy technique.)

SOFT-TISSUE INCISIONS FOR SMALL SEGMENT ANTERIOR MANDIBULAR DENTO-OSSEOUS SURGERY

One-Stage Procedure

A one-stage surgical technique is generally used to reposition anterior mandibular segments when adequate interdental bone is present at the osteotomy sites to permit completion of the osteotomies through both cortices from the labial side.

Horizontal Incision (Fig. 22–20)

Excellent access may be gained to the osteotomy sites through a horizontal incision extending anteriorly above the mental nerve in the second premolar region to cross the

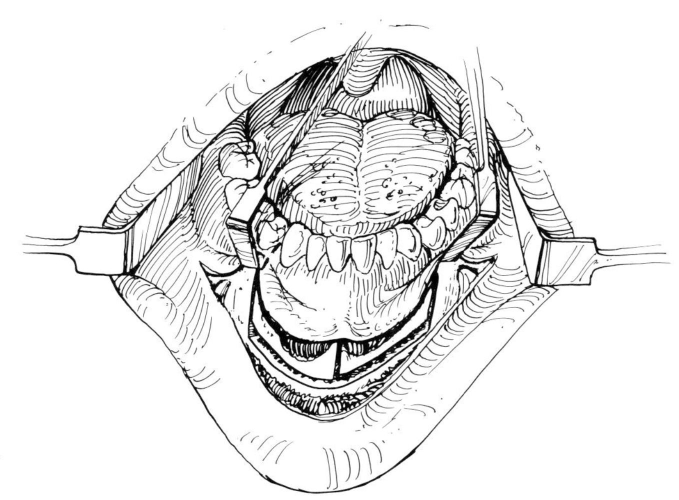

Figure 22–20. Horizontal incision. (See text for details.)

lip between the depth of the labial vestibule and the wet line, and extending above the mental nerve on the opposite side. This incision is carried obliquely down to bone through the mentalis muscles. The mucoperiosteum along the superior margin of the incision is elevated, exposing the bone over the apices of the mandibular anterior teeth and the interdental bone at the site of the proposed vertical osteotomies. Only minimal mucoperiosteal elevation should be accomplished on the segment to be mobilized. The mucoperiosteum may be elevated more extensively on the stable segment because it has a broad intact vascular pedicle from the contiguous bone and attached soft tissue. Where two adjacent segments are to be mobilized, the mucoperiosteum along the site of the vertical osteotomy should be preferentially elevated from the larger segment to maximize the soft-tissue attachment to the smaller segment. Generally, it is unnecessary to elevate the mucoperiosteum above the level of the attached gingiva.

The vertical osteotomy may be performed under direct visualization with a rotating instrument or oscillating saw up to the level of the attached gingiva. At this point, the osteotomy is completed by malleting a very fine osteotome into the interdental osteotomy site to split the crestal alveolar bone. Preservation of the integrity of the attached gingival cuff and a maximal amount of soft tissue to the interdental crestal bone is desirable in all cases. It is particularly important when the dento-osseous segments are to be separated. Such movements may cause devascularization and devitalization of the crestal bone, osteonecrosis, sequestration, and subsequent periodontal defect formation. Consequently, it is desirable to maintain the marginal attached gingiva intact and obtain the necessary relaxation by stretching the tissue between the segments after undermining the mucoperiosteum on the adjacent non-mobilized segment.

When an interdental ostectomy is performed to close an interdental space, it is desirable to elevate the tissue over the crest of the ridge to facilitate optimal visualization of the surgical site and more accurate removal of bone at the alveolar crest. When a small amount of bone is to be excised between two teeth, the segments are mobilized and separated before excising bone from the margins of the contiguous teeth. Care should be taken to preserve the integrity of the marginal gingival cuff around the teeth adjacent to the ostectomy. As the segments are juxtaposed, redundant soft tissue may produce a periodontal problem. Periodontal defects may be alleviated transversely by excising an elliptically shaped piece of tissue from the crest of the ridge without compromising the integrity of the marginal gingival cuff.

Modified Horizontal Incision (Fig. 22–21 *A* and *B*)

A modification of the horizontal incision may be necessary when an osteotomy is made between closely spaced teeth to facilitate separation of the teeth more than a few millimeters. Sufficient interdental gingiva may not be present to completely cover the crest of the ridge over the ostectomy site. As a result, interdental crestal bone may become exposed. If sufficient interdental crestal bone remains around the teeth adjacent to the osteotomy, healing occurs uneventfully. However, when minimal crestal bone remains or the space must be expanded more than stretching of the attached gingiva will permit, a modified incision may be utilized. The incision is utilized only when a mobilized segment is to be separated from a stable segment — not when two mobilized segments are to be separated from one another.

The incision is begun at the interdental papilla between the teeth to be separated and extended toward the stable segment. It is carried obliquely down through the attached gingiva into the mucoperiosteum. The tissue on the vestibular side of the incision is undermined so that it is advanced with the mobilized dento-osseous segment. A similar flap may also be developed on the lingual side of the ridge. It may be necessary to incise periosteum at the distal end of the flaps to permit adequate advancement without tension. The buccal and lingual flaps are advanced along the line of the incision and the attached gingiva is sutured over the crest of the ridge to obtain primary closure.

Horizontal Incision with Vertical Extension (Fig. 22–22)

For additional access and more direct visualization of the crestal alveolar bone, vertical incisions may be made over the proposed osteotomy sites, extending from the horizontal incision to the free gingival margin. This incision should not be used when segments are to be separated. A small amount of adjacent mucoperiosteum is elevated to

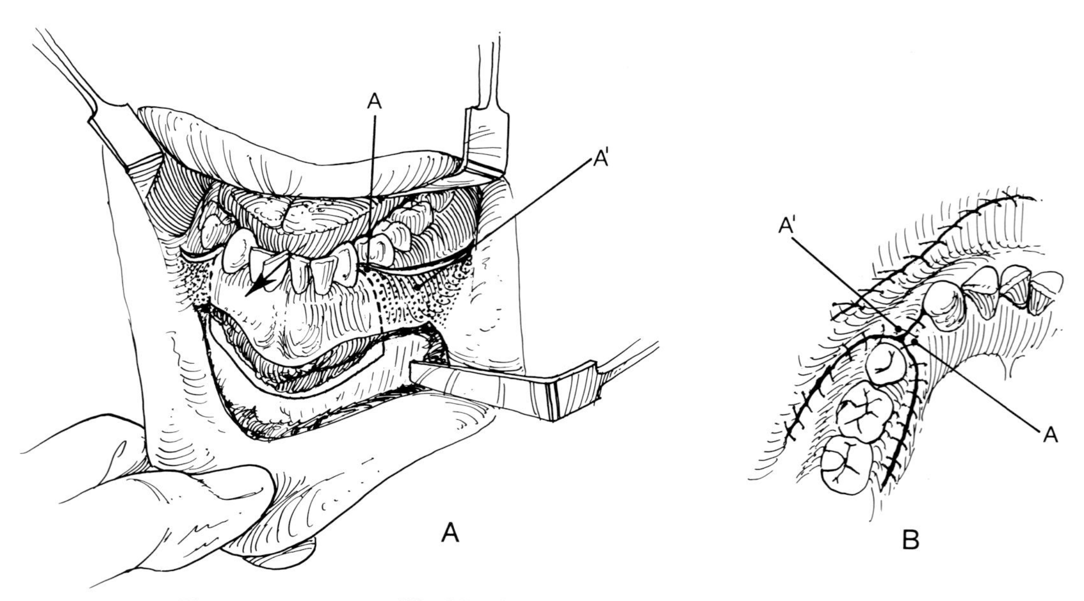

Figure 22–21. Modified horizontal incision. (See text for details.)

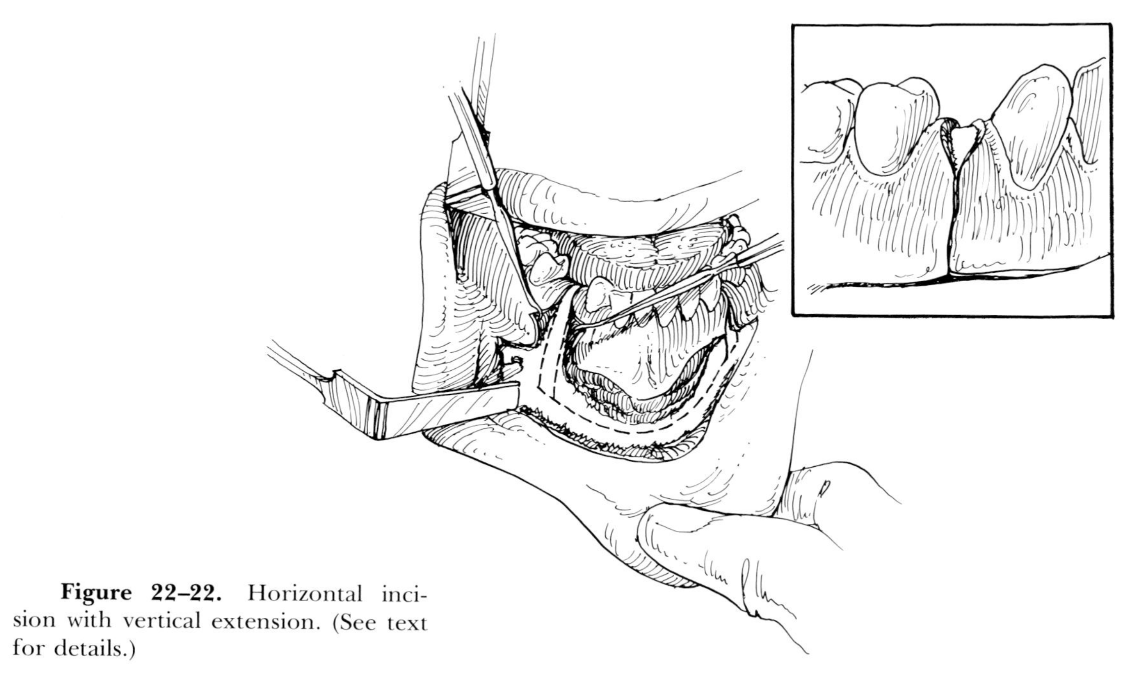

Figure 22–22. Horizontal incision with vertical extension. (See text for details.)

expose the bone at the osteotomy site and to permit transection of the crestal bone under direct visualization. Unless an ostectomy is performed, it is desirable to maintain as much bone as is possible at the crest of the ridge in order to preserve the integrity of the periodontium. Sectioning the interseptal crestal alveolar bone with an osteotome is the key to accomplishing this. Interruption of the blood flow along the buccal soft-tissue pedicle by multiple vertical incisions appears to be clinically insignificant when pedicled mucoperiosteum and gingiva remain attached to the segment or segments to be repositioned.

Vertical Incision (Fig. 22–23)

Even though the access provided by vertical incisions alone is not as good as that provided by a horizontal incision, they do permit maintenance of continuous vertical

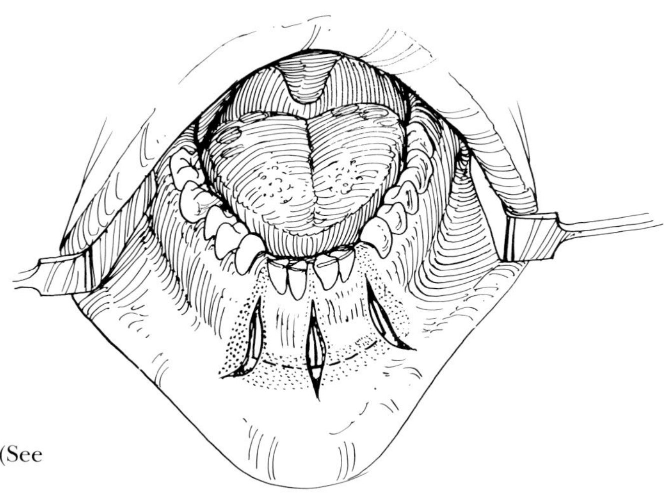

Figure 22–23. Vertical incision. (See text for details.)

buccal vascular pedicles to the mobilized segments. These buccal vascular pedicles are particularly valuable when mobilizing small dento-osseous segments involving one or two teeth, or larger segments with severe interdental crowding. Severe interdental crowding reduces the blood flow from the lingual pedicle to the buccal cortex and soft tissues because of the reduced area of interdental bone and soft tissue through which the blood may flow. In these situations, elimination of a vascularized buccal soft-tissue pedicle may compromise the blood supply to the buccal cortex and overlying soft tissues. Therefore, when vertical incisions are utilized, great care should be taken to maximize the soft-tissue attachment to the buccal aspect of the segment.

Two-Stage Procedure (Fig. 22–24)

The anatomic factors which make interdental osteotomies in a single stage difficult and potentially problematic include lingual tori, severely crowded teeth, and rotated and tipped teeth with apices in close approximation. When these problems are present a two-stage procedure is indicated to prevent damage to the roots of closely spaced teeth. The lingual osteotomies are accomplished as a part of the first stage because better access can be obtained from the buccal aspect for completion of the osteotomies during the second stage. An envelope flap is generally reflected around the necks of the teeth on the lingual aspect of the mandible and undermined inferiorly to provide access for the intended lingual osteotomies. These osteotomies are carried just through the lingual cortex to prevent damage to the roots of adjacent teeth. Generally, it is only necessary to perform the vertical osteotomies, as the horizontal osteotomy is easily completed from the buccal aspect. After waiting four to five weeks for the lingual tissues to reattach to the segments, the second stage of the procedure is accomplished through a horizontal vestibular incision.

Posterior mandibular dento-osseous surgery may be carried out through incisions similar to those used for anterior surgery. In the molar region, the horizontal incision at the depth of the buccal vestibule provides excellent access and visualization while maintaining a large soft-tissue pedicle to the buccal aspect of the segment. The muco-

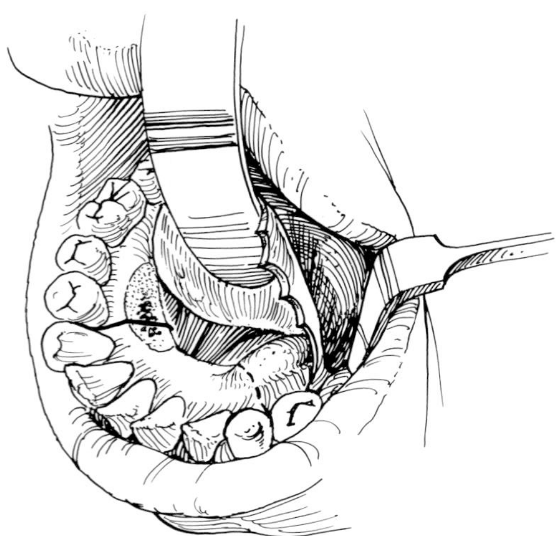

Figure 22–24. Two-stage procedure. (See text for details.)

periosteum may be judiciously elevated over both ends of the segment to provide access for completion of the vertical osteotomies. Sufficient buccal and lingual mucoperiosteum may be elevated from the stable segment to permit movement of the mobilized segment into the desired position (as described in the section dealing with surgical repositioning of posterior dento-osseous segments).

Premolar dento-osseous segments are surgically repositioned through the same type of horizontal incision used in the molar region. Care must be taken to extend the incision above the mental nerve to avoid damage to this structure. Vertical incisions may be utilized in conjunction with the horizontal incision in the premolar and molar region to provide additional access to the osteotomy site.

A clinical example of the use of a horizontal incision to move premolar segments is shown in Figure 22–25 *A* to *D*, in Case 22–3.

CASE 22–3 (Fig. 22–25)

C.J., a 24-year-old veteran, was referred by his general dentist for consideration of a surgical procedure to reduce the width of the mandibular anterior edentulous space so that a more physiologic mandibular fixed bridge might be fabricated. The six anterior mandibular teeth had been avulsed in an automobile accident six months previously.

EVALUATION

Esthetics

Frontal. Prominent maxillary anterior teeth when smiling and in repose; tongue appeared through edentulous mandibular space during talking.

Profile. Prominent lips, acute nasolabial angle (84°), deficient labiomental fold, anteroposterior chin deficiency.

Cephalometric Evaluation

1. Maxillary and mandibular protrusion (SNA = 94°, SNB = 90°)
2. Maxillary dentoalveolar protrusion (*1* to NA = 37° and 15 mm)

Occlusal Analysis (Fig. 22–25*A*)

Dental Arch Form. Maxilla and mandible symmetrical.

Dental Alignment. Good alignment, proclined maxillary anterior teeth.

Dental Occlusion. Class III malocclusion bilaterally, missing right and left mandibular central and lateral incisors, canines, and right second molar teeth.

TREATMENT PLAN (Fig. 22–25 *D*)

1. Mandibular subapical osteotomies in second premolar–first molar interspace and 11 mm midline ostectomy closed by medial rotation of the segments to:
   a. Narrow and round anterior mandibular arch to accommodate retracted anterior maxillary segment.

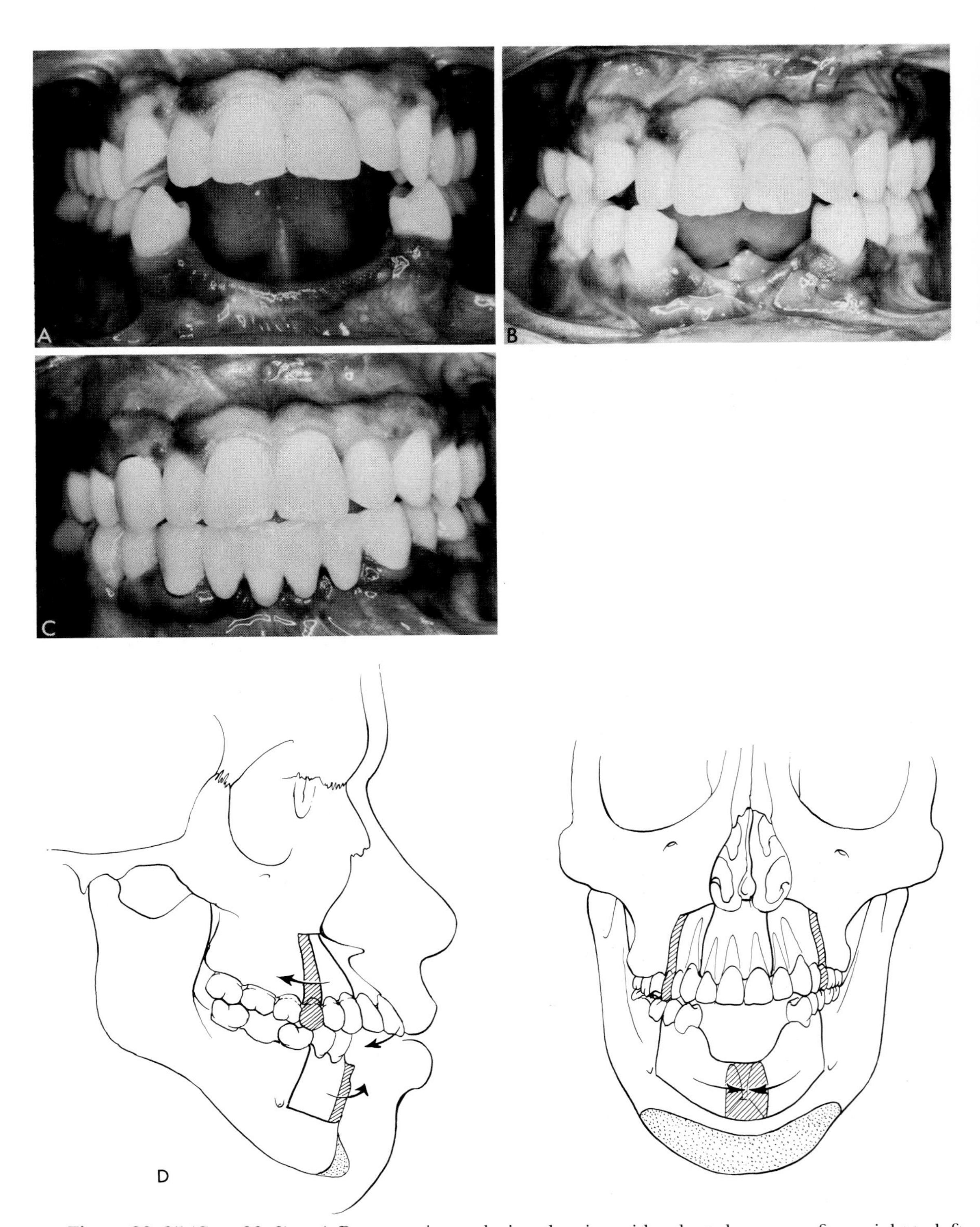

Figure 22–25 (Case 22–3). *A,* Preoperative occlusion showing wide edentulous space from right to left 1st premolar teeth. *B,* Two-month postoperative view after surgical procedures illustrated in *D* showing narrowed edentulous space and uprighted maxillary anterior teeth. *C,* After restoration of edentulous space with fixed bridge. *D,* Schematic illustration of surgical plan: bilateral mandibular subapical osteotomies with midline ostectomy with rotation of segments to close ostectomy site and reduce width of edentulous space; three-piece anterior maxillary osteotomy with extraction of 2nd premolar teeth to permit retraction and uprighting of anterior teeth; Proplast augmentation genioplasty (stippled area).

b. Bring first premolars into position for conversion into canines when crowned for bridge abutments.
c. Permit placement of anterior bridge with shorter edentulous span.

2. Extract maxillary second premolar teeth and perform 7 mm wide transpalatal ostectomy through extraction sites and two anterior maxillary interdental osteotomies to permit eight anterior maxillary teeth to be rotated inferiorly and posteriorly repositioned (7 mm) to:
a. Reduce proclination and prominence of maxillary anterior teeth.
b. Bring maxillary canines into occlusion between mandibular premolars (mandibular first premolar to be prosthetically converted into a canine form resulting in a class I cuspid occlusion).
c. Retract upper lip.

Augmentation genioplasty (7 mm) with Proplast to:
a. Increase chin prominence.
b. Improve labiomental fold.

Restoration of mandibular edentulous spaces with fixed bridges.

FOLLOW-UP

Subjective

The patient complained of numbness and tingling over his lower lip and chin. These altered sensations resolved over a 9-month period.

Objective

There was minimal postoperative swelling. Intermaxillary fixation was released after two weeks. The acrylic splint was left wired to the mandibular teeth for an additional two weeks. The arch bars served as retainers until they were removed 10 weeks postoperatively. Periodontal pockets developed with associated loss of interdental bone between the mandibular first molars and second premolars. These defects were probably due to excessive bone removal during interdental osteotomies. Periodontal bone grafting is planned to correct these defects. All segments developed excellent stability, and with the narrowed anterior mandibular edentulous space a strong, esthetic fixed bridge was fabricated without difficulty.

Surgeons: Kevin L. McBride, Dallas, Texas and Michael Zide, New Orleans, Louisiana. *Restorative dentistry:* William B. Currie, Dallas, Texas.

ANTERIOR SPACING

Maxillary interdental spacing is commonly associated with certain dentofacial deformities such as bimaxillary protrusion or horizontal maxillary excess. In adults, partially edentulous spaces are commonly associated with congenitally missing lateral incisors, extraction sites, and traumatically avulsed anterior teeth. Dental asymmetry and tipping of contiguous teeth may occur as a consequence of these missing teeth and result in an unesthetic smile.

The axial inclination and length of the teeth are assessed by direct visualization and palpation of the bone encasing the teeth to be moved and the adjacent immobile teeth.[7] These findings are correlated with periapical radiographic studies. Indicated

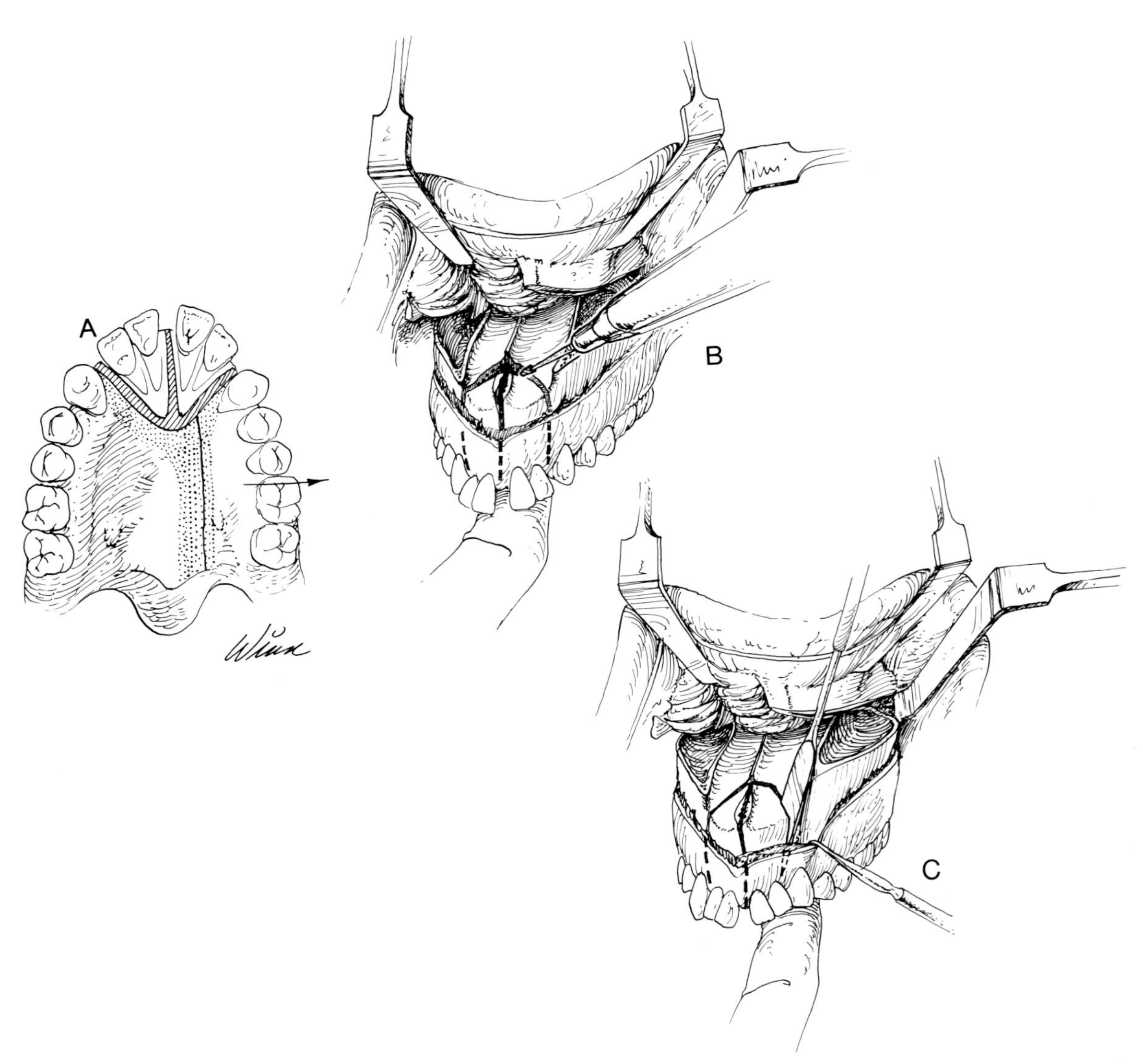

Figure 22–26. Segmentalized Le Fort I maxillary osteotomy to simultaneously close interincisal diastema, level maxillary occlusal plane, and expand maxilla (four-segment Le Fort I osteotomy). *A* and *B*, Plan of surgery: level maxillary occlusal plane by bilateral interdental ostectomies in the canine lateral incisor interspaces; midline ostectomy to close space between central incisors; parasagittal osteotomy to facilitate expansion of maxilla. *C*, Spatula osteotome is malleted into canine–lateral incisor interdental space to transect interradicular and interseptal bone; broken lines indicate planned interdental osteotomy sites.

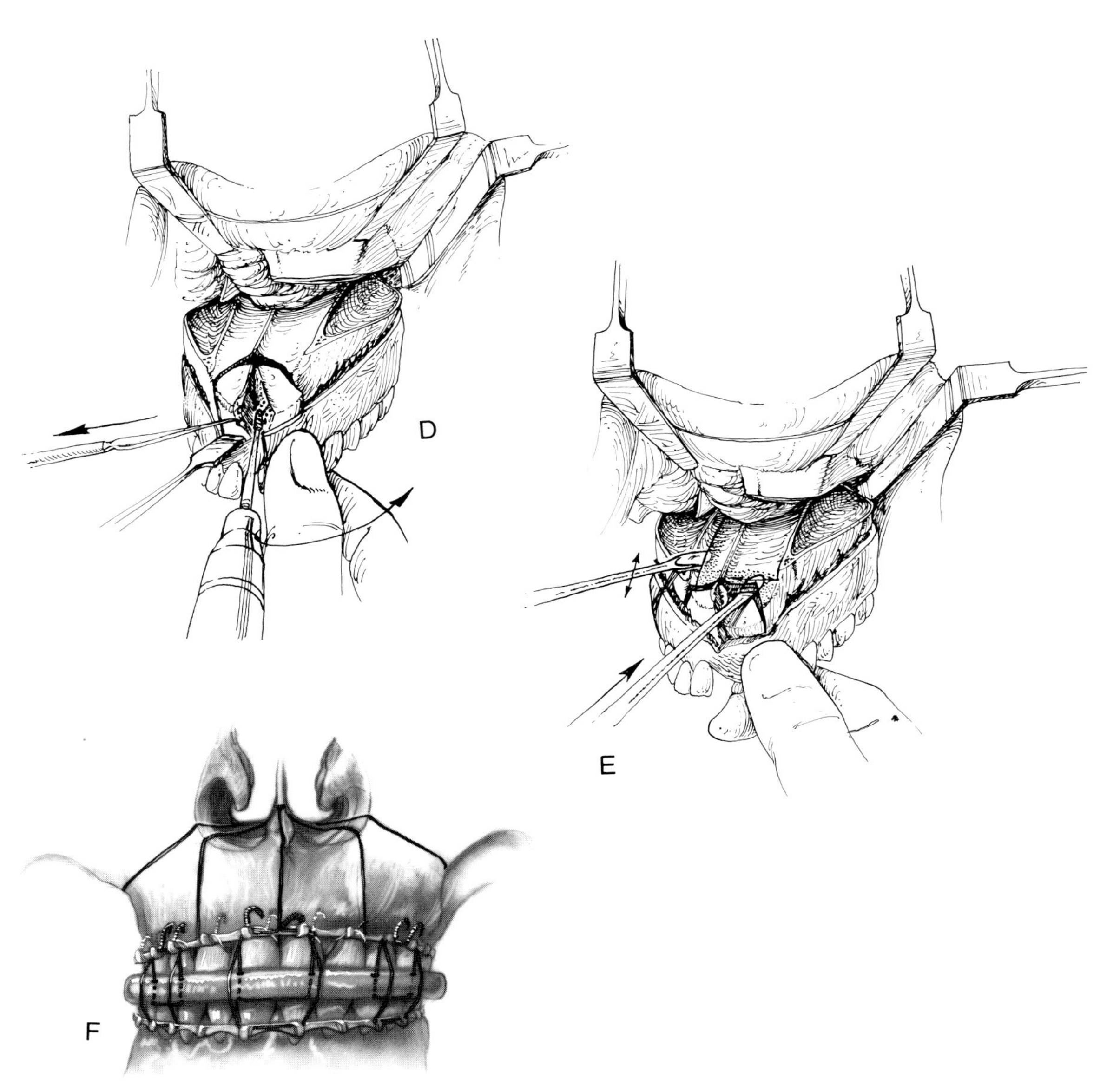

Figure 22–26 *Continued.* *D,* Dento-osseous segments are digitally manipulated to separate the margins along the midline osteotomy; with the segments separated, the midline ostectomy is accomplished under direct vision with a fissure bur. *E,* Palatal mucosa is freed from the edges of the large palatal segment to facilitate superior repositioning of the two incisor segments and lateral movement of posterior segment without detaching palatal tissue from the smaller segments. *F,* The mobilized segments are placed into the preoperatively determined occlusal relationship with the aid of an interocclusal splint. The segments are then fixed by ligating the arch bar lugs to the interocclusal splint.

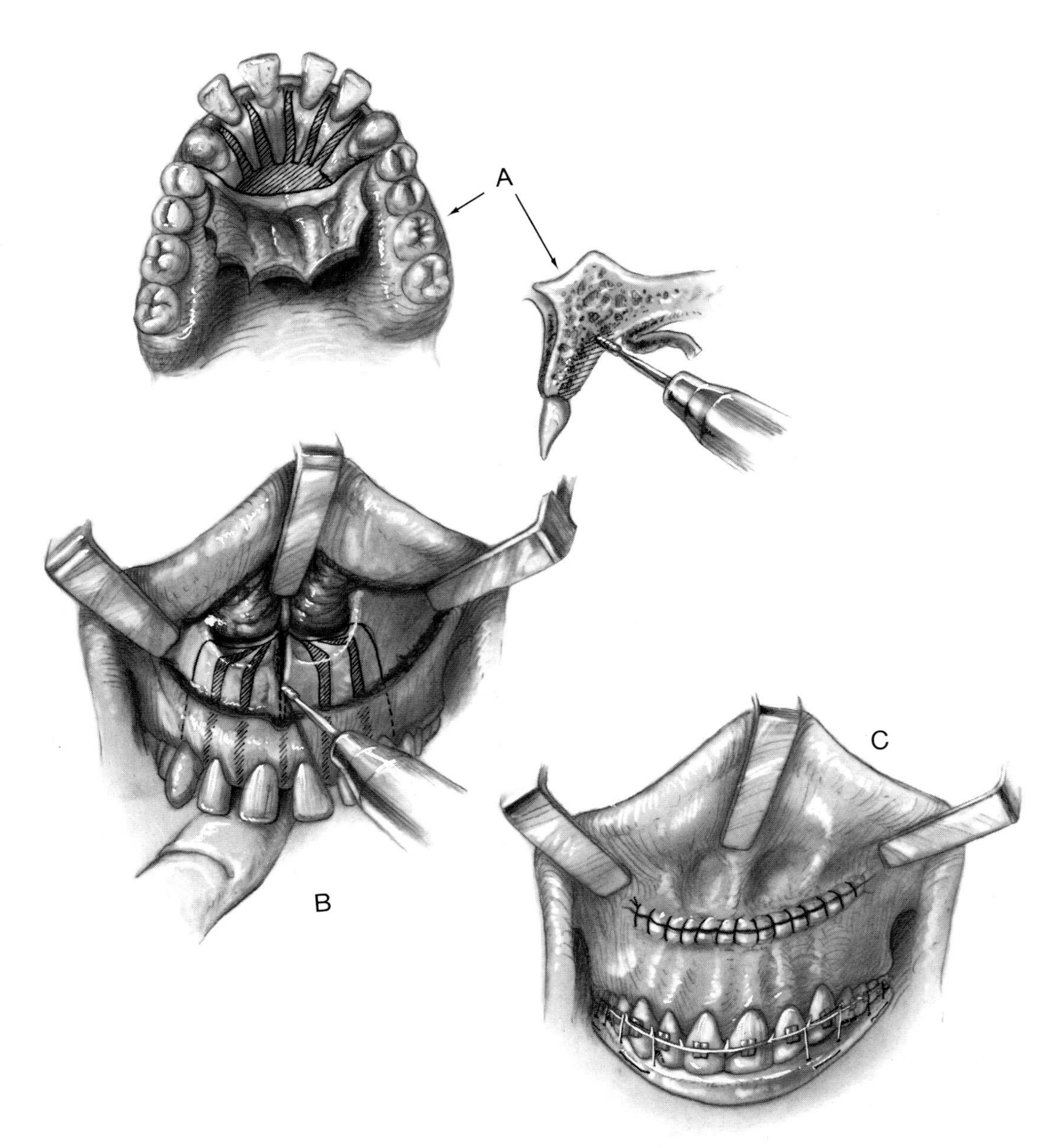

Figure 22–27. Immediate repositioning of maxillary anterior teeth by two-stage procedure; interincisal spacing is associated with lack of space between the 1st premolars and rotated canine teeth. *A, (1st Stage)* After a palatal mucoperiosteal flap is raised, lingual interdental ostectomies are made with a fissure bur. *B, (2nd Stage)* The inferior margin of a horizontal incision in the depth of the labial-buccal sulcus is undermined and retracted to expose the planned vertical interdental osteotomy and ostectomy sites. *C,* The mobilized segments are placed into the preoperatively determined occlusal relationship with the aid of an acrylic occlusal wafer splint. The segments are fixed by ligating the brackets on the dento-osseous segments to an orthodontic arch wire.

vertical interdental osteotomies or ostectomies are made with a 701 or 703 fissure bur in a straight handpiece (Fig. 22–26 *A* to *F*) (size of bur depends on size of interdental space) or with an oscillating or sagittal type saw.[27-29] Midline and canine–lateral incisor bone cuts are extended to and through the palatal cortical plate. Intraoperative periapical radiographs may serve as directional guides and provide additional orientation while performing interdental and subapical osteotomies.

Interdental osteotomies can usually be made safely with a fissure bur, an oscillating saw, or reciprocating saw blade in a single-stage procedure. When the use of a bur or saw is not feasible because of inadequate interradicular spacing, a sharp spatula osteotome is malleted between the teeth after etching the planned bony incisions into the labial bony plate. Wherever feasible, the labial cortical bone is partially osteotomized prior to sectioning the bone with an osteotome. Digital pressure on the palatal mucosa indicates when the saw, bur, or osteotome has transsected the palatal cortices.[7] This is important so as not to badly damage or strip palatal mucoperiosteum, the principal blood supply to the mobilized dento-osseous segments. The removal of small segments of interdental and subapical bone (when indicated) is accomplished with the use of a fissure bur *after* the dento-osseous segments have been made freely movable with digital pressure. Direct visualization of both sides of the osteotomized bone facilitates instrumentation of the lingual and interproximal areas, prevents excessive removal of interdental bone, and lessens the possibility of damage to the contiguous teeth.

Great care must be exercised to maintain a palatal soft tissue pedicle to the repositioned segments, which are placed into a preoperatively determined occlusal relationship with the aid of an acrylic occlusal wafer. Preoperative planning is usually not accurate enough to place the dento-osseous segments precisely into the planned position after the interdental ostectomies are accomplished. The splint must be repeatedly tried in place to determine when the desired amount of interproximal bone has been removed from both the mobilized and stable segments to allow the planned alignment of the teeth. Finally, the splint is fixed to the teeth with interdental wires for three to eight weeks. This method of fixation usually obviates the need for immobilization of the mandible.

Various modifications in the design of the soft-tissue and bone incisions have been made to facilitate treatment of the individual case. When crowded, closely spaced teeth without interradicular spacing must be repositioned, a two-stage technique may be indicated. In the first stage, lingual interdental ostectomies are made through a palatal mucoperiosteal flap (Fig. 22–27). Four or five weeks later, after the raised soft tissue flap has reattached and become revascularized to the underlying bone, the necessary labial and buccal bone cuts are made and the dento-osseous segments placed into the desired position. Such two-stage techniques are also useful where there is excessive palatal exostosis which is inaccessible from a labiobuccal approach, where there are multiple widely spaced teeth, and when rotational movements are necessary. By significantly reducing the operating time, the two-stage procedure may allow certain complex dentoalveolar surgical procedures to be accomplished with local anesthesia as an office procedure.

Figures 22–28 and 22–29 demonstrate closure of anterior maxillary interdental spaces by segmental dentoalveolar surgery.

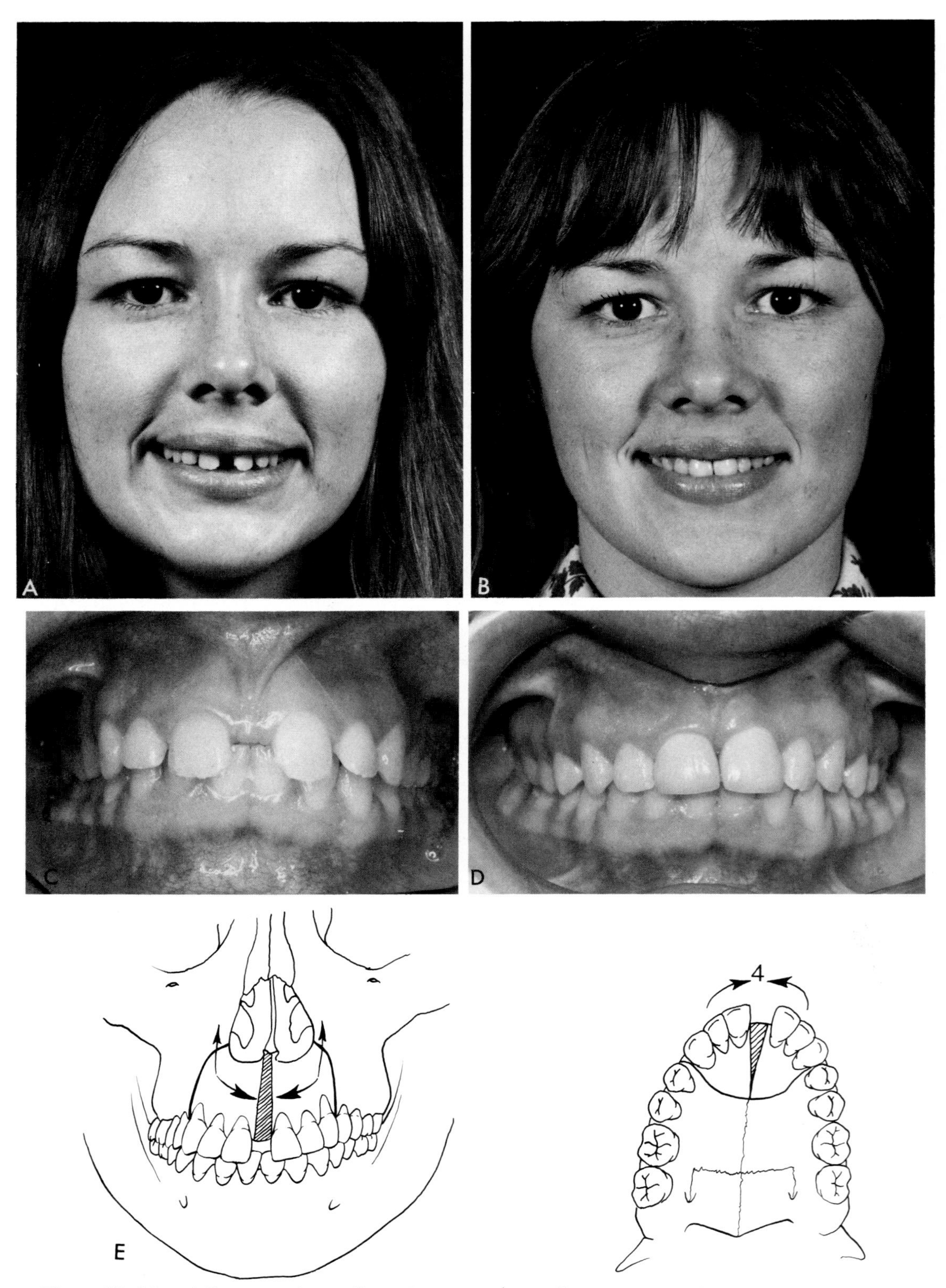

Figure 22–28. *A,* Preoperative smile, *B,* Postoperative smile. *C,* Preoperative Class I malocclusion with 4-mm interincisal diastema in 24-year-old woman. *D,* Postoperative occlusion after surgical closure of 4-mm diastema by anterior maxillary osteotomy and interincisal osteotomy *(E)* and placement of jacket restorations on central incisors. *E,* Schematic view of surgical procedure used to correct overbite and interincisal diastema. (Surgery by Timothy A. Turvey and William H. Bell.)

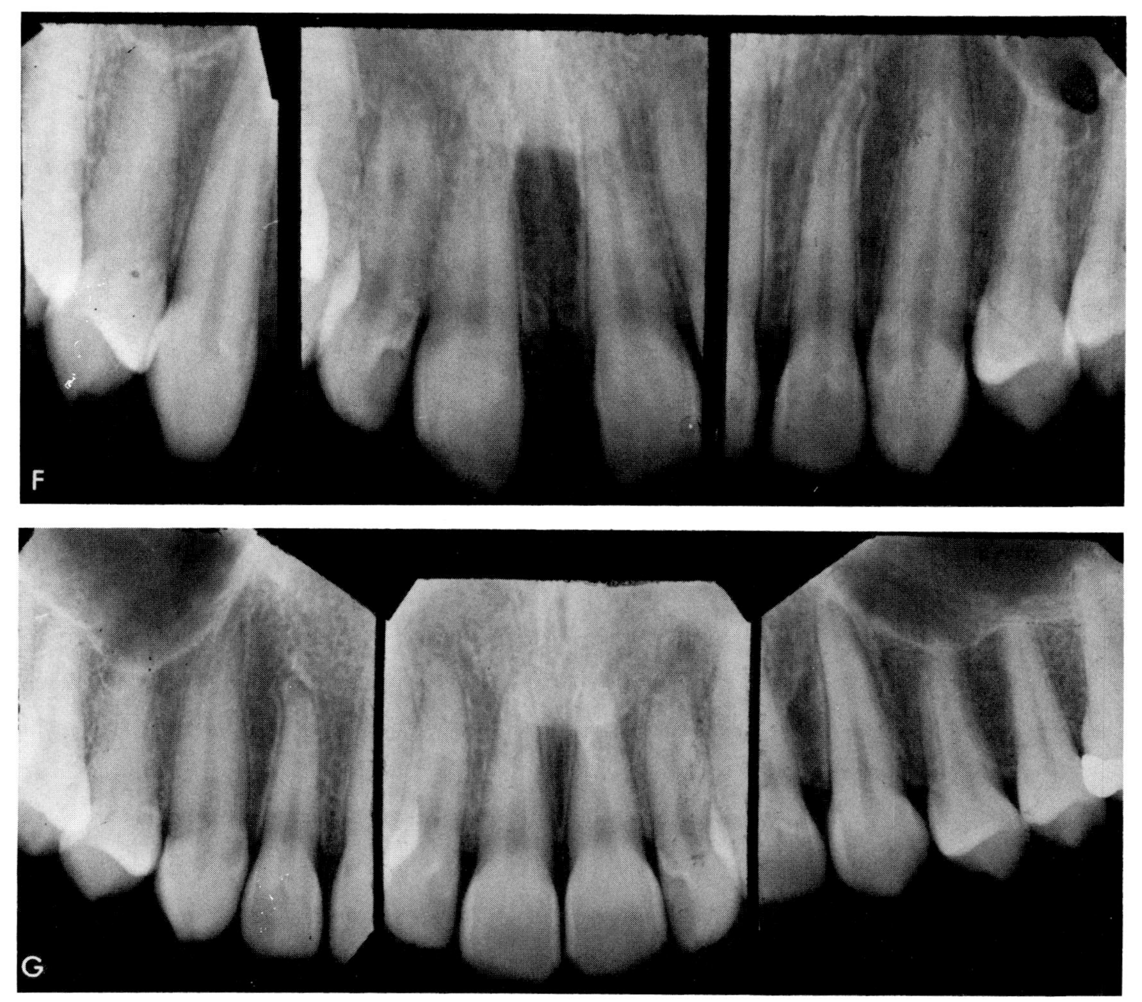

Figure 22–28 *Continued.* *F,* Preoperative periapical radiograph. *G,* Postoperative periapical radiograph showing apposition of teeth and consolidation of osteotomized bone in interdental osteotomy sites with minimal loss of interseptal bone three years after surgery.

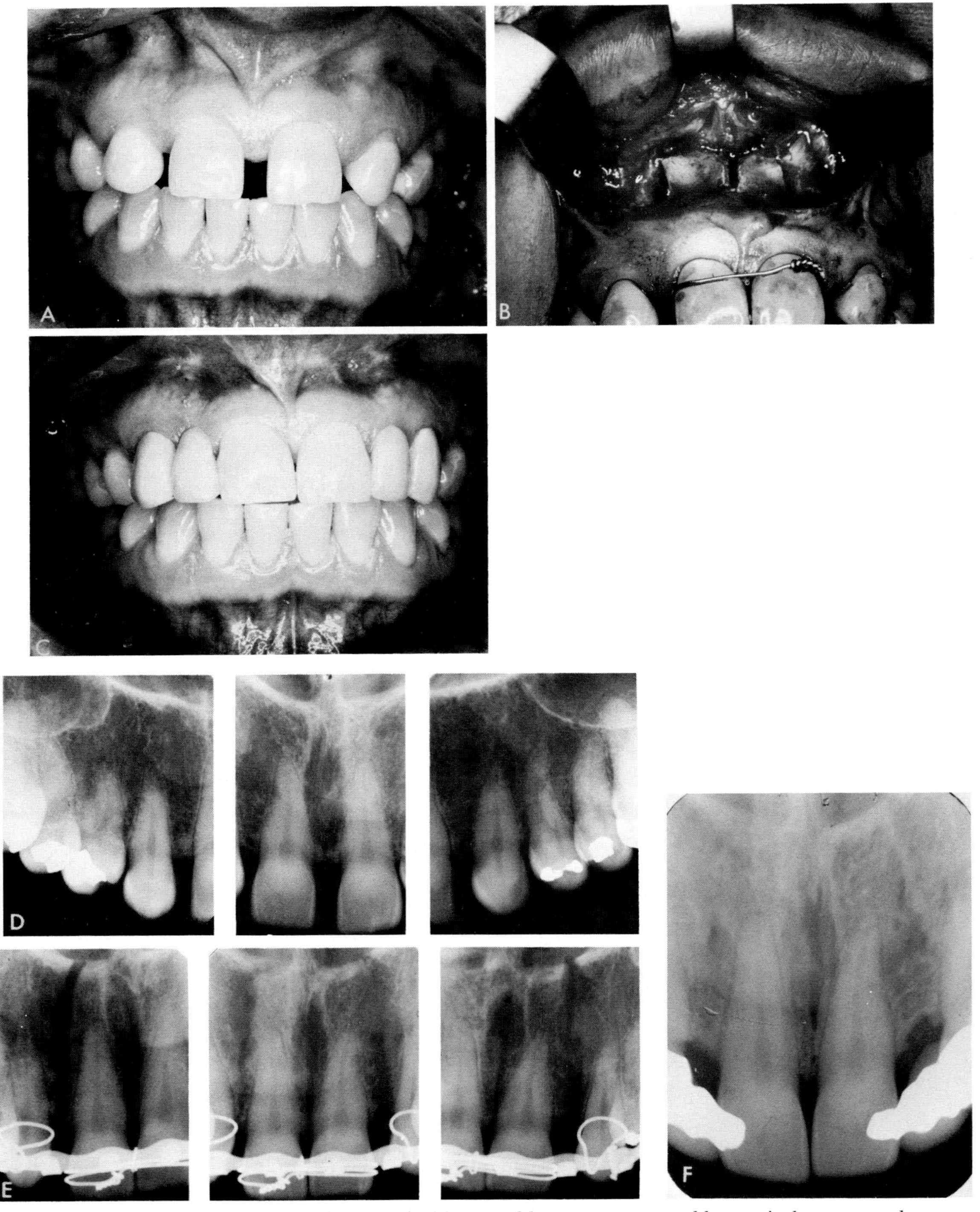

Figure 22–29. *A,* Interincisal diastema in 38-year-old woman corrected by vertical ostectomy between central incisors and vertical osteotomies in canine–central incisor interspaces. *B,* Central incisors are juxtaposed after dento-osseous segments were surgically repositioned through horizontal incision in depth of labial vestibule. (See Fig. 22–27 for details of surgical techniques.) *C,* Occlusion after canines were retracted distally with removable appliances and edentulous spaces restored with fixed bridges. *D,* Preoperative radiograph showing interdental spacing and congenitally missing lateral incisors. *E,* Immediate postoperative radiographs showing osteotomy sites. *F,* Apposition of teeth and consolidation of osteotomized bone with minimal loss of interseptal bone five years after surgery. (Surgery by William H. Bell.)

Posterior Maxillary Surgery to Open or Close Interdental Spaces

Anterior repositioning and uprighting of second and third molar teeth following the premature loss of first molar teeth are sound and predictable procedures which can obviate the need for prosthetic replacement of first molar teeth.[14, 17, 25] Conversely, maxillary posterior teeth can be repositioned posteriorly to gain space for a pontic. The efficiency of a fixed bridge can be significantly increased by surgically decreasing the distance between abutment teeth. These surgical procedures are accomplished as single-stage posterior maxillary osteotomies or in combination with anterior maxillary or Le Fort I osteotomy.[15]

Surgical Technique

Selection of the most appropriate surgical technique to reposition the posterior maxilla or small posterior maxillary dentoalveolar segments is based upon the planned positional change and anatomy of the individual patient's palatal vault. (See Chapter 8 for details of surgical techniques.) When the principal clinical objective is space closure without concomitant vertical reduction, or sectioning of the medial antral wall is not feasible because of a relatively small space between palatal root apices and the nasal floor, a direct approach to both the palatal and buccal aspects of the posterior maxilla may be necessary[17] (Fig. 22–30).

Success with this type of surgery is possible and predictable when the surgery is properly designed and executed and the segment is pedicled to palatal or labiobuccal gingiva and mucoperiosteum. Horizontal or vertical incisions in the buccal vestibule provide adequate access and visualization for the planned horizontal subapical osteotomies. The margins of the inferior flap may be undermined to gain access for a planned vertical bone incision. A transverse palatal bone incision can usually be accomplished from the buccal aspect with fissure burs and finely tapered osteotomes. Curved osteotomes may be used to accomplish the parasagittal palatal bone incision when there is sufficient space between the apices of the mobilized teeth and the nasal floor. When this is not feasible, a parasagittal palatal mucosal incision opposite the planned osteotomy site (bone incision is extended into nasal cavity) is made to facilitate the bone incision. When osteotomies are made between closely spaced teeth, the interdental bone cuts are made last with thin finely tapered osteotomes which fracture the interradicular and crestal alveolar bone.[14]

The movement of small posterior maxillary dentoalveolar segments which have contiguous anterior and posterior edentulous spaces is easily accomplished. The necessary transverse palatal osteotomies are readily made from the buccal aspect through the vertical osteotomy sites (Fig. 22–31).

Text continued on page 1625

Figure 22–30. Surgical technique for immediate repositioning of anterior and posterior maxillary dento-osseous segments. *A,* Procumbent maxillary anterior teeth associated with Class II malocclusion and low mandibular plane angle; cross hatched area indicates ostectomy site; solid line illustrates planned vertical and horizontal ostectomies. *B,* A midpalatal incision is placed from the junction of the hard and soft palates extending anteriorly to within 5 to 10 mm. of the interdental papilla. The tissues are undermined to the alveolar process allowing identification of the greater palatine artery and foramen. If necessary the dissection is extended posteriorly around the distal part of the tuberosity to the approximate junction of the tuberosity and palatine bone and pterygoid plates. This undermining may be performed using a double-ended curette maintaining attachment of the mucoperiosteum to the alveolar process. A fissure bur is used to make a U-shaped palatal bone incision into the nasal cavity without cutting through the nasal mucosa. Parasagittal placement of the osteotomy facilitates closure of the palatal mucosa over bone. The osteotomy is extended as far posteriorly as necessary to meet the vertical osteotomy behind the most posterior segment to be mobilized. The palatal cuts are completed anterior to the greater palatine foramen using a cross-cut fissure bur. When the transverse osteotomy is performed across the palate, a periosteal elevator or narrow malleable retractor is placed to protect the nasal mucosa. (Interdental bone incisions indicated by broken lines; palatal bone incisions indicated by solid line.) *C,* The incisions are terminated at least 5 mm above the alveolar crest (and attached gingiva if feasible) to ensure continuity of the periodontium. The anterior incisions are carried superiorly into the height of the vestibule and mucosal surface of the upper lip. This provides access to the piriform aperture and permits reflection of the nasal mucosa from the floor and the lateral wall of the nose and separation of the nasal septum from the nasal process of the maxilla. Margins of labial vertical incision are raised and retracted to expose planned interdental osteotomy site and piriform rim; proposed interdental osteotomy is etched into interproximal bone with fissure bur. Care is taken to avoid elevating more periosteum than is necessary to provide access for the bone incisions. *D,* Interdental osteotomy accomplished with oscillating saw blade, superiorly to the piriform aperture. *E,* Vertical interdental osteotomy of cortical alveolar bone only (1) above lateral incisor apex; bone incision is deepened into spongiosa. *F,* Osteotome malleted first into inter-radicular area until the tip of the instrument makes contact with the transverse portion of the U-shaped palatal bone cut; spatula osteotome is then malleted into lateral incisor canine interseptal area to fracture the crestal alveolar bone.

See illustration on the opposite pages.

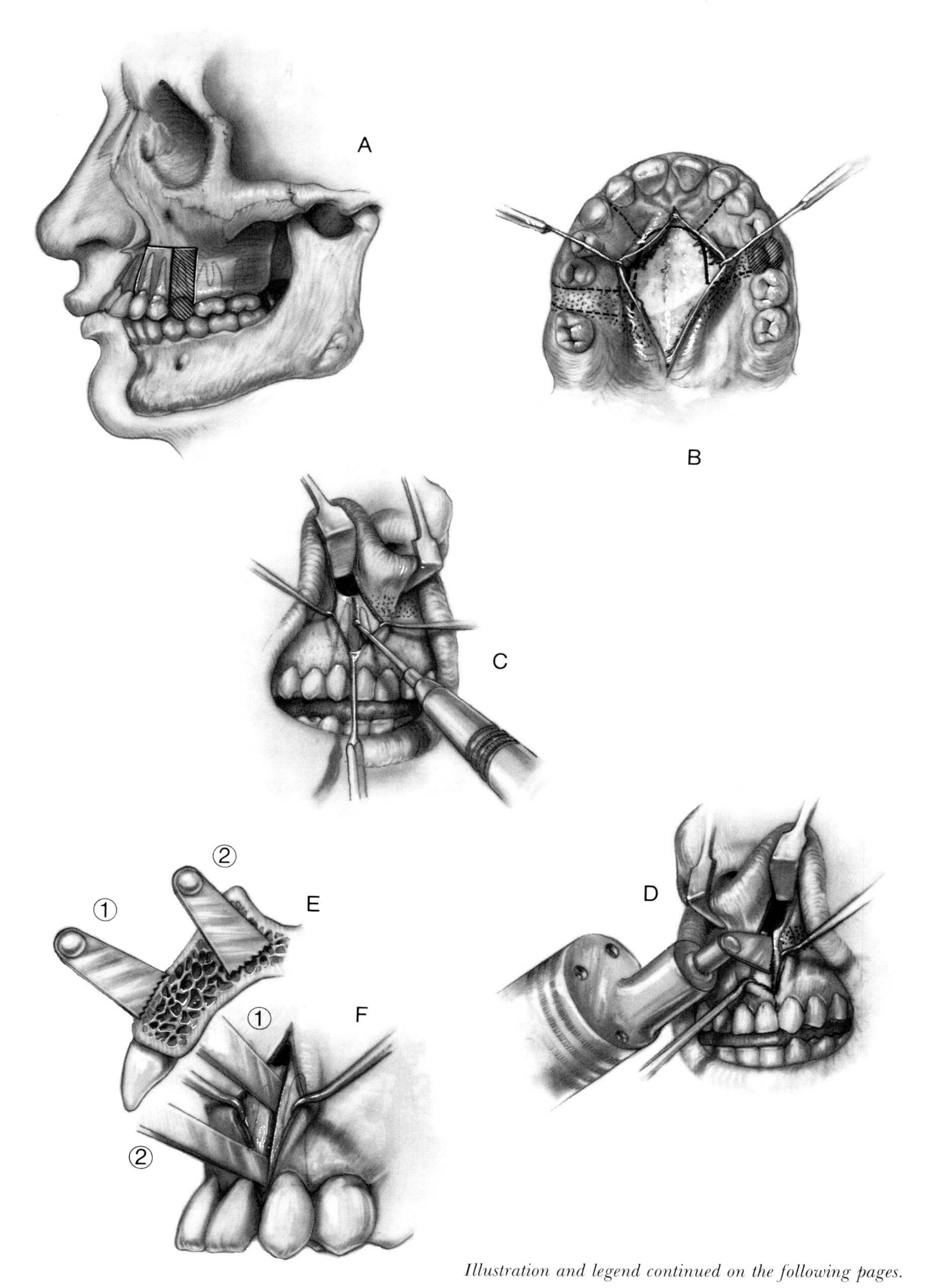

Illustration and legend continued on the following pages.

Figure 22–30 *Continued.* *G,* Bilateral vertical incisions are placed opposite the 2nd premolars. After a flap is reflected subperiosteally to expose the planned posterior vertical ostectomy sites, a measured segment of bone is excised; finger is positioned on palate to feel oscillating saw blade transect bone without injuring palatal mucosa; subperiosteal tunneling between anterior and posterior vertical incisions. *H,* Excision of bone from opposite 2nd premolar area; after subperiosteal tunneling between anterior and posterior vertical incisions, a horizontal osteotomy is made between piriform aperture and posterior vertical ostectomy site with small reciprocating saw blade. This horizontal bone cut is performed 5 to 8 mm. above the apices of the teeth and is carried through the lateral wall of the maxilla and the triangular buttress of bone at the piriform aperture. *I* and *J,* A thin osteotome is then malleted into the interseptal and inter-radicular areas of the posterior vertical osteotomies until the tip of the instrument makes contact with the parasagittal palatal osteotomies. With digital pressure and careful manipulation of the osteotome, the dento-osseous segments are mobilized and tipped medially and inferiorly. Now a thin, curved osteotome can be gently malleted through the lateral nasal wall to completely separate the segments from their bony attachments. Note the close relationship between molar root apices and nasal floor and low palatal vault. *K,* The maxillary segments are placed into a prefabricated occlusal splint. The segments should be sufficiently mobile to permit digital alignment since the adherent palatal mucoperiosteum has been elevated. Intermaxillary fixation is accomplished, temporarily permitting insertion of interosseous wires in the region of the maxillary zygomatic buttress and suspension wires. The suspension wires are secured, maintaining bony alignment, and where bony deficits exist along the lateral wall bone grafts are inserted and the interosseous wires secured. The patient is released from intermaxillary fixation to permit grafting of palatal defects and suturing of the palatal flaps. Alignment of the alveolar segments is maintained during this time by wiring the segments to the splint. Following closure of the palatal flaps, the patient is placed into intermaxillary fixation or, if mandibular surgery is to be performed, the splint is used to maintain the maxillary segmental alignment until mandibular surgery is complete.

See illustration on the opppsite page

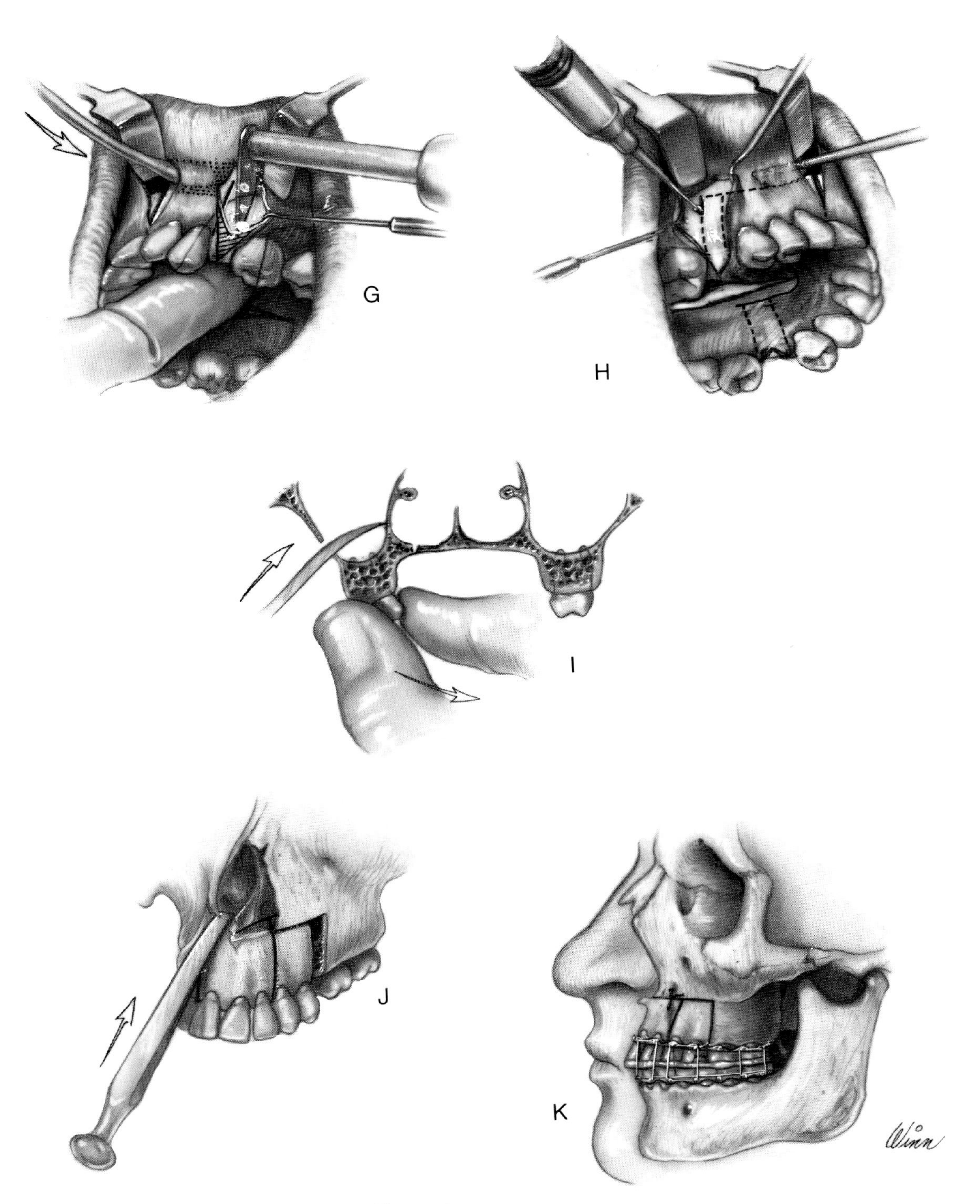

Figure 22–30. *Continued.*

Figure 22–31. Correction of supererupted posterior teeth and closure of edentulous first molar space by posterior maxillary osteotomy (Kufner or Schuchhardt technique). *A,* Preoperative deformity: inadequate posterior interarch space, supererupted posterior teeth, and edentulous first molar space. Plan of surgery: posterior maxillary osteotomy to increase posterior interarch space and close edentulous space. Cross-hatched areas indicate the intended osteotomy and ostectomy sites; broken line indicates the soft-tissue incision: arrows indicate directional movements of posterior maxillary segment. Visualization of the vertical ostectomy site may be facilitated by a vertical incision over or immediately anterior to the planned ostectomy site. To maximize the soft-tissue pedicle, only the anterior margin of the incision is detached from the bone to be mobilized. After the dento-osseous segment is repositioned, the buccal mucosa along the vertical incision is trimmed to eliminate redundant tissue. *B* and *C,* The medial wall of the maxillary sinus is sectioned between the palatal roots and the nasal floor with a curved osteotome passed through the bony window created by the horizontal ostectomy. The integrity of the palatal mucosa is preserved by carefully malleting an osteotome against the surgeon's finger, which is positioned at the juncture of the horizontal and vertical walls of the palate. *D,* Optional technique: buccal ostectomy of posterior lateral maxilla accomplished through horizontal incision only. The tuberosity is separated from the pterygoid plate with an osteotome. *E,* Posterior maxillary dentoalveolar segment pedicled to palatal mucosa and buccal gingiva is downfractured.

See illustration on the opposite page

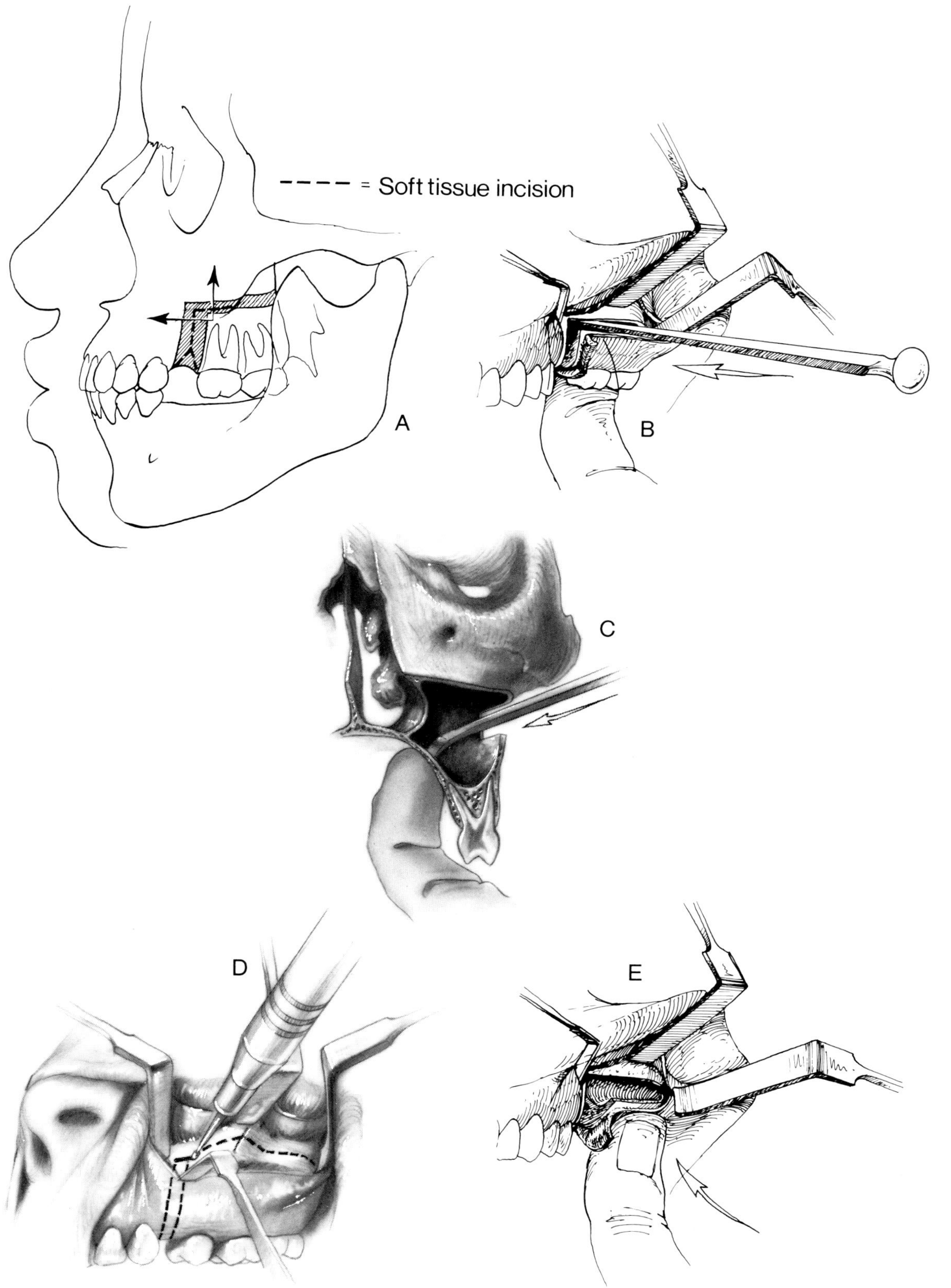

Illustration and legend continued on the following page

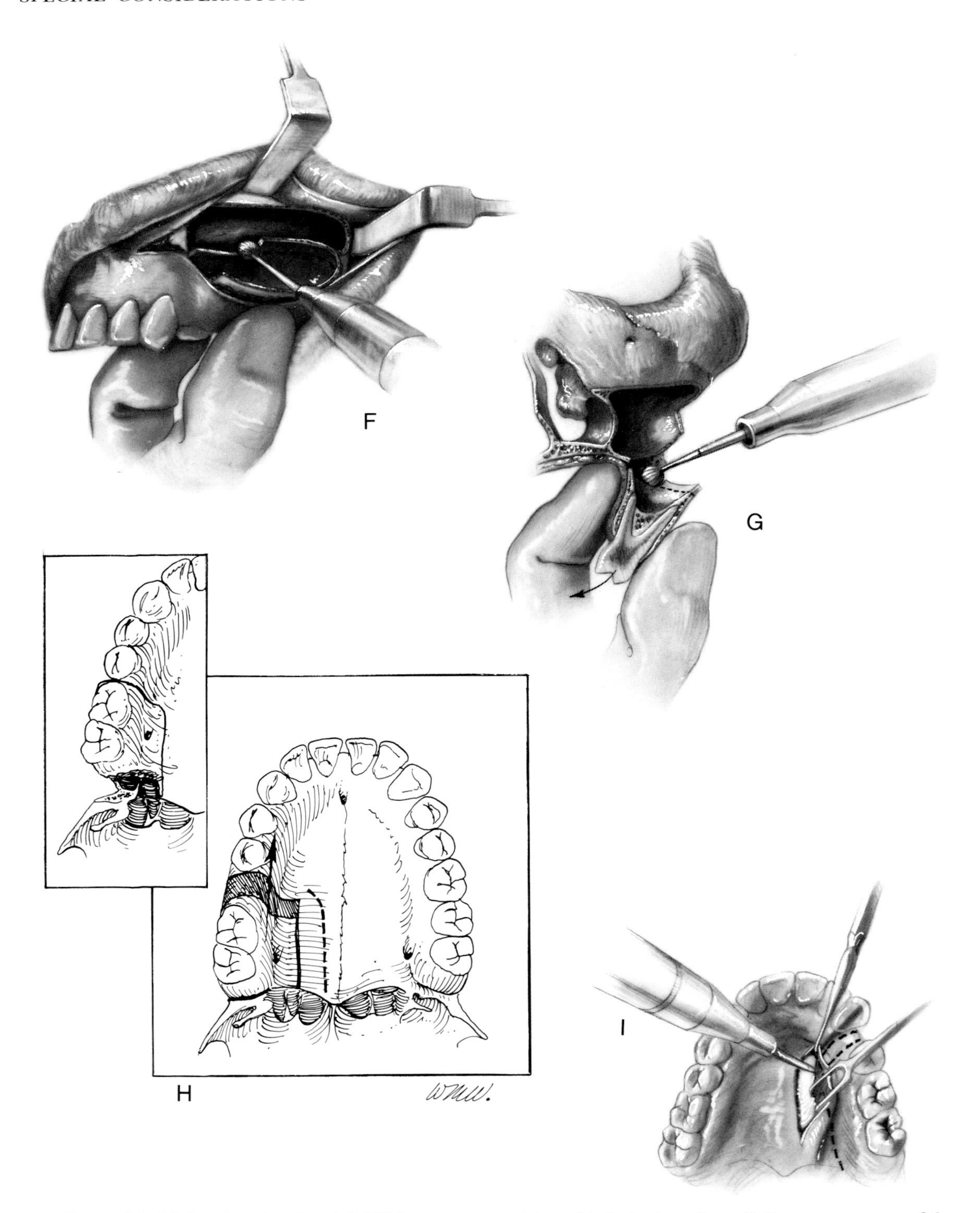

Figure 22–31 *Continued.* *F* and *G*, With segment positioned inferiorly and medially, an ostectomy of the superior, medial, and posterior aspects of the segment is accomplished. *H*, Posterior dento-osseous segment is moved anteriorly to close edentulous space; broken line indicates optional parasagittal soft-tissue incision to facilitate sectioning of palatal bone when there is insufficient space between the palatal root and floor of nose. *I*, With use of optional incision, parasagittal palatal osteotomy is made through retracted wound margins of palatal incision. (For further details of surgical technique, see Figures 8–45, 8–46, and 8–47.)

Interdental Crowding

Minimal interdental crowding in the adult may be tolerated if it does not constitute an esthetic problem. This is particularly true when crowding exists in the mandibular arch. Moderate to severe crowding should generally be corrected to improve the esthetic result as well as to improve the periodontal-anatomic relationship. Crowding contributes to plaque accumulation and increases the difficulty of maintaining good oral hygiene. Very mild crowding can be corrected prosthetically without creating a deleterious periodontal condition. It is difficult, however, to crown crowded teeth without creating a large interdental contact area with little space below it for the interdental papilla. Not only does this produce a poor esthetic result but the difficulty encountered with oral hygiene contributes to periodontal disease. Correction of interdental crowding by immediate repositioning of one-tooth and two-tooth dento-osseous segments has limitations when employed as the sole treatment entity owing to potential periodontal damge.

The combined surgical-orthodontic approach to correction of crowding in adults is particularly useful in cases where maxillary or mandibular anterior teeth need to be uprighted and flared but the labial plate of bone is so thin that a pure orthodontic technique would tend to push the roots of the teeth through this plate of bone. In the combined technique orthodontic bands or brackets are applied to the teeth preoperatively. One- or two-stage interdental osteotomies may then be performed, depending upon the degree of crowding present. If osteotomies are performed, the teeth are immediately repositioned and immobilized with a previously contoured heavy arch wire. If osteotomies are performed the orthodontic appliances may be activated immediately after completion of the single- or double-stage procedure.

In slight to moderate crowding problems, surgery may provide an effective expeditious method of correction when it is combined with orthodontics. Speed and precision are important elements of this therapeutic method.

The combined surgical-orthodontic approach to correction of crowding in adults is particularly useful in cases where the problematic area is confined to the anterior part of the maxillary or mandibular arch, and the maxillary and mandibular posterior segments are relatively harmonious. Historically, crowding has been corrected entirely by orthodontics after extraction of premolar teeth in both arches and retraction of anterior teeth into the extraction spaces. Unfortunately, this necessitates extraction of teeth in both arches and sometimes undesirable retraction of teeth in the normal arch. The final occlusion may be satisfactory, but the soft-tissue facial esthetic result may be compromised. Treatment of similar problems without extractions is precluded by the relatively small amount of bone supporting the incisor teeth.

Anterior crowding is commonly associated with mandibular dentoalveolar retrusion. Similar problems are frequently manifest in the maxillary arch where anteroposterior deficiency is associated with cleft lip–palate patients or in individuals with congenitally missing canines or premolars. In these patients, where there is already insufficient support for the facial soft tissues adjacent to the deficient arch, extraction of premolar teeth may tend to compromise facial esthetics even more. When there is minimal to moderate crowding of the anterior maxillary and mandibular teeth and extractions are contraindicated, subapical osteotomy techniques may be used to advance the anterior teeth to improve their relationship to basal bone, give additional support to the upper or lower lip, and increase arch length.[6] The resultant increased

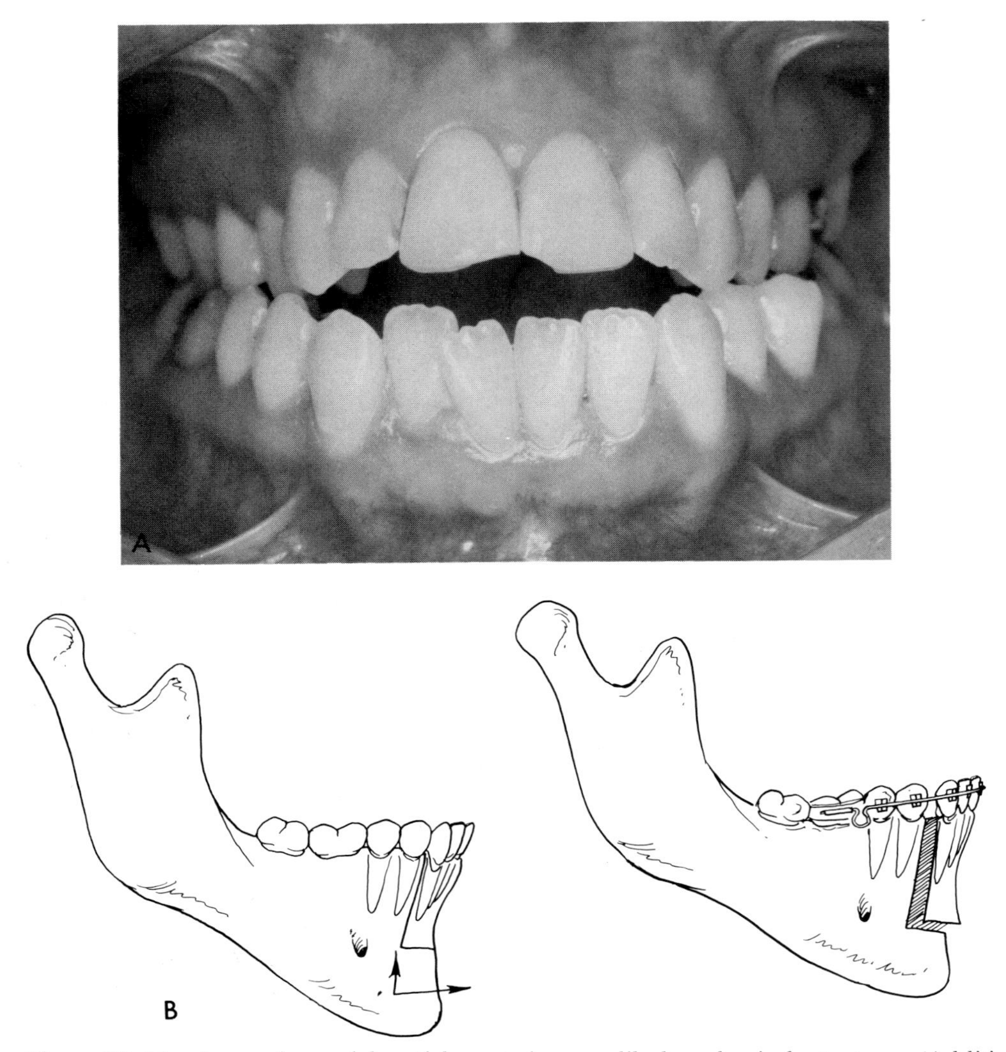

Figure 22–32. Increasing arch length by anterior mandibular subapical osteotomy. (Additional details of this technique are illustrated in Chapter 10). An increase in mandibular arch length to permit correction of mild to moderate anterior dental crowding without extraction of teeth may be accomplished by anterior mandibular subapical osteotomy. The mobilized six-tooth anterior mandibular segment is advanced to establish space bilaterally between the canine and 1st premolar teeth. Sufficient space is established to permit retraction of the canine and incisor teeth and to correct the crowding without extraction or flaring of the incisors. Simultaneous correction of occlusal plane abnormalities and uprighting of flared incisors may be accomplished. The anterior mandibular segment may be advanced at the time of surgery approximately 1.5 to 2 at the gingival margin without creating a periodontal defect. Additional space may be gained by placing a coil spring between the canine and 1st premolar teeth. During the postoperative period this will slowly expand the interdental space while maintaining periodontal health. The amount of advancement may be controlled via a ligature from the canine to premolar brackets. *A,* Preoperative appearance. Patient with anterior mandibular dental crowding, open bite, and reverse occlusal curve. Correction of the anterior mandibular crowding without extraction of premolar teeth was desirable owing to the lack of maxillary dental crowding. *B,* Surgical treatment plan demonstrating location of the osteotomies and direction of segmental movement. The cross-hatched area represents the amount of space to be developed between the segments after increasing arch length and uprighting the incisors.

arch length will facilitate postsurgical orthodontic treatment of crowded and malaligned teeth without extraction of premolars (Fig. 22–32). (See Chapter 10, Mandibular Deficiency for further details of surgical procedure to increase arch length.)

A surgical orthodontic approach can be considered which permits correction of the crowding and associated malocclusion by concentrating upon the abnormal arch. The technique consists of anterior subapical osteotomy within the crowded arch, without extraction of teeth, to advance a six- or eight-tooth dento-osseous segment. The advancement creates space at the osteotomy site and increases arch length, thereby facilitating orthodontic retraction of teeth in the advanced segment with resolution of

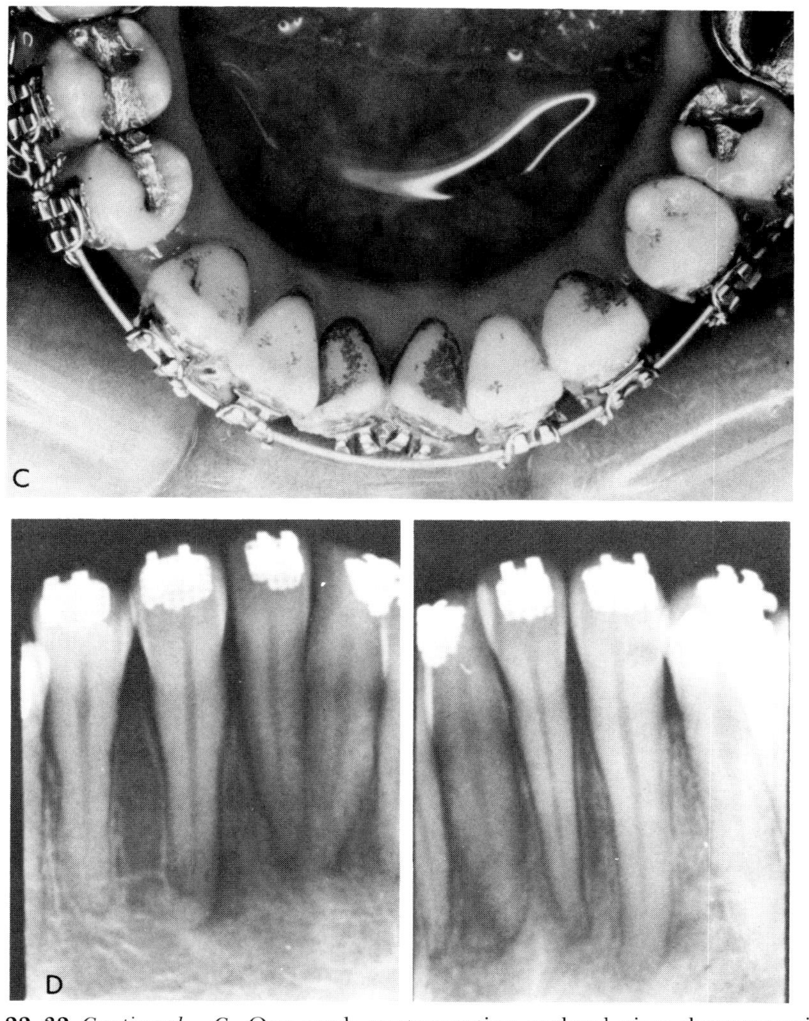

Figure 22–32 *Continued.* *C,* One-week postoperative occlusal view demonstrating the increased arch length and interdental spaces resulting from advancement of the six-tooth anterior segment. There is good periodontal health and integrity of the marginal gingiva. Additional controlled expansion of the space may be achieved by enlarging omega loops incorporated into the arch wire anterior to the molar band. *D,* Preoperative periapical radiographs of the planned osteotomy sites between the canine and 1st premolar teeth.

Illustration and legend continued on the following page

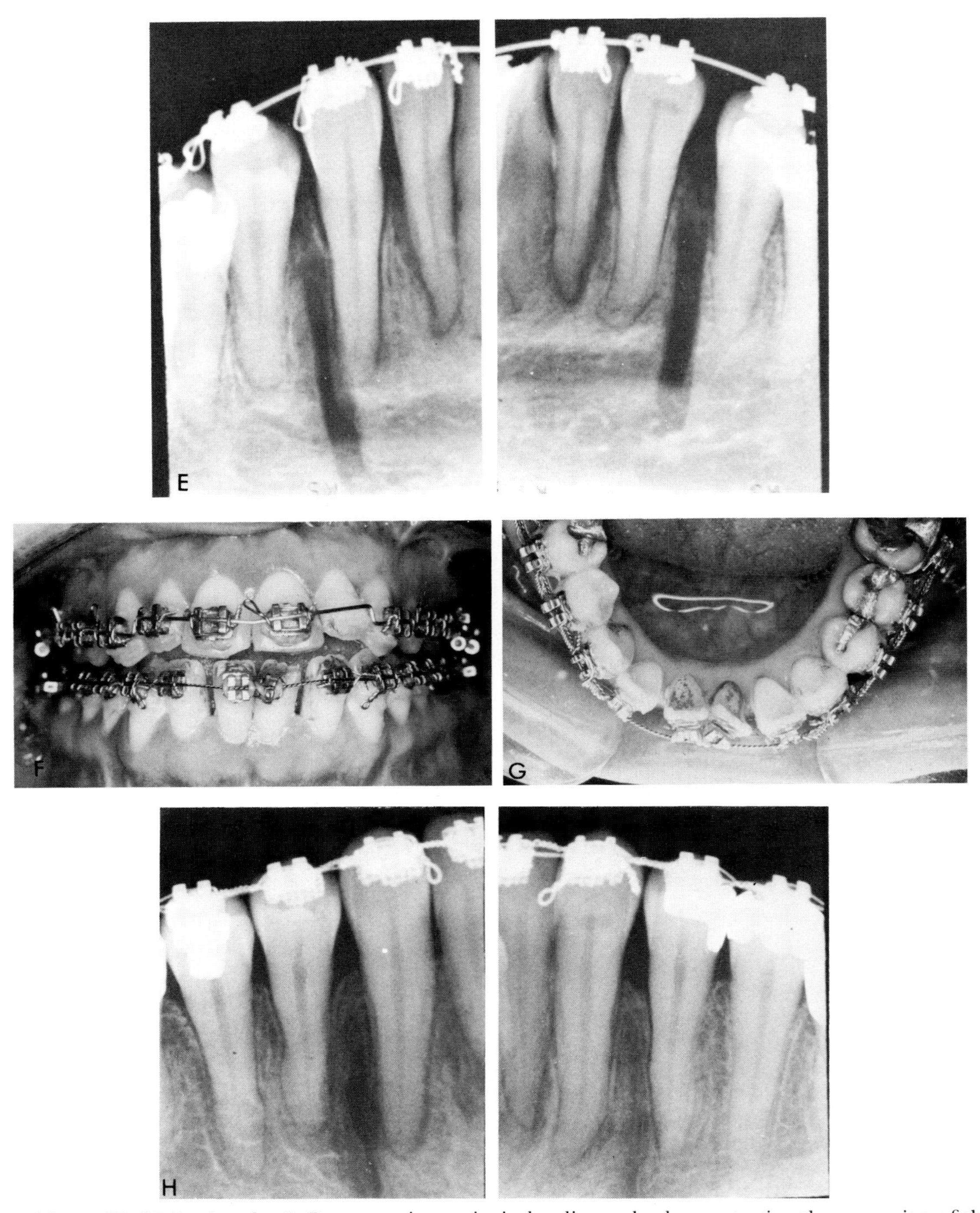

Figure 22–32 *Continued.* *E,* Postoperative periapical radiographs demonstrating the expansion of the segments and maintenance of interdental crestal bone adjacent to each tooth. *F,* and *G,* Four-month postoperative occlusion demonstrating closure of interdental spaces and correction of anterior dental crowding. *H,* Five-month postoperative periapical radiograph demonstrating consolidation of bone in interdental space and maintenance of normal interdental crestal bone height. (Surgeon: Kevin L. McBride, Dallas, Texas. Orthodontics by Frank Miller, Rockwall, Texas.)

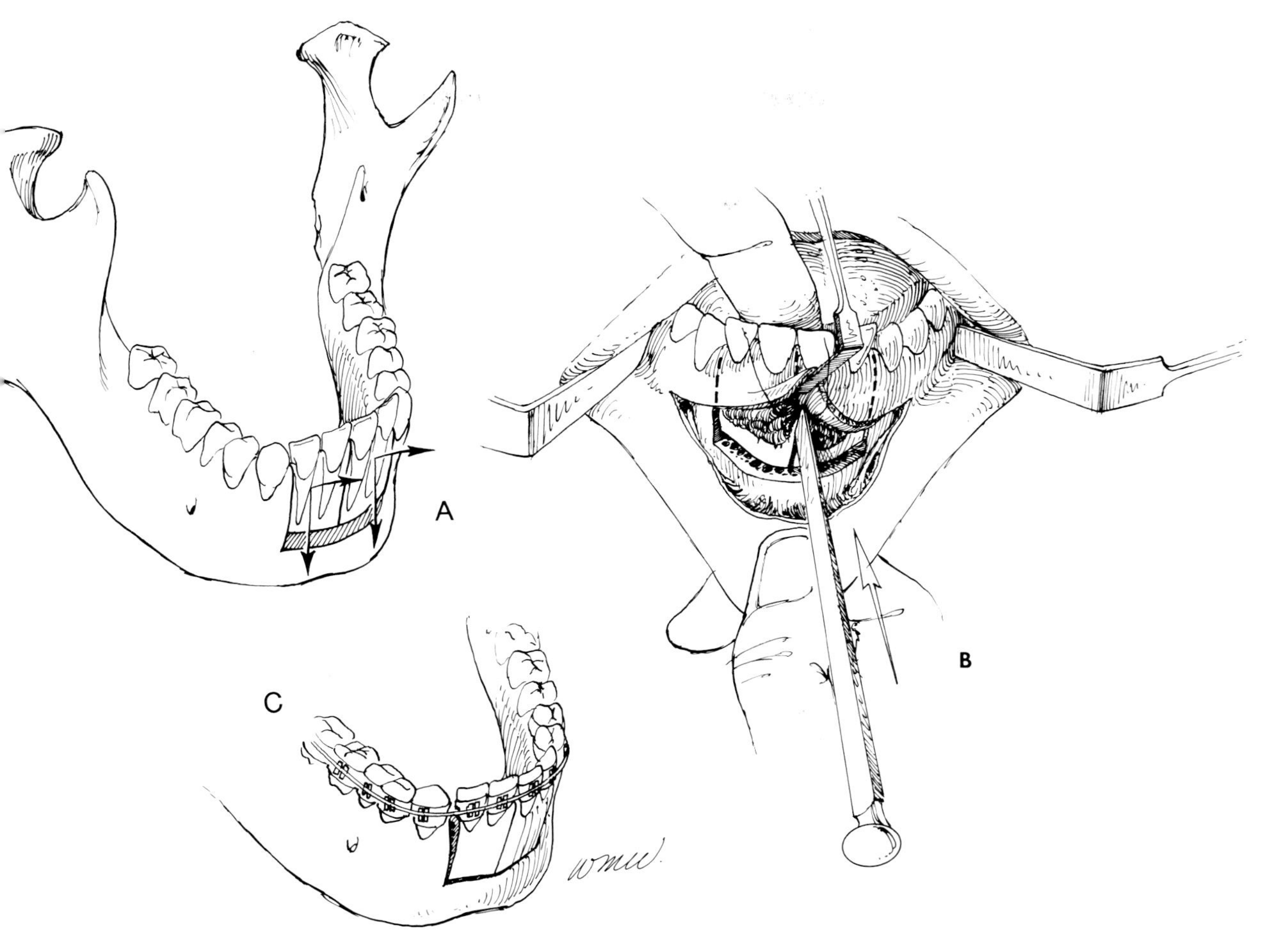

Figure 22–33. Leveling occlusal plane with anterior mandibular subapical osteotomy. *A,* Mandibular anterior subapical osteotomy with intrusion of supererupted anterior teeth may be employed to rapidly level an excessive mandibular occlusal curve. Simultaneous flaring or uprighting of the incisors may be accomplished. The specific occlusal deformity will dictate the number of interdental osteotomies, their location, and the appropriate direction and amount of segmental movement. This diagram illustrates correction of excessive mandibular occlusal curvature and retracted incisor teeth by simultaneous inferior repositioning and flaring of the four mandibular incisors in two segments. The cross-hatched area represents the amount of horizontal ostectomy and inferior repositioning of the incisors. *B,* A horizontal incision is utilized extending from the right 1st premolar to the left 1st premolar. The incision is made approximately 5 mm anterior to the depth of the labial mental fold and carried down through periosteum at the level of the proposed horizontal osteotomy. Care is taken to avoid damage to the branches of the mental nerve. The mucoperiosteum is elevated over the planned horizontal osteotomy sites while maintaining maximal soft-tissue pedicle to the mobilized segments. The horizontal ostectomy is performed, utilizing an oscillating saw or large bur. The inferior portions of the vertical osteotomies are performed with an oscillating saw or small bur while palpating the lingual mucoperiosteum to detect perforation of the lingual cortical plate. The bur or saw cut is carried to within 3 or 4 mm of the interdental crestal bone margin. The remaining bone is transected with a fine osteotome. The segments are mobilized until they can be repositioned into the planned location without tension on the soft-tissue pedicle. *C,* The segments are secured in their new position with a previously contoured mandibular arch wire or arch bar. It may be desirable to provide additional stabilization for the segments with transosseous wires along the horizontal osteotomy site or by securing an occlusal acrylic stent to the mandibular arch wire. Intermaxillary fixation is generally unnecessary. The incision is closed in layers with resorbable suture.

the crowding and malocclusion. The amount that the segment is to be advanced is determined preoperatively by the Bolton Analysis. If adequate interdental bone exists at the osteotomy site, the segment may be advanced immediately and stabilized with a heavy archwire and direct transosseous or circum-mandibular wiring. This approach is particularly useful when advancement of only a few millimeters is required bilaterally. If minimal interdental bone exists, or if advancement of more than a few millimeters is required, it is probably desirable to advance the segment posteroperatively by utilizing an orthodontic expansion appliance similar to that used for rapid palatal expansion. Slow postoperative advancement has the additional advantage of simplifying surgery because good periodontal integrity is maintained around the teeth adjacent to the osteotomy site during the expansion process. The segment is stabilized with an orthodontic appliance secured to the teeth prior to surgery. No transosseous or circum-mandibular wiring is utilized.

The advanced dento-osseous segment may be manipulated orthodontically to close the spaces at the osteotomy site while eliminating the crowding and coordinating the maxillary and mandibular arches. Additional soft-tissue facial support is gained from the advanced dento-osseous segment. Similar techniques can be used anywhere in the maxillary or mandibular arches to increase the arch length to facilitate correction of crowded and malaligned teeth or eruption of impacted teeth. Posterior maxillary or mandibular segments can be moved posteriorly to increase arch length and facilitate correction of malaligned or crowded anterior teeth in clinical situations where extractions are contraindicated.

Simultaneous leveling of the occlusal plane, by intrusion or extrusion of anterior dento-osseous segments, and increases in arch length may be accomplished with anterior mandibular subapical osteotomies (Fig. 22–33). This approach may produce substantial savings of time compared to treatment by orthodontics alone.[6]

ROTATED TEETH

Rotated teeth create problems in several different ways. By altering the normal marginal ridge relationship, rotation creates an abnormal contact area, and food impaction may develop. Rotations may produce intra-arch spacing problems by either increasing or decreasing the space occupied by a normally positioned tooth. Subsequent crowding of adjacent teeth, alteration of the normal tooth-bone-gingival architecture, and traumatic occlusal interference may occur. Rotated teeth are generally unesthetic because they create irregularities and asymmetries in the normal arch form.

Prosthetic or Orthodontic Correction

Minor rotations need not be corrected if they do not present an esthetic problem, form occlusal prematurities, or contribute to periodontal disease. When correction is desired it can be accomplished prosthetically or orthodontically. The prosthetic approach has the advantage of shorter treatment time and excellent stability. It does, however, sacrifice healthy tooth structure and may produce a somewhat compromised esthetic result. On the other hand, the orthodontic approach conserves tooth structure and produces an optimal esthetic result, but it is more time-consuming and has a greater propensity for relapse. In cases of moderate to severe rotation it is difficult to achieve an optimal result prosthetically. Not only is a good esthetic result difficult to achieve but the resultant abnormal crown form tends to contribute to periodontitis through the accumulation of plaque. The orthodontic rotation of teeth in adults may be technically difficult, time-consuming, and fraught with a tendency toward relapse. These problems may be reduced through the use of judicious complete interdental and subapical osteotomies. Surgery reduces the resistance of rotation caused by the cortical bone. Transection of transalveolar fibers and transseptal periodontal fibers tend to minimize relapse.

Surgical Correction of Rotated Teeth

The direction and magnitude of rotation of a dento-osseous segment must be considered carefully because of anatomic limitations to correction by surgery alone. In general, surgical techniques are used an an adjunct to orthodontic or restorative procedures. When orthodontic treatment is not available or is precluded by grossly aberrant tooth position, surgery may be an alternative method for correcting rotated teeth.

Interdental osteotomies should be performed through both the buccal and lingual cortical plates, with enough bone width removed to prevent impingement of the cut edges against one another as the dento-osseous segment is rotated. A complete subapical osteotomy connecting the two vertical interdental osteotomies is made simultaneously to achieve passive mobility of the dento-osseous segment.

The design of the soft-tissue incisions is based upon the direction and magnitude of movement and axis of rotation of the tooth to be repositioned (Fig. 22–34, *A* and *B*). The available space between the tooth or teeth to be rotated and the contiguous teeth, and the anatomy of the palatal vault are additional important considerations. Figure 22–34, *A* and *B* illustrates some of these technical considerations associated with surgical correction of rotated teeth by dentoalveolar surgery. Complete correction of the rotation by surgery alone may not be feasible unless there are continguous edentulous spaces. Indeed, excessive rotation may be impossible to correct by surgery alone (Fig. 22–35).

Simulation of the planned movements by model surgery and acetate overlay templates will indicate whether or not the surgical procedure is feasible, the amount of bone removal necessary, the osseous gaps to be created by surgery, and if there is a need for bone grafting of osseous defects. Autogenous particulate bone marrow grafts from the ilium or cancellous bone from other ostectomies are used to minimize loss of periodontal bone support.[33] Based upon these findings, an appropriate technique is selected (Fig. 22–34, *A* to *F*). Although it is ideal to design the bony and soft-tissue incisions to have the largest possible dento-osseous segment with a maximal soft-tissue pedicle, this is not necessarily feasible or desirable when surgically rotating a dentoalveolar segment (Fig. 22–34, *A* and *B*). The larger the segment the greater the bone reduction necessary to eliminate interferences as the segment is rotated. Because attached gingiva has more strength than free buccal mucosa, the more attached gingiva available on the buccal aspect of the segment to be mobilized, the less danger there is in compromising the circulation during manipulation.

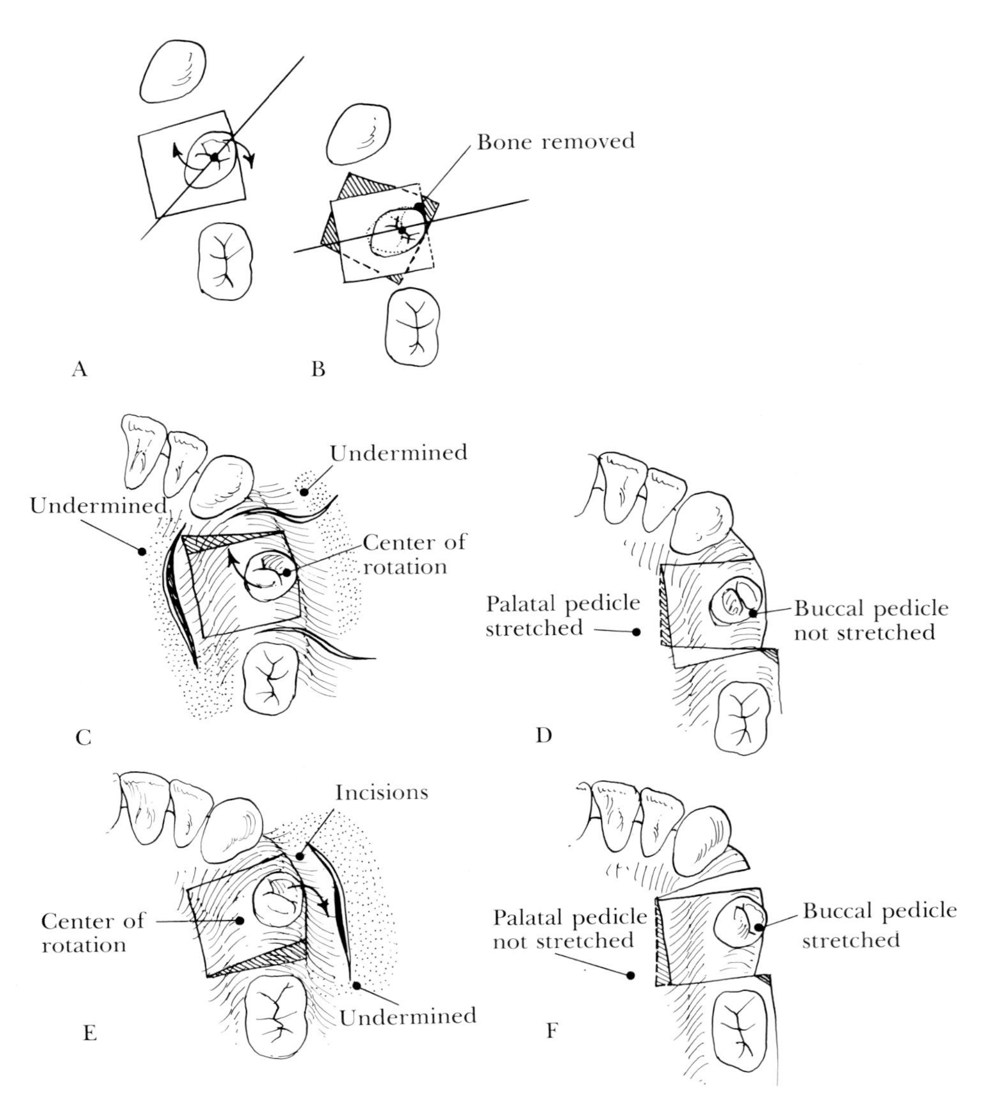

Figure 22–34. Surgical correction of a rotated tooth by dentoalveolar surgery. *A,* Rotated second premolar tooth associated with missing first molar and first premolar teeth. Solid lines indicate planned interproximal osteotomies; arrows indicate directional movement of segment; interproximal osteotomies are made 2 to 3 mm. away from root of the tooth to be repositioned and the contiguous teeth; axis of rotation is located in center of the tooth. *B,* Amount of bone removal necessary (cross-hatched area) to accomplish rotational movement and prevent impingement of the osteotomized margins against one another as the tooth is rotated. Axis of rotation is located in center of tooth. Movements can be stimulated with acetate overlays and model surgery. *C* and *D,* Surgical technique to maximize soft-tissue attachment to buccal aspect of dento-osseous segment when large rotational movement of palatal aspect of segment is necessary and palatal pedicle will be stretched; vertical incisions are placed opposite the planned interdental osteotomy sites and extend from the mucogingival junction superiorly to the depth of the vestibule and mucosal surface of the lip. Margins of vertical incisions are raised and retracted to expose planned interdental osteotomy and ostectomy sites. Margins of parasagittal palatal incisions are undermined to facilitate rotational movement of dentoalveolar segment; strippled areas indicate where mucoperiosteum has been detached to facilitate rotational movement and passive mobility. *E* and *F,* When the center of rotation is toward the palatal aspect of the segment, the inelastic palatal pedicle is minimally stretched; margin of horizontal incision is raised and retracted to allow necessary osteotomies.

When the planned rotation is small, any one of several basic surgical techniques for immediate respositioning of small dentoalveolar segments is feasible. When considerable rotation is needed and the axis of rotation is toward the buccal, the dento-osseous segment is pedicled primarily to the labial-buccal soft tissue (Fig. 22–34, *C* and *D*). The extensibility of this tissue, in contrast to the relatively inelastic palatal mucosa, allows rotational movement and passive repositioning of the dento-osseous segment. When there is a relatively small movement of the palatal aspect of the segment, the palatal pedicle is minimally stretched (Fig. 22–34, *E* and *F*).

CASE 22–4 (Fig. 22–35)

B.L., a 20-year-old man, was referred by his private dentist for surgical repositioning of two rotated, palatally displaced maxillary teeth prior to the construction of a left posterior fixed prosthesis.

Occlusal Analysis (Fig. 22–35, *A, B*)

Dental alignment and occlusion: Palatal crossbite of maxillary left canine and second premolar teeth, 45 degree rotation of second premolar, 15 degree rotation of canine, Class I molar, and canine.

TREATMENT PLAN

1. Maxillary interdental osteotomies anterior and posterior to left canine and second premolar teeth (Fig. 22–35 *E, F*) to:
   a. Round maxillary arch and correct constriction.
   b. Correct crossbite.
   c. Rotate maxillary left second premolar into better position.
   d. Equalize edentulous spaces to maximize the benefit of the second premolar as a pier for fixed prosthetics.
2. Fixation with an acrylated arch bar wired to the maxillary teeth only (Fig. 22–35 *G*).
3. Restoration of edentulous spaces with a fixed prosthesis.

FOLLOW-UP

Subjective

The patient had no postoperative complaints, was discharged from the hospital on the first postoperative day, and returned to work three days postoperatively.

Objective

Postoperative edema was minimal and there was essentially no postoperative pain. On the first postoperative day the patient was permitted to carefully eat soft foods. Healing during six weeks of fixation with the acrylic splint was uneventful, and immediately upon removal of the splint the osteotomized segments were found to be clinically stable and fixed prosthetics was begun. Periapical radiographs demonstrate excellent bone consolidation at the osteotomy sites after six months (Fig. 22–35 *I*).

Surgeon: Kevin L. McBride, Dallas, Texas. *Restorative dentistry.* Claude Ricks, Loma Linda, California.

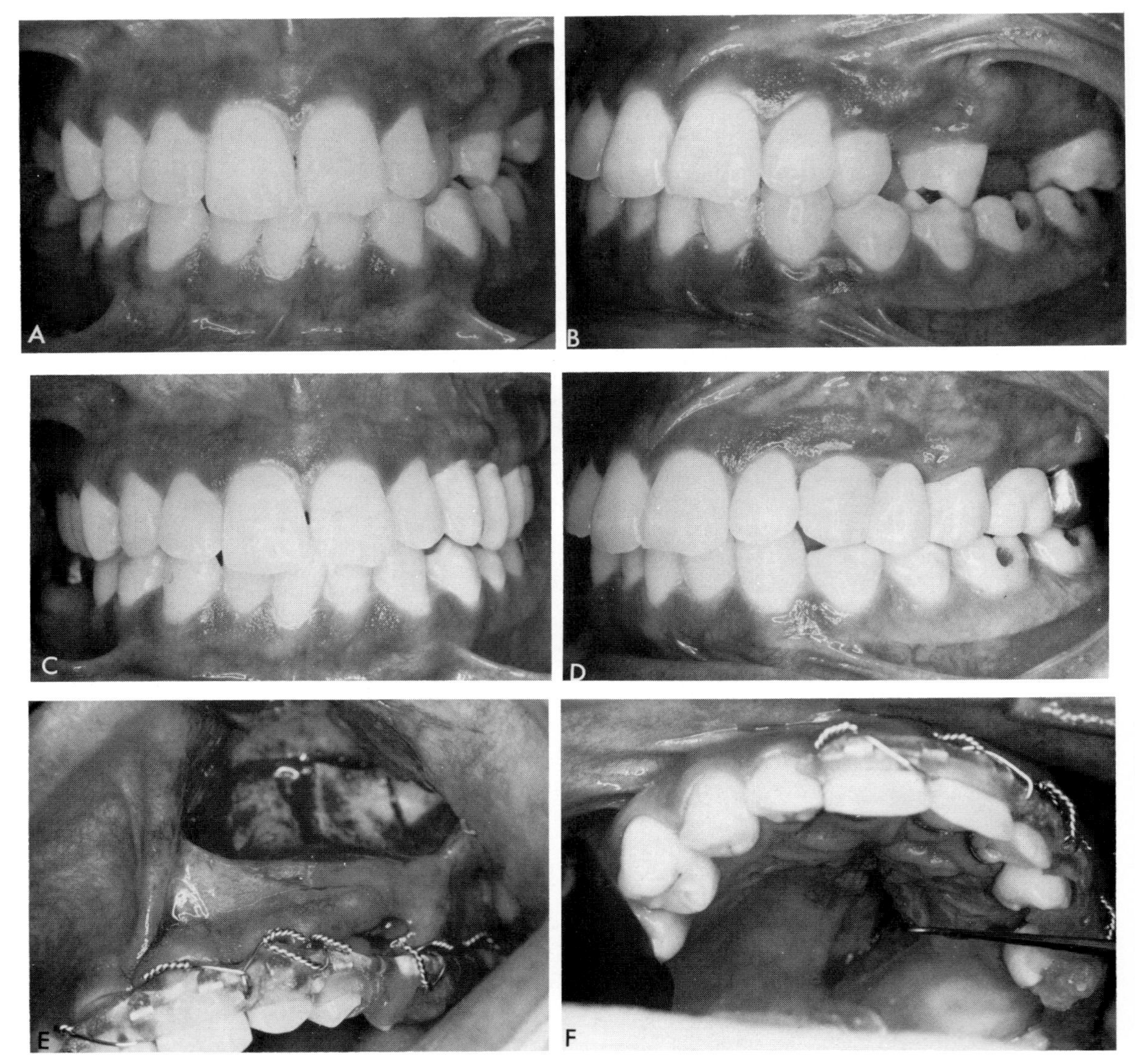

Figure 22–35 (Case 22–4). *A* and *B,* Preoperative occlusion showing maxillary left canine and second premolar rotation and palatal crossbite. *C* and *D,* Occlusion after subapical osteotomies around canine and second premolar with correction of crossbite and partial correction of rotation. Restoration of edentulous spaces with fixed bridge. *E* and *F,* Lateral and palatal incisions to facilitate osteotomies. *G,* Stabilization of repositioned dento-osseous segments with acrylated arch bar — mobilized teeth retained out of occlusion to eliminate occlusal trauma and permit less tooth reduction during crown preparation. *H,* Occlusal view showing improved lateral position of canine and 2nd premolar teeth and partial correction of rotations. *I,* Six-month postoperative radiographs showing consolidation of bone at interdental osteotomy sites.

See illustration on the opposite page.

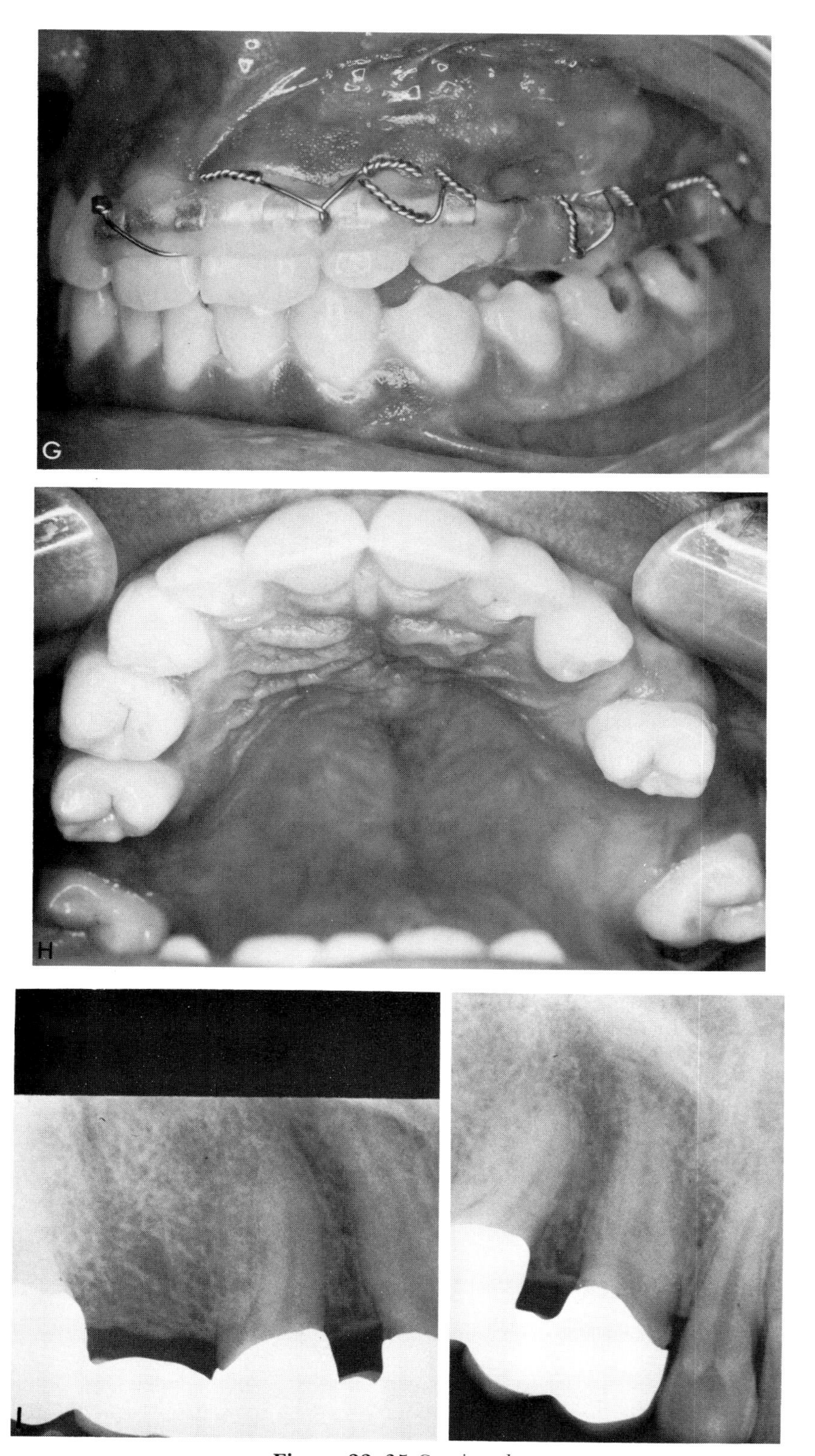

Figure 22–35 *Continued.*

ANKYLOSED TEETH

Ankylosed teeth are problems to the patient and restorative dentist because the individual tooth fails to erupt into a normal occlusal relationship with the opposing arch. As a consequence, there is shifting of the adjacent teeth, supereruption of the opposing teeth, and crowding around the ankylosed tooth. Periodontal defects are the hallmarks

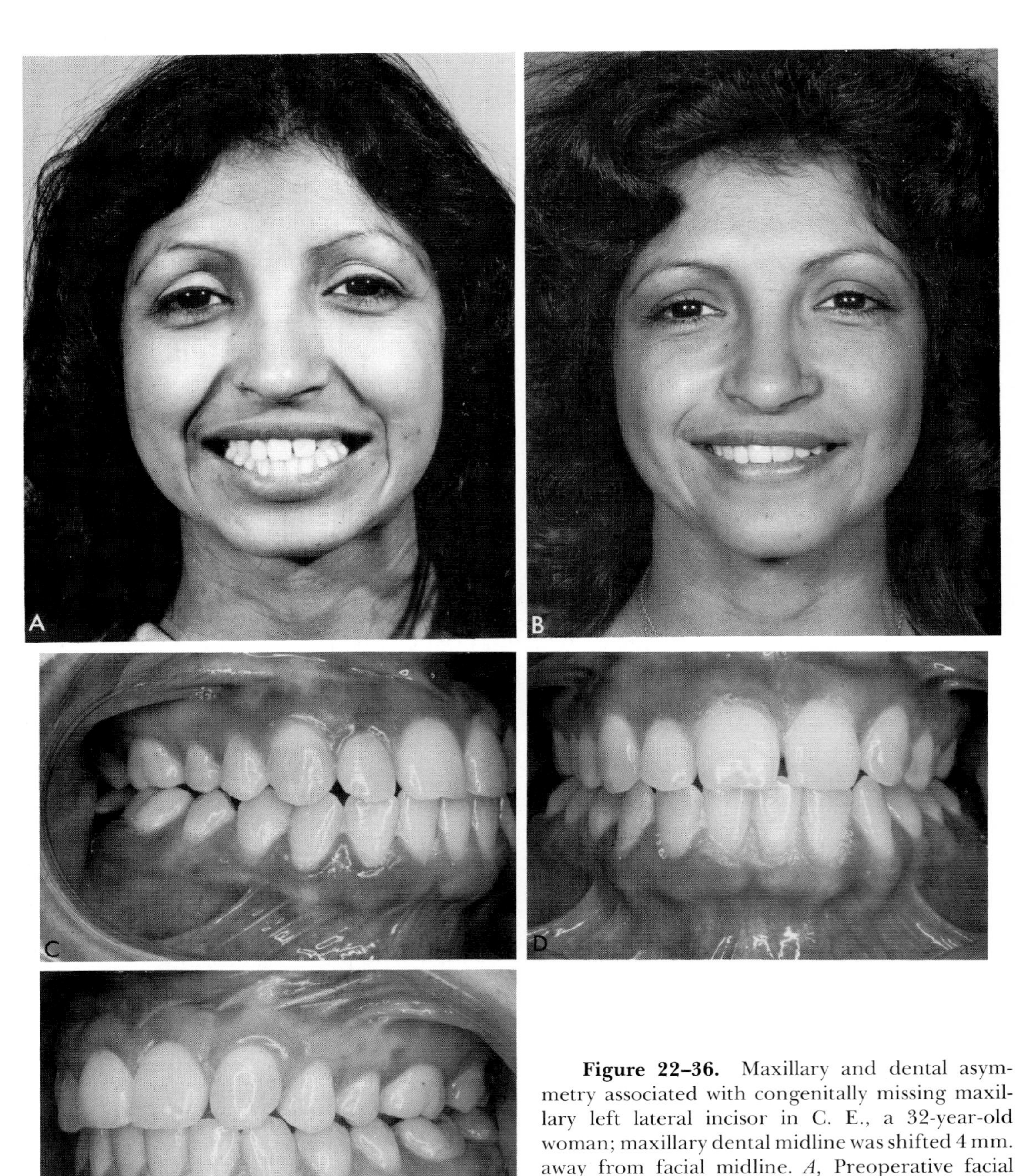

Figure 22–36. Maxillary and dental asymmetry associated with congenitally missing maxillary left lateral incisor in C. E., a 32-year-old woman; maxillary dental midline was shifted 4 mm. away from facial midline. *A*, Preoperative facial appearance. *B*, Postoperative facial appearance sion before surgery. (Surgery by Barry Acker and William H. Bell.)

of such teeth. Prosthetic restoration of the tooth without surgical repositioning of the ankylosed tooth and uprighting of the adjacent teeth compromises the restorative dentist's efforts. Because orthodontic movement of ankylosed teeth is usually not possible without some type of surgical intervention, ankylosed teeth in adults are repositioned by surgical means after complete interdental and subapical osteotomies (Fig. 22–36).

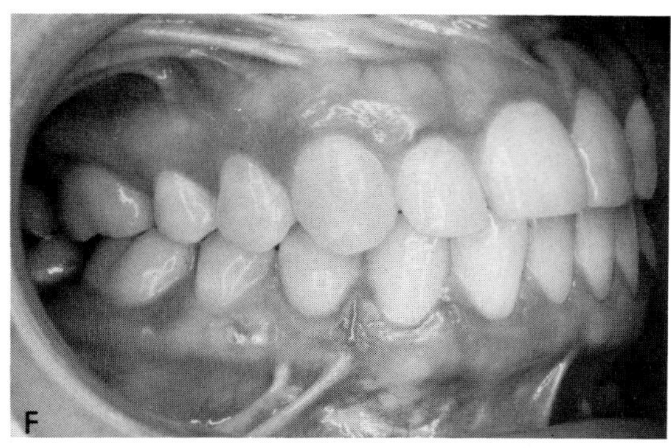

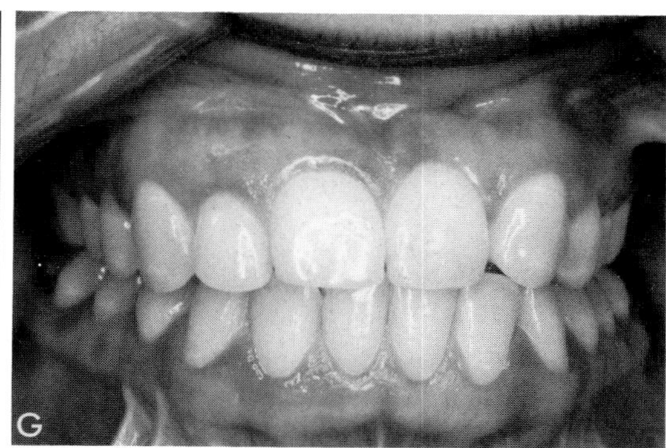

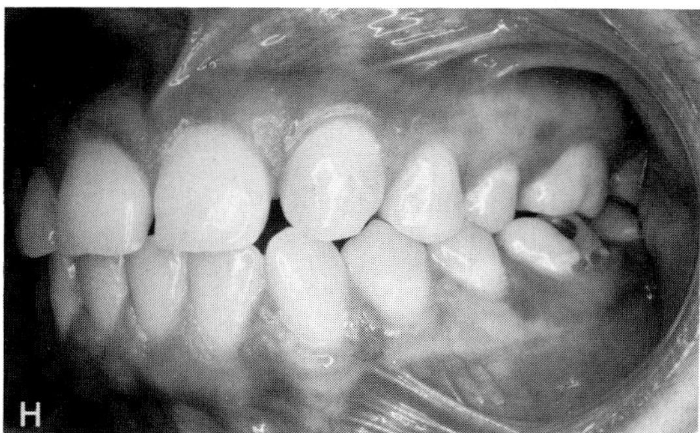

Figure 25–36 *Continued.* *F–H,* Occlusion after surgical procedure illustrated in *I. I,* Schematic view of Le Fort I osteotomy (four segments) to correct maxillary dental and skeletal asymmetry; broken line indicates facial midline; solid lines indicate osteotomy sites; arrows indicate directional movement of maxillary segments, which were predominantly rotational; maxilla was sectioned into four segments (one-tooth, three-tooth, four-tooth, and five-tooth dento-osseous segments) to achieve best possible interdigitation of teeth. Final occlusal result was achieved by restorative dentist, who jacketed the left canine tooth to stimulate the missing lateral incisor and reshaped the left first premolar tooth to resemble the contralateral canine.

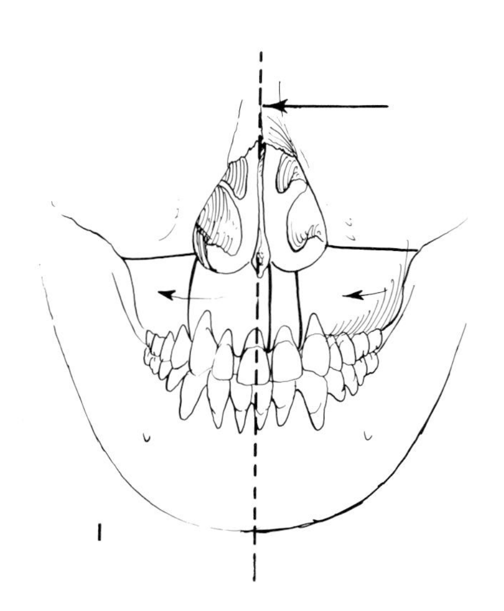

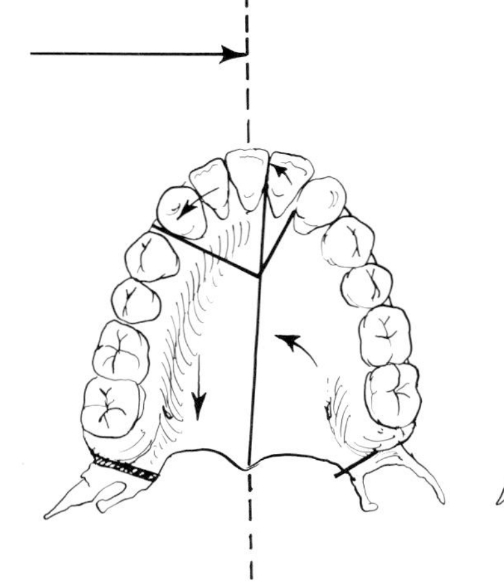

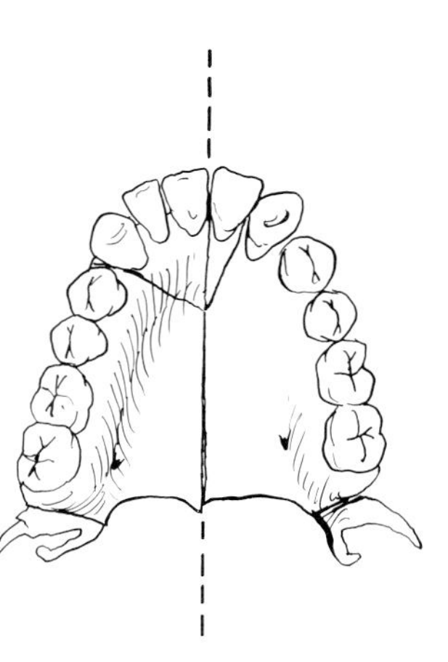

Surgical Techniques for Immediate Repositioning of Ankylosed Tooth (Fig. 22–37)

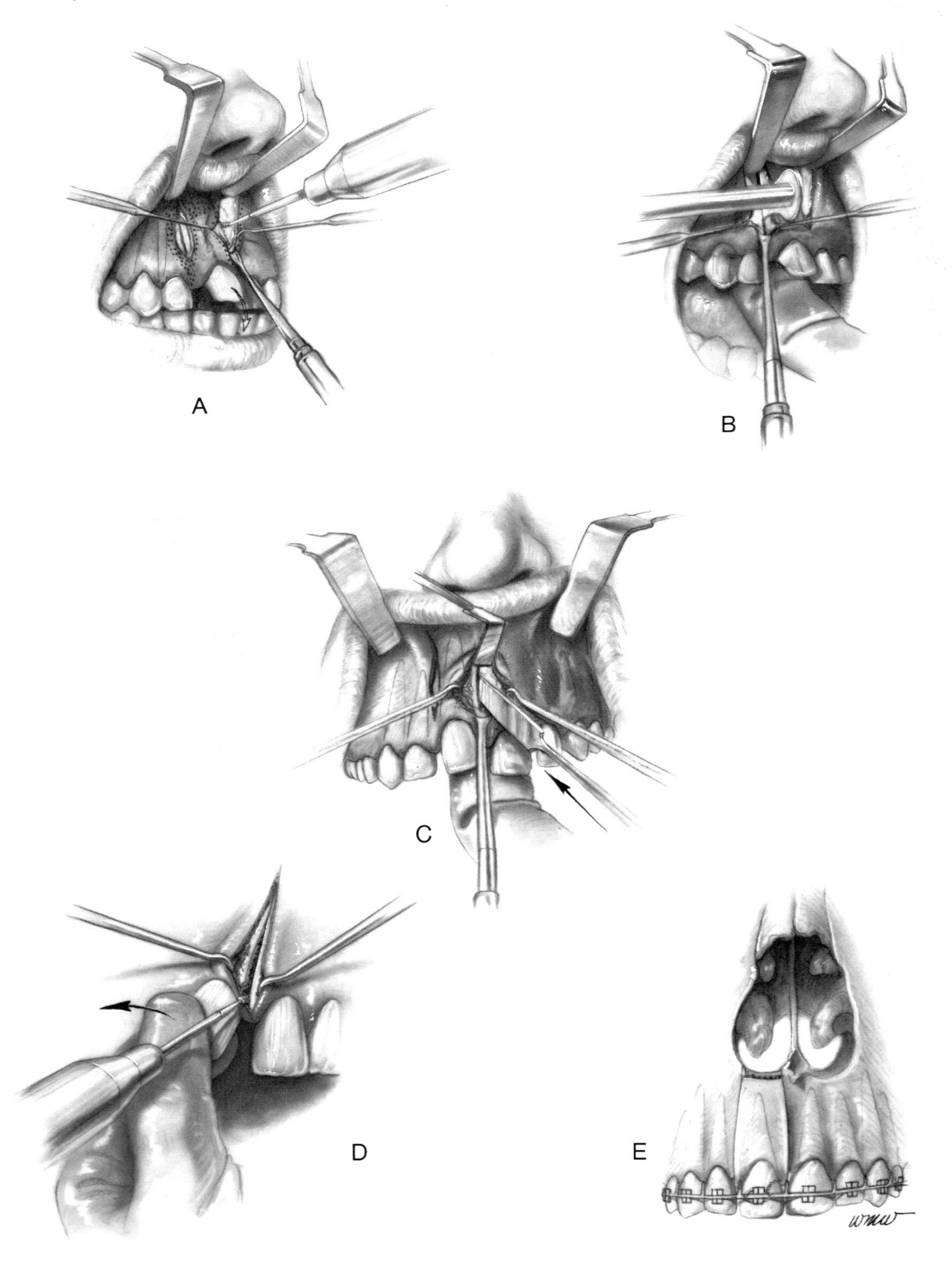

Figure 22–37. Surgical techniques for immediate repositioning of ankylosed tooth. *A,* Vertical incisions are placed opposite the planned interdental osteotomy sites. Incisions are carried superiorly into the depth of the vestibule and mucosal surface of the upper lip. This provides access to the piriform aperture and permits reflection of the nasal mucosa from the floor of the nose. Margins of labial vertical incisions are raised and retracted to expose planned interdental osteotomy sites and piriform rim; stippling indicates areas of detached gingiva and mucoperiosteum. Proposed interdental osteotomy is etched into interproximal bone with fissure bur. Care is taken to avoid elevating more periosteum than is necessary to provide access for the bone incisions. *B,* Interdental osteotomy accomplished with oscillating saw blade superiorly to the piriform aperture; nerve retractor is placed inferiorly to facilitate visualization and prevent injury of attached gingiva by saw blade. Finger is positioned on palate to feel oscillating saw blade and transect bone without injuring palatal mucosa. Superiorly, the interdental osteotomy is deepened into the spongiosa; more inferiorly, the interdental osteotomy is made through the cortical alveolar bone only. *C,* Osteotome is malleted into inter-radicular area until the osteotome transects the palatal bone; the osteotome is then malleted into the interseptal area between the central incisors to fracture crestal alveolar bone. Digital pressure on the palatal mucosa indicates when the osteotome has transected the palatal cortex. This is important so as not to badly damage or strip palatal mucoperiosteum, the principal blood supply to the mobilized dental-osseous segment. *D,* The removal of small segments of interdental and subapical bone (when indicated) is accomplished with the use of a fissure bur *after* the dento-osseous segment has been made freely movable with an osteotome and digital manipulation. Direct visualization of both sides of the osteotomized bone facilitates instrumentation of the lingual and interproximal areas, prevents excessive removal of interdental bone, and lessens the possibility of damage to the contiguous teeth and periodontium. Great care must be exercised to maintain a palatal soft tissue pedicle to the mobilized segments. *E,* The mobilized segment is placed into the preoperatively determined occlusal relationship with the aid of an acrylic occlusal wafer. The segment is then fixed by ligating the bracket on the dento-osseous segment to an orthodontic arch wire. This method of fixation obviates the need for immobilization of the mandible and allows the free gingival margin to be sutured into its normal position.

ADULT MALOCCLUSIONS

Prosthetic Considerations in Interarch Relationships

Crossbite

Prosthetic restoration of single or multiple teeth in buccolingual crossbite may be problematic for the restorative dentist.[17] Such conditions frequently receive compromised treatment by over- or under-contouring crowns; by restoration of the teeth in crossbite, which may be unesthetic or lead to cross-arch occlusal interference; or by endodontic filling of healthy teeth followed by post crowns in an attempt to compensate for the transverse disparity. Crossbites may predispose to periodontitis because of the abnormal occlusal relationship and may necessitate extraction of noncarious teeth to facilitate fixed or removable prosthetic appliances. Cross-arch or balancing occlusal interferences may exist in unrestored teeth and, when combined with primary occlusal traumatism, can lead to periodontal failure.

Orthodontic correction of crossbite may range from routine to impossible. A single anterior tooth in lingual crossbite may be corrected with a simple appliance incorporating a bite block and palatal finger spring. On the other hand, a full posterior unilateral palatal crossbite may present the orthodontist with an impossible task. To position the teeth in an acceptable occlusal relationship by conventional orthodontics, it may be necessary to ignore the tenet of tooth placement over the center of the ridge and move the teeth close to the buccal or lingual cortices, thus making them even more susceptible to periodontal destruction. These problems are alleviated by surgical repositioning of maxillary basal bone by posterior maxillary osteotomy. This is a very predictable procedure which increases arch length and width.

Single-stage or two-stage repositioning of dento-osseous segments affords the restorative dentist the opportunity to formulate a treatment plan that will allow restoration of the teeth in an ideal buccolingual relationship to minimize the chance of prosthetic or periodontal failure. (See Case 5 and Figure 22–38.) Prior to surgical repositioning of small dento-osseous segments, it is desirable to orthodontically correct tooth rotations and achieve sufficient interdental space in the planned interdental osteotomy site. Following orthodontic alignment, periapical or occlusal radiographs or both are necessary to determine the exact position for the osteotomy.

CASE 22–5 (Fig. 22–38)

G.B., a 41-year-old veteran, was referred by his general dentist for a surgical procedure to correct his malocclusion, prior to fabrication of crown and bridge restorations.

EVALUATION

Esthetics

Frontal. Constricted maxilla with inadequate maxillary tooth exposure and canted occlusal plane when smiling (Fig. 22–38*A*).

Profile. Slight flatness in infraorbital and nasal base regions (Fig. 22–38 *B*).

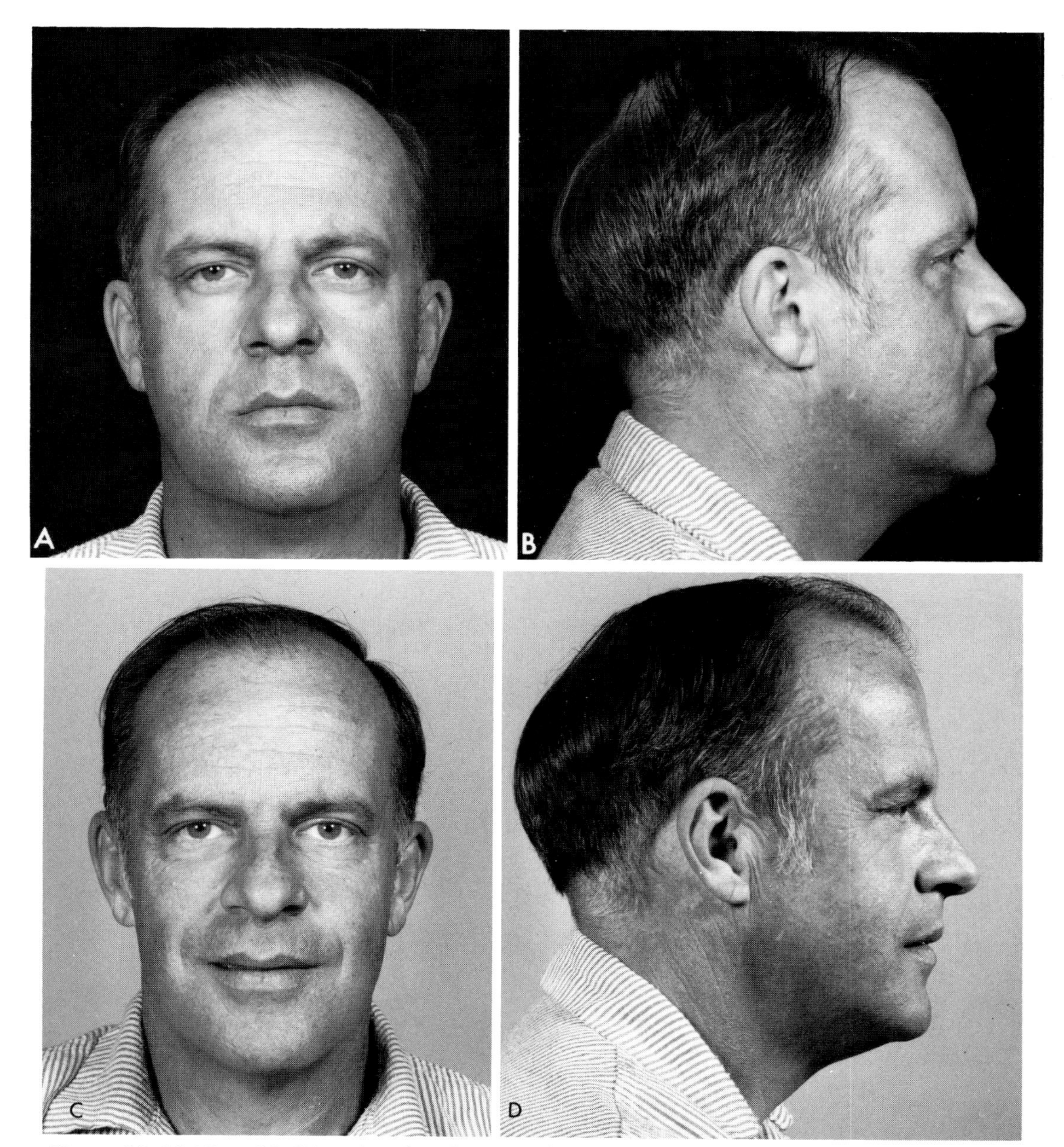

Figure 22–38 (Case 22–35). *A* and *B*, Preoperative appearance. *C* and *D*, Appearance 1 year after surgical procedures illustrated in *I*.

Illustration and legend continued on the following page

Cephalometric Evaluation

1. Relative maxillary deficiency — SNA = 81°, SNB = 82°

Occlusal Analysis (Fig. 22–38 *E, F*)

Dental Arch Form. Maxilla and mandible symmetric; maxilla constricted with left cuspid and first premolar outside of arch.

Dental Alignment. Anterior maxillary crowding and mandibular interdental spacing.

Dental Occlusion. Class III malocclusion bilaterally; total maxillary palatal crossbite with exception of left cuspid and first premolar; missing maxillary right first and second molars and left second molar teeth; missing mandibular right first and left second molar teeth. Mandibular dental midline 2 mm to the right of facial midline. Poor occlusal interdigitation. Premature centric relation contact producing 2 mm anterior slide into centric occlusion.

TREATMENT PLAN (Fig. 22–38 *I*)

Le Fort I osteotomy in three segments to advance (2.5 mm) and expand (5 mm) the maxilla to:

1. Correct anterior and posterior crossbites.
2. Level the occlusal plane.
3. Correct the maxillary left lateral–cuspid tooth alignment.

Dental restorations.

FOLLOW-UP

Subjective

Postoperatively the patient had no complaints and required no medication for pain.

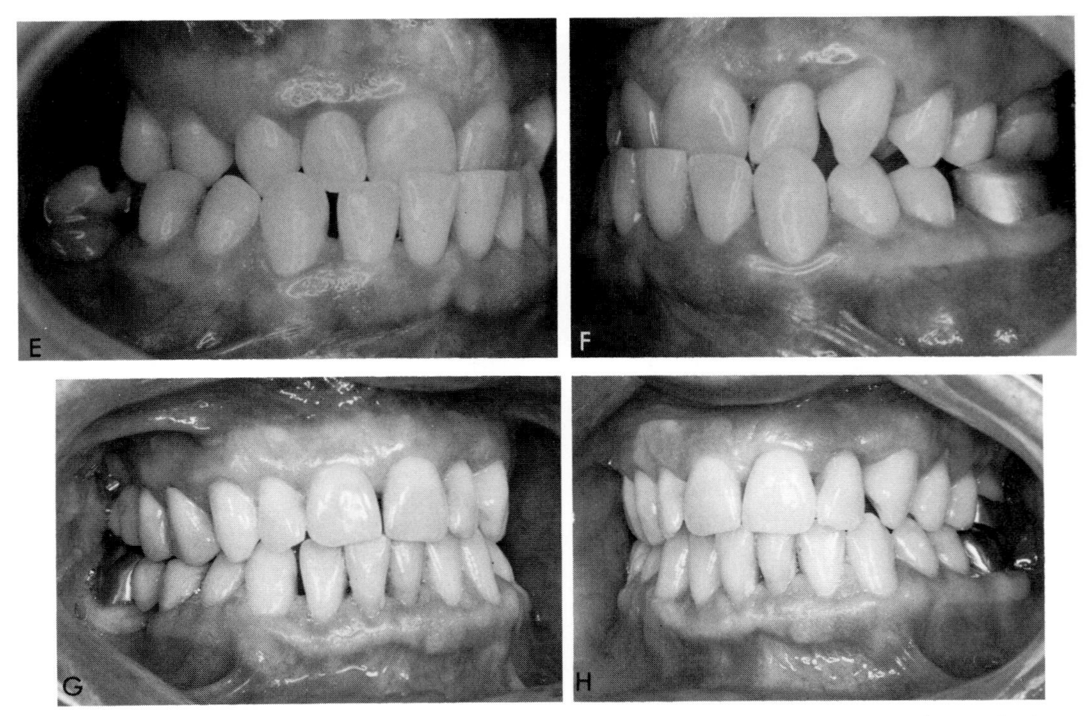

Figure 22–38 *Continued.* *E* and *F*, Preoperative occlusion. *G* and *H*, Postoperative occlusion after restoration of edentulous spaces with fixed bridges.

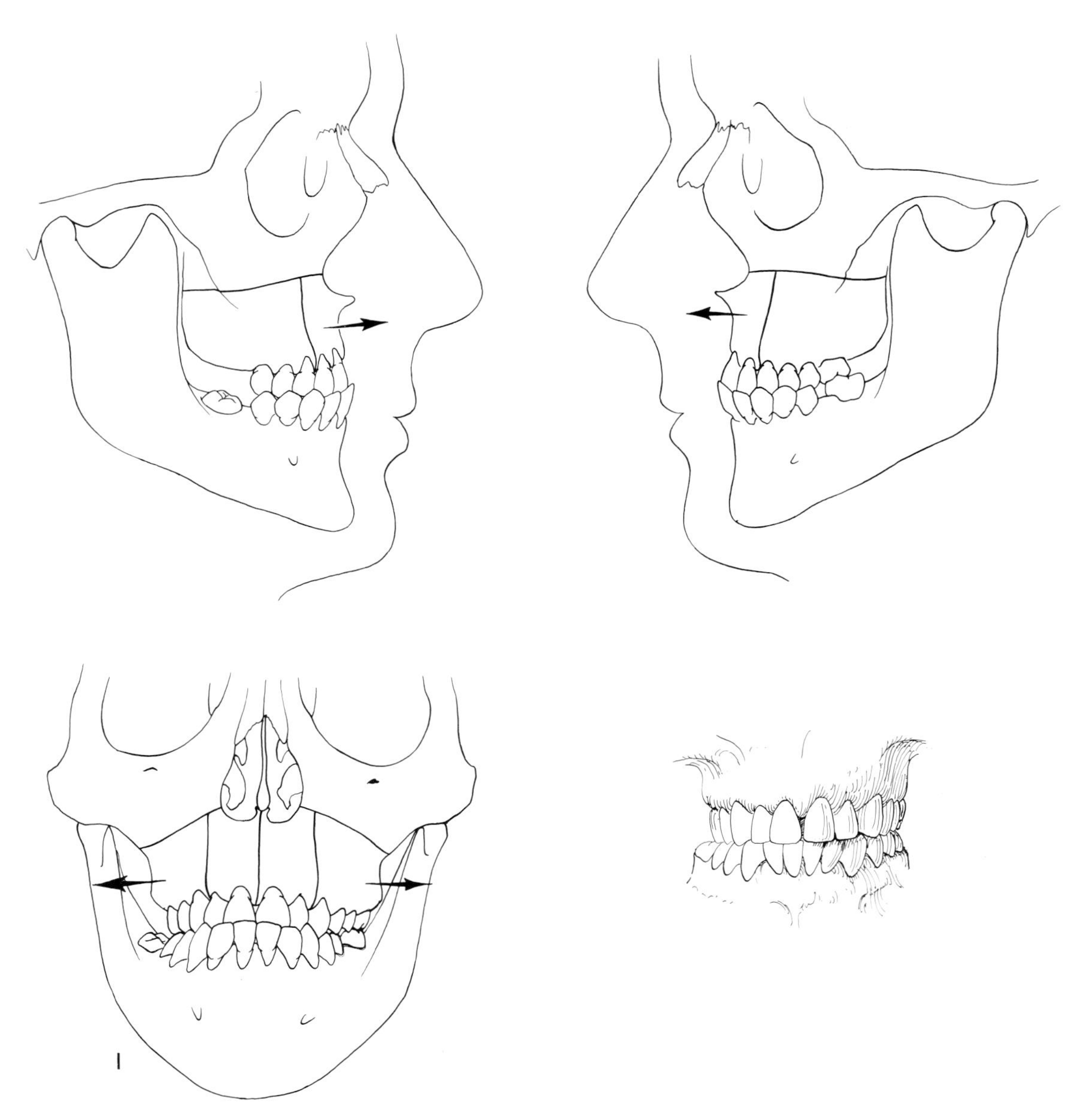

Figure 22–38 *Continued.* *I,* Schematic illustration of surgical treatment: Le Fort I osteotomy in three pieces with advancement and expansion.

Objective

Postoperative course and healing were uneventful. Intermaxillary fixation was released three weeks postoperatively. Manipulation revealed 1 mm vertical mobility at this time. Elastic intermaxillary fixation was maintained for 15 to 18 hours per day for the next three weeks. Good clinical union without mobility was present six weeks postoperatively. In order to establish good cuspid interdigitation bilaterally the maxillary midline was shifted 3 mm to the right, which placed the dental midline about 2 mm to the right of facial midline. This was not ideal, but was a minor compromise compared to the major mandibular surgical or orthodontic treatment needed to prevent this from occurring.

COMMENTS

Surgery provided the most rapid means of establishing normal dento-osseous and occlusal relationships prior to restorative dental procedures. Elimination of the crossbite and Class III malocclusion permitted restoration of the occlusion to a state of functional harmony by establishing balancing contacts and greatly improving functional contacts. Proper tooth interdigitation also removed premature occlusal contacts and poor sluice-ways, thereby eliminating these potentially destructive influences on the periodontium.

Owing to the minimal maxillary anterior movement, profile esthetics were essentially unchanged. Frontal esthetics were improved slightly during smiling as a result of the expanded maxillary arch; however, the lip-tooth relationship remained unchanged because of the adynamic upper lip.

Surgeons: Kevin L. McBride and Craig Williams, Dallas, Texas. *Restorative dentistry:* Claude Ricks, Loma Linda, California.

Because surgical techniques designed to reposition small dento-osseous segments should maintain maximal palatal or lingual bone and soft tissue attachment, the segments are often pie-shaped and preclude a large movement or rotation of greater than a few degrees. Various designs of soft-tissue incisions are described for repositioning small dento-osseous segments. The bone incisions for single-stage procedures are usually accomplished through vertical or horizontal incisions. When parasagittal palatal incisions are necessary, they are usually made in concert with vertical buccal mucosal incisions.

Using a bur or oscillating saw, osseous incisions are carried through cortex and medullary bone to a point about 5 mm above the interdental bone crest. The crestal interseptal bone is divided with a fine tapered osteotome. Care is taken to bisect the interdental septae at the height of the alveolus to preclude fracturing cortical bone away from the roots of teeth. In clinical practice, however, this is frequently not possible. When the interdental crestal bone is split with an osteotome, it does not have a discernible effect on the periodontium.

Fixation of small dento-osseous segments is accomplished with a preformed acrylic appliance, a heavy rectangular arch wire, or an acrylated arch bar.

Large dento-osseous segments are repositioned by the classic techniques of posterior maxillary osteotomy or anterior maxillary and mandibular osteotomy (Chapter 8).[17, 18, 34, 36, 38] The vascular pedicle to posterior mandibular segments may be more tenuous because of the lack of muscle attached above the mylohyoid muscle and the proximity of the inferior alveolar neurovascular bundle to the subapical bone cut. The basic principle of maximizing bone and soft-tissue attachment to the mobilized segment apply. Stabilization of a multiple-tooth dento-osseous segment may require a more rigid appliance, suspension wire, and, indeed, in some cases intermaxillary fixation.

Morbidity associated with the procedure is principally related to devitalization of teeth, mechanical damage to teeth, or injury to the periodontium. Devitalization of teeth and bone may occur if the circulation to the segment is severely compromised. The possibility of this occurring is minimized by careful preoperative planning and execution of surgery. Mechanical damage to the teeth themselves may occur, but because of the periodontal vascular plexus and the great propensity of the cementum to repair itself, it does not necessarily cause a clinical problem. Such problems can be prevented by preoperative orthodontics to widen interdental spaces, and careful identification of tooth roots intraoperatively so that the osteotomy is placed and directed as planned. Primary or secondary damage to the periodontium is probably the most common problem associated with repositioning small dento-osseous segments. As noted above, fractures of the interdental septae which do not maintain a soft-tissue pedicle can devascularize and devitalize the supporting bone and eventuate in avascular necrosis, sequestration, and loss of bone.

The use of segmental procedures to correct crossbites of all types provides a predictable and relatively uncomplicated means of correcting many adult malocclusions. (See Case 22–6 and Fig. 22–39.)

CASE 22–6 (Fig. 22–39)

A 17-year-old female (T.J.) was initially seen for treatment of carious mandibular first molar teeth. She complained of her malocclusion for which she desired correction. A problem list was formulated from the appropriate records.

PROBLEM LIST

Esthetics

Frontal. Deficient nasolabial and nasomaxillary areas.
Profile. Obtuse and deficient nasolabial area (Fig. 22–39 *A*); disharmony between upper and lower lips because of everted lower lip; prominent lower face.

Cephalometric Analysis

Mandibular plane angle (SN to GoGn = 31°); upright maxillary incisors; SNA = 80° SNB = 82°; ANB = –2°.

Occlusal Analysis (Fig. 22–39 *C*)

Arch Form. Maxilla and mandible U-shaped; low palatal vault.
Alignment. Crowded and retroclined maxillary anterior teeth.
Occlusion. Anterior crossbite; Class I malocclusion; 2 mm anteroposterior discrepancy between centric occlusion and centric relation.

TREATMENT PLAN*

1. Extraction of carious mandibular first molar teeth and subsequent prosthetic replacement.
2. Interdental osteotomy of palatal cortical bone between the four anterior maxillary teeth.
3. Presurgical orthodontic treatment: banding of posterior maxillary teeth.
4. Anterior maxillary interdental osteotomies to:
   a. Correct the anterior crossbite.

---

*Orthodontic treatment by Peter Paulus, Fort Worth, Texas; surgery by Larry Snider, Denver, Colorado.

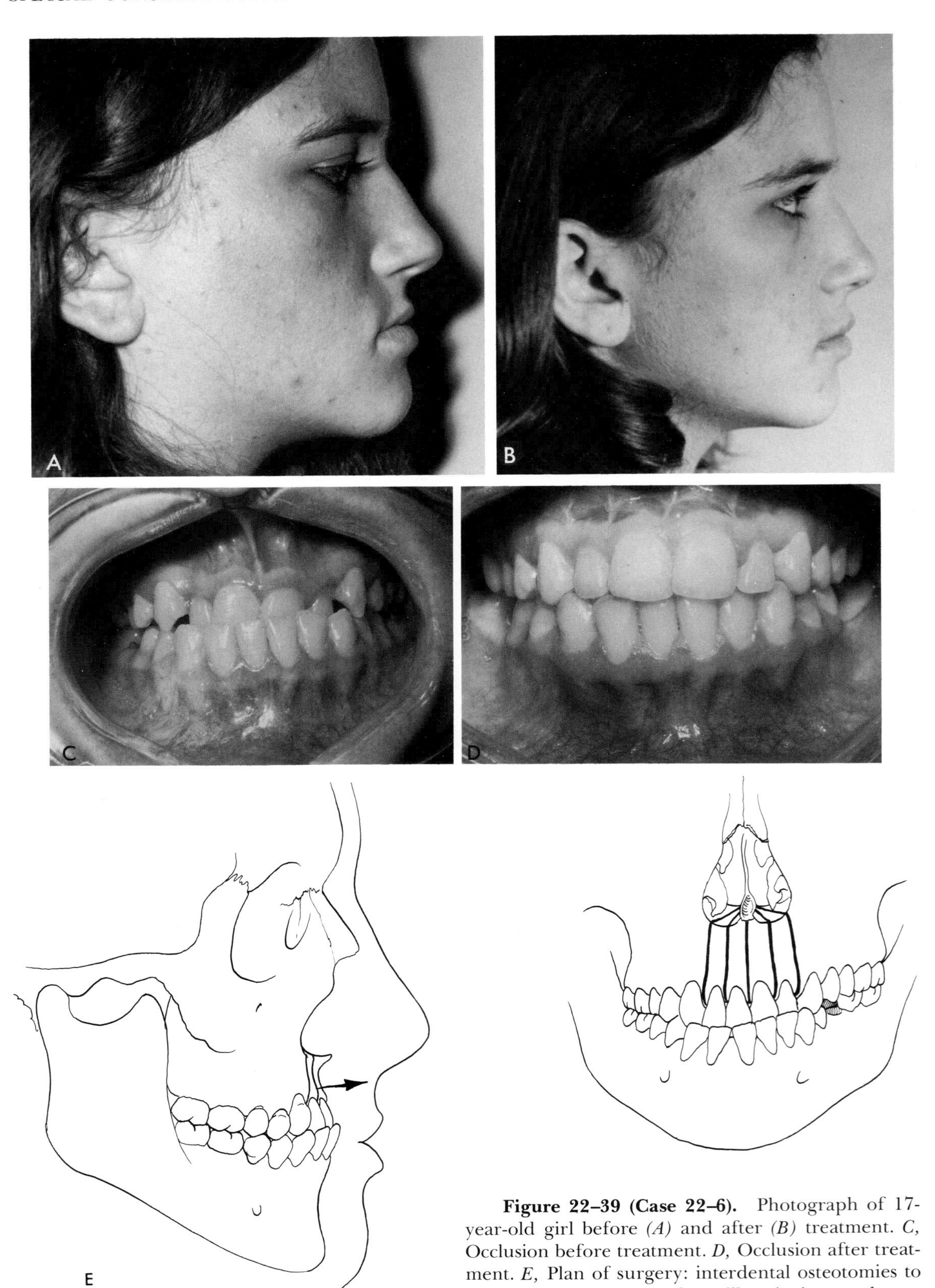

Figure 22–39 (Case 22–6). Photograph of 17-year-old girl before *(A)* and after *(B)* treatment. *C,* Occlusion before treatment. *D,* Occlusion after treatment. *E,* Plan of surgery: interdental osteotomies to facilitate repositioning of maxillary incisor teeth.

b. Achieve harmony between centric relation and centric occlusion.
c. Reduce lower facial prominence.
d. Reduce the obtuse nasolabial angle and increase prominence of upper lip.

5. Postsurgical orthodontic treatment: banding of the maxillary incisor teeth and placement of a labial arch wire to align the incisor teeth.

FOLLOW-UP

Subjective

The palatal and labial interdental osteotomies were accomplished in two stages to decrease the possibility of injury to the closely aligned anterior maxillary teeth (Fig. 22–39 *E*). The incisors were mobilized and repositioned at the second stage of surgery. With the crossbite corrected, the mandible could assume a stable centric and class I canine relationship. (Fig. 22–39 *D*).

Objective

Healing was uneventful and associated with minimal postoperative morbidity. The splint that was ligated to the maxillary arch was removed after two weeks. The maxillary incisor teeth were then banded and active orthodontics was carried out for two months to effect the necessary alignment of the maxillary incisor teeth. Within two months after the dento-osseous segments were repositioned, the segments were stable. A 12-month postoperative radiographic study has shown no loss of crestal alveolar bone in the interdental osteotomy sites or resorption of the roots of the repositioned maxillary incisor teeth.

Transverse and Anteroposterior Interarch Relationship in Partially Edentulous Patients

The importance of tooth position in a denture is stressed by all prosthodontists. Every attempt is made to place the prosthetic teeth directly over the residual ridge. Denture instability and secondary bone resorption are a predictable result of compromised occlusion or tooth position necessitated by abnormal ridge relationships in a transverse or anteroposterior direction. Because of the documented pattern of alveolar resorption in edentulous or partially edentulous patients, the anteroposterior ridge relationship may become Class III while the transverse relationship is altered so that the mandibular ridges are lateral to the maxillary ridges. Since denture stability depends on resistance to vertical and lateral stress, an ideal transverse and anteroposterior relationship of the arches results in a more functional and less destructive prosthesis. A very common indication for anterior mandibular subapical osteotomy occurs in individuals whose natural teeth function against a complete upper denture. The resultant Class III ridge relationship can be improved by surgical retraction of the mandibular anterior teeth and/or advancement of the edentulous maxilla by Le Fort I osteotomy. (See Case 22–7 and Fig. 22–40.)

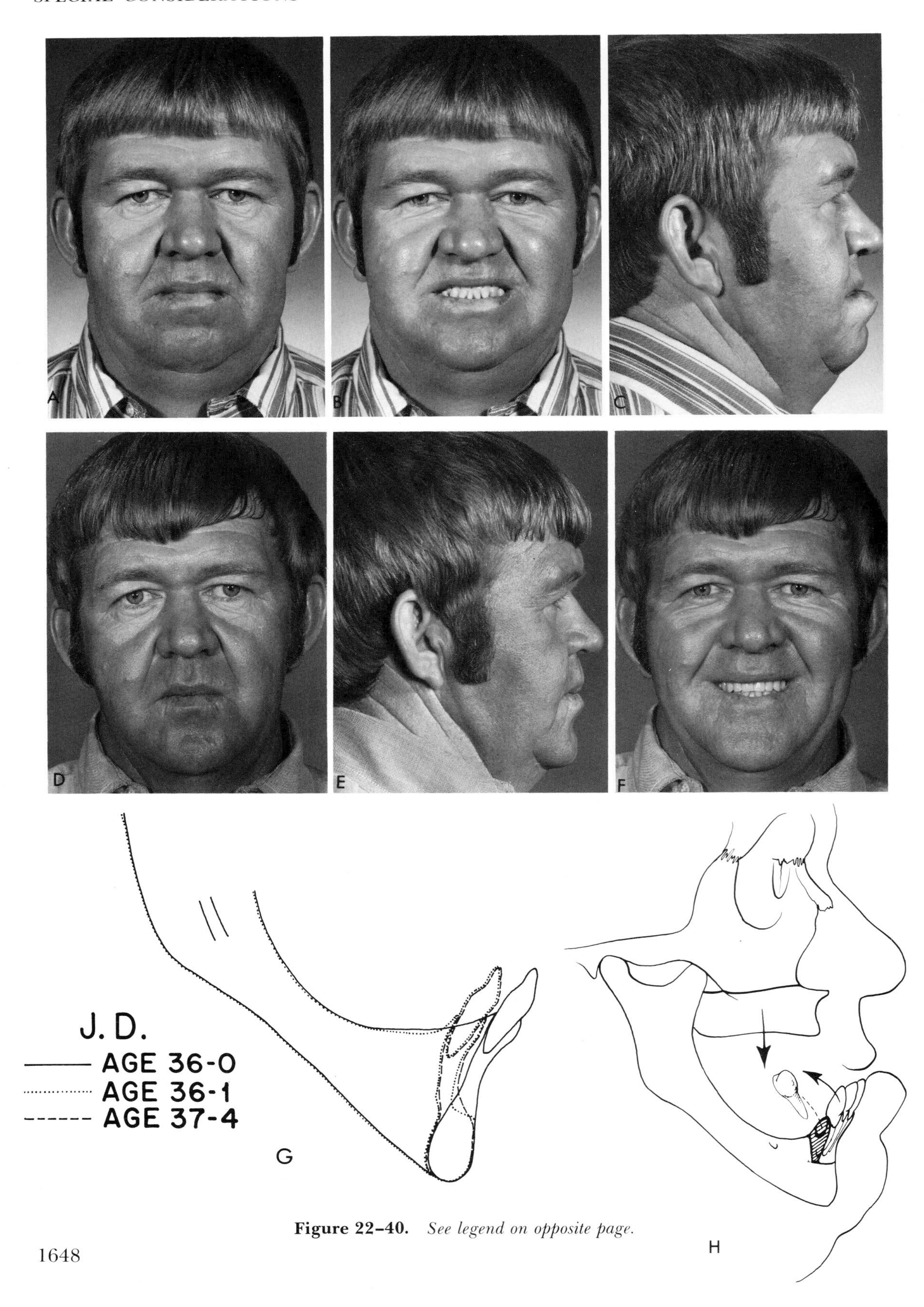

Figure 22–40. *See legend on opposite page.*

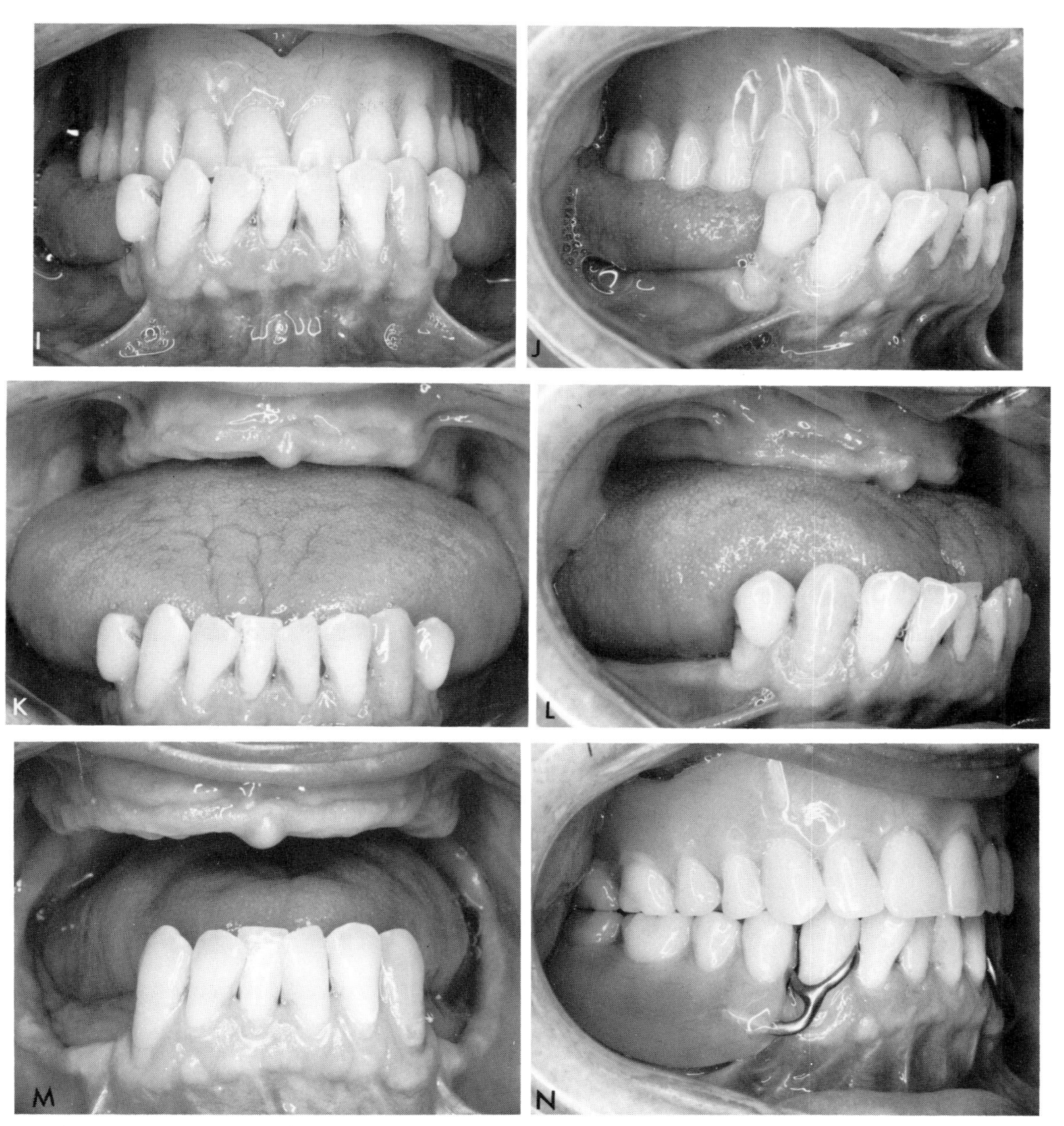

Figure 22–40 (Case 22–7). *A–C,* Facial appearance at age 36. *D–F,* Postoperative appearance after surgical procedures depicted in *H* and replacement with complete maxillary and partial mandibular prostheses. *G,* Composite cephalometric tracings before, 1 month after, and 15 months after mandibular subapical osteotomy *(H),* demonstrating stability. Mandible superimposed over mandible, registered at symphysis and mandibular canal. *H,* Schematic illustration of surgery: Le Fort I osteotomy and mandibular subapical osteotomy; arrows indicate positional changes. *I* and *J,* Preoperative relationship between mandibular anterior teeth and maxillary alveolar ridge; excessively large tongue was chronically postured against mandibular anterior teeth. *K* and *L,* Preoperative relationship between mandibular anterior teeth and maxillary denture; amorphous mass of tongue protruding into posterior interarch space. *M,* Maxillomandibular relationship after subapical osteotomy, Le Fort I osteotomy, interpositional bone graft, and partial glossectomy; tongue "fits" passively in oral cavity. *N,* New full maxillary and partial mandibular prostheses in place.

CASE 22–7 (Fig. 22–40)

J.D., a 36-year-old man, was referred by a prosthodontist for evaluation of his maxillary and mandibular ridge relationship prior to construction of a maxillary complete denture and a mandibular partial denture. Fifteen years prior, the patient had been treated for mandibular prognathism by extraoral mandibular vertical ramus osteotomies. Gradual and progressive postsurgical changes compromised the surgical result. Because only photographic and panographic records of the previous treatment were available it was difficult to ascertain exactly what changes occurred after surgery and whether these constituted skeletal or dental relapse. The remaining maxillary teeth were apparently extracted and replaced with a complete denture to compensate for the anteroposterior jaw disparity. A problem list was developed from clinical and radiographic studies and from the patient's esthetic and functional concerns.

PROBLEM LIST

Esthetics (Fig. 22–40 *A, B, C*)

Frontal. Bilateral symmetry and acceptable harmony between the upper, middle, and lower facial thirds; prominent nasolabial folds and a deficient paranasal region.

Profile. Frontal bossing with a deep nasofrontal fold; retrusive-appearing infraorbital rims and malar eminences; acute nasolabial angle; prominent lower lip, prominent and unesthetic chin-neck angle with excessive submental fullness.

Cephalometric Evaluation

Anterior facial height of 131 mm; disparate height between the upper and lower face (53 mm/78 mm); high mandibular plane angle = 40; SNA = 79; SNB = 88; ANB difference = –9; ratio of lower incisor to NB to pogonion to NB = 10/5; vertical dimension of the maxillary anterior alveolus (ANS to height of alveolus) = 13 mm, maxillary-mandibular anteroposterior discrepancy = –11 mm.

Occlusion (Fig. 22–40 *I*)

Dental Arch Form. Maxillary and mandibular arches oval and symmetric; severely atrophic edentulous maxillary alveolus with a low palatal vault.

Dental Alignment. Minimal crowding of mandibular anterior teeth; multiple missing posterior teeth.

Dental Occlusion. Full Class III maxillo-mandibular relationship; bilateral transverse discrepancy of posterior segments (maxilla smaller than mandible); excessively large tongue in all dimensions, which protruded between the edentulous ridges and pressed firmly against the mandibular anterior teeth.

DIAGNOSIS

1. Maxillary hypoplasia and severe maxillary atrophy.
2. Mandibular prognathism.

3. Macroglossia.
4. Mutilated dentition.

TREATMENT PLAN (Fig. 22–40 *H*)

1. Periodontal treatment.
2. Partial glossectomy to reduce the size of the tongue to within normal limits.
3. Anterior mandibular subapical osteotomy with posterior repositioning of the anterior segment to:
   a. Improve the $\overline{1}$ to NB and NB to Po ratio to approximately 1:1; reduce prominence of lower lip and mandibular anterior teeth, and produce relative increase in chin prominence.
   b. Improve the anteroposterior (Class III) maxillomandibular relationship and thereby decrease the amount of maxillary advancement necessary to achieve harmony between the dental arches.
4. Le Fort I type maxillary osteotomy with inferior repositioning of the maxilla 8 mm and anterior repositioning of the maxilla 5 mm; iliac crest corticocancellous interpositional bone graft to the maxilla to:
   a. Increase the height of the atrophic maxillary alveolus.
   b. Establish a functional Class I maxillary-mandibular relationship prior to prosthetic replacement of teeth.
   c. Improve shallow paranasal region.
5. Corticocancellous onlay bone graft augmentation of paranasal region to:
   a. Decrease prominence of nasolabial folds.
   b. Improve upper lip to nasal alae relationship.
6. Prosthetic replacement of missing teeth with complete maxillary denture and mandibular partial denture.

RESULTS

Subjective

The surgery was accomplished in two stages. The mandibular subapical osteotomy and partial glossectomy were performed first; two months later, the maxillary surgery was performed. Minimal facial pain and decreased function were noted after both procedures. Prosthetic restoration of the missing teeth was facilitated by the improved maxillomandibular ridge relationship, lower incisor to basal bone relationship, and increased maxillary bone mass.

Objective

Healing was uneventful following both procedures. Glossectomy resulted in minimal tongue edema. The small amount of tongue swelling may have been related to the use of pre- and postoperative Solu-Medrol. The use of a preformed mandibular splint precluded the need for intermaxillary fixation. Following maxillary surgery, no fixation or traction appliances were used. The patient was discharged on the third postoperative day after both procedures. Six weeks after maxillary surgery, maxillary and mandibular prostheses were constructed. Facial esthetics was improved by reducing lower lip prominence and increasing the prominence of the paranasal and infraorbital regions. (Fig. 22–40, *D, E,* and *F*). The maxillomandibular relationship was improved from a Class III (−11 mm) to a Class I (−1 mm) interarch relationship; additionally, the magnitude of the posterior crossbite was reduced. The size of the maxilla was increased to allow for construction of a well-fitting, full denture prosthesis. A three-year clinical and cephalometric follow-up reveals minimal resorption and positional change of the maxilla, stability of the repositioned anterior mandibular dentoalveolar segment, and a normally functioning tongue.

COMMENT

Despite the fact that the patient's old treatment records were incomplete, a retrospective study of available records and clinical findings indicated that there was concomitant skeletal and dental relapse after the initial mandibular ramus surgery. The propensity for skeletal relapse after surgical correction of "high angle" prognathic patients is supported by clinical experience. In this particular case the mandibular movement was also associated with postsurgical proclination of the mandibular anterior teeth as a consequence of the patient's very large tongue, which he chronically postured between his teeth anteriorly and laterally during rest and swallowing. The "keyhole" technique of partial glossectomy was utilized to reduce the overall size of the tongue — specifically its anteroposterior and *lateral* dimensions. After surgery the tongue appeared normal in size and seemed to "fit" into the patient's oral cavity. The patient no longer postured his tongue between his teeth. Despite the fact that myofunctional or speech therapy was not used before or after surgery, there was apparent improvement in the patient's speech.

The improved maxillomandibular relationship should decrease the amount of bone resorption in the anterior maxilla where natural teeth function against a full upper denture. To date, three years after surgery, there has been minimal resorption and positional change of the repositioned maxilla.

Mandibular prognathism is usually not a "pure" dentofacial deformity. It is not infrequently associated with varying degrees of maxillary deficiency in the anteroposterior plane of space. This patient's absolute mandibular prognathism was accentuated by his absolute maxillary deficiency. Treatment planning should include consideration of the osseous movements which will most improve the esthetic balance of the face. This patient's class III maxillomandibular relationship could have been corrected by advancing the maxilla, retropositioning the mandible, or a combination of maxillomandibular surgery, or by mandibular subapical osteotomy. Because this patient manifested a very obtuse chin-neck angle, retracting the mandible may have worsened his frontal appearance by creating a larger submental "pouch" effect. Moreover, there would have been no change in the labiomental region and overall facial esthetics would not have been significantly improved even if paranasal augmentation were added. Conversely, maxillary advancement combined with paranasal augmentation would significantly improve the patient's middle face esthetics. Additionally this would reduce the amount of anteroposterior maxillomandibular discrepancy. By retracting the mandibular anterior segment by anterior mandibular subapical osteotomy, a class I ridge relationship was achieved in addition to improving the lower lip to chin relationship.

Surgeon: William H. Bell, Dallas, Texas.

Various surgical procedures can be used to expand, narrow, raise, lower, retract, or advance the anterior or posterior parts of the maxilla or mandible to facilitate restoration of the partially edentulous patient. It is usually possible to stabilize the edentulous or partially edentulous segment with direct transosseous wires which remain in place below the prosthesis. When and if they cause irritation to the overlying mucosa with the prosthesis in place, they are easily removed with local anesthesia. Because of its propensity for relapse the anteriorly repositioned edentulous maxilla must frequently be stabilized by bone grafting.

INADEQUATE INTERARCH SPACE

Inadequate interarch space is one of the most common clinical problems confronting the dental practitioner and defies treatment without surgery. The restorative dentist is frequently faced with the problems of restoring the posterior occlusion after supereruption of maxillary posterior teeth into an edentulous space created by premature loss of mandibular posterior teeth. The super-eruption results in decreased interarch space and an aberrant occlusal plane. Such problems preclude restoration of the edentulous space without surgical repositioning of the supererupted teeth. If the edentulous space is restored without modification of the maxillary teeth, destructive occlusal interferences will develop. In addition, the reduced vertical space available for the prosthesis will compromise the design of the prosthesis. As a consequence, periodontal disease may develop around the abutment teeth. A moderate amount of supereruption requires extensive reduction of the maxillary occlusal surfaces to level the occlusal plane. Such modifications will result in short clinical crowns with poor occlusal form and a subsequent need for full crown restoration or endodontic therapy.

When the edentulous spaces have persisted for years, marked maxillary supereruption will occur to the extent that the maxillary teeth occlude with the mandibular edentulous ridge. In these cases it is impossible to reduce the maxillary occlusal surface sufficiently to re-establish the proper occlusal plane or to create adequate interarch space for a prosthesis. In previous years, cases of this type have been treated by extracting the supererupted maxillary posterior teeth, extensive alveolectomy, and subsequent replacement of the maxillary and mandibular teeth with a prosthesis. A vast improvement in the final occlusal and periodontal result can be achieved by superiorly repositioning the supererupted maxillary teeth by surgery. Although 15 mm is generally conceded to constitute an adequate posterior interarch space, there is really no practical limit to which the posterior maxillary dentoalveolar segment can be moved superiorly.

Small dento-osseous segments may also be superiorly repositioned to re-establish a more normal occlusal plane. They can be repositioned buccally or palatally to improve the medial-lateral occlusal relationship. Intermaxillary fixation is unnecessary because adequate stability can be obtained by ligating the mobilized dento-osseous segment to the adjacent teeth with an acrylated arch bar, cast metal splint, arch wire, or direct banding of a tooth contained within the mobilized segment to an adjacent tooth or pontic. Generally, there is adequate clinical union within four to six weeks, at which time the stabilizing appliance is removed and the restorative procedures are initiated.

It is not uncommon for the restorative dentist to encounter patients with edentulous maxillary and mandibular posterior areas and insufficient space between the ridges to permit restoration of the occlusion with removable partial dentures. A lack of vertical interarch space in such cases may be due to a reduced vertical dimension associated with a deep bite, attrition of the remaining anterior teeth, or excessive fibrous tissue over the maxillary bony ridge. In mandibular prognathism, the ramus is positioned anteriorly relative to the maxillary tuberosity, and may preclude normal restorative procedures. Methods used to increase the posterior interarch space in such cases include removal of soft tissue, alveoloplasty, and alveolectomy. All these procedures, however, result in removal of tissue that the edentulous patient cannot afford to lose.

In addition to restoring function and esthetics, the prosthodontist should make every effort to preserve remaining structures such as attached fibrous tissue and alveolar bone. This may be accomplished by surgically repositioning part or all of the edentulous area by segmental maxillary or mandibular osteotomy. Generally, a maxillary procedure is easier to perform and preserves the mandibular bone, which has a higher rate of resorption. An adequate interarch space may be obtained by a single-stage surgical procedure to facilitate fabrication of more efficient prosthetic appliances.

Surgical Correction

Adult patients with supererupted posterior teeth usually have numerous other associated interarch and intra-arch problems which can be solved by simultaneous movement of the anterior and posterior parts of the maxilla. This surgery is routinely accomplished as a Le Fort I osteotomy.[15, 30, 37] (See Case 22–8 and Fig. 22–41.) Isolated posterior maxillary osteotomies are predictable and stable procedures which are occasionally indicated to increase the posterior interarch space or level the maxillary occlusal plane to facilitate restoration of the occlusion with fixed or removable prosthetic appliances. (See Case 22–9 and Fig. 22–42.)

When superior movement of the posterior maxilla is the dominant objective, the Kufner technique, which is accomplished from a buccal approach, provides access to the superior aspect of the posterior maxilla to raise the posterior maxillary teeth and increase the interarch space.[25] Simultaneously, the segment may also be advanced, retracted, narrowed, or expanded.

When the dentoalveolar segment to be repositioned is small, the bony and soft-tissue incisions are carefully designed so that the mobilized segment is as large as possible to maintain a maximal soft-tissue pedicle. (See Case 22–10.) In selected patients superior repositioning of premolar and first molar teeth can be accomplished under local or general anesthesia as an office procedure. (See Case 22–10 and Fig. 22–43.)

The mobilized dento-osseous segment, pedicled to palatal and buccal soft tissue, is keyed into the preoperatively planned occlusal relationship with the aid of a strong acrylic occlusal wafer or processed Gunning-type splint with minimal extension into the sulcus. If there is a large space between the buccal horizontal bone incisions, bone grafting is indicated to facilitate union and help stabilize the repositioned posterior segment. The repositioned posterior segment is fixed with an orthodontic arch wire or arch bar to the interocclusal splint or Gunning-type splint, which is ligated to the remaining teeth with interdental wires. When an isolated posterior maxillary segment is repositioned, intermaxillary fixation is usually unnecessary with the use of an acrylic splint. When the entire maxilla is repositioned, however, a processed Gunning-type splint and intermaxillary fixation are used to maintain the desired interarch space. Either the splint or transitional prosthetic appliance is continually maintained in place to preserve the planned posterior interarch space. Retention may be accomplished by immediate restoration with a fixed or removable prosthesis. In most cases, however, it is more desirable to use a transitional prosthetic replacement or splint until the mobilized segment is consolidated and stable. During the period of time necessary for the maxilla to stabilize, and while the permanent prosthesis is being fabricated, the patient wears an interocclusal splint or transitional prosthesis continually to maintain the desired interocclusal space.

Supereruption of mandibular anterior teeth results in decreased anterior interarch space and an aberrant occlusal plane. The restorative dentist is again confronted with the difficult task of restoring the occlusion. Such problems may preclude proper restoration of the maxillary or mandibular occlusal planes without surgical repositioning of the supererupted mandibular anterior teeth. Mandibular subapical or body osteotomies provide a predictable and stable means of treating these difficult problems. (See Cases 22–11, 22–12, and 22–13 and Figs. 22–44, 22–45, and 22–46 which illustrate the use of surgical procedures to level the maxillary and mandibular occlusal planes.)

CASE 22–8 (Fig. 22–41)

D.C., a 37-year-old woman, had the facial and dental characteristics commonly associated with bimaxillary dental protrusion. She sought treatment to improve the contour of her face and the function of her teeth.

EVALUATION

Esthetics

Frontal. Excessive exposure of the maxillary incisors with the lips relaxed or when smiling; protrusive upper and lower lips (Fig. 22–41 *A, B*).

Profile. Excessive facial convexity associated with an acute nasolabial angle and contour-deficient chin (Fig. 22–41 *C*).

Cephalometric Evaluation (Fig. 22–41 *G*)

1. Vertical maxillary excess associated with increased lower anterior facial height.
2. Marked facial convexity; proclined maxillary and mandibular anterior teeth.
3. 13 mm lip incompetency.

Occlusal Analysis

Dental Arch Form. Maxilla and mandible were symmetric.

Dental Alignment. Proclined maxillary incisors with interincisal diastema.

Mandible — proclined incisors; multiple missing posterior teeth.

Dental Occlusion. Supereruption of maxillary posterior teeth with inadequate posterior interarch space (Fig. 22–41 *J, K, L*).

TREATMENT PLAN

1. Superior repositioning of maxilla in three segments by Le Fort I osteotomy (7 mm in anterior; 10 mm in posterior) (Fig. 22–41 *R*), to reduce exposure of teeth and gingiva, shorten facial height, and decrease interlabial gap.
2. Surgical repositioning of posterior maxillae superiorly (10 mm) to increase posterior interarch space.
3. Anterior maxillary and mandibular ostectomies in first premolar areas to reduce facial convexity and lessen proclination of anterior teeth.
4. Extraction of mandibular incisors and preparation of alveolus for partial denture.
5. Augmentation of contour-deficient chin with 6-mm thick alloplastic implant (Proplast).
6. Replacement of missing teeth with partial dentures.

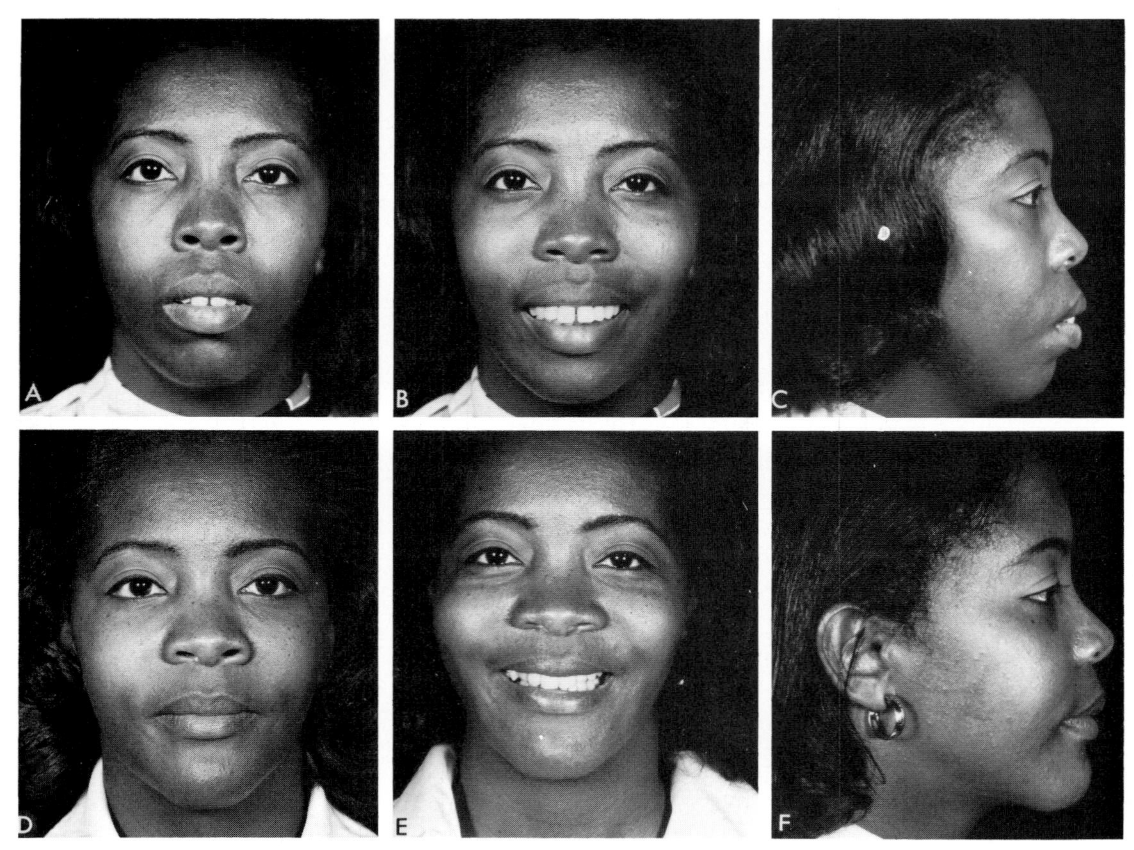

Figure 22–41 (Case 22–8). *A–C,* Preoperative appearance of a 37-year old woman. *D–F,* Appearance after maxillary and mandibular surgical procedure illustrated in *R*.

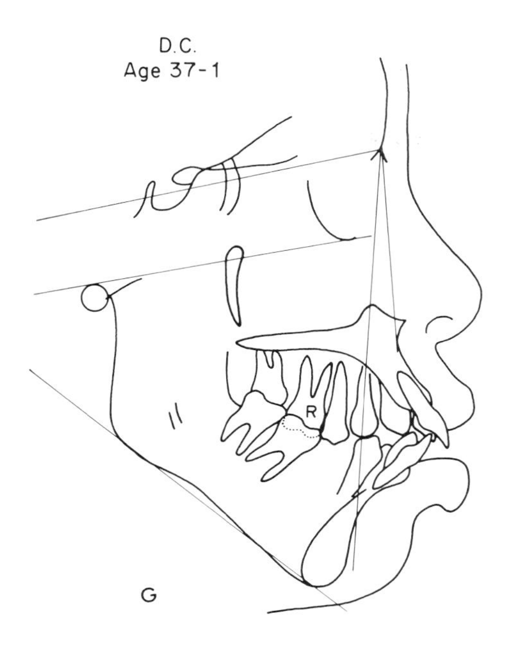

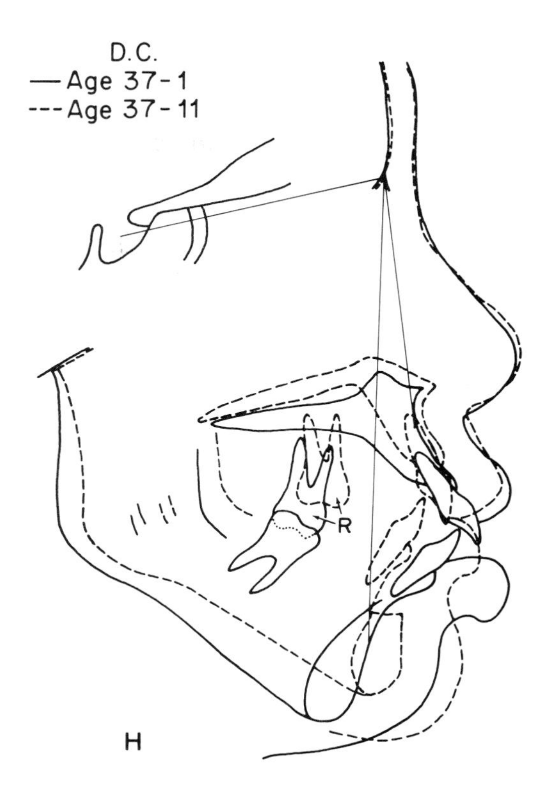

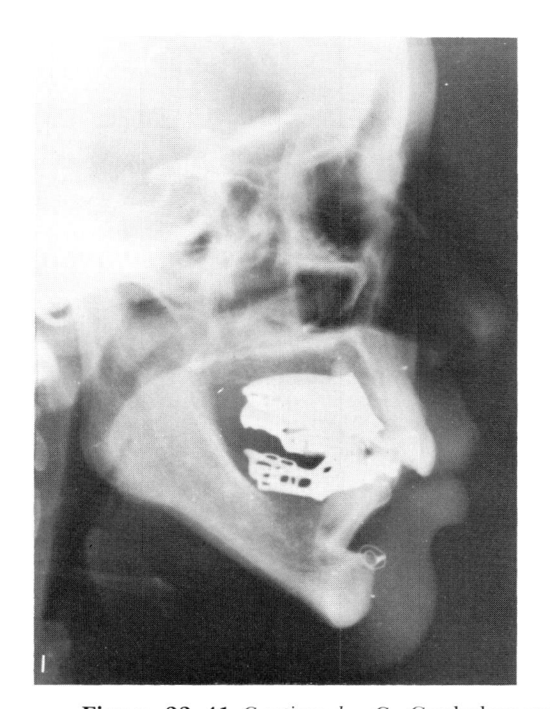

Figure 22–41 *Continued.* *G,* Cephalometric tracing (age 37 years, 1 month) before treatment. *H,* Composite cephalometric tracing before (*solid line,* age 37 years, 1 month) and 10 months after (*broken line,* age 37 years, 11 months) surgical intervention. *I,* Cephalogram taken 5 years after surgery; there was virtually no positional change of the maxilla or maxillary teeth based upon composite postoperative cephalometric radiographs, which were superimposed on bone markers placed at time of surgery.

Illustration and legend continued on the following page.

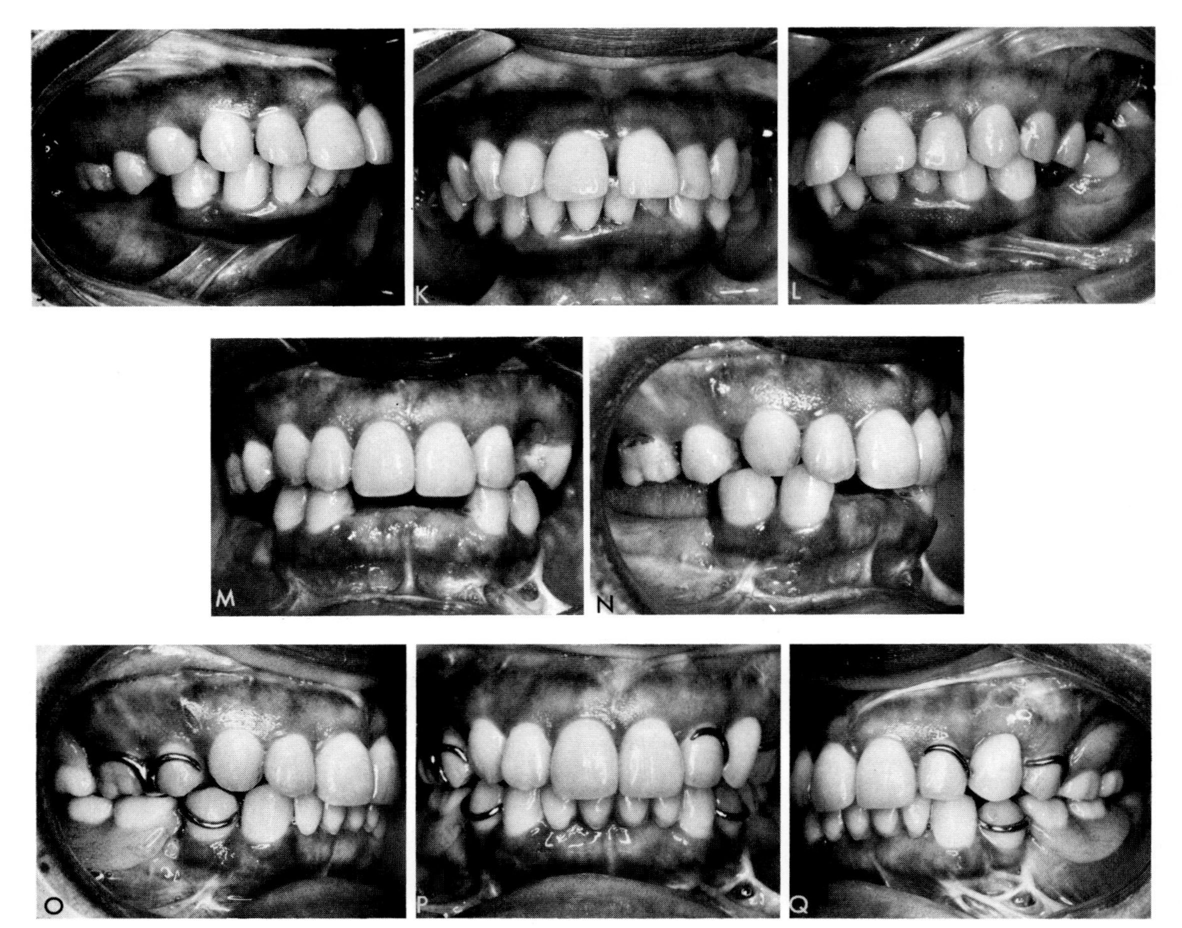

Figure 22–41 *Continued.* *J–L,* Occlusion before surgery. *M* and *N,* Occlusion immediately after surgery. *O–Q,* Occlusion after replacement of missing teeth with removable prostheses.

Illustration and legend continued on the following page.

FOLLOW-UP

Subjective

Postoperative healing was uncomplicated and associated with minimal pain. All mobilized and repositioned segments were clinically firm when intermaxillary fixation was discontinued five weeks after surgery.

Objective

By superior movement of the posterior maxillary dentoalveolar segments, sufficient interarch space was achieved to replace the missing maxillary and mandibular teeth with removable prostheses (Fig. 22–41 *O, P,* and *Q*). Facial harmony and a serviceable occlusion were achieved after four months of treatment. Postoperative clinical and cephalometric studies five years after surgery have revealed virtually no movement of the superiorly repositioned maxilla or anterior part of the mandible. There was minimal bony resorption below the onlayed Proplast implant.

Surgeon: William H. Bell, Dallas, Texas. *Resorative dentistry:* Irby Hunter, Dallas, Texas.

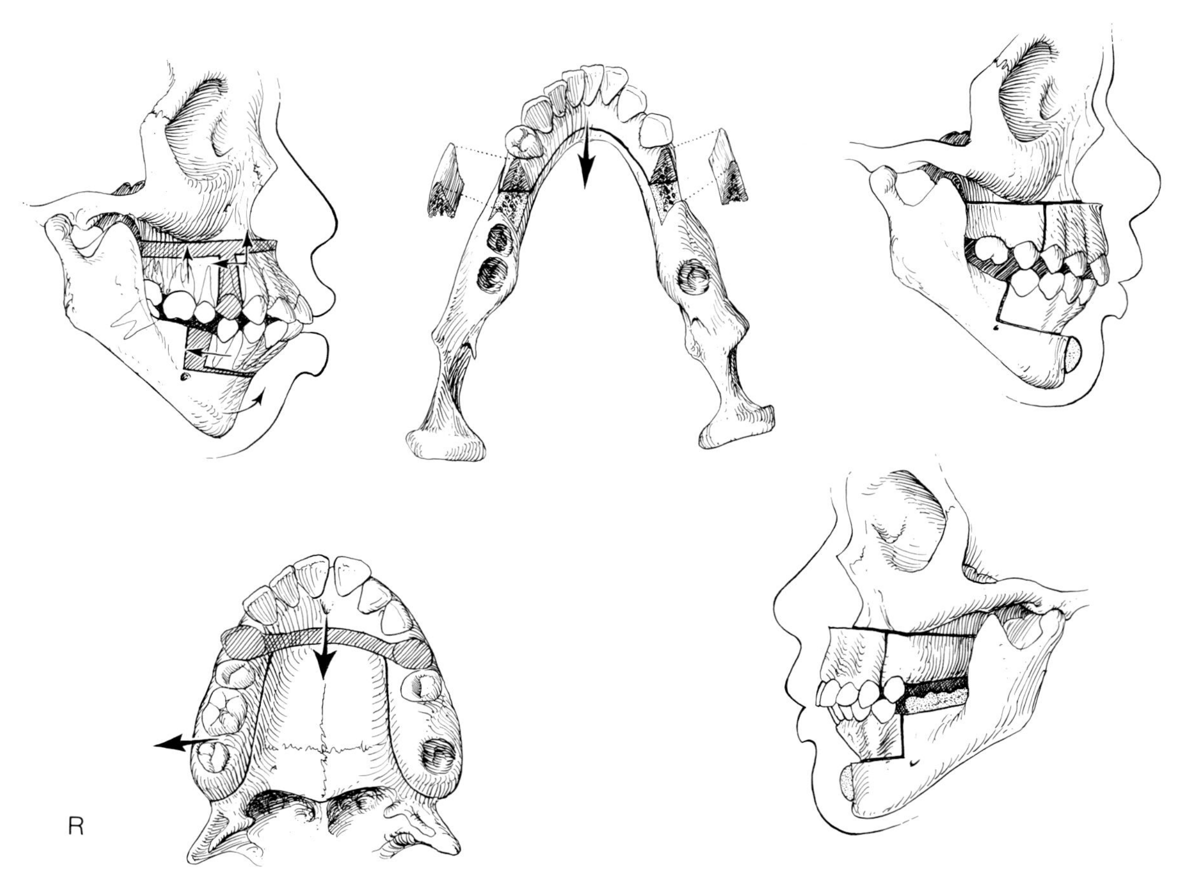

Figure 22–41 *Continued.* *R,* Diagrammatic plan of maxillary and mandibular surgery. Modified Le Fort I osteotomy was used to reposition the maxilla superiorly; 6-mm. vertical segments of bone were excised bilaterally from the maxillary and mandibular 1st premolar regions; the chin was augmented with a 6-mm. thick alloplastic implant (Proplast).

CASE 22–9 (Fig. 22–42)

M.B., a 31-year-old woman, had the facial and dental characteristics commonly associated with mild bimaxillary dental protrusion. She was referred by her general dentist to increase the left posterior interarch space, where the maxillary posterior teeth had supererupted into contact with the mandibular alveolar ridge. The following problem list was developed from an evaluation of her clinical records.

PROBLEM LIST

Esthetics

Frontal. Normal tooth exposure when in function and repose.
Profile. Mild facial convexity consistent with norms for black race.

Cephalometric Evaluation

1. Slight proclination of maxillary anterior teeth.
2. Lip competency with lips in repose.

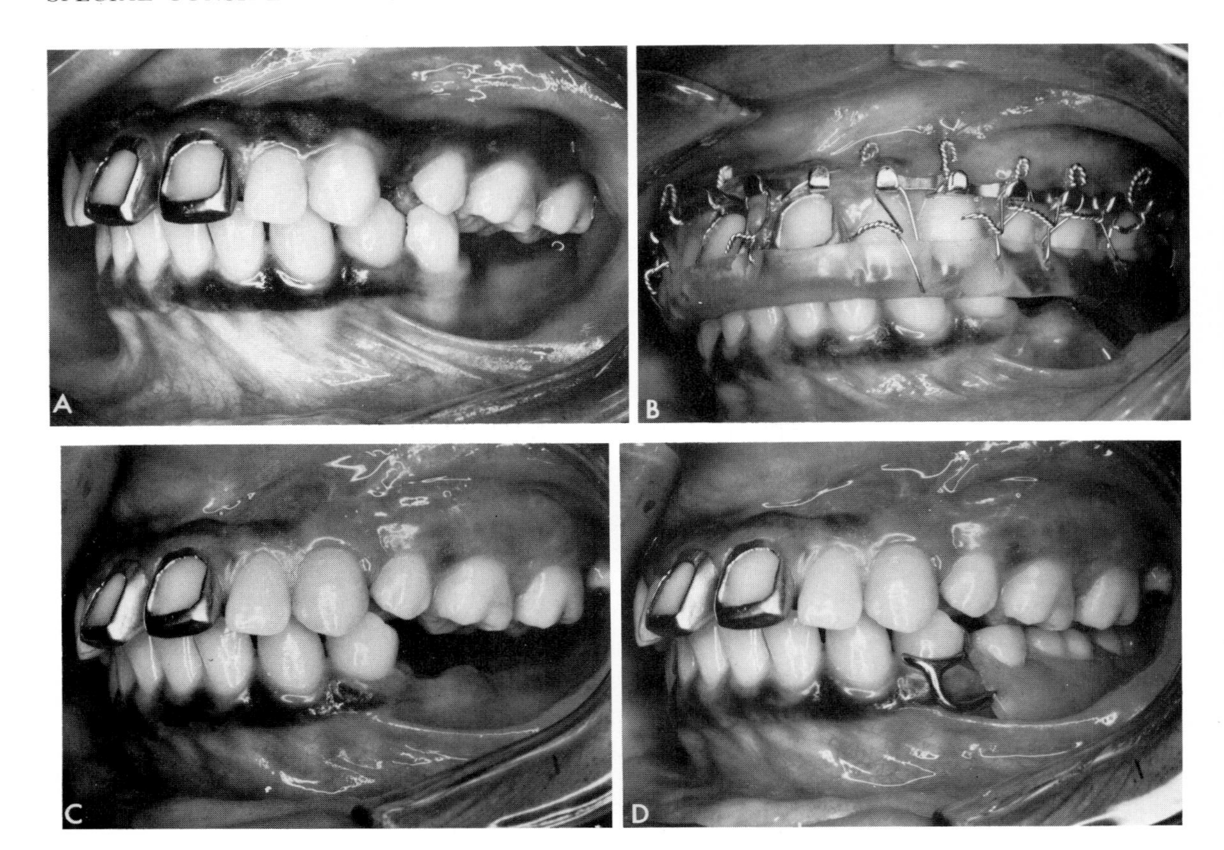

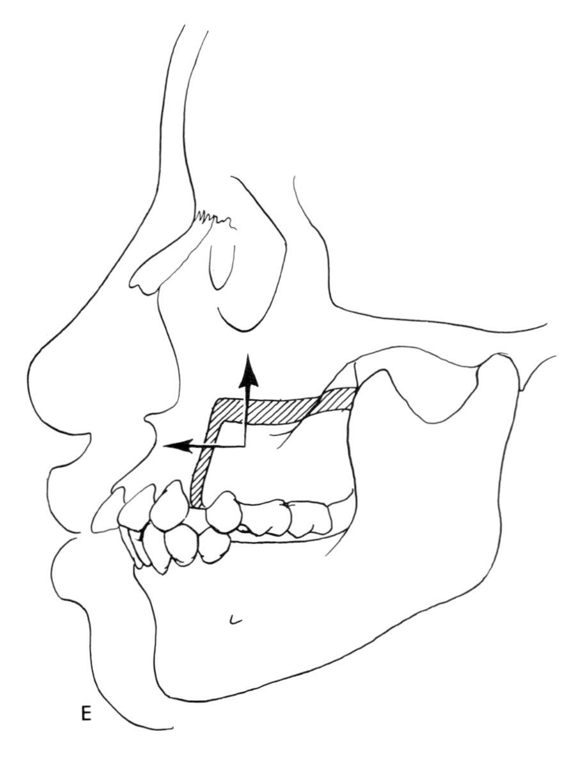

Figure 22–42 (Case 22–9). *A,* Preoperative occlusion. *B,* Repositioned posterior maxillary dentoalveolar segment fixed to acrylic splint with interdental wire ligatures. *C,* Postoperative interarch space. *D,* Replacement of missing mandibular posterior teeth with removable prosthesis. *E,* Schematic view of bony incisions for posterior maxillary osteotomy (arrows indicate positional changes).

Occlusal Analysis (Fig. 22–42 *A*)

Dental Arch Form. Maxilla and mandible symmetric.

Dental Alignment. Anterior maxillary interdental spacing; 3 mm space between maxillary left canine and second premolar tooth secondary to previous extraction; missing mandibular left posterior teeth.

Dental Occlusion. Supereruption of maxillary left second premolar and molar teeth into mandibular left posterior edentulous space, precluding replacement of the missing teeth because of inadequate posterior interarch space.

TREATMENT PLAN

1. Repositioning of left posterior maxilla (second premolar and molar teeth) superiorly 5 mm to increase posterior interarch space, anteriorly 3 mm to close residual interdental space, and medially 2 mm to improve the transverse maxillary tooth to mandibular arch relationship (Fig. 22–42 *E*).
2. Replace missing mandibular left posterior teeth with partial denture.

TREATMENT

The left posterior maxillary dentoalveolar segment was repositioned by a single-stage posterior maxillary ostectomy, as shown in Figure 22–42 *E* (after Kufner technique). The palatal and buccal bone incisions were all accomplished from a buccal approach without the use of palatal mucosal incisions (Fig. 22–42 *E*). The repositioned segment was fixed with a prefabricated acrylic splint, which also maintained the desired interarch space. The splint was suspended from an arch bar with interdental wires (Fig. 22–42 *B*). Intermaxillary fixation was not used.

RESULTS

Subjective

The postoperative course was uncomplicated and associated with minimal pain and swelling. The use of a prefabricated acrylic splint ligated to an arch bar precluded the need for intermaxillary fixation. The repositioned segment was slightly movable when the splint was removed seven weeks after surgery. By superior movement of the posterior maxillary dentoalveolar segment, sufficient interarch space was achieved to replace the missing mandibular teeth with a removable prosthesis (Fig. 22–42 *D*). Impressions were taken the following day for fabrication of a partial denture prosthesis to replace the missing left mandibular posterior teeth. During the three-week period of time necessary to fabricate the lower partial denture, the previously used interocclusal splint was replaced and suspended from the upper arch bar to assure that the desired interarch space would be maintained and to prevent inferior movement of the segment. A serviceable and functional interarch relationship was achieved and maintained by this surgical and prosthetic treatment. There has been no discernable movement of the superiorly repositioned posterior maxillary dentoalveolar segment over a 30-month period of postoperative follow-up.

Surgeon: William H. Bell, Dallas, Texas. *Restorative dentistry:* James H. Williams, Dallas, Texas.

CASE 22–10 (Fig. 22–43)

Supereruption of maxillary right second premolar tooth into mandibular right posterior edentulous space of a 50-year-old lady, M. C.

TREATMENT PLAN

1. Reposition right maxillary second premolar dento-osseous segment superiorly 4 mm to level maxillary occlusal plane.
2. Replace missing maxillary teeth with fixed prosthesis; replace missing mandibular teeth with partial denture.

Plan of Surgery (See Figure 22–43 and legends.)

Surgeon: William H. Bell, Dallas, Texas. *Resorative dentistry:* Richard G. Bendele, Dallas, Texas.

Figure 22–43 (Case 12–10). Supereruption of maxillary right second premolar tooth into mandibular right posterior edentulous space of 50-year-old woman. *A,* Plan of surgery: semilunar incision is made through mucoperiosteum in depth of buccal vestibule. The planned vertical osteotomies are made 3 mm. away from the second premolar tooth to increase the size of the dento-osseous segment. Cross-hatched area indicates planned subapical ostectomy; broken lines indicate planned vertical interdental osteotomies. Four mm. of bone are excised from the lateral maxilla above the root apex of the second premolar tooth. *B,* The mucoperiosteum along the inferior margin of the incision is elevated to expose the bone over the apex of the maxillary second premolar tooth and the interdental bone at the site of the proposed vertical osteotomies. The mucoperiosteum is minimally elevated away from the segment to be mobilized to maximize its soft-tissue pedicle. The mucoperiosteum can be elevated more extensively from the contiguous bone that remains stable because it has a broad vascular pedicle from the contiguous bone and the attached mucoperiosteum. Stippling indicates areas of detached gingiva and mucoperiosteum. Vertical interdental osteotomies are accomplished with a fissure bur; nerve retractor is placed inferiorly to facilitate visualization and prevent injury of attached gingiva. *C,* The medial wall of the maxillary sinus is sectioned between the palatal root and the nasal floor with a curved osteotome passed through the bony window created by the previously made horizontal buccal ostectomy. The integrity of the palatal mucosa is preserved by carefully malleting an osteotome against the surgeon's finger, which is positioned on the palatal mucosa at the juncture of the horizontal and vertical parts of the palate. *D,* A spatula osteotome is malleted interproximally to fracture the crestal alveolar bone and palatal bone until the tip of the instrument makes contact with the previously made parasagittal palatal osteotomy. The downfractured segment pedicled to palatal mucoperiosteum is then repositioned superiorly and fixed at the planned level with an interosseous wire and by fixing the repositioned tooth to the adjacent pontic.

See illustration on the opposite page.

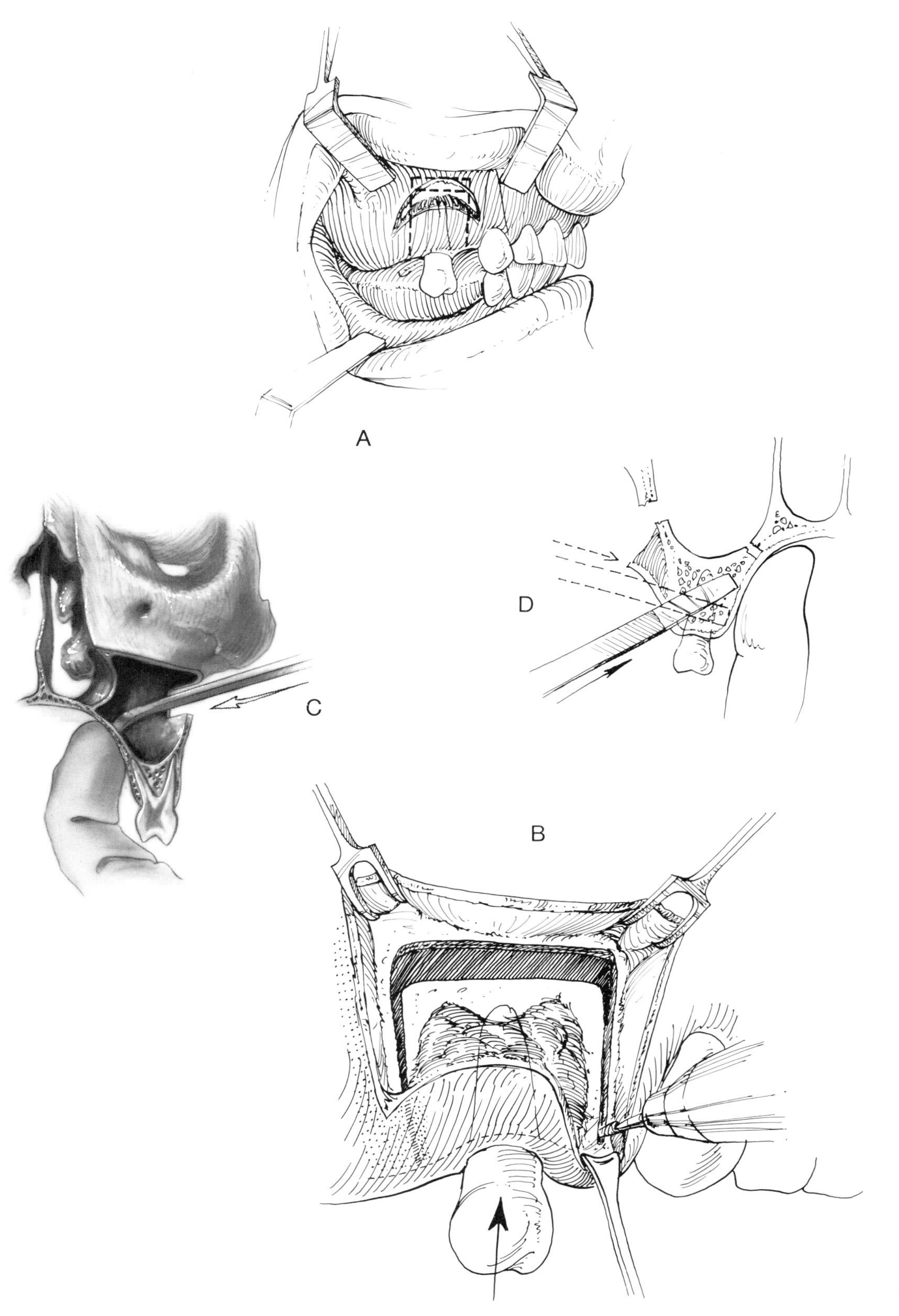

Illustration and legend continued on the following page.

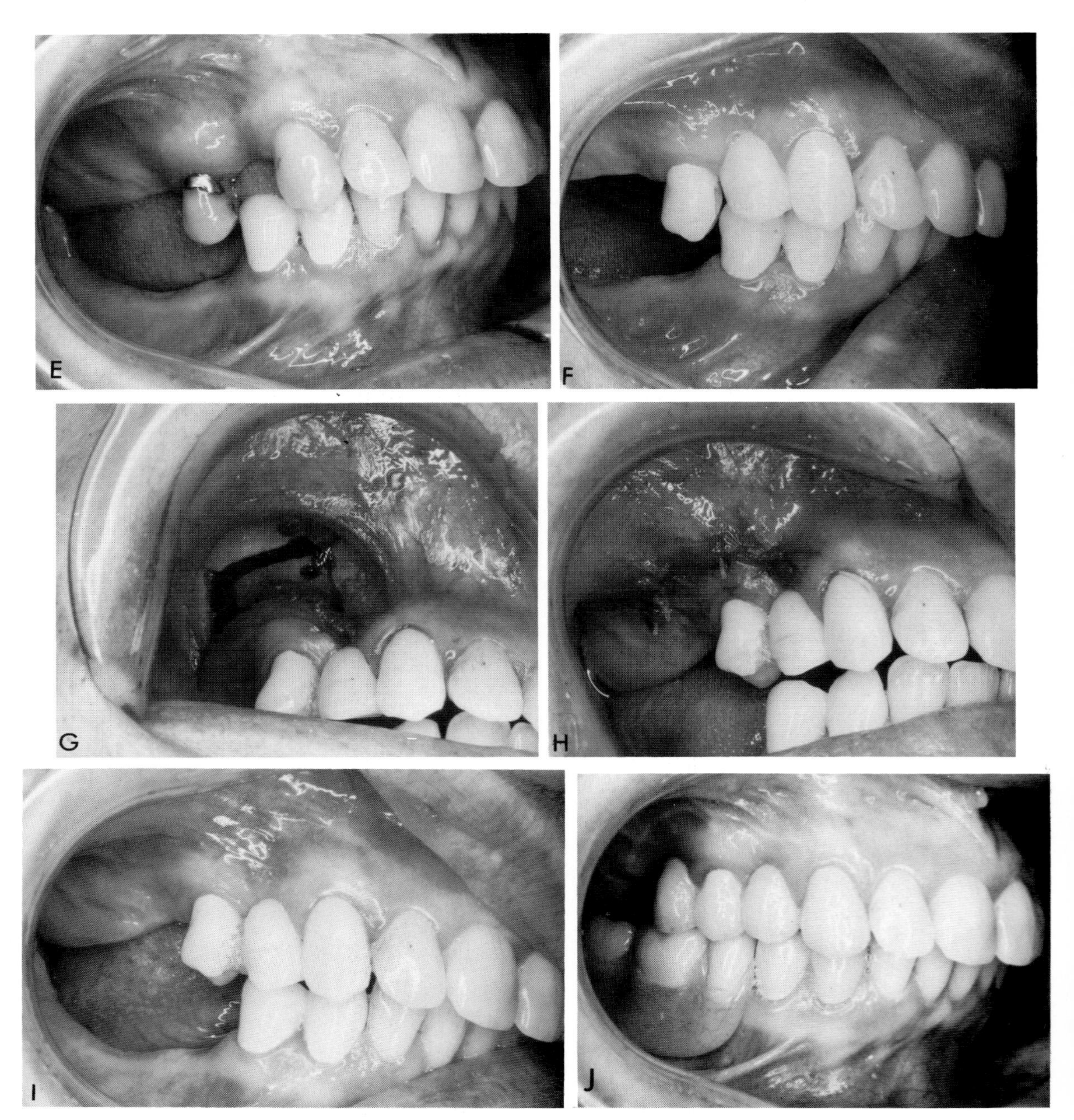

Figure 22–43 *Continued.* *E,* Preoperative occlusion, supererupted maxillary right second premolar tooth. *F,* Temporary pontic attached to canine tooth was used to fix the second premolar tooth into the desired position at the time of surgery. *G,* Fixation of repositioned dento-osseous segment at time of surgery. *H,* Mobilized segment was placed into the preoperatively determined occlusal relationship by fixing the crown of the tooth to the adjacent pontic. *I,* Repositioned segment remained fixed to adjacent pontic as healing occurred and while additional restorations were completed. *J,* Final occlusion.

CASE 22–11 (Fig. 22–44)

C.W., a 31-year-old man, sought treatment to improve his facial esthetics and function of his mutilated malocclusion.

EVALUATION

Esthetic Analysis (Fig. 22–44, *A* to *C*)

Frontal. Narrow nose; lack of tooth exposure when smiling; facial and chin asymmetry; short face.
Profile. Decreased facial height; short and retropositioned chin.

Cephalometric Analysis

Decreased lower anterior facial height (vertical maxillary deficiency).
Low mandibular plane angle.

Occlusal Analysis (Fig. 44,*G*)

Dental Arch Form. Maxillary arch: partially edentulous and too wide; analysis was based upon the occlusal relationship that was achieved when the models were hand-articulated into a simulated corrected Class I canine and molar relationship.
Dental Alignment. Maxilla: edentulous from right first premolar to left second premolar.
Mandible: minimal crowding; missing second premolars.
Dental Occlusion. Class II malocclusion with buccal crossbite; excessive curvature of mandibular curve of Spee secondary to supereruption of mandibular anterior teeth; lack of anterior interarch space; mandibular anterior teeth were retroclined and positioned distally relative to their supporting basal bone.

PROBLEM LIST

1. Vertical maxillary deficiency (short face) and horizontal maxillary excess (buccal crossbite).
2. Buccal crossbite.
3. Supererupted mandibular anterior teeth; lack of anterior interarch space; excessive curvature of mandibular occlusal plane.
4. Short, asymmetric and retropositioned chin.
5. Maxillary and mandibular edentulous spaces.

TREATMENT PLAN (Fig. 22–44 *K*)

1. Inferior repositioning of maxilla in two segments by Le Fort I osteotomy and interpositional autogenous bone graft (6 mm in anterior; 3 mm in posterior) (Fig. 22–44 *K*) to increase exposure of teeth and increase facial height.
2. Surgical narrowing of maxilla (5 mm in anterior, 3 mm in posterior) to correct buccal crossbite and decrease width of anterior edentulous space (Fig. 22–44 *K*).

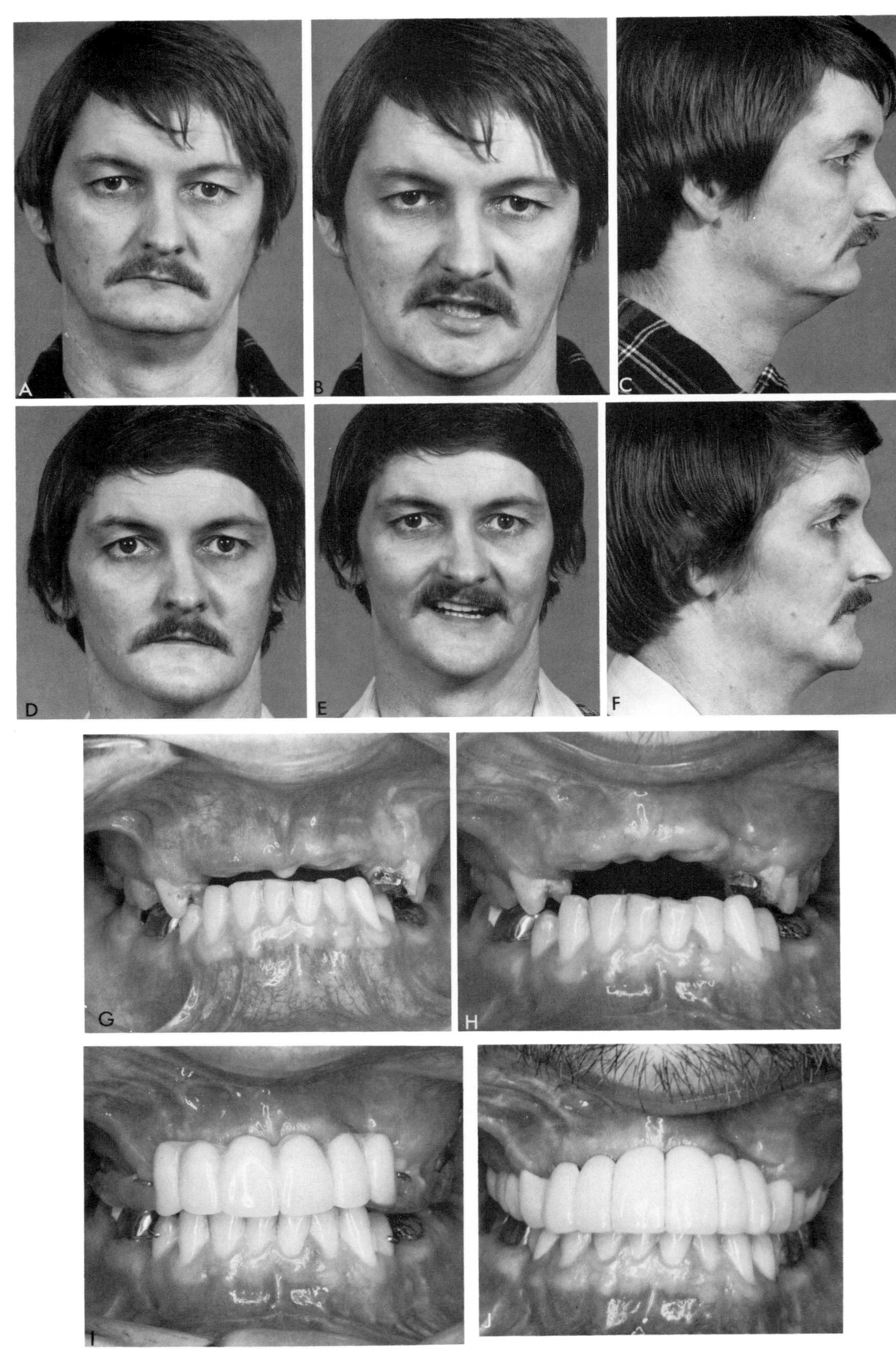

Figure 22–44. *See legend on the opposite page.*

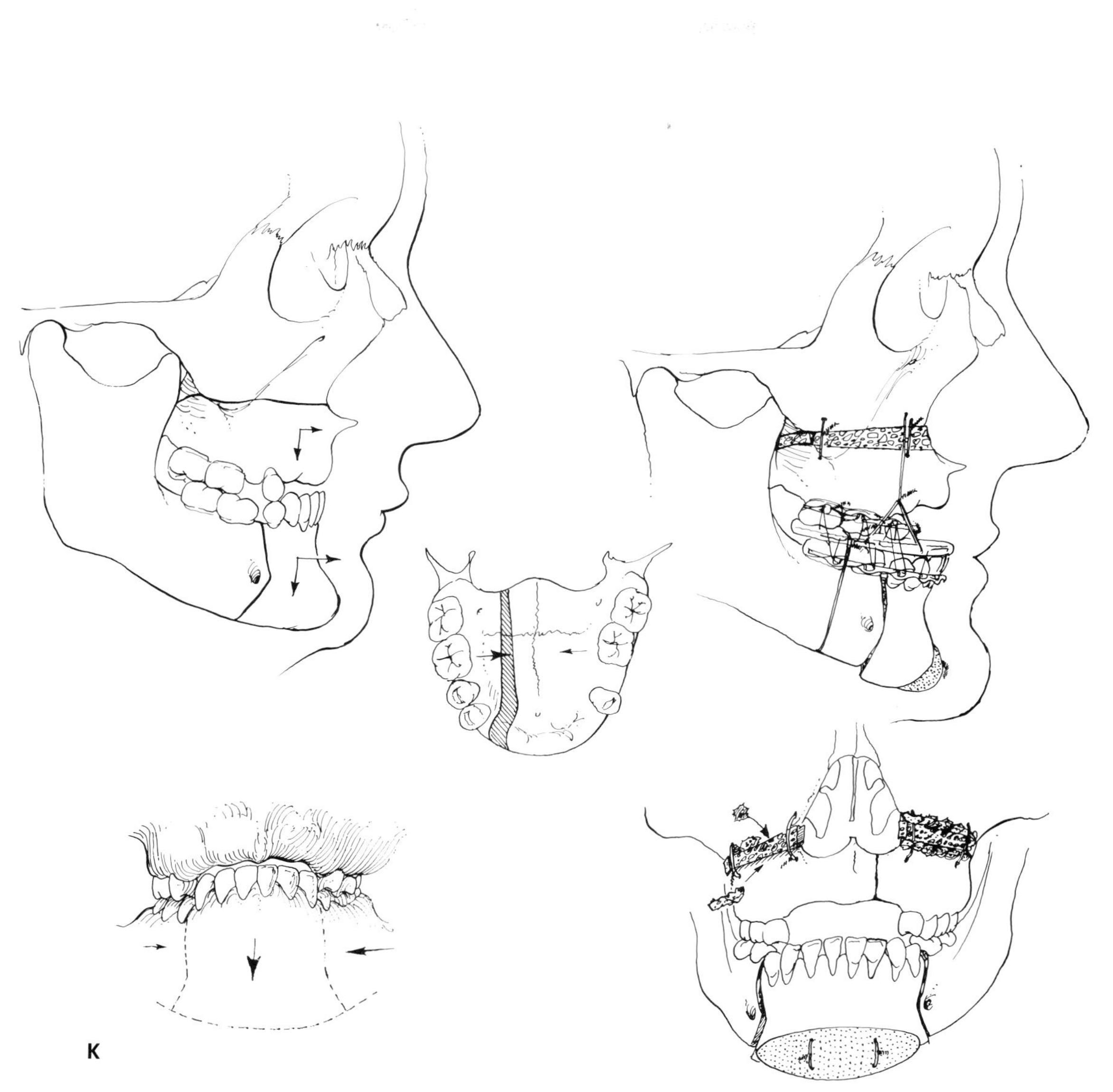

Figure 22–44. *A–C.* Facial appearance before treatment: short face and lack of tooth exposure. *D–F,* Facial appearance after treatment: increased facial height, improved smile line, and increased chin prominence. *G,* Occlusion before treatment: lack of anterior interarch space, buccal crossbite. *H,* Occlusion after surgery: increased anterior interarch space, correction of buccal crossbite. *I,* Occlusion with transitional prosthesis in place. *J,* after restorative dentistry. *K,* Surgical treatment plan.

3. Anterior mandibular body osteotomies (Fig. 22–44 *K*) to lower anterior portion of mandible, level mandibular occlusal plane, increase anterior interarch space, procline mandibular anterior teeth, and increase lower anterior facial height.
4. Augmentation of contour–deficient and asymmetric chin with 5 mm thick alloplastic implant (Proplast) (Fig. 22–44 *K*).
5. Replacement of missing anterior teeth with fixed prosthesis; jacket restorations of mandibular premolars.

FOLLOW-UP AND COMMENT

Subjective

Postoperative healing was uncomplicated and associated with minimal pain. All the surgical procedures were accomplished in a single stage. When intermaxillary fixation was discontinued five weeks after surgery, all the repositioned segments were clinically firm. The patient continued to wear a transitional prosthesis for approximately two months, during which time his occlusal and skeletal relationships were monitored clinically and with periodic cephalometric radiographs. Final restoration of his occlusion by fixed prosthetic appliances was facilitated by increasing the anterior interarch space, correcting the buccal crossbite, and improving the inclination of the mandibular anterior teeth. Inferior repositioning of the maxilla improved the smile line, increased the face height and corrected the buccal crossbite. Interocclusal harmony was easily accomplished with fixed prosthetic restorations with the mandible and maxilla in a stable relationship. Permanent restorations were undertaken only after cephalometric and clinical studies indicated occlusal and skeletal stability were achieved.

Surgeon: William H. Bell, Dallas, Texas. *Restorative dentistry:* Charles R. Williams, Dallas, Texas.

CASE 22–12 (Fig. 22–45)

This 49-year-old woman, A.R., was referred by her general dentist for surgery to correct her maxillomandibular relationship prior to prosthetic rehabilitation. The patient also desired treatment for chronic pain in her temporomandibular joints which had been associated with headaches and cervical pain for approximately five years.

EVALUATION

Esthetics (Fig. 22–45 *A, B, C*)

Moderate exposure of the maxillary anterior teeth and gingiva in repose and when smiling; large but narrow nose; face appeared relatively short; retropositioned mandible; everted lower lip; deep labiomental fold.

Cephalometric Analysis (Fig. 22–45 *G*)

Maxillary and mandibular deficiency; skeletal type class II malocclusion; SNA = 73.5°; SNB = 70°; ANB = 3.5°; High mandibular plane angle (SN–GoGn = 45°) associated with short ramus height.

Occlusal Analysis (Fig. 22–45 *I*)

Dental Arch Form. Maxillary arch: tapered and constricted; mandibular arch: V-shaped.

Dental Alignment. Mutilated malocclusion with multiple missing and malaligned teeth; multiple maxillary interincisal diastemas.

Dental Occlusion. Class II malocclusion bilaterally; excessive curvature of mandibular occlusal plane; deep bite with mandibular incisors biting into palatal mucosa; overbite = 8mm; overjet = 11mm; generalized periodonitis.

TREATMENT PLAN

1. Periodontal treatment.
2. Le Fort I osteotomy to raise (5 mm, anterior only), advance, and widen maxilla to:
   a. Reduce exposure of incisor teeth.
   b. Reduce prominence of nose.

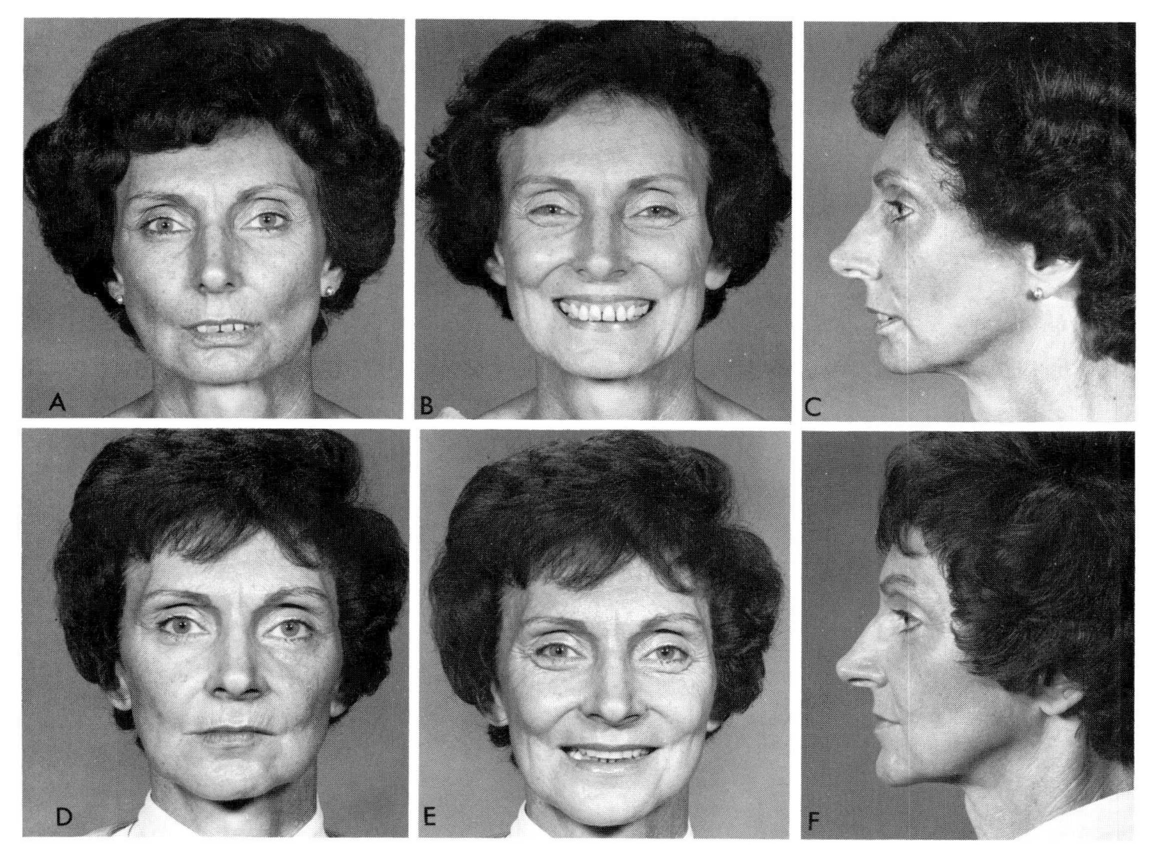

Figure 22–45 (Case 22–12). *A–C,* Preoperative appearance of 49-year-old woman. *D–F,* Postoperative facial appearance.

Illustration and legend continued on the following page.

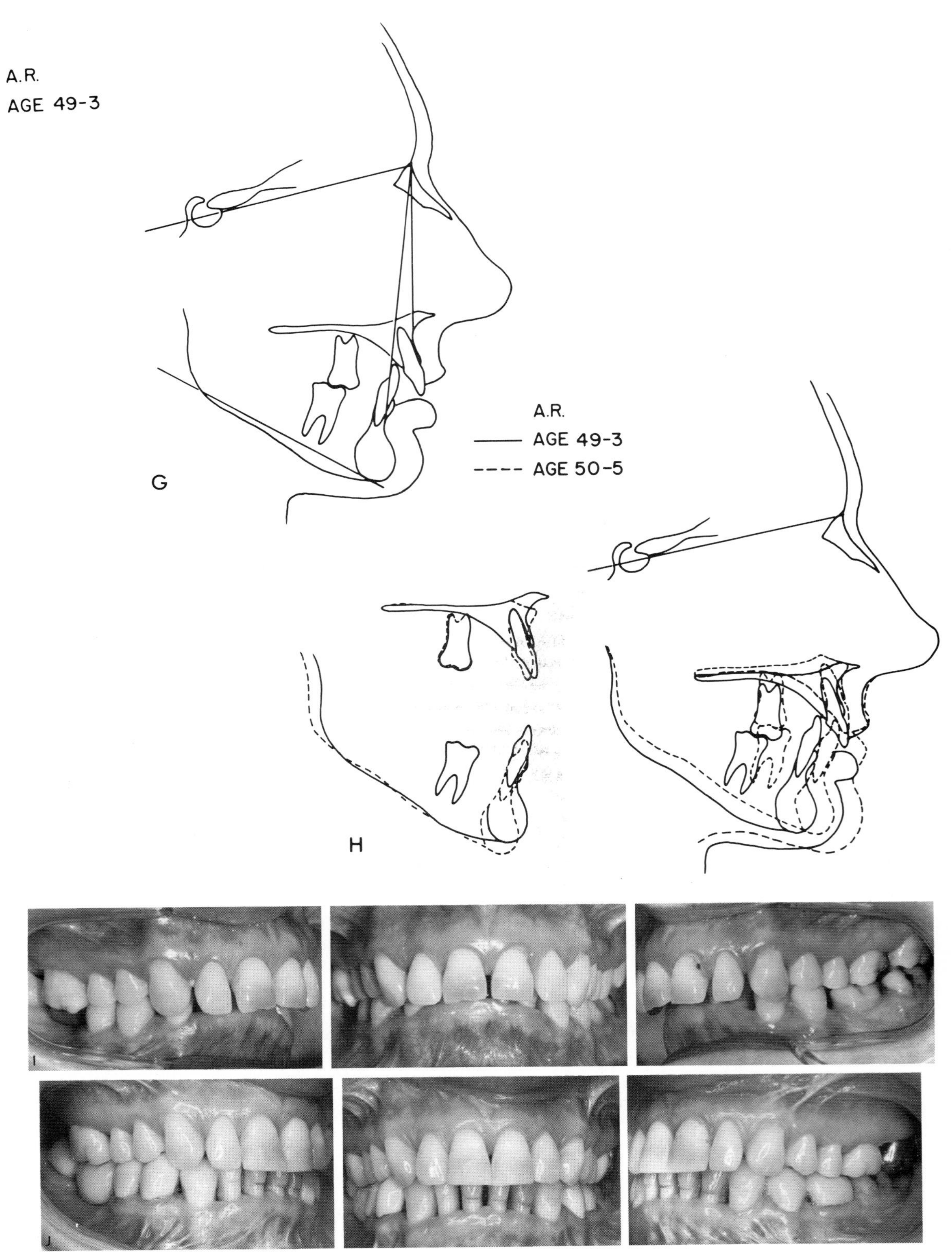

Figure 22–45 *Continued.* *G,* Cephalometric tracing before treatment (age 49 years, 3 months). *H,* Composite cephalometric tracings before (solid line) and after (broken line) treatment. *I,* Pretreatment occlusion. *J,* Post-treatment occlusion.

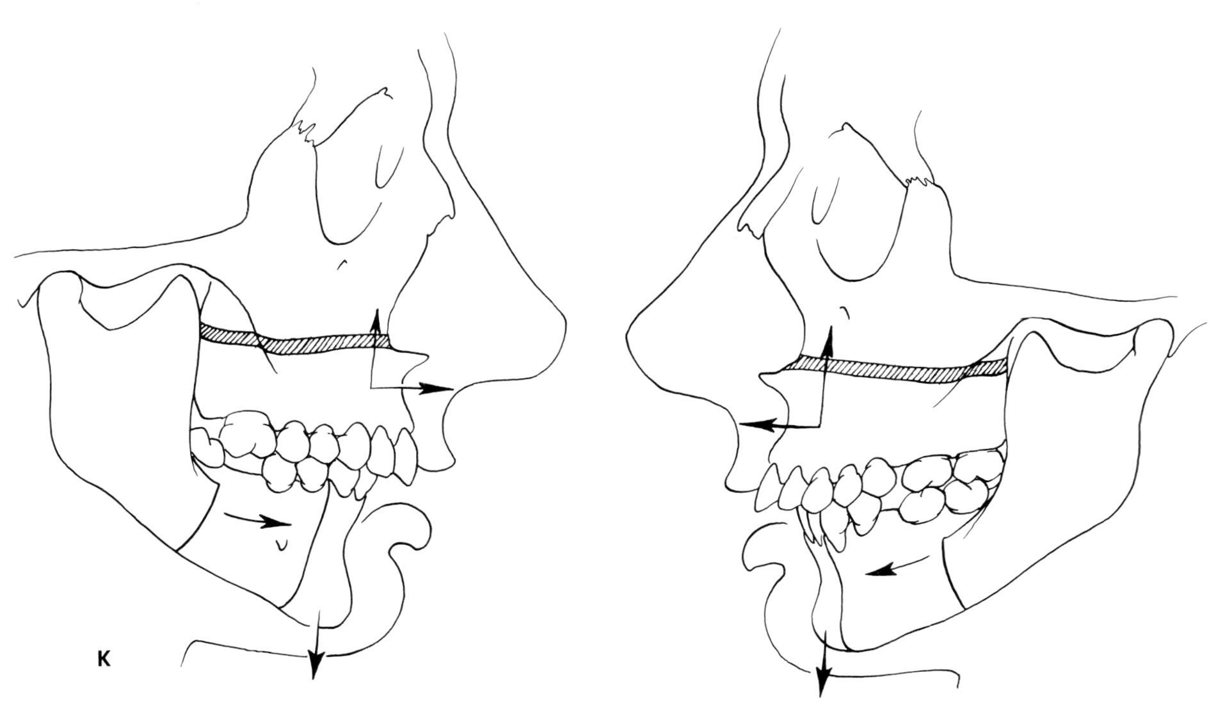

Figure 22–45 *Continued.* *K,* Diagrammatic plan of maxillary and mandibular surgery: Le Fort I osteotomy to raise, advance, and widen maxilla; sagittal split ramus osteotomies to advance mandible; anterior mandibular body osteotomy to level mandibular occlusal plane.

3. Mandibular advancement (8 mm) by sagittal split ramus osteotomies to achieve maxillomandibular harmony (Fig. 22–45 *K*).
4. Anterior mandibular body osteotomy (Fig. 22–45 *K*) in canine-premolar interdental spaces to lower anterior teeth 4 mm and level mandibular occlusal plane.
5. Possible reduction genioplasty after mandibular advancement.
6. Possible rhinoplasty if nose appeared too prominent and narrow after maxillary and mandibular surgery.
7. Restoration of residual malocclusion with fixed partial and jacket restorations to replace missing teeth and close interdental spaces in maxillary and mandibular arches.
8. Left temporomandibular joint arthroplasty if planned treatment did not effectively control the degenerative joint disease symptoms.

FOLLOW-UP

Subjective

The maxillary and mandibular surgical procedures (excluding genioplasty) were accomplished simultaneously without complications (Fig. 22–45 *K*). Postoperative healing was routine and associated with minimal pain and swelling. All the mobilized and repositioned segments were clinically stable when intermaxillary fixation was discontinued six weeks postoperatively. Restoration of the patient's mutilated malocclusion was completed within another three months by fixed restorations.

Objective

Facial balance (Fig. 22–45 *D, E, F*) and a functional occlusion (Fig. 22–45 *J*) were achieved after six months of treatment. Postoperative clinical and cephalometric studies 24 months postoperatively revealed virtually no movement of the superiorly repositioned maxilla or anteriorly repositioned mandible (Fig. 22–45 *H*). The patient continues to have intermittent myofascial and temporomandibular joint pain which has been adequately managed by conservative therapy. Arthroplasty is a viable alternative should the pain become intolerable to the patient.

COMMENT

The general dentist was the keystone around which a plan of therapy was evolved. Such a plan considered esthetics, function, and stability. The magnitude of the occlusal deformity and age of the patient do not preclude treatment of adult patients with dentofacial deformities. Orthognathic surgery is an effective means of sparing many adults with mutilated malocclusions the fate of partial or complete dentures.

Surgeon: William H. Bell, Dallas, Texas. *Restorative dentistry:* Charles R. Williams, Dallas, Texas.

CASE 22–13 (Fig. 22–46)

L.P., a 34-year-old veteran, was referred by his general dentist for correction of his malocclusion prior to restorative dental procedures.

EVALUATION

Esthetics

Frontal. Unesthetic lower third of face due to prominent lips with redundant tissue on the upper lip, constricted anterior mandible, deep labial mental fold, and inadequate tooth exposure during smiling (Fig. 22–46 *A*).

Profile. Deficient chin projection, procumbent lower lip, long upper lip, deep labial mental fold, and excessive prominence of upper lip (Fig. 22–46 *B*).

Cephalometric Evaluation

Maxillary protrusion—SNA = 96 degrees, $\underline{1}$–NA = 18 degrees, mandibular dentoalveolar protrusion—SNB = 90 degrees, $\overline{1}$–NB = 51 degrees, and inadequate chin protrusion.

Occlusal Analysis (Fig. 22–46 *E* to *J*)

Dental Arch Form. Maxilla rounded and symmetrical, mandible asymmetrical with constriction of left premolar region.

Dental Alignment. Anterior maxillary interdental spacing, mandibular left premolar supereruption with medial positioning.

Dental Occlusion. Class I cuspid occlusion on the right and Class II cuspid occlusion on the left, anterior deep bite extending from right cuspid to left second premolar with supereruption of left maxillary first and second premolars, which were in complete crossbite.

TREATMENT PLAN (Fig. 22–46 *K*)

1. Six tooth anterior maxillary subapical osteotomy with superior repositioning (6 mm) to:
   a. Correct deep anterior bite.
   b. Improve upper tooth to lip relationship (after excision of redundant upper lip tissue).
2. Left posterior maxillary ostectomy with superior repositioning (5 mm) to:
   a. Correct supereruption of left maxillary premolar teeth.
   b. Increase inter-ridge space to accommodate partial denture.
3. Augmentation genioplasty utilizing horizontal sliding technique to improve chin projection and insertion of Proplast implant to fill in labial mental fold.
4. Extraction of unrestorable maxillary left second premolar and mandibular left third molar teeth.
5. Restoration of carious lesions and restoration of mandibular edentulous spaces with fixed partial denture and fabrication of maxillary removable partial dentures.
6. Mandibular subapical ostectomy around left first and second premolar teeth with inferior and lateral repositioning to:
   a. Correct premolar crossbite.
   b. Level the occlusal plane.
7. Upper lip reduction cheiloplasty to eliminate redundant tissue.

FOLLOW-UP

Subjective

At 24 hours postoperatively the patient was comfortable and required no additional medication for pain. He noted paresthesia over the vermillion border of the upper lip. This resolved in approximately three weeks. Paresthesia over the chin resolved in approximately three months. There was no altered sensation in the lower lip vermillion border.

Objective

Minimal space existed between the roots of the mandibular left cuspid and first premolar teeth. An osteotomy could not be completed at this site; consequently a simple buccal corticotomy was performed. The horizontal ostectomy below the premolar teeth and the vertical osteotomy behind the second premolar teeth were completed through the lingual cortical plate. A thick occlusal acrylic stent was fabricated to open the bite sufficiently to permit correction of the premolar crossbite via elastic traction on the left mandibular premolar teeth. Following correction of the crossbite, it was felt that inferior repositioning of this two-tooth segment could be readily accomplished by reducing the thickness of the acrylic stent. After four weeks of elastic traction there was minimal movement of the premolar segment. Intermaxillary fixation was removed and a left mandibular lingual mucoperiosteal flap was elevated and a

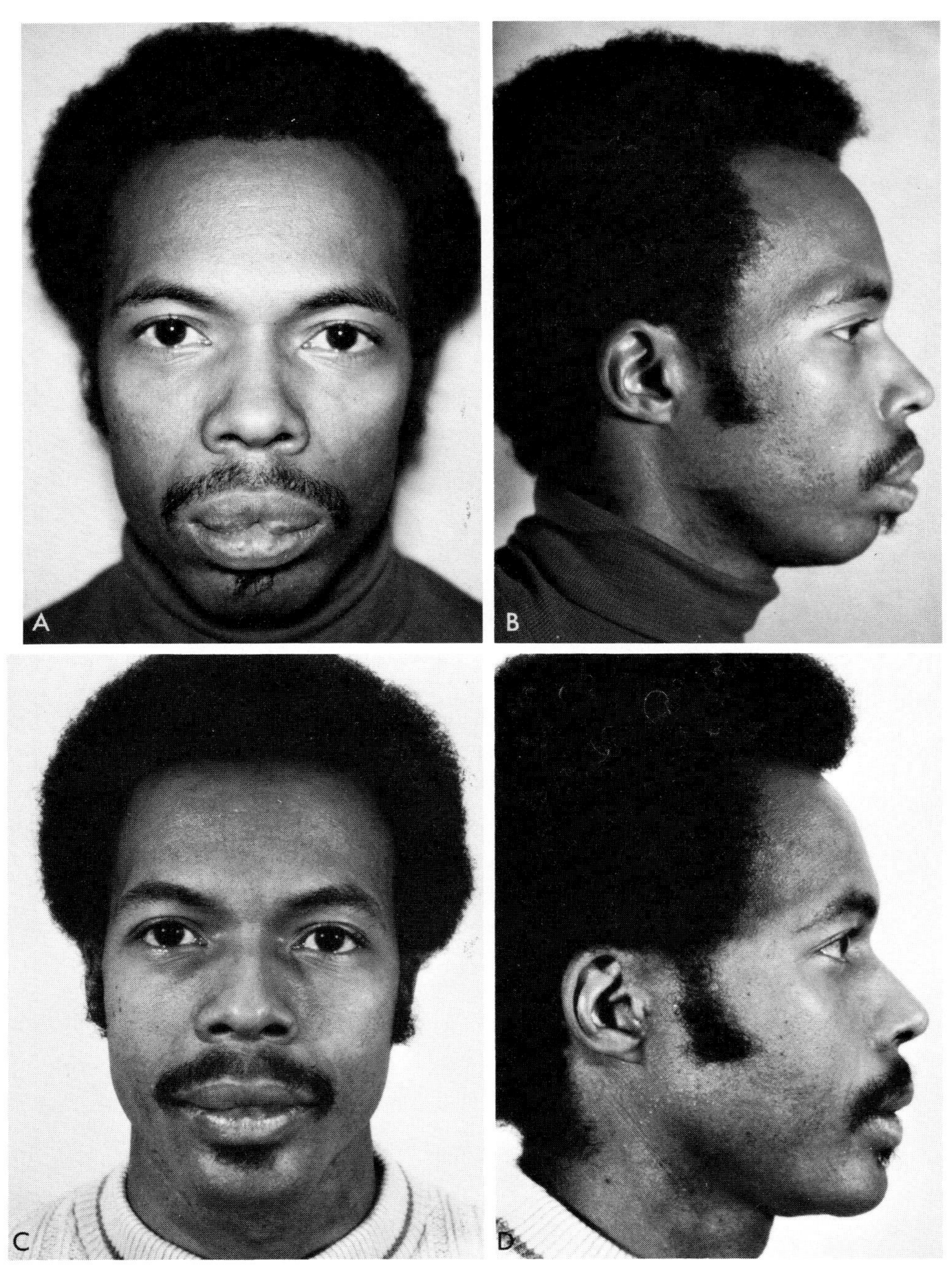

Figure 22–46 (Case 22–13). *A* and *B*, Preoperative facial appearance of 34-year-old man. *C* and *D*, One year postoperative appearance after surgical procedures illustrated *(K)* and completion of dental restorations.

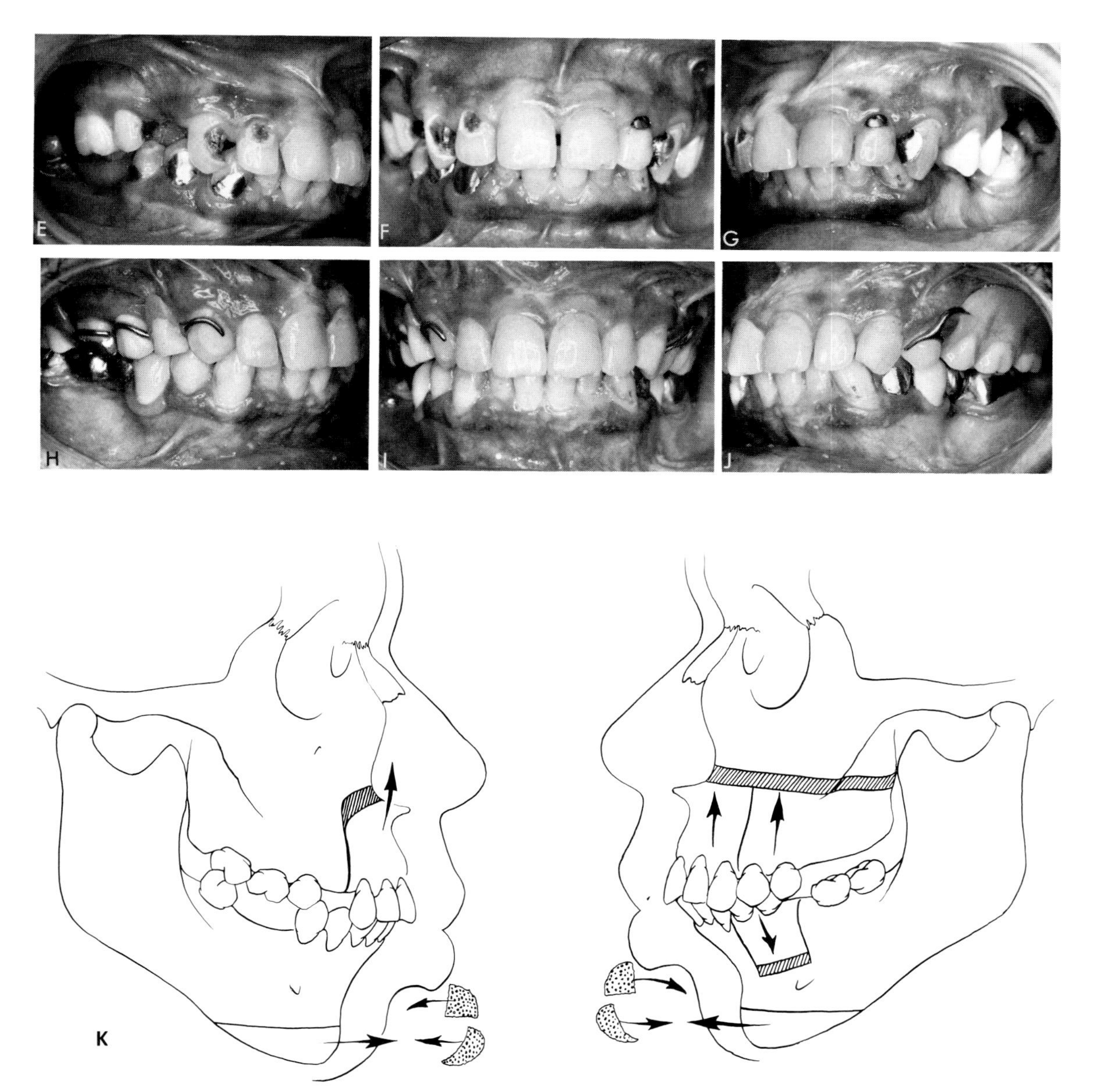

Figure 22–46 *Continued.* *E–G,* Preoperative occlusion. *H–J,* One year postoperative occlusion after prosthetic replacement of missing teeth. *K,* Schematic illustration of surgical plan: anterior and left posterior maxillary ostectomy, left mandibular subapical ostectomy around premolar teeth, augmentation genioplasty with horizontal sliding osteotomy and Proplast implants (stippled structures). Arrows indicate direction of segmented movement.

corticotomy was performed between the cuspid and first premolar teeth. Firm digital pressure mobilized the premolar segment, which was manually repositioned laterally and inferiorly. The acrylic stent was removed and intermaxillary fixation utilizing elastic traction was applied without a stent. Intermaxillary fixation was maintained for one additional week after which maxillary and mandibular Hawley retainers were inserted and worn 24 hours a day for the next two months.

Good clinical union of all segments was noted eight weeks postoperatively. The prosthetic and restorative dental procedures were carried out without difficulty, producing a good occlusal and esthetic result.

Eleven months postoperatively it was noted that the cheiloplasty had produced only a fair result, as there was some asymmetry to the upper lip and persistence of redundant tissue. Consequently a second reduction cheiloplasty was performed; on both occasions the tissue in the upper lip was soft connective tissue and salivary gland tissue, which made it difficult to determine the amount of tissue to be removed. The secondary procedure improved the appearance of the upper lip; however, 22 months postoperatively there was still evidence of redundant upper lip tissue.

Evaluation of frontal facial esthetics 22 months postoperatively revealed good balance in most respects; however, the chin appeared to be very narrow and would have benefited from some lateral mandibular augmentation. The patient was satisfied with the result and desired no additional surgery.

Surgeons: Kevin L. McBride, Dallas, Texas and Francis Collins, Seattle, Washington. *Restorative dentistry:* Claude Ricks, Loma Linda, California.

COMPLICATIONS

Varied occlusal deformities in the anterior and posterior parts of the maxilla and mandible have been successfully corrected by surgically repositioning small dento-osseous segments. Devitalization and subsequent loss of teeth and bone has been rare. Periodontal problems have usually been a consequence of injudicious instrumentation or treatment planning. External root resorption, internal resorption, and ankylosis, stigmata commonly associated with transplanted teeth, were not observed. These findings were attributed to the fact that circulation to the mobilized dento-osseous segments was maintained continuously. The judicious use of a sharp thin spatula osteotome, small fissure burs, and a thin oscillating or reciprocating saw blade (especially useful for sectioning the thicker parts of bone) has minimized bone loss associated with interalveolar osteotomies. A 1 or 2 mm loss of crestal alveolar bone observed in some of the interdental osteotomy sites is more likely the consequence of surgical technique and not vascular ischemia. The excessive removal of interseptal and interradicular bone causes protracted bone healing and has a destructive effect upon the periodontium.

When dentoalveolar segments are made freely mobile by complete transsection of the bone, and the final occlusion is properly balanced, the prognosis for stability after dentoalveolar surgery is excellent. Ten-year follow-up studies of a number of the patients illustrated in this chapter have revealed minimal positional change. The condition of the periodontium of most of these adults was not significantly different from the condition that existed at the time of surgery. Speed of treatment and elimination of long-term retention appliances are additional advantages of orthognathic surgery and segmental osteotomies.

REFERENCES

1. Banks, P.: Pulp changes after anterior mandibular subapical osteotomy in a primate model. J. Max-Fac. Surg. *5*(1):39–48, February, 1977.
2. Barton, P. R. and Rayne, J.: The role of alveolar surgery in the treatment of malocclusion. Brit. Dent. J. January, 1969.
3. Bell, W. H.: Revascularization and bone healing after anterior maxillary osteotomy: A study using adult rhesus monkeys. J. Oral Surg. *27*:249, April, 1969.
4. Bell, W. H.: Surgical-orthodontic treatment of interincisal diastemas. Am. J. Orthodont. *57*:158, Febuary, 1970.
5. Bell, W. H.: Correction of skeletal type anterior open bite. J. Oral Surg. *29*:706–714, 1971.
6. Bell, W. H.: Increasing mandibular arch length by subapical osteotomy. Am. J. Orthodont.
7. Bell, W. H.: Immediate surgical repositioning of one- and two-tooth dento-osseous segments. Int. J. Oral Surg. *2*:265–272, 1973.
8. Bell, W. H. and Levy, B. M.: Healing after anterior maxillary osteotomy. J. Oral Surg. *28*:728–734, 1970.
9. Bell, W. H.: Correction of the short-face syndrome — vertical maxillary deficiency: A preliminary report. J. Oral Surgery *35*:110, February, 1977.
10. Bell, W. H., Creekmore, T. D., Alexander, R. G.: Surgical correction of the long face syndrome. Am. J. Orthodont. *71*:40–67, 1977.
11. Bell, W. H. and Finn, R. A.: Healing after posterior mandibular subapical osteotomy. J. Oral Surg. (In Press).
12. Bell, W. H. and Levy B. M.: Revascularization and bone healing after posterior maxillary osteotomy. J. Oral Surg. *29*:313, May, 1971.
13. Bell, W. H. and Levy, B. M.: Revascularization and bone healing after maxillary corticotomies. J. Oral Surg. *30*:640, September, 1972.
14. Bell, W. H. and McBride, K.: Immediate surgical repositioning of anterior and posterior maxillary dento-osseous segments. J. Oral Surg. *34*:943–947, October, 1976.
15. Bell, W. H. and McBride, K.: Correction of the long face syndrome by Le Fort I osteotomy. A report on some new technical modifications and treatment results. Oral Surg., Oral Med., Oral Path. *44*:493–520, October, 1977.
16. Bell, W. H., Schendel, S. A. and Finn, R. A.: Revascularization after surgical repositioning of one-tooth dento-osseous segments. J. Oral Surg. *36*:757, October, 1978.
17. Bell, W. H. and Turvey, T. A.: Surgical correction of posterior crossbite. J. Oral Surg. *32*:811, November, 1974.
18. Bell, W. H.: Correction of maxillary excess by anterior maxillary osteotomy. J. Oral Surg. *43*:323–332, March, 1977.
19. Burk, J. L., Provencher, R. F., and McKean, T. W.: Small segmental and unitooth ostectomies to correct dento-alveolar deformities. J. Oral Surg. *35*:453, June, 1977.
20. Cunningham, G.: Methode sofortinger Regulierung von anomalen Zahn-stellungen. Oester-Ung Vjschr Zahnheilk *10*:455, 1894.
21. Köle, H.: Corticalisschwaechung zur Untersteutzung bei der Kieferorthopaedischen Behandlung. Fortschr Kiefer Gesichtschir *4*:208, 1958.
22. Köle, H.: Surgical operations on the alveolar ridge to correct occlusal abnormalities. Oral Surg. *12*:515–529, 1959.
23. Kretz, H., Cited by Reichenback, E., Köle, H., and Brueckl, H.: Chirurgische Kieferorthopaedie. Leipzig, Barth Verlag, p. 184, 1965.
24. Kretz, R.: Die chirurgische Immediatregulierung der Prognathie. Dtsch. Zahnheilkd. Vol. 81, Leipzig, 1931.
25. Kufner, J.: Nove notedy chirurgickeho leceni otevreneho skusu. (New methods of surgical treatment of open bites). Cslka. Stomat. *60*:5, 1960.
26. McBride, K., and Bell, W. H.: Immediate repositioning of posterior mandibular dento-alveolar segments. J. Oral Surg. (in press).
27. Merrill, R.: Corticotomy techniques. A.S.O.S. Clinical Congress Current Concepts in Oral Surgery. March, 17–20, 1973, Philadelphia, Pennsylvania.
28. Mehnert, H.: Die interalveolare Osteotomie im Oberkiefer. Dtsch Zahn Mund Kieferheilkd *61*:289, November, 1973.
29. Merrill, R. G. and Pedersen, G. W.: Interdental osteotomy for immediate repositioning of dental-osseous elements. J. Oral Surg. *34*:118, February, 1976.
30. Obwegeser, H. L.: Surgical correction of small or retrodisplaced maxillae: the 'dish-face' deformity. Plast Reconstr Surg *43*:351, April 1969.
31. Poswillo, D. E.: Early pulp changes following reduction of open bite by segmental surgery. Int. J. Oral Surg. *1*:87, 1972.
32. Rhinelander, F. W. and Baragry, R. A.: Microangiography in bone healing: I. Undisplaced closed fractures. J. Bone Joint Surg. *44-A*:1273, October, 1962.
33. Schallhorn, R.: The use of autogenous hip marrow biopsy implants for bony crater defects. J Periodont *39*:145, May, 1968.
34. Schuchardt, K.: Experiences with the surgical treatment of some deformities of the jaws: prognathia, micrognathia, and open bite. *In* Wallace, A. B. (ed.), International Society of Plastic Surgeons, Transactions

of Second Congress, London, 1959. Edinburgh, E. and Livingstone, S., page 73, 1961.
35. Ware, W. H. and Ashamalla, M.: Pulpal response following anterior maxillary osteotomy. Am. J. Orthodont. *60*:156–164, 1971.
36. Wassmund, M.: Frakturen und Luxationen des Gesichtsschadels. Berlin, 1927.
37. Willmar, K.: On Le Fort I osteotomy. Scand. J. Plast. Reconstr. Surg., Suppl *12*, 1974.
38. Wunderer, S.: Erfahrungen mit der Operativen Behandlung Hochgradiger Prognathien, Dtsch. Zahn-Mund-Kieferheilkd. *39*:451, 1963.

NEW HORIZONS

Section IV

Chapter 23

TERATOLOGIC DEVELOPMENT OF DENTOFACIAL AND CRANIOFACIAL DEFORMITIES

David Poswillo

Craniofacial malformations have aroused the curiosity of man since the first graphic records of cave dwellers were carved in their sandstone walls. The Babylonians have recorded prophetic announcements on their clay tablets based on the birth of an infant with cleft lip. Sculptured images of facial clefts, hemifacial microsomia, and the Treacher Collins syndrome are found in the "potato pots" of Central and South America and in the pre-Columbian terra cottas of the New World (Fig. 23–1). But it was not until the seventeenth century that Geoffrey St. Hilaire[16] changed the emphasis of interest in deformity from the historical and anatomic to the scientific investigation of causal mechanisms.

To enter life as a structurally normal individual, the human fetus must overcome at least two major hazards: noxious genetic influences and environmental trigger agents. Either or both of these may upset the delicately balanced timetable of morphogenesis, which is telescoped into a short span of 60 days between the twenty-fifth and eighty-fifth days of development. Although it has not yet proved possible to determine the degree to which specific factors adversely influence prenatal development, certain general observations have emerged. Fraser[2] has proposed that a minority of craniofacial malformations have a major environmental cause and a minority have a major genetic cause. However, it is believed that majority of malformations

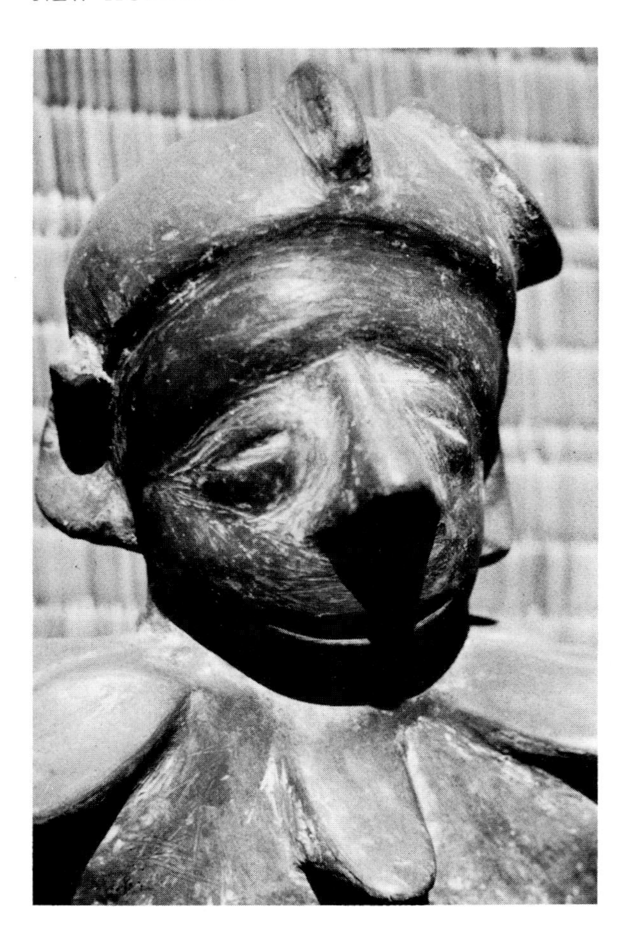

Figure 23–1. Pre-Columbian carving in terra cotta of Treacher Collins facies.

result from complex interactions between genetic predispositions and subtle factors, perhaps cumulative, in the intrauterine environment. This is generally known as the polygenic multifactorial hypothesis; that is, the instability or unsuitability of genes at many different loci may be influenced by additional environmental factors to such a degree that a departure from the programmed plan of normal morphogenesis occurs.

CAUSES OF CRANIOFACIAL DEFORMITY

Craniofacial Deformity with a Major Genetic Cause

Gross chromosomal aberrations capable of causing a genetic imbalance are responsible for a few well-known and easily identified craniofacial syndromes. These patients usually possess multiple malformations comprising a distinctive pattern that constitutes a clinical entity. Accumulated knowledge of these syndromes can be utilized in evaluating the patient and in providing specific management and prognostic and genetic counseling.

Gross Chromosomal Abnormality. Down syndrome (or trisomy 21) is the best known of the gross chromosomal abnormalities. It involves the presence of an extra G chromosome, generally referred to as number 21. The pathogenesis of this condition is directly related to the altered genetic control of morphodifferentiation produced by the extra chromosome with its superfluity of genes. Other recognized syndromes having a chromosomal pathogenesis are rare, but the classification includes Patau syndrome (trisomy 13–15), cri du chat syndrome (partial deletion of the short arm of B-group chromosome 5), and Edwards syndrome (trisomy 18).

Single Mutant Genes. In man, some mutant genes are responsible for deformities of the craniofacial complex. Dominant mutant genes are usually received from one affected parent. The gametes of the affected person have an equal chance of transmitting, or not transmitting, the mutant gene to the next generation. This means that the affected parent has an equal chance of transmitting the disorder to the children, but the unaffected children can never pass on the disorder. The Treacher Collins syndrome (mandibulofacial dysostosis) is an example of an autosomal dominant condition (Fig. 23–2). Expression of this malformation varies greatly among members

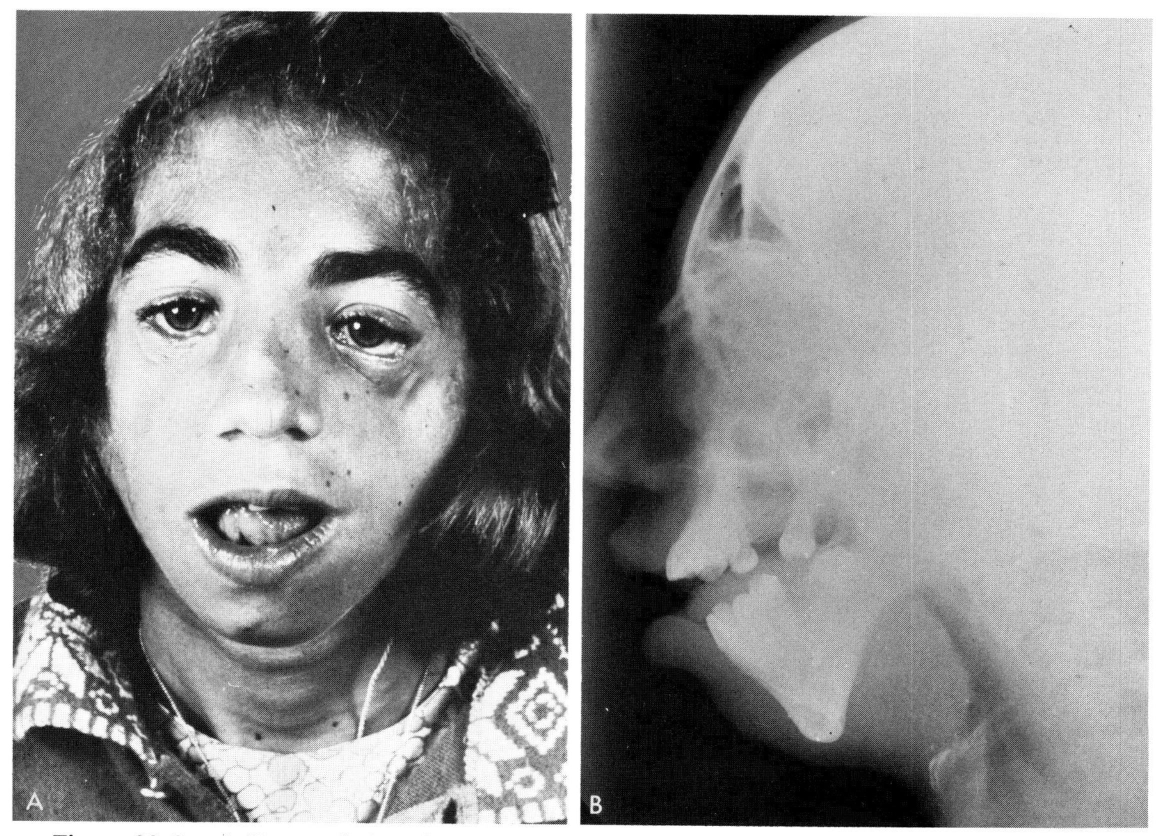

Figure 23–2. *A*, Human facies of Treacher Collins syndrome showing antimongoloid slope of eyes, malar hypoplasia, lower lid colobomata, and open bite. *B*, Lateral jaw radiograph of patient in *A*, showing characteristic concavity of lower border of mandible.

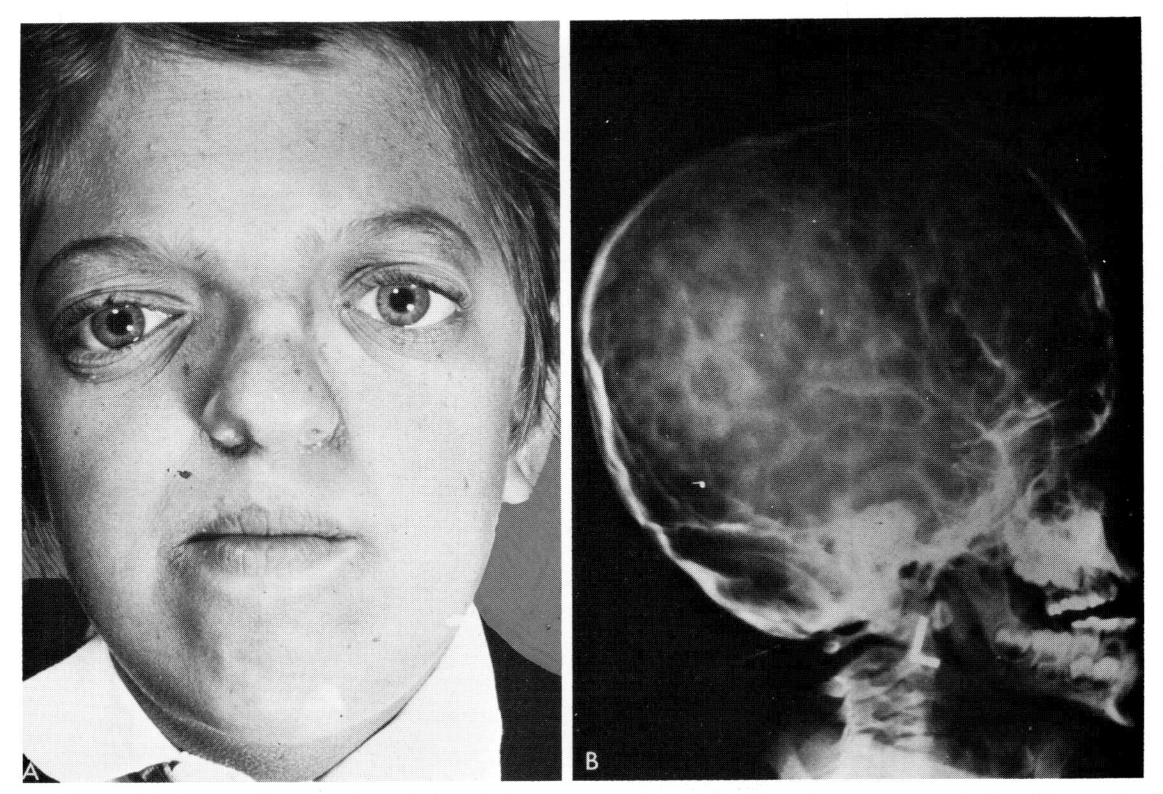

Figure 23–3. *A*, Characteristic facies of Crouzon syndrome. *B*, Digital markings in skull radiograph of patient in *A*; note maxillary hypoplasia.

of the same family. This variability is a clinical feature of autosomal dominant traits. Other well-known autosomal dominant traits inducing craniofacial deformity are Crouzon syndrome (craniofacial dysostosis) (Fig. 23–3), Apert syndrome (acrocephalo-syndactyly) (Fig. 23–4), cherubism, and cleft lip and/or palate with paramedian lip pits (Fig. 23–5).

Autosomal Recessive (Paired Mutant Genes). Some genetically determined malformations are recessive and require that the mutant gene to be present in double dose in an individual (the homozygous state) before the trait is expressed in the form of a defect. Hurler syndrome (mucopolysaccharidosis I) is an example of such a condition producing abnormal facial features (Fig. 23–6).

X-linked Inheritance. The term *X-linked* means sex-linked; that is, that the mutant gene is located on the X chromosome. The pattern of transmission is from women who are carriers to half their daughters (who also become carriers) and half their sons (who are therefore affected). Father-to-son transmission does not occur in either the dominant or the recessive X-linked condition. There are relatively few X-linked dominant traits affecting the facial skeleton. The oro-facial-digital syndrome characterized by frontal bossing, facial clefts, and dental crowding is one example of the X-linked dominant condition. The oto-palato-digital syndrome is probably an X-linked recessive condition with characteristic facial abnormalities.

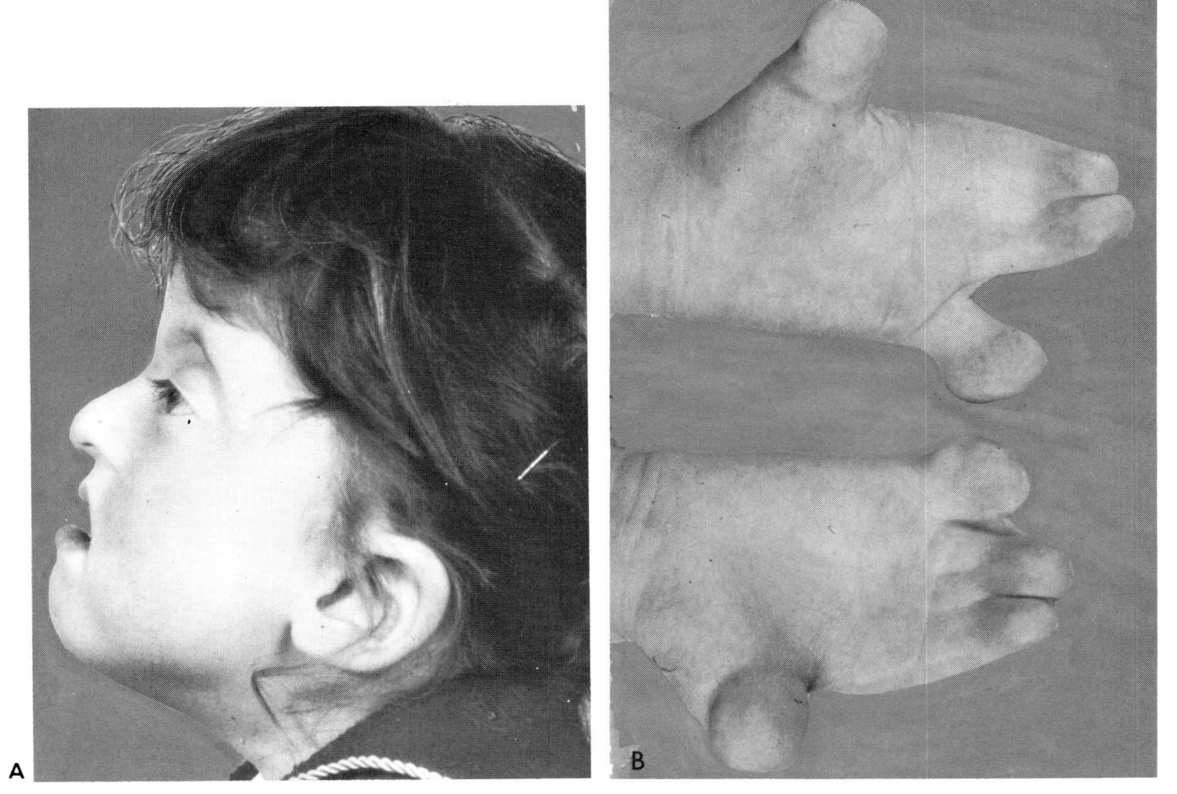

Figure 23–4. *A*, Lateral face characteristic of Apert syndrome. *B*, Syndactyly found in association with acrocephaly in same patient.

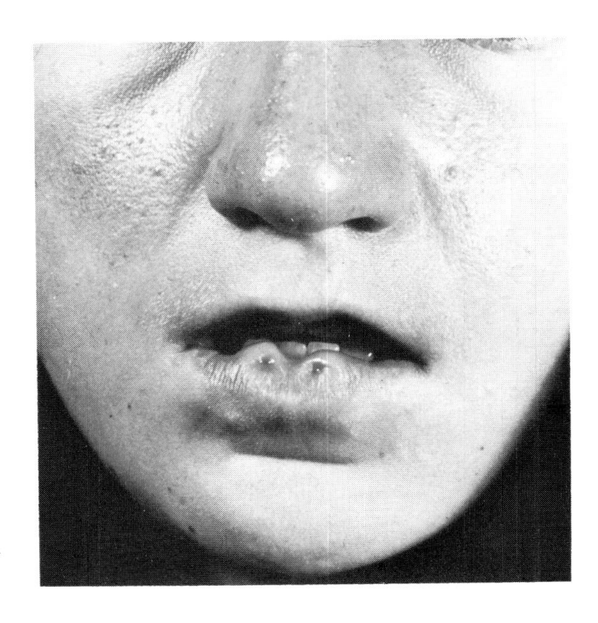

Figure 23–5. Congenital lip pits, also associated with cleft palate.

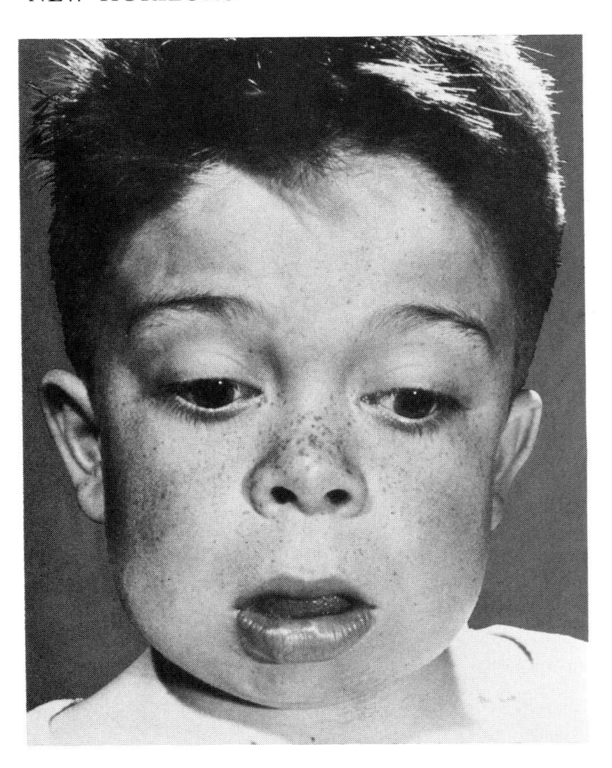

Figure 23-6. Characteristic "gargoylism" found in Hurler syndrome.

Environmental Agents of Major Effect Causing Craniofacial Deformity

It is surprising how few environmental agents have been positively identified as causing facial deformity in man. Many teratogens have been shown to be capable of inducing cleft lip and cleft palate in animal models, but there is very little evidence that the majority of these teratogens have a similar effect in causing human malformation.

Although many forms of maternal medication have been suspected of teratogenicity at one time or another, very few have been implicated as teratogens of major effect. Aminopterin and some other cancer chemotherapeutic agents that interfere with DNA synthesis lead to gross malformation if the fetus survives the abortifacient activity of the drug. Frontal bossing and cleft palate have been observed in offspring of mothers treated by these drugs. Thalidomide, taken very early during embryogenesis (between days 20 and 25), frequently leads to the development of otomandibular defects closely comparable with hemifacial microsomia. Defects in the outer and middle ear, malar bone, and ramus of the mandible have been observed in a large proportion of children in Germany and the United Kingdom whose mothers had taken thalidomide. Tetracyclines are also teratogenic. They have been shown to affect the differentiation of developing teeth and also to produce discoloration of the forming hard tissues. Whether they can affect skeletal and visceral morphogenesis is as yet unresolved. Anticonvulsant drugs such as phenytoin, trimethadione, and paramethadione are suspected of causing cleft palate in the offspring of epileptic mothers. Although the incidence of these facial clefts is higher in the anticonvulsant-treated group than in the population at large, positive identification of the teratogen has yet to be established.

Hydrocortisone analogs are also suspected of inducing clefts of the palate. Again, the picture is not clear, for many normal children have been born to mothers treated by corticosteroid drugs in the critical first trimester of pregnancy.

Viral agents such as rubella and cytomegalovirus are known teratogens. When they are acquired by the fetus from the mother, malformations of the eyes, ears, and heart may result. Other viral agents such as herpes simplex, vaccinia, varicella, and variola may cause serious fetal disease but have not as yet been known to lead to structural malformations.

Ionizing radiations have induced microcephaly and cleft palate in liveborn offspring whose mothers had been exposed to therapeutic or accidental pelvic irradiation during the first ten weeks of pregnancy (Fig. 23–7).

The role of maternal metabolic disease in the etiology of congenital defects of the head and face is still unclear. Diabetes mellitus has been shown to increase the likelihood of fetal loss and also to increase the incidence of malformation in offspring to about three times that found in offspring of nondiabetic mothers. The incidence of facial clefts is much higher in children of mothers with a family predispostion to diabetes. Even now, after many years of monitoring factors influencing pregnancies that resulted in deformed offspring, it is not easy to state with assurance what caused a solitary malformation in an otherwise normal individual. The etiology of a single malformation is less specific than that of a recognized pattern of multiple malformation, such as is seen in Down syndrome, in which chromosomal aberration is obviously the predominant factor.

Multifactorial Polygenic Causes of Craniofacial Deformity

At present there is apparently little evidence to show that the causative agent of most of the common craniofacial malformations such as cleft lip and/or palate, man-

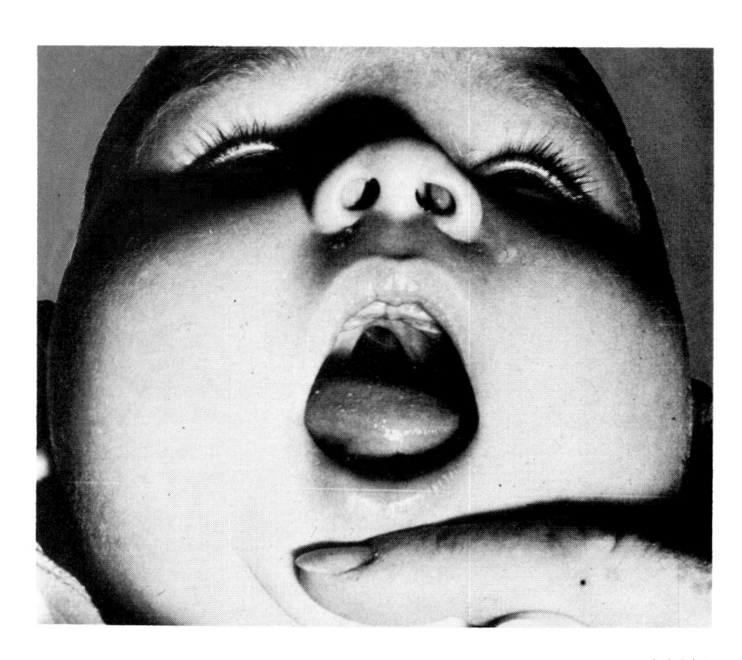

Figure 23–7. Cleft posterior palate in child affected by maternal pelvic irradiation in sixth week of intrauterine life.

dibular prognathism, and maxillary hypoplasia is either a single genetic factor or a major environmental teratogen. Many genetic factors may combine with environmental stimuli to advance the pattern of morphogenesis past the threshold that divides normal from abnormal development. Obviously, the genotype of both mother and fetus is of considerable importance in determining the vulnerability of the fetus to environmental teratogens. There is some evidence that the hormonal balance of the mother can influence the incidence of genetically determined deformities in the offspring. Maternal age, the position of the fetus in the uterus, and even the sex of the fetus may be significant in determining whether or not it is affected by environmental teratogens. At present one can only speculate on how genetically determined factors may modify the activity of teratogenic agents and vice versa. Until a great deal more is learned about the actual mechanisms of malformation, it will be difficult to define the etiology of common craniofacial disorders such as cleft lip and palate in more precise terms than "being caused by polygenic multifactorial inheritance."

MODEL SYSTEMS FOR CRANIOFACIAL STUDIES

Alexander Pope's adage, "the proper study of mankind is man," holds true for many facets of human inquiry. Unfortunately, studying the causal mechanisms of craniofacial malformation in the human species is not easy. It is essential for the developmental pathologist to investigate the sequence of events leading to deformity if he is to establish concrete data concerning the pattern of malformation. The agents that may cause malformation are probably numbered in the thousands, but the sites at which they operate and the mechanisms that they initiate are probably very few. Thus, there seems to be no reason for postulating different sites of primary action and different causal mechanisms for either teratogenic or causal factors. Both environmental agents and genes behave as initiators and set in motion mechanisms that affect similar developmental pathways in the dysmorphogenetic process. For these reasons, studies in animal species may contribute valuable information concerning the site and mode of action of teratogenic agents. When animal models of human malformations can be found, either with spontaneous or induced defects, detailed investigation of the pathogenesis of the animal deformity should hopefully shed light on the human counterpart.

Principles of Teratogenesis

In the last ten years, experimental teratology has produced considerable information derived from animal experiments that help to establish the principles of teratogenesis. Some of the important concepts derived from these studies are as follows:

When a pregnant mammal is exposed to a teratogenic agent, the end product of its action, both in type and incidence, will apparently be determined by the dose of the agent and the time at which it was administered. Timing is of more importance than dosage because there is a strictly limited period during which any organ is potentially vulnerable to the effects of a teratogen. During this teratogen-sensitive period, there is a critical phase of intense susceptibility to malformation. This critical period is probably determined by the degree of mitotic activity in the parts undergoing differentiation. Even so, in nature wide variation exists among teratogenic agents, even when these are administered at the same time. This may be explained, in part, by the time taken for the teratogen to become biologically active in the embryonic system. Agents such as trypan blue are slow-acting teratogens. These agents are stored in the yolk sac and probably cause cleft palate and other facial malformations in the rat embryo by impairment of embryonic nutrition. On the other hand, ionizing radiation, which has a direct effect on mitotic activity in the embryo, probably triggers off the causal mechanism in hours rather than days. Even in the most grotesque monsters, animal or human, normal development predominates over malformation. To maintain scientific perspective, the experimental pathologist must always remember that from the biologic point of view malformation represents a "near-miss" rather than a reproductive failure. Most teratogens act in a narrow dose zone; to exceed the dose induces fetal death, to fall short permits normal development. It is between these ever-looming traps that the experimentalist must steer in attempts to produce and study phenocopies of human facial deformity.

Spontaneous Animal Models of Craniofacial Deformity

Although much emphasis has been placed on the induction of abnormalities by teratogenic agents, numerous spontaneous defects of the craniofacial regions in animals have also been described. Achondroplasia, for example, is found in dog breeds such as the boxer and the dachshund. Just as cleft lip and palate are among the most common structural anomalies known to affect man, so too are they found with considerable frequency in domestic and laboratory animals. Spontaneous cleft lip and/or cleft palate occurs in about 10 to 15 per cent of all offspring in A strain mice. If there is an inbred susceptibility to such malformations, the incidence may be increased very considerably by administering teratogenic substances such as cortisone acetate to the dam between day 11 and day 13 of pregnancy (Fig. 23–8). Adjusting the malformation rate to near 100 per cent deformity permits serial study of those daily changes that distinguish normal from abnormal morphogenesis in the A strain mouse. Cleft lip and/or palate also occurs spontaneously in both boxer dogs and dachshunds. Again, the incidence of deformity may be increased by adding environmental teratogens such as excessive vitamin A to the diet. There are many advantages to having spontaneous animal models of craniofacial malformation that may be manipulated by teratogenic agents. For example, by establishing an incidence of 100 per cent cleft lip and palate in the A strain mouse by using teratogens such as cortisone or salicylate, the causal mechanism of malformation may be studied from the period of early development of the facial process until the time of parturition. Thus, a sequential pattern of events can be established and the pathogenesis of that particular malformation elucidated. By manipulating the incidence of malformation to 50 per cent normal and 50 per cent deformed, the postdifferentiation changes in growth and development in both the normal and deformed littermates may be evaluated and compared. Studies of this kind contribute much to our understanding of the origin and effects of facial malformation.

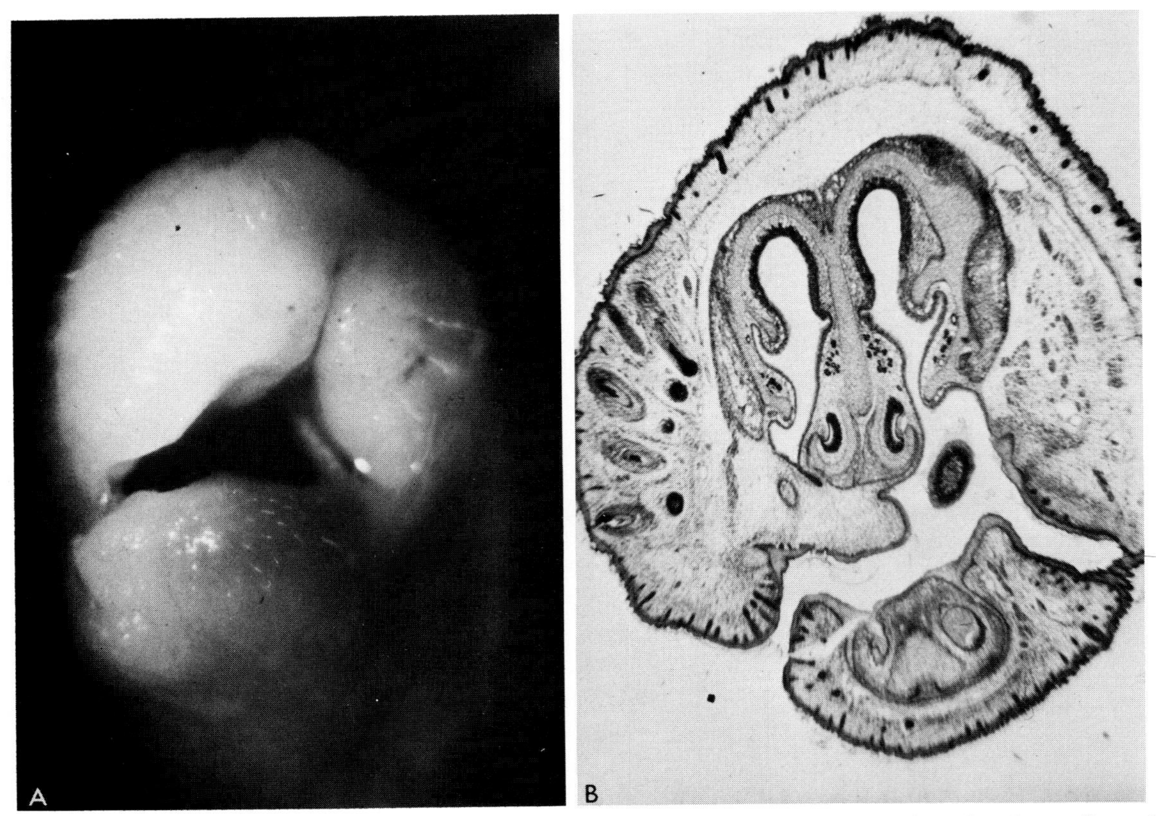

Figure 23–8. *A*, Cleft lip and palate in A strain mouse. *B*, Frontal section through *A*, showing unilateral defect of palate with tongue in cleft.

The spontaneous occurrence of human patterns of malformation in animals that survive birth and weaning provides an opportunity for the experimentalist to study the effects of reconstructive procedures on both normal and affected specimens. This provides comparative data that can be assessed against data from the unoperated controls. In this way valuable information about the effects of surgical procedures on growth and development of the craniofacial complex may be obtained, and new biologic methods of reconstruction can be planned and assessed.

Unfortunately, providing spontaneous/manipulated animal models of cleft lip and palate for surgical and growth studies is far from easy. Rodent models seldom survive birth; the rat or mouse selectively destroys the deformed neonates, and even cross-fostering or hand-rearing techniques have met with little success. Dogs and monkeys, on the other hand, can be reared to maturity and provide good material for further biologic investigation. The major drawback with the most readily available of these models, the dachshund dog, is that the structural malformation of cleft lip and palate is superimposed on the genetic growth disorder of achondroplasia. It is by no means certain that growth and development studies of malformations in this species, even when well-controlled, will provide relevant information about similar malformations in man (Fig. 23–9). Although the monkey, a near-human primate, is structurally similar to man, the incidence of spontaneous cleft lip and palate is so low in established colonies that it is presently no more than a rare curiosity. Such models

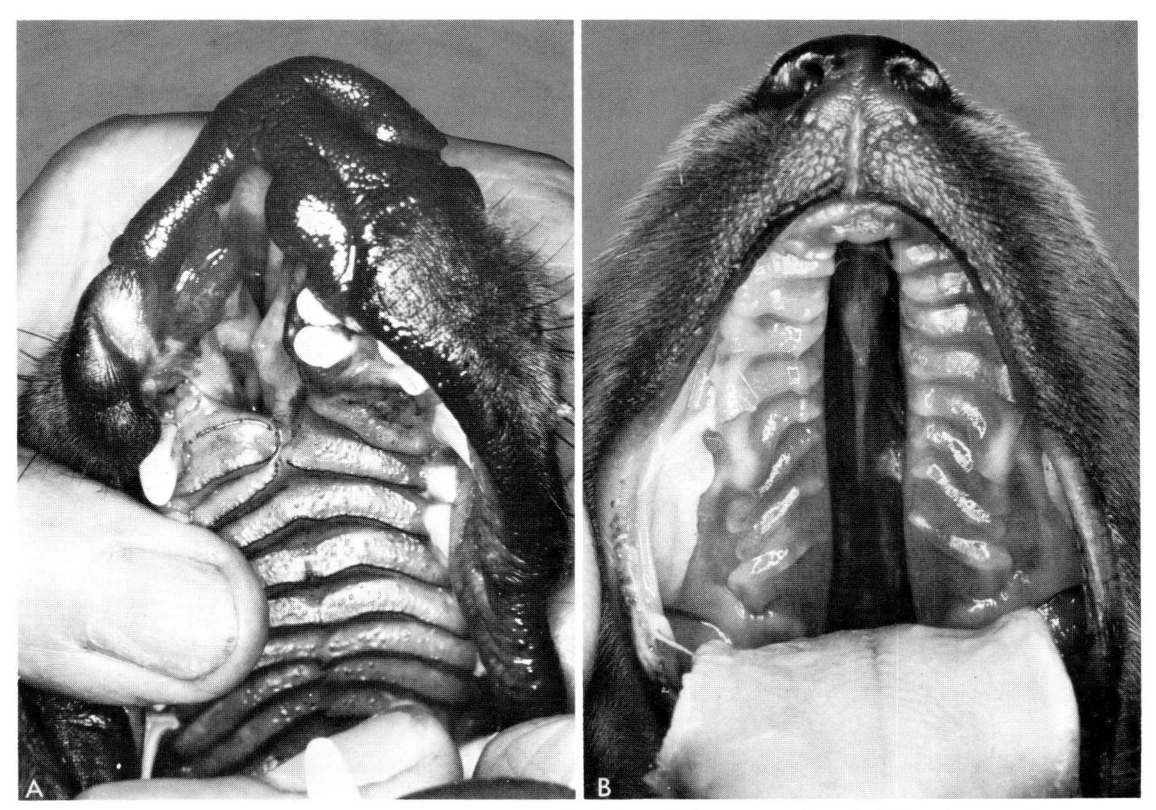

Figure 23–9. *A*, Cleft lip and alveolus in dachshund dog. *B*, Isolated cleft palate in dog.

would offer almost everything that the experimental maxillofacial surgeon could desire, but there seems little likelihood at this stage of establishing a colony with a high incidence of these facial clefts.

Induced Animal Models of Craniofacial Deformity

It is in the field of experimentally induced models of facial deformity that the most vigorous fundamental and applied biologic research will most likely be conducted. In the past decade, experimental teratologists have observed teratogen-induced patterns of malformation in the mammalian species (from rodent to near-human primate) that correspond closely to specific malformations in man. Some of the model systems developed have provided insights into the pathogenesis of malformations such as cleft lip and palate, isolated cleft palate, the Pierre Robin anomaly, submucous cleft palate, hemifacial microsomia, and the Treacher Collins syndrome. In addition, comparison of the pathogenesis of the animal malformation with the clinical defects and changes coincident with growth in man has revealed important information concerning the probable response of the deformities to reconstructive surgery at different stages of postnatal development. Hopefully, this field of biologic investigation will be studied in greater detail by maxillofacial surgeons. Therefore, a brief review is given of the useful induced-animal models of facial defects that are currently known to teratologists.

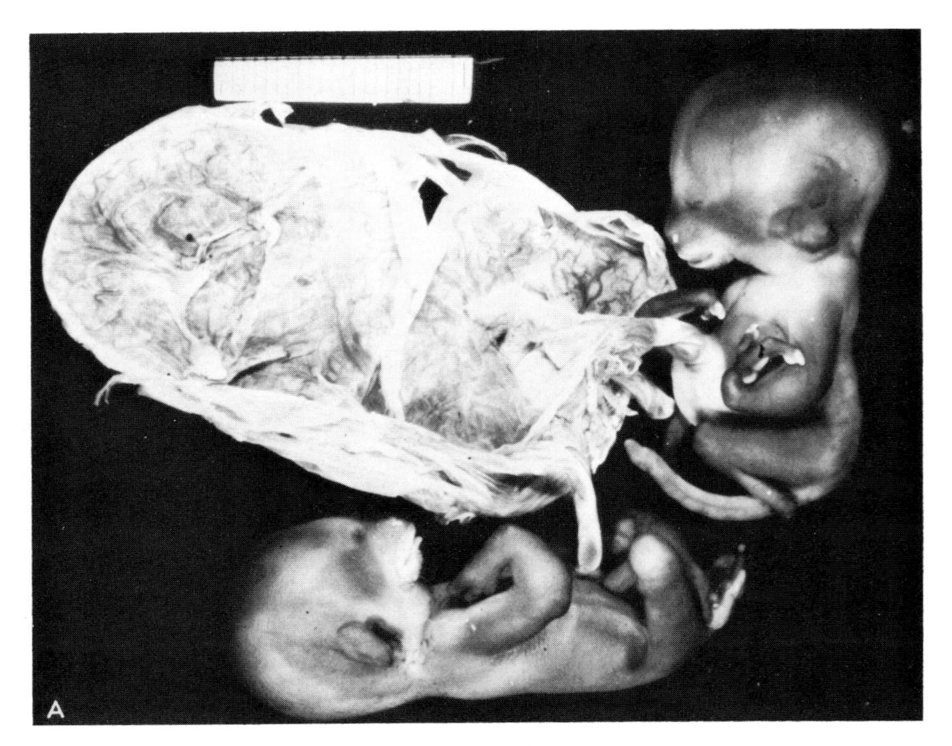

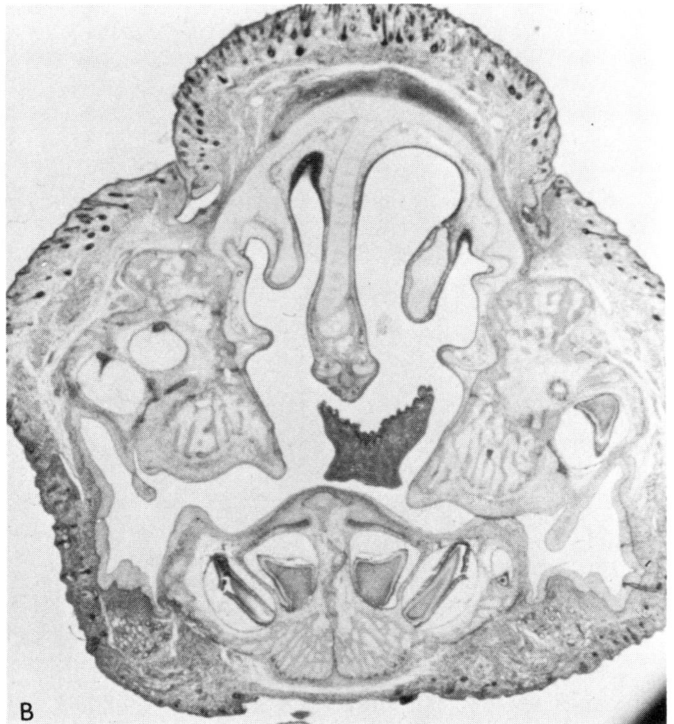

Figure 23–10. *A*, Marmoset twins affected by irradiation, showing variable defects of ears, mandible, and limbs. *B*, Frontal section through face of one twin, showing bilateral cleft palate.

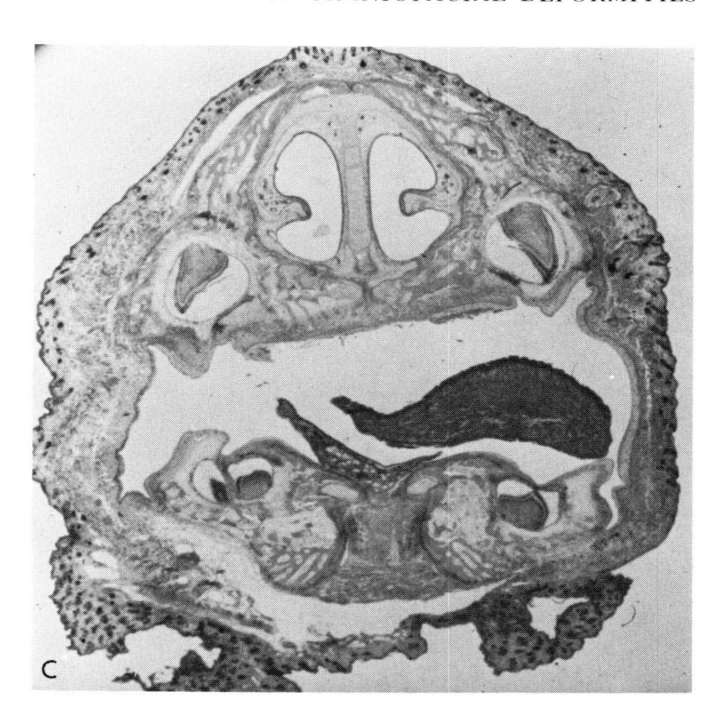

Figure 23–10 *Continued.* *C,* Frontal section through palate of other twin, showing normal palate.

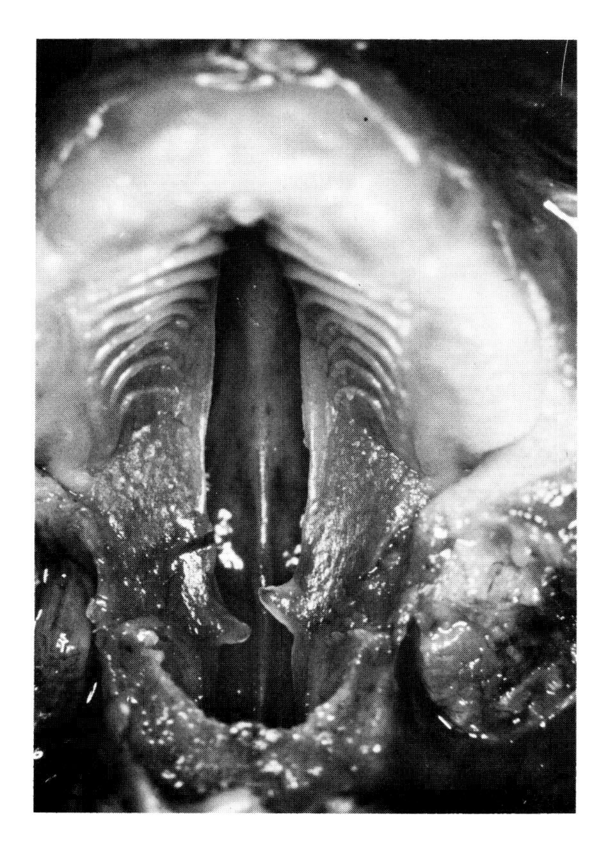

Figure 23–11. Isolated cleft palate induced in macaque fetus by hypervitaminosis A. (Photograph by courtesy of Dr. James G. Wilson.)

Cleft Lip and Alveolus

The antibiotic hadacidin, when given intraperitoneally to the pregnant Wistar rat on day 11 of development, induces cleft lip and alveolus. Lejour[6] has shown that the cleft arises from interference with programmed cell death in the vicinity of the nasal fin adjacent to the primitive nares. The extensive necrotic area in the primary palate leads to defective repair by the isthmus mesenchyme, and complete cleft of the lip and alveolus or cleft lip with Simonart's band can be induced by this mechanism. Only a proportion of these embryos survive to full term, and there is no record of any of these rodents being reared to maturity.

Cleft Lip and Palate

Trasler[18] has demonstrated that salicylates administered to A strain mice induce unilateral or bilateral clefts of the lip and palate. The predetermined shape of the face in this strain predisposes to cleft formation by reducing the pressure between the median nasal process and the lateral nasal process while mesenchymal penetration is attempting to take place. Subsequent growth forces apply traction to the faulty union, with the resultant onset of clefts characterized by residual tags of tissue on the nasal aspect. When the median process is abnormally large and unstable, the tongue becomes trapped on the nasal aspect. Thus restricted in the future nasal cavity, the tongue fails to descend into the floor of the mouth in time for the vertical palatal shelves to move to their final horizontal position. Therefore a sequence of events is established that links clefts of the lip and alveolus with clefts of the posterior palate.

In addition to their value in determining the pathogenesis of cleft lip and palate, these animal models may yield much information on both the selective laterality in this condition (that is, the pronounced left-sided incidence of unilateral cleft lip and palate) and the associated fetal growth changes. Although there are no reports of weaning of rodents with these defects, this could possibly be achieved by cross-fostering or hand-rearing under optimum conditions of animal husbandry. If weaning could be achieved, growth and development studies of the operated, nonoperated, and normal lip/palate could be conducted. Such studies would yield information of considerable value when compared with information concerning the natural history of the cleft lip and palate defect in man.

Isolated cleft palate has been produced in laboratory animals with monotonous regularity by a wide range of teratogens, many of which have little or no relevance to human situations. Nonetheless, by studying the effect on the developing palate of such widely differing substances as cortisone, vitamin A, lathyrogens, and busulfphan, it has been possible to obtain a great deal of information about the sequential changes that are involved in palate closure and the ways in which isolated cleft palate may arise. Serial studies of causal mechanisms in embryos affected by teratogens have revealed that cleft palate may result from defective mesenchymal activity in the palatal shelves proper, with the consequence of the shelves being too small for contact and fusion, or from some other interference with the potential for shelf elevation. Postural immobilization of the tongue between the palatal shelves at the expected time of palatal closure, whether induced by mechanical means such as amniocentesis or by pharmacologic techniques such as cortisone dosage, results in a molding defect of the palate that resembles the Pierre Robin anomaly in man. There is no reliable evidence to date to show that failure of fusion of the shelves is responsible per se for cleft palate, nor has it ever been demonstrated that mesenchymal penetration fails to take place after epithelial fusion. Rupture of the fused palate has been proposed as a causal mechanism of cleft palate, because of the finding of epithelial remnants in the margins of the cleft shelves.[5] However, it has never been proved that the epithelial pearls are derived from the process of shelf fusion followed by mechanical rupture, although there is some evidence to suggest that the epithelial remnants arise from programmed autolysis of the epithelial seam along the shelf margin prior to contact of the palatal plates. The information concerning the pathogenesis of isolated cleft palate that has been obtained from causal mechanism studies on animal models with induced clefts of the posterior palate has been reviewed by Poswillo.[13]

For many years workers have attempted to produce isolated cleft palate in laboratory primates "on demand." Poswillo[10] has shown that this can be achieved in the macaque and marmoset monkey by at least two techniques that are known to produce cleft palate in man. These results have stemmed in part from improved techniques for timing pregnancy in nonhuman primates,[8] and partly from a better understanding of the timing of normal primate palatogenesis.

Pelvic irradiation of the pregnant monkey with 300 rads on day 40 of development can induce cleft palate without embryolethality. The offspring can be delivered by cesarean section, hand-reared, and studied. Both the neonates and growing infants are amenable to surgery, orthodontic treatment, and other rehabilitative procedures. This technique for study of cleft palate can be utilized in the marmoset, in which it has been shown that by reducing the teratogenic irradiation dose to 250 rads, it is possible to induce cleft palate in one cotwin and not the other. Multiple births are frequent in the marmoset (twins being found in about 50 per cent of pregnancies) and offer the possibility of many varied studies in the fields of experimental surgery and growth analyses (Fig. 23–10).

Isolated cleft palate can also be induced in the macaque monkey by the oral administration of water-soluble vitamin A at the rate of 25,000 IU per kilogram from day 35 to day 45 of development. Although the incidence of multiple births in this species is low, the animal model of cleft palate has potential advantages for explorative surgical techniques because of the size of the neonate and the easy access to the oropharynx. The production of near-human models of cleft palate in various primate species can open up entirely new fields of investigation in the discipline of craniofacial anomalies (Fig. 23–11).

Submucous Cleft Palate and Bifid Uvula

These microforms of isolated cleft palate have received little attention from the laboratory investigator, yet their rate of incidence in man is remarkably high (bifid uvula, 1 in 100; submucous cleft palate, 1 in 1200). It has been demonstrated that administration of anticonvulsants such as phenobarbital or phenytoin to mice can induce cleft palate in 15 per cent and submucous cleft palate in 5 to 15 per cent of offspring, with the remainder showing no structural abnormality. This animal system

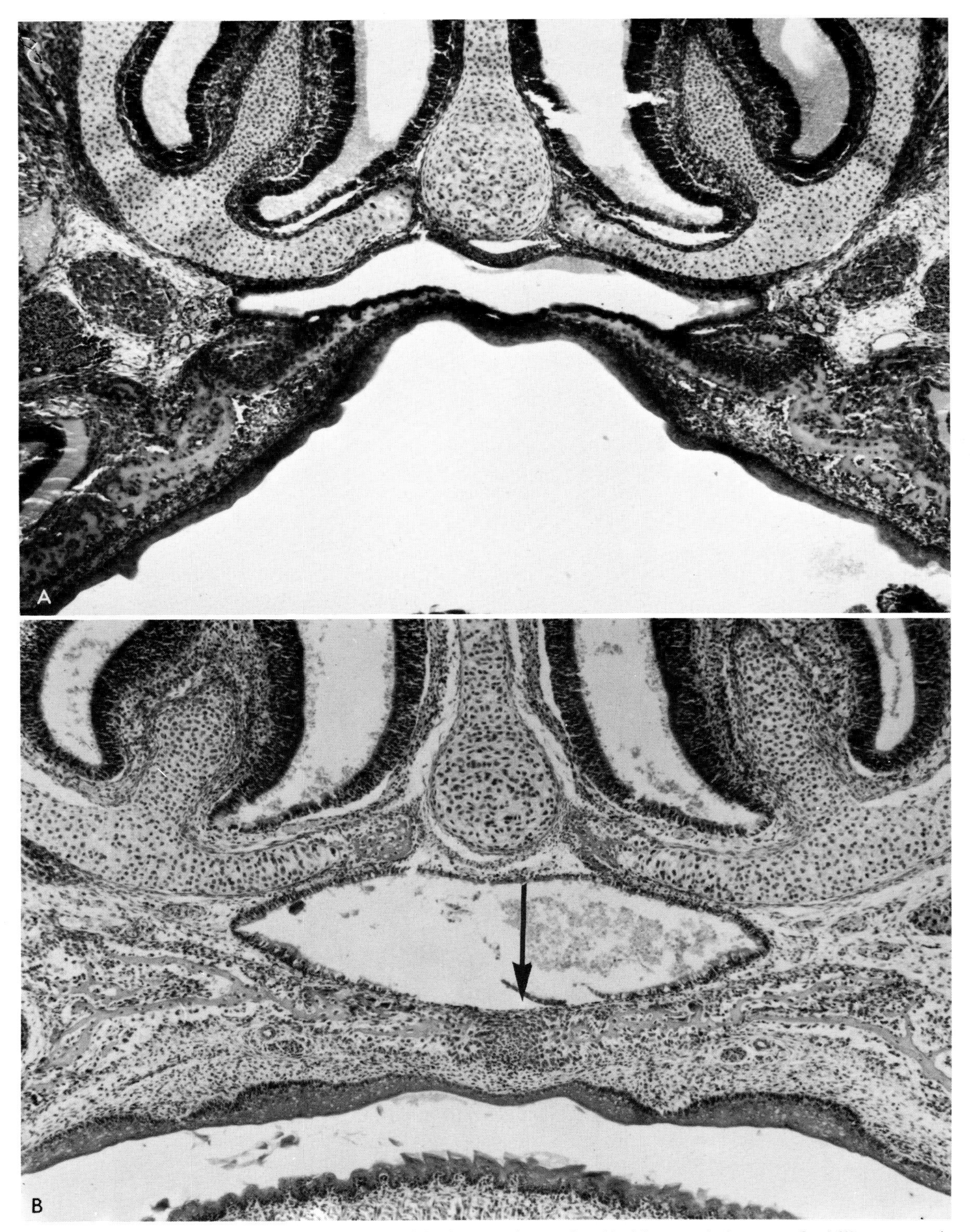

Figure 23–12. *A*, High-arched palate; thin, incomplete palatal bridge; and absence of midline suture in mouse with induced submucous cleft palate. *B*, Normal palate and median suture in littermate of mouse in *A*.

has provided an excellent opportunity to investigate the pathogenesis of submucous cleft palate and to compare the defective offspring with both the normal littermates and those with isolated cleft palate.[12] The mechanism of teratogenesis has been shown to involve interference with mesodermal differentiation in the bridge of the posterior palate, and the centripetal gradient of differentiation that extended from the nasopalatine foramen to the uvula was disturbed by the teratogen during and after palate closure.

The animal studies emphasized that the teratogen-sensitive period for palatogenesis should be regarded as extending from day 45 to day 85 in man, the time span required for completion of the palatal bony bridge and for muscle differentiation in the velum. Rodent models with submucous cleft palate can be reared to maturity and provide an animal system for studies concerning surgical repair and velopharyngeal closure. Although the rodent does not possess a uvula, many structures in the rat palate do lend themselves to studies related to man (Fig. 23–12).

Mandibular Prognathism

An animal model of prognathism, especially in a near-human primate, could provide excellent material for controlled studies on experimental surgical procedures. Mandibular prognathism has been induced by hyperthermia in the marmoset *Callithrix jacchus*. It is possible that just as nonconcordant twin models for cleft palate can be produced in the marmoset by irradiation, similar models could be developed for the study of prognathism in these animals. Further work in this field could lead to interesting studies of animal models of a deformity that is relatively common in man[15] (Fig. 23–13).

Harvold and associates converted macaque monkeys into mouth breathers by raising the bite of the posterior teeth of these animals and progressively occluding the nasal airway.[3] Over a 15-month period, marked changes in the appearance of the tongue were observed, with the tongue becoming thinner at the back, bulkier in the middle, and more pointed at the tip. Changes also occurred in the dental arches and in facial height. While face height increased slightly, the gonial angle opened by four degrees and the mandible lengthened by 1 or 2 mm. The lower anterior teeth extruded slightly, and the overall effect was an induced lowering of the mandible.

Similar experiments in rhesus monkeys, in which a mild skeletal Class III relationship was established by the use of gold onlays on the buccal segment teeth, were reported by Elgoyhen and associates.[1] After six months it was found that changes had taken place in many areas of the craniofacial complex to produce a mild mandibular prognathism.

Although these onlay experiments have induced less severe changes than would customarily be treated by surgical means, they demonstrate the possibility of influencing growth and development toward the abnormal state. The changes in the experimental animals were small, but they were statistically significant. Further attention to interceptive techniques such as these during the growth period could possibly lead to other primate models of facial disharmony.

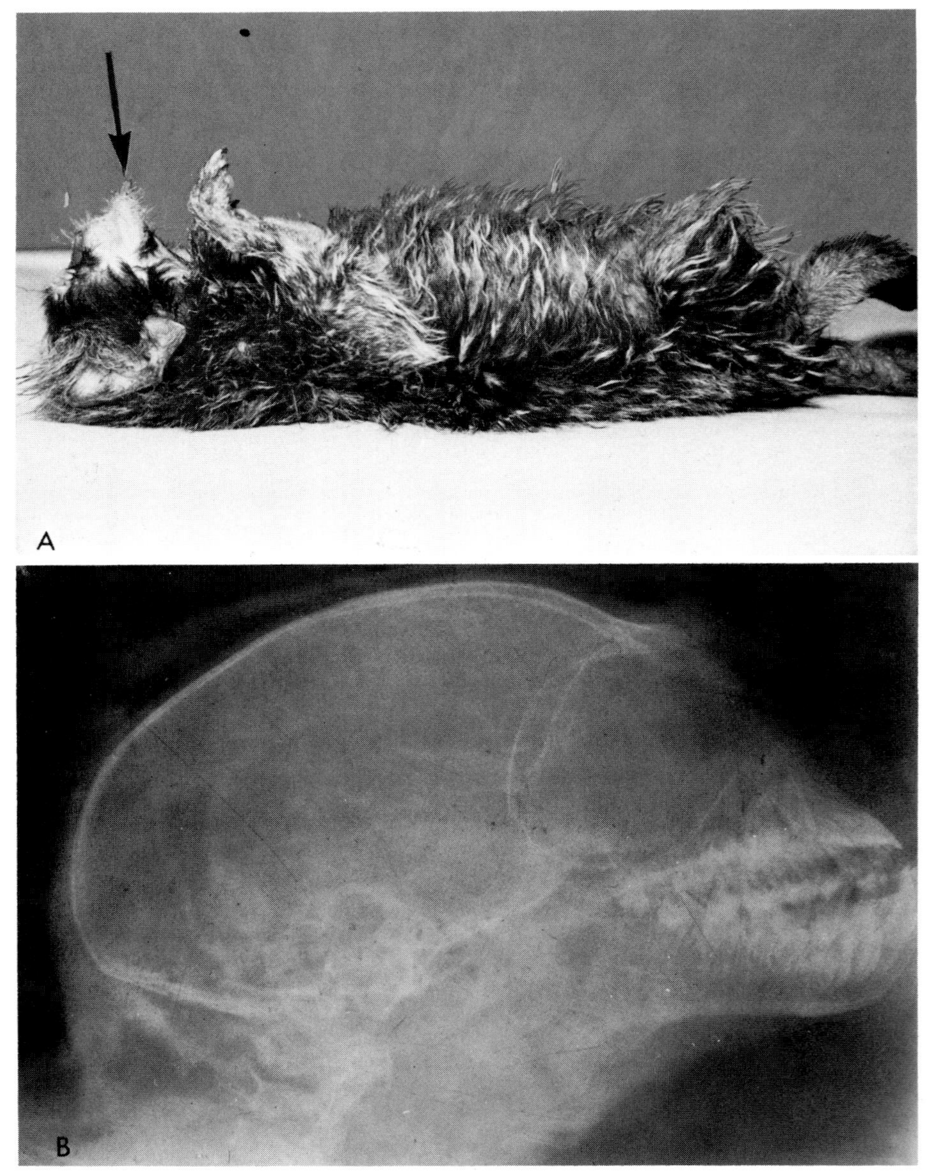

Figure 23–13. *A*, Mandibular prognathism induced in marmoset by hyperthermia. *B*, Radiograph of prognathous mandible in same animal.

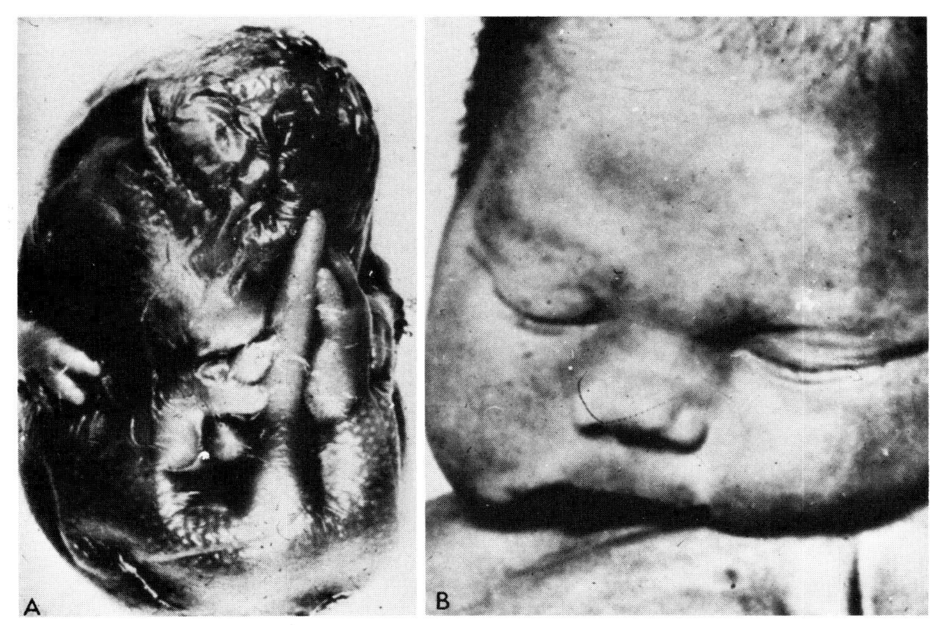

Figure 23–14. Rat model of postural molding defect of jaw with concomitant cleft palate (*A*) compared with human Pierre Robin anomaly (*B*).

Mandibular Retrognathism

A convincing animal model of the Pierre Robin anomaly, with or without cleft palate, has been demonstrated in laboratory rodents[8] (Fig. 23–14). The postural molding defects of the jaws offer opportunities to study growth and development of these deformities and the effects of early reconstructive procedures on the amelioration of microgenia.

Anterior Open Bite

Despite a plethora of orthodontic and surgical techniques for the correction of severe open bite, much remains to be learned about this condition, which could perhaps be deduced from animal models. Severe anterior open bite can be achieved in the macaque monkey by two simple methods. The first involves hand-rearing the infant monkey from birth with a child's feeding bottle. On this regimen the animal develops a thumb-sucking habit, which continues until maturity, and as a consequence, severe open bite develops spontaneously. The same condition can be induced in the adolescent and mature monkey by bilateral condylotomy by the blind Gigli saw technique. An immediate and progressive loss of vertical dimension of the jaws results, followed by gagging on the posterior teeth and anterior open bite. Although there are variations in the maxillomandibular deformity in these two distinct models, both lend themselves to surgical, orthodontic, and growth studies in animals that are morphologically similar to man (Fig. 23–15).

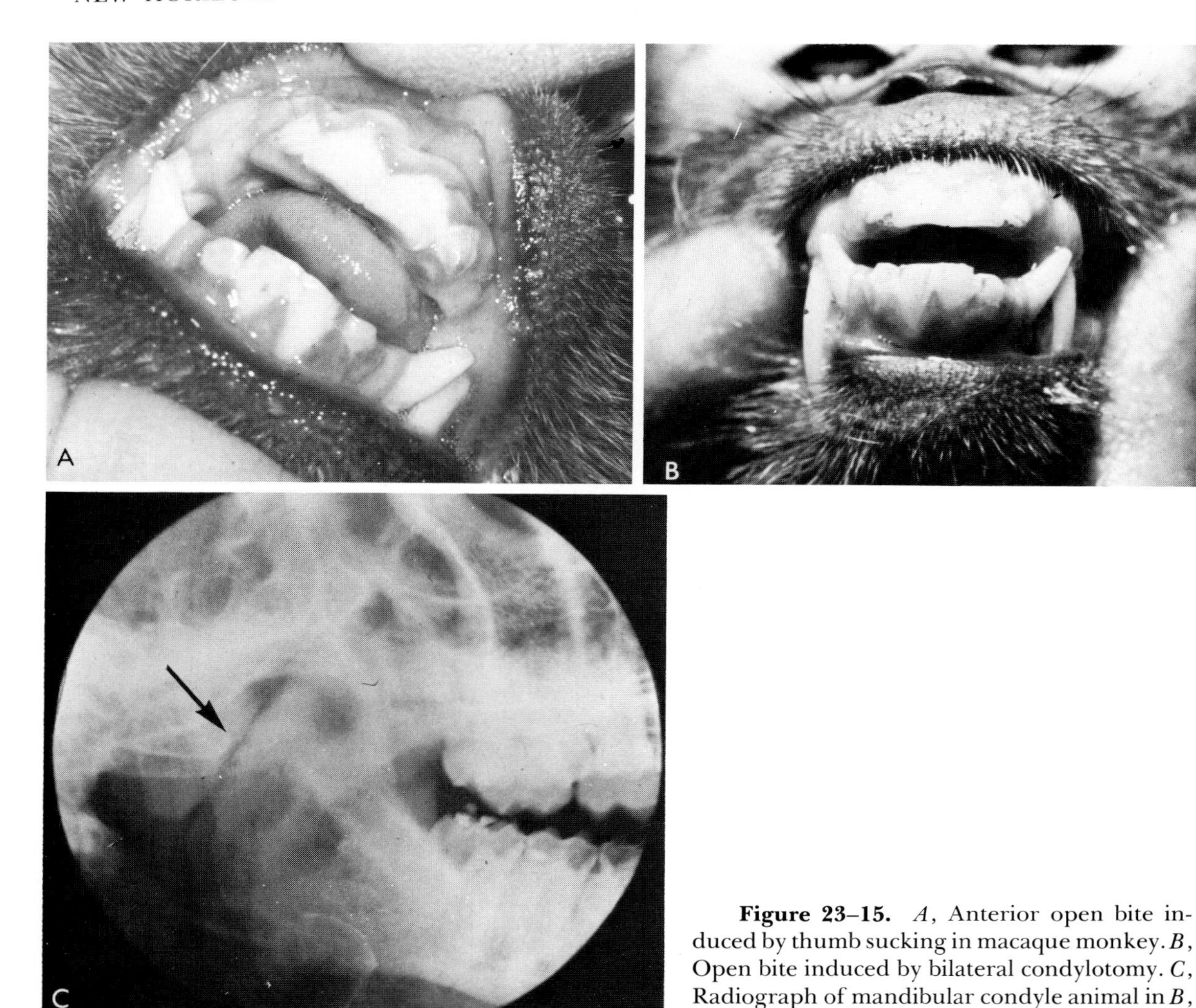

Figure 23–15. *A*, Anterior open bite induced by thumb sucking in macaque monkey. *B*, Open bite induced by bilateral condylotomy. *C*, Radiograph of mandibular condyle animal in *B*, showing condylotomy bone section.

Animal Models of Rare Major Craniofacial Malformations

Although the major congenital deformities of the craniofacial complex are much less common than the minor deformities (cleft lip and palate, prognathism, and open bite), they are no less significant in human terms and offer a greater challenge to the reconstructive surgeon. Malformations such as hemifacial microsomia, Treacher Collins syndrome, and Apert and Crouzon syndromes all have features that are of great interest to those concerned with the reconstruction of facially deformed individuals. The development of animal models of these conditions could fill a very real need, both by increasing awareness of the pathogenesis of these serious disorders and by relating the mechanism of malformation to the timing and type of reconstructive surgery. To date, models of both hemifacial microsomia and Treacher Collins syndrome have been described, which are of interest to all concerned with the clinical management of these deformities.[11]

Hemifacial Microsomia

In the mouse, the characteristic defects of hemifacial microsomia have been induced by the antifolate drug triazine. The causal mechanism of malformation was shown to be closely related to the formation of a hematoma arising from the junction of the ventral pharyngeal and hyoid arteries at the equivalent of day 32 of human development. These anastomosing vessels form the stapedial arterial system in man, and the hematoma spreads from these vessels into differentiating tissues in the vicinity of the developing structures of the outer and middle ear, malar bone, and condyle and ramus of the mandible. The process of morphodifferentiation is considerably disturbed by this event, and the ultimate morphologic development of the affected parts varies according to the degree of initial damage to differentiating mesenchyme and the ability of the affected tissues to repair and to catch up with the program of differentiation (Fig. 23–16).

In a similar way, thalidomide given to the macaque or marmoset monkey between days 20 and 25 of development results in otomandibular dysostosis (a variant of hemifacial microsomia) that is induced by an identical causal mechanism. Because offspring can be hand-reared without undue difficulty, the monkey model, in particular, provides excellent material for studies of the growth and development of faces affected by focal necrosis during early embryogenesis. It also permits the study of reconstructive surgical procedures[9] (Fig. 23–17).

Treacher Collins Syndrome

The bilaterally symmetric deficiencies of the orbit, malar region, maxilla, and mandible that are found with variable expressivity in the Treacher Collins syndrome in man can be reproduced in the Wistar rat by dosing the pregnant dam with 75,000 to 100,000 IU of vitamin A on day 8.5 of development. Whereas the syndrome in man is genetically induced, the teratogenic agent that induces the defects in this animal model probably sets in motion a causal mechanism similar to that in man. Analysis of the causal mechanism in sequential studies of the affected rat embryo shows that vitamin A acts by killing large areas of neural crest cells that are destined to migrate to the first and second branchial arches. The consequences of this selective destruction of ectomesenchymal cells are twofold.

First, the necrotic cavity in the neural crest is filled by inflow of the adjacent tissues, and the otic placode "floats" up from second arch into the region of the first arch and relocates the eventual ear over the angle of the jaw (Fig. 23–18). Second, the volume of mesenchyme in the first and second arches is greatly reduced. The mesenchyme that is there, partly derived from the surviving neural crest cells and partly from the lateral plate mesoderm, is insufficient to provide normal facial morphologic development. Although the basic design of the face is closely comparable to the normal facial design, the mesenchymal insufficiency determines that the fullness of form that is found in normal facial scaffolding is lacking. This diminution in form becomes obvious in the studies of fetal and postnatal facial development that can be conducted on these animal models.

A near-human primate model of Treacher Collins syndrome has not yet been described, but one may soon be available. The response of the *Macaca irus* and mar-

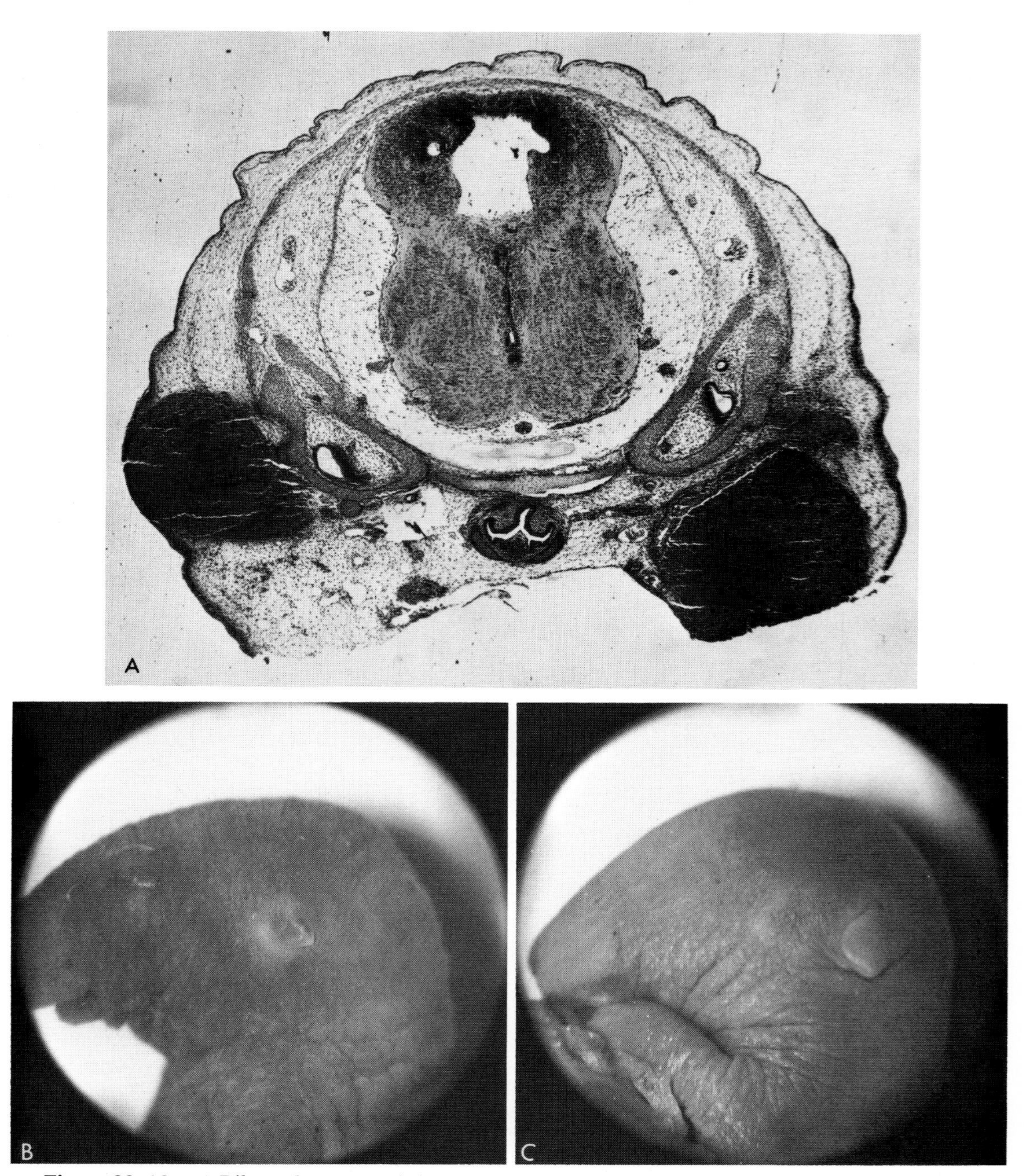

Figure 23–16. *A*, Bilateral asymmetric hematomas induced in otomandibular region to produce mouse model of first arch syndrome. *B*, Ear and jaw defects in mouse model of hemifacial microsomia (compare with *C*). *C*, Normal ear-jaw relationship in mouse.

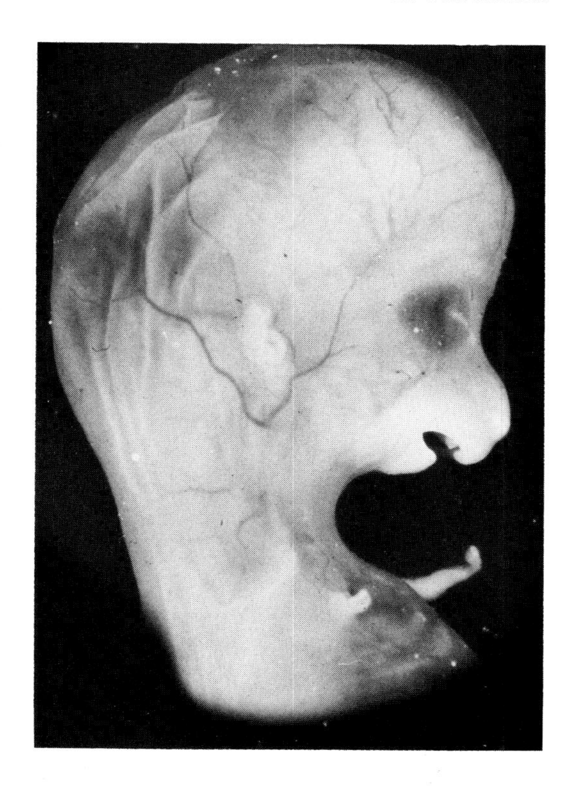

Figure 23–17. Thalidomide-induced defects of ear, jaw, and upper limbs in macaque monkey.

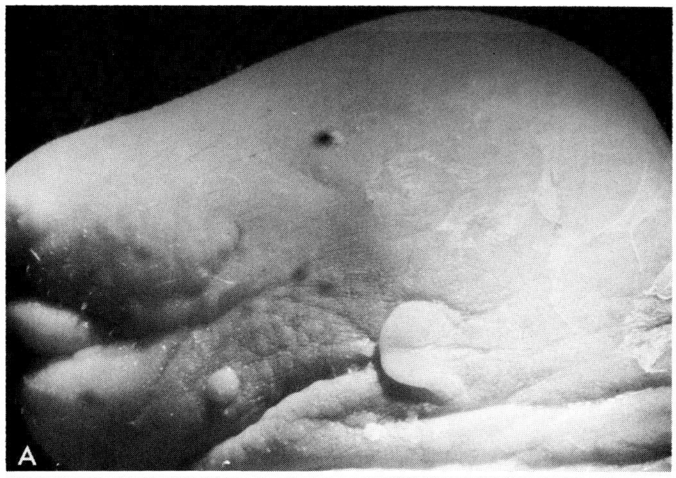

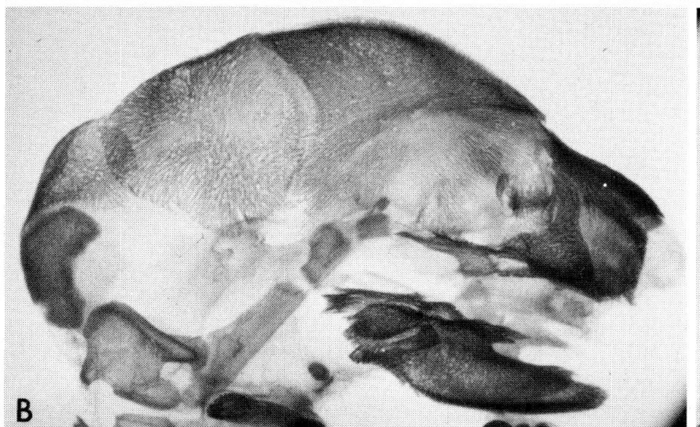

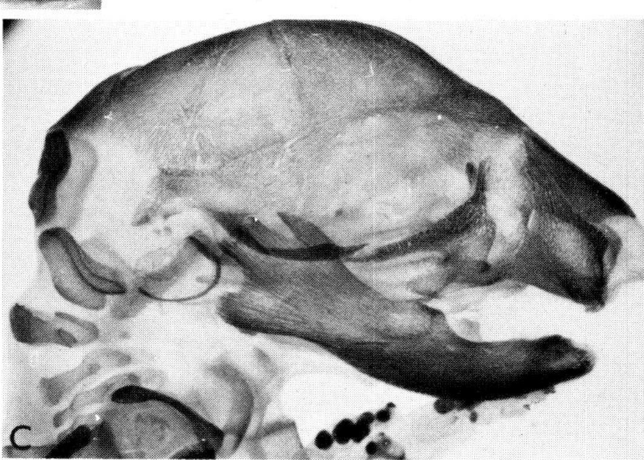

Figure 23–18. *A*, Abnormal shape and position of external ear and deficiency of malar region in rat model of Treacher Collins syndrome. *B*, Skeletal defects of ramus of mandible and zygomatic arch in rat model of Treacher Collins syndrome. *C*, Normal rat skeleton (compare with *B*).

moset embryo to the teratogenic effect of hypervitaminosis A prior to palate closure closely parallels the effect in the rat. The administration of equivalent doses of vitamin A to the pregnant monkey on approximately day 20 of development may, hopefully, produce effects comparable to those seen in the rat model of the Treacher Collins syndrome.

EXTRAPOLATION OF ANIMAL STUDIES TO MAN

The ultimate goals for each human malformation are complete, rational understanding of the pathogenesis; complete prevention in the foreseeable future; and improved therapeutic rehabilitation of the affected individual. Despite the liberal attitudes regarding termination of pregnancy that have been introduced in many parts of the world in recent years, there is still very little possibility that research into the mechanisms of dysmorphogenesis can be carried out on human embryos living in their maternal environment. For this reason alone, animal experiments will continue to provide much of the information necessary to understand the etiology and pathogenesis of craniofacial malformations. But the experimentalist will always be conscious of the care and reservation that must be emphasized when comparing observations in one species with those in another. The extrapolation of findings in lower mammals to conditions found in man requires an even higher degree of skill and caution. Kalter[4] has provided a rational basis for attempts at extrapolation that cannot at present be improved upon. He states that when the malformations observed in the experimental animal and in man are closely comparable in their structural characteristics and when it can be shown that in both cases a comparable pathway of abnormal development has been followed, even in part, there exists a basis for careful extrapolation between the species.

Growth and Development Studies

The determination of normal influences on growth and development of the embryo and fetus will inevitably assist in understanding the abnormal. On the other hand, one may argue, as Tolstoy did, that while this remark is very apt, the truth is really the opposite; i.e., by a study of malformation one can most readily learn the truth about normal growth and development. Whichever way the subject is argued, it seems reasonable that the comparative study of animal models of both normal and abnormal development will make a profound contribution to our knowledge of patterns of growth in man. Other things being equal, the closer the animal model is to man in both metabolism and structure, the more valid will be the extrapolation of the results of research.

The laboratory techniques available for study of growth and development of the fetus, be it normal or abnormal, are many and varied. Using model systems previously described for the induction of deformity in animals, one can monitor the sequential changes in craniofacial form by static techniques such as embryoctony or by dynamic studies such as the incorporation of radiopaque dyes into the amniotic cavity to assist in radiographic interpretation of structural changes. Incorporating vital stains into the amniotic fluid can enable their incorporation in the developing skeleton and assist in deciphering patterns of adaptive and remodeling responses in both normal and abnormal embryos after pathologic preparation of the specimens. Fiber endoamnioscopy in the marmoset and macaque monkey allows direct observation of the growth changes in the developing fetus. In addition, exteriorization of the embryo or fetus into the peritoneal cavity without detaching it from the placenta permits observation, over a limited period, of growing offspring nourished by the maternal vasculature. Studies such as these can yield considerable information about the prenatal changes that distinguish growth behavior in normal and abnormal conceptuses.

Postnatal growth and development may be studied by metrical and radiologic serial observations, thus permitting comparison of the normal and abnormal specimens at many different stages of maturation. Many of the vital stain techniques applicable to prenatal studies may be carried out by incorporating agents such as tetracycline or alizarin red-S into bone at significant periods of growth. Thus, the effects of surgery, sham surgery, and unoperated conditions may be compared and evaluated over selected periods ranging from hours to months or years. Apparatus for serial cephalometric radiologic investigation of rodents and primates has been described and may be used singly or in combination with vital dyes and other histopathologic techniques. There are a wide range of studies that may be conducted on the animal models of malformation. Twin studies can be particularly appropriate, and many of these will provide significant information about the expected response in man.

Animal Models for Prenatal Diagnosis and Fetal Surgery

Among the frontiers of surgery during the past decade has been the development of increasingly sophisticated techniques for the intrauterine diagnosis of fetal defects in man and the application of general surgical principles to fetal surgery in other mammals. It is therefore conceivable that certain fetal anomalies such as facial clefts and postural molding defects of the jaws, such as are found in the Pierre Robin syndrome, could be corrected by direct surgical intervention well before birth. Surgery in utero during the early part of the third trimester of pregnancy offers the fetus the major advantage of postoperative recovery in an ideal environment. The intrauterine repair of facial wounds is relatively free from scarring and would be greatly beneficial in the repair of clefts of the lip. On the other hand, these potential advantages must be balanced against the hazards, among which is excessive loss of amniotic fluid. It is well known that a small loss of amniotic fluid, such as occurs in amniocentesis, is well tolerated, but the sudden loss of a larger volume may disturb fetal cardiovascular dynamics. Also, it must be shown that the potential for postnatal growth and development is not seriously impaired by fetal surgery. These studies are essential before the feasibility of such procedures is decided, and they must be conducted on the animal model long before attempts are made to repeat them in man (Fig. 23–19).

Pilot studies on the method of wound healing in utero were conducted on the rat fetus and have been followed by additional investigations in the *Macaca irus* monkey.[17] It has been shown that in this species direct visualization of fetal structures can be

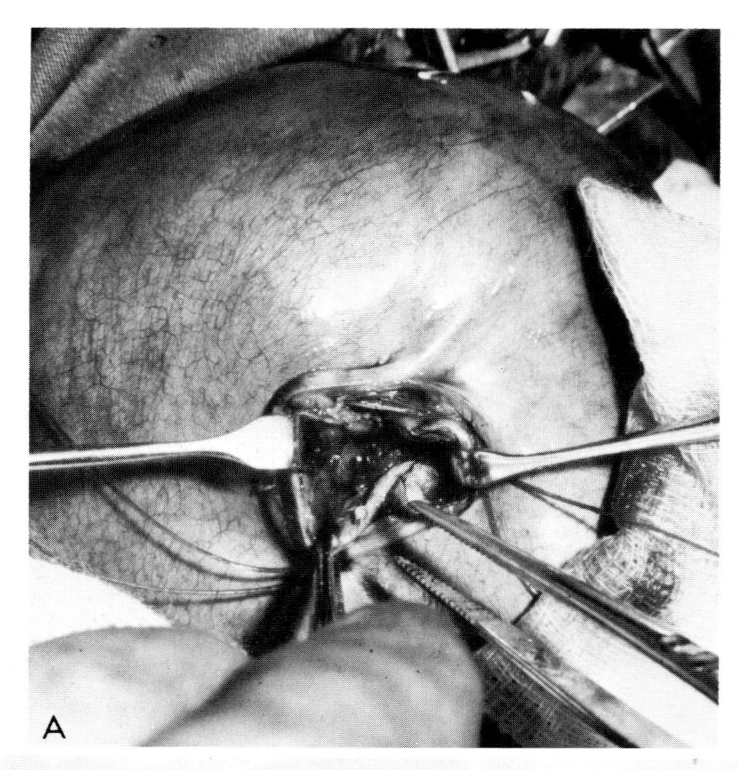

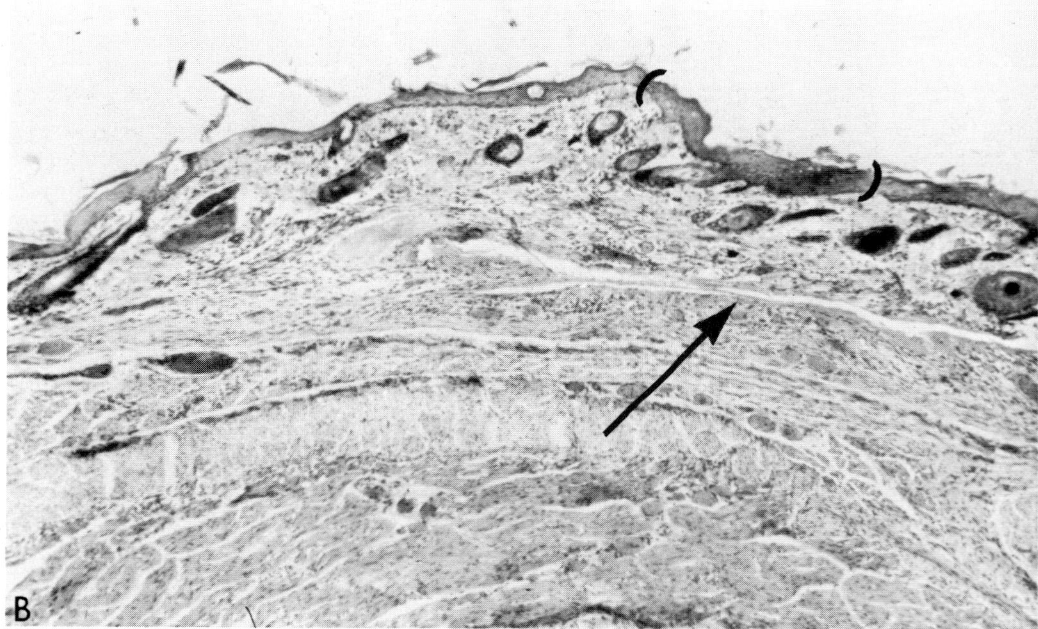

Figure 23–19. *A*, Surgical approach to intrauterine operation on lips of macaque monkey. *B*, Site of repair of facial tissues six weeks after surgery. No scar tissue is seen, but suture track (arrow) indicates site of previous surgery (between brackets).

obtained without excessive loss of amniotic fluid. In addition, surgical procedures can be carried out under direct vision and the fetus returned to the uterus for repair of the operated tissues, subsequently to be born at full term. Tissue repair is excellent, and signs of repair on the skin of the monkey fetus subjected to various surgical procedures around the face and jaws are almost invisible. Early results suggest that although there is some reduction in growth rates of the operated offspring (by comparison with unoperated animals), this deficiency is made up by six months of age and that beyond this age normal growth and development percentiles are maintained. Many clinical investigators believe that the most potent weapon available for reducing the problem of craniofacial malformations is a process of intrauterine screening that may lead to precise prenatal diagnosis of defects. Once this is achieved, the decision as to whether to terminate the pregnancy or to attempt fetal correction or amelioration of the anomaly then becomes clouded by difficult technical and ethical considerations. Whatever the future, it is mandatory that experiments using the animal model be employed with skill and tenacity in an effort to advance the state of the art on this new horizon of reconstructive surgery.

The Predictive Value of Animal Models

While considering the possibilities of prevention and intrauterine reparative surgery on the one hand, the experimentalist must also weigh the value of research in the field of improving the prognostic capabilities of the reconstructive maxillofacial surgeon. Before the surgeon can be assured of the perfection of his operative techniques, he must know the optimum time for surgical intervention and the response of a particular type of growth disorder to the various surgical techniques available. In this situation the animal model of malformation is of the utmost assistance. It has already been suggested that comparative growth studies of twin primates with unoperated and operated cleft lip and palate could be of immense value in predicting the response of humans to similar procedures. In addition, variations in experimental design could shed light on the optimum combinations of time and technique to be utilized for perfection in surgical reconstruction. Similar predictive information has been gained from studies of the pathogenesis of other malformations. For example, identification of those cases of microgenia and isolated cleft palate that arise from postural molding restraint in utero can assist the surgeon to time his reconstructive procedure based on a predicted "catch-up" growth potential. When the defect is a deformation induced by mechanical pressures, the most serious stigmata of deformity are found to diminish quite rapidly once birth has taken place and the restraining force is released.When operative procedures are delayed until catch-up growth has been achieved, surgical techniques are more easily applied and the ultimate repair is facilitated. The application of a biologic approach to the clinical management of neonatal Pierre Robin anomaly has eliminated mortality, reduced morbidity, and enhanced the final functional rehabilitative procedures.[8]

The similarity of the anomalies of hemifacial microsomia and the Treacher Collins syndrome has led many surgeons to believe that the approach to reconstruction should be similar for both entities. Disappointing and disparate clinical results in this field have left other surgeons wondering how and why the response to surgical reconstruction can be so unpredictable. This dilemma has been resolved to a considerable degree by the analysis of animal models of hemifacial microsomia and the Treacher Collins syndrome. When serious deficiencies of the masticatory muscles and skeleton coexist in those with hemifacial microsomia, it has been shown that early and severe damage to the developing functional periosteal matrix has occurred. In such cases early reconstructive surgery is frequently unable to restore the functional matrix of musculoskeletal elements. Consequently, growth of the affected side remains static, while the unaffected or less involved side continues to grow at a different rate. Thus, in the severely affected patient operative reconstruction prior to the cessation of growth on the unaffected side can at best provide a temporary solution to the dyssymmetry. As growth proceeds, the disparity between the two sides again becomes apparent and following surgical procedures may even be increased by the contraction on tissues that are less than ideal for tension-free coverage of the rebuilt skeleton. In less severe cases it is often possible to maintain the symmetry achieved by static reconstruction during the growth period by use of myofunctional therapy and postoperative orthodontic treatment.

In the Treacher Collins syndrome, however, there is distortion of the musculoskeletal elements of the functional matrix, but symmetrical motor units are not completely absent. When reconstruction is based on the restitution of contour to the deficient areas of the facial skeleton, the functional matrix is redesigned or modified but is still capable of sustained symmetric growth. Thus, the prospects for lasting benefit from early (prepubertal) facial reconstruction of Treacher Collins patients are good, and there should be continuing amelioration of the facial deformity in patients thus treated.[14]

It is probable that the development of additional animal models of prognathism and retrognathism, first and second arch malformations, and deformities of the cranial vault of the Crouzon type will provide new fields for exploring the effects of variations in timing and type of surgical reconstruction. Such models may greatly enhance predictability of the response of these conditions to surgical measures. Under such circumstances the prognostic capabilities of the surgeon will be improved, and the treatment of the handicapped individual will be advanced immeasurably.

PREVENTIVE ASPECTS OF RESEARCH INTO CRANIOFACIAL ANOMALIES

At the present time in the western world one child in forty is born with a congenital malformation sufficiently gross to be recognizable at birth. Many of these malformations affect the structures of the head and neck. Children who start life with a birth defect are doubly handicapped. Not only do they have to overcome all the disadvantages, both physical and emotional, of the deformity itself, but there remain all the hazards of disease and disorder that affect every individual throughout life. The eventual aim of all who work in the field of researching or treating deformities must be to prevent the defects, whether they are structural or biochemical. In order to do this, it is essential to find the cause. Congenital malformations, like most other serious events in this world, are multifactorial in origin. That the causes are multiple and complex is probably of great concern to genetic counselors, but this offers a strong ray of hope to those who study the mechanisms of malformation as a means to their prevention. The aim of preventive teratology coincides with the objects of preventive medicine — to seek and eliminate those etiologic factors that are manageable and amenable to removal at will. At present this research is in its infancy, and few successes can be claimed. As the environment in which man lives and reproduces is better understood and as the agents that may affect the structural development of the embryo are identified and eliminated, the incidence of polygenic multifactorial deformities of the craniofacial complex should be reduced. This will, of necessity, be a slow process, but the continued expansion of mammalian experimental teratology should hopefully make a major contribution to the ultimate prevention of birth defects.

Selection of "At Risk" Families

Although the need to identify all environmental teratogens is not being disputed, present evidence indicates that the cause of congenital malformations in a considerable proportion of individuals is influenced by their genetic predisposition. Despite remarkable advances in our knowledge of how genes can affect structural development, very little is known of the detailed mechanisms and forces by which they exert their action. About 5 per cent of congenital conditions are caused by chromosomal anomalies, and there appears to be no early prospect of preventing the fresh chromosome mutations that are responsible for most malformations. Nonetheless, epidemiologic studies have shown that more than 50 per cent of the infants with Down syndrome are born of mothers over 35 years of age. When a family history of Down syndrome exists, karyotype studies make it possible to identify mosaicism and warn the prospective parents of the risk factor. Culture of amniotic fluid cells removed early in pregnancy may establish a definitive diagnosis of chromosomal disorder and permit the alternative of termination of the pregnancy. However, cases of this type are rare, and prevention of many cases of malformation by the identification and removal of any single causative factor is unlikely. The most hopeful prospects appear to be the identification of specific factors underlying the proven associations of deformity with environmental factors such as geographic and seasonal variables or social class. If even in a proportion of cases familial predisposition to cleft lip and palate can be positively linked to facial shape, attention to factors such as adequate diet and housing, the elimination of pharmacologic agents in the first trimester of pregnancy, and the reduction of stress in those families identified as "at risk" may play an important role in the prevention of deformity.

Genetic Counseling

Genetic counseling is as old as mankind; primitive tribes introduced strict consanguinity laws to control the genetic stability of their children. It is becoming increasingly obvious that better-trained, rather than more, genetic counselors are needed to work in the field of preventive teratology. In the future, the success of counseling may possibly be enhanced by elucidating additional causal mechanisms of specific malformation. In this way, causal agents that react with genetic susceptibility may eventually be identified and removed from the maternal and embryonic environment. Complete elimination of all the factors in a multifactorial situation is probably beyond the bounds of possibility, but it may be sufficient simply to move the distribution of the developmental variables in the direction of increased resistance to dysmorphogenesis. Until such a state of knowledge is reached, counseling will be concerned more with the establishment of risk figures, particularly the risk of recurrence. Empiric risk figures for various types of families with histories of craniofacial deformity are now readily available.[19] These tables indicate, for example, that in a family with one child and a first-degree relative of either parent affected by cleft lip and palate, the risk to an additional child is approximately one in ten. The evaluation of each child with a craniofacial malformation should involve a genetically oriented family study. On the basis of this examination a risk figure can often be determined, and the parents can thus be informed. In the occasional family that carries an abnormal gene with a high risk of recurrence of a serious malformation, knowledge of this may lead to the decision to avoid the risk of reproduction.

The confidence that the parents and the deformed child have gained through association with their surgeon often leads them to request his opinion concerning genetic risk factors. When such requests are made, the surgeon who is familiar with both the risk tables (Table 23–1) and the nature and family history of the deformity is in an excellent position to act as genetic counselor. This is an obligation that can be met with confidence by the surgeon to the great benefit of all parties concerned.

For each human disorder there are ultimate goals. For craniofacial deformity these are the rational understanding of the pathogenesis of malformation, the eventual application of effective preventive measures, and finally the application of therapy to provide normal function and appearance for the affected individual. It is toward these goals that multidisciplinary research workers in the field of dentofacial deformity are working, united by their common aim so aptly expressed by the father of facial surgery, Gaspare Tagliacozzi, in 1589:

> We restore, repair, or make whole those parts of the face which Nature omitted, or which Fortune has taken away; not so much that they may delight the eye, but that they should buoy up the spirit and help the mind of the afflicted.

TABLE 23–1. Empiric Recurrence Risk for Common Craniofacial Malformations

Incidence	*Risk*
One parent affected with:	*Risk of affected child*
Autosomal dominant condition	50%
Autosomal recessive condition	25%
Multifactorial polygenic condition:	
Cleft lip with or without cleft palate	4.3%
Cleft palate alone	6.0%
Unaffected parents with one child affected with:	*Risk of further affected children*
Autosomal dominant condition	Negligible
Autosomal recessive condition	25% each child
Cleft lip with or without cleft palate	5.0%
Cleft palate alone	2.0%

REFERENCES

1. Elgoyhan JC, Moyers RE, McNamara JA, Riolo ML: Craniofacial adaptation to protrusive function in young rhesus monkeys. Am J Orthod *62*:469, 1972.
2. Fraser FC: Causes of congenital malformations in human beings. J Chron Dis *10*:97, 1959.
3. Harvold EP, Vargercik K, Chierici G: Primate experiments on oral sensation and dental malocclusions. Am J Orthod *63*:494, 1973.
4. Kalter H: Teratology of the Nervous System. Chicago: University of Chicago Press, 1968, p. 9.
5. Kitamura H: Epithelial remnants and pearls in the secondary palate in the human abortus. Cleft Palate J *3*:240, 1966.
6. Lejour M: Pathogène des fentes labiomaxillaires provoquees chez le rat par l'hadacidine. Arch Biol (Liege) Supp 1, 1970.
7. Phillips IM, Grist SM: The use of transabdominal palpation to determine the course of pregnancy in the marmoset. J Reprod Fert *43*:103, 1975.
8. Poswillo D: the aetiology and surgery of cleft palate with micrognathia. Ann Roy Coll Surg Engl *43*:61, 1968.
9. Poswillo D: The pathogenesis of the first and second branchial arch syndrome. Oral Surg *35*:302, 1973.
10. Poswillo D: Orofacial malformations. Proc Roy Soc Med *67*:343, 1974.
11. Poswillo D: Otomandibular deformity: pathogenesis as a guide to reconstruction. J Maxillofac Surg *2*:64, 1974.
12. Poswillo D: The pathogenesis of submucous cleft palate. Scand J Plast Reconstr Surg *8*:34, 1974.
13. Poswillo D: Causal mechanisms of craniofacial deformity. Br Med Bull *31*:101, 1975.
14. Poswillo D: The pathogenesis of the Treacher Collins syndrome (Mandibulo-facial dysostosis). Br J Oral Surg *13*:1, 1975.
15. Poswillo D, Nunnerley H, Keith J, Sopher D: Hyperthermia as a teratogenic agent. Ann Roy Coll Surg Engl *55*:171, 1974.
16. St Hilaire EG: Philosopie Anatomique des Monstruosities Humaines. Paris: Rignoux, 1822.
17. Sopher D: Future prospects for fetal surgery. *In* Berry C, Poswello DE (eds): Teratology: Trends and Applications. New York: Springer-Verlag, 1975, pp 165–180.
18. Trasler DG: Pathogenesis of cleft lip and its relation to embryonic face shape in A/J and C57/B1 mice. Teratology *1*:33, 1968.
19. Woolf CM: Congenital cleft lip: a genetic study of high propositi. J Med Genet *8*:65, 1971.

Chapter 24

NEUROMUSCULAR ASPECTS OF VERTICAL MAXILLARY DYSPLASIAS

Richard A. Finn,
Gaylord S. Throckmorton,
William J. Gonyea,
David R. Barker,
and William H. Bell

The need for surgery to correct vertical dysplasias of the facial skeleton has been recognized for centuries. As techniques were developed to shorten the face either by Le Fort I osteotomy[12, 73] or by combined anterior and posterior maxillary osteotomies,[11, 72, 75] surgeons were able to reposition major portions of the midface in order to establish facial harmony and balance. Recent success with surgical procedures designed to lengthen or shorten the face has been reported.[13, 61] Thus, major changes in the vertical dimension of the face can be safely made as a result of enormous technological gains in surgery.

Despite the clinical success obtained to date, only one study[61] has dealt with stability following the superior repositioning of the maxilla, and very little information has been gathered to document the stability of surgical procedures to lengthen the face. The postoperative movement associated with shortening of the long face tended to be in the direction that the maxilla was moved. The mean follow-up, however, was only 14 months, and thus, information relative to long-term stability is not available. Willmar[73] and Bell[13] have reported on short-term follow-ups in patients who were treated with Le Fort I osteotomy and bone grafting in order to lengthen short faces. Thus, the potential for relapse following the surgical correction of short or long faces is difficult to assess at this time, and the permanency of such procedures must await long-term follow-up studies.

One reason suggested for relapse following surgical manipulation is the supposed inviolability of the freeway space or interarch distance.[15, 24, 68] Encroachment upon this zone has generally been described as intolerable to the patient, i.e., the full denture wearer. Some studies suggest that the mandibular rest position remains constant throughout life.[7, 24, 44, 53, 54, 64, 65, 69, 70] The assumption is made that increasing or decreasing freeway space will result in overclosure of the mandible or inadequate vertical dimension because of the apparent inability of the mandible to assume a new rest position. The philosophy of the dental profession with regard to freeway space can be summarized by a quote from Heartwell's book on complete dentures: "Failure to provide adequate freeway space does not allow the muscles that elevate the mandible to complete their contraction. The muscle will continue to exert force to overcome this obstacle, and as a result, the supporting tissues will be resorbed until the proper distance is returned."[32]

On the other hand, the contention has been made that neuromuscular changes associated with loss of the dentition or gradual abrasion of the teeth result in adjustment of the mandibular posture to maintain a constant freeway space.[19, 38] In a 30-year longitudinal study in adults, Büchi[17] found that facial height (N-Gn) increased 3 mm, whereas the relationship between centric occlusion and postural rest did not change. This could indicate a delicate balance between vertical facial skeletal changes and neuromuscular adaptations in order to maintain a constant interarch distance. Such stability of the freeway space indicates neuromuscular changes, but similar adaptations in the neuromuscular system resulting from abrupt repositioning of the jaw bones have not been clearly demonstrated. However, it has been observed clinically that following the surgical correction of the long face syndrome, the freeway space is approximately the same, thus indicating a new mandibular rest position. Likewise, although the excessive preoperative freeway space is lessened following surgery to correct vertical maxillary deficiency, it appears as though the mandible assumes a new rest position. Such ability of the neuromuscular system to apparently change as a result of new conditions is imperative if long-term stability is to be obtained in these patients. Although certain studies[25, 66] have demonstrated the dynamic nature and adaptability of skeletal muscle, the ability of jaw muscles to adapt to a new mandibular rest position remains an unanswered question.

Nonetheless, one of the factors suggested as being responsible for skeletal relapse is abnormal function of the perioral and masticatory muscles that apply abnormal forces on the facial skeleton. Three aspects of muscle function are related to the force applied by a muscle: (1) the morphology of the muscle, (2) the activity of the muscle, and (3) the mechanics of the musculoskeletal system. There are basically two mechanisms by which muscle function could produce relapse of facial surgery. First, the jaw muscles of persons with vertical maxillary dysplasias could be abnormal in terms of any or all of the three aspects just listed. Surgical correction of skeletal relations may have no effect on these abnormal jaw muscles, which continue to produce abnormal forces and thus relapse. Second, repositioning of the maxilla could alter function of normal muscle by stretching or shortening the muscles, altering the direction of the muscle action, or changing the mechanical advantage of the muscles. The muscle may adapt to these changes by changing its activity patterns or by changing its morphologic characteristics, or both. If the muscles cannot adapt successfully, they may produce relapse.

Thus, in order to understand the consequences of altering vertical jaw relationships, two basic questions must be answered.

1. Are the jaw mucles in a person with vertical maxillary dysplasia abnormal?
2. How are the various aspects of muscle function altered by surgical alteration of maxillary height?

In order to answer these questions, we have begun a study of muscle function in patients with vertical maxillary dysplasias. The study examines three aspects of muscle function: (1) muscle morphology; (2) muscle activity, as measured during isometric bites at particular force levels; and (3) muscle mechanics, as determined by comparing the mechanical advantage of the jaw muscles.

The patients participating in these studies were all patients of the Oral Surgery Department, the University of Texas Health Science Center at Dallas. They were classified as to facial type using standard diagnostic procedures and normal preoperative work-ups.

MUSCLE MORPHOLOGY

Understanding the function of human skeletal muscle is complicated by the fact that each muscle consists of a heterogeneous population of fiber types that differ in their structural, physiologic, and chemical characteristics. In man, two general types of fibers are recognized.[8, 19, 20] Type I fibers have a slow speed of contraction, a low specific activity of myofibrillar adenosinetriphosphatase (ATPase), and a poorly developed glycolytic enzyme system but a highly developed oxidative system with large numbers of mitochondria. These fibers exhibit little or no fatigue.[21] Type II fibers can be further subdivided into Type II-A and II-B fibers, depending upon their capacity for oxidative metabolism.[19] Type II-A fibers have large numbers of mitochondria and total oxidative activity and are more resistant to fatigue than are Type II-B fibers, which have few mitochondria. These different types of fibers are distributed in a heterogeneous manner throughout a muscle. The ratio of Type I to Type II fibers varies from muscle to muscle and from species to species in homologous muscles, evidently depending upon the function of each specific muscle.

Procedure

Muscle samples were taken from the deep masseter muscle in three subjects in each of the following groups: patients with long face syndrome, patients with short face syndrome, and human cadavers with normal facial morphology. The muscle samples were taken from the patients during corrective surgery, using a specifically designed biopsy needle 3 mm in diameter. The needle removed approximately 10 to 20 mg of tissue.

After the muscle samples were removed, they were mounted in tragacanth gum on a cork disk and rapidly frozen by immersion in Freon cooled with liquid nitrogen. Transverse serial sections are then cut at 8 μ on a cryostat (20° C.) and mounted on coverslips by thawing. The serial sections were then stained by four methods: (1) alkaline-stable myosin ATPase with preincubation at pH 9.4,[30] (2) acid-stable ATPase with preincubation at pH 4.3,[30] (3) nicotinamide adenine dinucleotide tetrazolium reductase (NADH-TR) activity,[52] and (4) α-glycerophosphate dehydrogenase (α-GPD) activity.[71] The muscle fibers were then typed and their diameters measured. In this preliminary study, only the control tissue was subtyped as to Type II-A or II-B fibers, all others were typed as to Type I or II fibers only.

Results

Figures 24–1 and 24–2 provide the muscle fiber distribution and fiber size in the control patients. These parameters can be compared with those from the long-faced and short-faced patients. The control values for fiber diameter in this study were similar to those found by Serratrice and associates[63] for the deep portion of the human masseter muscle. In the short-faced patients there was a dramatic reduction in the main diameter of the Type II (fast-twitch) fibers when compared with that from control subjects (Figs. 24–3 and 24–4). On the other hand, both Type I (slow-twitch) and Type II (fast-twitch) fibers from the masseter of the long-faced patients had undergone hypertrophy when compared with control diameters (Figs. 24–5 and 24–6).

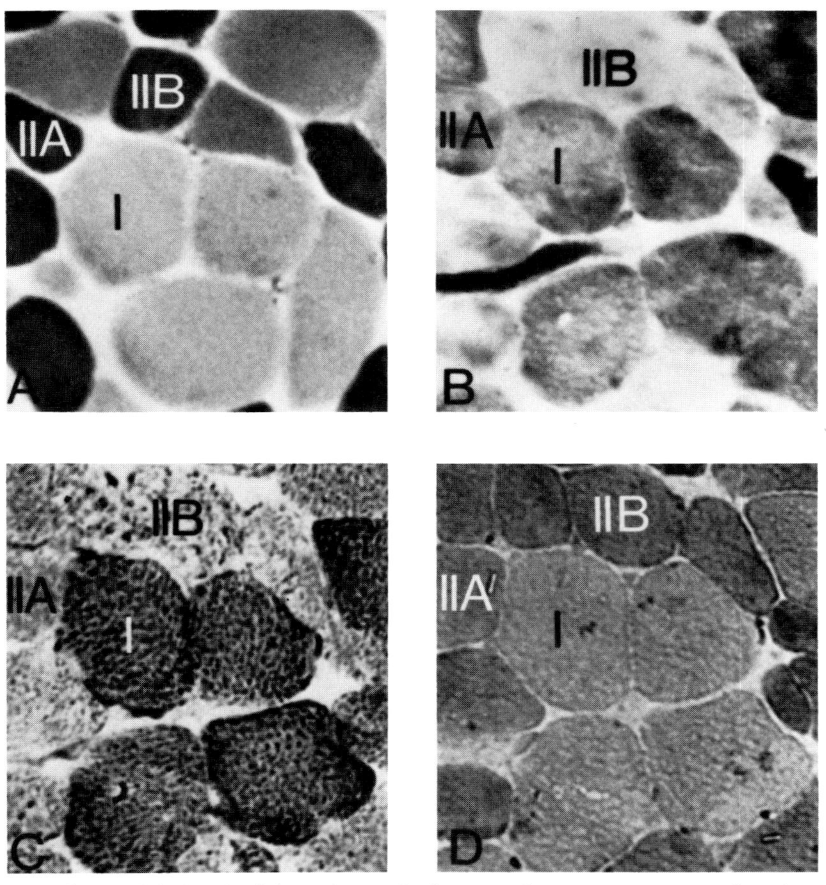

Figure 24–1. Serial sections of a human deep masseter muscle taken from a control subject and processed histochemically to demonstrate the three fiber types, (×350). *A*, ATPase, alkaline preincubation; *B*, ATPase, acid preincubation; *C*, NADH-TR activity; and *D*, α-GPD activity.

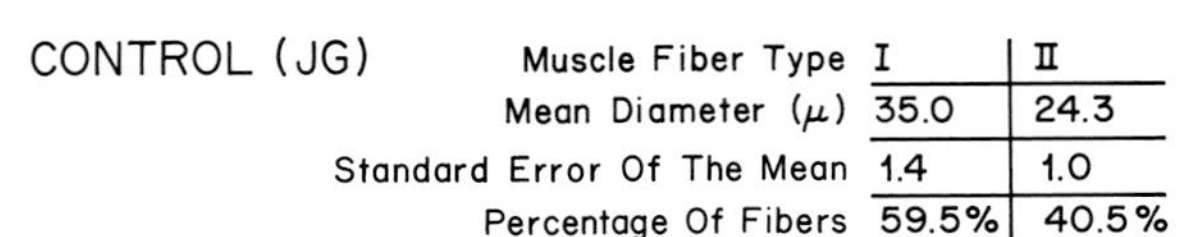
CONTROL (JG)

Muscle Fiber Type	I	II
Mean Diameter (μ)	35.0	24.3
Standard Error Of The Mean	1.4	1.0
Percentage Of Fibers	59.5%	40.5%

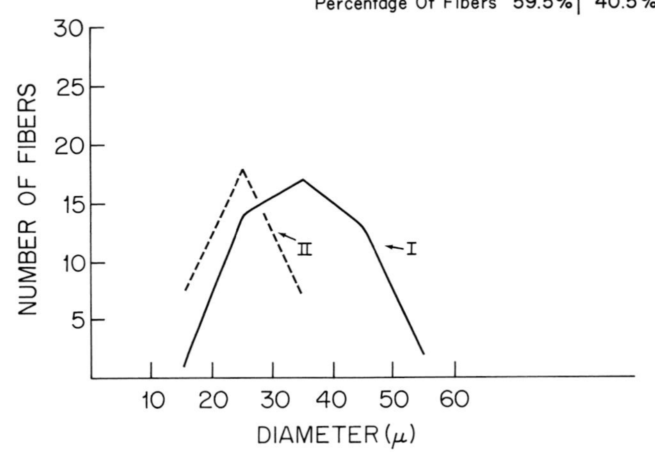

Figure 24–2. A histogram constructed from the biopsy taken from the control subject in Figure 24–1. The Type I (slow twitch) fibers were found to be larger than the Type II (fast twitch) fibers.

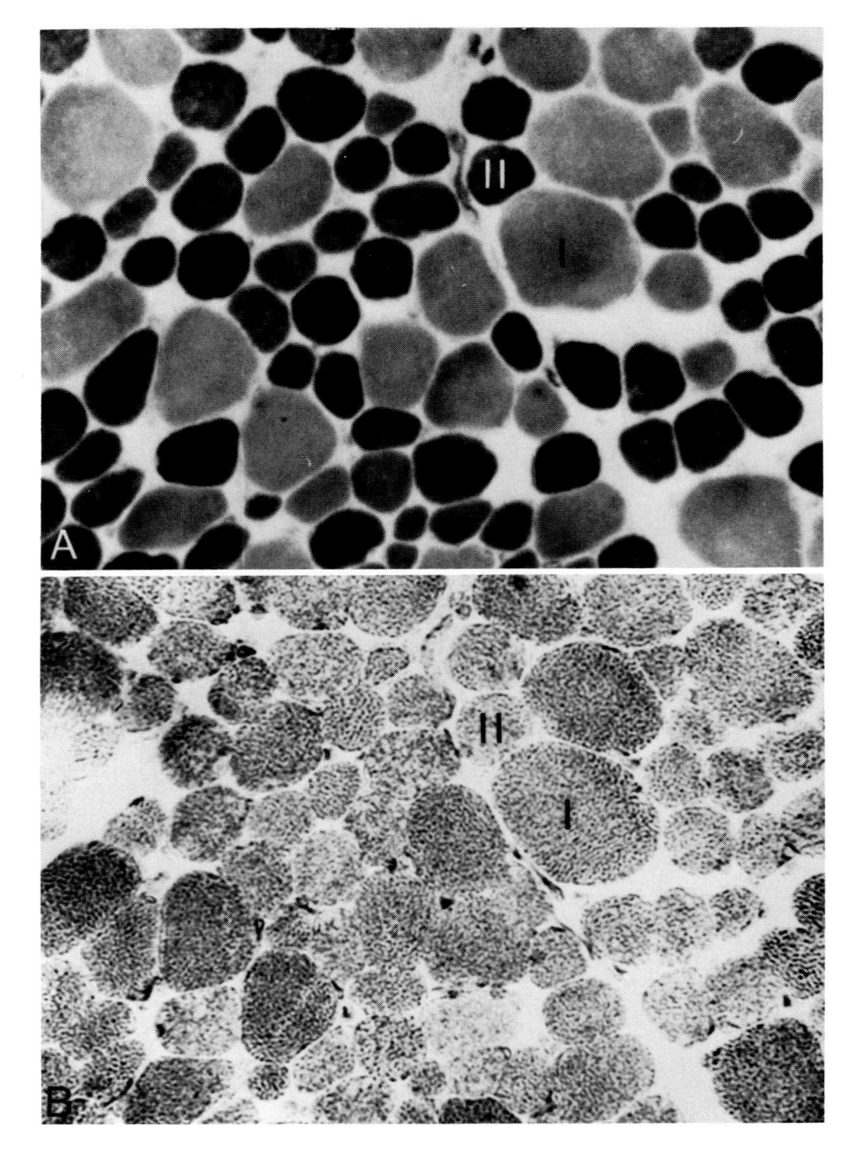

Figure 24–3. Serial sections of a biopsy from the deep masseter muscle taken from a short-faced patient. It can be seen that the Type II fibers are extremely small when compared with those from the control (×350). *A,* ATPase, alkaline preincubation, and *B,* NADH-TR activity.

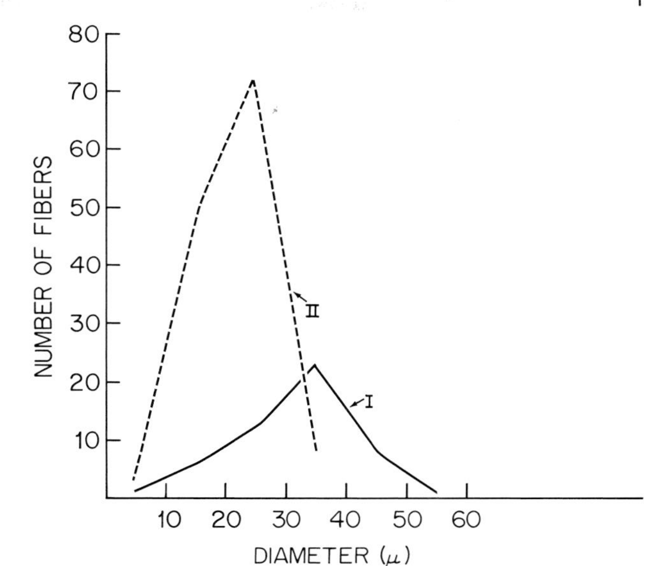

Figure 24–4. The histogram was constructed from the biopsy of the short-faced patient in Figure 24–3. It exhibits an unusually large distribution of Type II fibers with most of these fibers being abnormally small or atrophic.

MUSCLE MECHANICS

Orthognathic surgical procedures designed to reposition the entire maxilla or any of its component parts principally affect the muscles by changing the position of the muscle insertions relative to their origins and to the teeth. This may result in stretching or shortening of the muscle fibers, altering the direction of the muscle action, and changing the mechanical advantage of the muscles. One might expect these changes to require a corresponding change in muscle activity or morphology in order to maintain normal masticatory forces.

Changes in Muscle Length

The tension that a muscle produces has two components: active tension and passive tension. Active tension is the result of the contractile proteins, actin and myosin, within the muscle fibers under direct nervous stimulation. Passive tension results from stretching the connective tissue of the muscle and tendon. The work of Blix[14] showed that active tension is greatest at the resting length of the muscle. Thus, it decreases if the muscle is lengthened or shortened. Passive tension is 0 at resting length and increases as the muscle is lengthened. Thus, when muscle is stretched, as the jaw adductors are in surgical lengthening of the face, one would expect the active tension to decrease and the passive tension to increase.

Several workers[6, 18] have shown that when an entire muscle is stretched 20 to 30 per cent beyond its resting length, the amount of active tension produced by the muscle is altered. This functional limit to stretching may be caused either by rupturing of the connective tissue components of the sarcolemma or by damage to the individual contractile

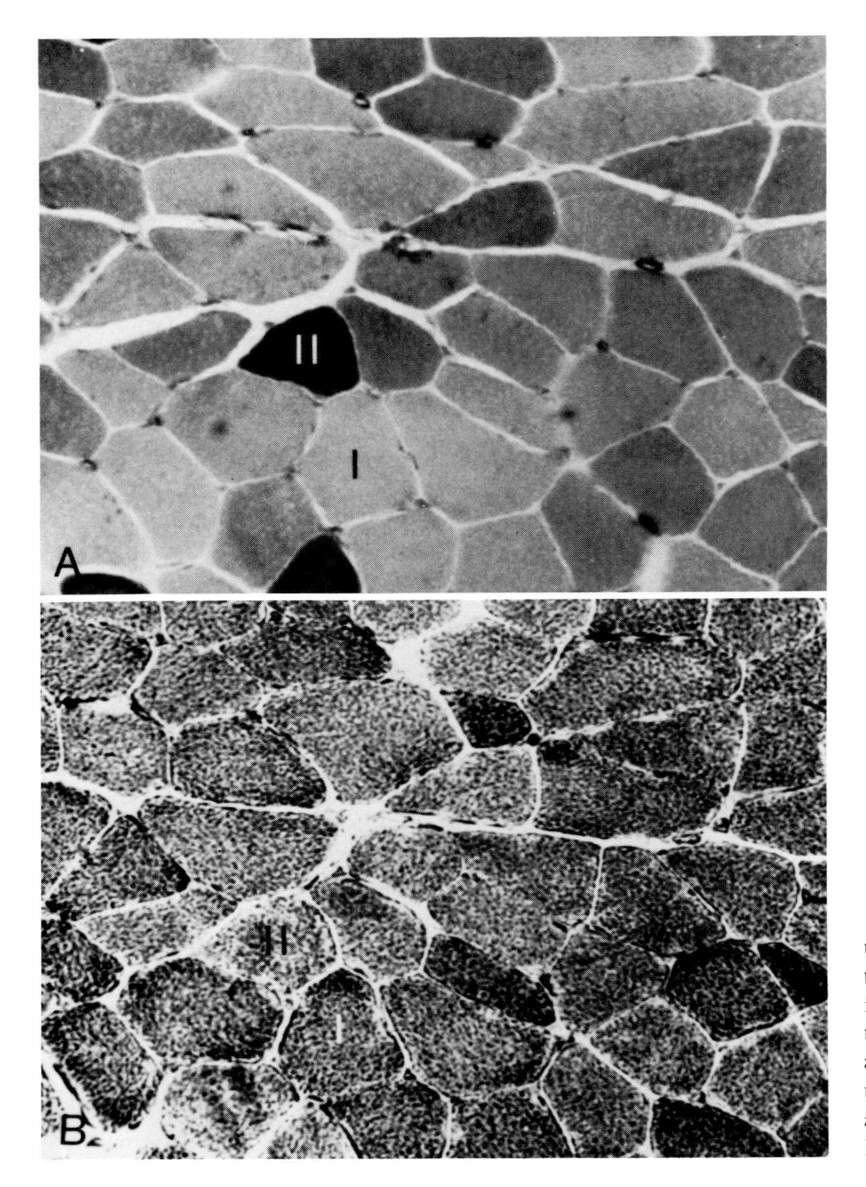

Figure 24–5. Serial sections of a human deep masseter muscle taken from a long-faced patient. Both fiber types have a much larger diameter than those from control tissue (×350). *A*, ATPase, alkaline preincubation, *B*, NADH-TR activity.

units. Studies to date have not determined which mechanism is responsible for the phenomenon, however, this limit to stretching does not occur in isolated single muscle fibers.[26, 27]

It should be remembered, however, that these were acute studies and that their results may not apply to surgical situations in which the muscles are immobilized for several weeks, during which time they are able to adapt to their new lengths. Several studies[25, 66] have shown that immobilized limb muscles can adapt to new lengths in as little as 2 weeks. This is accomplished by adding or removing sarcomeres at the ends of the muscle fibers and thus lengthening or shortening the muscle. The studies also showed that lengthened muscles had the same passive length-tension properties as normal muscle. However, muscles immobilized in the shortened position showed considerable increase in passive length-tension properties.

Work by McNamara and associates[43] suggests that jaw muscles are also adaptable.

LONG FACE (DA)

Muscle Fiber Type	I	II
Mean Diameter (μ)	44.4	33.1
Standard Error Of The Mean	1.1	1.2
Percentage Of Fibers	57.1%	42.9%

Figure 24–6. The histogram was constructed from the biopsy taken from the long-faced patient in Figure 24–5. It exhibits both Type I and Type II fiber hypertrophy.

The masseter muscles in monkeys were lengthened by inserting metal appliances into the oral cavity, thus opening the bite. The muscles gradually adapted to establish a new resting length. Although muscle fiber lengths were not determined in this study, the muscles presumably were lengthened by the serial addition of sarcomeres, as in the limb muscles.[25, 66]

Changes in Mechanical Advantage

The human mandible functions as a lever (Fig. 24–7) in which the fulcrum is the temporomandibular joint, the jaw-elevating muscles apply a force distal to the fulcrum, and the load is applied to the teeth distal to the muscle insertions (see Hylander[33] for a review of the lever action of the human mandible). The jaw-elevating muscles, tem-

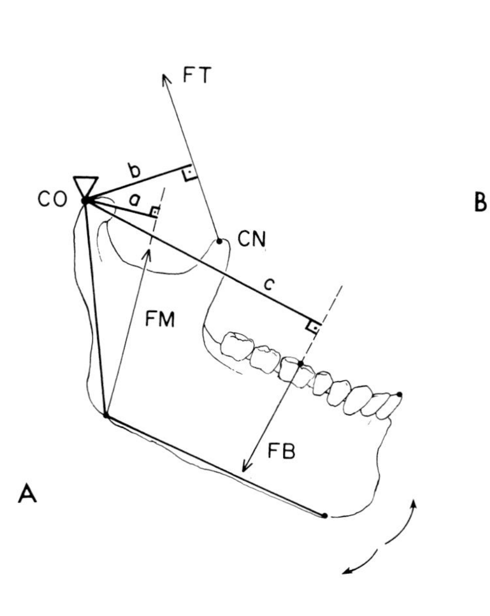

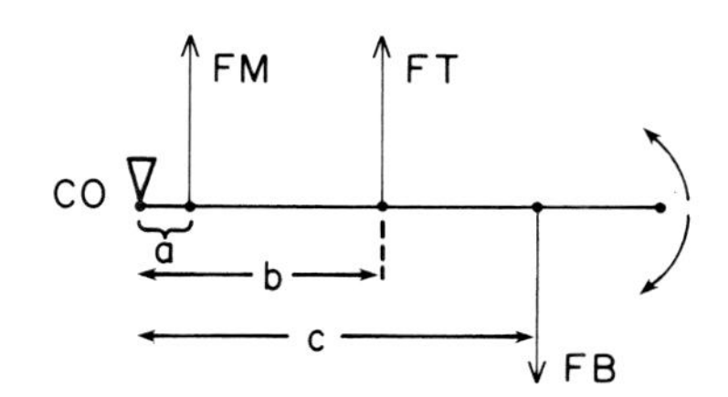

Figure 24–7. The human mandible functioning as a class III lever. *A*, two-dimensional model of mandibular system shown in *B*. Stylized lever system: *CO*, condyle and fulcrum; *CN*, coronoid process; *FB*, bite force vector; *FM*, muscle force vector for masseter; *FT*, muscle force vector for temporalis; (*a*) moment arm for masseter; (*b*) moment arm for temporalis; and (*c*) moment arm for bite force.

poralis and masseter, tend to produce a counterclockwise rotation of the mandible (when viewed from the right). This tendency to produce rotation is termed *torque*. The strength of the torque is the product of the strength of the muscle force (FM, FT, respectively) times the perpendicular distance (termed *moment arm*) of the muscle from the condyle (line segments a and b, respectively).

$$\text{torque} = \text{force times perpendicular distance to condyle}$$

Thus, the torque produced by the temporalis is $FT \times b$.

When the person is biting down on an object, i.e., an isometric bite (for example, when biting on the bite force gauge), the object that is being bitten produces a torque that is equal to, but opposite in direction, to the sum of the torques produced by the jaw-elevating muscles. This torque is the product of the bite force or load (FB) times its moment arm (line segment c). The total torque applied to the jaw is 0 because the bite force torque cancels exactly the muscle force torques. Thus, there is no movement of the jaw in the isometric bite.

The mechanical advantage of a muscle is the ratio of the moment arm of the muscle to the moment arm of the load.[5]

$$\text{Mechanical advantage} = \frac{\text{perpendicular distance from condyle to muscle}}{\text{perpendicular distance from condyle to load}}$$

For the temporalis, the mechanical advantage would be distance b divided by distance c.

The mechanical advantage of a muscle can be altered by changing the distance of the muscle from the condyle or changing the distance of the point of bite from the condyle, or both. For example, the mechanical advantage of the jaw-elevating muscles is greatly reduced by moving the point of bite from the molars to the incisors because of the increase in the length of the moment arm of the load.

Surgical alteration of maxillary height changes the perpendicular distance of the position of bite and, to a lesser extent, of the muscles from the condyle, thus having an effect on the mechanical advantage of the jaw muscles. To examine this effect, a model was developed that mimics the changes in positions caused by surgical corrections of long and short faces.

Procedures

Mean values were obtained from Schendel and associates[61, 62] and Opdebeeck and Bell[56] for the following points on 41 long-faced and 42 short-faced computerized cephalometric tracings: S, N, condylar summit, tip of coronoid process, gonion, menton, mesiobuccal cusp of upper first molar, and incisal edge of upper central incisor. In addition, the position of the electromyographic electrodes recording from the temporalis and masseter muscles (points T and Ms, respectively) was estimated in accordance with the insertion positions utilized during actual experiments. These points were plotted on graph paper, and the moment arms for the bite forces at the molars and the forces produced by the masseter and temporalis muscles were drawn in (Fig. 24–8).

The mechanical advantage of each muscle could then be calculated and the values

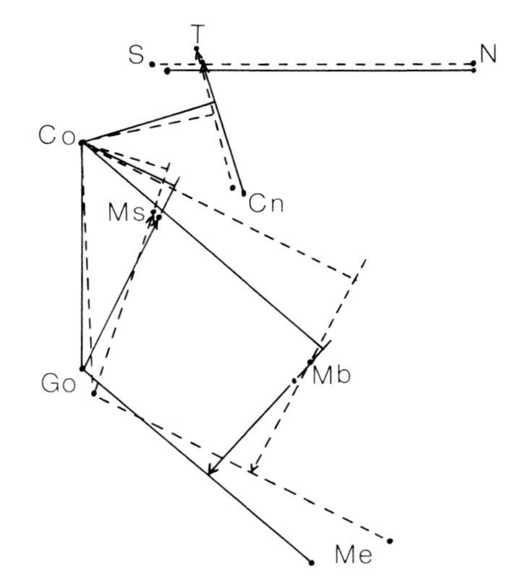

Figure 24–8. Comparison of muscle mechanics of mean long (solid lines) and short faces (broken lines). *S*, sella; *N*, nasion; *Co*, condyle summit; *Cn*, tip of coronoid process; *Go*, gonion; *Me*, menton; *Mb*, mesiobuccal cusp of upper first molar; *Ms*, position of electrode in masseter muscle; and *T*, position of electrode in temporalis muscle. To simplify superimposition *S-N* is drawn horizontal here.

compared between the long-faced group and the short-faced group. The mechanical advantage of the temporalis muscle was determined to be 0.428 for long face and 0.438 for short face. Corresponding values for the masseter muscle were 0.318 for long face and 0.295 for short face.

To determine the effect of changes in maxillary height, the bite point (mesiobuccal cusp of upper first molar) was moved upward (for the long-faced model) and downward (for the short-faced model) relative to S-N. Then the resultant rotation of the mandible was plotted, and the new moment arms were measured (Figs. 24–9 and 24–10).

Notice that the two mesiobuccal cusps move away from each other during autorotation of the lower jaw. Thus, the mechanical advantage becomes different for the upper and lower molars in their new positions. In the present study, the molar bite point is assumed to be at the position of the upper molar.

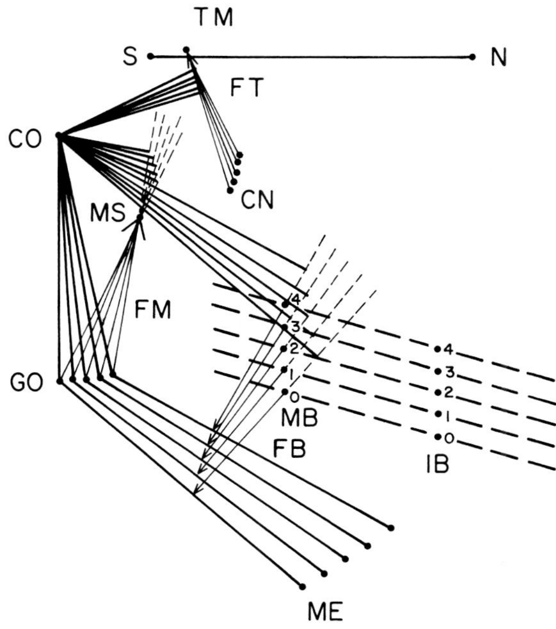

Figure 24–9. Changes in mechanics of the temporalis and masseter muscles with shortening of the maxilla. *FT*, line of action of temporalis muscle; *FM*, line of action of masseter muscle; *FB*, line of action of bite force.

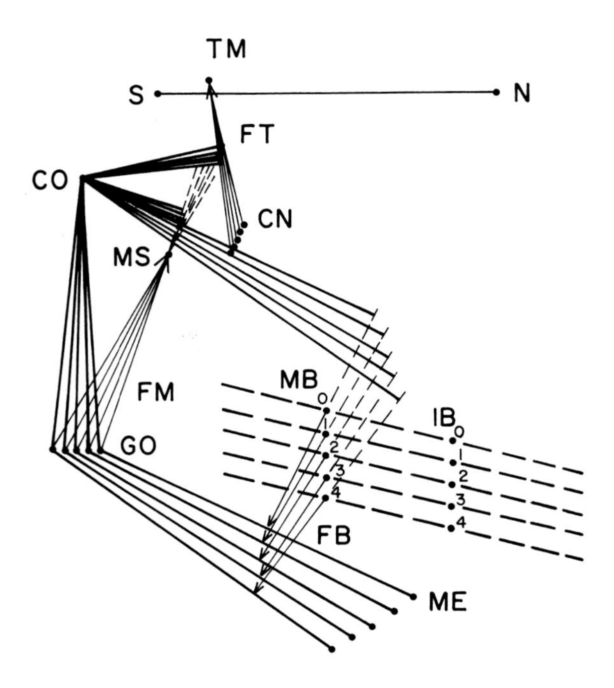

Figure 24–10. Changes in mechanics of the temporalis and masseter muscles with lengthening of the maxilla. *FT*, line of action of temporalis muscle; *FM*, line of action of masseter muscle; and *FB*, line of action of bite force.

Results

The major effect of raising or lowering the maxilla is to change the distance between the point of bite and the condyle. Thus, if the maxilla is raised, the distance between the molars and the condyle is decreased, and the mechanical efficiency of the muscles will tend to be increased. Since the insertions of the temporalis and masseter muscles are closer to the condyle than the molars, the amount of movement of these points during autorotation is less than the movement at the molars. Thus, the moment arms of the muscles are less affected by the rotation than is the moment arm for bite load. The model suggests that the maximum amount of lengthening or shortening of the muscle is approximately 10 per cent of its total length.

As the maxilla is raised (Fig. 24–9), the moment arm for the temporalis muscle is lengthened slightly, whereas the moment arm for the masseter is shortened slightly. The reverse is true if the maxilla is lowered (Fig. 24–10). The effect of these changes on mechanical advantage is shown in Figure 24–11. As the maxilla is superiorly repositioned for correction of the long face, the moment arm for the temporalis muscle increases approximately 2.5 per cent for each 5 mm of maxillary elevation. The moment arm for the bite force correspondingly decreases. The result is an increased mechanical advantage for the temporalis muscle. (We could expect decreased temporalis muscle activity for a given bite force after this procedure.) The moment arm for the masseter muscle decreases at approximately the same rate as that of the bite force. Thus, the mechanical advantage of the masseter is not changed by this procedure. This trend is continued in the correction of maxillary deficiency. Although the short face usually has a slightly higher mechanical advantage in the temporalis muscle, this advantage decreases as the maxilla is lowered. Again, the advantage of the masseter muscle undergoes little change.

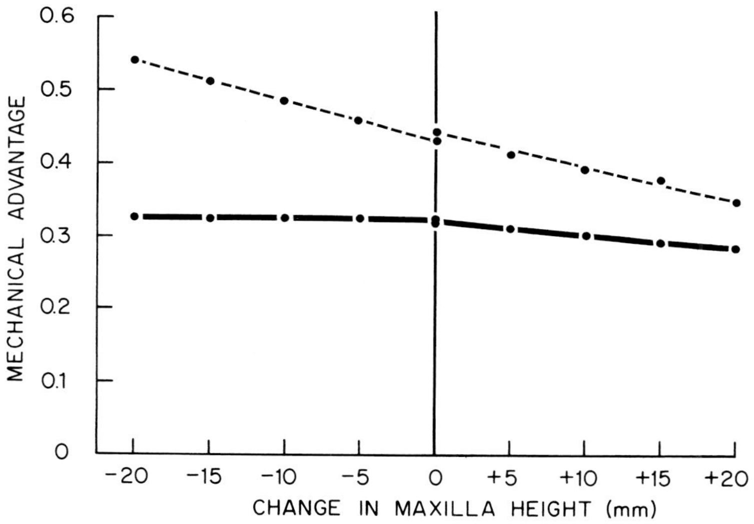

Figure 24–11. Effect of changing maxillary height on mechanical advantage. The broken line represents the temporalis muscle and the solid line represents the masseter muscle. To the left of O the maxilla is being shortened to correct long face syndrome. To the right of 0 the maxilla is being lengthened to correct short face syndrome.

MUSCLE ACTIVITY

Myopotentials produced by depolarization and repolarization of muscle cells or fibers are the source of the electrical changes recorded on electromyography (EMG). The functional unit of striated muscle is the motor unit, consisting of a motor neuron, its axon and terminal branches, and all of the muscle fibers supplied by that axon. By the use of amplifiers and recording machinery, the electrical activity of muscles can be monitored and evaluated. The electromyogram has not been utilized to study patients with vertical dysplasias of the facial skeleton, but because of electronic refinement and a better understanding of normal muscle physiology, we can better employ EMG as a tool to elucidate neuromuscular response to corrective jaw surgery.

In 1949, Robert Moyers[49] became the first individual to seriously establish EMG as a valuable tool for studying the muscles of mastication while using the method to analyze Class II malocclusions. Orthodontists became very intrigued with this new research tool and began using it to study their patients.

As numerous articles were published, it became increasingly clear that results reported were not consistent. Inexperienced electromyographers, with admirable zeal but with lack of basic knowledge, were jeopardizing the credibility of the technique by reporting conflicting results. Most of the early studies[1, 3, 22, 28, 29, 31, 37, 39, 48-51, 55, 57] and much of the more recent research[47, 74] have compared groups of individuals with similar malocclusions but have failed to establish a characteristic EMG pattern for any given malocclusion.

More recently, the aim of EMG investigations has been directed toward facial morphology rather than malocclusions.[2, 4, 34, 35, 46, 67] The error in comparing patients with similar malocclusions is due to differing facial morphologic characteristics. The point is exemplified by comparing a Class II long face syndrome with open bite and a Class II patient with vertical maxillary deficiency. The dental malocclusions in the sagittal plane are comparable, but the dentofacial deformities are completely distinct. Thus, the grouping of patients according to similar skeletal disfigurements is more appropriate for EMG experiments.

Several authors[4, 34, 35, 46] have reported that as gonial angle decreases, the EMG activity increases in the mandibular elevator muscle group (masseter and temporalis) during maximal isometric contractions. Although bite force values were not reported in their studies, the elevated EMG activity in short-faced type patients is consistent with our data and can be at least partially explained by the muscle atrophy noted in our group. Others[58, 60] have demonstrated a strong tendency for persons with small gonial angles, parallel jaw bases, rectangular profiles, and short faces to produce very large bite forces with an anticipated increase in electromyographic activity of the mandibular elevators. Ingervall[34] stated that persons with short faces tended to have elevated EMG activity in the masseter and temporalis muscles during functional maneuvers such as swallowing or chewing and in rest position. Furthermore, in a longitudinal clinical assessment of alveolar bone loss in denture wearers,[67] the short-faced individuals had four times the alveolar bone loss over the same period of time as patients with normal vertical facial height. The increased bite force capacity of these patients was offered as an explanation for this phenomenon.

Despite the similarities mentioned, considerable controversy exists concerning the exact relationship between muscle forces and facial morphology. If subtle changes in muscles are to be noted following surgery, it is important to appreciate the possible explanations for the apparent contradictions.

The lack of a controllable clinical situation is probably the primary factor resulting in inconsistent EMG results in previous studies. Patient selection (adult versus child) and maneuvers performed by the patients were usually dissimilar in most of the studies. Furthermore, acquisition of data in terms of types of electrodes, amplification, filtering, and storage was not the same in the majority of the previous studies. Evaluation of the records, however, is probably the most abused aspect of electromyography.[9] Disciplined qualitative and quantitative analysis of good records taken in a controllable setting by an experienced electromyographer is the key to obtaining reliable EMG information.

Thus, with all of the factors just mentioned in mind, a clinical electromyographic investigation was designed to identify differences in groups of patients and controls and possible changes in muscle activity subsequent to surgery to correct vertical facial heights. Rigid parameters (i.e., isometric bites of designated force on a strain gauge and topographic accuracy of reinsertion of electrodes) were established to facilitate the identification of the most subtle alteration in the neuromuscular system.

Preliminary Study

The Patients

This clinical electromyographic investigation was designed to identify possible differences in muscle activity between groups of long-faced open bite patients prior to surgery, short-faced patients prior to surgery, and normal controls. To date, five short-faced patients, eight long-faced patients, and four controls have been examined. The experiment was performed with each patient just prior to surgery. The controls were tested three times approximately one week apart.Two trials were conducted for each control experiment; whereas, only one trial was utilized for patients.

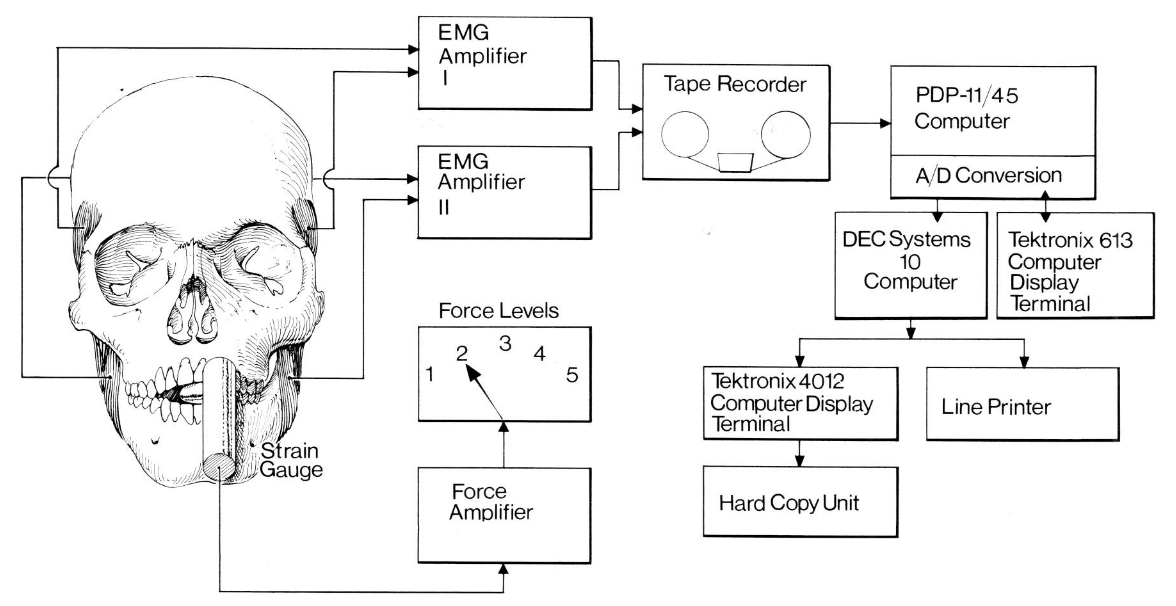

Figure 24–12. Flow diagram for recording of electromyography of the jaw muscles during isometric bites. (See text for explanation of figure.)

Experimental Procedure (Fig. 24–12)

Monopolar fine-wire electrodes were inserted bilaterally into specific locations within the deep masseter and temporalis muscles. A line was drawn on both sides of the patient's face corresponding to Frankfort horizontal (portion to infraorbitale). For insertion into the temporalis muscle, the needle was introduced 3 cm anterior to the tragus of the ear and 2 cm superior to Frankfort horizontal. The point of insertion of the masseter muscle was 2 cm anterior to the tragus and 2 cm inferior to the reference line. The depth of insertion was one-half inch. The fine wire electrodes were connected to insulated lead wires by slipping the wires into the coils of small steel springs at one end of the leads. Reference electrodes were placed bilaterally over the angle of the jaw, and a ground electrode was placed at the chin. The EMG signals were amplified by an electroencephalograph machine (Grass Model 8–16) with a frequency response of 5 Hz to 10 KHz. The amplified signals were recorded on a four-channel AM tape recorder (Teac A 33405) with a frequency response up to 24 KHz for storage and subsequent analysis.

Each experiment consisted of eight bites: four incisor bites (10, 15, and 20 kg and maximum) and four right molar bites (20, 30, and 40 kg and maximum). Some long-faced patients could not do all the bites. Bite force was determined using a strain gauge device similar to that described by other workers.[23, 40] The force was displayed to the patient on a large scale as the subject attempted to maintain a constant force for 5 seconds.

The recorded EMG signals were played into a PDP 11/45 minicomputer where they were digitized and displayed in real time onto a Tektronix 613 graphics terminal. While viewing the incoming data, the investigator initiates actual data acquisition, whereupon 4 seconds of data are acquired and held for visual approval before being transferred[59] to the DEC System-10 computer for further processing and analysis. Thus, a qualitative analysis and the possibility of rejection of the EMG signals were performed before the data reached the analysis phase. This visual evaluation of the signals, made with the knowledge of the techniques employed, is a crucial step to properly monitor and prevent total quantitation of the data regardless of its quality and content. Careful disciplined balance between qualitative and quantitative evaluation of the records was maintained at all times.

Results

The computer calculates 18 parameters from the EMG signal. To date, we have compared only the total area under the EMG curve among the three groups. Total area is the parameter thought most likely to correspond to force generated by the muscle during isometric contraction.[10, 36, 41, 45] Within our controls we were able to establish correlation between the integrated EMG and bite force for each muscle at a significance level of $P < 0.05$. Furthermore, we correlated per cent increase in bite force and per cent increase in integrated EMG at a significance level of $P < 0.001$.

BITE FORCE. The short-faced group was characterized by being able to generate the highest bite forces. One patient had a maximum molar bite of 100 kg. None had lower than normal bite forces. These results are in agreement with those of Sassouni[60] and Ringqvist.[58]

The long-faced group had great difficulty doing the incisor bites. Only one of the patients could generate normal incisor bites. The others either had greatly weakened incisor bites or could not do incisor bites at all. In addition, half of the group had lower than normal molar bite forces.

The two groups could be statistically separated by mean maximum incisor and molar bites at a significance level of $P < 0.05$. The average maximum incisor bite for the short-faced group was 29.2 kg and 14.8 kg for the long-faced group. The mean maximum molar bite was 72.0 kg and 30.5 kg for the short- and long-faced groups, respectively.

EMG VALUES. In order to compare the EMG results with the two-dimensional mechanical model, the areas under the total EMG curve were combined to give one value for both temporalis and both masseter muscles. The means for these values for each group are presented in Table 24–1. The short-faced group had the highest EMG activity during molar bites. They also tended to have higher EMG activity during incisor bites, but there was more variability. These results are in agreement with those of Algren and associates,[4] Ingervall,[34] Ingervall and Thilander,[35] and Möller.[46] If short-faced individ-

TABLE 24–1. EMG Area (in mv-seconds) vs. Molar Bite Force

Muscle	*Group*	*20 kg*	*30 kg*	*40 kg*	*50 kg*
Temporalis	Short-faced	952	1045	1448	–
	Control	554	809	1065	2639
	Long-faced	453	740	798	1414
Masseter	Short-faced	723	986	1273	–
	Control	512	780	1012	1593
	Long-faced	500	783	728	1106

uals do have muscle fiber atrophy, as suggested by the morphologic studies, this could explain the higher than normal EMG values.

The long-faced group tended to have lower than normal EMG values during molar bites (Table 24–1). There were no comparable values for incisor bites. If long-faced individuals do have muscle fiber hypertrophy, as suggested by the morphologic studies, this could explain the lower than normal EMG values.

DISCUSSION AND CONCLUSIONS

Muscle tone in the orofacial region may be influenced by psychic input and by proprioceptive stimuli through peripheral receptors in the periodontal ligament, muscle spindles, temporomandibular joint, gingiva, tongue and palate. The postural activity for certain muscles of mastication can be altered as an adaptive response to experimentally induced alterations of vertical facial height. Studies by McNamara[42] have shown that the functional length of a muscle can be transiently influenced by feedback through the central nervous system without anatomic changes within the muscle itself. The apparent adaptation of the masticatory muscles to increasing or decreasing facial height, without a discernible change in the freeway space, may be mediated through a feedback mechanism within the central nervous system. Decreasing vertical facial height (Fig. 24–13) by Le Fort I osteotomy shortens the muscle fibers and alters the orientation of the masseter and temporalis muscles. On the other hand, increasing vertical facial height by LeFort I osteotomy (Fig. 24–14) and interpositional bone grafting has the opposite effect of stretching the muscle fibers in addition to altering the orientation of the masseter and temporalis muscles. Alterations in jaw biomechanics, muscle morphology, and muscle activity along with adaptive changes within the central nervous system apparently occur to alter the postural position of the mandible and allow restoration of a freeway space

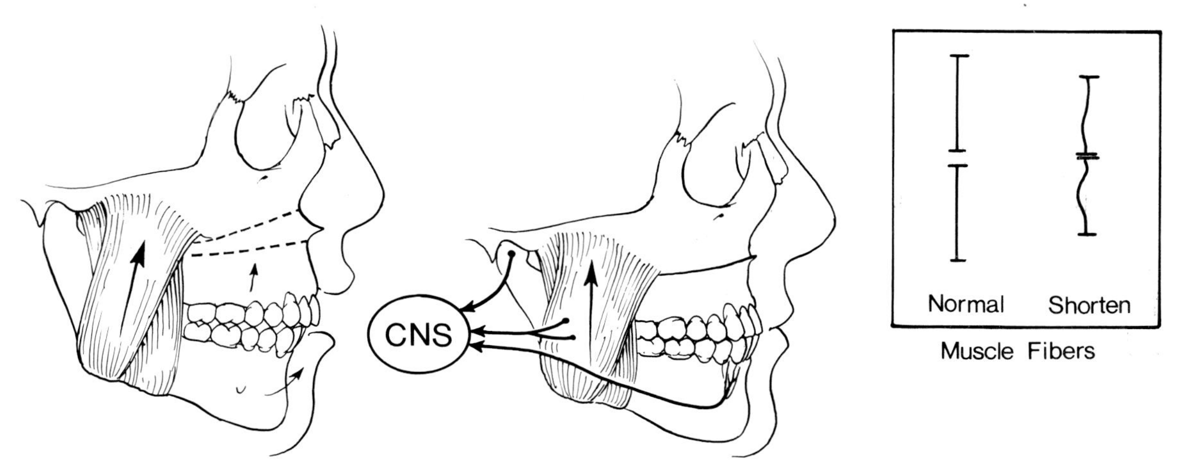

Figure 24–13. Neuromuscular adaptation to decreasing facial height by Le Fort I osteotomy. CNS indicates central nervous system; small arrow indicates counterclockwise rotation of mandible superiorly and anteriorly; large arrow indicates orientation of masseter muscle before and after surgery; proprioceptive stimuli by sensory receptors in the periodontal ligament, muscle spindles, and temporomandibular joint.

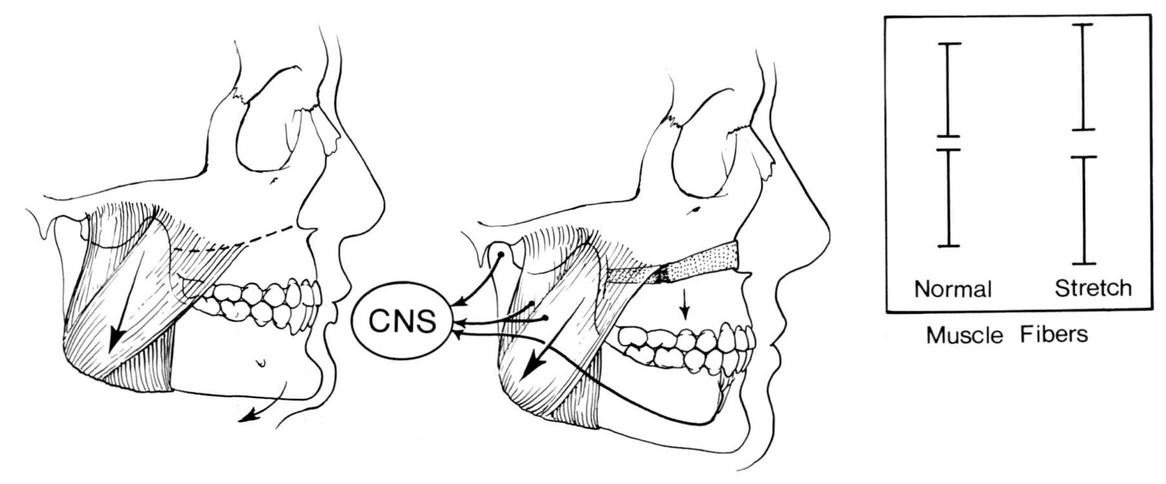

Figure 24–14. Neuromuscular adaptation to increasing facial height by Le Fort I osteotomy and interpositional bone graft. CNS indicates central nervous system; stippled area indicates interpositional bone graft; small arrow indicates clockwise rotation of mandible inferiorly and posteriorly; large arrow indicates orientation of masseter muscle before and after surgery; proprioceptive stimuli by sensory receptors in the periodontal ligament, muscle spindles, and temporomandibular joint.

comparable to that which existed before surgery. Also, such physiologic alterations are possible and plausible explanations for clinical stability after surgical alteration of vertical facial height. Additional experimental studies are needed to elucidate the postsurgical adaptation of the muscles of mastication by way of the central nervous system feedback mechanism.

The results of these preliminary studies suggest that patients with vertical maxillary dysplasias have abnormal jaw muscles, with atrophy of muscle fibers in the short-faced patients and muscle fiber hypertrophy in the long-faced patients. Since the force that a muscle fiber can generate is proportional to the cross-sectional area of the fiber, short-faced patients must recruit more muscle fibers to generate the same bite force as long-faced patients. This is reflected in the higher electromyographic activity of the muscles in short-faced patients. The differences in morphology apparently mask the relatively small differences in mechanical advantage between the two groups.

The morphologic and mechanical differences, however, do not explain the great disparity in maximum bite force between the two groups. Recent observations[25a] indicate that an increase in the total number of muscle fibers (hyperplasia) due to fiber splitting can be induced by exercise in animals. It has been suggested,[60] and it has been our clinical observation, that short-faced patients have larger than normal masseter muscles. The simultaneous observation of atrophic muscle fibers with large bite forces would suggest that these patients have an increase in the total number of muscle fibers in the masseter muscle.

The mechanical model predicts the differences in mechanical advantage of the temporalis muscle to be altered by corrective surgery with anticipated concomitant changes in muscle activity if muscle fiber size is not altered. Studies of these and additional patients following corrective surgery are just beginning. These studies will determine the effect of changing mechanical advantage, whether the muscle fibers adapt to the altered position of the muscles, and how these changes affect the electromyographic activity of the muscles during isometric bites.

REFERENCES

1. Ahlgren J: An electromyographic analysis of the response to activator therapy. Odont Rev *11*:125, 1960.
2. Ahlgren J: Mechanism of mastication. Acta Odont Scand *24*(Suppl):44, 1966.
3. Ahlgren J: Form and function of Angle Class III malocclusion. A cephalometric and electromyographic study. Tr Eur Orthodont Soc 77, 1970.
4. Ahlgren J, Ingervall B, Thilander B: Muscle activity in normal and post-normal occlusion. Am J Orthod *64*:445, 1973.
5. Alexander R: Animal Mechanics. Seattle: University of Washington Press, 1968, pp. 13–15.
6. Bahler AS, Fules JT, Zierler KL: The dynamic properties of mammalian skeletal muscle. J Gen Physiol *51*:369, 1968.
7. Ballard CF: A consideration of the physiological background of mandibular posture and movement. Dent Pract *6*:80, 1955.
8. Bárány M: ATPase activity of myosin correlated with speed of muscle shortening. J Gen Physiol *50*:197, 1967.
9. Basmajian JV: Muscle Alive, ed 3. Baltimore: Williams & Wilkins, 1974.
10. Bayer H, Flechtenmayer C: Ermunding und aktion spannung bei der isometrischen muskel-contraktion des menschen. Arbeitsphysiol *14*:261, 1950.
11. Bell WH: Correction of skeletal type anterior open bite. J Oral Surg *29*:706, 1971.
12. Bell WH: Le Fort I osteotomy for correction of maxillary deformities. J Oral Surg *33*:412, 1975.
13. Bell WH: Correction of the short face syndrome — vertical maxillary deficiency: A preliminary report. J Oral Surg *35*:110, 1977.
14. Blix M: Die Länge und die Spannung des Muskels. Skand Arch Physiol *5*:150, 1895.
15. Boos RH: Intermaxillary relations establishing by biting forces. JADA *27*:1192, 1940.
16. Büchi EC: Anderungen der Korperform beim Erwachsenen Menschen. Anthropologishe Forschungen Anthrop. Gesell. Heft 1, Horn Wien, 1950.
17. Büchi EC: Anderungern der Korperform beim Erwachsenen Menschen. Anthropologishe Forschungen Anthrop. Gesell. Heft 1, Horn Wien, 2, 1954.
18. Carlson FD: Kinetic studies on mechanical properties of muscle. *In* Remington JW (ed); Tissue Elasticity. Washington DC: Am Physiol Soc 1957, pp 55–72.
19. Close RI: Dynamic properties of mammalian skeletal muscle. Physiol Rev *52*(1):139, 1972.
20. DuBowitz V, Pearse AG: A comparative histochemical study of oxidative enzyme and phosphorylase activity in skeletal muscle Histochemie *2*:105, 1960.
21. Edström L, Kugelburg E: Histochemical composition, distribution of fibers and fatigability of single motor units. J Neurol Neurosurg Psychiat *31*:424, 1968.
22. Ekholm A, Siirilä H: Elektromyografisia tutkimuksia musculus pterygoideus lateral iksen toimiun asta. Suam Hammasloak Toim *56*:89, 1960.
23. Garrett FA, Angelone L, Allen WL: The effect of bite opening, bite pressure, and malocclusion on the electrical response of the masseter muscles. Am J Orthodont *50*:435, 1964.
24. Gillis RR: Establishing vertical dimension in full denture construction. JADA *28*:433, 1941.
25. Goldspink G, Tabary C, Tabary JC, Tardieu C, Tardieu G: Effect of denervation on the adaptation of sarcomere number and muscle extensibility to the functional length of the muscle, J Physiol *236*:733, 1974.

25a. Gonyea W., Ericson GC, Bonde-Petersen F: Skeletal muscle fiber splitting induced by weight lifting exercise in cats. Acta Physiol Scand *99*:105, 1977.

26. Gordon AM, Huxley AF, Julian FJ: Tension development in highly stretched vertebrate muscle fibers. J Physiol (London) *184*:143, 1966.
27. Gordon AM, Huxley AF, Julian JF: The variation in isometric tension with sarcomere length in vertebrate muscle fibers. J Physiol (London) *184*:170, 1966.
28. Greenfield BE, Wyke BD: Electromyographic observations on some of the muscles of mastication. J Anat (London) *89*:578, 1955.
29. Grosfeld O: Changes in muscle activity patterns as a result of orthodontic treatment. Tr Eur Orthodont Soc *41*:203, 1965.
30. Guth L, Samaha FJ: Procedure for the histochemical demonstration of actomysin ATPase. Exp Neurol *28*:365, 1970.
31. Haralabakis V: Electromyographic analysis of a series of 50 treated posterior crossbites. Tr Eur Orthodont Soc *40*:206, 1964.
32. Heartwell C: Syllabus of Complete Dentures. Philadelphia: Lea & Febiger, 1968.
33. Hylander WL: The human mandible, lever or link? Am J Phys Anthro *43*:(2):227, 1975.
34. Ingervall B: Facial morphology and activity of temporal and lip muscles during swallowing and chewing. Angle Orthod *46*(4):372, 1976.
35. Ingervall B, Thilander B: Facial morphology and masticatory activity. J Oral Rehab *1*(2): 131, April, 1974.
36. Inman VT, Ralston HF, Saunders JB, Feinstein B, Wright EN Jr: Relation of human electromyogram to muscular tension. Electroenceph Clin Neurophysiol *4*:187, 1952.
37. Jarabak JR: Electromyographic analysis of muscular and temporomandibular joint disturbances due to imbalance in occlusion. Angle Orthod *26*:170, July, 1956.
38. Kazis H: Complete mouth rehabilitation through restoration of lost vertical dimension. JADA, *37*:19, 1948.
39. Liebman FM, Cosenza F: Evaluation of electromyography in the study of the etiology of

malocclusion. J Prosth Dent *10*:1065, 1960.
40. Linderholm H, Wennström A: Isometric bite force in children and its relation to body build and general muscle force. Acta Odont Scand *29*:563, 1971.
41. Lippold OCJ: The relation between integrated action potentials in human muscle and its isometric tension. J Physiol *117*:492, 1952.
42. McNamara JA: Neuromuscular and skeletal adaptations to altered function in the orofacial region. Am J Orthodont *64*:578, 1973.
43. McNamara JA, Carlson DS, Yellich GM: Posttreatment adaptations to orthognathic surgery. Presented at Third International Congress for Orthodontics, Munich, Germany, November, 1977.
44. Mershon JV: Possibilities and limitations in the treatment of closed bites. Int J Orthodont *23*:581, 1937.
45. Milner-Brown HS, Stein RB: The relation between the surface electromyogram and muscular force. J Physiol *246*:549. 1975.
46. Möller E: The chewing apparatus. Acta Physiol Scand *69*(1)Suppl:280, 1966.
47. Moss JP: An electromyographic investigation of certain muscle activities associated with malocclusion of the teeth. PhD thesis, University of London, 1971.
48. Moss JP, Greenfield BE: An electromyographic investigation and survey of Class II cases. Br Soc Study Orthodont Tr 147–156, 1965.
49. Moyers RE: Temporomandibular muscle contraction patterns in Angle Class II division I malocclusions: An electromyographic analysis Am J Orthod *35*:837, 1949.
50. Moyers RE: An electromyographic analysis of certain muscles involved in temporomandibular movement. Am J Orthod *36*:481, 1950.
51. Moyers RE: Some recent electromyographic findings in the orofacial muscles. Tr Eur Orthodont Soc *32*:225, 1956.
52. Movikoff AB, Shin W, Drucker J: Mitochondrial localization of oxidate enzymes. Staining results with two tetrazolium salts. J Biophys Biochem Cytol *9*:47, 1961.
53. Niswonger ME: The rest position of the mandible and the centric relation. JADA *21*:1572, 1934.
54. Niswonger ME: Obtaining the vertical relation in endutulous cases that existed prior to extractions. JADA *25*:1842, 1938.
55. Okun JH: Electromyographic study of Class II cases during orthodontic treatment. Am J Orthod *48*:474, 1962.
56. Opdebeeck H, Bell WH: The short face syndrome. Am J Orthod *73*:499, 1978.
57. Perry HT: Functional electromyography of the temporal and masseter muscles in Class II division I malocclusion and excellent occlusion. Angle Orthod *25*:49, 1955.
58. Ringqvuist M: Isometric bite force and its relation to dimensions of the facial skeleton. Acta Odont Scand *31*:35, 1973.
59. Saffer SI, Mishelevich DI, Fox SJ, Summerar VB: NODAS — The network-oriented data acquisition system for the medical environment. Proceedings of the National Computer Conference *46*:295, 1977.
60. Sassouni V: A classification of skeletal facial types. Am J Orthod *55*:109, 1969.
61. Schendel SA, Eisenfeld JH, Bell WH, Epker BN: Superior repositioning of the maxilla: Stability and soft tissue osseous relations. Am J Orthod *70*:663, 1976.
62. Schendel SA, Eisenfeld J, Bell WH, Eplser BN, Mishelevich DJ: The long face syndrome: Vertical maxillary excess. Am J Orthod *70*:398, 1976.
63. Serratrice G, Pellissier TF, Vignon C, Baret J: The histochemical profile of the human masseter. J Neurol Sci *30*:189, 1976.
64. Sicher H: Oral Anatomy. St. Louis: C. V. Mosby, 1949.
65. Silverman SI: Denture prosthesis and the functional anatomy of the maxillo-facial structures. J Prosth Dent *6*:305, 1956.
66. Tabary JC, Tabary C, Tardieu C, Tardieu G, Goldspink G: Physiological and structural changes in the cat's soleus muscle due to immobilization at different lengths by plaster casts. J Physiol *224*:231, 1972.
67. Tallgren A: Alveolar bone loss in denture wearers as related to facial morphology. Acta Odont Scand *28*:251, 1970.
68. Tallgren A: Changes in adult face height. Acta Odont Scand *15*:(Suppl 23), 1957.
69. Thompson JR: The rest position of the mandible and its significance to dental science. JADA *33*:151, 1946.
70. Thompson JR, Brodie AG: Factors in the position of the mandible. JADA *29*:925, 1942.
71. Wattenberg LW, Leong JL: Effects of coenzyme Q_{10} and menadione on succinate dehydrogenase activity as measured by tetrayolium salt reaction. J Histochem Cytochem *8*:296, 1960.
72. West RA, Epker BN: Posterior maxillary surgery: Its place in the treatment of dentofacial deformities. J Oral Surg *30*:562, 1972.
73. Willmar K: On Le Fort I osteotomy. Scand J Plast Reconstr Surg Suppl 12, 1974.
74. Witt E: Kilferwinkel und Kaumuskulatur. Fortschr der Kieferorthopadie, *24*:295, 1965.
75. Wolford LM, Epker BN: The combined anterior and posterior maxillary osteotomy. J Oral Surg *33*:842, 1975.

Chapter 25

COMPUTER-BASED RESEARCH STUDIES ON THE CORRECTION OF DENTOFACIAL DEFORMITIES

J. Eisenfeld and D. J. Mishelevich

Computer methods have been used successfully in research studies in which cephalometric analysis is applied. This is especially true when the studies include a large sample of patients. Typically, the research team is not likely to know in advance which of the cephalometric parameters are most important in explaining a morphologic phenomenon. Therefore, they will initially select a large number of variables to be analyzed. Thus, the research design will call for the measurement and statistical analysis of several thousand parameters, which may be achieved most efficiently with the aid of a computer, both in terms of data input and calculation. The use of the digital computer for mathematical and statistical purposes as described in this chapter is well known. Less well known are the use of digitizing devices to input experimental data and the use of computer graphics to present results in the form of line drawings rather than numbers that have to be analyzed in tabular form or perhaps subsequently plotted by hand. Hand calculations require a great deal of time and are subject to error. The computer also provides a degree of standardization in the definition of variables as well as consistency in their measurement. Computer application tends to challenge the researchers to be as precise as possible in defining their objectives and expressing their ideas. Probably the most important advantage to be gained from use of computers is the suggesting of new approaches, new ideas, and new methods for observing results as well as techniques for their follow-up. In addition, the computer also provides a convenient record-keeping facility. An entire study may be stored on a tape in such a manner that the complete study or any part of it may be readily and economically accessible.

This chapter is primarily concerned with the use of computer methods in cephalometric studies. The literature contains some good discussions of computers in dental science, in particular the survey articles by Solow,[14] and Walker and Kowalski[16] and the symposium papers by Biggerstaff and Wells,[2] Krogman,[8] Savara,[11] and Walker.[15] The studies of our own, which are discussed in this chapter, were performed in collaboration with members of the Division of Oral Surgery of the Department of Surgery of the Southwestern Medical School component of The University of Texas Health Science Center at Dallas, Drs. William H. Bell, Stephen A. Schendel, John J. Dann, III, Heidi Opdebeeck, and Bruce W. Epker.

RECENT STUDIES

The Long Face Syndrome

Clinicians tend to classify patients into groups and then attach labels to these groups. However, groups are not always defined precisely enough to avoid confusion, as there may be several different labels attached to the same group. For example, the literature reports patients with "maxillary alveolar hyperplasia,"[6] "vertical maxillary excess,"[17] and "skeletal open bite."[10] It is natural to ask if these diagnostic labels refer to the same group or to different groups. In order to answer this question and, in fact, to research the entire subject, these terms must be clearly differentiated. To do this a retrospective study based on cephalometric analysis is usually performed, in which researchers collect a sufficiently large number of cephalometric radiographs belonging to patients having a common dysmorphology that is clinically recognizable to the research team. Such an effort was carried out by Schendel and associates,[13] which resulted in their description of a morphologic group labeled the long face syndrome group, having two subgroups — the open-bite group and the not-open-bite group. These groups are defined mathematically in terms of the statistics of the most relevant cephalometric parameters. Moreover, the two subgroups are presented schematically by means of computer drawings. The graphic mathematical model that evolved over a period of time using the lateral view is shown in Figure 25–1. The model now has 220 points that can be obtained from the lateral view radiographs used in the studies (to be described later). The computer drawings were instrumental in detecting the existence of two morphologically distinct groups.

Computer drawings have played an important role in studies of craniofacial morphology. Their main advantage is in their expression of statistical information, i.e., by means of images. Basically, computer drawings are simply polygons in which the vertices are anatomic points. In the long face syndrome study, only 22 anatomic points were used in the construction of the computer drawings (Fig. 25–2). However, in the studies to be discussed in this chapter, additional points were used in the construction of the computer drawing, thereby producing computer drawings that closely simulate a tracing of a cephalometric radiograph (Figs. 25–3 and 25–4).

Stability and Soft-Tissue Osseous Relations

It is important to measure and document the success of any surgical procedure. This includes recording the long-term condition of the patient, i.e., the stability of the surgical procedure, and predicting the soft-tissue changes that will be caused by surgi-

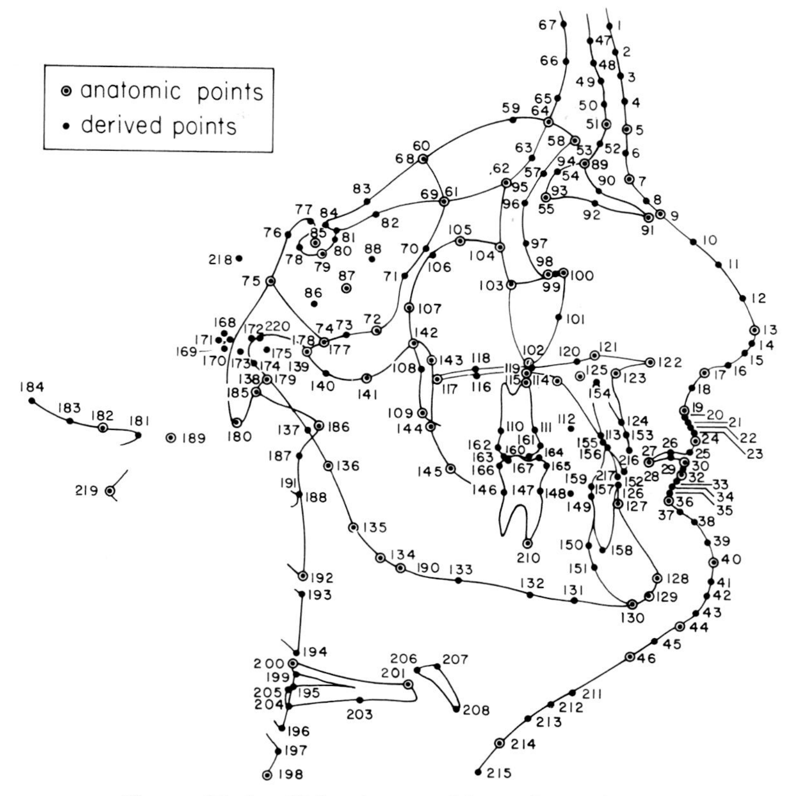

Figure 25-1. 220-point graphic mathematical model.

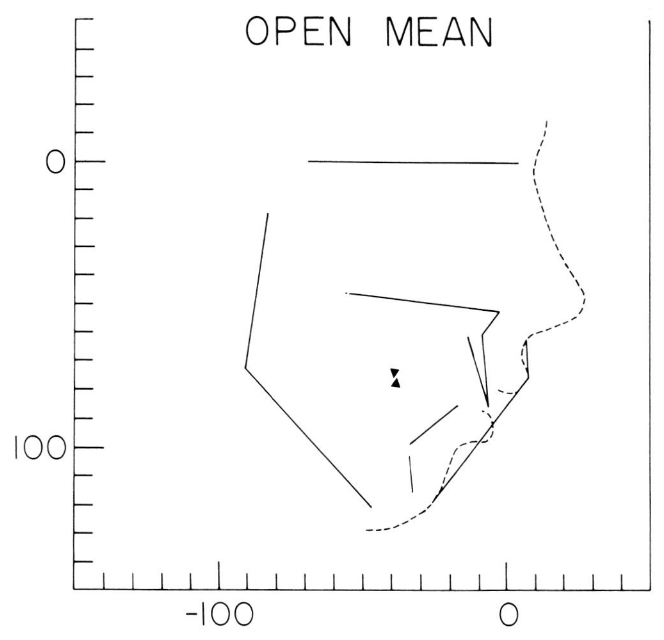

Figure 25-2. Computer drawing of the average long face, open-bite patient based on the 220-point model that was used in the long face syndrome study.

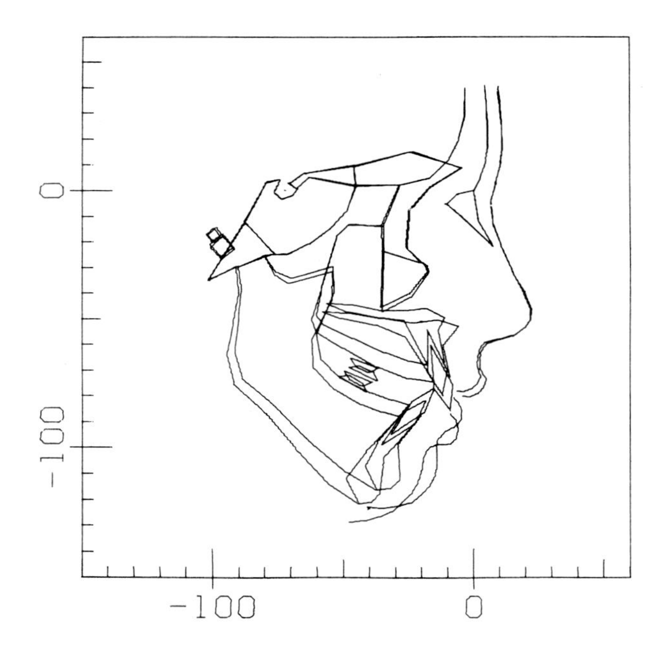

Figure 25–3. Composite of presurgical and recall averaged computerized faces showing surgical soft-tissue and osseous changes in the vertical maxillary excess group. This drawing is based on a 180-point model used in the study pertaining to superior repositioning of the maxilla.

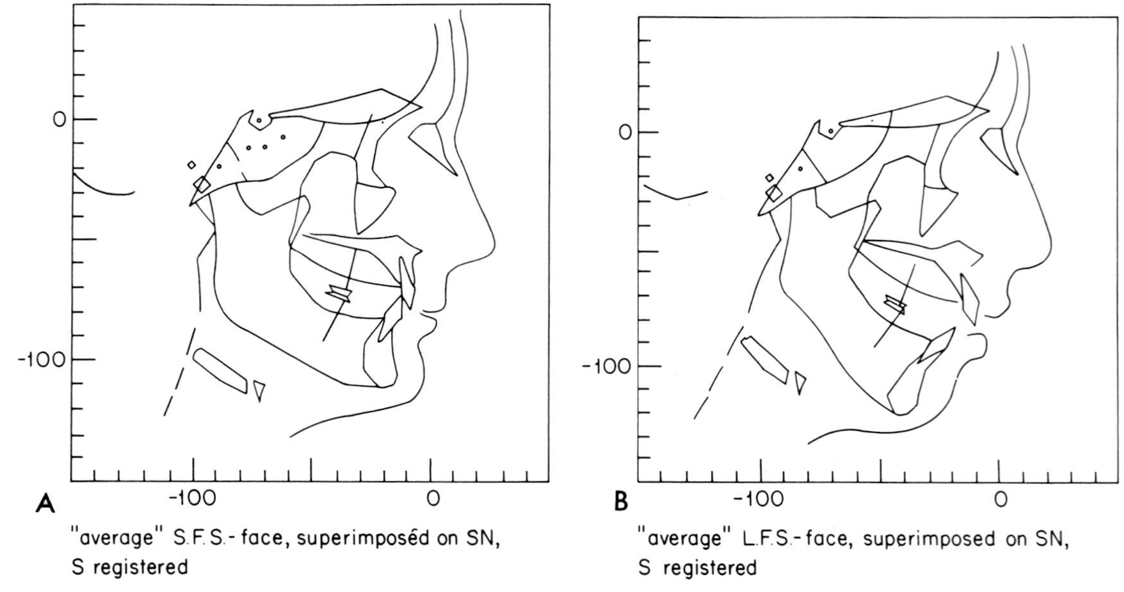

Figure 25–4. Comparison of short-faced (*A*) and long-faced (*B*) patients. These drawings are based on the 220-point model (Fig. 25–1) used in the short face study.

cally induced osseous displacement. Procedures have both critical functional and cosmetic components, as illustrated in the following case of superior repositioning of the maxilla. A study was performed by Schendel and co-workers[12] that utilized the data of 30 patients. The computer was used to measure the cephalometric variables and perform the statistical calculations. By means of regression analysis, mathematical equations were obtained to predict certain soft-tissue changes resulting from repositioning of the underlying hard tissue. For purposes of analysis, the patient population was divided into subgroups. For example, one subgroup was comprised of adult Caucasian patients judged to have vertical maxillary excess. Computer line drawings were constructed that depicted the average presurgery, postsurgery, and recall cephalograms for this subgroup. By superimposing these computer cephalograms, one may assess not only the average amplitude of change that occurred in each anatomic point but also the direction of change. In other words, computer drawings make possible the evaluation of the "vector of change" because the drawings present a two-dimensional perspective. In contrast, a table of statistical results is unidimensional. It is clearly not visual and does not communicate the direction, as well as the magnitude, of change.

The Short Face Syndrome

A study was performed by Opdebeeck and associates[9] to define and analyze a group of patients whose morphologic characteristics were almost opposite to those of the long face group. As in the long face study, the researchers sought to: (1) identify the important cephalometric parameters, (2) obtain their statistical properties, and (3) represent the average patient by means of computer drawings. However, this study includes an additional component that was not present in the long face study. Since there are two groups with opposing morphologic characteristics, it is natural to seek the underlying morphogenic mechanisms that cause the formation of at least one of the two extremes. In fact, there is a temptation to analyze all patients as a compromise between the long-faced and the short-faced patients (Fig. 25–4) to suggest a morphologic transformation that will produce the long face as opposed to the short face. Conceivably, by means of further studies and computer drawings it may be possible to mathematically determine this morphologic transformation. The long face and short face studies probably have generated more questions than they have answered, but this is the nature of research. In addition, the computer has played an important role in the generation of new research questions.

Soft-Hard Tissue Correlation and Computer Drawings for the Frontal View

Cosmetics has always been a major concern in the correction of dentofacial deformity. The relationships between the hard-tissue matrix and the soft-tissue drape are a topic of considerable interest to clinicians. It seems natural to first study such

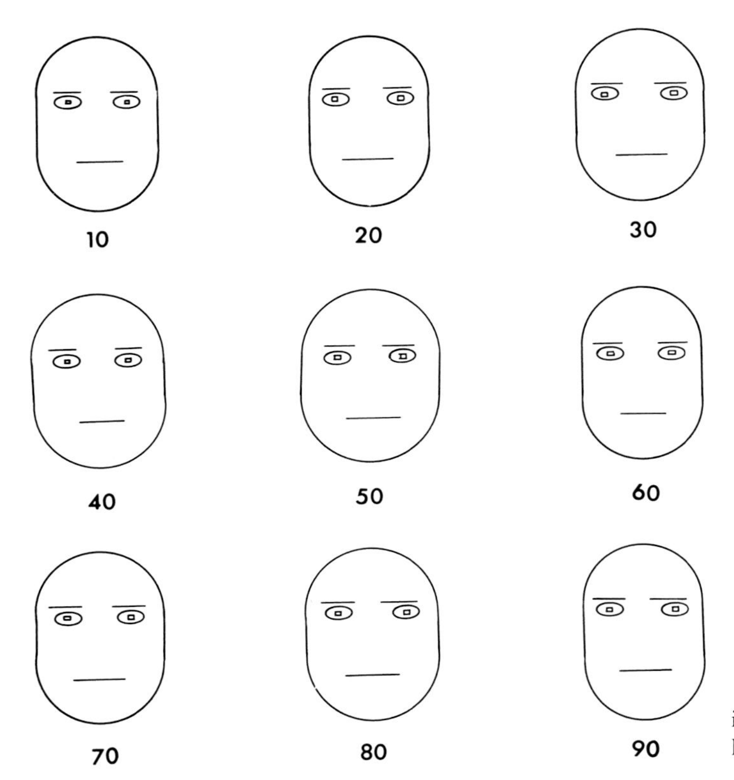

Figure 25–5. Computer drawings for the frontal view based on hard-tissue parameters.

relationships in normal individuals before proceeding to the abnormal group. Moreover, the frontal view is more important for cosmetic considerations, since this is the view by which patients see themselves most often.

Attempting to utilize mathematical formulas to determine the hard-tissue/soft-tissue relationship that would be valid for every individual may be an overly ambitious project. On the other hand, there are certain soft-tissue variables that may be strongly correlated to a subset of hard-tissue variables. The study by Eisenfeld and associates[5] has suggested that such correlations do indeed exist. Moreover, the study also demonstrates how a computer may be programmed to draw a soft-tissue matrix based on the hard-tissue data. Sample frontal-view computer drawings are illustrated in Figure 25–5. The computer drawings used by Eisenfeld and co-workers[4] are based on regression analysis and are entirely different types of computer drawings than were previously discussed when outlining projects that were concerned with the lateral aspect. In the previous projects the computer drawing is a mechanism utilized to discriminate and define subgroups of patients, whereas in this application the computer drawing is used as a device for treatment planning prediction. A primary long-range goal is to create a system in which the clinician can, in essence, peform one or more alternative procedures on the computer-based mathematical model. The alternative functional and cosmetic results (perhaps as a function of time) can be generated on a computer graphics facility to be evaluated by the clinicians and the patient. Thus, the appropriate choice of procedure can be made on the basis of first operating on the model prior to attempting an actual operation on the patient.

MATHEMATICAL MODEL OF A CEPHALOGRAM

In order for a computer to perform mathematical operations on a cephalogram, it is necessary to translate the cephalogram into a set of numbers that represent the coordinates of the relevant anatomic points. The manner in which this translation is performed is based on a mathematical model of the cephalogram. The choice of a mathematical model is an important consideration, as it may significantly affect the resarch project.

The model must contain all the anatomic points that are necessary for the determination of the appropriate cephalometric parameters. A model is essentially a number drawing. For purposes of visual esthetics the model may include points that are not anatomically defined (e.g., see points 1 through 4 in Figure 25–1). Such points are called derived points and should not be used in the calculation of cephalometric parameters. The location of each point in the model is determined by its x-y coordinates. The choice of the coordinate has no effect on the drawing process, but it does affect the construction of "averages." The optimum choice of the coordinate system depends on the specific study. The origin chosen should be a stable point, and the horizontal axis should be chosen to coincide with a stable plane.

Digitizing the Cephalogram

In order to record the desired components of a cephalogram in the computer memory system, a tracing is first made of the cephalogram, indicating all the points on the model. Then the tracing is placed over a digitizer tablet (Fig. 25–6), which is

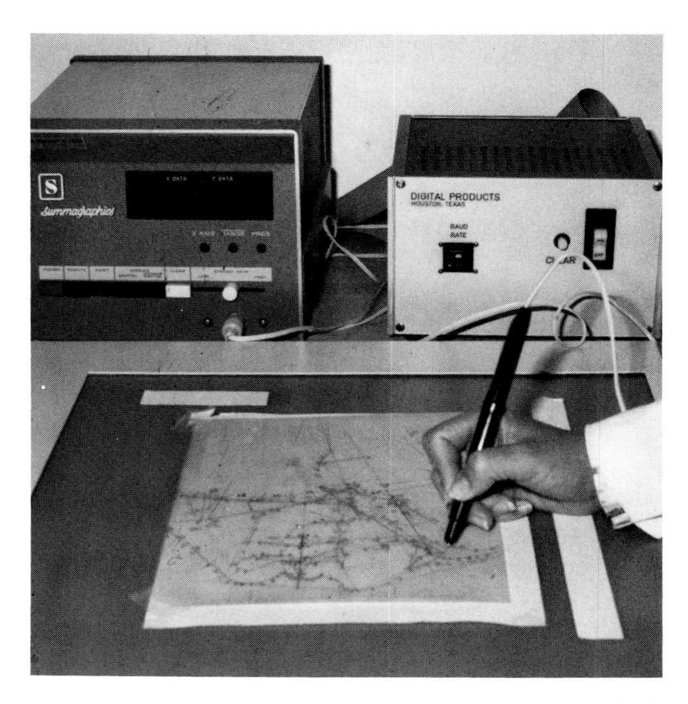

Figure 25–6. Digitizing the cephalogram.

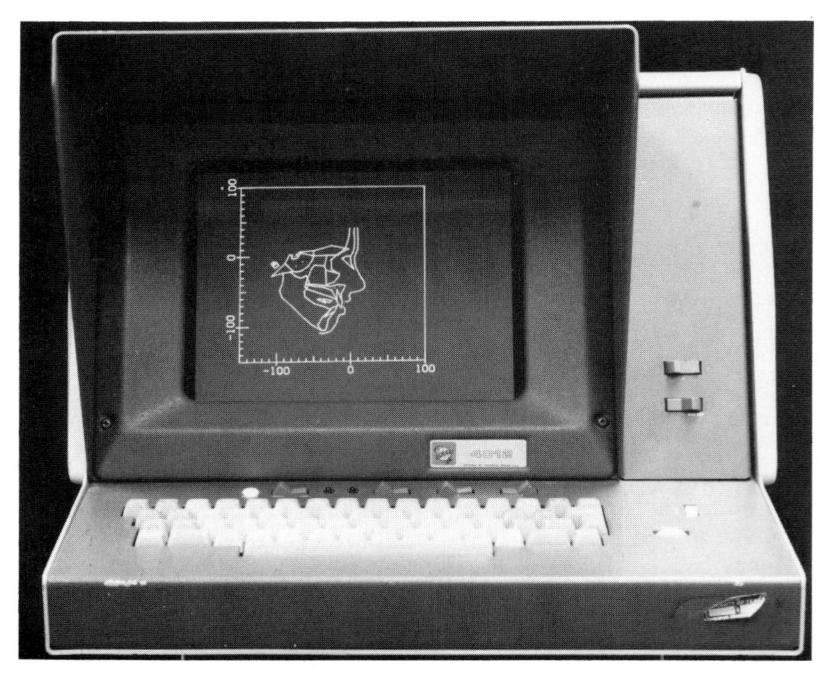

Figure 25–7. A cathode ray tube (CRT) display terminal.

normally connected to an interactive computer terminal (Fig. 25–7). The terminal may be either a cathode ray tube (CRT) display, essentially a television set with a keyboard, or a hardcopy device, one that produces paper output. The orientation of the tracing with respect to the tablet is not a matter of concern because the cephalogram will be "standardized" later. Most digitizers are equipped with a stylus or pen-like object. When the needle of the stylus touches a point on the tablet, a switch is closed and the x-y coordinates (with respect to the digitizer tablet) are recorded.

A typical digitizer is shown in Figure 25–6. The tablet surface is normally backlighted to facilitate the process. In such cases, the digitizing could be done from the cephalogram radiograph itself, but this is discouraged because of both data point definition and recording of the points actually digitized to permit checks of accuracy and reproducibility. Two types of recording methods used are those employing either sound or local position sensing. In the first type, the stylus point emits a sound pulse (e.g., from a spark gap), and the position is recorded from the linear microphones placed along the coordinate axes. When using some digitizers, it is important not to rest the hand on the tablet, as this may disturb the sound pulse. In the second type, a grid of wires is embedded in the tablet surface, and coupling is detected between the stylus point and the localized grid coordinates. The operator begins with a point in the model and touches each point in succession with the tip of the stylus needle until the last point is reached. Then he proceeds to the next cephalogram. Thus, each cephalogram is translated into a sequence of pairs of numbers, i.e., the x-y coordinates of the model points. Such a sequence is called a file, and each file must be given a name. The operator should be familiar with the instructions for the computer operating system. Some digitizers record the digitized points on paper tape that must then be delivered to a location having a paper tape reading facility, perhaps in the computer center.

It is advisable to check the digitizing process for each facial diagram by displaying the computer drawing to detect obvious data input errors. This can significantly reduce frustration later. There is no question that the resultant output is only as good as the initial input.

Cephalometric Measurements

A computer program MEASUR[3] has been programmed to calculate any distance, angle, or projection on a plane that may be determined by the points in the model. In particular, for the model presented in Figure 25–1, the following planes may be defined: the sella-nasion plane by points 85 and 89, the palatal plane by points 117 and 122, and the mandibular plane by points 134 and 130. The mathematical definitions are consistent with clinical evaluations of these planes. The occlusal plane is usually more difficult to define by means of a computer algorithm or formula. One choice is the line drawn through the point equidistant from the incisor tips (points 156 and 152) and the point equidistant from the molar cusps (points 160 and 164).

We emphasize that the application of MEASUR is not restricted to the model presented in Figure 25–4 and may be applied to any model with the appropriate modifications in dimension statements in the FORTRAN language program.

COMPUTER GRAPHICS

Computer drawings may be viewed interactively on a line-drawing Tektronix 4012 computer graphics display, such as a relatively inexpensive model of the 4000 series Tektronix bistable storage cathode ray tube device, or plotted on a hardcopy device (in our studies a Calcomp digital drum plotter with an 11-inch bed). The computer program SHORT I[1] connects the points to produce the computer drawing illustrated in Figure 25–1.

An important consideration is that a computer terminal can be used in one's office, laboratory, or residence and that access to a complete computer set-up is not always necessary. Connections to a computer can be via hardwired or telephone connection. A standard telephone can be used that is equipped with a special device called an acoustic coupler, which has a cradle to hold the telephone headset. The acoustic coupler turns computer electrical logic signals into sound and vice versa so communication can be accomplished. Interactive computing, also called time sharing, permits many operators to be connected to a given computer at one time and to use it simultaneously.

The graphics program provides the option of superimposing faces. This feature might be used to evaluate changes resulting from surgery, either a binary pre- and postoperative comparision or at several points of time postoperatively to provide the basis for a longitudinal analysis of procedure stability. Another application might be to construct an "average" cephalogram for a patient representing a morphological group. In order to construct an average cephalogram one simply averages the x-y pairs contained in the computer files corresponding to the individual cephalograms in the group. However, prior to performing the averaging process, the x-y coordinates in each file must be measured with respect to a common coordinate system. For example, the origin might be at the S point, and the horizontal axis might be chosen to be the S-N line. The computer program MEASUR (discussed previously) permits one to specify the coordinate system in order that valid averages and comparisons can be performed.

COMPUTER APPLICATIONS

AS A TEACHING AID. We have previously indicated that a cephalogram may be viewed interactively on a screen. It is possible to design a program that would permit an individual to request changes in the hard-tissue matrix. The computer program could be designed to construct a cephalogram that not only contains the requested changes but also indicates other significant correlated changes that occur in in vivo hard- and soft-tissue structures. Thus, a student could gain a wealth of experience by experimenting with computer-simulated surgery. In addition, by providing appropriate longitudinal data on which to base a model, dynamic growth patterns could also be amply demonstrated.

SELECTION OF PROCEDURE. As indicated in the previous sections, longitudinal studies of anatomic stability can be performed with the techniques described. This can be done by the clinician's employing a computer graphics (line-drawing) terminal and using a light pen (a device that by detecting light can determine to which point on the display screen a person is pointing). In this way various procedures can be performed, almost as one could use surgical instruments, and the result can be viewed. Even longitudinal stability can be assessed based on the mathematical model, thus providing even more impetus for refinement of this model as more data are acquired. Light pens work on so-called refresh display computer graphics terminals on which images can be displayed continuously but in which changes and movement are permitted without having to erase and redraw the figure each time a change is made. Such devices are more expensive than the less costly models of the 4000 Series Tektronix CRT units previously mentioned.

CHOOSING A FACE. Although esthetics is typically a very important concern to the patient, he frequently has difficulty predicting his new appearance after treatment. A computer program may allow a patient to view new (and perhaps alternative) images on a screen, and he may even be given some choice as to what he prefers. Of course, the patient should be told that computer predictions are not perfect.

INTERACTION OF MUSCLES. Thus far only anatomic correlates have been discussed, but functional relationships with respect to the muscles of mastication also exist. The mechanical forces generated by the muscles influence not only development due to growth but also the stability of operative procedures as well. These mechanical forces have electrical correlates in the electromyograph (EMG). We are beginning additional collaborative studies with members of the Division of Oral Surgery of the Department of Surgery of the Southwestern Medical School, the University of Texas, with investigators from the Departments of Cell Biology and Neurology being added at a later date. These studies will evaluate EMG, mechanical force, and anatomic interrelationships using computer graphic techniques. Other investigators, such as Ingervall and Thilander,[7] have begun work pertaining to the relationship between facial morphology and masticatory muscle activity. The computer graphics and mathematical modeling techniques may significantly aid such investigations.

CONCLUSION

A number of oral surgery and orthodontic problems have been shown to be amenable to computer investigations, not only in the field of statistics but in areas of mathematical modeling and computer graphics as well. To an accelerating extent, computing power will be brought into the user's own environment by the use of timesharing or in some cases by minicomputers or microprocessors. Thus, the presence of computer terminals in one's office, laboratory, home, or other areas will become increasingly common. We project that the routine clerical and investigatory uses of the computer will be realized in the not-too-distant future.

REFERENCES

1. Barker DR, Eisenfeld J, Mishelevich DJ: A computer graphics program for analysis of craniofacial morphology. MCRC Report, Medical Computer Sciences Resources Center, University of Texas Health Science Center at Dallas, Dallas, Texas, 75235.
2. Biggerstaff RH, Wells JA: Computerized analysis of the occlusion in the postcanine dentition. Am J Orthod, *61*:245–254, 1972.
3. Dana K, Eisenfeld J, Mishelevich DJ: A computer program for analysis in craniofacial morphology. Computer Programs in Medicine, *9*:56–62, 1979.
4. Eisenfeld J, Barker DR, Mishelevich DJ: Iconic representation of the human face with computer graphics. Comput Graphics *8*:9–11, 1974.
5. Eisenfeld J, Mishelevich DJ, Dann JJ III, Bell WH: Soft-hard tissue correlations and computer drawings for the frontal view. Angle Orthod *45*:267–272, 1975.
6. Hall HD, Roddy SC Jr: Treatment of maxillary alveolar hyperplasia by total maxillary osteotomy. J Oral Surg *33*:180–188, 1975.
7. Ingervall B, Thilander B: Relation between facial morphology and activity of the masticatory muscles. J Oral Rehab *1*:131–147, 1974.
8. Krogman WM: Use of computers in orthodontic analysis and diagnosis: A symposium. Am J Orthod *61*:219–220, 1972.
9. Opdebeeck HM, Bell WH, Eisenfeld J, Mishelevich DJ: Comparative study between the SFS and LFS rotation as a possible morphogenic mechanism. Am J Orthod *74*:509–521, 1978.
10. Sassouni V: A classification of skeletal facial types. Am J Orthod *55*:109–123, 1969.
11. Savara BS: The role of computers in dentofacial research and the development of diagnostic aids. Am J Orthod *61*:231–245, 1972.
12. Schendel SA, Eisenfeld J, Bell WH, Epker BN: Superior repositioning of the maxilla: Stability and soft tissue osseous relations. Am J Orthod *70*:663–674, 1976.
13. Schendel SA, Eisenfeld J, Bell WH, Epker BN, Mishelevich DJ: The long face syndrome — Vertical maxillary excess. Am J Orthod *70*:398–408, 1976.
14. Solow B: Computers in cephalometric research. Comput Biol Med *1*:41–49, 1970.
15. Walker GF: A new approach to the analysis of craniofacial morphology and growth. Am J Orthod *61*:221–230, 1972.
16. Walker GF, Kowalski CJ: Computer morphometrics in craniofacial biology. Comput Biol Med *2*:235–249, 1971.
17. West RA, Epker BN: Posterior maxillary surgery: Its place in the treatment of dentofacial deformities. J Oral Surg *30*:562–575, 1972.

Chapter 26

BIOLOGIC REGULATORY MECHANISMS RELATED TO DENTOFACIAL DEFORMITIES

Harold C. Slavkin

Craniofacial development is a complex process requiring sequential integration of the numerous biologic steps that lead to the formation of the human face. This process has been a source of fascination and an object of intensive study since early in scientific history. "Experiments in nature," the often grotesque congenital malformations that involve the human face, require complex treatment procedures that are both lengthy and costly and necessitate a sophisticated cadre of professional clinicans to achieve habilitation of the patient.

Congenital malformations of the head and face, often referred to as craniofacial anomalies, represent variations on normal craniofacial development. Mutant genes are a common etiologic agent, but extrachromosomal or epigenetic factors can induce a far broader spectrum of birth defects. In contrast to *congenital craniofacial anomalies,* which result directly from gene mutations or intrauterine insults (*i.e.,* the malformation of the face resulting from chemical agents administered to the mother during critical stages of fetal development), *acquired malformations* of the head and face represent the numerous aberrations caused by physical injuries during postnatal growth, development, and maturation.

Attention in this chapter is focused primarily upon the mechanisms by which the mutant gene produces clinically manifested congenital craniofacial anomalies and upon biomedical research designed to find methods for early detection and subsequent efficacious intervention. Some of the heritable craniofacial anomalies examined in this chapter are common; many are very rare. The extremely rare anomalies are important out of

I wish to thank all my colleagues who graciously contributed references, illustrative suggestions, advice, and criticisms for this chapter. I am extremely grateful to Ms. Kari Chandler for painstaking assistance with the bibliography that made my task immeasurably easier and for typing of the manuscript. I wish to especially thank Mr. Pablo Bringas, Jr., for his illustrations. Many of the concepts described have become better understood by the author through research supported, in part, by research grants DE–02848, DE–03569, and DE–03513, and training grants DE–00044, DE–00134, and DE–07006 from the National Institute of Dental Research, United States Public Health Service.

proportion to their rate of occurrence, for they teach us much about biologic regulation of normal craniofacial development. For example, the details of numerous biochemical processes, of the clotting of blood, and of the functions of alkaline phosphatase in bone and dentin metabolism first became known through "experiments of nature" in which a specific molecular reaction was faulty because of an inborn error in metabolism resulting from a gene mutation. Studies of congenital craniofacial anomalies continue to provide fascinating clues about the nature of cell differentiation, morphogenesis, metabolic regulation, hormonal control mechanisms, immunologic processes, neoplastic transformation, and other fundamental biologic mechanisms.

A large literature describing the etiology and treatment of congenital and acquired craniofacial deformities has accumulated. It is frequently opinionated, contradictory, and confusing. Subtle yet significant distinctions between congenital and acquired deformities have all too often been ignored. Recently, biomedical research concerning congenital craniofacial anomalies, inherited variations, metabolic abnormalities, developmental and molecular biology, and developmental endocrinology and immunology has significantly expanded. The consequent expansion in knowledge made it necessary to integrate new data and concepts derived from animal and human experiments and to communicate them to the clinician.

This chapter presents highlights from an expanding matrix of new biologic knowledge to acquaint the reader with the myriad complex congenital and acquired craniofacial anomalies and the many new modalities of therapy. The constraints of space and time make it necessary to exclude numerous contributions from the enormous quantity of literature from which this information was drawn. The curious reader may independently pursue many of the major topics included by referring to the pertinent monographs, recent reviews, and proceedings of recent colloquia that are cited at the conclusion of the chapter.

LEVELS OF BIOLOGIC ORGANIZATION

During the early part of the twentieth century, analyses of the causes of death in infancy and early childhood indicated that relatively few deaths were due to congenital abnormalities. With the advent of pediatric preventive medicine, nutrition, and immunology, and the exponential rise in the number of effective drugs available, the number of deaths from such causes as infection has decreased remarkably in the United States.[75, 108] But even though craniofacial anomalies in newborn infants are rarely life-threatening, the effects of this class of major birth defects on the development and maturation of the individual and on the resources of society are profound.

Throughout history, many writers have sought explanations for the genesis of congenital malformations. William Harvey, for example, concluded that disturbances of embryogenesis resulted directly from teratologic phenomena. Researchers have identified numerous causes of birth defects in birds, in animals, and — more recently — in primates, including human beings.[18, 19, 21, 22, 35, 36, 39, 42, 48, 53, 54, 61, 67, 84, 87, 90, 92, 98, 108, 109, 122, 124, 125] Administering *or* withdrawing simple or complex molecules, and even ions, produces widely varying developmental defects. The *time* of administration or withdrawal has been found to be a major factor. There are critical periods, especially the first trimester of gestation, when small amounts of a variety of substances initiate aberrations in morphogenetic processes within the embryo. *Very different trace elements, cations, or molecules, and even environmental stresses, can induce identical effects on fetal development.* In evaluating causes of craniofacial anomalies, both genetic determinants ("predisposition") and environmental factors may be considered.[16, 18, 32, 34, 35, 36, 48, 51, 52, 53, 72, 78, 84, 90, 98, 101, 103, 122]

Metazoan embryos are unique in many ways. Consider the organization of the mammalian embryo to be like a symphony. A relatively few different molecules, or "notes," can be arranged into an impressive array of unique macromolecules, or "melodies." These, in turn, interact to form subcellular organelles (themes), which compose the structure that we call the cell. Individual cells form discrete aggregates termed *tissues,* which interact to form *organs.* Spatial, temporal, and functional properties of individual organs have evolved into a complex network of integrated *organ systems,* each dependent upon others for many types of regulation. An integrated organ system like the human face has functional properties that derive its individual organs as well as functional

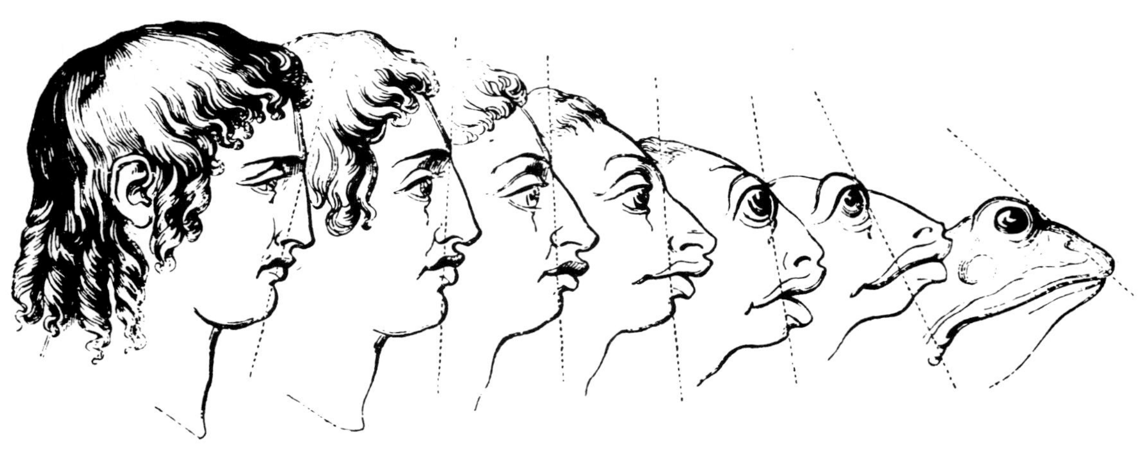

Figure 26–1. The genesis of the human face.

properties that are the product of the integrated system: the embryo becomes much more than the sum of its parts by the conclusion of the third trimester (Fig. 26–1).

Cellular Organization

Living cells exist in many different circumstances and display many biochemical and structural differences. But even though our biosphere is characterized by vast diversity, a basic pattern of organization common to all cells does exist. This enables the student of biology to utilize experimental data derived from very disparate organisms, such as bacteria, hydras, amoebas, sea urchins, frogs, chicks, mice, and human beings.

The fundamental level of organization possessed by all living cells is a continuous molecular barrier, or cell membrane, that separates the interior of the cell from the immediate microenvironment. The two major classes of cells are distinguished by the nature of their intracellular environment.[14, 20, 24, 102] *Basically, all cells in our biosphere can be classified as either prokaryotic or eukaryotic.*

Prokaryotic Cells

Prokaryotic cells (*pro* = primitive, *karyon* = nucleus) are found in all bacteria and in blue-green algae. As their name indicates they have no membrane-limited subcellular organelles, e.g., nuclear envelope, mitochondria, Golgi apparatus, endoplasmic reticulum, lysosomes, and so forth.[29, 44, 58, 76, 94–97] The biologically active molecules are randomly dispersed throughout the cytoplasm.

The prokaryote *Escherichia coli* is one of the simplest bacteria and is so far the best understood. It is a normal inhabitant of the intestinal tract of man, is an aerobic organism as is man, is composed of the same classes of biologically significant molecules as man, and possesses molecules that function much as they function in man. It is fascinating that *Escherichia coli* evolved approximately 1.5 billion years *before* man. At present, the most reliable estimate of the age of the earth is 4.6 billion years, and *Escherichia coli* evolved some 3 to 3.5 billion years ago!

A remarkable discovery has been DNA recombinant technology.[13, 27, 58, 64, 105] For example, messenger ribonucleic acid (mRNA) for mammalian insulin has been physically isolated. The mRNA has been used to fabricate an artificial structural gene for insulin in a test tube (i.e., *in vitro*). The artificial gene for insulin has been inserted into the chromosome of *Escherichia coli* and this prokaryotic cell (e.g., a bacterium), then synthesized biologically active mammalian insulin.

Eukaryotic Cells

Unlike prokaryotic cells, eukaryotic cells contain conspicuous membrane-limited subcellular organelles throughout the cytoplasm (*eu* = true, *karyon* = nucleus). The organization of the eukaryotic cell as visualized with transmission electron microscopy and as studied by molecular biologists is exquisite in detail. Transmission electron photomicrographs shown in Figures 26–2 through 26–7 highlight the most distinctive characteristics of several mammalian cells. Table 26–1 compares the genetic apparatus of prokaryotic and eukaryotic cells.

Text continued on page 1752

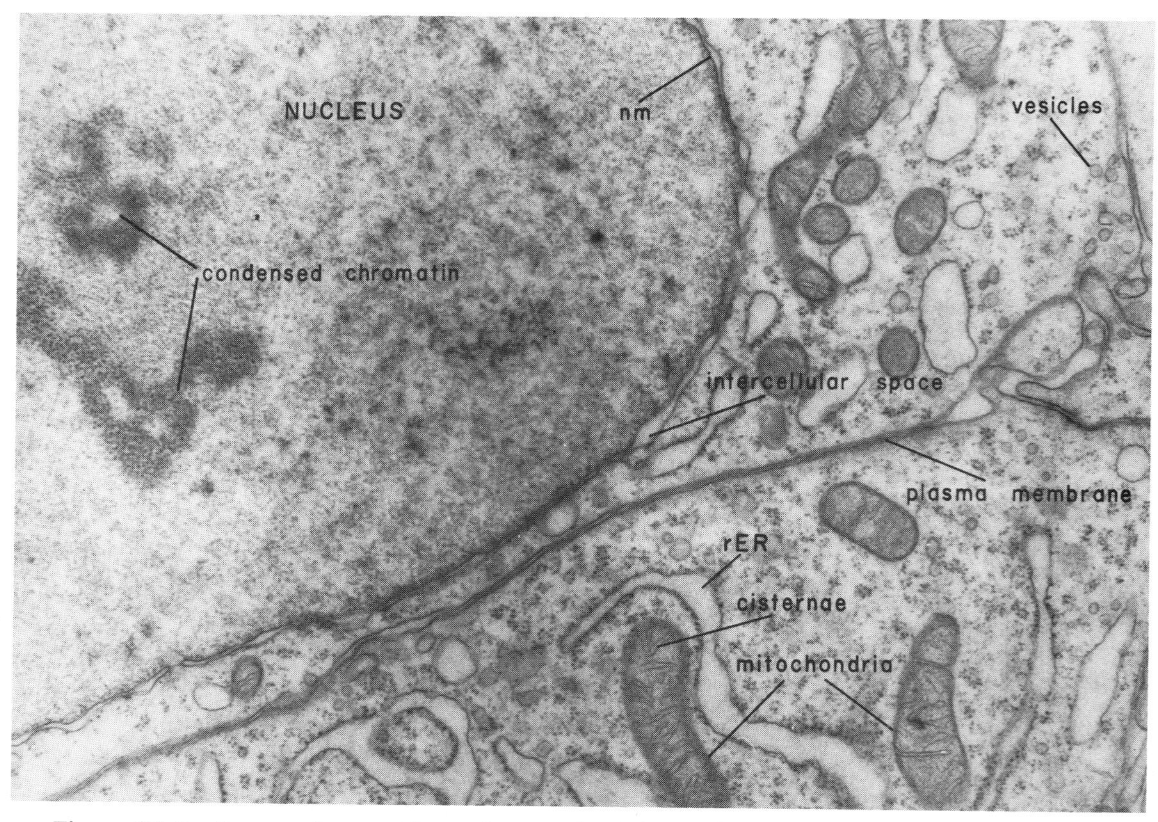

Figure 26–2. Survey electron photomicrograph of the nuclear region of embryonic inner enamel epithelial cells. Transcription of unique sequences of genes in the DNA results in transcripts (mRNAs), which are transported from the nucleus, through the nuclear membrane (nm) to the rough endoplasmic reticulum (rER).

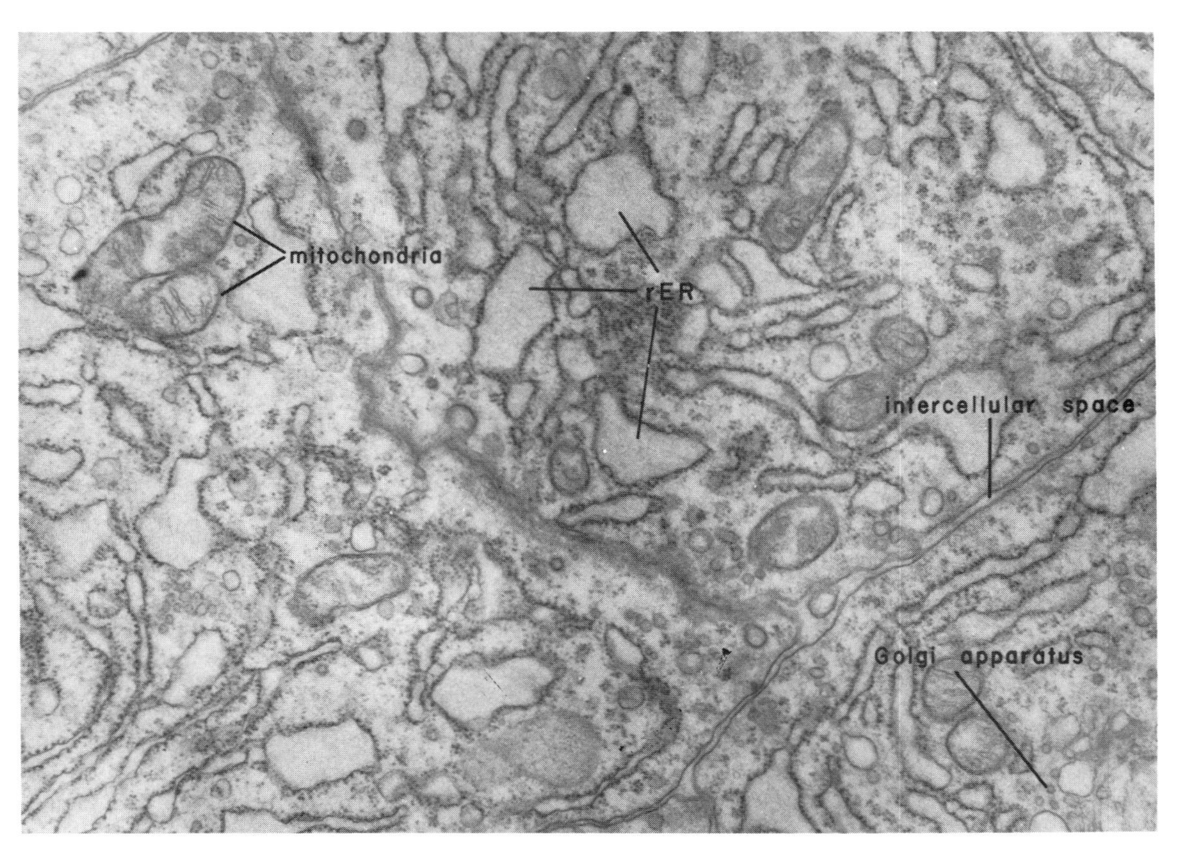

Figure 26–3. Survey electron photomicrograph of the subnuclear region of the cells shown in Figure 2 illustrating the intracellular organelles related to chemical energy production (i.e. oxidative phosphorylation producing ATP in the mitochondria), the polysomes associated with translation, and the Golgi apparatus in which newly synthesized proteins are glycosylated.

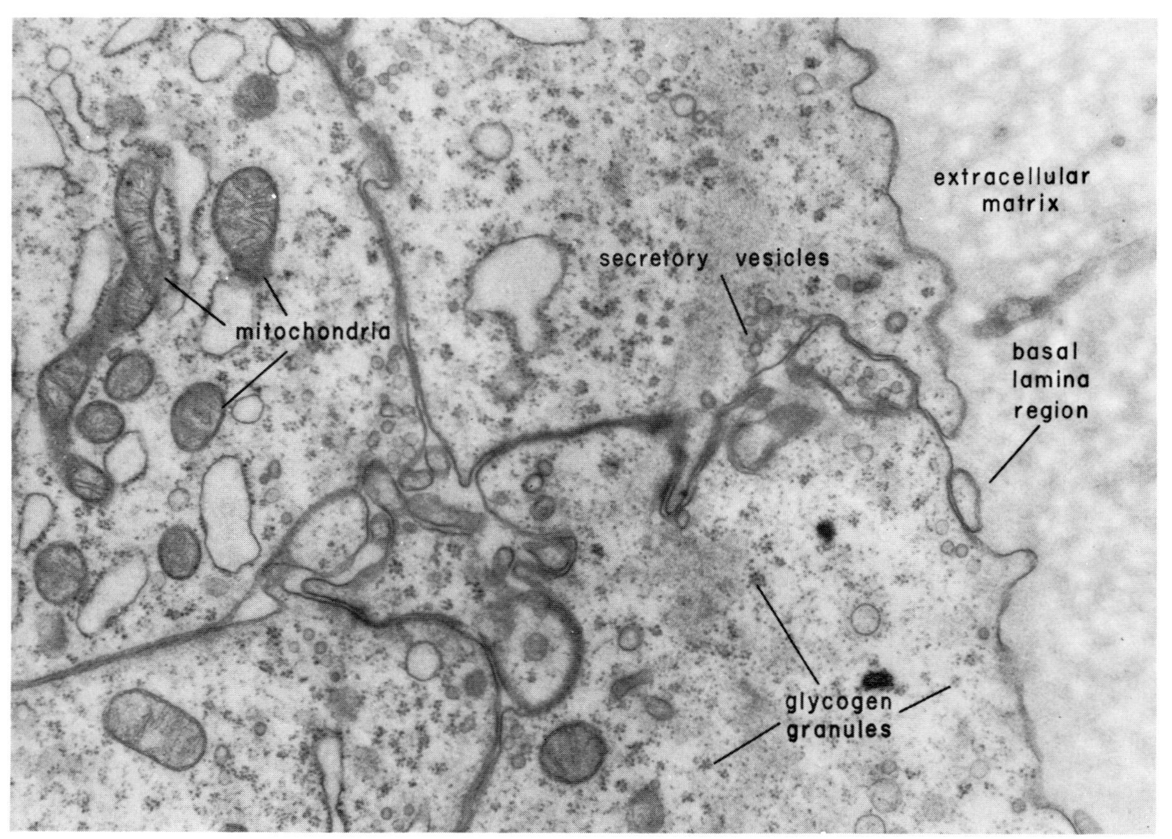

Figure 26–4. Survey electron photomicrograph illustrating the secretory region of the inner enamel epithelial cells. Glycosylated proteins are packaged in secretory vesicles derived from the Golgi and are transported toward the plasma membrane adjacent to the extracellular collagenous matrix.

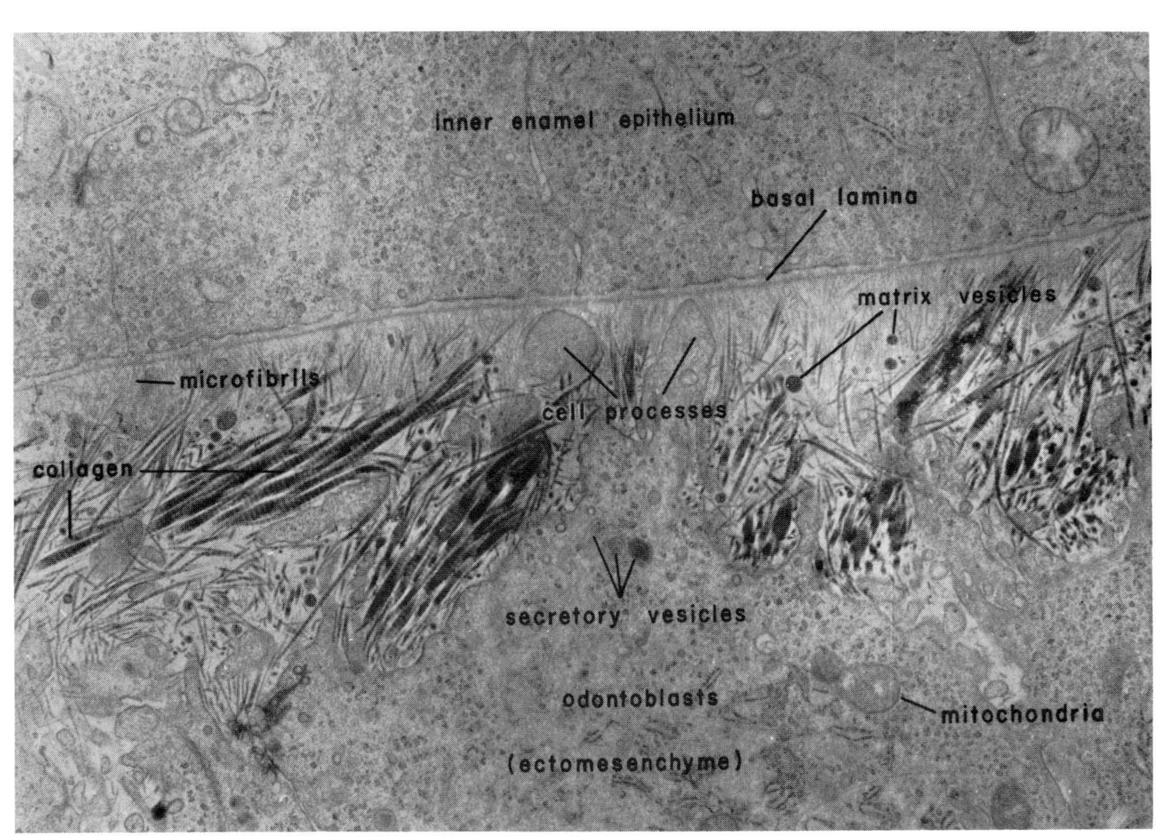

Figure 26–5. A series of interdependent interactions between ectodermally derived epithelium and cranial neural crest-derived mesenchyme result in tooth development characteristic of many epidermal organ systems in a connective tissue matrix interface between heterologous tissue interactants.

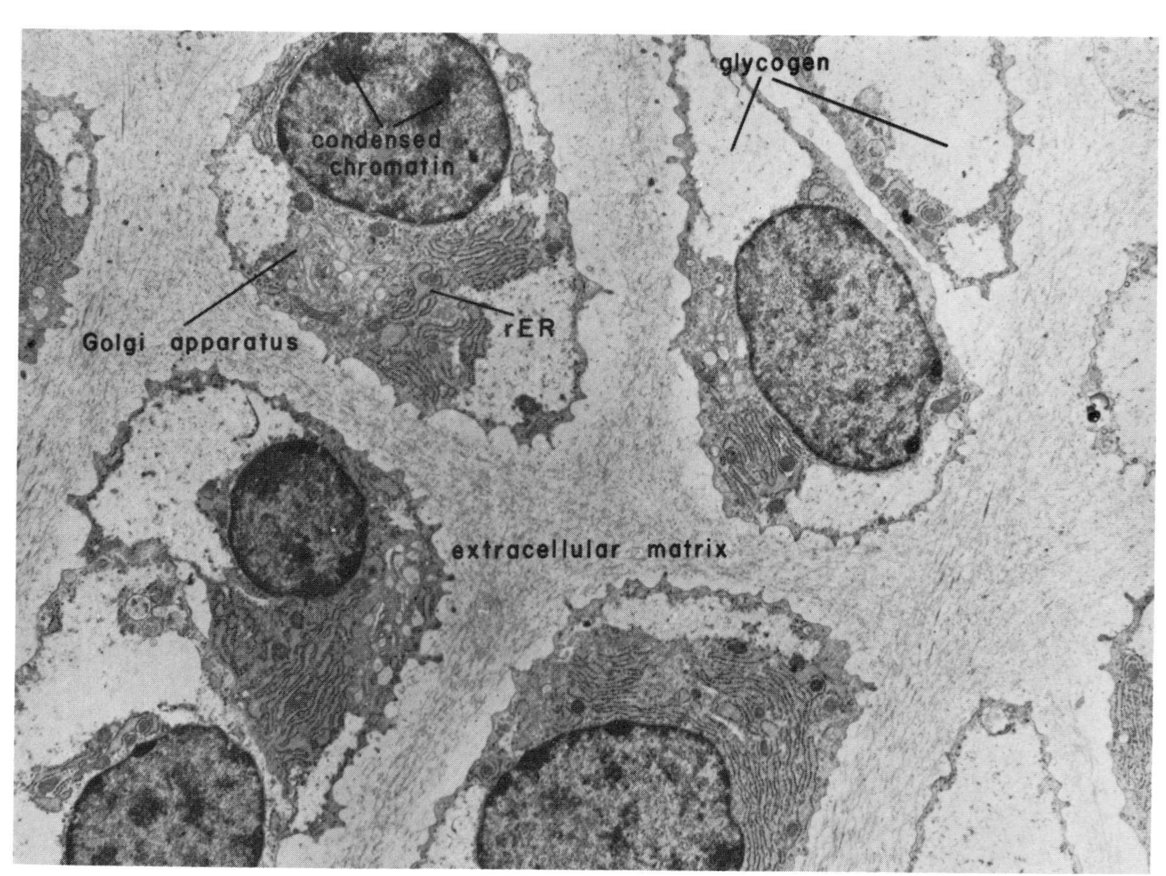

Figure 26–6. Cranial neural crest cells are the progenitors for many different cell types involved in craniofacial biology. Crest cells differentiate into Meckels' cartilage found in the developing mandible. The polygonal chondroblasts synthesize and secrete type II collagen [$\alpha(II)_3$], proteoglycans, hyaluronic acid, and other major constituents of the cartilaginous extracellular matrix.

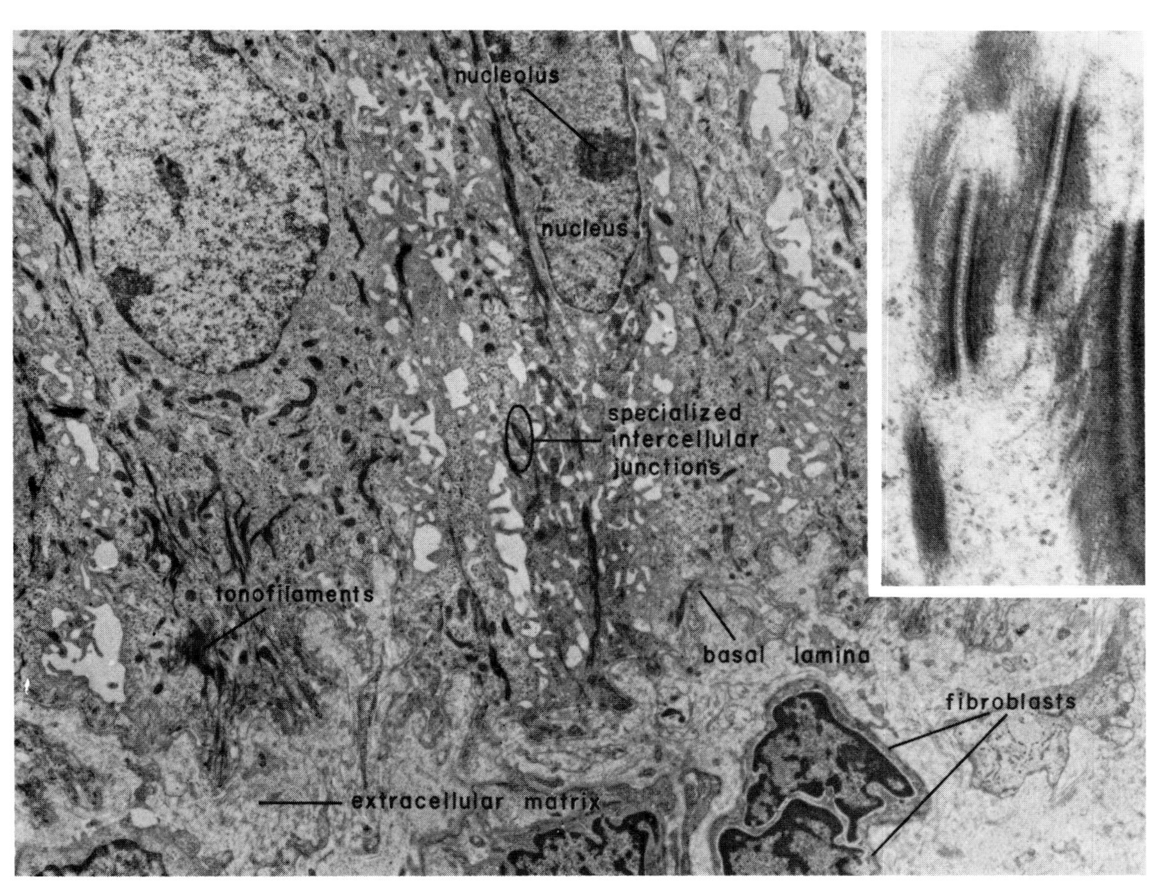

Figure 26–7. Survey electron photomicrograph of the gingival sulcus "non-keratinized" epithelium and adjacent connective tissue stroma. The insert illustrates the characteristics of the desmosome specialized intercellular junction found within the epithelia.

TABLE 26–1. Comparison of the Complexity of the Genetic Apparatus in Prokaryotic and Eukaryotic Cells

	Escherichia coli	*Human*
DNA		
	0.02×10^{-12} gm/cell	7×10^{-12} gm/cell
	Single copy of genes	Frequent, multiple, repeated gene sequences
PROTEIN		
		Histone (basic) protein 1 gm/gm DNA
	Small concentration of acidic protein	Nonhistone protein (acidic) 0.1 to 1.5 gm/gm DNA
RNA		
	Nascent mRNA	Up to 0.15 gm/gm DNA—nascent mRNA and other RNA types
GENE REGULATION		
	Discrete alterations with single stimulus	Simple stimuli generation; multiplicity of cascading effects

It is very important that we appreciate the differences between prokaryotes and animal cells, which are eukaryotes. All too often, we integrate microbial genetics with eukaryotic cell genetics and ignore the profound structural and functional differences that are so important in understanding the mechanisms that regulate developmental processes.

LEVELS OF BIOLOGIC REGULATION

Biologic regulation of human development ranges in scale from molecular interactions through cell and tissue reactions to human evolution.[2–6, 10, 13, 24–28, 52, 97, 114] It can be examined by means of x-ray diffraction, electron microscopy, and the wrong end of a telescope. This discussion highlights the significant advances of the last decade toward an understanding of the molecular biology of craniofacial development.

Gene Regulation of Biosynthesis

The human ovum contains a maternal inheritance that includes mitochondria, plasma membranes, numerous other subcellular organelles, and 23 chromosomes. The sperm contributes an additional 23 chromosomes that integrate with the maternal inheritance during fertilization to assemble into the *genotype* of the organism. The

TABLE 26-2. Genetic Information: Base Pairings of Nucleic Acid Biosynthesis*

DNA → DNA	*DNA → RNA*
A–T	A–U
G–C	G–C
C–G	C–G
T–A	T–A

*The gene is deoxyribonucleic acid (DNA). DNA contains information determined by the precise sequence of purine (adenosine [A] and guanine [G]) and pyrimidine (cytosine [C] and thymidine [T]) nucleotide bases in the gene. DNA forms the template from which other nucleic acid molecules of precise structure can be synthesized. The purine of the DNA chain will only base pair with the pyrimidine bases, and the pyrimidine of the DNA chain will only base pair with the purine bases. The obligatory base pairings are described in this table. The constraints of base pairing specificities allow specific genes to determine the nucleotide or base sequences in synthesized complementary molecules of DNA or RNA. Replication defines DNA-directed synthesis of complementary DNA molecules as during cell division in which the mother cell will produce two identical daughter cell progeny (DNA → DNA). The *transfer* of information from DNA to RNA involves no change of language (nucleotide → nucleotide) and is called *transcription*. *Translation* describes the transfer of information from RNA to a polypeptide (protein) and involves *new* language (nucleotide → amino acid).

inheritance of a human being is determined by information carried on these 23 pairs of chromosomes, which are estimated to contain 20,000 to 40,000 different gene pairs. Each subsequent division of the cell gives rise to additional daughter cells, each of which contains the genotype complement of deoxyribonucleic acid (DNA). Each cell in the forming embryo contain the identical quantity of DNA. The DNA in any individual somatic cell contains the complete genetic inheritance of the human race! The inherited genetic code is transcribed into specific messages in the form of ribonucleic acids: transfer RNA (tRNA), ribosomal RNA (rRNA), and messenger RNA (mRNA). Messenger RNA can then be translated into unique sequences of amino acids called proteins. Many of the proteins are enzymes that regulate highly specific organic reactions taking place within cells. The central point to remember is that all the basic instructions for the molecular composition of a human being come from the inherited DNA. (See Tables 26–2 and 26–3.)[2, 8, 12, 14–15, 24–29, 37, 38, 65, 76, 80]

TABLE 26-3. The Genetic Code: Example of the Biochemical Language*

DNA (Codons)	→	*RNA (Codons)*	→	*Amino Acids*
AAA		UUU		Phenylalanine
AAC		UUG		Leucine
GAA		CUU		Leucine
ACC		UGG		Tryptophan
GGT		CCA		Proline
CCG		GGC		Glycine

*The complementarity between DNA and the tRNA codons that are specific for amino acids is shown. Note that there are two or more codons for many of the amino acids, as indicated for leucine in the table.

If one reflects upon developmental biology, however, this information is but partially useful. What are the instructions that transform an egg into a frog, a chick, a mouse, or a man? What commands form, bilateral symmetry, integration of discrete organ systems, or vascularization throughout the embryo?

Some of the most fascinating questions in modern biology, and in clinical medicine and dentistry, concern the regulation of gene activity in differentiated cells. What causes genes to turn "on" and "off" in an orderly fashion during the precise temporal stages of embryogenesis? Once genes are "on," what determines how many copies of gene products are made? How many copies are made per unit of time and for how long? What causes a stem cell to differentiate into a mature, functional cell type or organism? Conversely, what changes lead to congenital malformations, neoplasia, or the failure of wounds to heal?

Understanding of three aspects of embryogenesis can help in integrating the findings of molecular biology with descriptive embryology. These are (1) the *synthesis* of molecules, (2) the *timing* of synthesis, and (3) the *localization* of individual cells and their intracellular synthetic activities. The role of DNA in protein biosynthesis has been well documented, but the functional significance of DNA in the processes of timing and of localization remains as yet obscure.[8, 10, 14, 20, 24, 28, 29, 38, 43, 44, 46, 52, 76, 103, 123, 124]

Several types of predictable gene regulation are found in higher organisms: (1) *quick* "on and off" synthesis of enzymes in response to hormonal stimuli; (2) *slow,* reversible differentiation of a quiescent tissue activity, as in the induction of lactation in the mammary gland; and (3) *stable,* highly differentiated, *restricted* response to environmental influences (as contrasted with the more numerous options available to an immature stem cell). Currently available evidence indicates that either (1) the inherited DNA is for the most part "off" or repressed, and discrete, unique sequences of DNA (individual cistrons or genes) become transcriptively active to participate in protein biosynthesis; or (2) the entire inherited DNA is essentially "on" or derepressed, and the intensity of specific sets of genes is amplified or increased in relation to the somewhat "dormant" activity of adjacent cistrons during differentiation, as a rheostat can transmit increasing levels of light.[10, 28, 29, 31, 37, 38, 43, 65, 76, 118]

Control of biosynthesis implies much more than control of gene expression. Which genes are transcribed and what are the processes by which DNA transcripts (messenger ribonucleic acids or mRNAs) are subsequently translated into unique proteins (*i.e.,* "one gene . . . one messenger RNA . . . one protein")? These are crucial questions. It is necessary as well as advantageous to describe and understand gene expression in terms of how individual genes are selectively transcribed within the nucleus and how the transcription products reach the cytoplasm and are translated into proteins.

Regulation at the Chromosomal Level

The DNA of animal cells is associated with basic proteins (histones) and acidic proteins (nonhistones) in specific units, the *chromosomes.* The chromosomes can be easily identified as discrete structures at metaphase, when transcription is minimal. They increase in size and then become morphologically diffuse during interphase, when most transcription occurs (Fig. 26–8).

All genetic mapping of mammalian cells is described in terms of chromosomal units, which presumably function in the intact cell or organism as a linear array of sequenced

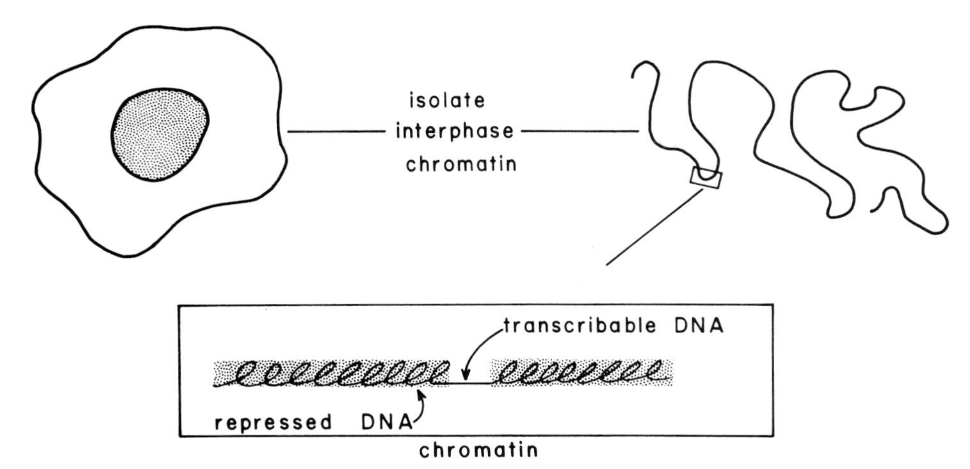

Figure 26–8. Illustrated model of chromatin indicating the condensed regions represented as a supercoil stabilized with basic proteins (histones) considered to be repressed DNA (a nucleosome). Also shown are the extended or transcriptively active regions. Gene derepression involves the synthesis of one or more species of RNA by transcription. Derepression is also related to physical displacement of histones and resulting conformational changes within chromatin.

genes. The exact spatial arrangement of the DNA in each chromosome is not yet clear. A chromosome consists of a fiber or strand of chromatin, called a chromatid, composed of a DNA double helix associated with basic and acidic proteins and believed to be about 30 Å thick. In addition to the chromatid fiber there is a structure that suggests supercoiled or condensed sections about 200 Å thick, and adjacent regions of extended chromatin. Although the matter is still controversial, it is believed that there is one chromatid per chromosome. The sum of the chromosomes (46 chromosomes in humans) contains the total genetic inheritance.

The structure of each gene is subject to variation. Variant genes within a specific locus is called *alleles.* Variations of chromosome content are introduced by recombination, in which genetic material is exchanged between homologous chromosomes in the course of the pairing that occurs during meiosis.

Chromosomes vary in biologic activity. Some are relatively repressed and appear to contain but a few transcriptively active genes. The Y chromosome in the male is an example, as is one of the two X chromosomes of the female. There are also position effects within and among chromosomes. In the process of *translocation,* a piece of one chromosome will break off and attach to another, causing whole segments to be inserted in new positions within the same chromosome or on another homologous or heterologous chromosome.[12, 24, 108] This is a possible mechanism of *mutation,* by which a unique sequence of genes from one chromosome is shifted into a different position on another chromosome. If the translocated sequence is attached to a functioning chromosome, it may become functional in the new site. On the other hand, if the translocated sequence is positioned in a new location, it can become inactive and may serve to repress the entire chromosome. The ability to predict the developmental significance of translocation during embryogenesis should be achieved in the next few years.

Whereas our recent attention can become focused upon the extraordinary advances being made in "genetic engineering," one should also fully appreciate the remarkable strides being taken toward understanding fundamental chromatin structure and function.[27, 28, 58, 64–65, 80, 94, 112, 115, 124] Traditionally, it has been generally assumed that gene structure and function in eukaryotic cells are regulated in the same way as in prokaryotes. Although early data suggested that this might be the case, many features of eukaryotic chromosomes seem today to be incompatible with procaryotic models of gene activity. A major "unsolved problem" is the acquisition of knowledge necessary to formulate an accurate representation of differential gene activity in human cells.

Both bacterial and eukaryotic chromosomes are based on a single DNA double helix. The total genome in eukcaryotic chromosomes is 100 to 1000 times larger than that found in *E. coli.* A variable amount of the DNA, on the order of 50 per cent, appears to consist of unique sequences of nucleotides that are present only once in the genome (Table 26–1). These unique sequences of nucleotides are assumed to represent structural genes. This implies an information content in a mammalian cell about 500 times greater than in *E. coli*, that is, the amount of information is equal to about 1 million genes coding for the proteins of 20,000 molecular weight.[27] The remainder of the DNA in mammalian cells consists of repetitive sequences of bases that occur in families, each containing some 10s or 100s of thousands of nonidentical but very similar members, the functions of repetitive classes of DNA are not fully understood.[29, 102, 103] Finally, whereas the *E. coli* chromosome consists essentially of naked and functional DNA, the mammalian chromosome contains at least as much permanently associated protein as DNA, histone, and nonhistone acidic proteins (Table 26–1).

It is now known that DNA synthesis and histone protein synthesis are both confined to the S phase of the cell's life cycle.[25] Functions of histones include the maintenance of chromatin structure as well as to repress DNA-dependent RNA synthesis. It was tentatively suggested that DNA to histone ratios might vary as a function of transcription, histone concentrations might be reduced in areas of high DNA-dependent RNA synthesis. This is not the case. In fact, the DNA to histone ratio is constant in tissues actively synthesizing RNA as well as in tissues containing condensed chromatin not synthesizing RNA. Since early 1977, a fascinating and new model of chromatin structure has emerged that partially explains a great deal of often perplexing information — the *nucleosome.*[58]

The structure of chromatin is based upon a repeat unit, termed *the nucleosome,* which consists of a set of eight histone molecules complexed with about 200 base pairs of DNA.[58] The set of eight histones consists of two each of the four types of histones (H2A, H2B, H3 and H4). In addition, a fifth histone, H1, is found associated with most but not all nucleosomes. The DNA component of the nucleosome is made of a *core* region of 140 base pairs and a *linker* region of 15 to 100 base pairs, dependent upon cell type. In three dimensions, the DNA is wrapped in some as yet undetermined manner *around* the set of eight histones, forming a spherical particle visualized at 100 Å in diameter. These nucleosome particles lie in close apposition along the entire length of a chromatin fiber, including yeast and mice and human chromatin. X-ray diffraction studies, transmission electron microscopy, enzyme studies, hydrodynamic measurements and, perhaps the most compelling evidence, actual isolation and crystallization of the nucleosome have all provided consistent evidence.[58] The existence of nucleosomes is now firmly established. Although not as yet unequivocal, the nucleosome would appear to be the smallest structural unit with chromatin.

The "search" for molecules with the capacity for regulation of specific genes in eukaryotic chromatin continues.[12] Variations in gene expression occur throughout the cell cycle, however, the most pronounced differences in transcription are observed between the S phase (the period of DNA synthesis) and mitosis.[10, 27, 28, 115] One intriguing possibility are the nonhistone acidic proteins as specific gene regulators. These proteins range from 10,000 to 150,000 molecular weight and exhibit significant structural and possibly functional heterogeneity. These proteins may themselves provide differential gene regulation as a function of their size, charge, or rates of synthesis or possibly serve as chromatin "receptors" for epigenetic factors such as steroid-receptor complexes to enhance or amplify DNA-dependent RNA synthesis.

It is known that DNA configuration is not altered by histone binding, whereas major DNA conformational alterations can be caused by polyanionic molecules such as nonhistone proteins or chromosomal RNAS. Perhaps the result of interactions between polyanionic molecules and a particular nucleosome might be to provide an approach for an RNA polymerase molecule to a now accessible region of chromatin, the search continues.

Finally, recent advances in molecular biology now indicate that the process of transcription is even more complex than previously anticipated. The central dogma of molecular biology had repeatedly indicated that DNA → RNA → protein; "one gene → one protein." It was assumed that a continuous sequence of nucleotides within DNA "encoded" the inherited information (i.e., structural gene) for a specific gene product (Table 26–2). In the last three years (1977–1980) the details of this process have proved to be much more complex than initially assumed because of the unexpected discovery that unique structural genes in eukaryotes are encoded as *discontinuous genes* within DNA rather than as continuous nucleotide sequences as originally assumed.[64] Current evidence suggests that many mammalian "genes" are arranged in the DNA in at least two discontinuous nucleotide sequences per "gene" separated from one another by interrupting segments of DNA termed *intervening nucleotide sequences*. One obvious "unsolved problem" is how this interrupted genetic information is processed into a functional mRNA and subsequently translated into the specific gene product. It is postulated, that some of these intervening sequences (e.g., those associated with beta-globin genes) are transcribed into hnRNA in the nucleus and then excised at a subsequent step prior to leaving the nucleus as a functional mRNA for globin. It is assumed that very precise nucleases cleave out segments of the entire nucleotide sequence found in the hnRNA. Following cleavage, the functional nucleotide sequences characteristic of the gene product are "spliced together" so that the triplet codons at either end of the excision will then join in exact phase for translation. Why "discontinuous genes?" One suggestion has been that *discontinuous genes* provide a plausible mechanism for exceedingly rare mutations to occur through evolution in a relatively short period of time.[46]

Regulation at the Cytoplasmic Level

Mitochondria are maternal inheritances, as are unique "masked messenger RNAs," certain cytoplasmic receptors for hormones, and many of the subcellular organelles contained within the ovum.[20, 24] In experiments with frogs, nuclei have been isolated from highly differentiated cells and transplanted into unfertilized ova, and a functioning frog has repeatedly been produced by such experimentation.[43] The maternally inherited cytoplasmic constituents regulate the heterologous nuclei to express gene activities analogous to those associated with normal frog embryogenesis. Somatic cell hybridization experiments have also indicated that heterologous nuclei will function in cells that have been enucleated. Regulation over gene expression at the cytoplasmic level is now well appreciated and has been found to influence transcription and translation, as well as secretion of proteins.[15, 33]

Regulation at the Cellular Level

It is impossible to do more than mention the enormous number of available examples of regulation at the cellular level. Cell division and the morphologic characteristics acquired by cells are mediated by small, relatively ubiquitous molecules such as adenosine 3′:5′-cyclic phosphate (cyclic AMP), hormones, simple ions (calcium, potassium, sodium, magnesium, and so forth), physical qualities of the microenvironment (temperature, pH, osmolarity), and the density of cell populations.[5, 6, 25, 31, 48–52, 66, 68, 82, 85]

Regulation at the Multicellular Level

One of the fascinating and significant properties of metazoan (*i.e.,* multicellular) organisms is the organization of cells into cell types and the formation of derived tissue

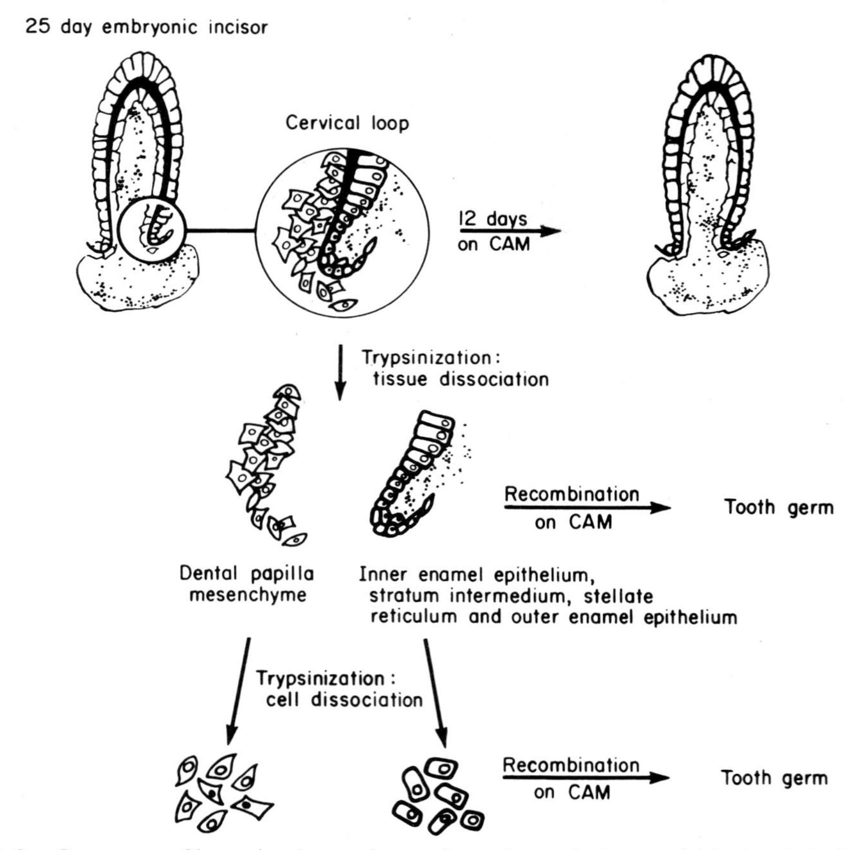

Figure 26–9. Summary of investigations using embryonic tooth tissues which clearly indicate that both tissues are required for morphogenesis. Reciprocal epithelial-mesenchymal interactions are required for tooth morphogenesis. Moreover, the mesenchyme tissue contains organ-specific instructions. Dental papilla mesenchyme determines tooth shape and form (44).

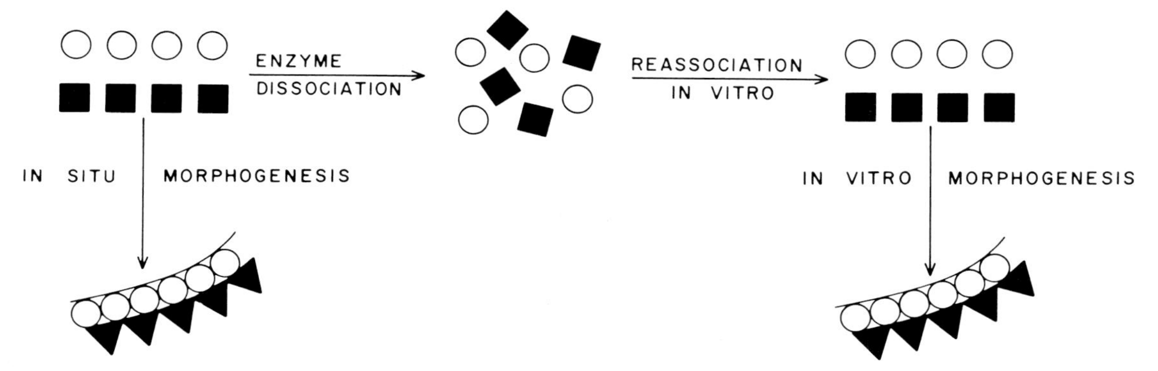

Figure 26–10. Diagram of heterotypic cell re-association experiments. Various organ systems consist of two different types of tissues (e.g. epithelium and mesenchyme). Organ fragments can be dissociated into cell suspensions. Under suitable environmental conditions, the isolated cells re-synthesize their respective cell surface ligands, recognize "self" and "non-self," and interact to form new tissue and subsequently organ reconstructions.

types that interact to form organs. Organogenesis occurs when two embryologically different tissue types interact to form a specific organ, *e.g.,* epithelial-mesenchymal interactions lead to development of teeth (Fig. 26–9), and development of the pancreas, salivary glands, skin, and mammary glands. Organs have been experimentally dissociated into tissue types, and in turn, tissues have been dissociated into cell suspensions. In suitable artificial tissue culture environments, the individual cells resynthesize their phenotypic surface molecules, recognize "self" (homotypic) and "nonself" (heterotypic), and reassociate to form functioning tissues (Fig. 26–10) and organs demonstrating characteristic cytology. The reader is encouraged to explore selected references for an increased appreciation of cell and tissue interactions related to morphogenesis.[7, 11, 16, 26, 45, 49, 50, 52, 55–57, 62, 79, 81, 91, 93, 95–99, 104, 107, 120, 121, 123]

It is by no means clear how presently known molecular events can explain all these phenomena. As one examines the published literature, moving from the molecular biology of prokaryotic cells to the biologic level of cell, tissue, and organ interactions within complex mammalian embryos, information becomes less precise and, all too often, unavailable.

GENE EXPRESSION: TRANSCRIPTION AND TRANSLATION

Transcription

It is now possible to describe organizational levels and important functional attributes of chromatin (Table 26–4). Chromatin consists of DNA, histones, nonhistone proteins, and RNA in the proportions of 1 to 1 to 0.5 to 0.05.[94, 115] The ratio of DNA to histone does not appear to vary from cell to cell in the same species.[115] The process by which cells synthesize new DNA is called *replication.* Cells must synthesize DNA if they are to divide and give rise to two daughter cells, each of which must contain as much

TABLE 26-4. The Criteria and Results Which Clearly Indicate That Human Chromatin Contains Both Structural and Functional Heterogeneity*

1. Limited transcription as measured by RNA–DNA hybridization methods.
2. Template activity is less than isolated DNA to an extreme extent.
3. Circular dichroism spectrum comparisons of chromatin, DNA, sheared DNA, and BrdU-substituted DNA indicate two or more conformations of DNA.
4. Transmission electron microscopic observations indicate variable widths: thicker (100 to 200 Å) and thinner (30 to 50 Å) strands or fibers.
5. Thermal denaturation profiles indicate that DNA has several conformations dependent upon the association of proteins. Basic proteins associated with nucleic acids stabilize DNA and repress gene transcription.

*Generalizations stated in this table were formulated from recent evidence.[12, 29, 38, 124]

DNA as the original single cell. DNA is replicated during the S phase of cell generation. New histones are synthesized in the cytoplasm; they move to the nucleus, complexing with the nascent DNA to form chromatin for the daughter cells. Researchers find it quite significant that the nonhistone, acidic proteins occur in a broad range of proportions in different tissues and organs (many are tissue-specific and can be used to identify, or "fingerprint," tissue).

The inherited DNA contains several types of regions. First, there are regions of structural genes for proteins, for example polypeptide chains that comprise phosphoproteins of collagen, bone and dentine, proline hydroxylase, lysyl oxidase, and so forth. These structural genes are believed to be represented once or possibly twice in each haploid set (23 chromosomes) of DNA.[29, 59] Structural regions are believed to be unique, nonrepetitive sequences, but the genes that code for histone proteins are a rare exception to this generality. The histone genes are repeated as often as a thousand times in the DNA. The second type of region within DNA consists of those genes that code for tRNAs and rRNAs. These genes are repetitive, redundant sequences of nucleotides that form a small percentage of the total DNA. The rRNA genes are condensed in the nucleolar region, whereas the tRNA genes are associated with chromatin dispersed throughout the nucleus. The third type of region consists of highly repetitious gene sequences, which are generally very short and are relatively comparable. The molecular weight and the nucleotide base composition of these sequences suggest that they do not code for meaningful peptides and are probably never transcribed or translated.[10, 12, 14, 34, 58, 94, 115]

Properties Unique to Eukaryotic Cells

The properties unique to the organization of eukaryotic genetic material should be summarized. The DNA of eukaryotic cells (1) is organelle-restricted and is generally found in the nucleus, although small amounts are also contained within the mitochondria, (2) contains many redundant nucleotide sequences, and (3) is closely associated with a large number of both basic and acidic proteins. The DNA in eukaryotic cells is also unique in that *most of the DNA is never transcribed* but is permanently repressed or "off." It is assumed that histones "insulate" the genes from being activated and transcribed. Nonhistone (acidic) proteins may participate in the actual regulation of specific genes.

Briefly consider the highlights of transcription. In eukaryotic cells, genes are transcribed into rapidly labeled RNAs that are degraded before they ever leave the nucleus.[28, 94] These *heterogeneous nuclear RNAs* (HnRNAs) are extremely large — much too large to code for proteins of normal size.[8, 60, 65] The pool of very large RNAs also contains the mRNAs. Recent data have disclosed that the nuclear mRNAs contain a polyadenylate-rich sequence of 120 polynucleotides.[28] The poly A sequence is not found in tRNAs or rRNAs. The heterogeneity of rapidly labeled HnRNAs and the specificity of the mRNA poly A sequences suggest several additional sites for the regulation of transcription and translation. Specific nucleases may serve to regulate what leaves the nucleus.[115] Certain classes of mRNAs might be affected, and such regulations could also be cell-type specific and time-dependent, perhaps playing a critical role during embryogenesis.[28]

Recently, researchers have proposed models for the mechanisms by which unique sequences of polynucleotides (i.e., genes) are activated, transcribed, and then translated. The diagram in Figure 26–11 illustrates genes for mRNA, tRNA, and rRNA being transcribed and translated. In "native" chromatin, the genes are obviously not arranged in the manner illustrated; the diagram conveys only the essential steps of a complex series of biochemical processes. Many of these steps are now considered to be rate-limiting sites for regulation.[24] Also, one must not forget the possibilities for control at the level of DNA replication associated with cell division.[31]

Transcription (DNA → RNA) results in synthesis of the primary gene product. It is known, for example, that in the case of ribosomal RNA (rRNA), the primary gene product (the transcript) is much larger than the functional rRNA in the cytoplasm; the rRNA is step-wise degraded in the nucleus into fragments, which eventually recombine in the cytoplasm. The total processing requires about an hour. It is also important to note that the RNAs discussed in this context are associated with proteins and are actually ribonucleoproteins that exist as discrete particles that can be visualized as ribosomes or polysomes (Tables 26–3 and 26–4).

Processing of tRNA appears to involve a comparable sequence of events, i.e., larger tRNAs are degraded to smaller functional isoaccepting tRNA molecules involved with the transport of specific amino acids to the site of translation associated with the ribosomes in the cytoplasm. Nucleotide base modifications are essential in controlling rRNA and tRNA transcription, processing, and function, with specific enzymes being required.

Translation of Genes

Several salient steps of translation take place in the cytoplasm of the animal cell. The mRNA, in concert with protein factors and trinucleotides, combines with the 40S ribosomal subunit.[14, 28, 30, 60] It has been suggested that this recognition site is an important regulatory position for the control of gene expression in animal cells. The specific recognition of certain messages representing structural genes could serve as either positive or negative regulation, i.e., for amplification of translation or for inhibition. In the cytoplasm, amino acids are added to the transfer RNA by tRNA-specific synthetases and, with the addition of protein factors and energy, the process of translation proceeds: that is, essential or nonessential amino acids are sequenced to determine the physical and chemical properties of the resulting protein molecules. Regulation of cell differentiation

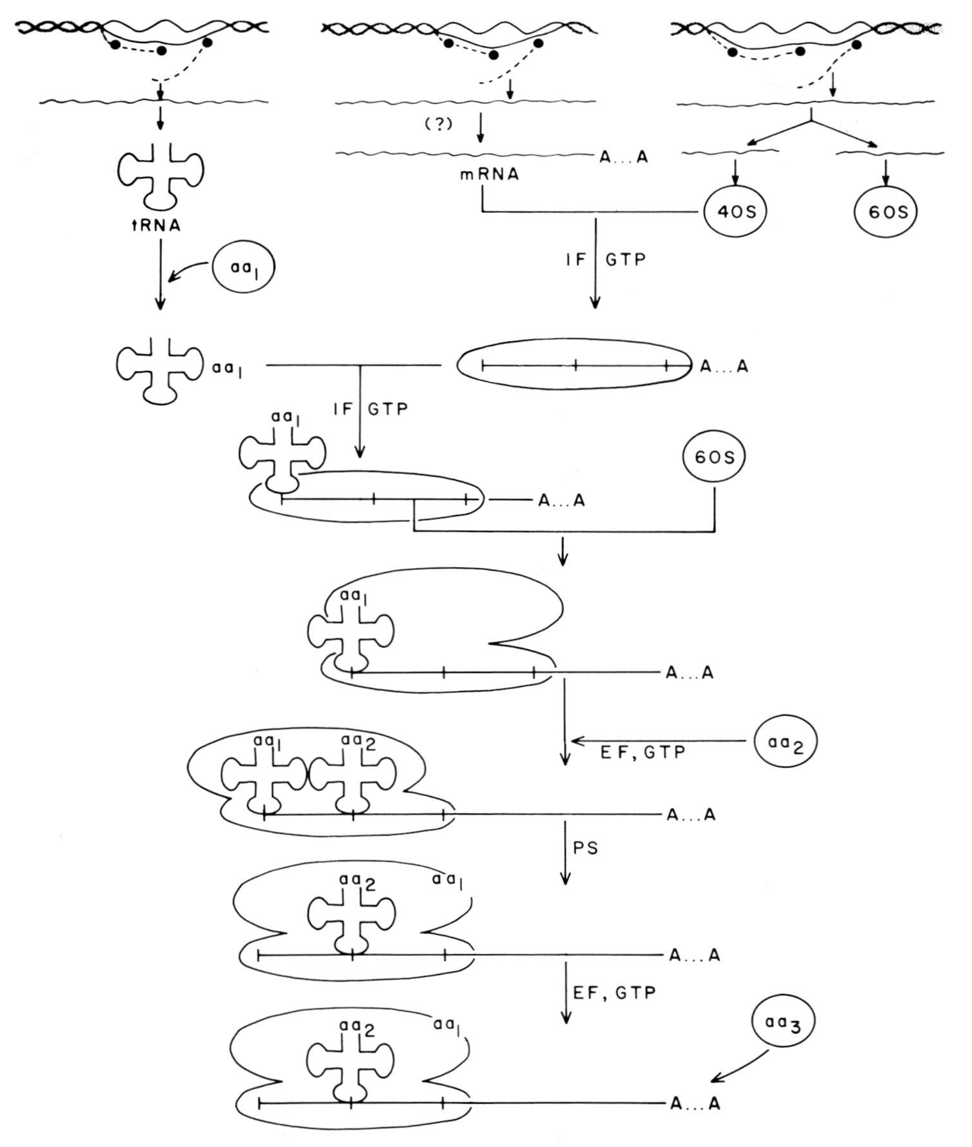

Figure 26–11. Diagrammatic representation of the sequential events in transcription and translation. Transcription of three cistrons (genes) are indicated for transfer RNA (tRNA), messenger RNA (mRNA) and ribosomal RNAs (rRNA). The diagram illustrates the subsequent fate of each nascent gene product as it leaves the nucleus and collectively interacts as an element in mRNA translation along with several cytoplasmic factors as shown. DNA, DNA, and DNA represent genes coding for tRNA, mRNA and rRNAs, respectively. Not indicated in this diagram are the complex mechanisms by which discrete regions of the DNA (i.e. the total inherited genotype of the organism) are initially activated and then become transcriptively active regions of the DNA. Therefore, following gene activation and gene de-repression, RNA polymerase (0--0---) is involved in the nascent synthesis of the various RNA molecules during transcription. Individual amino acids are indicated as aa_1, aa_2, and aa_3. The transcript mRNA is adenylated with an appreciable extension of polyadenylic acids (up to 120 nucleotides) (A . . . A). IF, initiation factors: GTP, guanosine triphosphate; EF, elongation factors; PS, peptidyl synthetase. The small and large ribosomal RNA subunits are shown as 18S and 28S, respectively. The 40S and 60S are the small and large ribosomal subunits associated with ribosomal proteins *per se.* This diagram is a composite of research in eukaryotic protein biochemistry which required almost 25 years of active research to acquire from the scientists throughout the world.

may also reside at the level of tRNA specificities. It is notable that in differentiated cells such as erythrocytes, the pattern of tRNAs is modulated to reflect the requirements of certain tRNAs for translation of specific codons, as in the message for hemoglobin.[60] Since the genetic code for tRNAs is redundant, there is more than one tRNA codon for each amino acid, and thus it is possible that a codon may occur which is recognized only by a minor group of the total tRNA pool. By regulating the level of that specific tRNA, one could regulate the rate of peptide chain synthesis at this limiting point along the message. This regulation could, for example, exert profound influence toward asymmetry in the forming face (Table 26–4).

When the completed protein chain is separating from the codon, termination must occur in response to other protein factors. Therefore, termination of polypeptide chain synthesis is quite a significant point of regulation. Cyclic AMP, small hormones, specifications, or drugs (i.e., teratogens) could enhance or retard the release of incomplete polypeptide chains, creating significant qualitative alterations in craniofacial development during embryogenesis. Another level of control is at the point of the functional expression of translation: the completed protein. Protein folding probably occurs at the time that synthesis is completed. Proteins in animal cells have finite decay rates that vary from minutes to days. Protein folding, protein to protein interactions, post-translational modifications of newly synthesized proteins (e.g., glycosylation, phosphorylation, sulfation), and hormonal alterations of the limiting membranes around lysosomes (e.g., subcellular organelles containing proteolytic enzymes) could each influence the fidelity of translation and the rates of protein degradation.[104]

CONGENITAL MALFORMATIONS

Chromosomal Aberrations

Until approximately twenty years ago, it was not recognized that chromosomal aberrations could be responsible for congenital anomalies in humans. During this notably short time, the fields of pediatrics, hematology, genetics, biochemistry, and developmental biology have converged to produce new knowledge.[34, 40, 41, 75, 77, 80, 81, 108] Although it is now possible to conduct sophisticated biochemical experiments using tissue-culture simulations of human organs, much of our information has been derived from studies of abnormal people and from increasingly refined clinical techniques.[7, 17, 21, 34, 36, 39, 40–42, 47, 59, 69, 70–74, 86, 89, 92, 100, 106, 110, 114]

Generally, the new knowledge has evolved from the following steps: (1) a new investigational technique is discovered; (2) the technique is applied to human malformations; (3) one or more causes of specific malformations are illuminated through the use of the technique; (4) the information is applied clinically to provide more accurate diagnosis and treatment of the malformation; and (5) the frequency of the malformation is reduced.[47]

In human beings, meiosis results in the formation of the gametes. The primordial germ cells contain two sets of 23 chromosomes (46 chromosomes in all), one set inherited from each parent. Except for the XY sex pair in males, each member of a set has its homologue in the other set. The second meiotic division achieves the formation of cells each containing a single set of single-stranded chromosomes. At fertilization, two cells fuse to form a zygote in which the diploid number of chromosomes characteristic of the species is restored.

Human chromosomes are usually studied during the metaphase period of cell division (mitosis). Recent advances in cytogenetics have made it possible to visualize homologous pairs of human chromosomes and arrange them according to size to make a display called a *karyotype.* Each metaphase chromosome consists of a pair of chromatids held together at the centromere. The position of the centromere in relation to the center of the chromosomes indicates morphologic variance (e.g., metacentric, submetacentric, acrocentric, or telocentric). Every chromosome in a normal set can readily be assigned to one of seven groups, labeled A to G in order of decreasing size. The normal karyotype for humans indicates a pattern and a specific number of chromosomal pairs in each of the seven groups. Variations in number of chromosomes per group (additions or deletions), additional morphologic modifications of the chromosomes (e.g., satellite structures or bodies), and varying rates of formation during mitosis can be used to characterize normal and abnormal craniofacial development. For example, the chromosomes of a significant percentage of patients with Down's syndrome possess an unbalanced translocation with extra G material.[40–43, 102, 110, 117]

Down's syndrome is a major example of autosomal trisomy that probably results from meiotic nonsegregation (i.e., an abnormal gametal distribution of homologous chromosomes). It is a relatively common malformation that occurs in about 1 of 660 live neonates. Although the syndrome was first described in 1866 by J. L. H. Down, it was only after the advent of human karyotyping (about 1956 to 1959) that a chromosomal abnormality was found to be involved. The condition is too well known to require an extensive description.[102]

Table 26–5 shows several of the more common clinical signs associated with Down's syndrome. The incidence of this autosomal trisomy does not vary among racial groups, yet maternal age has a critical influence on the frequency of the syndrome. Whereas the disorder occurs in 1 of 1000 infants born to women aged 30 to 32, it occurs in 1 of 300 children born to women aged 35 to 37, 1 of 100 born to mothers aged 40 to 44, and 1 of 50 born to women aged 45 and older. Many of the most serious congenital anomalies that are manifested in the craniofacial complex follow a similar pattern.[21, 22, 54, 74, 89]

Malformations represent a broad spectrum of phenotypic variations resulting from a diversity of inborn or environmental mechanisms affecting human embryogenesis. During a specific time in morphogenesis, a single event can irreversibly alter development, yet not be followed by secondary effects (Table 26–6). Such a situation would not usually be associated with a single gene factor but rather would be multifactorial: the result of multiple abnormal factors associated with genes and with the environment.

TABLE 26–5. Major Clinical Signs Appearing in More Than 50 Per Cent of Patients with Down's Syndrome

Mental retardation	Prominent ears
Slanting eyes	Small teeth
Hyperextensible joints	Curved fifth finger
Flat occiput	Short, broad hands
Red cheeks	High-arched palate
Flat nose bridge	Narrow palate
Small nose	Fissured lips

TABLE 26–6. Selected Examples of Human Disorders in Which a Deficient Activity of a Specific Protein Has Been Demonstrated

Human Disorder	*Abnormal Protein*
Ateliotic dwarfism	Growth hormone
Childhood diabetes	Insulin
Analbuminemia	Albumin
Classic hemophilia (type A)	Factor VIII (antihemophilic factor)
Albinism	Tyrosinase
Tay-Sachs disease	Hexosaminidase A
Phenylketonuria	Phenylalanine hydroxylase
Immunoglobulin-deficiency diseases	Immunoglobulins
Gout	Hypoxanthine–guanine phosphoribosyl
Vitamin D–resistant rickets	Cholecalciferase[a]

[a]Specific assays not performed.

Conversely, the presence of a single defective gene could cause a multitude of malformations that would sequentially affect morphogenesis in a variety of tissues at different critical times. An example would be Tay-Sachs disease, which is caused by a single gene defect that produces abnormal lipid accumulation in neurons, deterioration of motor function, mental retardation, seizures, and death. Many aspects of Down's syndrome also suggest that only a few genes are responsible for the numerous abnormalities that are observed (Table 26–7).

Polygenic Effects

Studies of genetic mutations and aberrations in animals have been useful tools for proving the mechanisms by which development and differentiation are regulated.[49] However, the most sophisticated models of genetic regulation came from studies using prokaryotic cells and viruses. In the chromosomes of eukaryotic cells, the genes exhibit positional effects; the phenotypes of individuals heterozygous for two mutant genes differ when the two mutations are located on the same chromosome and when they are on different homologues. The intricate mechanisms regulating the organization and sequential regularity of the complex series of processes involved in craniofacial morphogenesis offer a staggering puzzle to the biologist studying craniofacial development.

What controls the order of events during cell division? What limits the blastula and initiates gastrulation? What mediates the initiation of organogenesis throughout the embryo after gastrulation? What influences the spatial and temporal "sense" of homologous and heterologous cell populations? Obviously single genes or constellations of genes are operant throughout these critical phases of craniofacial development.

Many craniofacial anomalies are congenital malformations representing a broad spectrum of phenotypic variations resulting from diverse etiologic mechanisms.[7, 21, 34, 40–42, 48, 57, 61, 83, 84, 87, 109, 111, 113, 125] Skeletal defects of the craniofacial complex can be caused by single-gene defects or by intermittent or multifactorial developmental processes, or they can occur as part of a chromosomal anomaly syndrome.[90, 102]

The etiology of most congenital craniofacial malformations is as yet unknown. The major indications that genetic factors are involved are derived from pedigree (family)

TABLE 26–7. Examples of Inherited* Congenital Anomalies in Humans That Involve Severe Craniofacial Malformations

Congenital Anomaly	*Clinical Characteristics*	*Biochemical Defects*	*Genetic Pattern*
Ehlers-Danlos Syndrome	Moderate bone malformations; no mental retardation; extreme hyperelasticity and fragility of skin; hyperextensibility of joints; ectopia lentis (micro-hemorrhages of retina); rupture of aorta and large arteries.	No detectable Type III collagen synthesis and secretion; possibly defect in collagen cross-linking mechanism (e.g., lysyl oxidase).	Autosomal dominant
Hunter's Syndrome (Mucopolysaccharidosis II)[a]	Marked skeletal deformities with "gargoyle-like" facial appearance; moderate mental retardation; dwarfism; deafness; no corneal opacity.	Dermatan and heparan sulfate excesses in urine	X-linked recessive
Hurler's Syndrome (Mucopolysaccharidosis I)[a]	Major skeletal deformities with large head and prominent ridge along the sagittal suture, hypertelorism, thick lips; large tongue; diastemas with peg-shaped teeth; hypertrophic gingiva; severe mental retardation; corneal opacities; hyperostosis; "boot-shaped" sella turcica.	Dermatan and heparan sulfate excesses in urine; decreased β-galactosidase in tissues.	Autosomal recessive
Marfan Syndrome	Excessive length of long bones (dolichostenomelia); arachnodactyly; long, narrow face (i.e., "El Greco painting"); highly arched palate; joint weaknesses; no mental retardation; prognathism.	Defect in elastin and collagen cross-linking.	Autosomal dominant
Morquio's Syndrome (Mucopolysaccharidosis IV)[a]	Severe skeletal deformities with prominent maxilla; broad mouth; short nose; diastemas; defective enamel; corneal opacities; no mental retardation.	Excess keratan sulfate, chondroitin 4/6 sulfates in urine and in tissues.	Autosomal recessive

*The methods for distinguishing separate genetic entities include demonstration of different modes of inheritance or different linkage relationships and the study of offspring produced by the marriage of two persons with a recessively inherited disorder. Further, it becomes quite evident that heterogeneity of genetic diseases is a corollary of the axiom that the phenotype is not an indication of the genotype.

[a]The current terminology for "mucopolysaccharidosis" has been revised. Acid mucopolysaccharides are now called glycosaminoglycans (GAG) and include hyaluronic acid, chondroitin, chondroitin 4-sulfate, chondroitin 6-sulfate, dermatan sulfate, heparan sulfate, and heparin.

studies, but these must be applied cautiously, because socioeconomic traits are often superimposed on genetic predispositions. Classic mendelian single-factor analyses often prove frustrating to the population geneticist. Recently, theories of polygenic causation have been advanced. A "multifactorial etiology" assumes that genetic factors and environment exert interdependent influences upon morphogenesis at crucial stages in the development of the human embryo. For example, the various intramembranous flat bones that form the skull are not yet fused at birth. The age at which the sutures close varies. Premature ossification of the sutures of the skull, or craniostenosis, causes gross aberrations of growth. Does hyaluronic acid normally prevent or retard mineralization in connective tissue matrices? If so, the hyaluronic acid has perhaps been degraded too soon, inducing a complex process of collagen synthesis and formation of matrix vesicles, thereby causing the premature ossification of the fontanelles.

In Apert's syndrome, or acrocephalosyndactyly, pronounced underdevelopment of the midfacial region, a brachycephalic head with a high, prominent forehead, mental retardation, ankylosis of many of the joints, (often) anomalies of the vertebral column, and syndactyly are generally present. What developmental sequence was affected? How many genes were mutated or repressed? How many cell divisions were in error? How many enzymes were synthesized too late?

A relatively common malformation, which has several forms, is the cleft defect. It may occur as an isolated cleft lip, a cleft lip and palate, or a cleft defect in combination with other congenital malformations.[90] It is thought that when the cleft defect occurs alone, it is caused by a relatively simple fusion failure in the oral-facial-cranial tissues. As part of the morphogenesis of the human facial region, the oral cavity forms from two lateral structures that grow toward the midline and fuse at approximately the seventh to eighth weeks of fetal development.[87] The palate forms from the maxillary palatal shelves and the lip from the nasal processes. This fusion must occur while the skull and the remainder of the face are also growing; the temporal aspect is critical.[34] Any factor that retards morphogenesis and inhibits fusion of the palate and lip could produce a cleft defect. Even if these structures continue to grow toward the midline, fusion is aborted if it does not occur by the eighth week of embryogenesis.

Cleft lip and palate may also occur as secondary problems in a more severe congenital malformation disorder. The formation of the face and palate depends upon the prior normal development of the anterior midline, or prechordal mesoderm. This is a complex process that is under polygenic control and is subject, of course, to errors in transcription and translation, and to post-translational modifications. Timing is crucial. The process should be completed by three and a half to four weeks of development if subsequent development of the face and forebrain is to be normal.

A similar problem occurs with the development of the posterior embryonic neural tube, which develops from a plate of tissue that folds over and closes, eventually forming the central nervous system, the brain, and the spinal cord. A congenital malformation syndrome that includes an open spine or undeveloped brain suggests failure of this mechanism of morphogenesis. Anencephaly, or absence of the cranial vault above the orbital regions, is the result of such a failure in the cephalad portion of the neural tube.[40, 41, 90] The face and other aspects of the craniofacial complex may be affected secondarily, producing anomalies of the eyes, forehead, and ears. Such malformations may be produced mechanically by edema and distention resulting from the primary defect and may not be true developmental anomalies. Faulty morphogenesis in a caudad portion of the neural tube produces a child with meningomyelocele. As in anencephaly, the overlying skeleton is involved—in this case spina bifida is present. The severity of this malformation is highly variable, with the least affected child having only an enclosed skeletal defect. In more severe cases, an open lesion affects spinal cord function below the level of the defect.

For normal development to occur, both the anterior and posterior portions of the embryonic neural tube must be completely formed by 28 days of gestation.[15, 20, 40–42, 53, 63, 90, 98, 109, 118] But why does the neural tube fail to close? Numerous processes including cell migration, cell adhesion, contact inhibition, glycoprotein synthesis, programmed cell death, cell division, and ectodermal-mesodermal interactions may be implicated in this failure.

Environmental Versus Inherited Influences

Almost thirty years ago, animal experiments were initiated that subsequently demonstrated that different strains of mice would respond quite distinctly to the teratogenetic action of cortisone, which produced cleft palate.[32, 33, 35, 53, 87, 90] It was elegantly demonstrated that the highest incidence of cortisone-induced cleft palate, regardless of mouse strain, was produced by injecting pregnant mice with 2.5 mg of cortisone four times daily, beginning on the eleventh day of gestation.[29, 42] If one uses the A/J strain of mice, it is possible to produce cleft palate in 100 per cent of the offspring.[16, 35] In contrast, other strains of mice, when given comparable injections of cortisone, display only modest susceptibility (12 to 20 per cent) to this craniofacial anomaly.[42] Because of the ease of bioassay and the ease of determining whether a cleft palate had formed, this approach could be applied to studies of genetics, embryology, and immunogenetics related to experimental teratology.

More recently, Bonner designed a method for determining what contributions to embryonic development are made by intrauterine environment as opposed to the genotypic characteristics intrinsic to the embryo.[16] Bonner's method employed blastocyst transplantation. Embryos from a highly resistant strain were explanted to pseudopregnant foster females possessing a high predilection for producing cleft-palate offspring when injected with cortisone. The converse experimental transplantation protocol could also be used to test the results of placing highly susceptible embryos within highly resistant maternal environments. These data, as well as an enlarging literature, clearly indicate that the maternal influence has a major effect on the resistance or susceptibility (or both) of the forming embryo.[16, 21, 32, 35, 53, 82] However, the data also suggest that genetic or intrinsic factors within the embryo also contribute, and these must be examined.

Such experimentation can explore a variety of aspects of developmental biology, such as examining the offspring of reciprocal crosses between two strains of inbred mice that are identical genetically. The incidence of cleft palate in hybrid mice can also be determined. These studies can be extended further by localizing unique cortisone receptor proteins within cell cytoplasm.[33, 104] Differences in the binding of cortisone within specific populations of cells may be correlated with cleft palate formation in the mouse model and, perhaps, in the human embryo.

Using the principles of mendelian genetics, it is possible to produce highly defined congeneic strains of mice.[71, 84] Congeneic hybrid mice can be produced so that they are genetically identical at the 99.9 per cent confidence limit, with the exception of the major histocompability complex termed H-2 in mice (HL-A in man).[17-19] By the use of such methods, it becomes readily possible to determine the relative contributions of both mother and father to the susceptibility of the embryo during development. In A/Jax mice, for example, steroids induce cleft palate in almost all fetuses. If a female A/Jax mouse is mated with a C57BL/6 male, steroids induce cleft palate in almost all offspring.[18] In the reciprocal mating, using an A/Jax father and a C57BL/6 mother, steroids induce 18 to 22 per cent clefting—a frequency comparable with the C57BL/6 relative resistance to steroid-induced cleft palate.[98, 101–103] What A/Jax maternal characteristics are associated with susceptibility to steroid-induced cleft palate?

The MHC (major histocompatibility complex) haplotype of the A/Jax strain is $H\text{-}2^{a}$, whereas the haplotype of the C57BL/6 strain is $H\text{-}2^{b}$.[101–102] In congeneic-hybrid studies, cortisone- or triamcinolone-induced cleft palate was found to be associated with the specific $H\text{-}2^{a}$ haplotype of the mother. If the mother is $H\text{-}2^{a}$ and is given a teratogen, the developing embryo is "at risk." If the mother is $H\text{-}2^{b}$, the embryo is relatively resistant to teratogen-induced cleft palate under comparable experimental conditions.[101, 102]

Which chromosome contains the MHC in mice? Which locus? What are the functions of the structural genes located within this region. The H-2 complex is located on chromosome 17, locus IX. The H-2 complex contains (1) genes for the immune response, (2) genes for complement, (3) genes for androgen hormone receptor proteins, (4) genes for the histocompatibility antigens located on the histocompatibility antigens located on the outer cell surfaces of all somatic cells, (5) genes for the differentiation alloantigens functional during organogenesis in the embryo, and (6) genes that mediate B- and T-cell interactions associated with immunity. Only a handful of genes have been identified within this complex, which contains several hundred genes, however.

The $H\text{-}2^{a}$ haplotype confers susceptibility to steroid-induced cleft palate in mice. Moreover, the maternal haplotype appears to specifically affect susceptibility in mice. One can easily predict that rigorous H-2 typing before reproduction would facilitate the prediction of pregnant animals "at risk." Further, the selection of mouse strains for drug testing must carefully consider the H-2 haplotype before dose-response data and frequency-of-birth-defect data can be interpreted. The results of drug studies in mice can be significantly altered, based on the selection of mouse immunogenetics. Although these studies are promising, it is not yet known what gene or genes are implicated in maternal effects on steroid-induced cleft palate in the A/Jax strain. It is reasonable to predict, however, that the hematopoietic and reticuloendothelial systems should be highly responsive to steroid treatment in A/Jax mice. These animals should also be highly susceptible to immunodeficiency diseases and should have a reduced life span. This is indeed the case.[101, 102]

It is reasonable to postulate that a significant correlation could be established between the human mother's HL-A haplotype and relative susceptibility to teratogen-induced congenital craniofacial malformations. HL-A typing of females before pregnancy might provide important data that could offer the means with which to predict and possibly prevent such congenital deformities. In humans the MHC is located on chromosome 6 and consists of three closely linked loci—HL-A-A, HL-A-B, and HL-A-C. The distribution of HL-A genes in the population can be measured on three levels of biologic organization: (1) phenotype frequencies, (2) gene frequencies, and (3) haplotype frequencies.[19]

Numerous diseases, including juvenile diabetes, congenital heart defects, myasthenia gravis, multiple sclerosis, ankylosing spondylitis, cleft palate, periodontal diseases, optic neuritis, and Hodgkin's disease, have been associated with HL-A.[102] Whereas some of these "associations," such as that between ankylosing spondylitis and HL-A-B27, are quite strong, most of the associations between HL-A and diseases are highly equivocal.[102] Perhaps the most obvious technical difficulty in establishing definitive correlations rests on the nature of the techniques used in HL-A typing and the formidable degree of genetic heterogeneity. It is tempting, however, to entertain the notion that the HL-A complex located on chromosome 6 may represent part of an even larger system conferring relative susceptibility or resistance through inheritance patterns for a large number of somewhat different human diseases.

It should be further emphasized, especially since the information from the mouse studies is so provocative, that much more knowledge is necessary to elucidate the mechanism(s) of H-2-disease associations in mice and HL-A-disease associations in humans. The anticipated data should include those from epidemiologic studies, family studies with multiple occurring disease, studies of concordant and discordant monozygotic twins with and without disease, gene-mapping studies, and a great deal of fundamental cellular, molecular, and developmental biology.

The emerging data suggest (1) that maternal inheritance has a strong influence; (2) that histocompatibility loci in the mouse (HL-A loci in humans) play a significant role, and (3) that maternal age is also a factor. The incidence of cleft palate steadily decreases with increasing parity. Parity correlates closely with maternal age, however, and it has been learned that as maternal age advances, the incidence of cleft palate increases. Obviously, there is a vast range of environmental sources that contribute to craniofacial anomalies, for example the parity, age, weight, and general health and nutrition of the mother (see Table 26–8).[9, 53, 90]

During the secondary development of the palate, the palatal shelves grow from the maxilla and rotate into positions on either side of the tongue. Although the physiologic relationships between palatal shelves, tongue, craniofacial complex, musculature, and forming brain are now appreciated, the specific causal relationships related to cleft palate formation have not yet been scientifically confirmed.[87, 90] As the palatal shelves approach one another, there are striking alterations in the cytodifferentiation of the several layers of epithelium that cover the mesenchyme of the palatal process (a neural crest derivative) (Fig. 26–12). During elevation, the medial edge of the epithelium of the palate contacts the epithelium of the tongue, but adhesion does not occur. Adhesion is a property of the cell surface of the medial palatal epithelium that is expressed *only* as the shelves approximate one another for epithelial fusion. What regulates the induction, transcription, translation, and post-translational modifications of the glycopeptides of the medial epithelium surface at a specific point in time and space?

Recent biochemical and morphologic studies suggest that the cell surface modifications occur prior to epithelial fusion and are mediated by "instructions" from the underlying palatal ectomesenchyme.[87, 90, 104] Findings of histochemistry and scanning electron microscopy suggest that relatively small glycoproteins are expressed along the fusing medial epithelial surfaces of the palatal shelves just prior to fusion. Gene expression, cell division, programmed cell death, epithelial-mesenchymal interactions, migrations of cranial neural-crest cells, tongue development, and the fidelity of the cyclic AMP, adenyl cyclase, and phosphodiesterase system are all interdependently influential in the palatal fusion process and the possible advent of cleft palate formation.[7, 16, 30, 31, 35, 42, 50, 51, 59, 62, 82, 85, 87, 90, 91, 98, 104, 107, 120, 121, 125]

In summary, congenital malformations can be produced by a variety of developmental mechanisms and etiologic agents. The extent of our understanding of these varies considerably. In some we can isolate the developmental step but are unable to distinguish a discrete factor that can be demonstrated to induce the craniofacial anomaly. In other situations, the etiologic factor is well known (cortisone for example), but the mechanism by which it influences the formation of cleft palate is not really understood. To the clinician, the practical questions are how to predict, prevent, and correct congenital malformations

TABLE 26–8. Examples of Teratogens That Produce Congenital Craniofacial Anomalies in Normal Individuals

Teratogen	*Mode of Action*
Vitamin A excess	Cofactor in several enzymatic processes
Riboflavin deficiency	Cofactor in several enzymatic processes
Lodoacetic acid	Inhibits glucose metabolism and succinate dehydrogenase
6-aminonicotinamide	Analogue of nicotinamide, cofactor in enzymatic processes
X-radiation	Distortion of thymine dimer formation; perturbation of DNA replication
Nitrogen mustard	Crosslinks thymine and guanine in DNA; perturbation of DNA replication and transcription
Hycanthone	Intercalates base pairs of DNA; inhibits transcription
Caffeine	Analogue of purines; perturbation of DNA synthesis
Diphenylhydantoin	Inhibits conversion of folic acid to biologically active derivatives
2,3-dimercaptopropanol	Chelating agent that inhibits microtubule protein assembly
β-aminopropionitrile	Inhibits lysyloxidase and thereby inhibits collagen crosslinking and fibrillogenesis
β-2-thienylalanine	Analogue to phenylalanine (essential amino acid)
Diazo-oxo-norleucine	Antagonist to glutamine; inhibits glycosaminoglycan and glycoprotein synthesis
Phenobarbital	Central nervous system depressant
Cortisone (glycocorticoid)	Inhibits protein synthesis, anti-inflammatory agent
Dexamethasone	Structural analogue of cortisone; inhibits protein synthesis; anti-inflammatory agent
Prednisolone	Structural analogue of cortisone; inhibits protein synthesis; anti-inflammatory agent

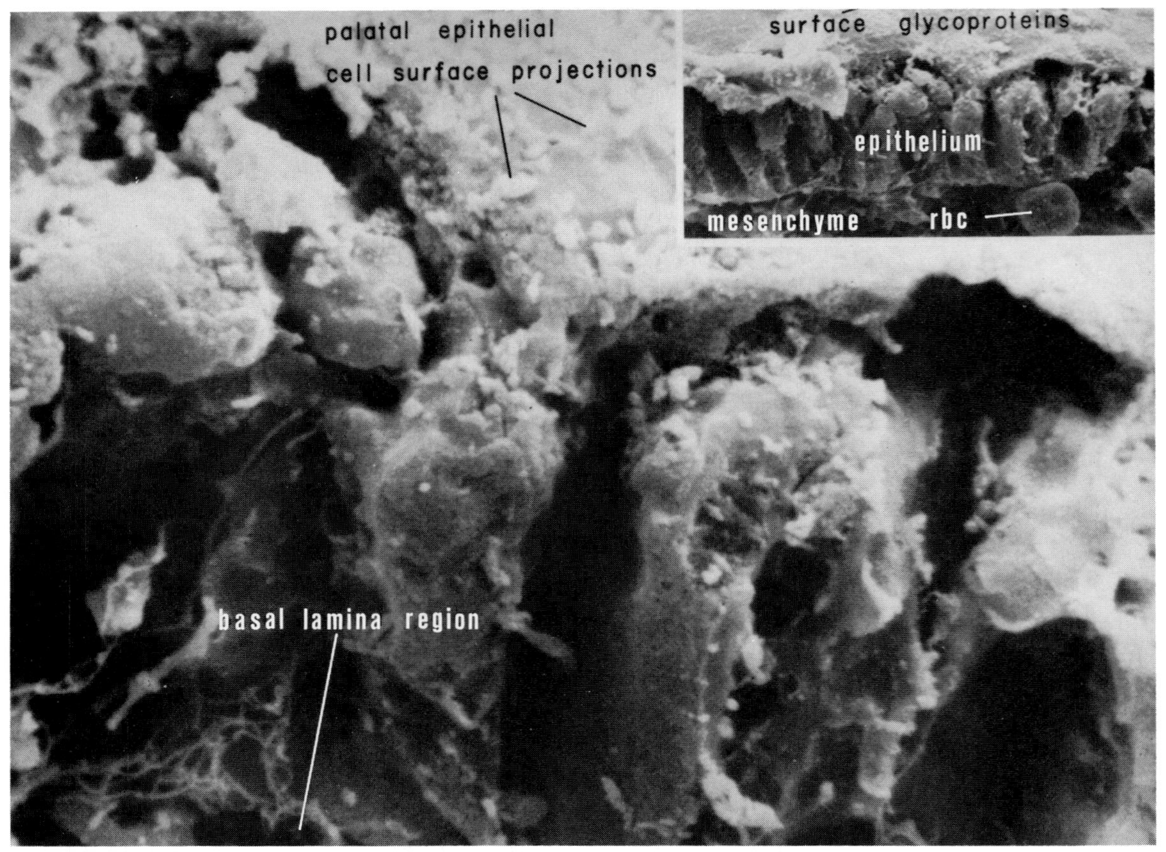

Figure 26–12. Scanning electron microscopy provides a unique opportunity to observe surface topography of biological specimens. Special fixation procedures and critical point freezing methods were used to prepare embryonic mouse palatal tissues during various stages of epithelial fusion. This survey photomicrography demonstrates the surface details of the epithelial and mesenchymal cells following closure.

in humans. Between the islands of knowledge, an ocean of ignorance is awaiting exploration.

Although much of the information needed will be derived from new and sophisticated scientific techniques, continued stimulation must be provided by careful thought and analysis of the malformation syndromes. Cooperative investigations by clinicians and research biomedical scientists should continue to improve our collective understanding of human congenital malformations.

ESSENTIAL CONCEPTS OF CRANIOFACIAL DEVELOPMENT

Molecular Heterogeneity

For many years it was assumed that many of the molecules that comprise connective tissues were homogeneous.[97] For example, one of the most abundant proteins in our body is collagen, which forms 25 per cent of our total body protein.[14] It had been assumed that collagen molecules found in various anatomic locations throughout the forming embryo and the subsequent growing and maturing animal were homologous. All collagens in vertebrates were believed to consist of two alpha-2 chains with only minor variations in amino acid composition. Since the recent discovery that the primary and secondary molecular structures of collagen are heterogeneous, various questions concerning the possible functions of collagen in developmental and physiologic processes have become more cogent.[97, 104]

Is a single cell type capable of synthesizing and secreting a variety of different collagen gene products? What extracellular matrix influences serve to regulate gene expression? How are extracellular environmental factors used to regulate intracellular synthesis? What is the functional significance of genetically distinct collagen species in the same organism? What is the function of collagen in morphogenesis? (For example, it is now well established that cartilage collagen differs from that found in skin and bone both in amino-acid sequence of the *alpha* chains and in their distribution within the triple helical collagen molecule.[97,104] Can a single cell secrete genetically distinct molecular species such as dentine-type and cartilage-type collagen?)

There is also increasing evidence that other types of *alpha*-chains that have not been detected in mature tissues are present in embryonic chick skin and in human fetal skin. It is distinctly possible that transitions of one type of collagen to another — analogous perhaps to the fetal-newborn transitions associated with hemoglobin biosynthesis — take place during developmental processes. At present, five different structural genes for collagen have been determined, and four different types of collagen have been isolated and characterized. In many instances, antibodies have been made that are specific to a particular type of collagen (see Table 26–9).

TABLE 26–9. Collagen Heterogeneity

Tissue	*Collagen Molecule*	*Collagen Type*	*Developmental Process*
Bone Cementum Dentine Gingiva Liver Lung Periodontal ligament Skin Spleen	$[\alpha 1\ (I)]_2\alpha 2$	Type I	Cementogenesis Fibrogenesis Osteogenesis Dentinogenesis
Cartilage	$[\alpha 1\ (II)]_3$	Type II	Chondrogenesis
Aorta Cementum Embryonic dermis Periodontal ligament Uterine leiomyoma	$[\alpha 1\ (III)]_3$	Type III	Fibrogenesis Cementogenesis
Basement membrane(s)	$[\alpha 1\ (IV)]_3$	Type IV (A, B, C)	Basal lamina formation

This new information can be utilized in considering the repair mechanisms operant in soft and skeletal tissues involved in dentofacial surgery. Intramembranous bone displays healing properties different from those of endochondral bone. Repair mechanisms in dentine, cartilage, intramembranous bones, long bones, gingival tissues, skin, and other areas important in treatment of craniofacial deformity may differ, in part because the collagens characteristic of each of these tissues are heterogeneous; they differ in composition and sequence of amino-acids, in degree of glycosylation and hydroxylation, and in the presence or absence of a nonhelical registration polypeptide that contains an essential amino acid (tryptophan) not found in the collagen molecule (Fig. 26–13).

The transcription, translation, and post-translational modifications of collagen synthesis and secretion have been thoroughly studied, and many of the temporal aspects have been learned (Fig. 26–14). For example, it requires 8 minutes to synthesize the collagen molecule in vitro, whereas studies dealing with intact cells and tissues indicate that it requires approximately 28 to 30 for the synthesis, intracellular transport, and secretion of collagen molecules in a variety of tissue types (Table 26–10).

For a fuller appreciation of the specificity of various connective tissues associated with the craniofacial complex and for an examination of the details regarding bone, cartilage, dentine, and soft-tissue repair and regeneration, the reader is encouraged to seek out primary sources.[9, 23, 45, 57, 62, 95, 96, 98, 104, 119]

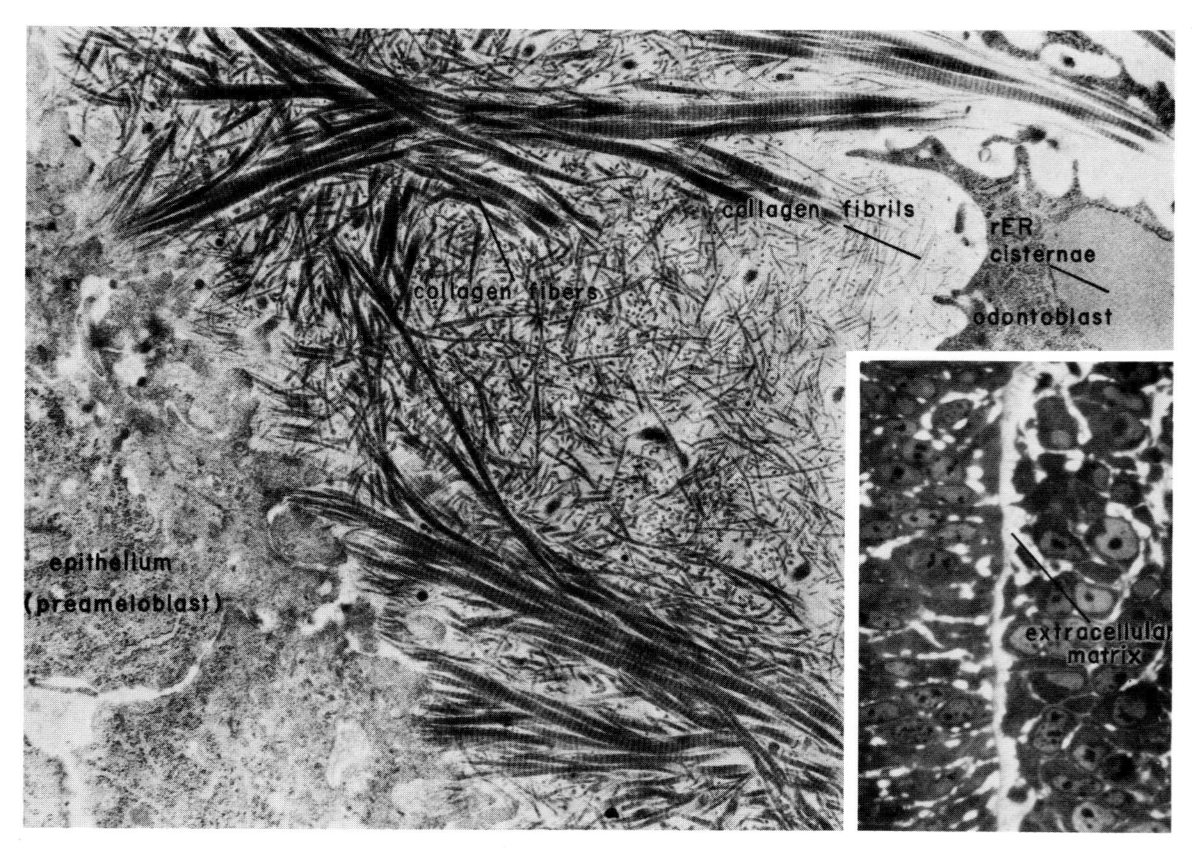

Figure 26–13. Embryonic mouse incisor dentinogenesis is illustrated at a specific stage of development just prior to dentine mineralization. The inner enamel epithelial cells synthesize and secrete Types I and IV preprocollagens whereas the mesenchymal cells make only Type I preprocollagen. Note the transitions during fibrilogenesis which collagen molecules form fibrils and fibrils form fibers.

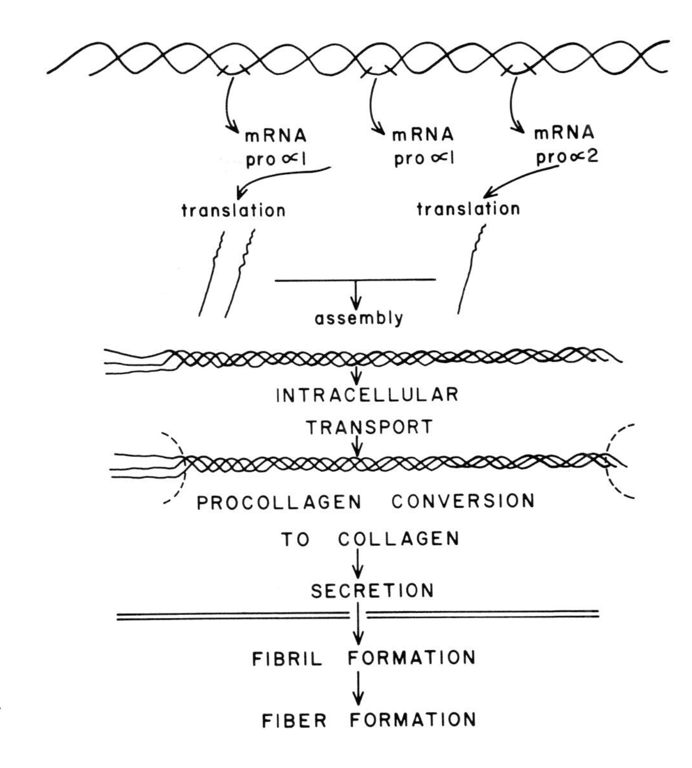

Figure 26–14. Diagram of Type I collagen biosynthesis.

Migrations of the Cranial Neural Crest Cells

The cranial neural crest cells in vertebrates give rise to a striking diversity of differentiated cells and tissues (Table 26–11). Because of the diversity of the derivatives and the extensive and precise distribution of cranial neural crest cells throughout the developing craniofacial complex during embryogenesis, this transitory and nomadic cell

TABLE 26–10. Genetic Regulation of Collagen Synthesis, Intracellular Transport, Secretion, and Extracellular Fibril Formation

Process	*Enzyme*
Selection of structural genes	?
Transcription	Multiple RNA polymerases, endo- and exonucleases
Translation of α-chain mRNAs	Translation enzymes
Hydroxylations	Peptidyl proline hydroxylase Peptidyl lysine hydroxylase
Molecular assembly	—
Helix formation	—
Glycosylations	Galactosyl transferase Glucosyl transferase
Procollagen-collagen conversion	Procollagen peptidase(s)
Cross-linking	Lysyl oxidase

TABLE 26-11. Derivatives of Cranial Neural Crest Cells*

Structure or Tissue	*Derivative*
Connective Tissues	Intramembranous bones (osteoblasts) Dental papilla (odontoblasts) Visceral cartilage (chondroblasts) Sclera and choroid optic coats Anterior trabecular cartilage Meckel's cartilage (mandibular) Maxillary processes Hyoid arch cartilages Corneal mesenchyme
Sensory Ganglia	Trigeminal (V) Geniculate (VII) Superior (root IX) Jugular (root X)
Parasympathetic (Cholinergic) Ganglia	Ciliary Ethmoid Sphenopalatine Submandibular Enteric System
Accessory Cells	Glia cells Schwann sheath cells
Pigment Cells	Melanophores in the iris

*Data obtained from[50, 51, 78, 90, 104]

population demands the interest and respect of clinicians and scientists engaged in biomedical research. Numerous investigators have used experimental analysis to enhance our understanding of the normal developmental fates of cranial neural crest cells and their patterns of migration and localization in the forming embryo.[50, 51, 52, 78, 121]

The neural crest cells function as essential components in the formation of many constituents in the craniofacial complex, including the connective tissue elements, the peripheral neurons, and the sensory ganglia. The cells derived from the cranial neural crest cells are unique. They apparently are capable of migrating from their point of origin to move in highly patterned formations into specific regions of the embryo, where they differentiate into biochemically and cytologically dissimilar cell types. Studies suggest that crest cell–derived, terminal cytodifferentiation is determined by time, positional information, and the extracellular microenvironment.

It is becoming increasingly evident that as the neural crest cells migrate through the forming cephalic region, they are profoundly influenced by environmental cues, such as collagen, glycosaminoglycans, ions, glycoproteins, and cell surface ligands. These cues partially determine the phenotype of the neural crest derivative. The acquisition and expression of these characteristics indicate that neural crest cells are involved in many of the fundamental problems currently being investigated in developmental biology.

Recent experiments have begun to reveal the nature of specific environmental influences that direct the migratory behavior of neural crest cells. Changes in the adhesive properties of the outer surface of the crest cells may play a major role in the aggregation of crest cells to form specific ganglia of the spine. The mechanisms of cell to cell recognition, possibly mediated by a glycosyltransferase, may influence the molecular basis of cell to cell interactions leading to specific morphogenetic processes, including the migrations of presumptive cells into the developing central nervous system, the forming brain, the forming eye, the forming maxillary and mandibular processes, and other structures.[91] The specificity of the extracellular environment may be very crucial.[49, 50, 78, 121] The specific types of collagen found in the extracellular matrix may be arranged in unique patterns to provide a substratum upon which cells may migrate toward specific locations.[87] Furthermore, the concentration of collagen and noncollagenous molecules such as hyaluronic acid, glycosaminoglycans, proteoglycans, or hyaluronidase also may influence cell migrations and subsequent cytodifferentiation.[45, 95–97]

On the basis of studies conducted on experimental mice embryos, it is clear that the cranial neural crest contributes extensively to structures in the oral and pharyngeal regions (see Table 26–11). Many kinds of cells are derived from this cell population. In some cases, there is evidence that the crest cells become progressively differentiated as they move past various structures toward their final destination. For example, crest cells migrating past the pharyngeal endoderm become preconditioned, so that when they come into contact with oral epithelium, they interact with it to produce a tooth organ, with crest cells forming the dental papillae (odontoblasts).

Tissue-Tissue Interactions

All organs in the forming embryo are derived from a sequential series of exquisitely timed interactions between dissimilar tissues that give rise to the unique characteristics of the organ system. It has been generally agreed that tissues in these forming organs follow a series of secondary embryonic inductions or epithelial-mesenchymal interactions (Fig. 26–15). In many of these instances, the mesenchymal tissue component is profoundly influential in determining the epithelial tissue phenotype. For example, when the dental papilla mesenchyme from a forming tooth rudiment is experimentally recombined with a nonoral epithelium, it will give rise to a forming tooth rudiment in which the nonoral epithelium will express the morphologic characteristics of amelogenesis (Fig. 26–16). Mesenchymal specificity instructed the epithelium to express a very specialized phenotype. The molecular mechanism by which the mesenchyme instructs the adjacent epithelium appears to be intrinsic in properties associated with the basement membrane or extracellular matrix that is interposed between the two dissimilar tissue interactants (Fig. 26–17). Macromolecules in the extracellular matrix, membrane-limited structures, or extremely close-range cell-cell interactions appear to mediate the mesenchymal-derived instruction upon the adjacent epithelium.

These same general relationships apply to the epithelial-mesenchymal interactions associated with formation of the palatal shelf. Palate formation, like tooth development, is the consequence of reciprocal, interdependent epithelial-mesenchymal interactions. These interactions have been demonstrated both *in vitro* and *in vivo,* and it has been discovered that properties of the mesenchyme associated with the forming embryonic palate have a profound effect on the acquisition of specific properties of the epithelium. If, for example, the lining epithelia of the palatal shelves do not express specific glycoproteins, presumed to be adhesive, just before the forming palatal shelves fuse at the

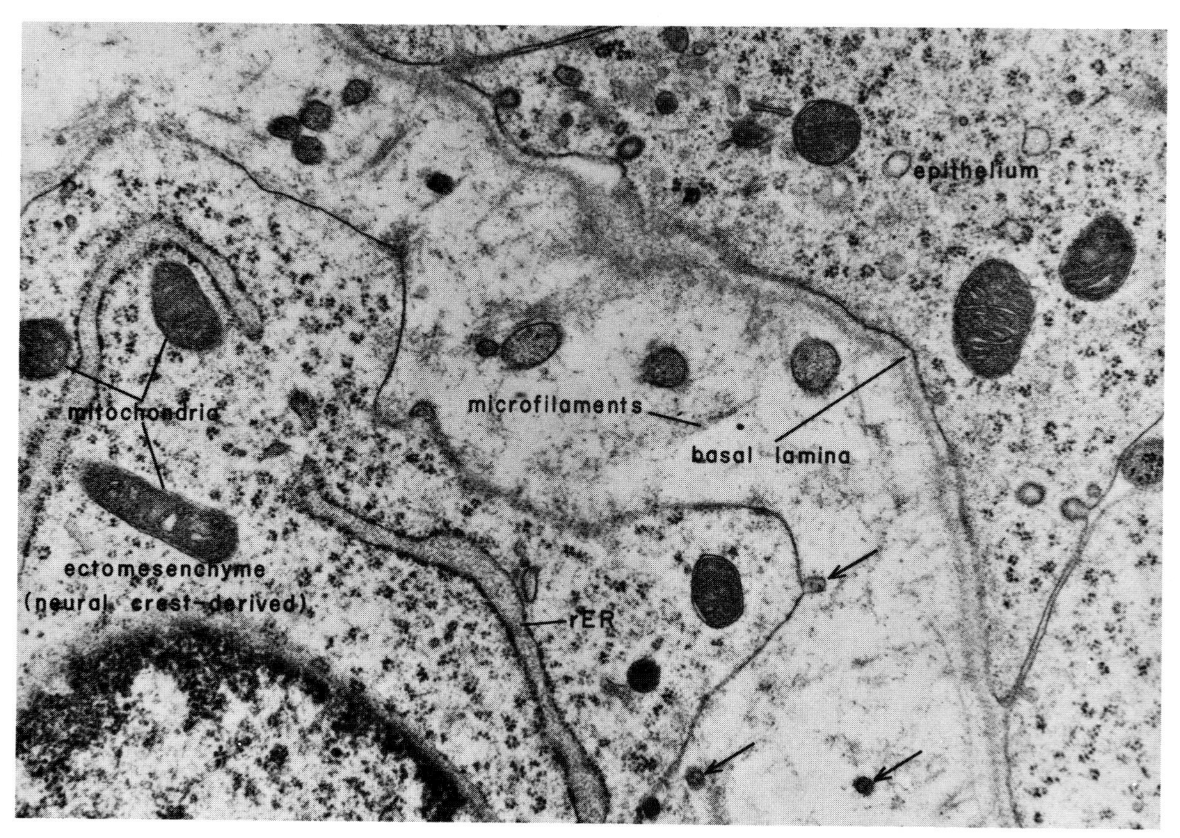

Figure 26–15. Epithelial-mesenchymal interactions associated with embryonic tooth formation *in situ*. Arrows indicate matrix vesicles derived from the ectomesenchyme cells. Possibly particulate, membrane-associated macromolecules mediate mesenchymal specificity.

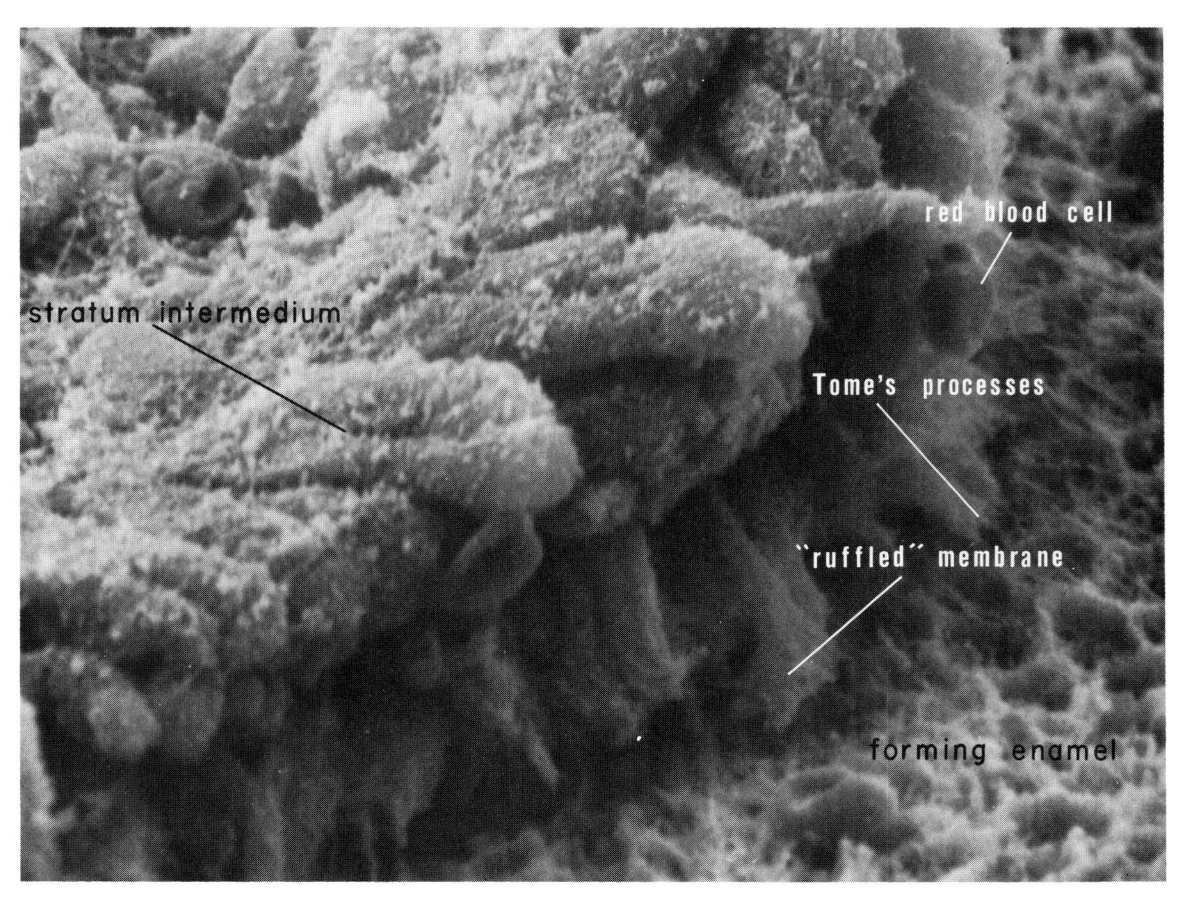

Figure 26–16. Scanning electron microscopy used to study the secretion of enamel proteins during embryonic rabbit tooth development.

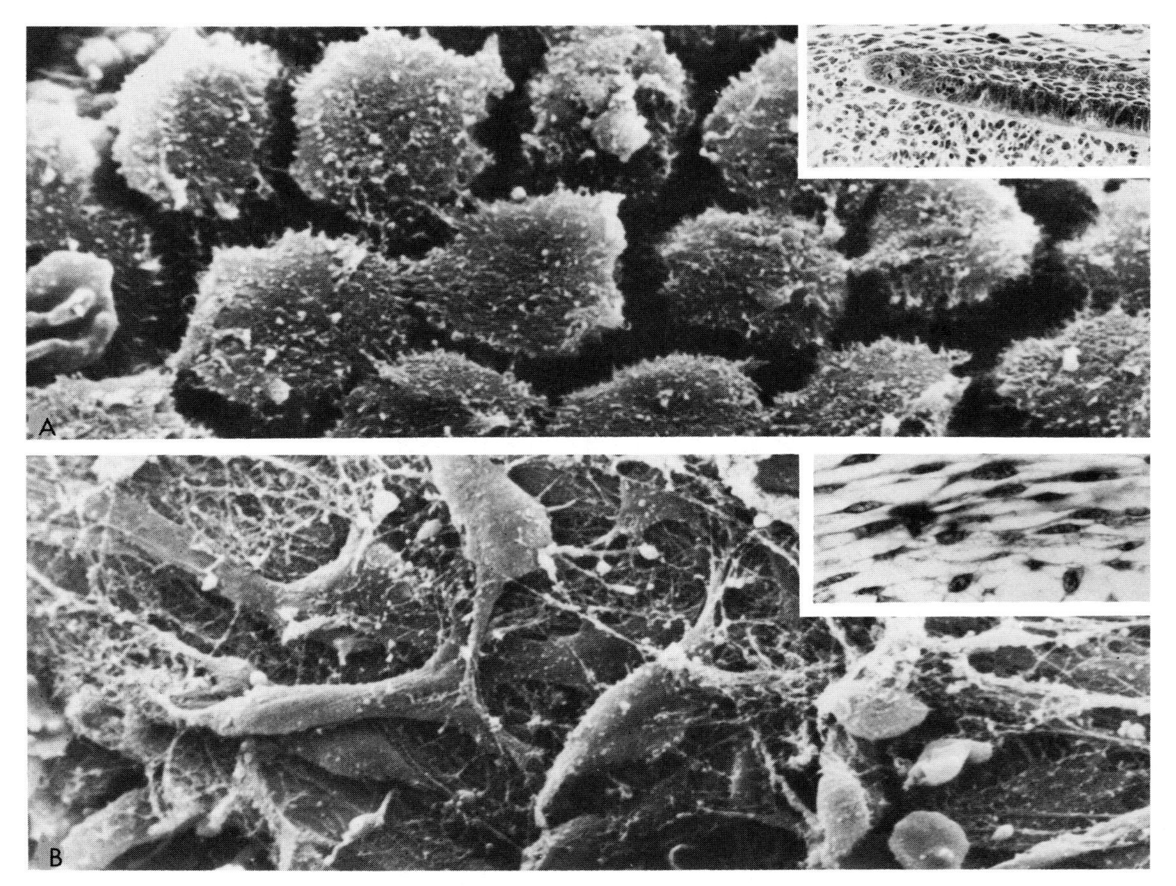

Figure 26–17. (A) Topographical characteristics of the epithelium during tooth development. *Insert* describes light microscopic criteria to study cell interactions. (B) Topographical characteristics of the mesenchyme during tooth development. Note the collagen fibers. *Insert* describes light microscopic criteria used to study homotypic and heterotypic cell interactions.

midline, overt palatal clefting is the consequence. The synthesis of mRNA for the specific glycoproteins associated with the outer cell surfaces of the epithelium may be impaired by certain teratogens during critical stages of craniofacial morphogenesis. Details of the relationships among teratogens, heterologous tissue-tissue interactions, immunogenetics, and palatal fusion are not as yet well understood. The thrust of research in this area should soon produce considerable useful evidence about these mechanisms.

CONCLUSIONS

The task of biomedical scientists, physicians, and dentists is to understand human biology and to apply research humanely and cautiously with respect for the individual human being. It is now quite evident that many common birth defects, such as cleft palate, pyloric stenosis, several types of congenital heart disease, and retinoblastoma can be treated by conventional surgical techniques. Most patients who receive surgical treatment for these disorders are normally habilitated and can lead relatively normal lives. Untreated patients with these congenital malformations, except for cleft palate, often die. Developed societies have enough surgeons to take care of these defects. All these conditions have a genetic etiology involving single or multiple sets of structural genes.

These congenital malformations occur five to twenty times as often in the children whose parents already have these diseases as they do in the general population. Congenital heart disease, pyloric stenosis, and cleft palate are all considered polygenic conditions that can be expected to double their rate of occurrence in about twenty generations or 500 years. Bilateral retinoblastoma is a dominant trait and can be expected to double its frequency rate (from 1 in 70,000 to 1 in 35,000) *in a single generation.*

Despite these findings, the dysgenic effects of modern dentistry and medicine have been exaggerated. Natural selection before birth, in the form of spontaneous abortions and genetic sterility, has not been significantly altered by modern clinical practice. Nevertheless, it is true that restoring patients with congenital disorders to full health and vigor, medically or surgically, leads to fertility and thus to transmission of harmful genes.

Rational plans for the prevention of most birth defects cannot be formulated as long as we do not understand the etiology of these diseases. Preventive measures such as immunization against rubella to prevent fetal birth defects and administration of rhesus (Rh) antibodies to prevent Rh hemolytic diseases constitute "high technology" of disease control. Moreover, it must be painfully acknowledged that a significant proportion of birth defects may not be explained by genetic or environmental factors or by genetic-environmental interactions. For instance, monozygotic twins share identical heredity and a very similar intrauterine environment, yet birth defects that appear to have a genetic etiology often occur in only one twin of an identical pair, suggesting that random factors may also play a part. The complex dynamics of early embryonic organ formation may allow appreciable chance errors even if all the genetic and environmental factors affecting development can be fully elucidated and controlled. For the prevention of most birth defects at present, we can only recommend that pregnancy be avoided too early or too late in life and that exposure to drugs, chemicals, x-rays, and infection be minimized.

Recent developments are raising new questions about the prevention and treatment of birth defects and research on these disorders. Among these problem issues that concern basic human values and ethics are genetic counseling, abortion for birth defects, withholding of complex treatment from individuals in some situations, population screening for genetic and other diseases, artificial insemination, and fertilization in vitro. Other concerns such as the dysgenic effects of modern medicine and new possibilities of cloning in gene therapy are remote but challenging. Each of these issues must be thoughtfully considered by the clinician on its own merits, and the immediate and remote consequences must be carefully evaluated.

For example, cloning of an animal means creating an organism that is genetically identical to the donor of a somatic cell nucleus implanted into an enucleated egg.[35] Cloning has been repeatedly and successfully accomplished in amphibians and has been discussed as a possibility for mammals. Recent developments in molecular biology make it possible to synthesize genes and cause the possibility of introducing genes into cells by viral transduction. Such advances have raised provocative discussions.

It must be observed that only defects in mendelian traits whose biochemistry is well understood can as yet be approached with gene therapy. At present, we know very little about the regulatory mechanisms of mammalian cells. Even though a gene whose mRNA can be isolated can be now manufactured relatively easily, its safe introduction into the nucleus of a highly specialized cell followed by normal function remains exceedingly problematical.

Awareness of the need to create forums for interdisciplinary communication and rapid dissemination of new knowledge and a desire on the part of the clinician and the biomedical research scientist to share ideas and approaches create a harmonization of our scientific, cultural, and ethical capabilities. It is becoming more and more plausible that results obtained from judicious biomedical research will introduce us to the threshold of a new era of better health and less human suffering.

REFERENCES

1. Andersen PF: Inheritance patterns for cleft lip and cleft palate. *In* Pruzansky S (Ed): Congenital Anomalies of the Face and Associated Structures. Springfield, Ill: Charles C Thomas, 1961, pp 123–133.
2. Apple MA: Potent inhibition of sarcoma virus RNA-directed RNA-DNA duplex synthesis and arrest of ascites murine leukemia and sarcoma in vivo by anthracyclines. Physiol Chem Physics *3*:307–318, 1971.
3. Apple MA: Reverse transcription and its inhibitors. Ann Rep Med Chem *8*:251–262, 1972.
4. Auerbach R: Development of immunity. *In:* Lash J, Whittaker JR (Eds): Concepts of Development. Stamford, Conn: Sinauer Assoc, 1974, pp 261–271.
5. Azarnia R, Larsen WJ, Loewenstein WR: The membrane junctions in communicating and noncommunicating cells, their hybrids, and segregants. Proc Nat Acad Sci *71*:880–884, 1974.
6. Balsamo J, Lilien J: Embryonic cell aggregation: kinetics and specificity of binding of enhancing factors. Proc Nat Acad Sci *71*:727–731, 1974.
7. Barry A: Development of the branchial region of human embryos with special reference to the fate of epithelial cells. *In*: Pruzansky S (Ed): Congenital Anomalies of the Face and Associated Structures. Springfield, Ill. Charles C Thomas, 1961, pp 46–62.
8. Bautz, EKF, Karlson P, Kersten H: Regulation of Transcription and Translation in Eukaryotes. New York: Springer-Verlag, 1973.
9. Bavetta LA: Nutritional aspects of embryogenesis. *In:* Slavkin HC, Vavetta, LA (Eds): Developmental Aspects of Oral Biology. New York: Academic Press, 1972, pp 1–10.
10. Bekhor I: Consideration of the molecular biology of developing systems. *In* Slavkin HC, Bavetta LA (Eds): Developmental Aspects of Oral Biology. New York: Academic Press, 1972, pp 11–34.
11. Bennet D, Boyse EA, Old LJ: Cell surface

immunogenetics in the study of morphogenesis. *In* Silvestri LG (Ed): Cell Interactions: Third Lepetit Colloquium. New York: American Elsevier, 1972, pp 247–263.
12. Biwas BB: Chromatin and ribonucleic acid polymerases in the eukaryotic cell. Sub-cell Biochem *3*:27–38, 1974.
13. Bobrow M: New ways to look at X inactivation. Nature *271*:505–506, 1978.
14. Bohinski RC: Modern Concepts in Biochemistry. Boston: Allyn and Bacon, 1973.
15. Bondy SC, Prasad KN, Purdy JL: Neuroblastoma: drug-induced differentiation increases proportion of cytoplasmic RNA that contains polyadenylic acid. Science *186*:359–361, 1974.
16. Bonner JJ: Method for evaluating intrauterine versus genetic influences on craniofacial anomalies. J Dent Res *53*:1313–1316, 1974.
17. Bonner JJ: Cell surface polymorphisms: theory describing the molecules which can direct development. Birth Defects: Original Article Series, 1979. (In press.)
18. Bonner JJ: The multifactorial problem of cleft palate: the research. Doctoral Dissertation, Graduate School of Arts and Sciences, University of Southern California, Los Angeles, 1976.
19. Bonner JJ, Thompson P, Holve LM, Ebbin AJ, Terasaki PI, Slavkin HC: HLA phenotype frequencies associated with cleft lip and/or palate. Tissue Antigens *12*:228–232, 1978.
20. Bonner JT: On Development: The Biology of Form. Cambridge: Harvard University Press, 1974.
21. Bosma JF (Ed): Development in the Fetus and Infant. DHEW Publ No. (NIH) 73–546. Bethesda, Maryland: US Dept of HEW, 1973.
22. Bosma JF (Ed): Development of the basicranium: a symposium. DHEW Publ No (NIH) 76–989. Washington: US Government Printing Office, 1976.
23. Boyde A, Jones SJ: Scanning electron microscopic studies of the formation of mineralized tissues. *In*: Slavkin HC, Bavetta LA (Eds): Developmental Aspects of Oral Biology. New York: Academic Press, 1972, pp 243–274.
24. Brachet J: Introduction to Molecular Biology. London: The English University Press Ltd. New York: Springer-Verlag, 1974.
25. Castor LN: Cell contact and cell division. *In* King TJ (ed): Developmental Aspects of Carcinogenesis and Immunity. New York: Academic Press, 1974, pp 43–64.
26. Coggin JH Jr, Anderson NG: Embryonic and fetal antigens in cancer cells. *In*: King TJ (Ed): Developmental Aspects of Carcinogenesis and Immunity. New York: Academic Press, 1974, pp 173–186.
27. Comings DE: Mechanisms of chromosome banding and implications for chromosome structure. Ann Rev Genet *12*:25–46, 1978.
28. Darnell JE, Jelinek WR, Malloy GR: Biogenesis of mRNA: genetic regulation in mammalian cells. Science *181*:1215–1221, 1973.
29. Davidson EH, Britten RJ: Organization, transcription, and regulation in the animal genome. Quart Rev Biol *48*:565–613, 1973.
30. Davies J: Errors in transplantation. *In* Hahn FE (Ed): Progress in Molecular and Subcellular Biology. New York: Springer-Verlag, 1969, pp 47–81.
31. De Terra N: Cortical control of cell division Science *184*:530–537, 1974.
32. Dostal M, Jelinek R: Sensitivity of embryos and intraspecies differences in mice in response to prenatal administration of corticoids. Teratology *8*:245–252, 1973.
33. Filburn CR, Wyatt GR: Developmental endocrinology. *In*: Lash J, Whittaker JR (Eds): Concepts of Development. Stamford, Connecticut: Sinauer Assoc, 1974, pp 321–348.
34. Ford CE: Chromosomal abnormality and congenital malformation. *In* Wolstenholme GEW, O'Connor CM (Eds): Congenital Malformations. Boston: Little, Brown & Co, 1960, pp 32–47.
35. Fraser FC: Experimental induction of cleft palate. *In* Pruzansky S (Ed): Congenital Anomalies of the Face and Associated Structures. Springfield, Ill: Charles C Thomas, 1961, pp 188–197.
36. Fraser FC: The multifactorial threshold concept — Uses and Misuses. Teratology *14*:267–280, 1976.
37. Frenster JH, Hernstein PR: Gene derepression. Physiol Med *288*:1224–1229, 1973.
38. Goldberger RF: Autogenous regulation of gene expression. Science *183*:810–824, 1974.
39. Goodman RM, Gorlin RJ: Atlas of the Face in Genetic Disorders. St. Louis: The CV Mosby Co, 1977.
40. Gorlin RJ, Goldman HM: Thoma's Oral Pathology, vol. 1. St. Louis: The CV Mosby Co, 1970.
41. Gorlin RJ, Goldman HM: Thoma's Oral Pathology, vol. 2. St. Louis: The CV Mosby Co, 1970.
42. Grabb WC, Rosenstein SW, Bzoch KR (Eds): Cleft Lip and Palate: Surgical, Dental and Speech Aspects. Boston: Little, Brown and Co, 1971.
43. Gurdon JB: The Control of Gene Expression in Animal Development. Cambridge: Harvard University Press, 1974.
44. Hahn FE: On molecular biology. *In*: Hahn FE (Ed): Progress in Molecular and Subcellular Biology. New York: Springer-Verlag, 1969, pp 1–4.
45. Hay ED: Cellular basis of regeneration. *In* Lash J, Whittaker JR (Eds): Concepts of Development. Stamford, Connecticut: Sinauer Assoc, 1974, pp 404–428.
46. Heddle JA, Althanasion K: Mutation rate, genome size and their relation to the rec concept. Nature *258*:359–361, 1975.

47. Heinonen OP, Stone D, Shapiro S: Birth Defects and Drugs in Pregnancy. Littleton, Massachusetts: Publishing Sciences Group, 1977.
48. Ingalls TH: Environmental factors in causation of congenital anomalies. *In*: Wolstenholme GEW, O'Connor CM (Eds): Congenital Malformations. Boston, Little, Brown and Co, 1960, pp. 51–66.
49. Johnson KE: Gastrulation and cell interactions. *In*: Lash J, Whittaker JR (Eds): Concepts of Development. Stamford, Conn: Sinauer Assoc, 1974, pp 128–148.
50. Johnston MC, Listgarten MA: Observations on the migration, interaction and early differentiation of orofacial tissues. *In*: Slavkin HC, Bavetta LA (Eds): Developmental Aspects of Oral Biology. New York: Academic Press, 1972, pp 55–80.
51. Johnston MC, Bhakdinaronk A, Reid YC: An expanded role of the neural crest in oral and pharyngeal development. *In*: Bosma JF (Ed): Oral Sensation and Perception Development in the Fetus and Infant. DHEW Publ No (NIH) 73–546, Bethesda, Md: US Dept of HEW, 1973, pp 37–52.
52. Johnston MC, Morris GM, Kushner DC, Bingle GJ: Abnormal organogenesis of facial structures. *In* Wilson JG, Fraser FC (Eds): Handbook of Teratology. New York: Plenum Press Publishing Corp, 1977.
53. Kalter H: Interplay of intrinsic and extrinsic factors. *In* Wilson JG, Workany J (Eds): Teratology: Principles and Techniques. Chicago: The University of Chicago Press, 1965, pp 57–80.
54. Kawamoto HK Jr: The kaleidoscopic world of rare craniofacial clefts: order out of chaos (Tessier classification). Clin Plast Surg *3*(4):529–572, 1976.
55. Koch WE: Tissue interaction during the in vitro odontogenesis. *In*: Slavkin HC, Bavetta LA (Eds): Developmental Aspects of Oral Biology. New York: Academic Press, 1972, pp 151–164.
56. Kollar EJ: Histogenetic aspects of dermal-epidermal interactions. *In*: Slavin HC, Bavetta LA (Eds): Developmental Aspects of Oral Biology. New York: Academic Press, 1972, pp 126–150.
57. Konigsberg IR, Buckley PA: Regulation of the cell cycle and myogenesis by cell-medium interaction. *In*: Lash J, Whittaker JR (Eds): Concepts of Development. Stanford, Conn: Sinauer Assoc, 1974, pp 179–196.
58. Kornberg RD: Structure of chromatin. Ann Rev Biochem *46*:931–994, 1977.
59. Krogman WM: The growth of the head and face studied craniometrically and cephalometrically, in normal and in cleft palate children. *In* Pruzansky S (Ed): Congenital Anomalies of the Face and Associated Structures. Springfield, Ill: Charles C Thomas, 1961, pp 208–236.
60. Lane CD, Gurdon JB, Woodland HR: Control of translation of globin mRNA in embryonic cells. Nature *251*:436–437, 1974.
61. Langman J: The influence of teratogenic agents on serum proteins. *In*: Pruzansky S (Ed): Congenital Anomalies of the Face and Associated Structures. Springfield, Ill: Charles C Thomas, 1961, pp 149–161.
62. Lash J: Tissue interactions and related subjects. *In*: Lash J, Whittaker JR (Eds): Concepts of Development. Stamford, Conn: Sinauer Assoc, 1974 pp 197–212.
63. Lash J, Whittaker JR (Eds): Concepts of Development. Stamford, Conn: Sinauer Assoc, 1974.
64. Leder P: Discontinuous genes. New Engl J Med *298*:1079–1081, 1978.
65. Lodish HF: Model for the regulation of mRNA translation applied to haemoglobin synthesis. Nature *251*:385–388, 1974.
66. Loewenstein WR: Cell-to-cell connections. *In* Silvestri LG (Ed): Cell Interactions: Third Lepetit Colloquium. New York: American Elsevier, 1972, pp 296–298.
67. McKusick VA, Ruddle FH: The status of the gene map of the human chromosomes. Science *196*:390–405, 1977.
68. McMahon D: Chemical messengers in development: a hypothesis. Science *185*:1012–1021, 1974.
69. McNamara JA (Ed): Control Mechanisms in Craniofacial Growth. No. 3 in Craniofacial Growth Series. Ann Arbor: University of Michigan Press, 1975.
70. Matthews DN: Experiences in major craniofacial surgery. Plast Reconstr Surg. *59*:163–174, 1977.
71. Melnick M, Bixler, D: Letter to the editor (re: Fraser FC, Teratology *14*:257, 1976). Teratology *18*:119–121, 1978.
72. Melnick M, Shields ED: Allelic restriction: a biologic alternative to multifactoral threshold inheritance. Lancet *1*:176–179, 1976.
73. Migeon B, Jelalian K: Evidence for two active X chromosomes in germ cells of female before meiotic entry. Nature *269*:242–243, 1977.
74. Mishimura H, Semba R, Tanimura T, Tanaka O: Prenatal Development of the Human With Special Reference to Craniofacial Structures: An Atlas. DHEW Publ No (NIH) 77–946, Washington: US Government Printing Office, 1977.
75. Motulsky AG: Brave new world? Science *185*:653–663, 1974.
76. Nemer M: Molecular basis of embryogenesis. *In*: Lash J, Whittaker JR (Eds): Concepts of Development. Stamford, Conn: Sinauer Assoc, 1974, pp 119–127.
77. Niu MC, Segal SS (Eds): The Role of RNA in Reproduction and Development. Proceedings of the AAAS Symposium, December 28–30, 1972. New York: American Elsevier, 1973.
78. Noden DM: The migratory behavior of neural crest cells. *In* Bosma JF (Ed): Oral Sensation and Perception Development in the Fetus and Infant. DHEW Publ No (NIH) 73–546, Bethesda, Md: US Dept of HEW, 1973, pp 9–33.
79. Nossal GJV: Lymphocyte differentiation and immune surveillance against cancer. *In* King TJ (Ed): Developmental Aspects of Carcinogenesis and Immunity. New York: Academic Press, 1974, pp 205–214.
80. Ohno S: Single gene translational control of

testosterone "regulon." *In* Silvestri LG (Ed): Cell Interactions: Third Lepetit Colloquium. New York: American Elsevier, 1972, pp 293–295.

81. Ottolengthi S, Lanyon WG, Paul J, Williamson R, Weatherall DJ, Clegg JB, Pritchard J, Pootrakul S, Boon WH: Gene deletion as a cause of α thalassaemia. Nature *251*:289–392, 1974.
82. Padilla GM, Cameron IL, Zimmerman A: Cell Cycle Controls. New York: Academic Press, 1974.
83. Peach R: Development of the trigeminal ganglion. *In*: Bosma JF (Ed): Oral Sensation and Perception Development in the Fetus and Infant. DHEW Publ No (NIH) 73–546, Bethesda, Md: Dept of HEW, 1973, pp. 69–74.
84. Penrose LS: Genetical causes of malformation and the search for their origins. *In*: Wolstenholme GEW, O'Connor CM (Eds): Congenital Malformations. Boston: Little, Brown and Co., 1960, pp 22–27.
85. Pitts JD: Direct interactions between animal cells. *In* Silvestri LG (Ed): Cell Interactions. Third Lepetit Colloquium. New York: American Elsevier, 1972, pp 247–263.
86. Pruzansky S: Cleft lip and palate: therapy and prevention. J Am Dent Assoc *87*:1048–1054, 1973.
87. Pourtois M: Morphogenesis of the primary and secondary palate. *In*: Slavkin HC, Bavetta LA (Eds): Developmental Aspects of Oral Biology. New York: Academic Press, 1972, pp 81–108.
88. Raff MC: Development and differentiation of lymphocytes. *In* King TJ (Ed): Developmental Aspects of Carcinogenesis and Immunity. New York: Academic Press, 1974, pp 161–172.
89. Riolo ML, Moyers RE, McNamara JA, Hunter WS: An Atlas of Cranifacial Growth. Ann Arbor: University of Michigan Press, 1975.
90. Ross RB, Johnston MC: Cleft Lip and Palate. Baltimore: Williams and Wilkins, 1972.
91. Roth S: A molecular model for cell interactions. Quart Rev Biol *48*:541–563, 1973.
92. Shapiro BL: The genetics of cleft lip and palate. *In*: Stewart RE, Prescott GH (Eds): Oral Facial Genetics. St. Louis: The CV Mosby Co, 1976.
93. Sidman RL: Cell interactions in developing mammalian nervous system. *In*: Silvestri, LG (Ed): Cell Interactions: Third Lepetit Colloquium. New York: American Elsevier, 1972, pp 1–13.
94. Simpson RT: Separation of transcribable and repressed chromatin. *In* Anfinsen CB, Schechter AN (Eds): Current Topics in Biochemistry — 1973. New York: Academic Press, 1974, pp 135–186.
95. Slavkin HC: Intercellular communication during odontogenesis, *In* Slavkin HC, Bavetta LA (Eds): Developmental Aspects of Oral Biology. New York: Academic Press, 1972, pp 165–201.
96. Slavkin HC: Intercellular communication during epidermal organ formation. *In*: Maibach HI, Rovec DT (Eds): Epidermal Wound Healing. Chicago: Year Book Medical Publishers, 1972, 331–321.
97. Slavkin HC (Ed): Proceedings of the Santa Cataline Island Colloquium. The Comparative Molecular Biology of Extracellular Matrices. New York: Academic Press, 1972.
98. Slavkin HC: Research frontiers in oral biology — genetic alterations in craniofacial anomalies. J Oral Surg *32*:333–342, 1973.
99. Slavkin HC: Tooth formation: a tool in developmental biology. *In*: Melcher AH, Zard GA (Eds): Oral Sciences Reviews. Copenhagen: Munksgaard, 1974.
100. Slavkin HC: Morphogenesis of the mandible: developmental, cellular and molecular biological considerations. *In* Whitaker LA (Ed): Symposium on Reconstruction of Jaw Deformities. St. Louis: The CV Mosby Co, 1978.
101. Slavkin HC: Congenital craniofacial malformations: identifying individuals at risk. Ear Nose Throat J *58*(1):7–20, 1979.
102. Slavkin HC: Developmental Craniofacial Biology. Philadelphia: Lea and Febiger, 1979.
103. Slavkin HC, Bonner JJ: Genetic control mechanisms during early oral facial development. *In*: Stewart RE, Prescott GH (Eds): Oral Facial Genetics. St. Louis: The CV Mosby Co., 1976, pp 1–45.
104. Slavkin HC, Greulich R (Eds): Second International Santa Catalina Colloquium: Extracellular Matrix Influences on Gene Expression. New York: Academic Press, 1975.
105. Smith M: The first complete nucleotide sequencing of an organism's DNA. Am Sci *67*:57–67, 1979.
106. Sperber GH: Craniofacial Embryology, ed 2. Dorchester, England: John Wright and Sons, 1976.
107. Spooner BS: Morphogenesis of vertebrate organs. *In* Lash J, Whittaker JR (Eds): Concepts of Development. Stamford, Conn: Sinauer Assoc, 1974, pp 213–240.
108. Stanbury JB, Syngaarden JB, Fredrickson DS: The Metabolic Basis of Inherited Disease. New York: McGraw-Hill Book Co., 1972.
109. Stark RB: Embryology, pathogenesis and classification of cleft lip and cleft palate. *In*: Pruzansky S (Ed): Congenital Anomalies of the Face and Associated Structures. Springfield, Ill: Charles C Thomas, 1961, pp 66–84.
110. Stewart R, Prescott GH (Eds): Oral Facial Genetics. St. Louis: The CV Mosby Co., 1976.
111. Subtelny JD: Studies of the configuration of the nasopharynx and palatal segments in children with clefts as they relate to embryologic studies. *In* Pruzansky S (Ed): Congenital Anomalies of the Face and Associated Structures. Springfield, Ill: Charles C Thomas, 1961, pp 198–205.
112. Temin HM, Kang C: RNA-directed DNA poly-

merase activity in uninfected cells. *In*: King TJ (Ed): Developmental Aspects of Carcinogenesis and Immunity. New York: Academic Press, 1974, pp 137–144.

113. Tenenhouse HS, Gold RJM, Kachra Z: Biochemical marker in dominantly inherited ectodermal malformation. Nature *251*:431–432, 1974.
114. Tessier P: The definitive plastic surgical treatment of the severe facial deformities of craniofacial dysostosis: Crouzon's and Apert's diseases. Plast Reconstr Surg *48*:419–520, 1971.
115. Thompson EB: Gene expression in animal cells. *In*: Anfinsen CB, Schechter AN (Eds): Current Topics in Biochemistry — 1973. New York: Academic Press, 1974, pp 187–218.
116. Tondury G: On the mechanism of cleft formation. *In* Pruzansky S (Ed): Congenital Anomalies of the Face and Associated Structures. Springfield, Ill: Charles C Thomas, 1961, pp 85–101.
117. Warkany J: Congenital Malformation: Notes and Comments. Chicago: Year Book Medical Publishers, 1971.
118. Wassermann GD: Molecular genetics and developmental biology. Nature New Biol. *245*:163–165, 1973.
119. Weinstock A: Matrix development in mineralizing tissues as shown by radioautography: formation of enamel and dentin. *In*: Slavkin HC, Bavetta LA (Eds): Developmental Aspects of Oral Biology. New York: Academic Press, 1972, pp 202–242.
120. Weiss PA: Dynamics of Development: Experiments and Interferences, Selected Papers on Developmental Biology. New York: Academic Press, 1968.
121. Weston JA: Cell interaction in neural crest development. *In*: Silvestri LG (Ed): Cell Interactions: Third Lepetit Colloquium. New York: American Elsevier, 1972, pp 286–292.
122. Wilson JG: Environment and Birth Defects. New York: Academic Press, 1973.
123. White E, Trump GN: Immunological determinants in development. *In* Slavkin HC, Bavetta LA (Eds): Developmental Aspects of Oral Biology. New York: Academic Press, 1972, pp 35–54.
124. Woese CR: The biological significance of the genetic code. *In* Hahn FE (Ed): Progress in Molecular and Subcellular Biology. New York: Springer-Verlag, 1969, pp 5–46.
125. Woollam DHM, Millen JW: The modification of the activity of certain agents exerting a deleterious effect on the development of the mammalian embryo. *In*: Wolstenholme GEW, O'Connor CM (Eds): Congenital Malformations. Boston: Little, Brown and Co, 1960, pp. 158–172.

INDEX

In this index, page numbers in *italics* indicate illustrations; those followed by t indicate tables. The abbreviation *vs.* indicates differential diagnosis.

INDEX

INDEX